NEUROPATHOLOGY
A reference text of CNS pathology

David ELLISON
MD PhD MA MSc MBBChir MRCP MRCPath

Consultant Neuropathologist,
Southampton University Hospitals Trust
Honorary Senior Lecturer,
Southampton University, UK

Leila CHIMELLI
MD PhD

Associate Professor,
Department of Pathology,
Medical School of Ribeirao Preto,
University of Sao Paulo, Brazil

Brian HARDING
MA DPhil BMBCh FRCPath

Consultant Neuropathologist,
Great Ormond Street Hospital for Children,
UK

Jim LOWE
BMedSci BMBS DM FRCPath

Honorary Consultant Neuropathologist,
University Hospital NHS Trust, Nottingham
Professor of Neuropathology,
University of Nottingham, UK

Seth LOVE
MBBCh PhD FRCP FRCPath

Consultant Neuropathologist,
Frenchay Hospital, Bristol
Professor of Neuropathology,
University of Bristol, UK

Gareth W ROBERTS
BSc PhD FRSA

Opine Consultancy,
Cambridge, UK

Harry V VINTERS
MD FRCP (C)

Professor of Pathology and Lab Medicine
Chief, Section of Neuropathology
Member, Brain Research Institute & Mental
Retardation Research Centre,
UCLA Medical Centre, USA

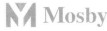 Mosby

London Chicago Philadelphia St Louis Sydney Tokyo

Project Manager	Richard Foulsham
Development Editor	Sue Hodgson
Cover Design	Paul Phillips
Layout Artists	Gisli Thor, Chris Read, Lara Last
Illustration	Jenni Miller, Lynda Payne, Mike Saiz
Production	Hamish Adamson
Index	Laurence Errington
Publisher	Fiona Foley

Copyright © 1998 Mosby International Ltd.

Published in 1998 by Mosby, an imprint of Mosby International Ltd.

Printed by Grafos S.A., Arte sobre papel, Barcelona, Spain.

ISBN 0 7234 2550 7

Set in 9.5pt Sabon.

Preface

The pace of change in neuropathology is such that it is increasingly difficult for the diagnostic pathologist to keep abreast of all fields in this exciting discipline. One has only to think of recent conceptual and diagnostic innovations in the field of neurodegenerative diseases, advances in our understanding of the molecular basis of brain tumors, recognition of the spectrum of CNS pathology associated with human immunodeficiency virus infection, and the correlation of neuropathologic findings with specific genetic defects in a wide range of disorders, for this conviction to be reinforced.

We recognize that the diagnostic pathologist is often under pressure to survey and distil a large amount of clinical, pathologic and molecular genetic information relating to diverse disorders, and usually within a very limited amount of time! Our aim has been to produce a reference book in which this information is presented in an integrated, rapidly accessible format. In a speciality like neuropathology, the practice of which depends primarily on morphology, a clear illustration is often worth more than a page of prose. Consequently, much of the information in *Neuropathology* is incorporated in a wealth of color illustrations, which number over 2500. But while illustrations are a key feature of this book, they are also accompanied by a large amount of clinical and scientific data previously available only from a variety of sources. Techniques for facilitating access to information have been incorporated in the layout of this book, which has benefited from the design expertise of Mosby. Illustrations and descriptions of pathology are arranged around color-coded boxes of information, each with its particular emphasis:

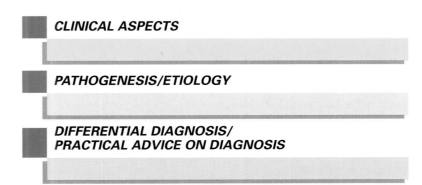

CLINICAL ASPECTS

PATHOGENESIS/ETIOLOGY

DIFFERENTIAL DIAGNOSIS/ PRACTICAL ADVICE ON DIAGNOSIS

Each section also contains many tables and diagrams which are designed to facilitate clinicopathological correlation, and to present key background facts.

Compromises have been inevitable to accommodate such a large amount of visual and factual information in a book of this size. It has not been possible to include some rare entities, and we have deliberately used an annotated style in the presentation of some data. We have restricted the number of references and most of these are to key review articles or to the larger neuropathology reference books.

The practice of neuropathology is reaping great rewards from recent scientific advances. We hope that this book conveys some of the excitement of these advances whilst also integrating them into a practical account of the current principles of neuropathologic diagnosis.

D.E.
S.L.

September, 1997

Acknowledgements

We have many people to thank. These include Fiona Foley, Sue Hodgson, Richard Foulsham, Pete Wilder, Lynda Payne and Hamish Adamson at Mosby International, without whose experience, expertise, constant cajoling and encouragement this enterprise would soon have foundered, and our families, who have been extraordinarily tolerant and supportive. We should also emphasize that this book has been a collaborative effort, involving not only the authors but also many colleagues, who provided advice and generously allowed us to use precious slides and photographs, and whose help is gratefully acknowledged.

The following figures have been reproduced or adapted from the listed sources. Their use is gratefully acknowledged.

2.3, 2.4, 2.5a, 2.7b, 2.12, 2.64c–e, 2.65 reproduced with permission from Graham DI and Lantos PL (1997) *Greenfield's Neuropathology* 6th Edn, Arnold, London.Volume I, pp. 457, 443, 456, 457, 459, 487, 480.

2.5a,b, 2.23a, 2.38a reproduced with permission from Reed GB et al. (1995) *Diseases of the Fetus and Newborn.* Chapman & Hall, London. Figures 30.16, 30.23, 30.30.

3.13b; 3.24; 3.30; 3.32a,b; 3.34; 3.35a; 3.38a,b,e; 3.40b; 3.46b; 3.48a; 3.53a; 3.58g, d; 3.64; 3.70a; 3.73a; 3.76a; 3.82b; 3.90a; 3.96a,b; 3.103; 3.104d,c; 3.107; 3.112b reproduced with permission from Graham DI and Lantos PL (1997) *Greenfield's Neuropathology* 6th Edn, Arnold, London.Volume I, pp 414, 418, 422, 425, 424, 428, 426, 431, 432, 435, 441, 440, 443, 447, 448, 450, 455, 507, 472, 485, 484, 487, 500.

4.5; 4.11; 4.13a; 4.14a,b; 4.15a,b; 4.18 and 4.20 reproduced with permission of Oxford University Press from *Hydrocephalus*: Schurr and Polkey (1983), Chapter 3.

4.9b reproduced with permission from Graham DI and Lantos PL (1997) *Greenfield's Neuropathology* 6th Edn, Arnold, London.Volume I, pp 505.

5.5a reproduced with permission from Harding B. (1990) *J Child Neurol* 5:273–87.

6.1a; 6.1b; 6.1c reproduced with permission from Harding B et al. (1986) *Brain* 109:181–206.

6.12a reproduced with permission from Graham DI and Lantos PL (1997) *Greenfield's Neuropathology* 6th Edn, Arnold, London. Volume II, p.566.

6.16a reproduced with permission from Graham DI and Lantos PL (1997) *Greenfield's Neuropathology* 6th Edn, Arnold, London. Volume II, p. 848.

7.8a reproduced with permission of Dr Susan Mayou and Dr Phillip McKee from McKee P (1996) *Pathology of the Skin*, Second edition. Mosby-Wolfe, London. p. 5.6.

9.8a,b,c reproduced with permission from Ikeda E and Hosoda Y (1993) *Clin Neuropathol* 12:44–48.

11.1 reproduced with permission from Teasdale G, Jennett B (1974) *Lancet* (ii): 81–83, copyright by The Lancet Ltd.

13.28 (a), 13.29, 13.49 reproduced with permission from Vinters, HV and Anders, KH (1990) *Neuropathology of AIDS*, CRC Press.

13.43 reproduced with permission from Anders KH et al. (1990–1991) *Pediatr Neurosurg.* 16:316–320.

13.54 (a) reproduced with permission from Farrell MA et al. (1995) *Acta Neuropathol.* 89:313–321.

17.12a reproduced with permission from Queiroz L et al. (1979) *Arq. Neuropsiquiatr.* 37:303–10.

18.2, 18.3 reproduced with permission from Martinez and Visvesvara (1997) *Brain Pathology* 7:583–98.

18.12, 18.42, 18.60 adapted with permission from Jeffrey HC and Leach RM (1991) *Atlas of Medical Helminthology and Protozoology*, pp. 20, 27, 42, by permission of Churchill Livingstone.

18.43a, 18.45 reproduced with permission from Colli BO et al. (1994) *Arq Neuropsiquiatr.* 52:166–186.

18.57 reproduced with permission of Dr JEH Pittella.

19.24 (a) reproduced with permission from Prineas JW (1985) *Handbook of Clinical Neurology*, Volume 3(4), Chapter 8, figure 22, by permission of Elsevier Science Publishers.

19.30 reproduced with permission from Cook SD (1990) *Handbook of Multiple Sclerosis*, Chapter 9, Figure 4b, by permission of Marcel Dekker, Inc.

22.33 reproduced with permission from Anders KH et al. (1993) *Human Pathology* 24: 897–904.

23.4b, 23.11b reproduced with permission from Graham DI and Lantos PL (1997) *Greenfield's Neuropathology* 6th Edn, Arnold, London. Volume I, p. 670, p. 699.

24.1 adapted with permission from Zevani M and Antozzi C (1992) *Brain Pathology* 2: 121–132.

25.3(a) reproduced with permission from Hargreaves RJ et al. (1988) *Neuropath Appl Neurobiol.* 14: 443–52.

31.20 adapted with permission of Dr RA Crowther from Crowther RA (1991) *PNAS USA* 88: 2288.

31.26, 31.27 adapted with permission from Braak et al. (1991) *Acta Neuropathologica* 82: 239–59.

31.30, 31.31 adapted with permission from Mirra et al. *Neurology* (1991) 41:479–86 (as republished in *Arch Pathol Lab Med* (1993) 117) American Academy of Neurology.

34.5 reproduced with permission of Teaching Support and Media Services, University of Southampton.

34.13 reproduced with permission from Kleihues P, Burger PC, Scheithauer BW (1993) *International Histological Classification of Tumors. Histological typing of tumors of the central nervous system,* Second edition. Berlin: Springer–Verlag.

35.2(a) adapted with permission from Watanabe et al. (1996) *Brain Pathology* 6:217–224.

35.27 adapted with permission from Short MP et al. (1995) *Brain Pathology* 5:173–9.

The box giving the survival rate of patients with oligodendrogliomas graded according to the St Anne/Mayo system (p. 36.1) quotes data with permission from Shaw et al. (1992) *J Neurosurg* 76: 428–434.

43.1 reproduced with permission from Kleihues P, Burger PC, Scheithauer BW (1993) *International Histological Classification of Tumors. Histological typing of tumors of the central nervous system,* Second edition. Berlin: Springer–Verlag.

Contents

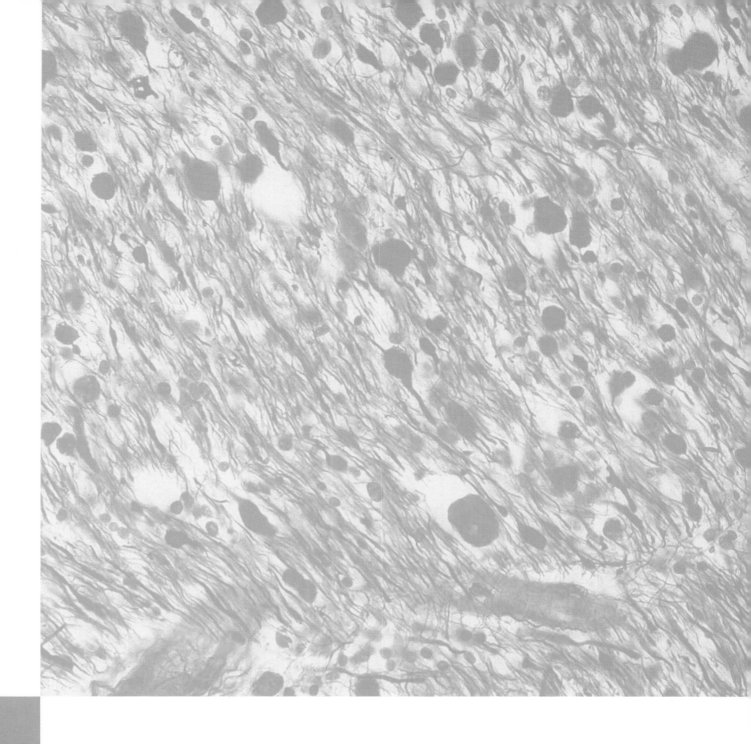

1 Pathologic reactions in the CNS

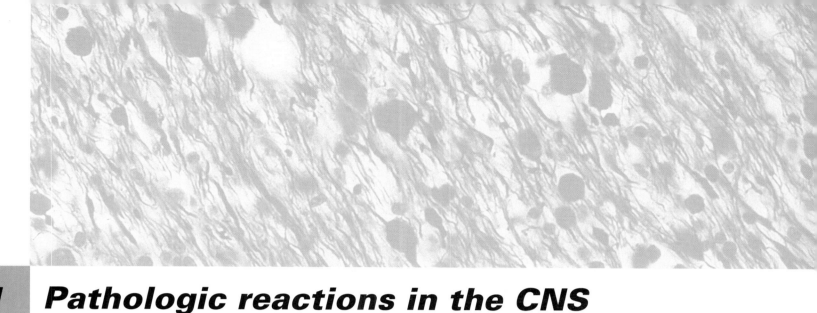

1 *Pathologic reactions in the CNS*

PATHOLOGIC RESPONSES IN NEURONS

NORMAL NEURONAL CYTOLOGY AND STAINING

The cytologic appearance of neurons varies depending upon their location. In general, neurons have moderate to abundant cytoplasm and a relatively large round nucleus with a prominent nucleolus. Projecting from the neuronal cell body are branching dendrites and a single axon. A range of tinctorial and immunohistochemical staining techniques are used for demonstrating neurons and their processes (**Fig. 1.1**).

ABNORMALITIES OF NEURONAL MORPHOLOGY

Axonal degeneration

Axonal degeneration is an inevitable consequence of death of the neuron of which it is a part. A severed or severely damaged axon undergoes distal degeneration without usually provoking death of the proximal part of the neuron, although this does undergo a series of structural and metabolic changes (i.e. axon reaction and chromatolysis, see below). Within days, the distal part of the axon fragments and the surrounding myelin sheath breaks up into ovoids. Over the course of the next 3 weeks or so, the axon and myelin debris are taken up by macrophages, which infiltrate the degenerating fiber tracts. Several methods can be used to demonstrate degenerating nerve fibers in the CNS. These include specialized silver impregnation techniques and stains for degenerating myelin and for lipid (**Fig. 1.2**). Marchi's method, and oil red O or other stains for neutral lipid are particularly useful. During the first 2–3 weeks after injury when most of the products of fiber degeneration are still extracellular, their demonstration by Marchi's method requires staining of unembedded tissue that has not fixed long in formalin. If there has been a longer period of time since the injury and much of the debris has been taken up by macrophages, Marchi's method can be used on frozen sections and the staining is not affected by the duration of formalin fixation. Stains for neutral lipid can be used to demonstrate degeneration of fiber tracts for several months after an injury and Marchi's method for several years.

Axon reaction and chromatolysis

Damage to the axon provokes a series of morphologic and biochemical changes in the neuronal cell body and these are collectively referred to as the axon reaction (**Figs 1.3, 1.4**). The changes include disruption and dispersion of Nissl bodies (chromatolysis) associated with rearrangement of the cytoskeleton and marked accumulation of intermediate filaments. The axon reaction is conspicuous in large neurons with axons that project into the peripheral nervous system and in some of the larger neurons with central projections. Chromatolysis is not visible on conventional light microscopy of small neurons or certain large neurons such as the cerebellar Purkinje cells, but changes can be demonstrated in these cells on electron microscopy and immunohistochemistry.

Histologic demonstration of neurons: techniques and comments concerning their applications
Conventional staining
Hematoxylin and eosin • Good for assessing general cytoarchitecture.
Nissl stain (e.g. cresyl fast violet) • Good for assessing general cytoarchitecture. Allows estimation of cell density in thick sections; may be combined with stains for myelin.
Axon silver impregnation techniques • Good for demonstration of axons and some neuronal inclusions. Used in conjunction with myelin stains to distinguish between demyelination and fiber degeneration.
Golgi stain • Allows visualization of fine detail of neuronal cell processes. A technically difficult stain to perform which depends on block impregnation.
Immunohistochemistry
Neurofilament proteins • Strongly expressed in perikaryal and axonal cytoplasm (in normal neurons, perikaryal neurofilament proteins are non-phosphorylated and axonal neurofilament proteins phosphorylated).
Neuron specific enolase • Strongly expressed in neuronal and axonal cytoplasm.
Synaptophysin • Detects neurosecretory vesicles, which are mainly located at synapses. Little staining of neuronal cell bodies.
PGP9.5 • An antibody to neuron-specific ubiquitin C-terminal hydrolase, which is abundant in neurons and neuronal cell processes.
Chromogranin A • Detects dense-core neurosecretory vesicles, which are sparsely distributed within the perikaryon of some neurons and concentrated at the synapses. Moderate staining of neuronal cell bodies.
Neurotransmitter-related • Detection of neurotransmitter substance or enzyme involved in its biosynthesis.

Fig. 1.1 Tinctorial and immunohistochemical staining techniques used for demonstrating neurons and their processes.

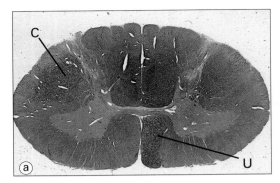
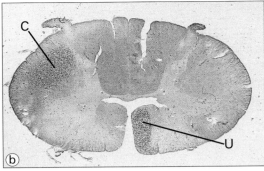

Fig. 1.2 Tract degeneration. Adjacent sections of cervical spinal cord 1 month after an infarct involving the internal capsule. The infarct has caused degeneration of the descending crossed (C) and uncrossed (U) corticospinal tract fibers. (**a**) Stained with oil red O. (**b**) Stained with Marchi's method.

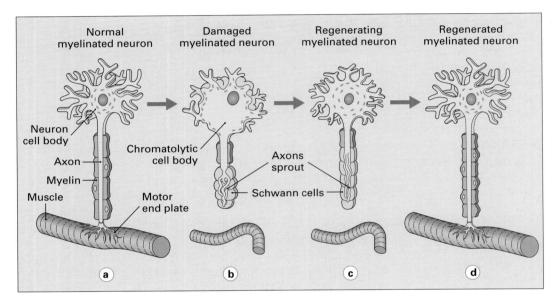

Fig. 1.3 Axon reaction. The changes that constitute the axon reaction have been most extensively investigated in anterior horn cells after peripheral nerve injury, as depicted in this figure, but neurons undergo similar alterations after injury to axons in the CNS. (**a**) A normal neuronal cell body is characterized by well-organized dendritic branches making synaptic contact with other neurons. Nissl bodies are prominent. (**b**) Following axonal damage there is degeneration of the peripheral axon. Dendrites that normally form synapses retract and synaptic contacts are lost. The rough endoplasmic reticulum becomes reorganized into small vesicular elements. The neuron inactivates genes coding for high molecular weight neurofilament protein (NFH) and switches on genes for peripherin. Neurofilaments and peripherin accumulate in the neuronal cell body. At this stage the neuronal cell body is swollen, shows only weak acidophilia, and lacks Nissl bodies. Denervated muscle fibers atrophy. (**c**) The axon regenerates in the peripheral nervous system (but not within the CNS). NFH synthesis is re-established with axonal elongation. (**d**) If the target tissue is reinnervated, the neuronal dendrites re-establish synaptic contact with other neurons and the normal cytologic appearance of the cell body is regained.

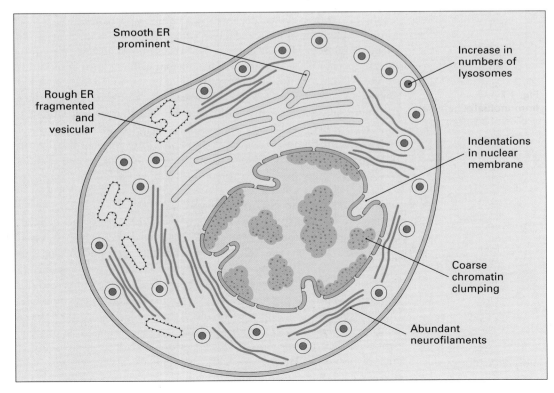

Fig. 1.4 Ultrastructural characteristics of the axon reaction. Several morphologic changes are seen in neurons after axonal damage.

Swollen neurons

Swollen or ballooned neurons are a feature both of the axon reaction and of a variety of diseases in which perikaryal changes occur independently of axonal damage (**Fig. 1.5**). Histologically they appear as swollen pale-staining cells with large, relatively clear nuclei (**Fig. 1.6**). Occasionally the cells contain small intracellular vacuoles. In conventionally processed tissues an artefactual lacuna is often present around the abnormal cell. Swollen or ballooned neurons can be demonstrated with several immunohistochemical markers (**Figs 1.7, 1.8**).

Trans-synaptic neuronal degeneration and olivary hypertrophy

Neurons within some nuclei in the CNS atrophy and degenerate in response to deafferentation. Examples are neurons in the lateral geniculate nucleus, which degenerate after optic nerve or tract lesions, and neurons in the pontine nuclei, which degenerate after interruption of descending frontopontine afferent fibers. Neurons in the inferior and accessory olivary nuclei undergo an unusual form of trans-synaptic degeneration after a destructive lesion (such as an infarct) of the ipsilateral central tegmental tract (**Fig. 1.9**). The olivary ribbon as a whole becomes thickened and neurons show marked enlargement, cytoplasmic vacuolation, and some dispersion of Nissl bodies. Olivary hypertrophy is associated with the development of palatal myoclonus in some patients.

Causes of ballooned neurons
Physiologic • Anterior horn motor neurons, with age
Pick's disease • Cortical and some basal neurons
Corticobasal degeneration • Cortical and some basal neurons
Pellagra • Spinal, brain stem, and cortical neurons
Prion disease • Cortical and some basal neurons
Alzheimer's disease • Rare cases show swollen cortical neurons

Fig 1.5 Causes of ballooned neurons.

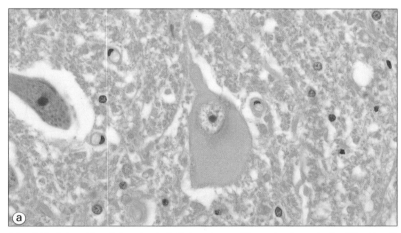

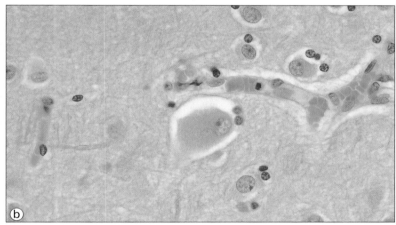

Fig. 1.6 A swollen (chromatolytic) neuron. The cytoplasm lacks Nissl bodies and is weakly eosinophilic. The nucleus is large and vesicular. (**a**) Example from the anterior horn of the spinal cord. (**b**) Example from the cerebral cortex in corticobasal degeneration (see chapter 28).

Immunohistochemical profile of swollen neurons
Neurofilament protein • Accumulation of highly phosphorylated high-molecular-weight neurofilament protein, which is normally restricted to the axon
αB-crystallin • Accumulation of αB crystallin, which is not normally expressed by neurons
Tau protein • Accumulation of abnormally phosphorylated tau protein by a proportion of swollen neurons in corticobasal degeneration and Pick's disease
Ubiquitin • Variably increased immunoreactivity for ubiquitin-protein conjugates
PGP9.5 • Variably increased immunoreactivity for this ubiquitin C-terminal hydrolase

Fig. 1.7 Immunohistochemical profile of swollen neurons.

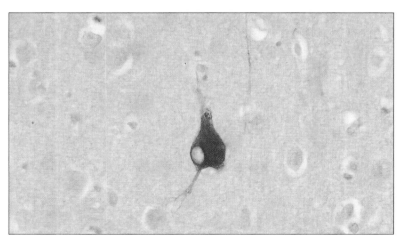

Fig. 1.8 αB-crystallin immunoreactivity. This is a characteristic feature of swollen neurons in most conditions. The protein is not, however, expressed by swollen neurons in pellagra (see chapter 21), suggesting that neuronal swelling in this disorder has a different mechanism.

Hypoxic cell change

Neurons are especially vunerable to damage from hypoxia, which causes the following distinctive histologic changes (**Fig. 1.10**) (see also chapter 8):

- microvacuolation (visible only at an ultrastructural level), due to swelling of endoplasmic reticulum and mitochondria
- shrinkage of the cell body and increasing cytoplasmic acidophilia
- condensation of nuclear chromatin and nuclear pyknosis
- later, disappearance of the nuclear chromatin, resulting in increased acidophilia of the nucleus, which appears to merge into the surrounding cytoplasm (nuclear 'drop out').

Histologic changes identical to these can be induced in neurons by hypoglycemia or by exposure to excessive amounts of excitotoxic neurotransmitters.

Cell stress proteins are expressed at an early stage of hypoxic injury and are demonstrable by immunohistochemical techniques.

Neurons in certain parts of the brain that are especially vulnerable to hypoxic damage are:

- pyramidal neurons in the CA1 field of the hippocampus
- pyramidal neurons in layers 3 and 5 of the neocortex
- purkinje cells in the cerebellum.

The pattern of regional susceptibility to hypoxia differs in infants from that in adults (see chapters 2 and 8).

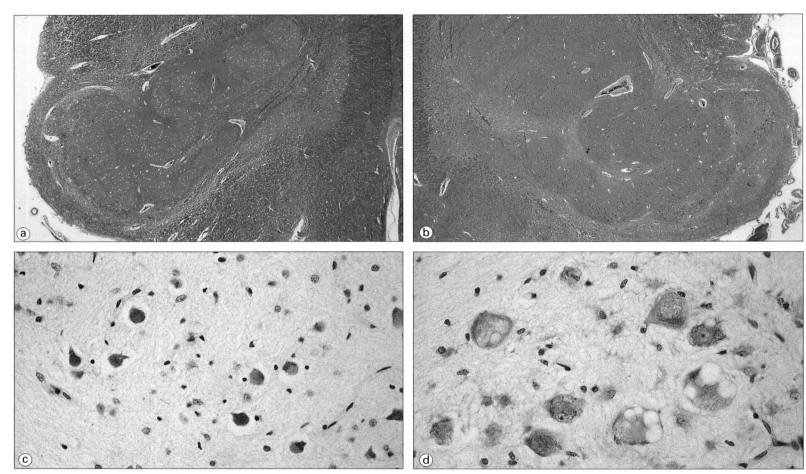

Fig. 1.9 Hypertrophy of the left olive due to a lesion involving the left central tegmental tract. (a) Normal right olive. **(b)** Hypertrophy of the left olive. The lesion involving the left central tegmental tract is not shown. Compare the normal-sized neurons in the right olive with the enlarged vacuolated neurons in the left olive. **(c)** Normal neurons of the right inferior olivary nucleus stained with cresyl violet. **(d)** Neurons of the hypertrophic lleft inferior olive are enlarged and vacuolated. (Cresyl violet)

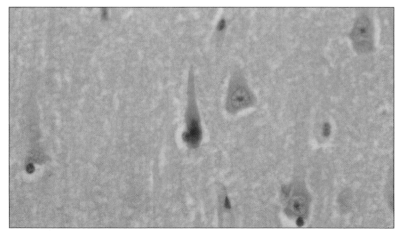

Fig. 1.10 Hypoxic cell change in neurons. Affected neurons become shrunken and eosinophilic. The nuclei become condensed and lose their crisp contours. In this illustration the neuron in the center is affected while surrounding neurons appear normal.

Ferrugination

Although dead neurons usually undergo liquefaction or are removed by phagocytosis they may instead become encrusted and replaced by mineral salts, a process termed ferrugination. This is particularly prominent in the infant brain in response to hypoxic-ischemic damage (**Fig. 1.11**).

NUCLEAR INCLUSIONS

Marinesco bodies

These are small spherical nuclear inclusions that are brightly eosinophilic and are often seen in adults in neurons of the substantia nigra (**Fig. 1.12a**). They may also occur in other neurons, such as the pyramidal cells of the hippocampus and neurons in the tegmentum of the brain stem.

Ultrastructurally, Marinesco bodies are composed of filaments with the same diameter as intermediate filaments, and may be derived from the nuclear lamins. They are immunoreactive for ubiquitin, an 8 kD polypeptide involved in the degradation of many abnormal or short-lived proteins (**Fig. 1.12b**).

Viral inclusions

Nuclear inclusions are a feature of infection by several viruses (see chapters 13 and 14), for example cytomegalovirus infection, which produces particularly striking nuclear inclusions (**Fig. 1.13**).

NEURONAL CYTOPLASMIC INCLUSIONS

Neuronal cytoplasmic inclusions can be divided into those composed of cytoskeletal elements, cytosolic inclusions, and membrane-bound inclusions.

CYTOSKELETAL AND FILAMENTOUS INCLUSIONS
Hirano bodies

These are brightly eosinophilic rod-shaped or elliptical cytoplasmic inclusions that may appear to overlap the edge of a neuron (**Fig. 1.14**). They are immunoreactive for actin, and actin-associated proteins.

Ultrastructurally, Hirano bodies consist of a regular lattice of multiple layers of parallel 10–12 nm filaments, the filaments in one layer being transversely or diagonally oriented with respect to those in the adjacent layers.

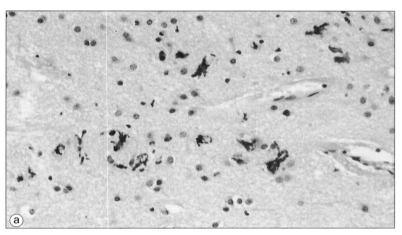

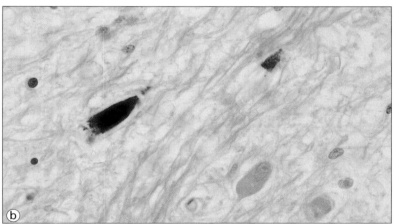

Fig. 1.11 Ferruginated neurons. Ferruginated neurons become encrusted in mineral deposits and appear dark purple in sections stained with hematoxylin and eosin. The mineral deposits contain both calcium and iron and can be stained by Perls' method and von Kossa's technique.

(a) Many ferruginated neurons in the cortex of a neonate who had hypoxic brain damage. Astroglial cells are not affected. **(b)** Higher power illustration of neurons replaced by mineral deposits.

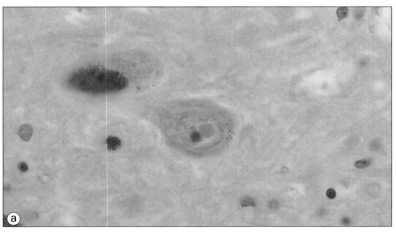

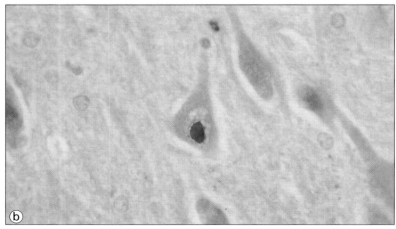

Fig. 1.12 Marinesco bodies. These intranuclear inclusions are visible in several neuronal groups. **(a)** Marinesco bodies are brightly eosinophilic intranuclear inclusions about the same size as a large nucleolus. **(b)** As shown here, they are strongly immunoreactive for ubiquitin.

Hirano bodies are most numerous in the CA1 field of the hippocampus. Their density in the stratum lacunosum increases until middle age and declines gradually thereafter, except in chronic alcoholics, in whom the density may continue to increase. In the elderly, the number of Hirano bodies increases in the stratum pyramidale, and they are particularly numerous in this region in Alzheimer's disease, Pick's disease, and Guam parkinsonism–dementia.

Eosinophilic thalamic neuronal inclusions

These are smaller than Hirano bodies, but are otherwise similar in shape and tinctorial staining characteristics. They occur in thalamic neurons in normal middle-aged and elderly individuals, but are commoner in patients with myotonic dystrophy.

Rod-like cytoplasmic inclusions

These eosinophilic cytoplasmic inclusions occur in large neurons of the caudate nucleus. The inclusions resemble loose bundles of twigs and, like the thalamic neuronal inclusions described above, are common in patients with myotonic dystrophy but are sometimes an incidental finding in elderly patients who do not have neurologic or muscular disease. The rod-like inclusions stain strongly with phosphotungstic acid/hematoxylin (**Fig. 1.15**).

Other filamentous neuronal inclusions

There are several other types of neuronal inclusion that comprise or include elements of the cytoskeleton and usually occur in the context of specific neurodegenerative diseases (**Fig. 1.16**). These inclusions are described in more detail and illustrated in the sections concerned with the relevant diseases.

CYTOSOLIC INCLUSIONS
Lafora bodies

These are composed of polyglucosans (polymers of sulfated polysaccharides) and are similar to corpora amylacea in composition and staining characteristics (see below). They are present in large numbers in Lafora's disease (see chapter 7), both in the CNS and in certain peripheral tissues such as sweat glands, liver, and skeletal muscle. The inclusions usually have a round core that is intensely periodic acid–Schiff (PAS)-positive (**Fig. 1.17**). Spicules of the core may radiate outwards, into a surrounding zone of less intensely PAS-positive material.

Eosinophilic inclusions in the inferior olives

A characteristic feature of aging is the development of ill-defined eosinophilic inclusions in the neurons of the inferior olivary nuclei. These inclusions are intensely immunoreactive with antibodies to ubiquitin (**Fig. 1.18**) and should not be confused with lipofuscin, which also accumulates with age (see below) and is particularly abundant in neurons of the inferior olivary nuclei.

MEMBRANE-BOUND CYTOPLASMIC INCLUSIONS
Colloid inclusions

Colloid inclusions are rounded eosinophilic inclusions that usually occur in neurons in the hypoglossal nuclei (**Fig. 1.19**), but may be seen in other large neurons, particularly in the elderly. Electron microscopy shows that these inclusions result from dilatation of the endoplasmic reticulum by amorphous material. The importance of recognizing colloid inclusions, which do not have any clinical significance, is that they are occasionally confused with inclusions that are clinically significant such as Lewy bodies, pale bodies, and hyaline inclusions of motor neuron disease (see chapter 27).

Bunina bodies

These are small beaded eosinophilic inclusions seen in motor neurons in motor neuron disease. Ultrastructurally they appear as electron-dense membrane bound bodies (see chapter 27).

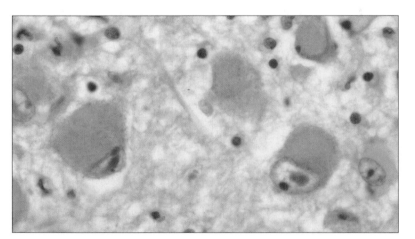

Fig. 1.13 Intranuclear cytomegalovirus inclusion. While several viruses cause intranuclear inclusions the most impressive are those caused by cytomegalovirus, here seen as eosinophilic intranuclear bodies.

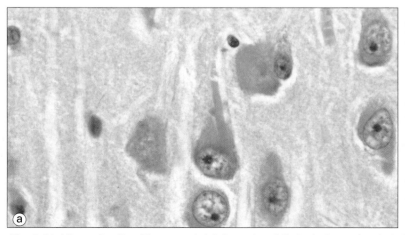
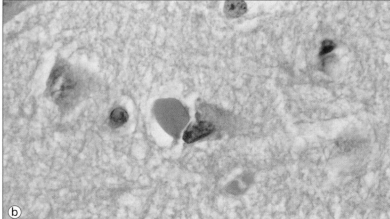

Fig. 1.14 Hirano bodies. These are brightly eosinophilic inclusions of varied shape. (**a**) The majority are small rod-shaped structures with rounded ends. (**b**) Others have a globular appearance.

Inclusions derived from the acid vesicle system

The acid vesicle system consists of endosomes, lysosomes, and lysosome-derived dense bodies.

Lipofuscin (**Fig. 1.20**) is produced by oxidation of lipids and lipoproteins within the lysosomal system. It appears as orange-brown granular material in sections stained with hematoxylin and eosin, is acid-fast (as demonstrated by the long Ziehl–Neelsen method), and autofluorescent under ultraviolet light. The granules are also sudanophilic and stain with PAS and Schmorl's stain. Lipofuscin accumulates with aging in neurons and glia, particularly in:

- the inferior olive
- the dentate nucleus
- pyramidal neurons in the cerebral cortex and hippocampus
- large neurons in the amygdala, thalamus, and hypothalamus
- motor neurons in the brain stem and spinal cord

The lipofuscin accumulation is increased in some neurodegenerative disorders such as Alzheimer's disease and motor neuron disease.

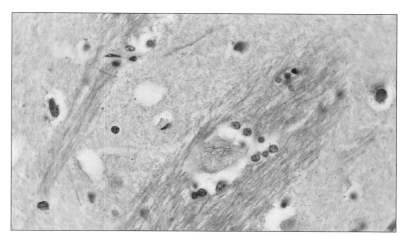

Fig. 1.15 Rod-like cytoplasmic inclusions in the caudate nucleus. These occur exclusively in large neurons in the caudate nucleus. The inclusions may be an incidental finding, particularly in the elderly, but are most common in myotonic dystrophy. (Phosphotungstic acid/hematoxylin) (Courtesy of Dr DA Hilton, Derriford Hospital, Plymouth)

Examples of inclusion bodies in specific conditions and diseases

Inclusion	Association	Main constituents
Lewy bodies	Aging, Parkinson's disease, dementia with Lewy bodies	Neurofilament protein and ubiquitin
Neurofibrillary tangles	Aging, Alzheimer's disease, progressive supranuclear palsy, post-encephalitic parkinsonism, Guam parkinsonism–dementia, myotonic dystrophy, subacute sclerosing panenecephalitis, Niemann–Pick disease type C, other rare disorders	Phosphorylated tau protein, ubiquitin
Pick bodies	Pick's disease	Neurofilament protein, phosphorylated tau protein, ubiquitin
MND inclusions	Motor neuron disease	Filaments of uncertain nature, ubiquitin

Fig 1.16 Examples of inclusion bodies in specific conditions and diseases.

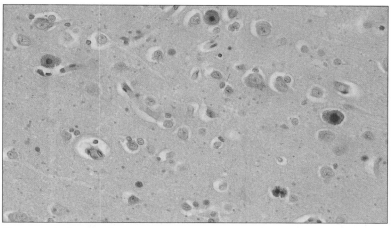

Fig. 1.17 Lafora bodies in both neurons and glia in the cerebral cortex. The strong affinity of the polyglucosans for PAS reagent is not affected by diastase digestion. Many of the inclusions consist of a deeply stained core surrounded by a concentric zone of less intensely PAS-positive material.

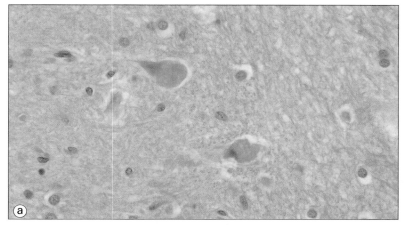

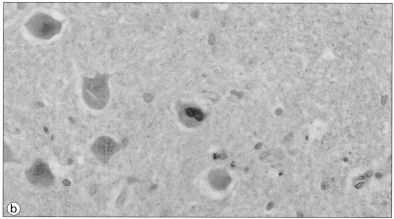

Fig. 1.18 Eosinophilic inclusions in the inferior olives. (a) There are ill-defined eosinophilic inclusions surrounded by lipofuscin in these inferior olivary neurons. **(b)** The inclusions are intensely immunoreactive with antibodies to ubiquitin.

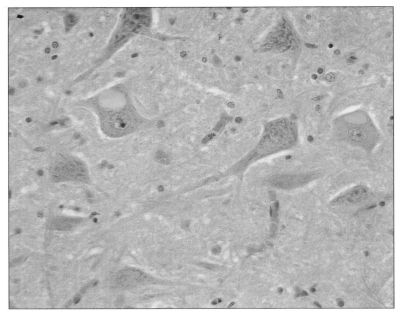

Fig. 1.19 Colloid (hyaline) inclusions in the hypoglossal nucleus. In this example, two neurons contain typical rounded, homogeneous, eosinophilic inclusions.

Granulovacuolar degeneration. This term describes the accumulation of vacuoles containing small round dense bodies (granulovacuoles) (Fig. 1.21). The dense bodies are ubiquitinated and react with antibodies to some epitopes of the microtubule-associated tau protein. The immuno-histochemical data have been interpreted as suggesting that the dense bodies are derived from partial degradation of tau protein within lyso-somes. Granulovacuolar degeneration is seen in normal aging after the sixth decade, predominantly in the hippocampal formation. Neurons in the CA1 field are most severely affected and, in descending order of severity, those in the prosubiculum, CA2, CA3, and CA4 fields less so. The density of hippocampal neurons showing granulovacuolar degeneration is increased in patients with Alzheimer's disease and Pick's disease, in whom granulovacuolar degeneration may also occur in neurons in the subcortical nuclei.

Storage products in neurometabolic diseases. The accumulation of material within the acid vesicle system is a feature of many neurometabolic diseases including the lysosomal storage disorders as well as certain other metabolic disorders caused by non-lysosomal enzyme defects. These disorders are considered in chapter 23.

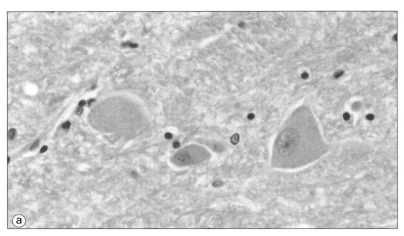
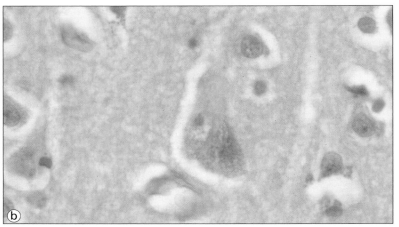

Fig. 1.20 Lipofuscin. This accumulates with age in neurons and glia. **(a)** It has a golden brown color in sections stained with hematoxylin and eosin. **(b)** Lipofuscin stains strongly with PAS.

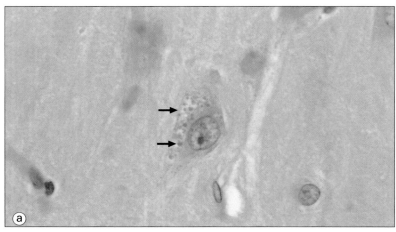
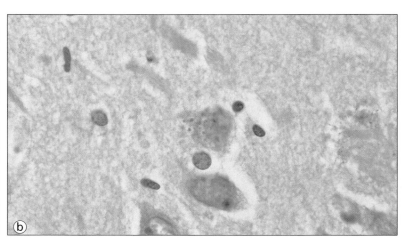

Fig. 1.21 Granulovacuolar degeneration. (a) These are small round basophilic bodies within otherwise clear vacuoles (arrows). They are mainly found in pyramidal neurons of the hippocampus. **(b)** The granules are often immunoreactive for ubiquitin.

STRUCTURAL ABNORMALITIES OF AXONS

AXONAL SPHEROIDS AND DYSTROPHIC AXONAL SWELLINGS

Spheroids are axonal swellings composed of neurofilaments, organelles, and other material that is normally conveyed along the axon by anterograde transport systems, but accumulates focally when these are impaired (**Fig. 1.22a,b**). Spheroids are a feature of axonal damage by diverse extrinsic insults, especially trauma (see chapter 11) and infarcts. There may be numerous axonal spheroids around the edge of an infarct.

The term 'torpedo' is applied to Purkinje cell axonal swellings, which are a feature of a wide range of metabolic and degenerative cerebellar diseases. These swellings appear as fusiform eosinophilic structures in the cerebellar granule cell layer (**Fig. 1.22c,d**). They are well demonstrated by silver impregnation (see chapter 29).

The axonal swellings that develop when axonal transport is disrupted by neuronal metabolic dysfunction are usually termed dystrophic (**Fig. 1.22e**). These occur in certain nutritional deficiencies (particularly vitamin E deficiency, see chapter 21) and inherited metabolic diseases (e.g. Niemann–Pick disease type C). Dystrophic axonal swellings are the principal pathologic abnormality seen in a group of conditions termed the neuroaxonal dystrophies (see chapter 33).

The term 'dystrophic neurite' is also used to describe neuronal processes within the grey matter that are distended by tau protein or other abnormal ubiquitinated material. These occur in several neurodegenerative diseases (**Fig. 1.23**).

Dystrophic axons that react strongly with antibodies to ubiquitin are a feature of ageing in the CNS, especially in the gracile and cuneate nuclei, the substantia nigra, the globus pallidus, and the anterior horns of the spinal cord.

In brains from people over 60 years of age, antibodies to ubiquitin label smaller dot-like structures in the neuropil of the cerebral cortex and in the white matter. These correspond to membrane-bound dense bodies in dystrophic neurites and foci of granular degeneration in myelin sheaths (**Fig. 1.24**).

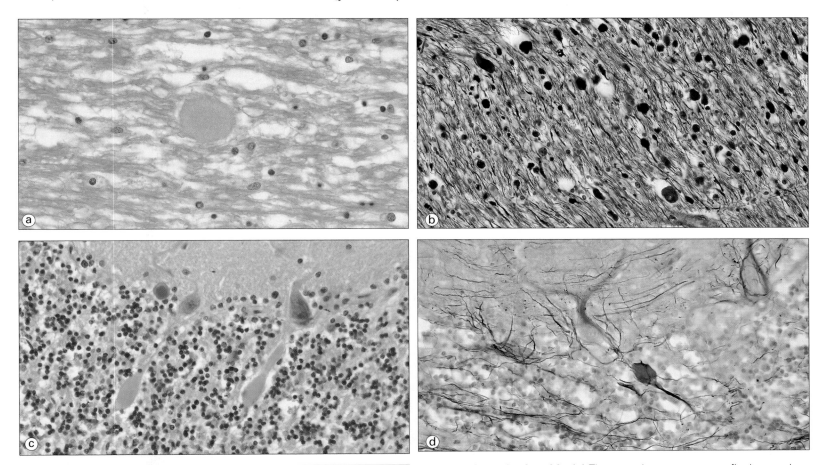

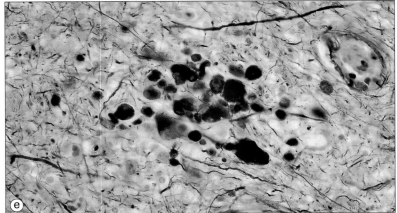

Fig. 1.22 Axonal spheroids. (a) These are homogeneous or finely granular, rounded, eosinophilic bodies. **(b)** They can be demonstrated with antibodies to neurofilament proteins or by axonal silver impregnation, as in this section through the centrum semiovale after head trauma that resulted in diffuse axonal injury with numerous spheroids. **(c)** Torpedoes are Purkinje cell axonal swellings seen in the granule cell layer of the cerebellum. They have a characteristic fusiform appearance, as shown here, and occur in conditions that cause cerebellar cortical atrophy with degeneration of Purkinje cells. **(d)** Torpedoes with a characteristic fusiform appearance. (Glees and Marsland silver impregnation) **(e)** Dystrophic axonal swellings are a feature of some metabolic diseases, as illustrated in this section of putamen from a patient with Niemann–Pick disease type C. (Palmgren silver impregnation)

PATHOLOGIC RESPONSES IN ASTROCYTES

Astrocytes are vital suppport cells of the nervous system. They can be demonstrated by a range of tinctorial stains and immunohistochemical techniques (**Fig. 1.25**) and undergo a range of structural changes in reaction to disease of the CNS.

SWELLING OF ASTROCYTES

This is a relatively rapid response to a wide range of stimuli. Acutely reactive astrocytes are swollen by hyalin eosinophilic cytoplasm and have enlarged vesicular nuclei (**Fig. 1.26**).

Dystrophic axons in aging and neurodegenerative diseases	
Condition	Dystrophic processes
Normal aging	• Neuronal processes accumulate dot-like ubiquitin-immunoreactive material (Fig 1.24).
Alzheimer's disease	• The swollen neuronal processes around amyloid plaques are termed dystrophic neurites. Many contain ubiquitinated proteins, with or without accumulation of tau protein (chapter 31).
Lewy body disease	• Abnormal neurites in affected brain regions can be detected by ubiquitin immunohistochemistry (chapter 28).
Huntington's disease	• Abnormal neurites in the cerebral cortex can be detected by ubiquitin immunohistochemistry (chapter 30).
Frontal lobe dementia	• Abnormal neurites in the cerebral cortex can be detected by ubiquitin immunohistochemistry (chapter 31).

Fig 1.23 Dystrophic axons in aging and neurodegenerative diseases.

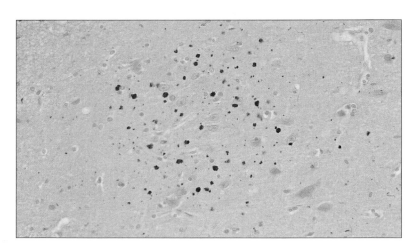

Fig. 1.24 Dot-like ubiquitin immunoreactivity in the temporal cortex in one of the pre-α cell clusters. The frequency and density of ubiquitin-immunoreactive dot-like bodies increases with age in both gray and white matter. This example shows dot-like bodies in the temporal cortex in one of the pre-α cell clusters.

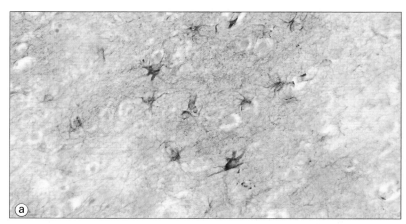

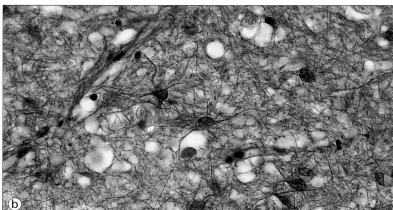

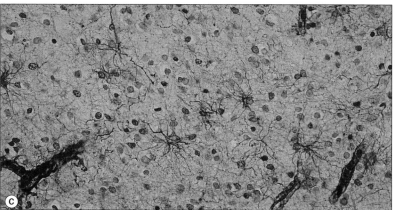

Fig. 1.25 Stains demonstrating astrocytes. (a) Astrocytes are often demonstrated by immunohistochemical staining for glial fibrillary acidic protein (GFAP). This reveals their stellate morphology as well as the blush-like staining of very fine processes in the neuropil. **(b)** Phosphotungstic acid–hematoxylin stain demonstrating astrocytes. **(c)** Holzer stain. This also demonstrates astrocytes, but is seldom used now because of the potential carcinogenicity of some of the reagents used in its preparation.

FIBRILLARY GLIOSIS

With time, reactive astrocytes proliferate and insinuate long cytoplasmic processes into the adjacent brain parenchyma. These processes contain bundles of glial intermediate filaments, which appear as fibrils in appropriately stained preparations; hence the term fibrillary gliosis. The abundance of glial intermediate filaments is readily demonstrated by immunostaining for GFAP. Two patterns of fibrillary gliosis are recognized:

- Isomorpic fibrillary gliosis in which the alignment of astrocyte processes conforms to the architecture of previously normal local tissues (**Fig. 1.27**). This occurs mainly in chronic degenerative conditions.
- Anisomorphic fibrillary gliosis in which there is a haphazard deposition of a meshwork of astrocyte processes (**Fig. 1.28**). This is typical of the gliosis that occurs in relation to destructive lesions.

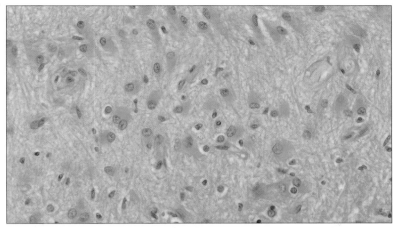

Fig. 1.26 Reactive astrocytes. Reactive astrocytes are enlarged and contain abundant homogeneous eosinophilic cytoplasm and open vesicular nuclei.

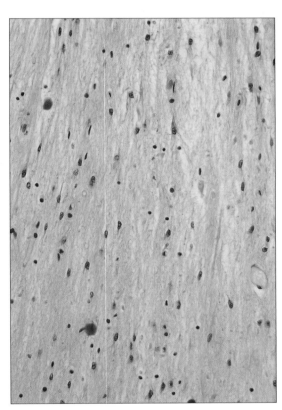

Fig. 1.27 Isomorphic astrocytic gliosis. The orientation of astrocyte processes conforms to that of cell processes in the underlying tissue. This pattern is characteristic of chronic degenerative conditions.

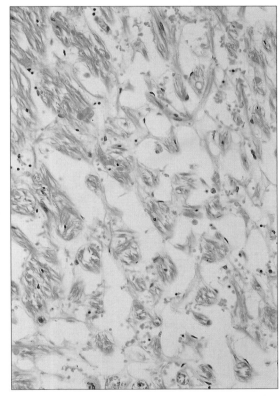

Fig. 1.28 Anisomorphic astrocytic gliosis. The haphazard orientation of astrocyte processes is typical of the glial scarring related to a destructive lesion such as an infarct.

ROSENTHAL FIBERS

Rosenthal fibers are inclusions that develop in astrocytes in chronic reactive and neoplastic proliferations. They are brightly eosinophilic structures of variable size and shape (**Fig. 1.29a,b**). On electron microscopy they contain admixed amorphous granular material and 10 nm diameter filaments (**Fig. 1.29c**). Immunohistochemistry reveals GFAP, αB-crystallin, 27 kD heat-shock protein, and ubiquitin at the periphery of the Rosenthal fibers (**Fig. 1.29d–f**), while the central hyaline region is generally unlabeled.

Rosenthal fibers are seen in longstanding reactive gliosis, especially when it occurs in the spinal cord, cerebellum, or hypothalamus. They are also a feature of pilocytic astrocytomas (see chapter 35). Rosenthal fibers are abundant in Alexander's disease (see chapter 6) and in giant axonal neuropathy (see chapter 33).

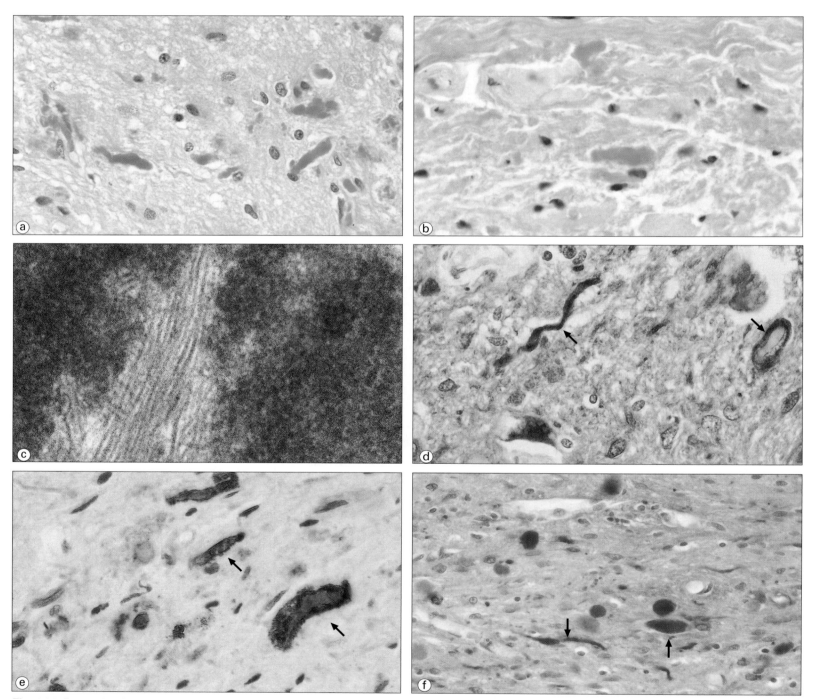

Fig. 1.29 Rosenthal fibers. (a) and **(b)** These fibers appear as brightly eosinophilic, rounded, elongated or carrot-shaped structures in hematoxylin and eosin-stained sections. **(c)** Electron microscopy revealing amorphous granular material and 10 nm diameter filaments within a Rosenthal fiber.

(d) Immunostain showing peripheral labeling (arrows) for GFAP.
(e) Immunostain showing peripheral labeling (arrows) for ubiquitin.
(f) Immunostain showing peripheral labeling (arrows) for αB-crystallin.

GRANULAR BODIES

Granular bodies are found in regions of chronic astrocytic gliosis, usually in conjunction with Rosenthal fibers. They are clusters of round eosinophilic granules within the cytoplasm of astrocytes (**Fig. 1.30**) and express GFAP as well as αB-crystallin. Ultrastructural examination reveals membrane-bound dense bodies.

TAU-REACTIVE GLIA

Tau protein has long been known to be the main constituent of neurofibrillary tangles, which are neuronal inclusions in Alzheimer's disease and several other disorders (see chapters 28, 29, and 31), but the recognition that glial cells can accumulate tau protein is a relatively recent finding. Several different types of tau-immunoreactive glial cell change have been described (**Figs 1.31, 1.32**).

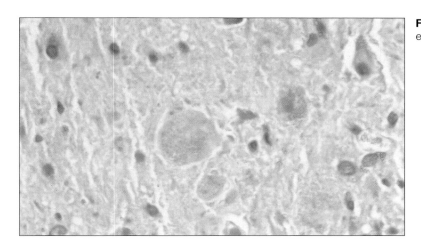

Fig. 1.30 Granular bodies. These are cytoplasmic clusters of rounded eosinophilic granules that vary in diameter.

Tau-reactive glial abnormalities		
Type	Association(s)*	Immunoreactivity
Glial fibrillary tangles	PSP, CBD, Pick's disease	Tau
Tufted astrocytes	PSP, Pick's disease	Tau
Thorn-shaped astrocytes	Several degenerative diseases	Tau
Interfascicular threads	PSP and CBD white matter (oligodendroglial inclusions)	Tau
Coils and threads	PSP, CBD	Tau
Astrocytic plaques	CBD	Tau
Glial cytoplasmic inclusions	Multiple system atrophy, CBD	Tau, ubiquitin, tubulin

*PSP – progressive supranuclear palsy
 CBD – corticobasal degeneration

Fig. 1.31 Tau-reactive glial abnormalities. This table lists the different types of tau-immunoreactive glial change, several of which are illustrated in Fig. 1.32. Others are illustrated in the relevant chapter.

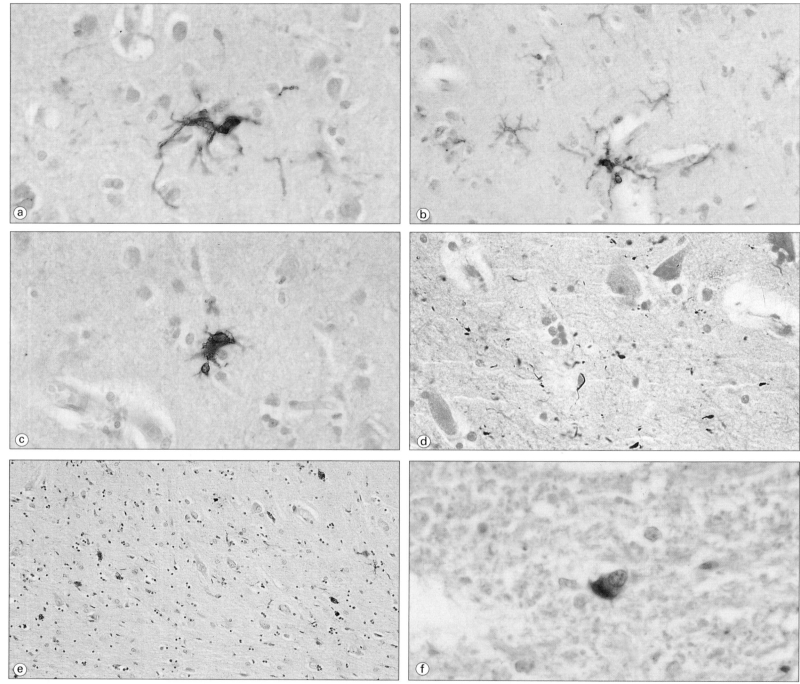

Fig. 1.32 Tau immunoreactivity in glial cells. This is usually seen in neurodegenerative diseases in which there is also a prominent accumulation of tau protein in neurons as inclusions. **(a)** Glial fibrillary tangles are stellate cells with an astroglial morphology. **(b)** Tufted astrocytes are a particular feature of progressive supranuclear palsy and corticobasal degeneration and are mainly seen in the cerebral cortex. **(c)** Thorn-shaped astrocytes have more abundant immunostained cytoplasm and blunt thorn-shaped processes and are found in many tau-related neurodegenerative diseases. **(d)** Coil-shaped bodies and threads occur mainly in progressive supranuclear palsy and corticobasal degeneration and can be detected by Gallyas silver impregnation. **(e)** The coil-shaped bodies and threads that occur mainly in progressive supranuclear palsy and corticobasal degeneration can also be detected by tau-immunostaining. **(f)** Glial cytoplasmic inclusions are seen in oligodendroglia and occur in large numbers in multiple system atrophy and in small numbers in corticobasal degeneration.

CORPORA AMYLACEA

Corpora amylacea are spherical inclusions, predominantly in astrocyte processes (**Fig. 1.33a,b**), although they occasionally occur within axons. They range from 10–50 μm in diameter, consist largely of polyglucosans and stain with hematoxylin, PAS, and methyl violet. Minor constituents include ubiquitin, heat-shock proteins, tau protein, complement proteins, and some oligodendrocyte proteins (i.e. myelin basic protein, proteolipid protein, galactocerebroside, and myelin oligodendrocyte protein). Ultrastructurally, corpora amylacea consist of densely packed 6–7 nm filaments that may be admixed with amorphous granular material and are not membrane bound.

Corpora amylacea increase in number with normal aging, particularly in subpial (**Fig. 1.33c**) and subependymal regions, around subcortical blood vessels, and in the spinal white matter. Their increase in number is greater in conditions where there has been atrophy and gliosis, including Alzheimer's disease and other neurodegenerative disorders.

The functions of corpora amylacea, if any, are not known. Suggestions include a role in the accumulation of inorganic materials from the blood and cerebrospinal fluid or in shielding immunogenic products of neuronal and oligodendroglial degeneration from lymphocytic recognition and autoimmune activation.

NUCLEAR CHANGES IN ASTROCYTES

Alzheimer type II astrocytes are seen in cortical and subcortical gray matter regions in liver failure. They have an enlarged vesicular nucleus with marginated chromatin, scanty cytoplasm, and little or no demonstrable GFAP (**Fig. 1.34**) (see also chapter 22).

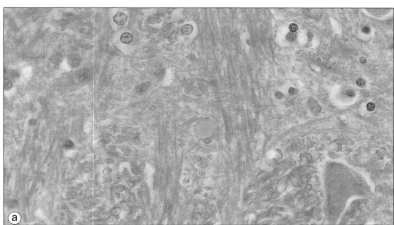

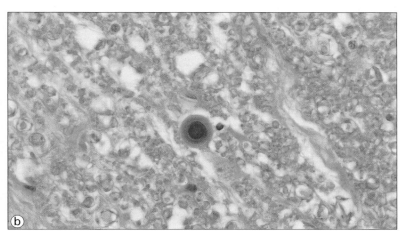

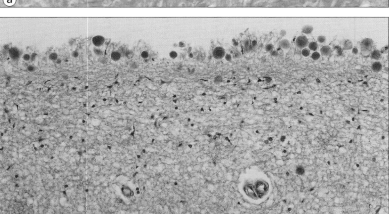

Fig. 1.33 Corpora amylacea. These are basophilic round bodies. (**a**) Some are only weakly basophilic. (**b**) Some, possibly more mature corpora amylacea, are more strongly basophilic and may consist of concentric lamellae of varying staining intensity. Some corpora amylacea contain tiny eosinophilic pockets of incorporated glial cytoplasm. (**c**) Corpora amylacea are relatively numerous in the subpial region.

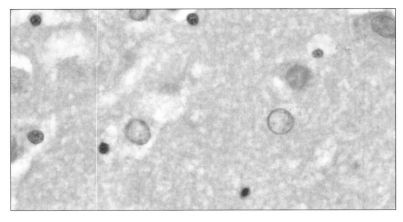

Fig. 1.34 Alzheimer type II astrocytes. These have enlarged empty-looking nuclei and virtually no discernible cytoplasm. The nuclei of Alzheimer type II astrocytes in the globus pallidus, dentate nucleus, and brain stem are often irregularly lobulated.

INCLUSIONS IN EPENDYMAL CELLS AND CHOROID PLEXUS EPITHELIUM

BIONDI BODIES

These are intracellular accumulations of amyloid fibrils in ependymal cells and choroid plexus epithelium. The number of Biondi bodies increases with age and they are consistently present in large numbers in the elderly. In choroid plexus epithelium the fibrils may be arranged in wispy strands or large cytoplasmic rings, which are also known as Biondi rings (Fig. 1.35). In ependymal cells the fibrils appear as irregular strands rather than rings. The fibrils consist of tightly packed bundles of straight 10 nm filaments, which stain with thioflavin S and less intensely with Sirius red or Congo red. They have been reported to react with an antibody to Aβ-amyloid.

Biondi bodies persist even after the autolysis of other tissues and their density in homogenates of choroid plexus has been used to provide a rapid indication of the age of an unidentified dead person.

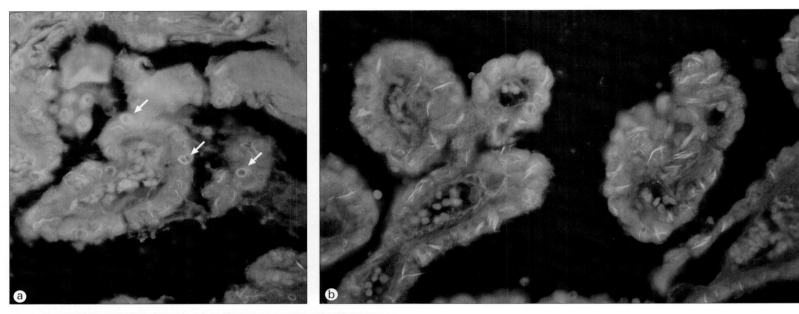

Fig. 1.35 Biondi bodies. In sections stained with thioflavin S, Biondi bodies appear as autofluorescent rings (arrows) or threads in the cytoplasm of choroid plexus epithelial cells (**a, b**) and ependymal cells (**c**).

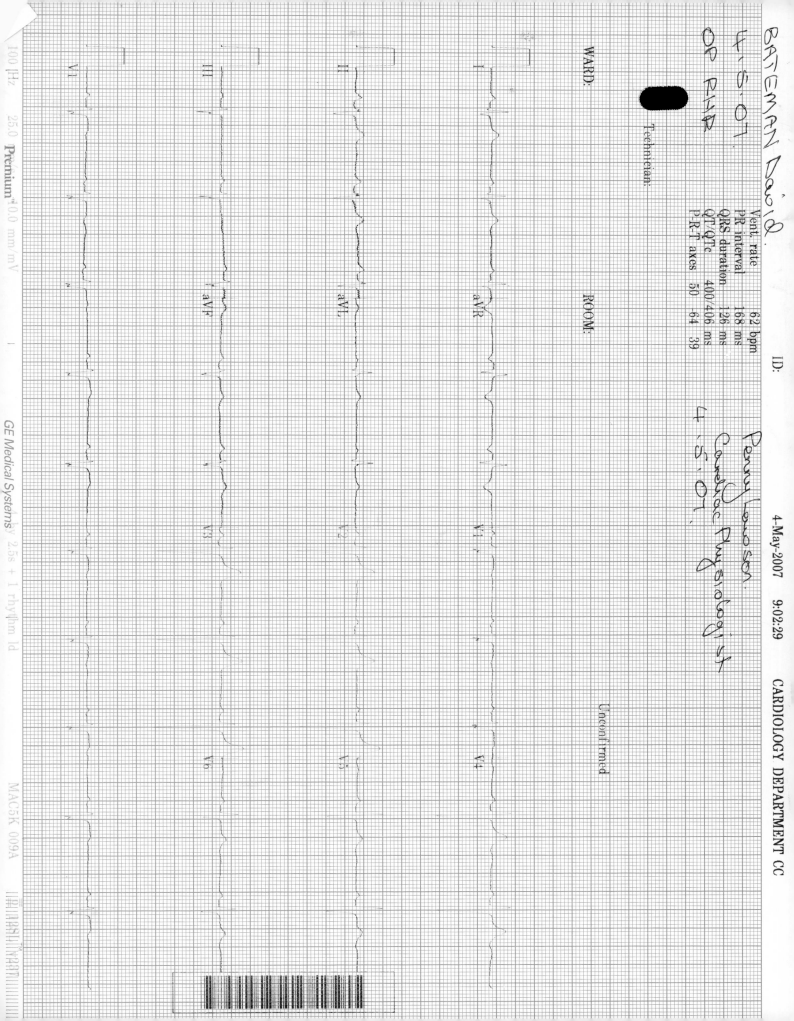

BATEMAN David.

4.5.07.

OP RHR

Vent. rate   62 bpm
PR interval   168 ms
QRS duration 126 ms
QT/QTc   400/406 ms
P-R-T axes   50 64 39

WARD: Technician: ROOM:

Penny Lawson.
Cardiac Physiologist
4.5.07.

Unconfirmed

ID: 4-May-2007   9:02:29   CARDIOLOGY DEPARTMENT CC

I   aVR   V1   V4

II   aVL   V2   V5

III   aVF   V3   V6

V1

PATHOLOGIC RESPONSES IN MICROGLIA

MICROGLIAL ACTIVATION AND ROD CELL FORMATION

Microglia are cells of monocyte lineage and are inconspicuous in the normal brain. They can be demonstrated by silver impregnation (**Fig. 1.36a**), but this has been largely superseded by immunohistochemical and lectin-binding techniques. The antibodies and lectins that label microglia are mostly those that react with monocyte–macrophage markers (**Fig. 1.36b**). Microglia in normal brain have been subdivided into:

- resident microglia, which undergo little turnover with hematogenous monocytes and occur within the CNS parenchyma, though they may abut blood vessels
- perivascular microglia, which occur within the perivascular basal lamina and undergo turnover with hematogenous monocytes

Microglial activation occurs in inflammatory conditions of the CNS, especially encephalitides, and involves:

- increased entry of hematogenous monocytes into the CNS (**Fig. 1.36c**).
- proliferation of resident microglia
- expression or secretion of a range of proteins most of which are concerned with antigen presentation and inflammation — these include major histocompatibility (MHC) class I and II antigens and several cytokines

In sections stained with hematoxylin and eosin, infiltrating monocytes or microglia can be recognized by their rod-shaped nucleus (see Fig. 1.36d). These 'rod cells' are a prominent finding in chronic infections such as general paresis (see chapter 16) and chronic viral encephalitides (see chapter 13).

In regions of tissue damage hematogenous monocytes infiltrate the CNS and phagocytose dead cells and necrotic debris. The accumulation of lipid material by phagocytic cells gives their cytoplasm a foamy appearance in paraffin-embedded material and they are therefore often described as foam cells or foamy macrophages.

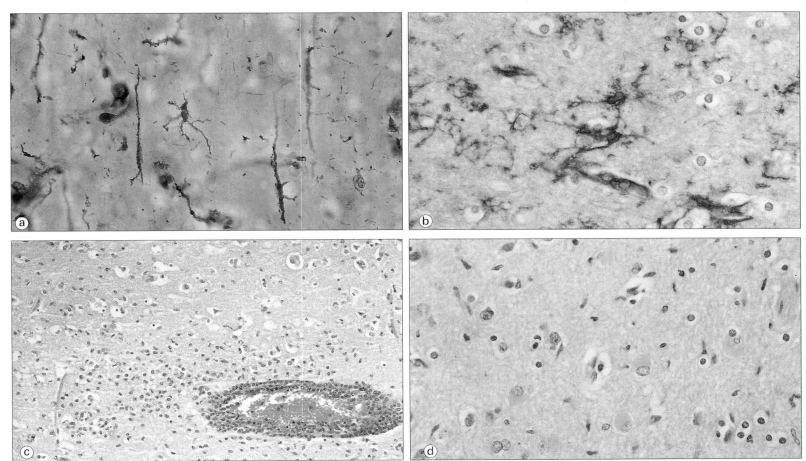

Fig. 1.36 Microglia. (a) Microglia can be detected by silver impregnation, as shown in this silver carbonate preparation from a patient with syphilitic general paresis. (**b**) The silver impregnation technique has been largely superseded by immunostaining for monocyte–macrophage markers such as CD68 or the lectin *Ricinus communis* agglutinin, as shown here. (**c**) There is perivascular cuffing and infiltration of the brain by hematogenous monocytes. (**d**) At higher magnification the infiltrating monocytes or microglia can be recognized by their rod-shaped nuclei.

MINERALIZATION IN THE BRAIN

Mineralization of the brain is common, especially in the basal ganglia, which show incidental vascular mineralization in 1–2% of the population as a whole and a much higher proportion of the elderly.

Deposits are most common and extensive in the globus pallidus, putamen, caudate nucleus, internal capsule, dentate nucleus, the lateral part of the thalamus, and the pineal. (Pineal mineralization has a different appearance and age distribution from that elsewhere in the brain and is considered separately, below).

Small deposits can be found in most parts of the brain. Foci of mineralization are deeply basophilic, and stain for calcium and, variably, for iron. Early mineralization takes the form of rows of small calcospherites lying along capillaries (**Fig. 1.37a**). These small deposits may enlarge to form large perivascular concretions (**Fig. 1.37b**). Larger deposits also

occur within the media of small and medium-sized arteries and veins (**Fig. 1.37c**). Large foci of mineralization are presumed to result from coalescence of smaller deposits (**Fig. 1.37d**).

Parenchymal calcospherites can be seen in a small proportion of pineal glands during the first decade. The frequency of pineal mineralization rises steeply during the second decade, but remains fairly constant therafter, although the deposits may undergo remodeling.

Brain mineralization is a feature of several diseases including disorders of calcium metabolism, some neurodegenerative disorders, mitochondrial encephalopathies, and viral and parasitic infections. The neuropathologic findings in these conditions are described in the relevant chapters.

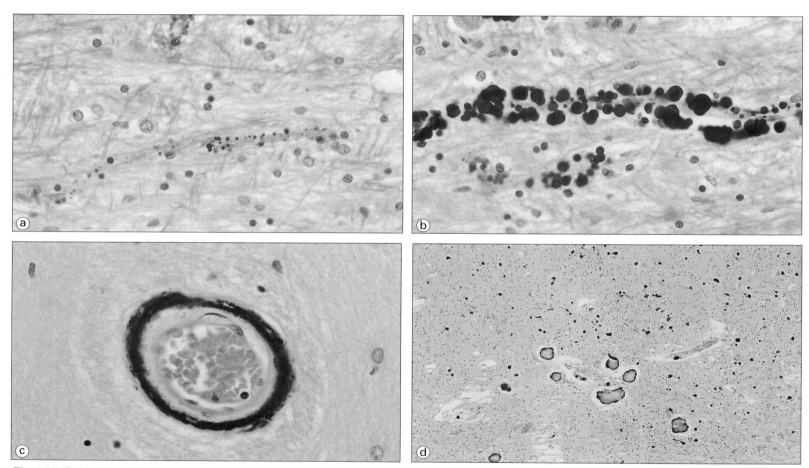

Fig. 1.37 Brain mineralization. (a) Early mineralization visible as punctate deposits along capillaries.
(b) Perivascular concretions form by enlargement of smaller deposits. **(c)** Medial mineralization in the wall of a small vessel. **(d)** Large parenchymal mineral deposits.

REFERENCES

Biondi G (1934) Zur Histopathologie des menschlichen Plexus chorioideus und des Ependyms. *Arch Psychiatr Nervenkr* **101**: 666–728.

Dickson DW, Wertkin A, Kress Y, Ksiezak Reding H, Yen SH (1990) Ubiquitin immunoreactive structures in normal human brains. Distribution and developmental aspects. *Lab Invest* **63**: 87–99.

Eriksson L, Westermark P (1990) Characterization of intracellular amyloid fibrils in the human choroid plexus epithelial cells. *Acta Neuropathol* **80**: 597–603.

Gehrmann J, Matsumoto Y, Kreutzberg GW (1995) Microglia: intrinsic immuneffector cell of the brain. *Brain Res Rev* **20**: 269–287.

Lantos P and Graham D (eds) (1997) *Greenfield's Neuropathology* (6th Edition). Arnold: London.

Davis RL and Roberston DM (eds) (1997) *Textbook of Neuropathology* (3rd edition) Baltimore: William & Wilkins.

Hirano A (1994) Hirano bodies and related neuronal inclusions. *Neuropathol Appl Neurobiol* **20**: 3–11.

Iwaki T, Iwaki A, Tateishi J, Sakaki Y, Goldman JE (1993) Alpha β-crystallin and 27-kd heat shock protein are regulated by stress conditions in the central nervous system and accumulate in Rosenthal fibers. *Am J Pathol* **143**: 487–495.

Love S (in press) Neuropathology of ageing (chapter 6). In MSJ Pathy (ed.) *Principles and Practice of Geriatric Medicine. Third edition.* Chichester: John Wiley & Sons Ltd.

Lowe J, Mayer RJ, Landon M (1993) Ubiquitin in neurodegenerative diseases. *Brain Pathol* **3**: 55–65.

Singhrao SK, Morgan BP, Neal JW, Newman GR (1995) Functional role for corpora amylacea based on evidence from complement studies. *Neurodegeneration* **4**: 335–345.

Tokutake S, Nagase H, Morisaki S, Oyanagi S (1995) X-ray microprobe analysis of corpora amylacea. *Neuropathol Appl Neurobiol* **21**: 269–273.

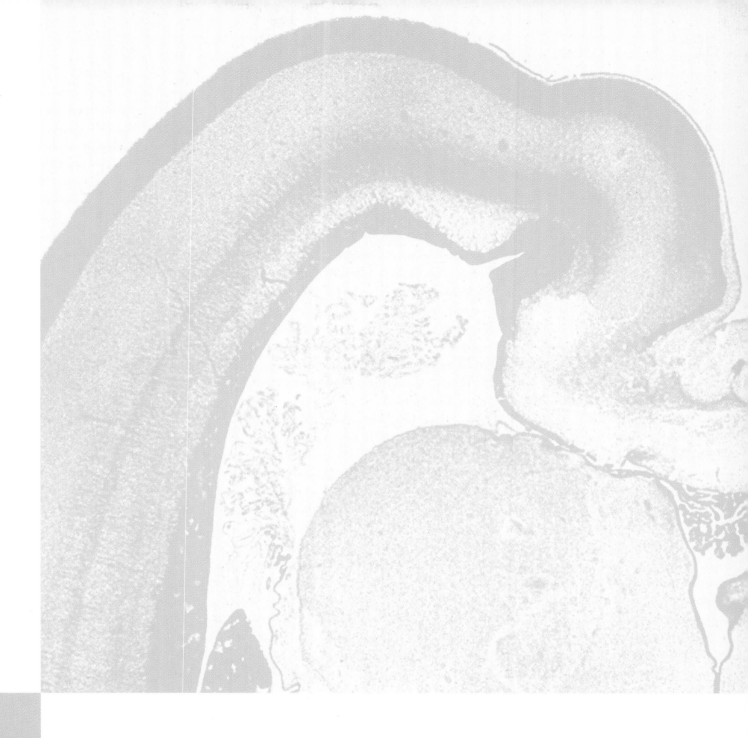

2 Pediatrics

2 Fetal and neonatal hypoxic–ischemic lesions

The most common neuropathology encountered in pediatric autopsies is that associated with hypoxia and/or ischemia. The great variety of lesions associated with these two pathologic processes, either alone or in combination, poses a special challenge to the histologist, whose principal task is to distinguish them from the rare inherited disorders with which they overlap morphologically. Unlike the static reactions of mature brains to acquired injury, fetal and neonatal pathologic reactions must be considered in the context of:

- The extraordinarily rapid growth and plasticity of the immature nervous system.
- The major changes in cell and tissue properties that occur during development.

The differences between the mature and the immature nervous system partly explain the enormous diversity of the morphologic changes associated with hypoxic–ischemic damage.

Present knowledge of embryology and developmental physiology allows a tentative chronology to be assigned to individual lesions (**Fig. 2.1**) although this remains relatively imprecise and extreme caution is needed in the forensic arena. Although some pathologic changes closely parallel those found in older individuals, others such as intraventricular hemorrhage, white matter necrosis, and marbling are unique to the perinatal period.

FETAL LESIONS

Tissue repair in the immature brain differs significantly from repair in the adult CNS. Macrophages are able to mount a phagocytic response early in the second trimester, while fiber-forming astrocytes are detectable only from 20 weeks' gestation. Consequently, resorption of necrotic tissue in the

PATHOGENESIS OF HYPOXIC–ISCHEMIC LESIONS

Possible pathophysiologic schema

Principal factors involved in the production of lesions

- **Cerebral blood flow:** This is much greater in the fetus than in adults, but the autoregulatory range is narrower. Regional differences in flow vary during development and affect the pattern of lesions.
- **Nature of the injury:** Determined by whether it is produced by local or global ischemia or hypoglycemia. Seizures influence the severity of the lesions.
- **Duration or repetition of the injury:** This affects the extent and number of lesions.
- **Selective vulnerability of neurons:** This depends on many factors, including the release of endogenous excitotoxic amino acids, the role of calcium-binding proteins, regional differences of perfusion, and the maturity of the neurons.
- **Timing of the injury is paramount:** Developmental changes affect the water content of the brain, the maturation of metabolic pathways, the location of watershed zones, the vulnerability of mature neurons, and the histologic response to injury (e.g. the macrophage response predates the astrocyte response and hypoxic change in immature neurons is karyorrhexis and not cytoplasmic eosinophilia).

CAUSES OF HYPOXIC–ISCHEMIC LESIONS

Maternal (intrauterine environment)

- Effects of severe maternal disease such as hemorrhage and shock (abruption), cardiac arrest, hypoxia (e.g. drugs, anesthetics), anemia
- Intrauterine infection
- Teratogens
- Smoking
- Trauma
- Disorders inherited from the mother
- Twins (particularly fetus papyraceous)

Placenta and cord

The placenta should be examined for hemorrhage, infarction, infection, and meconium staining. Pathologic factors include:

- Maternal hypertension, toxemia, diabetes mellitus, hematologic disease, sarcoid, autoimmune disease, neoplasia
- Short cord (tethering and placental separation)
- Long cord (knots, cord around neck)

Problems immediately postpartum

- Respiratory disease (obstruction, pulmonary insufficiency, neuromuscular disease)
- Congenital heart disease
- CNS malformations
- Metabolic disease (inherited or acquired)

first half of gestation occurs without any trace of glial repair, leaving a smooth-walled defect, which is often associated with disorganization of the surrounding cerebral cortex. This gives the false impression of a primary malformation rather than an acquired lesion. In contrast, destruction in the latter part of gestation engenders a brisk astrocytic response, resulting in ragged gliovascular cysts (**Fig. 2.2**).

HYDRANENCEPHALY
MACROSCOPIC AND MICROSCOPIC APPEARANCES
Much of the cerebral mantle is replaced by a thin translucent membrane. The hemispheres are cystic, and lack surface convolutions (**Fig. 2.3**). Inferior aspects of the temporal, occipital, and frontal lobes are usually spared, but sometimes only the hippocampi remain. The deep gray nuclei may be rotated outwards and the thalami are atrophied.

The membranous cerebral mantle comprises an outer connective tissue layer and an inner irregular glial layer which also contains mineralized neurons, debris, and hemosiderin-laden macrophages. The ependyma is usually absent. At the interface with surviving cerebral tissue, the inner glial layer runs into the molecular layer, covering it for a short distance, while adjacent cortex is usually disorganized, often with a pattern of polymicrogyria (**Fig. 2.4**).

BASKET BRAIN
MACROSCOPIC APPEARANCES
Basket brain is a rare intermediate state between porencephaly and hydranencephaly. It is characterized by extensive bilateral porencephalic defects, which leave only a thin strip of cingulate cortex connecting the frontal and occipital lobes.

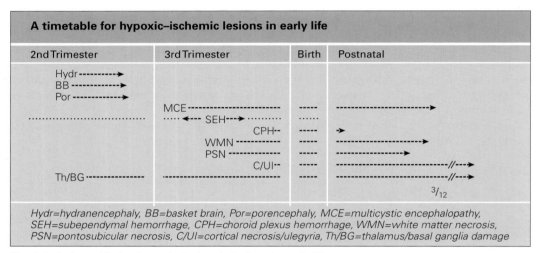

Fig. 2.1 A timetable for hypoxic–ischemic lesions in early life.

ETIOLOGY AND PATHOGENESIS OF FETAL HYPOXIC–ISCHEMIC LESIONS

Clinical associations
- Attempted abortion
- Maternal poisoning
- Attempted suicide
- Severe maternal hypoxia
- Anaphylactic shock
- Fetal infection
- Twinning

Clinical histories relate some smooth-walled defects to maternal disasters occurring between 18 and 27 weeks' gestation. Direct pathologic observations of the evolving lesion as early as 22 weeks' gestation show a central zone of destruction and disorganization with neuroblasts and macrophages surrounded by an early manifestation of polymicrogyria.

Features suggesting that pathogenesis is ischemia or infarction
- Symmetric lesions
- Lesions in carotid artery, anterior communicating artery, or middle cerebral artery territories. (Animal experiments using carotid block or ligation show that these territories are the preferred sites for ischemic lesions or infarction.) The surrounding polymicrogyria may represent exposure to a less intense ischemic penumbra.

HYDRANENCEPHALY

- Hydranencephaly is characterized by normocephaly at birth followed by excessive cranial growth in the first few months and a transilluminable head.
- Hydranencephaly is associated with minimal psychomotor development, spasticity, and epilepsy.
- Life span depends on the condition of the central gray matter. Severe involvement means impaired thermoregulation, sleep, sucking, and swallowing, and survival beyond the neonatal period is unlikely. If this region is preserved, the life span may be several years.

PORENCEPHALY AND SCHIZENCEPHALY
MACROSCOPIC AND MICROSCOPIC APPEARANCES

A porus is a smooth-walled defect in the cerebral mantle which is usually surrounded by an abnormal gyral pattern. It varies in depth from a slight indentation or fissure to a full-thickness breach of the hemispheric wall connecting subarachnoid space with ventricle. Pori tend to be bilateral, approximately symmetric, and situated over the Sylvian fissures or central sulci. Unilateral defects may be parasagittal, orbital, or occipital, and associated with abnormal convolutions, especially polymicrogyria, which are symmetrically placed in the contralateral hemisphere. Gyri surrounding the defect form irregular or radiating patterns (**Fig. 2.5**). The cortex around the porus is broken into islands or folded into polymicrogyria, which extends down into the cleft to meet the ventricular wall. The latter is denuded of ependyma, but covered by glial tissue, which extends a short

Clinical diagnosis of perinatal asphyxia

In labour	At delivery	Neonatal	Infancy
Signs of fetal distress: • abnormal fetal heart rate • meconium stained amniotic fluid	• maternal shock • APH • cord prolapse or around neck • placental infarct • abnormal Apgar • difficult ventilation • acidosis	• apnea • cyanosis • seizures • hypothermia • feeding difficulties • persistent vomiting • hypotonia or hypertonia	• cerebral palsy • seizure disorder • mental retardation

There is increasing evidence that most cases of cerebral palsy are associated with prenatal damage

Fig. 2.2 Clinical diagnosis of perinatal asphyxia.

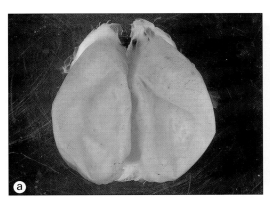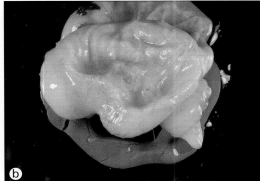

Fig. 2.3 Hydranencephaly in a twin of 22 weeks' gestation whose co-twin died at 17 weeks. (a) The bubble-like hemispheres photographed under water and viewed from above. **(b)** Removal from water allows the diaphanous membrane of the cyst wall to collapse. Damage is largely restricted to the internal carotid territory with sparing of the orbitofrontal cortex and inferior temporal and occipital lobes.

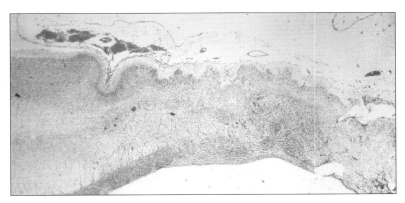

Fig. 2.4 Hydranencephaly. Thinned and irregularly folded polymicrogyric cortex forming a transition between surrounding normal cortex and the cyst wall. Same case as Fig. 2.3.

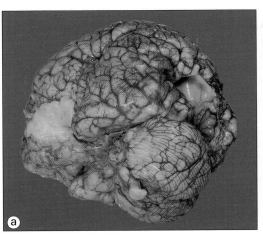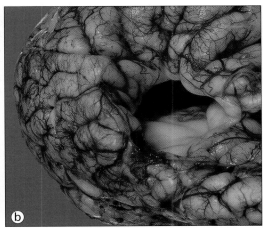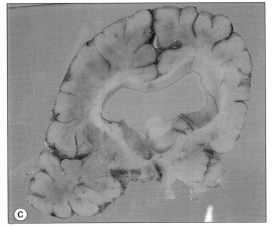

Fig. 2.5 Porencephaly. (a) Two unilateral pori are present. The shallow depression in the orbitofrontal cortex contrasts with the wide-mouthed full-thickness defect in the occipital lobe allowing communication between the subarachnoid space and the ventricle. **(b)** The surrounding convolutions have a radiating pattern. **(c)** Coronal section through the frontal lobes showing the extent of the anterior defect, which is lined by nodules of gray matter. The septum pellucidum is absent.

way over the adjacent gray matter (**Fig. 2.6**). Subependymal nodular heterotopia and partial or complete absence of the septum pellucidum are other features.

Extensive bilateral porencephalic clefts (**Fig. 2.7**) are sometimes termed schizencephaly, especially in the radiologic literature. Schizencephaly refers to an outmoded concept of circumscribed growth failure of the cerebral wall. The narrowness of the cleft with either closed or open lips was thought to differentiate malformed from acquired lesions, but clinical, morphologic, and experimental evidence favors a destructive origin for all these lesions.

MULTICYSTIC ENCEPHALOPATHY
MACROSCOPIC APPEARANCES

In contrast to the smooth-walled defects of hypoxic–ischemic lesions of early gestation, third trimester insults produce many cysts throughout large areas of cerebral white matter and deeper cortical layers (**Figs 2.8, 2.9**). Occasional cases are unilateral and circumscribed (**Fig. 2.10**), but most are extensive and bilateral. Bilateral multicystic encephalopathy is often associated with cystic necrosis in the basal ganglia and brain stem tegmentum (**Fig. 2.11**).

MICROSCOPIC APPEARANCES

A meshwork of thin gliovascular septa form numerous cysts containing lipid-laden macrophages. Global hemispheric necrosis (**Fig. 2.12**) is the term used to describe morphologically similar but particularly extensive cases following severe birth asphyxia and sudden hyperpyrexia and collapse in the postnatal period.

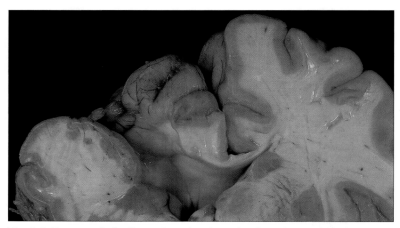

Fig. 2.6 Porencephaly. Coronal section through a frontal porus in a 48-year-old man. The cortical gray matter dips down into the cleft to meet the white gliotic ependyma. The cortical ribbon around the edge of the defect is irregularly thickened and disorganized. Courtesy of Dr T. Moss, Frenchay Hospital, Bristol.

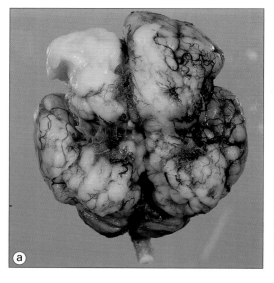
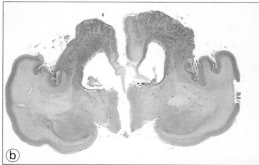
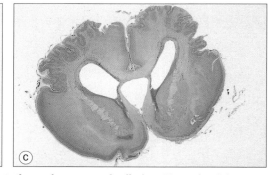

Fig. 2.7 Schizencephaly in a twin of 32 weeks' gestation, whose co-twin died at 19 weeks. (a) Bilateral porencephalic clefts centered on the middle cerebral artery territory. The hemispheres are viewed from above. **(b)** Coronal section at anterior thalamic level. The cortex in the center of the lesion is a completely disorganized mixture of neuroblasts and macrophages surrounded either side by polymicrogyric cortex. **(c)** Coronal section at striatal level. Polymicrogyric cortex from the anterior border of the cleft. (Luxol fast blue/cresyl violet)

PORENCEPHALY

The following are associated with porencephaly:
- Congenital hemiplegia
- Mental retardation
- Chronic neurologic handicap (i.e. bilateral spasticity and epilepsy), which is more severe in patients with bilateral defects

MULTICYSTIC ENCEPHALOPATHY

- Follows a history of reduced fetal movement, a twin dying *in utero*, or perinatal asphyxia.
- Causes abnormalities from birth that include seizures, hypertonia, irritability, abnormal cry, and microcephaly.
- Leads to death within weeks or months.

PERINATAL LESIONS

ACUTE HEMORRHAGE

Hemorrhage is the commonest pathology in fetal and neonatal brains. It can start in any intracranial compartment and rapidly spread elsewhere. The pathogenesis is multifactorial. The principal risk factors are immaturity, perinatal distress, and asphyxia, though a similar spatial distribution in still and live births also implicates antenatal factors. The variety of hemorrhages in the neonatal brain is shown in **Fig. 2.13**.

SUBDURAL HEMORRHAGE (SDH)

SDH is not related to asphyxia, but is closely related to perinatal distress. Excessive compression and distortion of the head during delivery can disrupt the superior cerebral bridging veins that drain into the sagittal sinus, or the veins to the transverse sinus. More rarely, the falx and sagittal sinus or the tentorium (**Fig. 2.14**) with the straight sinus or great vein of Galen are torn.

SUBARACHNOID HEMORRHAGE (SAH)

SAH (**Figs 2.15–2.17**) may manifest as:
- Petechial or diffuse extravasates.
- Massive localized temporal or occipital hematomas.
- Hemorrhage in the basal cisterns and cerebellar subarachnoid spaces.

Secondary SAH may follow SDH or ruptured intraparenchymal hematoma, or more frequently extension of intraventricular hemorrhage (IVH) through the fourth ventricular foramina. Primary SAH is also common in neonatal autopsies, especially in premature infants. Etiologic factors include hypoxia, capillary fragility, coagulopathy, and sepsis.

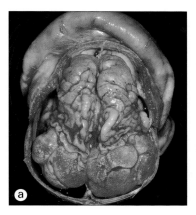
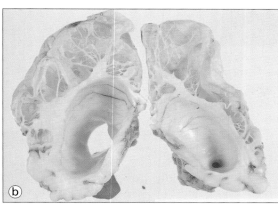

Fig. 2.8 Multicystic encephalopathy in a smaller first twin at 36 weeks' gestation. (a) Superior view of the brain within the skull. The convolutions are either massively cystically dilated or narrow and thin. **(b)** Coronal section showing dilated ventricles and replacement of much of the cortex and white matter by an irregular firm white cystic meshwork.

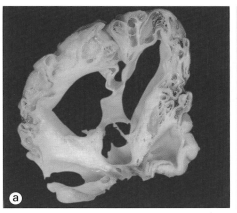
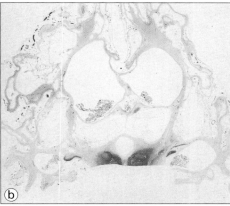

Fig. 2.9 Multicystic encephalopathy. (a) Tough gliovascular bands transform much of the deep cortex, white matter, and basal ganglia into a spongy mass. The thalamic nuclei are shrunken and extremely white. **(b)** Comparable histologic section from another patient showing that not only the cortex and white matter, but also the thalami and basal ganglia have been replaced by large cysts. (Luxol fast blue/cresyl violet)

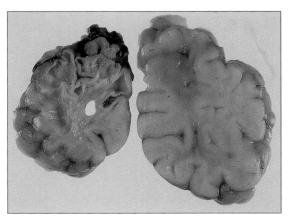

Fig. 2.10 Unilateral circumscribed form of multicystic encephalopathy. Destruction is restricted to the occipital lobe in one of a pair of conjoined twins.

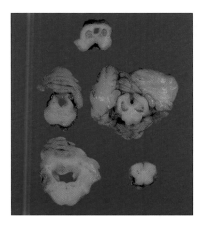

Fig. 2.11 Horizontal sections of the brain stem in multicystic encephalopathy. There is bilateral symmetric cystic destruction running down through the tegmentum.

SUBPIAL HEMORRHAGE (SPH)

SPH is often confused with SAH. It is a focal hemorrhage, which is usually temporal, parietal, or cerebellar, and occurs with or without other signs of bleeding. It is most common in asphyxiated premature infants, but also occurs in premature or term infants with respiratory distress syndrome or congenital heart disease (**Figs 2.18, 2.19**).

SUBEPENDYMAL GERMINAL PLATE/MATRIX HEMORRHAGE (SEH)
MACROSCOPIC AND MICROSCOPIC APPEARANCES

Acute SEH has variable appearances: small, multiple, and bilateral bleeds occur anywhere in periventricular matrix tissue (**Fig. 2.20**), including the roof of the fourth ventricle. Acute SEH is usually found in

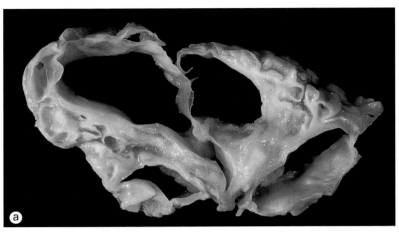

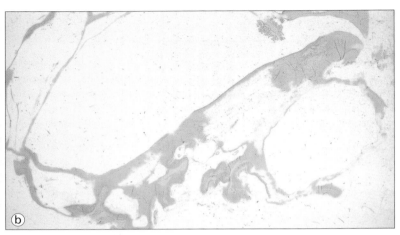

Fig. 2.12 Global hemispheric necrosis. (a) Extensive cystic destruction of the cortical white matter and basal ganglia following severe birth asphyxia. Courtesy of Dr T. Moss, Frenchay Hospital, Bristol. **(b)** Low-power section of the frontal lobe. (Luxol fast blue/cresyl violet)

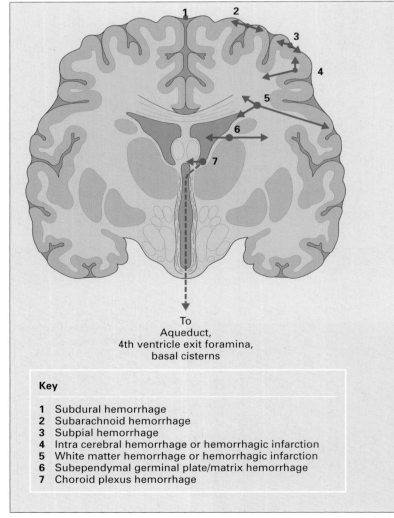

To
Aqueduct,
4th ventricle exit foramina,
basal cisterns

Key

1 Subdural hemorrhage
2 Subarachnoid hemorrhage
3 Subpial hemorrhage
4 Intra cerebral hemorrhage or hemorrhagic infarction
5 White matter hemorrhage or hemorrhagic infarction
6 Subependymal germinal plate/matrix hemorrhage
7 Choroid plexus hemorrhage

Fig. 2.13 Types of hemorrhages in neonatal brain.

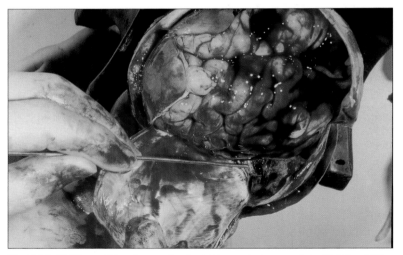

Fig. 2.14 SDH resulting from a tentorial tear at an unassisted birth at 35 weeks' gestation.

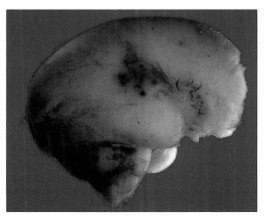

Fig. 2.15 Small petechial SAHs overlying the central sulcus in a 19-week fetus.

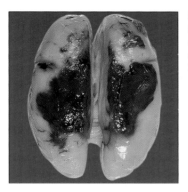

Fig. 2.16 Well-demarcated subarachnoid hematomas localized over parietal cortex. This was associated with a threatened abortion at 20 weeks' gestation.

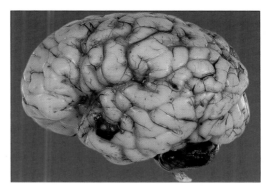

Fig. 2.17 A small localized SAH on the temporal pole as well as extensive basal SAH secondary to hemorrhagic white matter infarction. This occurred in a term infant with multiple congenital anomalies who was cyanosed at birth.

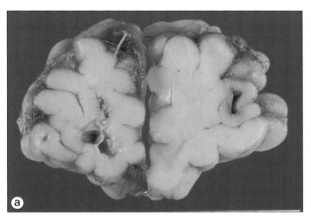

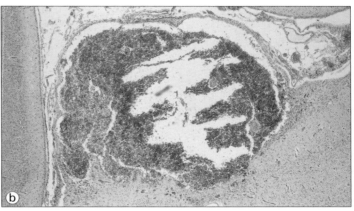

Fig. 2.18 SPH in a term infant with multiple congenital anomalies including cyanotic congenital heart disease. (a) Anterior coronal sections in the frontal lobes showing right-sided central white matter softening and several superficial hemorrhages. **(b)** Microscopy reveals an entirely intracortical bleed covered by pia.

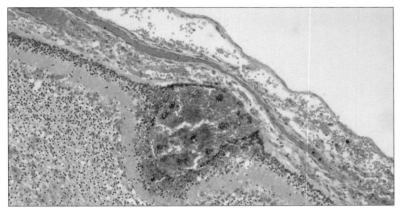

Fig. 2.19   SPH in the cerebellum in a term infant with congenital heart disease. This discrete hematoma displaces the external granular layer and lifts the pia.

GRADING OF SEH*

Grade	Distribution of hemorrhage
1	Confined to germinal matrix
2	Germinal matrix and lateral ventricle, but no ventricular dilatation
3	Germinal matrix and lateral ventricle, which is acutely distended by hematoma within the ventricle because hematoma has obstructed the aqueduct of Sylvius
4	As above with extension of hemorrhage into adjacent brain parenchyma

*Based on the grading scheme of Papile *et al.*

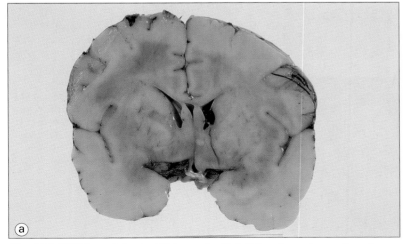

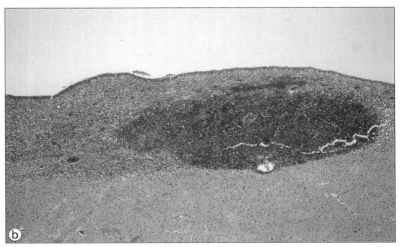

Fig. 2.20 SEH in an infant with hypoplastic left heart syndrome born by Cesarean section at 36 weeks' gestation who survived three days. (a) Small SEH that has remained within the matrix zone (grade 1) in the most typical position near the terminal vein close to the caudate nucleus and thalamus. **(b)** The small bleed remains *in situ* within the cellular matrix tissue. The ependyma is intact. No bleeding point can be ascertained.

SEH

- SEH is mainly seen in low birth weight premature infants under 34 weeks' gestation, but occasionally in term infants and rarely in still births as young as 12 weeks' gestation
- Most intraventricular hemorrhages (IVHs) in neonates are secondary to SEH.
- Commonly associated conditions include respiratory distress syndrome with hyaline membranes, congenital heart disease, hypernatremia, and coagulopathy.
- Hemorrhage begins between 6 hours and 8 days postpartum and in 60% of cases before 48 hours.
- The extent of SEH is variable: it may be a small asymptomatic bleed or a massive IVH heralded by circulatory collapse or a rapidly rising intracranial pressure.

PATHOGENESIS OF SEH

This is controversial, but the consensus opinion favors a combination of the following contributory factors:
- Persistence until 34 weeks of a large matrix zone containing a fragile microcirculation that lacks supporting stroma.
- Hypoxic stress leading to a failure of autoregulation and overperfusion and disruption of the microcirculation of the matrix zone, which receives a major proportion of total cerebral blood flow in premature infants.
- Focal endothelial cell necrosis.
- Poor hematosis, due to high levels of tissue plasminogen activator in the matrix.

the germinal zone over the head of the caudate and thalamus, at or just behind the foramen of Monro; hematoma may extend into the centrum semiovale, simulating or accompanying hemorrhagic infarction (**Figs 2.21–2.24**). Rapidly fatal bleeds burst through the ependymal lining, fill the ventricles, and spill into the basal cisterns and subarachnoid spaces. Ventricular dilatation results from tamponade or hematoma in the aqueduct, foramen of Monro (**Fig. 2.25**), or fourth ventricular outlets. Microscopic evidence of ruptured vessels, thrombosis, or infarcts within the densely cellular matrix is rare.

Several weeks after the initial bleed, the leptomeninges are stained green–brown and the ventricles contain organizing hematoma, macrophages, and granulation tissue. Hydrocephalus often occurs due to occlusion of the aqueduct by hematoma which organizes as a gliotic plug, fibrotic occlusion of the fourth ventricular outlets, or adhesive basal arachnoiditis.

CEREBRAL AND CEREBELLAR HEMORRHAGE

Common causes of cerebral hemorrhage are extension of SEH into periventricular white matter, massive IVH bursting through the ventricular wall (**Fig. 2.26**), or hemorrhage into areas of periventricular infarction (**Fig. 2.27**). Other sources include hemorrhagic middle cerebral artery territory infarction, and sinus thrombosis with venous infarction. Cerebellar hemorrhages may be petechial or large hematomas in the cortex or white matter (**Figs 2.29–2.31**), and are most often seen in low birth weight premature infants.

CHOROID PLEXUS HEMORRHAGE (CPH)

CPH is usually a coincidental finding in neonates and is occasionally responsible for massive IVH in term infants (**Fig. 2.28**).

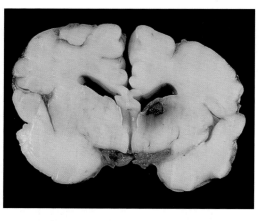

Fig. 2.21 *In situ* matrix zone hemorrhage. This occurred in an infant born by cesarean section for hydrops fetalis at 33 weeks' gestation who survived 10 days. The clot has retracted and organized.

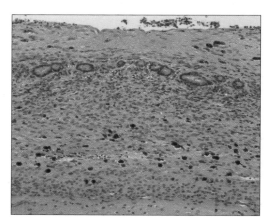

Fig. 2.22 SEH 1–2 weeks after the ictus. Hemosiderin-laden macrophages may be all that remains to indicate previous SEH. Note that the ependyma has been disorganized and glial tissue has overgrown ependymal canaliculi.

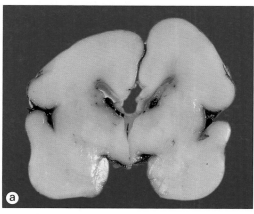

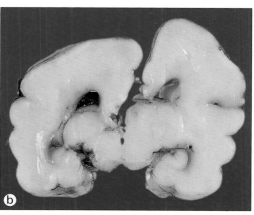

Fig. 2.23 Grade 2 SEH with intraventricular entension. This occurred in an infant born by cesarean section following antepartum hemorrhage at 26 weeks' gestation who had respiratory distress syndrome with hyaline membranes and survived three days. **(a)** This shows bilateral bleeds in the typical position. **(b)** The hemorrhage in the matrix tissue surrounding the right temporal horn has leaked into the ventricle.

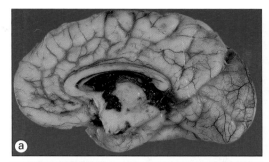

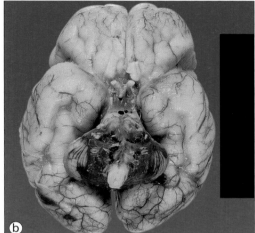

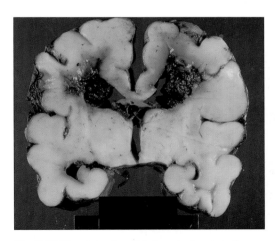

Fig. 2.24 Grade 3 SEH filling the ventricles. This occurred in a premature infant born at 30 weeks' gestation with tracheo-esophageal fistula and esophageal atresia, who developed respiratory distress syndrome and survived nine days. **(a)** Medial surface of the hemisphere. The septum has been removed. The large clot forms a cast of the ventricular system and aqueduct. **(b)** Blood has flushed through the fourth ventricular outlet foramina to fill the basal cisterns. Note the rusty staining of the temporal lobe due to an earlier SAH.

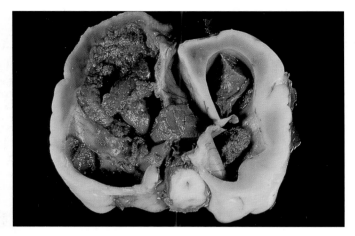

Fig. 2.25 Ventricular dilatation resulting from blockage of the foramen of Monro. This occurred in an infant born at 26 weeks' gestation with tracheo-esophageal fistula and esophageal atresia who survived three weeks. The clot has begun to retract and organize.

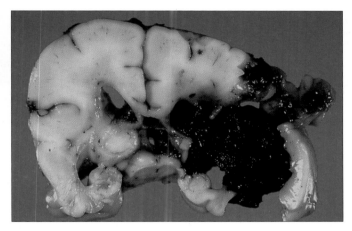

Fig. 2.26 Grade 4 SEH bursting out into the periventricular tissues. This occurred in an infant of 26 weeks' gestation treated with a laporotomy for perforating necrotizing enterocolitis. A grade 4 SEH sometimes reaches the cortical surface, as shown here.

Fig. 2.27 Coexistent matrix hemorrhage and hemorrhagic WMN. This occurred in an infant born by cesarean section at 33 weeks' gestation following pre-eclampsia and fetal distress, postnatal jaundice, hypoglycemia, and disseminated intravascular coagulation. He survived five days. Despite its misleading appearance this is not a grade 4 SEH.

Fig. 2.28 SAH due to CPH in a second twin born by cesarean section after cord prolapse at 37 weeks' gestation. The infant had necrotizing enterocolitis, disseminated intravascular coagulation, a cardiac arrest, and renal failure, and survived 15 days. **(a)** Massive SAH.

(b) The cause is evident as bleeding from the choroid plexus. There is also extensive softening of periventricular white matter, but no trace of SEH.

ACUTE WHITE MATTER LESIONS

WHITE MATTER NECROSIS (WMN)

WMN (synonym: periventricular leukomalacia) consists of focal or more extensive softenings in hemispheric white matter.

MACROSCOPIC APPEARANCES

Typical lesions manifest as yellow–white spots or cavities with a chalky white border. These measure up to several millimeters in diameter and may be single or multiple and unilateral or bilateral. They are situated in periventricular white matter anterior to the frontal horns, adjoining the lateral angles of the lateral ventricles, and in the temporal acoustic and optic radiations. WMN may also be invisible or evident as a diffuse area with soft consistency and a gray color. It occasionally presents as hemorrhagic softening in the subcortical, callosal, and capsular regions, producing extensive cavitation (**Figs 2.32–2.38**).

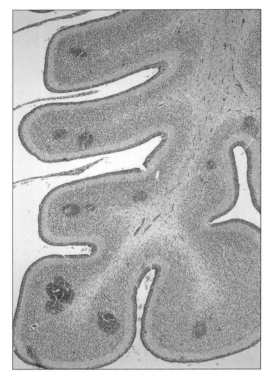

Fig. 2.29 Cerebellar hemorrhage. Numerous petechial hemorrhages in cerebellar cortex in a twin with congenital heart disease.

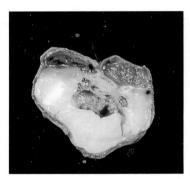

Fig. 2.30 Cerebellar parenchymal hemorrhages. There are a large dorsal hematoma and smaller matrix zone bleeds in the roof of the fourth ventricle in the same case as shown in Fig. 2.16.

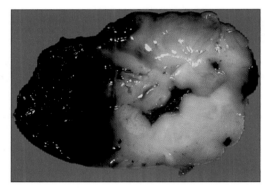

Fig. 2.31 Massive intracerebellar hemorrhage. Hemorrhage has obliterated one cerebellar hemisphere in the same case as shown in Fig. 2.17.

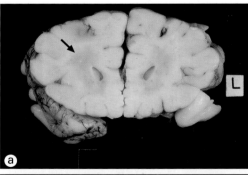
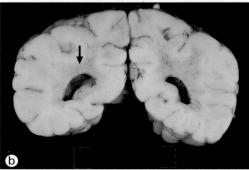

Fig. 2.32 WMN. In an infant born by cesarean section for fulminating pre-eclampsia at 31 weeks' gestation who suffered bronchial stenosis and pulmonary collapse and survived two months, small white spots and linear streaks (arrows) in the centrum semiovale indicate acute focal necosis. The lesions stand out against the rather congested white matter. **(a)** Frontal lobes. **(b)** Parietal lobes

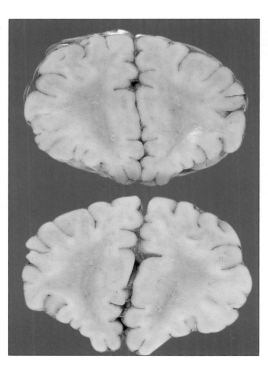

Fig. 2.33 WMN. Tiny necrotic foci in the frontal white matter have a central cavity surrounded by a chalky white rim. This is the same case as shown in Fig. 2.30.

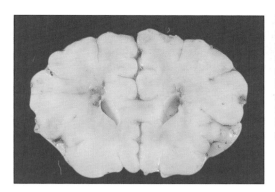

Fig. 2.34 WMN resulting in bilateral periventricular softening around the angles of the frontal horns. This occurred in an infant delivered at term who had congenital heart disease and survived ten days.

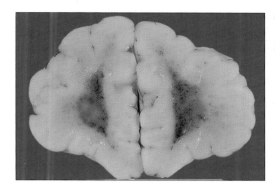

Fig. 2.35 WMN producing only a diffuse duskiness of the white matter. There are no focal lesions in this case, which is the same as that shown in Fig. 2.18.

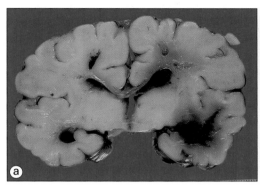

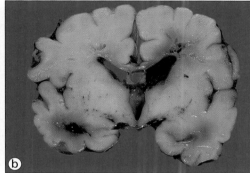

Fig. 2.36 WMN. This occurred in an infant born at 37 weeks' gestation with hypoglycemia and hyperinsulinemia due to nesidioblastosis who survived ten days. Irregular linear cavities fan out from the lateral angle of the ventricle into frontal and parietal white matter. There is also considerable IVH due to hemorrhagic softening of the temporal white matter.
(a) Coronal section at mid-thalamic level.
(b) Coronal section at anterior thalamic level.

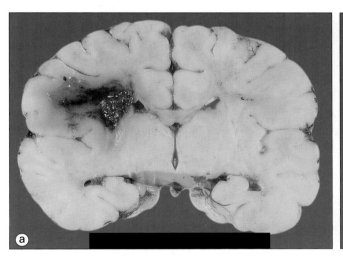

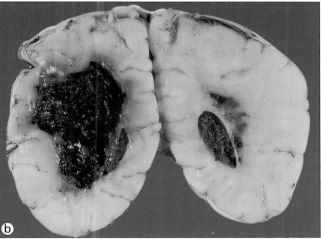

Fig. 2.37 WMN. Hemorrhagic softenings have resulted in huge intracerebral hematomas. **(a)** Coronal section at mid-thalamic level. **(b)** Coronal section through the occipital lobes. This is the same case as Fig. 2.35.

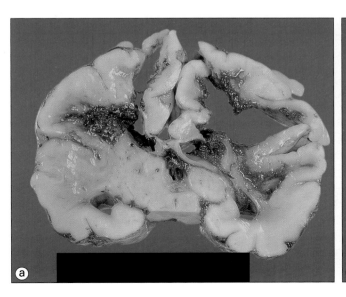

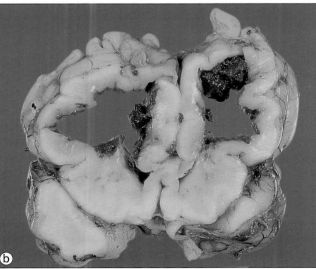

Fig. 2.38 WMN. This occurred in an infant born at 31 weeks' gestation with coarctation of the aorta and vena caval thrombosis who survived three weeks. Massive hemorrhagic necrosis and cavitation in the white matter of both hemispheres.
(a) Thalamic level.
(b) Striatal level.

MICROSCOPIC APPEARANCES

Soon after the insult, irregular zones of coagulative necrosis are surrounded by rings of intense eosinophilia. At a later stage, fragmented axons and axon balloons are seen at the periphery of the lesion, with microglia, reactive astrocytes, and macrophages. Alternative appearances include cavities surrounded by gliosis and mineralized axons and vessels; a gliotic and microcystic parenchyma with clusters of foamy macrophages; and (rarely) massive infarcts consisting largely of macrophages (**Figs 2.39–2.44**).

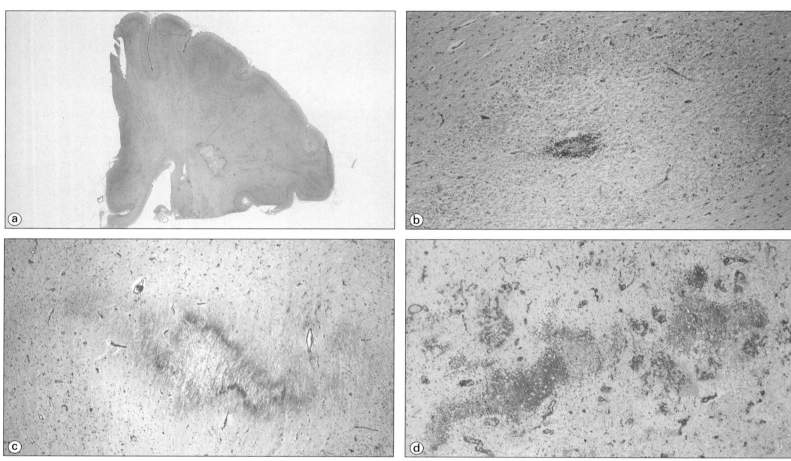

Fig. 2.39 Microscopic features of white matter necrosis. (a) With hematoxylin and eosin, the acute lesion (a focus of coagulative necrosis) is indicated only by a zone of pallor. In this case there is also a central petechial hemorrhage. **(b)** Periodic acid–Schiff (PAS) often outlines acute focal lesions more clearly, as shown here where it reveals a typical focus in the periventricular white matter of the frontal lobe. There was coexisting germinal matrix hemorrhage and polymicrogyria. This occurred in a twin born at 36 weeks' gestation who survived 12 days. **(c)** Luxol fast blue outlines acute focal lesions. Here there is central pallor surrounded by an irregular rim of accentuated staining. This occurred in an infant born at 33 weeks' gestation with multiple congenital abnormalities including congenital heart disease, who survived 13 days. **(d)** Occasionally, acute lesions are evident as ill-defined patches of increased PAS staining.

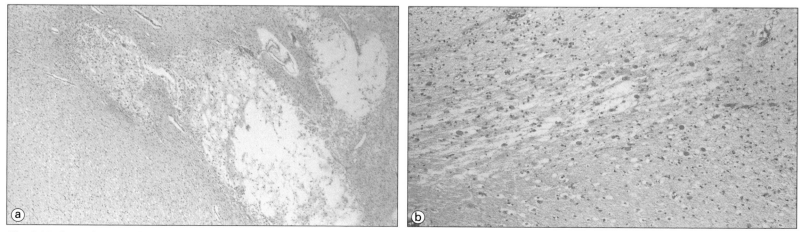

Fig. 2.40 Acute lesions of WMN. (a) Multiple foci of necrosis have coalesced within the central white matter (in the same case as shown in Fig. 2.38). **(b)** Focal necrosis within the corpus callosum is evident as a central cavity and macrophages surrounded by astrocytosis.

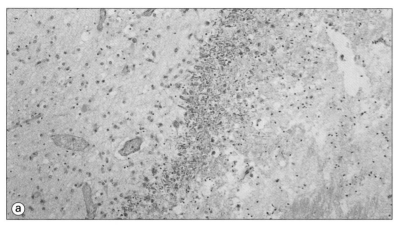

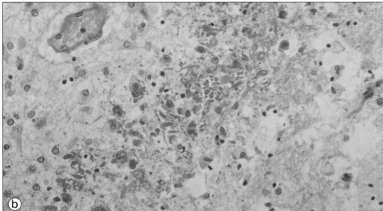

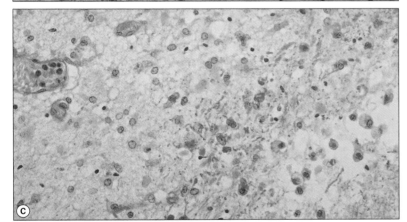

Fig. 2.41 WMN. Early course of the lesion. Within a few days there is marked cellular infiltration by foamy macrophages and reactive astrocytes around the necrotic focus that contains stick-like debris residual to either necrotic axons or vessels. (PAS) **(a)** Low power view of a necrotic focus surrounded by tissue debris and cellular infiltrate. (PAS) **(b)** Debris and reactive astrocytes at the edge of the lesion. (PAS) **(c)** Infiltrate of reactive astrocytes and foamy macrophages neighbouring the necrotic zone. (PAS)

Fig. 2.42 White matter necrosis. Indicated is the most widely held view of the pathogenesis of the focal softenings of white matter necrosis, by noting the correspondence between the most common position of these lesions in periventricular regions (shown in the right hemisphere) and the putative boundary zone between ventriculo-petal deep branches of superficially derived cerebral arteries and ventriculo-fugal arteries derived from lenticulo-striate and choroidal arteries.

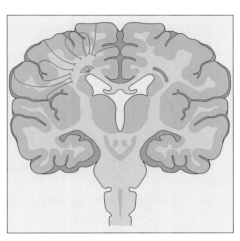

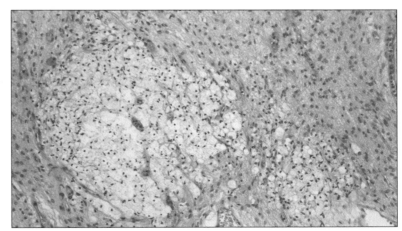

Fig. 2.43 WMN showing further organization of the lesion into nodular collections of lipid phagocytes associated with capillary proliferation. This occurred in an infant who survived three weeks.

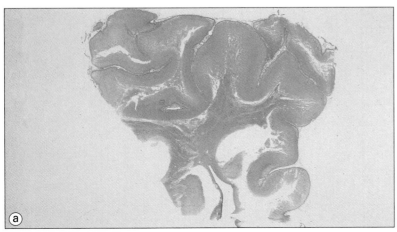

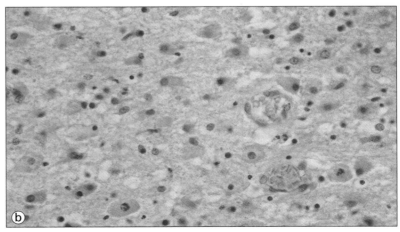

Fig. 2.44 Extensive WMN. If white matter destruction is very extensive soft friable tissue may appear autolysed at brain cut. This occurred in a term infant who was delivered by forceps after fetal distress in the second stage and who then developed seizures from six hours of age and survived one week. **(a)** Frontal lobe section. **(b)** Microscopy of this lesion. The white matter has been replaced by sheets of macrophages, some in mitosis.

■ *PATHOGENESIS OF WMN*

- The principal theory is that WMN results from impaired perfusion at the boundary zone between ventriculopetal and ventriculofugal arteries where the metabolic requirements of myelinating white matter are high (see Fig. 2.42).
- Other theories are that WMN results from neonatal sepsis and endotoxemia or increased anerobic glycolysis and an accumulation of lactic acid and free radicals.

■ *WMN*

- WMN affects approximately 5% of all hospital births and as many as 35% of low birth weight newborns.
- Associated conditions include respiratory distress syndrome with hyaline membranes in premature infants, congenital heart disease in term infants, septicemia, shock, intrauterine growth retardation with hypoglycemia, and meningoencephalitis.
- The lesions can be well demonstrated by ultrasound scanning.
- The initial manifestations are relatively non-specific but most surviving infants later develop spastic motor dysfunction.

OTHER PATTERNS OF WHITE MATTER DAMAGE

These are:

- Subcortical leukomalacia, which is focal necrosis preferentially sited beneath the deep sulci.
- Telencephalic leukoencephalopathy (**Fig. 2.45**), which is characterized by diffuse depletion of myelination glia, astrocytic proliferation and hypertrophy, karyorrhectic glial nuclei, and amphophilic globules. The hypertrophic reactive glia should not be confused with normal myelination glia, that have a smaller, more hyperchromatic nucleus and a more fusiform cytoplasmic profile (**Fig. 2.46**).

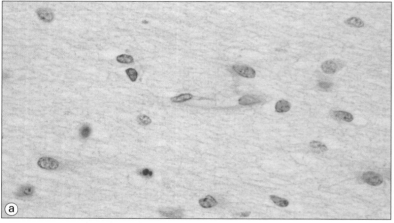

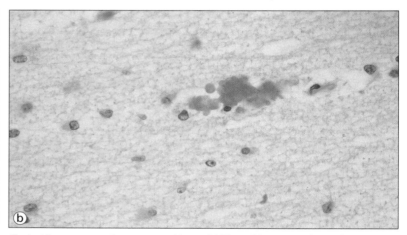

Fig. 2.45 Telencephalic leukoencephalopathy. This is characterized by poorly cellular white matter, loss of myelination glia, diffuse gliosis, karyorrhexis in glial nuclei, and amphophilic globules. **(a)** and **(b)** Histology from the corpus callosum of a one-month-old baby with severe congenital heart disease, cleft lip, and pituitary and adrenal hypoplasia.

Typical features are demonstrated here. (a) The white matter is poorly cellular, with loss of myelination glia, and diffuse gliosis. Some of the glial nuclei are karyorrhectic. (b) Amphophilic globules are also observed within the gliotic white matter.

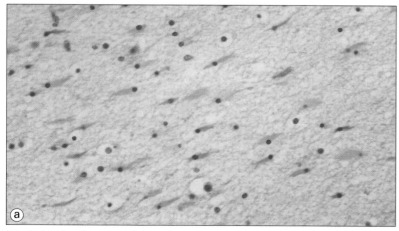

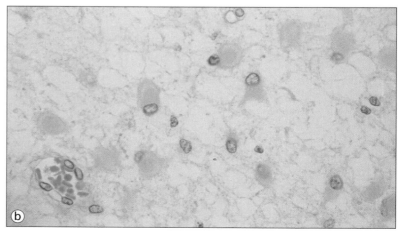

Fig. 2.46 Myelination glia and reactive gliosis in the neonatal brain. (a) Myelination glia have small round hyperchromatic nuclei eccentrically set in oval or elongated basophilic cytoplasm. **(b)** Astrocytic hypertrophy is less pronounced than in older subjects. Reactive astrocytes have an eccentrically placed nucleus and plump cytoplasm, often containing a central region of strong eosinophilia surrounded by an ill-defined, less intensely stained halo.

ACUTE GRAY MATTER LESIONS

CEREBRAL NECROSIS
MACROSCOPIC APPEARANCES

Diffuse cerebral edema may lead to flattened gyri and obliterated sulci, and occasionally there will be massive swelling with softening of the entire brain. A white or hemorrhagic ribbon of cortex contrasts with dusky congested white matter (**Figs 2.47, 2.48**). Smaller lesions may be scattered, restricted to an arterial territory, or localized in watershed regions. The depths of sulci are preferentially involved (**Fig. 2.49**).

MICROSCOPIC APPEARANCES

Very early lesions may exhibit only focal pallor in the cortical gray matter. Hypoxic–ischemic changes in immature neurons are characterized by nuclear pyknosis and karyorrhexis. Laminar or full-thickness necrosis also may be observed (see Fig. 2.49). Activated microglia, astrocytosis, foamy macrophages, and capillary proliferation are seen in lesions after survival

for several days (**Fig. 2.50**). Mineralized neurons are seen when survival exceeds two weeks (**Fig. 2.53**).

CEREBRAL NECROSIS

- Cerebral necrosis is the usual observation in term infants whereas hemorrhage and white matter lesions are typical of premature infants.
- Severe intrapartum difficulties, perinatal problems such as congenital heart disease, and vascular collapse are associated with cerebral necrosis.
- Neurologic sequelae include hypotonia, abnormal eye movements, problems with sucking and swallowing, seizures, and coma.

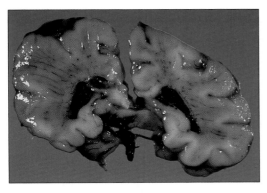

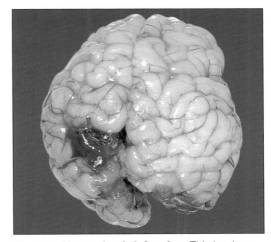

Fig. 2.47 Cerebral necrosis; the ribbon effect. Produced by severe hypoxia affecting both cortex and white matter, the paradoxically pale cerebral cortex stands out against the gray duskiness of the white matter. This occurred in an infant delivered by emergency cesarean section following a flat fetal tocograph trace at 38 weeks' gestation whose Apgar score was 1 at ten minutes. Autopsy one day later revealed recent colonic perforation with peritonitis.

Fig. 2.48 Hemorrhagic infarction. This is a less common manifestation of acute cerebral ischemia and occurred in an infant born at 33 weeks' gestation with jaundice, hypoglycemia, and renal failure.

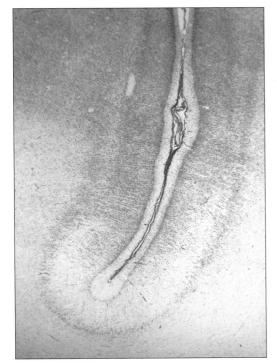

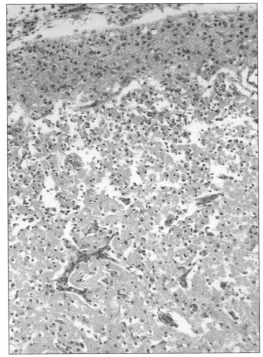

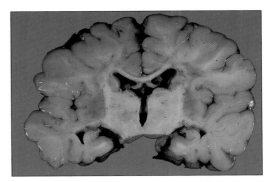

Fig. 2.49 Cortical necrosis preferentially situated in the depths of the gyri in a term infant.

Fig. 2.50 Organizing cortical necrosis with a pseudolaminar pattern. Astrocytic hyperplasia and hypertrophy in the superficial layers overlie a zone of lipid phagocytes and capillary proliferation.

Fig. 2.51 Prominent hypoxic–ischemic damage in the dusky putamina and shrunken mottled thalami. The grayish periventricular tissue indicates that white matter is also involved. This pathology was found in a six-month-old infant whose mother had hypertension in the third trimester and a spontaneous delivery at 36 weeks' gestation.

PONTOSUBICULAR NECROSIS

The undoubted association between necrosis of neurons in the pontine nuclei and the subiculum in neonates is uncommon, and does not usually occur in isolation from other hypoxic lesions (**Fig. 2.55**).

BASAL GANGLIA AND THALAMIC LESIONS

Hypoxic–ischemic damage in these regions varies from focal neuronal necrosis to large areas of infarction. The latter usually occurs in conjunction with widespread CNS involvement (**Fig. 2.51**). The initiating

injury may be postnatal, perinatal, or intrauterine. Damage to these regions also forms part of an extensive reticular core destruction of brain stem reticular formation and central gray nuclei which follows perinatal cardiac arrest (**Fig. 2.56**).

CEREBELLAR LESIONS

Although all cortical layers and dentate neurons (**Fig. 2.54b**) may be affected, the immaturity of Purkinje cells before 37 weeks' gestation means that they are less vulnerable to hypoxia than internal granular cells.

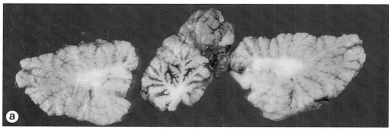

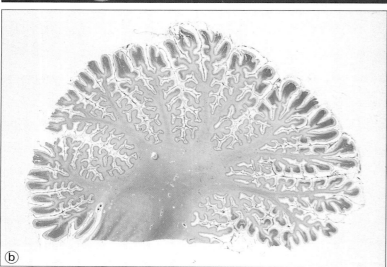

Fig. 2.52 Necrosis of the deep cerebellar cortex with sparing of only the more superficial parts of the folia. This is one particular pattern of selective vulnerability to hypoxia in neonates. **(a)** Cerebellum from a five-month-old infant delivered by cesarean section for fetal distress who had an Apgar score of 5 at ten minutes. **(b)** Cerebellum from a six-month-old infant delivered by emergency cesarean section for cord prolapse and multiple abnormalities including congenital heart disease. (Luxol fast blue)

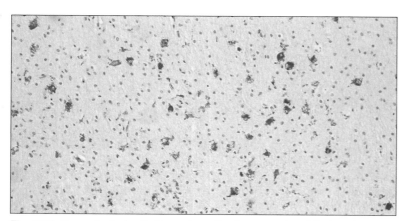

Fig. 2.53 Ferruginated cells (i.e. mineralized neuronal residua) and astrogliosis. These are prominent and regular features in necrotic thalamic nuclei. This is the same case as shown in Fig. 2.63b.

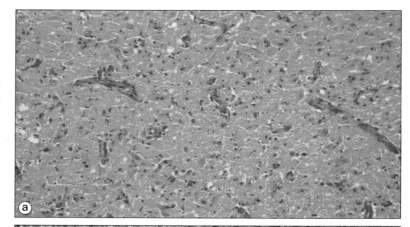

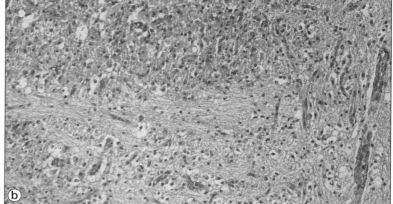

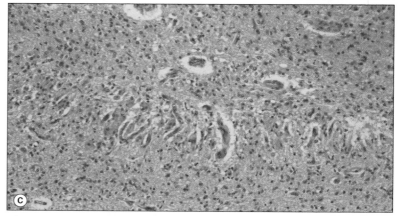

Fig. 2.54 Severe birth asphyxia resulting in extensive gray matter damage. This occurred in a six-day-old neonate who had no registrable heart rate on the monitor during delivery, an Apgar score of 4 at ten minutes, no spontaneous respiration, and later seizures and disseminated intravascular coagulation. There was diffuse cortical necrosis and widespread involvement of the basal ganglia, brain stem, and cerebellum. Subacute lesions show marked cellularity, prominent capillaries, neuronal loss, and the characteristic changes of hypoxia in mature neurons (i.e. cytoplasmic eosinophilia) in the remaining cells. **(a)** Subacute lesions in the substantia nigra. **(b)** Subacute lesions in the dentate nucleus. **(c)** Subacute lesions in pontine gray matter.

Various patterns of involvement are seen: diffuse, focal damage at the SCA/PICA watershed, or infarction of the deeper parts of the folia (**Fig. 2.52**).

BRAIN STEM LESIONS

Many brain stem structures are vulnerable to asphyxia, particularly the inferior colliculi, pontine nuclei, inferior olives, cranial nerve nuclei, and reticular formation (**Fig. 2.54**).

SPINAL CORD LESIONS

Two patterns of damage have been described:
- Infarction involving the central parts of the lumbosacral cord segments in premature infants.
- Diffuse necrosis affecting the ventromedial neurons in term neonates.

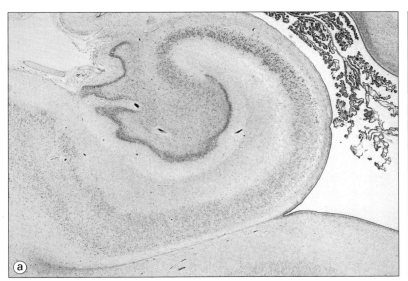

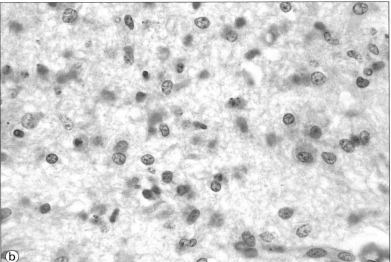

Fig. 2.55 Pontosubicular necrosis. This is the association between ischemic destruction of the subiculum and pontine nuclei. It is uncommon, and rarely occurs in isolation from more widespread hypoxic damage. **(a)** Low power view of Ammon's horn showing neuronal loss from Sommer's sector and subiculum. **(b)** Severe neuronal depletion and astrocytosis in the basal pontine nuclei. Karyorrhectic nuclei indicate ischemic neuronal necrosis because immature neurons have little cytoplasm and do not respond with the cytoplasmic eosinophilia characteristic of more mature cells. This is the same case as shown in Fig. 2.36.

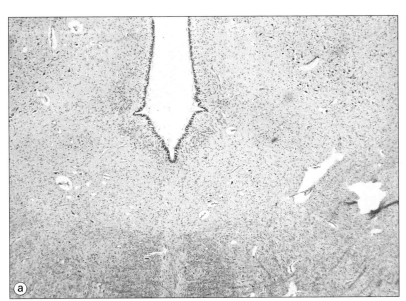

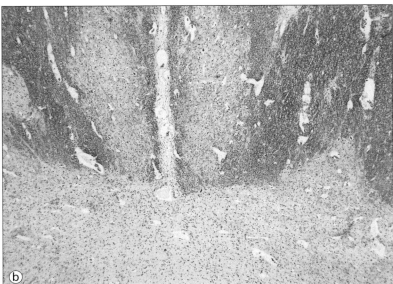

Fig. 2.56 Reticular core necrosis. Destruction was confined to thalamic and brain stem nuclei in this seven-week-old baby born at term with a true knot in the cord resulting in apnea and hypotonia and an Apgar score of 2 at ten minutes, seizures from 30 minutes, and later hypertonia and striking cranial nerve palsies. **(a)** There is marked neuronal loss and astrocytosis in the XII nucleus. **(b)** Marked neuronal loss and astrocytosis is also evident in the gracile and cuneate nuclei in the lower medulla. (Luxol fast blue)

CHRONIC LESIONS

POST-HEMORRHAGIC LESIONS
Periventricular cysts

Small bleeds within the germinal matrix become transformed by macrophage infiltration into unilocular or honeycomb subependymal cysts (**Fig. 2.57**). Longitudinal imaging studies have shown rapid resolution without neurologic deficit. Similar cysts have also been related to congenital infection.

POST-HEMORRHAGIC HYDROCEPHALUS

This is described in chapter 4.

POST-WHITE MATTER NECROSIS
White matter scars and cysts

The hallmarks of birth injury comprise two overlapping patterns (**Figs 2.58–2.60**):
- Sclerotic atrophy characterized by myelin loss, gliotic scars, macrophage clusters, and mineralized debris in the centrum semiovale and callosum, accompanied by ventricular dilatation.
- Unilocular or multilocular cysts traversed by gliomesodermal bands around the dorsolateral corners of the lateral ventricles.

In practice there is often a combination of white and gray matter scars.

POST-GRAY MATTER NECROSIS
Ulegyria and cortical marbling

Many factors influence the final pathology of gray matter necrosis including:
- The extent of edema.
- The extent of neuronal loss, cortical infarction, or involvement of neighboring white matter.
- Superadded effects of recurrent hypoxic episodes.

Extreme cases appear severely microcephalic with cysts and a thin, firm, white cortex (**Fig. 2.61**). The sparing of gyral crowns results in a mushroom-like appearance called ulegyria (Figs 2.61d, 2.62). Cortical scarring may be full-thickness or laminar. The glial scar is sometimes associated with hypermyelination (état fibromyélinique) (Fig. 2.61c); mineralized neurons and lipid-laden macrophages can remain *in situ* for many years.

STATUS MARMORATUS

Chronic lesions of the basal ganglia and thalamus are gliotic and/or cystic (**Fig. 2.62**); mineralized neurons are common, but marbling is rare. Marbling appears as irregular white mottling and shrinkage of the deep gray matter (**Fig. 2.63**) and is due to abnormal hypermyelination

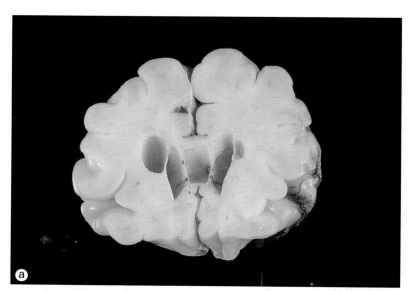

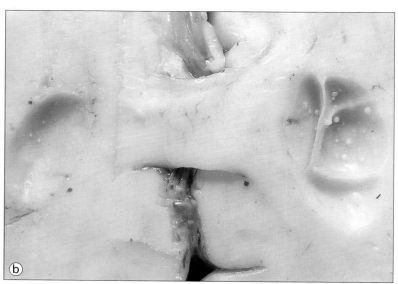

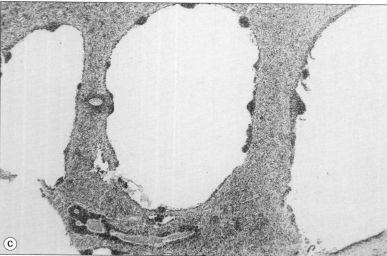

Fig. 2.57 Subependymal matrix cysts. (a) Unilocular or multilocular smooth-walled cysts hug the angles of the lateral ventricles. **(b)** Closer inspection may reveal tiny protrusions into the cavity as shown here. **(c)** Histologically, the tiny protrusions are residua of matrix tissue.

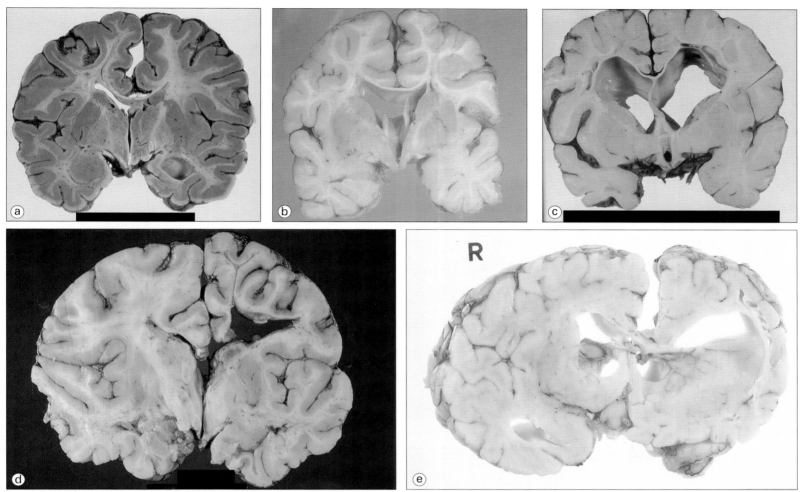

Fig. 2.58 Chronic lesions in white matter. These so-called hallmarks of birth injury have widely varying appearances. Both unilateral and bilateral lesions are usually accompanied by ventricular dilatation. **(a)** A partly cystic linear gliotic scar in the left frontal white matter above the dilated left frontal horn. **(b)** Bilateral gliotic white matter scars and small periventricular cysts. There is also marked ventriculomegaly. **(c)** Prominent cyst formation following the contours of the dilated frontal horns. **(d)** Extensive unilateral cystic destruction of the central and subcortical white matter in the frontal lobe. **(e)** Unilateral white matter atrophy and ventricular dilatation. Here the overlying cortex is also involved and shows ulegyria.

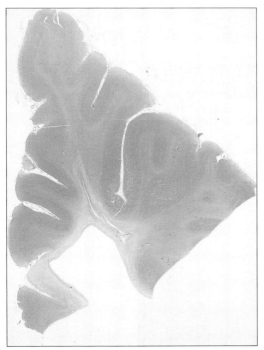

Fig. 2.59 Chronic slit-like defect in the frontal white matter. Ultrasound scanning in the perinatal period had shown a considerably larger area of cystic necrosis, which had dramatically reduced in size over several months.

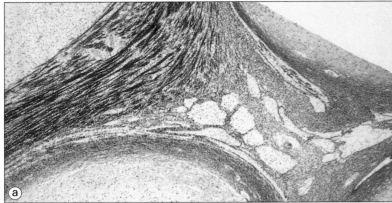

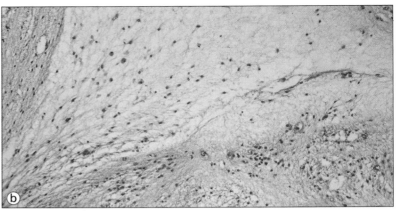

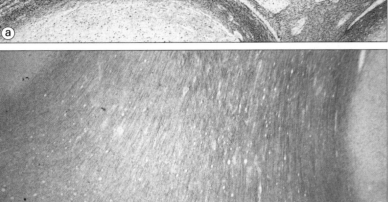

Fig. 2.60 Chronic longstanding white matter lesions. (a) Cyst formation in the central white matter of an eight-year-old girl. (Luxol fast blue/cresyl violet) **(b)** Dense gliosis surrounding a paucicellular area containing foamy macrophages in a 17-year-old man. **(c)** Poor myelination, which is the likely sequel to telencephalic leukoencephalopathy. (Luxol fast blue/cresyl violet)

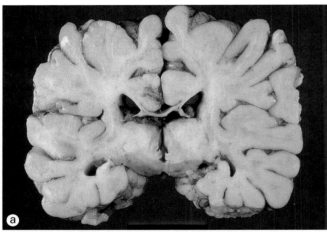

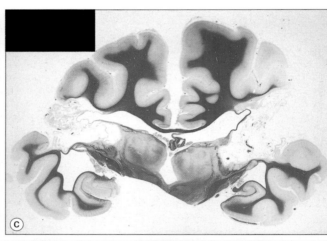

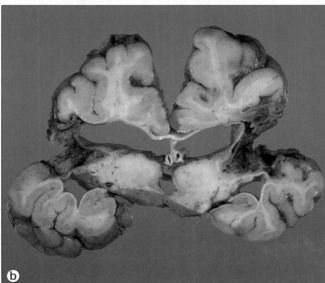

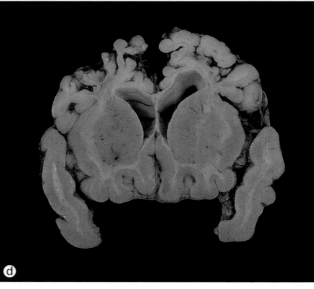

Fig. 2.61 Various patterns of chronic gray matter damage.
(a) Global atrophy following diffuse cortical involvement.
(b) Bilateral symmetric scars due to perinatal cortical infarctions restricted to the territory of the middle cerebral arteries in a 21-year-old man.
(c) Stained section from (b) showing irregular myelination (marbling) in the thalami and left superior temporal gyrus (état fibromyélinique).
(d) Severe cerebral atrophy with sparing of the crests of the convolutions producing mushroom-shaped gyri, termed ulegyria (compare with Fig. 2.52).

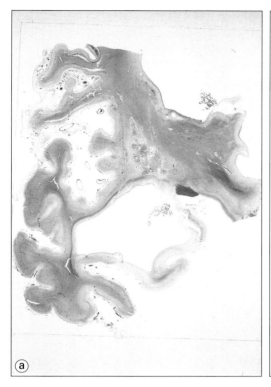

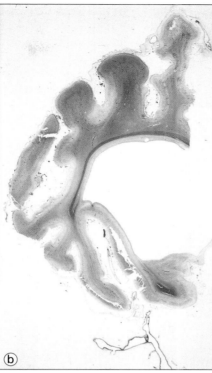

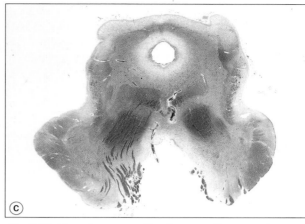

Fig. 2.62 Chronic gray matter damage. Severe and extensive gyral scarring or ulegyria, sclerotic atrophy of the thalamus, and cystic destruction of the lentiform nucleus and internal capsule are seen in a six-month-old infant, who was delivered by emergency cesarean section for cord prolapse and had multiple congenital abnormalities including tracheo-esophageal fistula, congenital heart disease, and a rudimentary limb. **(a)** Low power coronal section at anterior thalamic level. **(b)** Low power coronal section of temporal lobe. **(c)** Horizontal section of the midbrain showing secondary atrophy of the cerebral peduncles.

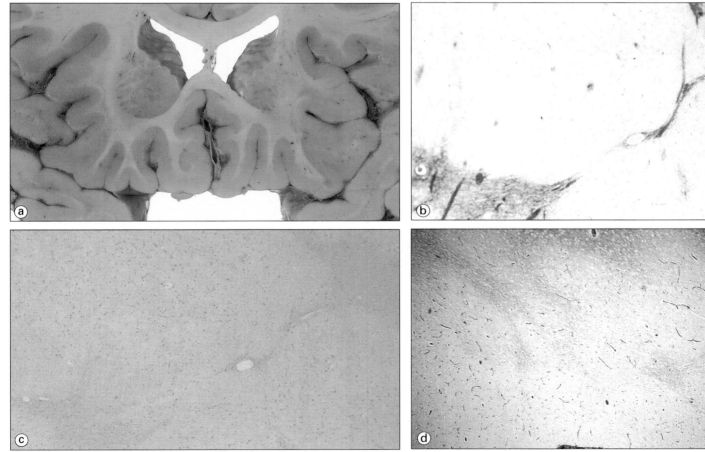

Fig. 2.63 Status marmoratus. (a) Coronal section at the level of the corpus striatum. Both striatal nuclei are shrunken, their dorsal surfaces abutting the ventricle are corrugated, while their cut surfaces show an irregular white mottling characteristic of marbling. **(b)** Microscopic appearance of marbling in the basal ganglia showing an excessive and abnormally situated myelination.

(Luxol fast blue/cresyl violet) **(c)** An adjacent microscopic section to (b) showing the close association between the hypermyelination and gliosis as demonstrated by GFAP immunoreactivity. **(d)** Similar aberrant myelination in the surviving cortex neighboring an infarcted area (état fibromyélinique).

in association with glial scars. There is evidence that the hypermyelination is, in part, due to the formation of myelin sheaths around astrocyte processes. Status marmoratus occurs after both prenatal and postnatal hypoxia, provided that the damage takes place before the onset of myelination at about six months postpartum.

UNILATERAL HYPERTROPHY OF THE PYRAMIDAL TRACT

An uncommon consequence of midgestational unilateral lesions involving sensorimotor cortex or internal capsule is hypotrophy of the ipsilateral corticospinal pathway and enlargement (reflecting excess fibers) of the contralateral tract (**Fig. 2.64**).

CROSSED CEREBELLAR ATROPHY

Rarely, extensive unilateral cerebral damage resulting from an intra-uterine or postnatal insult results in atrophy of the contralateral cerebellar hemisphere (**Fig. 2.65**). The histologic findings vary, and with them the suggested pathogenesis. Some cases show a simple reduction in hemispheric size following transneuronal atrophy of the ipsilateral pontine nuclei. A few show additional granule cell degeneration suggesting tertiary anterograde transneuronal degeneration.

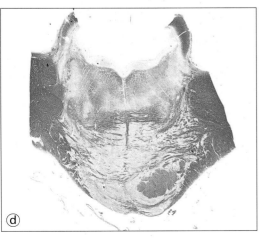
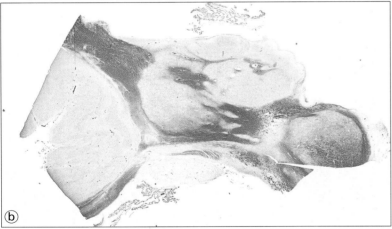
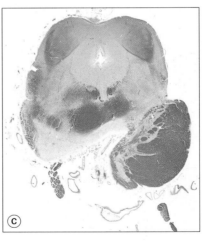
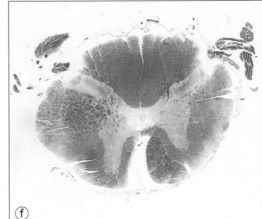
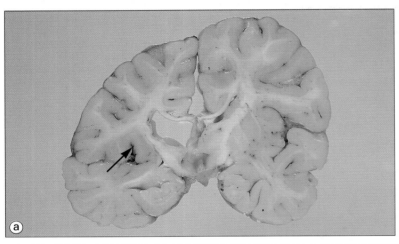
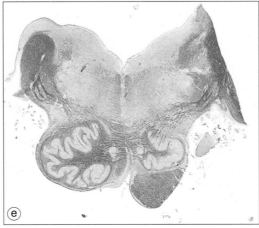

Fig. 2.64 Unilateral hypertrophy of the pyramidal tract in an 11-month-old girl. This infant had a gestational history of threatened miscarriage at eight weeks followed by recurrent maternal ill health. **(a)** Coronal section at the anterior thalamic level shows left-sided ventricular dilatation, atrophy of the thalamus, internal capsule, and lentiform nucleus, and polymicrogyria of the insula (arrow). **(b)** At a slightly more posterior level on the left side there is shrinkage of the internal capsule and atrophy with marbling of the left thalamus. **(c–e)** Horizontal sections through the brain stem showing ipsilateral (left) hypotrophy and contralateral (right) enlargement of the pyramidal tract. (c) midbrain, (d) mid-pons, (e) medulla. **(f)** In the cervical spinal cord the contrast between the pyramidal tracts is maintained in both crossed and uncrossed pathways.

KERNICTERUS

Kernicterus is selective yellow staining of deep gray matter and brain stem nuclei occurring in bilirubin encephalopathy (**Fig. 2.66**).

MACROSCOPIC AND MICROSCOPIC APPEARANCES

The subthalamic nucleus, globus pallidus, and lateral thalamus are characteristically affected. Other affected areas are the hippocampus CA2 field, lateral geniculate nucleus, the colliculi, the substantia nigra pars reticularis, the brain stem reticular formation, the cranial nerve nuclei, Purkinje cells, and the dentate and olivary nuclei (**Fig. 2.67**). The staining is best appreciated in unstained frozen sections, but remains for prolonged periods after formalin fixation. Yellow pigment is also visible in paraffin sections within the vacuoles of swollen cells. The accumulation of bilirubin causes neuronal necrosis and later mineralization and gliosis.

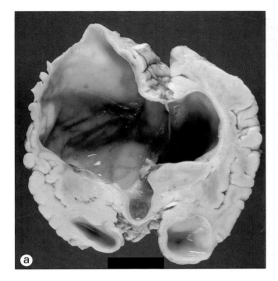

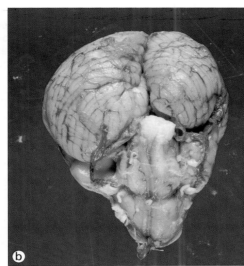

Fig. 2.65 Crossed cerebellar atrophy. Presentation in a five-month-old twin with ventriculomegaly detected ultrasonically at 32 weeks' gestation. **(a)** Coronal view of the hemispheres showing marked left ventricular dilatation, longstanding destruction of much of the hemispheric cortex and white matter, and thalamic atrophy. **(b)** There is obvious asymmetry of the hindbrain when viewed from below with ipsilateral (to the supratentorial damage) atrophy of the left pontine base and contralateral atrophy of the right cerebellar hemisphere.

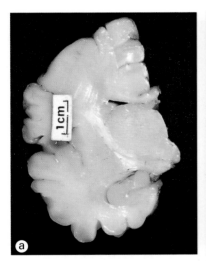
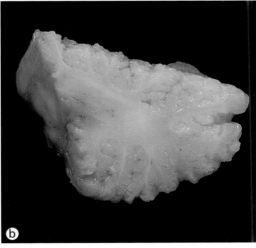
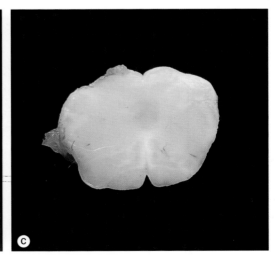

Fig. 2.66 Kernicterus. This is characterized by bright yellow staining of affected gray matter structures. **(a)** Hippocampus and subthalamic nucleus. **(b)** Dentate nucleus. **(c)** Inferior olives.

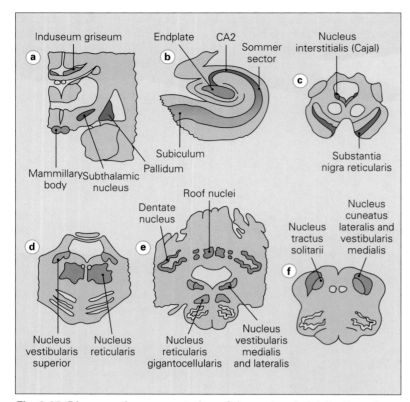

Fig. 2.67 Diagramatic representation of the regional distribution of lesions in kernicterus. (a) Coronal section at the level of the mamillary bodies. **(b)** Hypocampus. **(c)** Mid-brain. **(d)** Pons. **(e)** Cerebellum and upper medulla. **(f)** Lower medulla. Key: red, most vulnerable; pink, moderate vulnerability; beige, slight vulnerability.

PATHOGENESIS OF KERNICTERUS

- The accumulation of bilirubin is due to excessive production or insufficient conjugation and excretion. The unconjugated circulating form of bilirubin is toxic.
- The classic form of kernicterus in which the bilirubin level is at least 30 mg/dl follows hemolytic disease of the newborn and has largely been eradicated.
- Kernicterus is now observed in small preterm infants who have suffered asphyxia, acidosis, hypoglycemia or septicemia and in whom bilirubin levels may be as low as 10 mg/dl. Contributory factors are damage to the blood–brain barrier and reduced binding of bilirubin to albumin during treatment with certain drugs or following hepatic necrosis.

REFERENCES

Armstrong DD. Neonatal Encephalopathies. In: Duckett S, Malver PA (eds) *Pediatric Neuropathology* (1995). pp. 334–351. Baltimore: Williams and Wilkins.

Kinney HC, Armstrong DD. Perinatal neuropathology. In: *Greenfield's Neuropathology* (1997). pp. 537–600. London: Arnold.

Larroche JC, Encha-Razavi F. The Central Nervous System. In: Wigglesworth JS, Singer DB (eds) *Textbook of Fetal and Perinatal Pathology* (1991). pp. 778–842. Oxford: Blackwell Scientific Publications.

Papile LA, Burnstein J, Burnstein R, Koffler H. (1978) *J. Pediatr* **92**: 529–534.

Rorke LB. (1982) *Pathology of Perinatal Birth Injury*. New York: Raven Press.

3 *Malformations*

NEURAL TUBE DEFECTS: DYSRAPHIC DISORDERS

The following classification is based on present understanding of the development of the neural tube and axial skeleton (**Figs 3.1–3.3**).

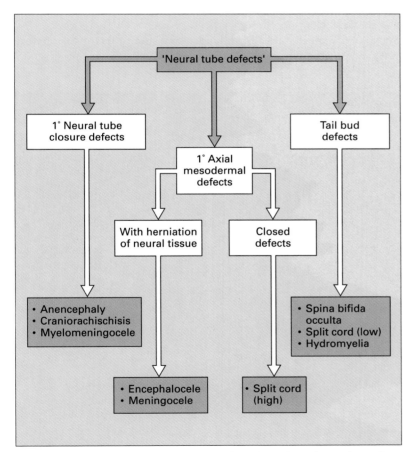

Fig. 3.1 **Classification of neural tube defects based on the embryonic tissues principally affected.**

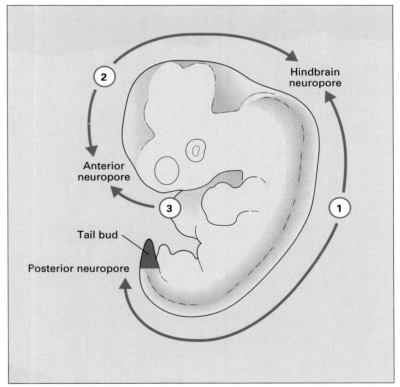

Fig. 3.2 **Primary and secondary neurulation.** There is a multisite mechanism of primary neural tube closure (i.e. primary neurulation) in the mouse and it is thought that there is a similar system in man. Closure begins at approximately 22 days after ovulation at closure site 1 (the future cervical/hindbrain boundary), and separately soon after at sites 2 (midbrain/forebrain junction) and 3 (rostral tip of forebrain). Fusion spreads bidirectionally from sites 1 and 2, and unidirectionally from site 3. About 26–28 days after ovulation cranial closure is completed at the anterior and hindbrain neuropores, and cord closure at the posterior neuropore at the upper sacral level. Caudal to this level all non-epidermal tissues are formed from the tail bud of multipotential stem cells (shaded red) by a process of differentiation and canalization (i.e. secondary neurulation).

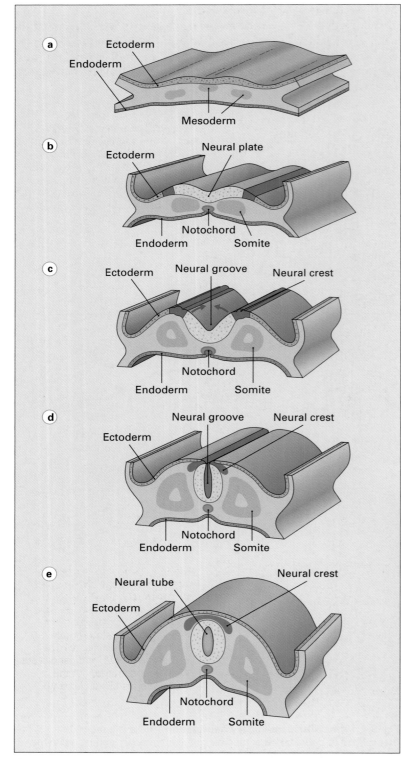

Fig. 3.3 Development of the neural tube and axial skeleton. (a) Induction of the neural plate from midline ectoderm occurs at around 16 days after ovulation. **(b, c)** From 18–20 days after ovulation, there is a gradual elevation of the lateral edges of plate to form the neural folds, and deepening of the longitudinal neural groove. Midline mesodermal tissue gives rise to both the centrally placed notochord and lateral somites. Neural crest arises at the boundary between the neural plate and ectoderm. **(d)** At about day 22, the neural folds start to close at the cervical/hindbrain boundary (see Fig. 3.2). **(e)** Fusion is completed to produce the neural tube. Soon after, the mesodermal somites migrate around the tube to produce the spinal vertebrae, skull vault, and occiput. The skull base and facial bones are derived from neural crest.

DEFECTS OF NEURAL TUBE CLOSURE

ANENCEPHALY

ANENCEPHALY

- is incompatible with independent existence
- is usually detected early in gestation by ultrasound scan
- is detected, as with all neural tube defects, by raised α-fetoprotein levels in maternal serum
- is more common in females
- is occasionally familial
- has an incidence up to ten times greater in Wales and Ireland than in France

MACROSCOPIC APPEARANCES

Anencephaly is characterized by replacement of most of the intracranial contents by a ragged, cavitated, vascular mass, the area cerebrovasculosa (**Fig. 3.4**). Remaining neural tissue usually includes the gasserian ganglia, distal parts of the cranial nerves, a variable amount of the medulla, and rarely a few cerebellar folia.

The skull shows various abnormalities including:
- an absent or hypoplastic skull vault
- a thickened and flat skull base
- shallow orbits so that the eyes protrude
- a shallow sella.

Spinal involvement varies from failure of fusion of the upper cervical vertebrae to craniorachischisis (**Fig. 3.5**).

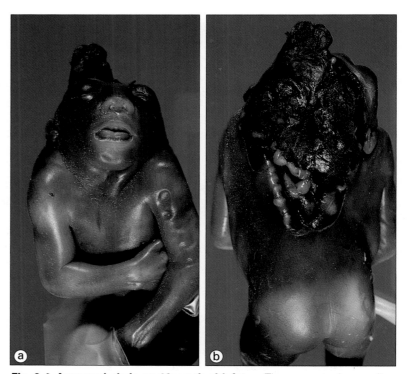

Fig. 3.4 Anencephaly in an 18-week-old fetus. The eyes are abnormally protuberant, the pinnae are low-set, and the neck is short. The calvarium is absent and the upper cervical vertebrae are not fused. The intracranial contents are a ragged vascular mass, the cerebrovasculosa. **(a)** Anterior view. **(b)** Posterior view.

Associated abnormalities are:
- a hypoplastic anterior pituitary
- absent intermediate and posterior lobes of the pituitary
- adrenal hypoplasia
- hypoplastic lungs
- a large thymus

MICROSCOPIC APPEARANCES

Histologically, the area cerebrovasculosa consists of an angiomatous mass of small blood vessels (**Fig. 3.6**) mixed with disorganized neuro-epithelial tissue, particularly glia, some neuroblasts or neurons, ependyma, and choroid plexus. Rarely, ependyma-lined cavities suggest forebrain ventricle.

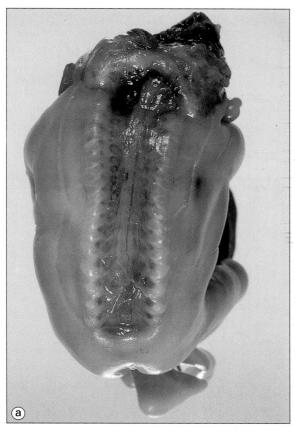

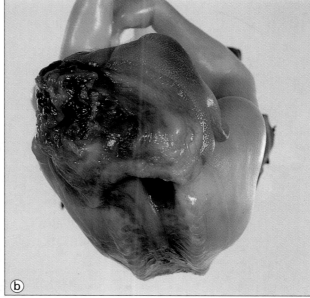

Fig. 3.5 Anencephaly with complete rachischisis in a 20-week-old fetus. The skull vault and vertebral arches are deficient, but the deformed skull base remains. **(a)** Viewed obliquely from behind. **(b)** Viewed from above.

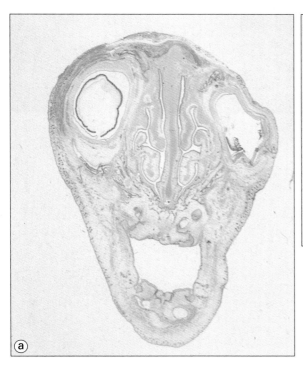

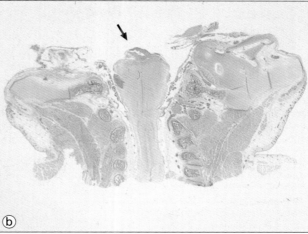

Fig. 3.6 Low-power frontal sections through the head in anencephaly. (a) Well-formed orbits are present, but central nervous system tissue is not apparent, only numerous thin-walled blood vessels. **(b)** The spinal cord, roots, and ganglia are well demonstrated, but the medulla ends blindly (arrow).

MYELOMENINGOCELE

Myelomeningocele (Figs 3.7, 3.8) is the herniation of spinal cord and meningeal tissue through a vertebral defect.

MYELOMENINGOCELE

- Myelomeningocele occurs at any level, but lumbosacral lesions are commonest. These are often associated with Chiari type II (Arnold–Chiari) malformation and hydrocephalus.
- A lesion above the twelfth thoracic vertebra is frequently associated with malformations in other systems and is more common in females.
- A lesion below the twelfth thoracic vertebra is more often solitary, shows a roughly equal sex distribution, and is associated with less severe neurologic sequelae.

MACROSCOPIC APPEARANCES

Macroscopically, a myelomeningocele is either:

- a cystic mass covered by a delicate membrane or skin, with the dilated hydromyelic cord floating within it, or
- a flat open lesion or myelocele, with a mass of vascular connective tissue and disorganized neural tissue, the area medullovasculosa, which becomes epithelialized after birth. Because the spinal cord is open posteriorly, the central canal opens directly onto the skin.

Other cord abnormalities (e.g. syringomyelia, hydromyelia, and split cord) are frequently found above the defect.

MICROSCOPIC APPEARANCES

Histologically, the epidermis overlying a myelomeningocele is atrophic (Fig. 3.9), lacking rete pegs and skin appendages, and often ulcerates. Beneath the epidermis there is fibrotic connective tissue, many dilated thin-walled vessels, and islands of glial tissue, which are sometimes accompanied by nerve cells and ependymal tissue.

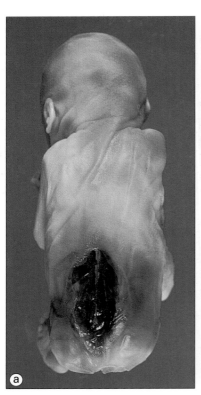
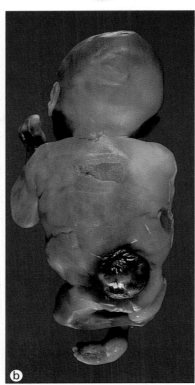
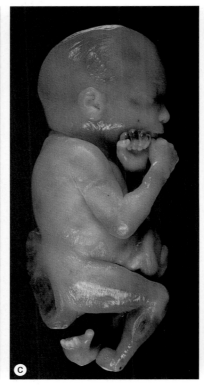
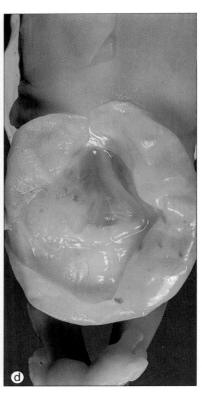

Fig. 3.7 Three examples of lumbosacral myelomeningocele in fetuses. (a) An open disc of vascular and neural tissue, or myelocele. **(b)** A closed cystic lesion. **(c, d)** Spina bifida cystica in combination with exomphalos, the closed cord floating within a myelomeningocele sac, viewed from the side in **(c)**, and viewed from behind, in **(d)**.

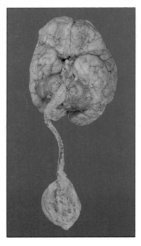

Fig. 3.8 Lumbosacral myelomeningocele in association with the Arnold–Chiari malformation. A tangled mass of cord tissue, peripheral nerves, and fibrous tissue opens to the exterior and blends with surrounding skin.

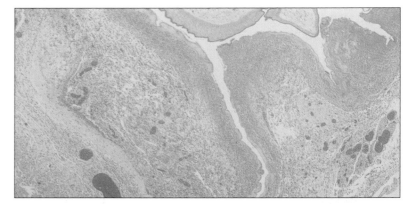

Fig. 3.9 Histology of a surgically excised myelomeningocele. The epidermis is atrophic and ulcerated and within the inflamed dermis there are many ectatic vessels and islands of glial tissue.

HERNIATION OF NEURAL TUBE THROUGH AXIAL MESODERMAL DEFECTS

ENCEPHALOCELE
Encephalocele is herniation of brain tissue through a skull defect (**Figs 3.10–3.16**) and is usually (75%) occipital. Rarer examples are parietal or fronto-ethmoidal.

MACROSCOPIC APPEARANCES
Small encephaloceles contain jumbled fragments of CNS tissue, but many are voluminous and include considerable parts of the hemispheres with ventricular cavities and sometimes hindbrain. Herniation is usually asymmetric, often leaving the intracranial contents skewed.

The leptomeninges covering the herniated tissue have a persistent fetal vasculature, an exuberant plexus of thin-walled sinusoids. Both intracranial and extracranial brain may show cortical migration defects such as heterotopias and polymicrogyria. Associated lesions include hippocampal and commissural anomalies, agenesis of cranial nerve nuclei, and partial absence of the cerebellum.

Occipital encephalocele may be associated with Meckel–Gruber syndrome (**Fig. 3.17**). Other neuropathologic findings include midline and hindbrain anomalies. Protrusion of meninges alone is termed a cranial meningocele (**Fig. 3.18**).

MECKEL–GRUBER SYNDROME

- shows autosomal recessive inheritance
- is characterized by occipital encephalocele, polycystic kidneys, hepatic fibrosis, and bile duct proliferation
- is associated with the characteristic dysmorphology of polydactyly, cleft palate, and microcephaly
- is a lethal condition

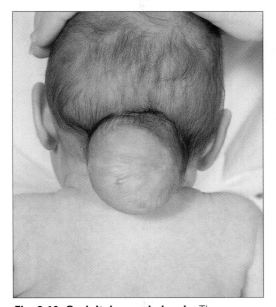

Fig. 3.10 Occipital encephalocele. The encephalocele is a fluctuant mass covered by skin, which is peripherally hairy but centrally shiny and thin.

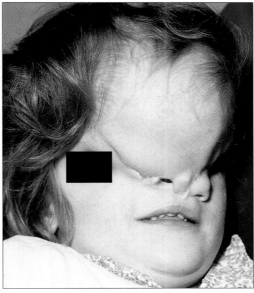

Fig. 3.11 Anterior encephalocele. This large swelling at the fronto-ethmoidal junction bulges out over the forehead and root of the nose and causes marked hypertelorism.

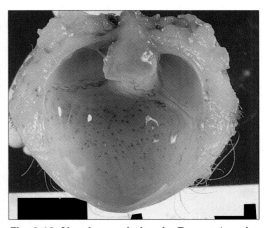

Fig. 3.12 Nasal encephalocele. Transection of a cystic polyp surgically excised from the nose revealed an ependyma-lined cavity containing a tuft of choroid plexus.

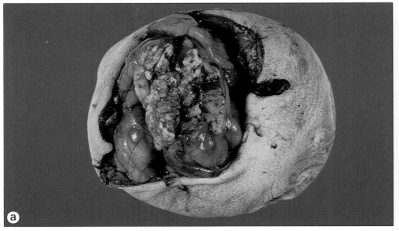 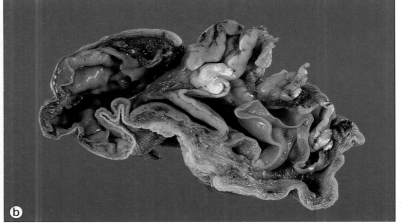

Fig. 3.13 Occipital encephalocele. Parts of both occipital horns and occipital poles fill the sac of this large surgical specimen. The cortex is markedly thinned and the lobes appear fused. Highly vascularized meninges are sandwiched between the cortical remnant and overlying skin. **(a)** Resection margin. **(b)** Section through the specimen.

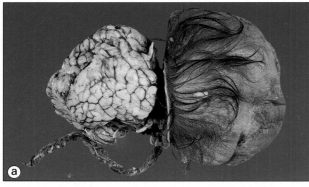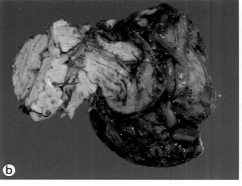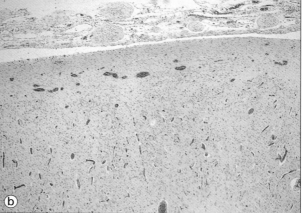

Fig. 3.14 Herniation due to a massive occipital encephalocele. The herniation is usually asymmetric. This occipital sac contains much of the posterior part of the left hemisphere as well as cerebellum. **(a)** Viewed from the left side. **(b)** Viewed through the midline. **(c)** A coronal section at the thalamic level appears very confusing at first. The smaller left hemisphere remnant is out of register with the right side and there is marked distortion of central structures.

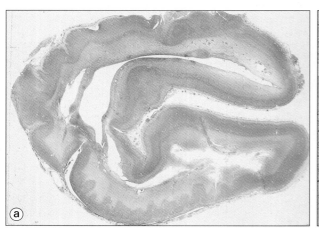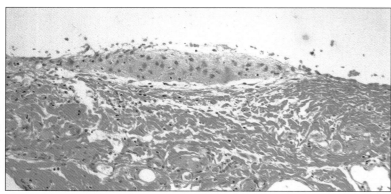

Fig. 3.15 Histology of a surgically excised encephalocele. (a) At low magnification, there is a recognizable cortical ribbon and ventricular cavity. The cortical ribbon has the undulating pattern of polymicrogyria, while heterotopic gray matter abuts the ventricular wall. (Luxol fast blue/cresyl violet) **(b)** At higher magnification the surface shows an excessively folded polymicrogyric cortex and numerous nodular glioneuronal heterotopias within the overlying leptomeninges.

Fig. 3.16 Surgically excised encephalocele. Some encephaloceles contain only small islands of glial tissue, which can be readily demonstrated with hematoxylin–van Gieson.

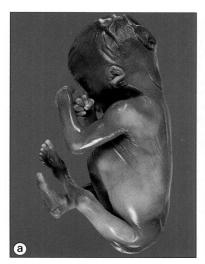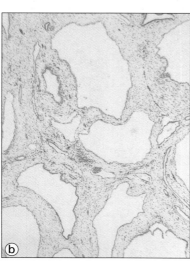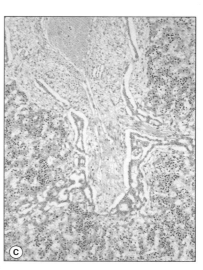

Fig. 3.17 Meckel–Gruber syndrome. The complex dysmorphology of this autosomal recessive syndrome includes **(a)** occipital encephalocele, **(b)** renal cysts, and **(c)** hepatic fibrosis with a striking bile duct proliferation.

MENINGOCELE

A meningocele is characterized by herniation of highly vascular arachnoid and dura through a vertebral defect with a covering of atrophic epidermis. It is most often lumbosacral. Although the cord remains within the spinal canal, it may show other anomalies such as hydromyelia, splitting, or tethering.

OCCULT SPINA BIFIDA

Occult spina bifida is the mildest form of neural tube defect and probably reflects failure of tail bud development or secondary neurulation.

MACROSCOPIC APPEARANCES

The cord may appear normal but often shows a distended central canal (hydromyelia) (**Fig. 3.19**), diastematomyelia (**Fig. 3.20**), or cord tethering (**Fig. 3.21**), all of which involve lower lumbar or sacral levels.

Although a closed lesion, occult spina bifida is often indicated by overlying tufts of hairy skin or lipomatous skin tags (**Fig. 3.22**). It may be associated with sacral, anorectal, and urogenital defects.

CHIARI MALFORMATIONS

Chiari defined three anatomic types of cerebellar deformity associated with hydrocephalus.

CHIARI TYPE I MALFORMATION

Chiari type I malformation is the herniation of a peg of cerebellar tonsil through the foramen magnum in the absence of an intracranial space-occupying lesion or preceding hydrocephalus (**Figs 3.23–3.25**).

CHIARI TYPE I MALFORMATION

- may be asymptomatic
- may present in infancy with neck pain, lower cranial nerve palsies, sleep apnea, or sudden unexpected death
- may present in adulthood with cerebellar ataxia, late-onset hydrocephalus, long tract signs, or symptoms and signs of syringomyelia
- is strongly associated with syringomyelia (Chiari type I occurs in 90% of patients with syringomyelia, including familial types)
- is associated with skeletal abnormalities including platybasia, suboccipital dysplasia, and Klippel–Feil anomaly (radiologic studies emphasize the small size of the posterior fossa and suggest that occipital dysplasia is a major pathogenetic factor)

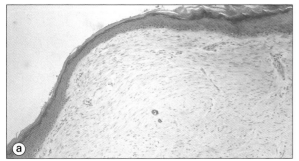
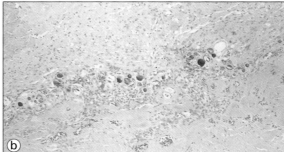

Fig. 3.18 **Cranial meningocele.** Cranial and spinal meningoceles have similar histologic features. **(a)** As with all dysraphic lesions the overlying epidermis is thin and atrophic. **(b)** Deeper in the fibrotic dermis there are islands of meningothelial cells, which may form whorls and psammoma bodies.

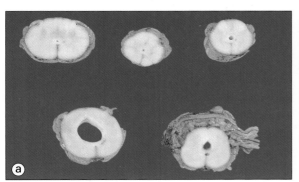
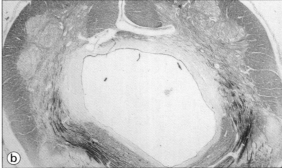

Fig. 3.19 **Hydromyelia. (a)** Horizontal sections of the cord showing marked dilation of the central canal at thoracic and lumbar levels. **(b)** Despite marked distension of the lumbar central canal the ependyma is virtually intact. (Luxol fast blue/cresyl violet)

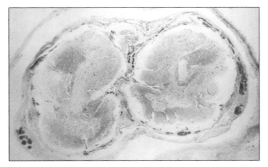
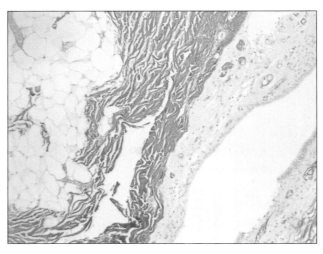

Fig. 3.20 **Diastematomyelia.** This is characterized by splitting of the cord into two hemicords separated by a median septum of fibrous meninges. This example is from a patient with Chiari type II malformation. (Luxol fast blue/cresyl violet)

Fig. 3.21 **Tethered cord.** Lower limb motor and sensory deficits and neuropathic bladder are the principal presenting signs of the tethered cord syndrome. Operative findings include a low conus and thickening of the filum, often in association with a lipoma, as shown in this typical surgical specimen, which comprises remnants of ependymal canal and lobules of mature adipose tissue. (Hematoxylin/van Gieson)

CHIARI TYPE II (ARNOLD–CHIARI) MALFORMATION

Chiari type II malformation combines herniation of the cerebellar vermis with malformation and downward displacement of the brain stem (**Figs 3.26–3.29**). The degree of cerebellar herniation varies from slight (in fetuses) to extensive, at which point the choroid plexus and tonsils may be included. The cerebellar tail is bound by fibrous adhesions to the dorsal surface of the medulla or occasionally is situated within the fourth ventricle. Folia in the herniated cerebellar tissue show neuronal loss, absence of myelinated fibers, and gliosis.

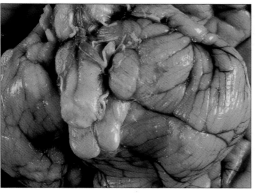

Fig. 3.22 'Fawn's tail'. A massive subcutaneous lipoma extending into a large skin tag (fawn's tail) associated with an occult spina bifida.

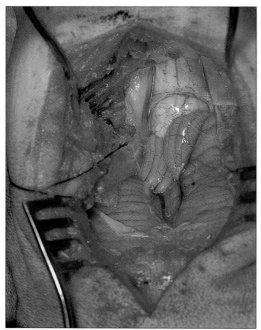

Fig. 3.23 Chiari type I malformation, posterior view. Both cerebellar tonsils are markedly but asymmetrically elongated into the spinal canal.

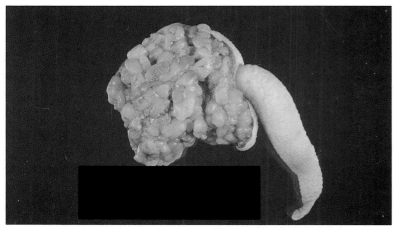

Fig. 3.24 Chiari type I malformation. In a 10-month-old child presenting with polydactyly, hemihypertrophy, and hemimegalencephaly plus polymicrogyria, a bifid tongue of tonsillar tissue extends 2.5 cm below the inferior olives.

Brain stem malformations include:
- fusion of the inferior colliculi, which gives a beak-like appearance to the quadrigeminal plate
- an indistinct pontomedullary junction and rod-shaped pons
- looping of the lower medulla over the cervical cord
- less frequently, dysplasias of cranial nerve nuclei, olives, and pontine nuclei.

Other findings include:
- an abnormal upwards course of the first six cervical spinal roots
- subependymal nodular heterotopias in the lateral ventricles
- disordered cortical lamination including polymicrogyria
- asymmetry or flattening of the cerebellar hemispheres, which may form a collar around the ventral medulla

CHIARI TYPE II MALFORMATION

- is almost invariably associated with a lumbosacral myelomeningocele
- is associated with craniolacunia, a shallow posterior fossa and enlarged foramen magnum, a wide tentorial hiatus and low tentorial insertion, a low torcula, and a short fenestrated falx
- is accompanied by hydrocephalus at birth in more than 80% of cases

PATHOGENESIS OF CHIARI TYPE II MALFORMATION

- Older theories attribute distortion of the cerebellum and brain stem to compression by hydrocephalic cerebral hemispheres or to traction from cord tethering, but these explanations cannot be sustained in the presence of an S-shaped brain stem deformity or the absence of spina bifida or hydrocephalus in a few cases.
- Disproportion between the growth of the posterior fossa and its contents is a more likely mechanism: the cerebellar weights and posterior fossa volumes are both reduced, and experimental vitamin A administration to pregnant hamsters induces a shortened basichondrocranium and reduced posterior fossa volume, suggesting that the neurologic anomalies are secondary to skeletal defects.
- A small posterior fossa could compress the developing medulla causing abnormalities of the pontine and cervical flexures and force the cerebellum to grow into the spinal canal during its relatively late growth spurt. This theory is consistent with observations in second trimester human fetuses who show only slight cerebellar herniation in association with major medullary abnormality.

CHIARI TYPE III

Chiari type III malformation is the rare cerebello-encephalocele through an occipitocervical or high cervical bony defect (**Fig. 3.30**). Associated brain stem deformities and lumbar spina bifida are reminiscent of those associated with Chiari type II malformation.

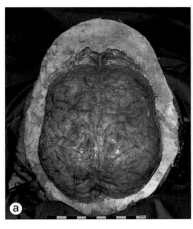

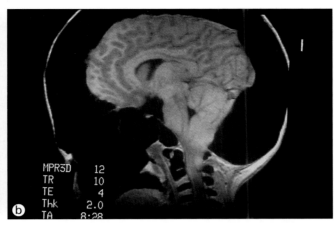

Fig. 3.25 Chiari type I malformation associated with craniosynostosis due to craniometaphysial dysplasia. (a) Superior view of the brain within the thickened skull. **(b)** MRI shows tonsillar herniation to the level of the second cervical vertebra. The brain, spinal cord, and roots are surrounded by a dark halo of massively thickened bone. (Courtesy of Dr K. Chong, Great Ormond Street Hospital for Children, London, UK)

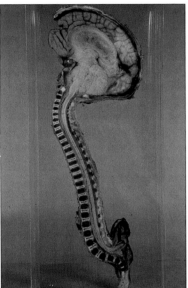

Fig. 3.26 Chiari type II (Arnold–Chiari) malformation. Midline section of the brain and cord within the skull and vertebral column, demonstrating the downward displacement of vermis and brain stem and beaking of the tectum. Chiari type II malformation is usually associated with a lumbosacral myelomeningocele and hydrocephalus, as illustrated here.

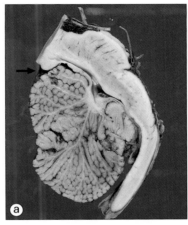 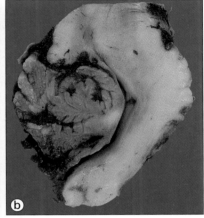

Fig. 3.27 Chiari type II malformation. Mid-sagittal sections of the hindbrain are most helpful when the diagnosis is not clear. **(a)** A tongue of vermis capped by choroid plexus extends down over the dorsal surface of the cervical cord. The lower brain stem is elongated and the tectum is beaked (arrow). **(b)** In this example, the lowest part of the medulla overrides the cord producing an S-shaped bend.

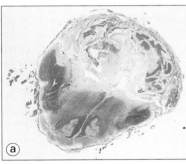 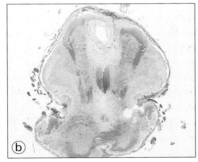

Fig. 3.28 Horizontal microscopic sections of herniated tissue in Chiari type II malformation. (a) Cerebellar vermis herniating over the medulla has markedly sclerotic folia. **(b)** A section through the region of the S-bend where low medulla overrides cervical cord. (Luxol fast blue/cresyl violet)

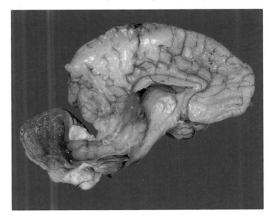

Fig. 3.30 Chiari type III malformation. There is herniation of cerebellum into an occipitocervical encephalocele.

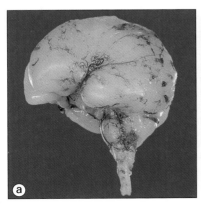 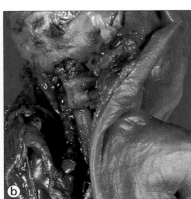 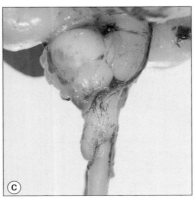

Fig. 3.29 Chiari type II malformation in three fetal brains. Brain stem elongation and downward herniation over the upper cord are obvious, but there is only slight herniation of the vermis. **(a)** The brain of a 14-week-old fetus viewed from the side. **(b)** 18-week-old fetus. The herniation is seen *in situ* after removal of the atlanto-occipital membrane and upper vertebral arches, which is the most reliable method for arriving at a necropsy diagnosis. **(c)** 20-week-old fetus, the hindbrain viewed from the side.

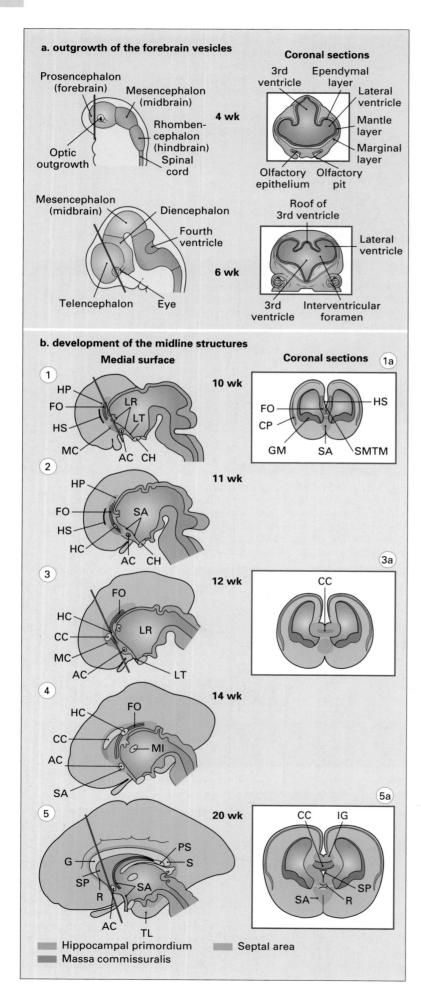

a. outgrowth of the forebrain vesicles

Prosencephalon (forebrain)
Mesencephalon (midbrain)
Rhomben-cephalon (hindbrain)
Optic outgrowth
Spinal cord

4 wk

Coronal sections

3rd ventricle
Ependymal layer
Lateral ventricle
Mantle layer
Marginal layer
Olfactory epithelium
Olfactory pit

Mesencephalon (midbrain)
Diencephalon
Fourth ventricle

6 wk

Telencephalon   Eye

Roof of 3rd ventricle
Lateral ventricle
3rd ventricle
Interventricular foramen

b. development of the midline structures

Medial surface

1
HP
FO
LR
LT
HS
MC
AC   CH

2
HP
FO
SA
HS
HC
AC   CH

3
FO
HC
LR
CC
MC
AC   LT

4
HC
FO
CC
MI
AC
SA

5
PS
G   S
SP
SA
R
AC
TL

Coronal sections

1a
FO   HS
CP
GM   SA   SMTM

10 wk
11 wk
12 wk
14 wk
20 wk

3a
CC

5a
CC   IG
SA   SP
R

■ Hippocampal primordium   ■ Septal area
■ Massa commissuralis

DISORDERS OF FOREBRAIN INDUCTION

Various interrelated hemispheric anomalies result from failures in outgrowth and separation of the forebrain vesicles and in the development of the commissures (**Fig. 3.31**). The hemispheric anomalies are associated with craniofacial anomalies (**Fig. 3.38**).

HOLOPROSENCEPHALY

Holoprosencephaly is expressed as variable degrees of failure in outgrowth and cleavage of the prosencephalic vesicles.

HOLOPROSENCEPHALY

- occurs sporadically, but is occasionally familial
- has an incidence of 1/16,000–30,000 births and 1 in 250 abortions
- is diagnosed during pregnancy by ultrasound scan, which reveals a monoventricular brain and fused basal nuclei
- results in stillbirth in its severest form, but liveborn have facial dysmorphism, psychomotor retardation, spasticity, apneic attacks, and disturbed temperature regulation

ETIOLOGY OF HOLOPROSENCEPHALY

- Holoprosencephaly is a heterogeneous group of conditions.
- Environmental factors include maternal diabetes mellitus, toxoplasmosis, syphilis, rubella, and fetal alcohol syndrome.
- Mechanical or chemical methods have been used to induce it experimentally.
- Genetic factors include autosomal recessive, autosomal dominant, and X-linked inheritance patterns. There are chromosomal aberrations in about 50% of cases. Trisomy 13 is most frequent (holoprosencephaly, occurs in 70% of cases of trisomy 13). Others include trisomy 18 and triploidy. Putative genes have been recognized at four sites: 21q22.3, 2p21, 7q36, 18pter-q11.

ALOBAR HOLOPROSENCEPHALY
MACROSCOPIC APPEARANCES

Alobar holoprosencephaly (**Figs 3.32–3.37**) is the severest form and is characterized by:
- a very small brain, monoventricular and undivided into hemispheres

Fig. 3.31 (a) Outgrowth of the forebrain vesicles. (b) Development of the midline structures. By 10 weeks gestation (1) the anlage of the anterior commissure (AC) appears in the ventral part of the lamina reuniens (LR) and the fornix (FO) appears in its dorsal part and grows dorsally with the hippocampal primordium (HP). In the floor of the interhemispheric fissure (1a) below the hemispheric sulcus (HS) the banks of a median groove, the sulcus medianus telencephali medii (SMTM) fuse into the massa commissuralis or commissural plate (MC), but the groove remains open below into the interhemispheric fissure. Soon after (2) the hippocampal commissure (HC) appears dorsal to the septal area (SA) and AC. By 12 weeks (3, 3a) the corpus callosum (CC) is forming in the MC and then grows caudally with the growth of the hemisphere. Around 14 weeks (4) as the hemisphere grows upwards and backwards a pocket forms in the SMTM below the CC. (5, 5a) As the CC grows and bends forwards and downwards into its genu (G) it covers the pocket in the SMTM, and finally the callosal fibres of the rostrum (R) grow through the MC so sealing the space which becomes the cavum septi pellucidi. LR lamina reuniens; LT lamina terminalis; CH optic chiasm; CP cortical plate; GM germinal matrix; IG Indusiom griseom; MI massa intermedia; S splenium of callosum; SP septum pellucidum; PS hippocampal commissure (psalterium); TL temporal lobe.

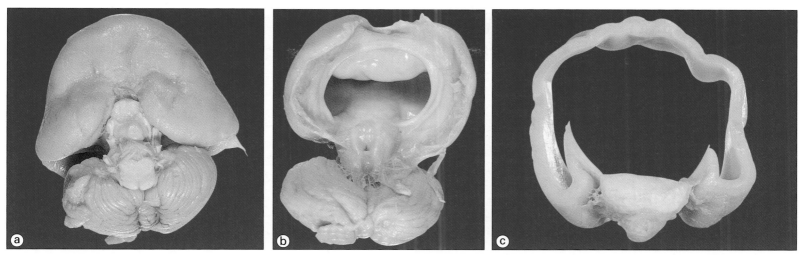

Fig. 3.32 Alobar holoprosencephaly. (a) Viewed from below, the small single fused holosphere is helmet shaped with minimal gyration, absent olfactory structures, and anomalous cerebral arteries, which run in shallow gutters. Although the hindbrain is relatively well preserved overall there is marked microcephaly and the total brain weight is 150 g at 18 months. **(b)** Lifting the holosphere forwards allows a view from behind into the single ventricular cavity. Around its margin runs the hippocampus in a complete arch, while in the floor are fused basal ganglia and thalamus. Just behind them is the quadrigeminal plate with the pineal and entrance to the aqueduct. Note the tattered remnant of the roof membrane at the lateral posterior edge of the holosphere. **(c)** A coronal section through the holosphere shows marked hydrocephaly, thin pallium, and fused thalami.

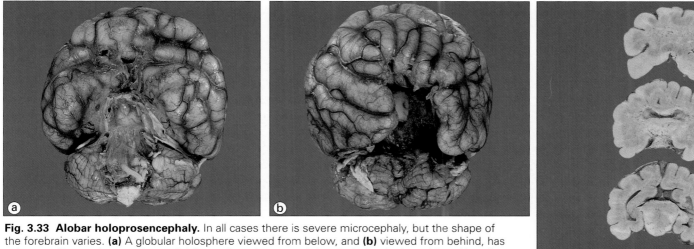

Fig. 3.33 Alobar holoprosencephaly. In all cases there is severe microcephaly, but the shape of the forebrain varies. **(a)** A globular holosphere viewed from below, and **(b)** viewed from behind, has only a small posterior membrane. **(c)** Coronal sections reveal the single forebrain and fused basal ganglia, but the ventricular cavity here is not dilated.

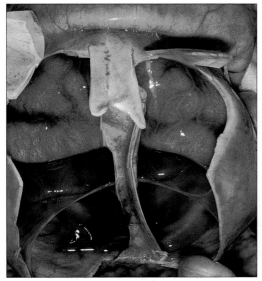

Fig. 3.34 Alobar holoprosencephaly. Viewed *in situ* within the skull the delicate cyst that covers the caudal part of the holosphere is well demonstrated.

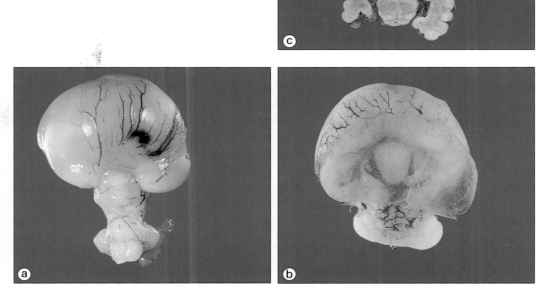

Fig. 3.35 Alobar holoprosencephaly in 17-week-old fetuses. (a) An inferior view of a horseshoe holosphere with olfactory aplasia and aberrant vessels radiating across the orbital surface. **(b)** A similar case seen from behind and photographed in water so that the cystic roof membrane billows out.

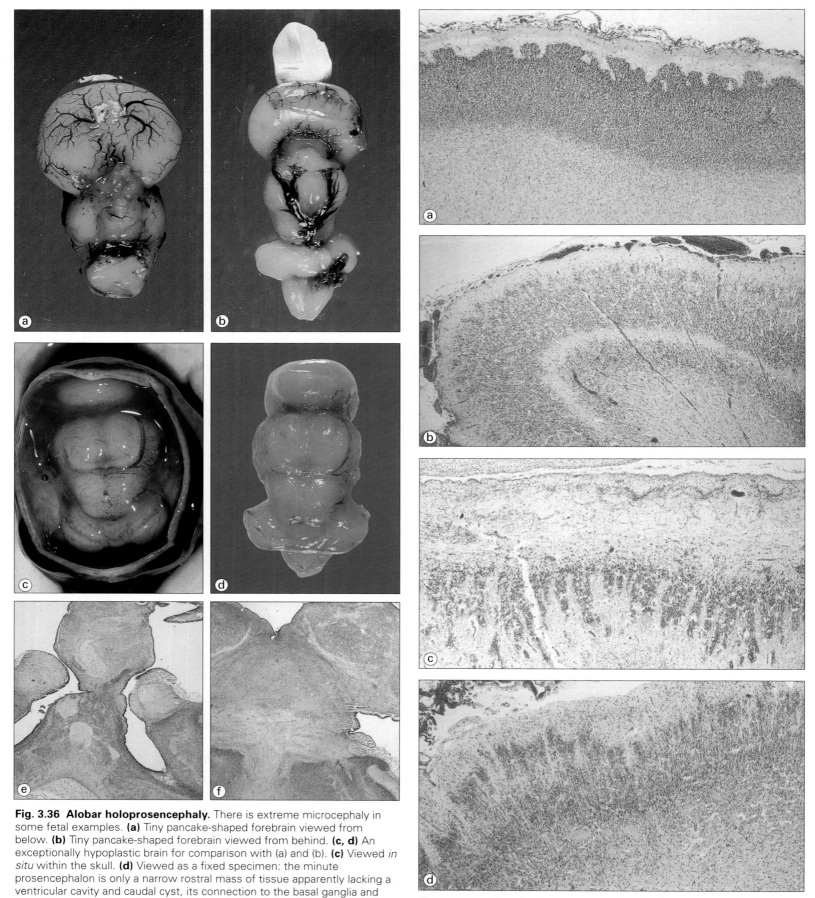

Fig. 3.36 Alobar holoprosencephaly. There is extreme microcephaly in some fetal examples. **(a)** Tiny pancake-shaped forebrain viewed from below. **(b)** Tiny pancake-shaped forebrain viewed from behind. **(c, d)** An exceptionally hypoplastic brain for comparison with (a) and (b). **(c)** Viewed *in situ* within the skull. **(d)** Viewed as a fixed specimen: the minute prosencephalon is only a narrow rostral mass of tissue apparently lacking a ventricular cavity and caudal cyst, its connection to the basal ganglia and fused thalamus being only a thin ventrally situated bridge. **(e, f)** Microscopic coronal sections through the central part of the specimen reveal bilateral hippocampi and lateral ventricular horns (e) opening into a cystic space lined by ependyma. (f) Note the fused midline thalamus and dorsolateral striata.

Fig. 3.37 Cortical dysplasias encountered in holoprosencephaly at microscopy. (a) Status verrucosus (Luxol fast blue/cresyl violet). **(b)** A four-layer cortex with segregation of the superficial layers. **(c)** Thick cords of neurons running across the pallium. **(d)** Similar cords as in (c) associated with deeply placed acellular zones or glomeruli.

- a globular or flattened holosphere with a bizarre convolutional pattern and no interhemispheric fissure, gyri recti, or olfactory structures.

The horseshoe-shaped dorsal surface of the holosphere continues posteriorly as a delicate membranous roof to the single ventricle, which attaches distally to the tentorium. A cavity is thus formed, which may be small or balloon into a dorsal cyst. In the floor of the ventricle are fused basal ganglia and thalami, from the lateral edges of which the hippocampus makes a continuous arch around the ventricle and attaches to the roof membrane. Corpus callosum and septum are absent. Holospheric white matter is minimal.

Craniofacial malformations are associated with alobar holoprosencephaly (**Fig. 3.38**). The face tends to predict the brain, particularly midfacial hypoplasia. The severest is cyclopia with fused orbits and eyes. Other anomalies include a proboscis (ethmocephaly), absent jaw (agnathia), fused ears (synotia, otocephaly), flat nose with a single nostril (cebocephaly), microphthalmia, hypotelorism, and occasionally hypertelorism.

Skeletal anomalies include a short narrow skull base, absent crista galli and lamina cribrosa, absent or shallow sella, and variable hypoplasia of nasal bones. The falx and sagittal sinus are also usually missing.

MICROSCOPIC APPEARANCES

There is histologic evidence of:

- neocortical hypoplasia with a relative lack of prefrontal association cortex and excessive allocortex
- cortical disorganization or disturbed neuronal migration such as polymicrogyria, superficial cortical segmentation, prominent perpendicular cords of cells, and more deeply placed aneuronal neuropilic glomerular structures.

The anterior part of the circle of Willis is anomalous. The anterior and middle cerebral arteries are replaced by forward directed branches of one or both internal carotids. Large choroidal arteries supply the dorsal cyst.

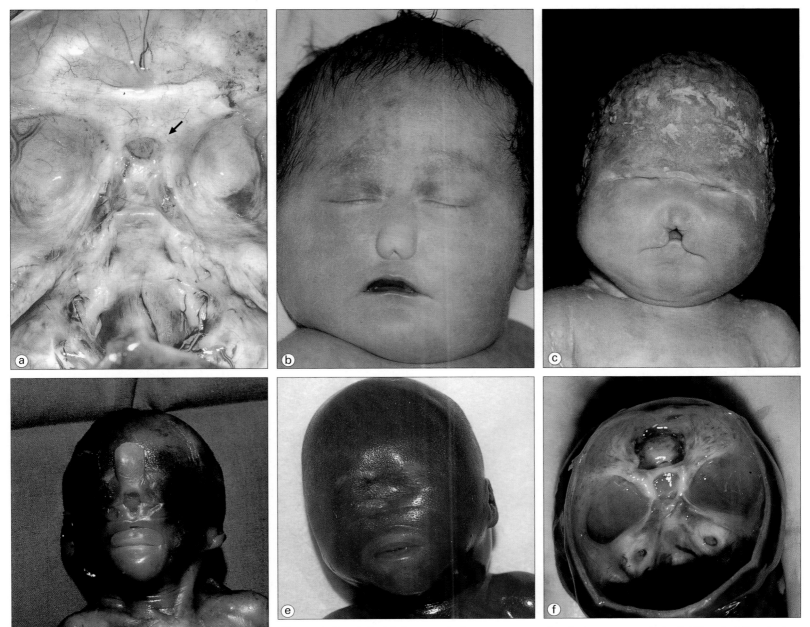

Fig. 3.38 Craniofacial dysmorphology accompanying holoprosencephaly. (a) The skull floor lacks an ethmoid plate and there is olfactory aplasia. In this case the optic nerves are hypoplastic (arrow). **(b)** Hypotelorism and cebocephaly with a single nostril. **(c)** Cleft lip and palate. **(d)** Cyclopia and proboscis in a case of trisomy 13. **(e)** External view of cyclopia and nasal pit in the case depicted in Fig. 3.36c–f. **(f)** Intracranial view of the single globe and minuscule anterior fossa in the case depicted in Fig. 3.36c–f.

SEMILOBAR HOLOPROSENCEPHALY

This lesion is intermediate between the alobar and lobar forms (**Fig. 3.39**). There are mild microcephaly, a partly formed shallow interhemispheric fissure, and some lobar structure with rudimentary temporal and occipital horns, but continuity of the cortex across the midline. Olfactory structures are usually absent.

LOBAR HOLOPROSENCEPHALY

Despite near normal brain size, normal lobe formation, and separated hemispheres, the cerebral cortex is continuous across the midline, at the frontal pole, or in the orbital region, or above the callosum (cingulosynapsis) (**Fig. 3.40**).

Olfactory bulbs and callosum may be absent or hypoplastic. Heterotopic gray matter may be found in the ventricular roof.

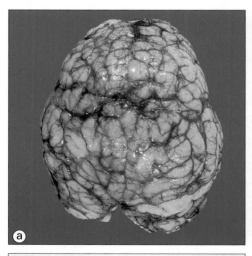

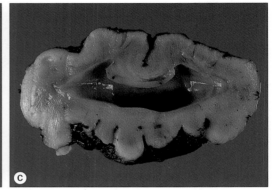

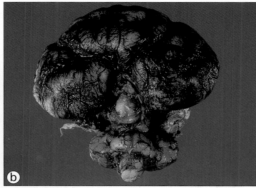

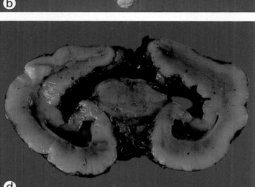

Fig. 3.39 Semilobar holoprosencephaly. (a) Superior view of brain within the skull showing anterior fusion and anomalous gyral pattern. **(b)** The fixed specimen viewed from below showing rudimentary temporal lobes. **(c)** In coronal sections there is a shallow interhemispheric fissure, but the cortical ribbon is continuous over the vertex and the orbital pallium is completely fused. **(d)** More posteriorly there is separation of the hemispheres.

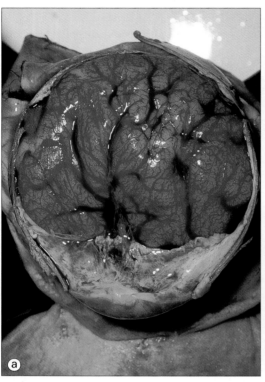

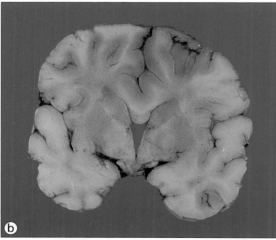

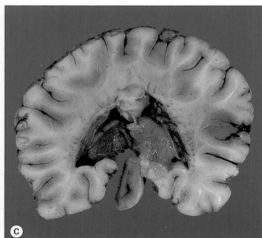

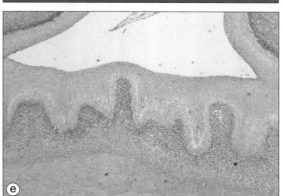

Fig. 3.40 Lobar holoprosencephaly. (a) There is gyral fusion over the central part of the hemispheres. **(b)** In coronal sections the cingulate cortex runs continuously across the midline over the corpus callosum (cingulosynapsis). Slung beneath the callosum is a nodular gray heterotopia. **(c)** Further back the hemispheres remain incompletely separated. A continuous parietal cerebral wall and no sagittal fissure are evident superiorly. The occipital horns and temporal lobes are quite distinct. **(d)** Cingulosynapsis in fetal brain. The fused cingulate cortex is thin and looped, reminiscent of polymicrogyria. **(e)** Close-up view of the polymicrogyric fused cingulum.

OLFACTORY APLASIA

This is characterized by absent olfactory bulbs, tracts, trigone, and anterior perforated substance and is associated with anomalous cortical convolutions and an absent gyrus rectus (**Fig. 3.41**). Olfactory aplasia is usually an incidental postmortem finding or associated with holoprosencephaly, callosal agenesis, septo-optic dysplasia, or Kallmann's or Meckel–Gruber syndrome. It is usually bilateral. Unilateral absence is exceptional.

ATELENCEPHALY AND APROSENCEPHALY

These rare syndromes manifest as microcephaly (Fig. 3.42) and show features common to both anencephaly and holoprosencephaly.

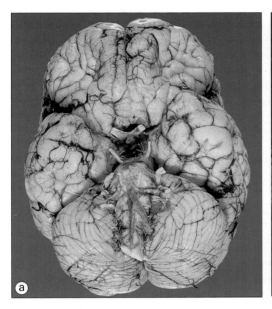
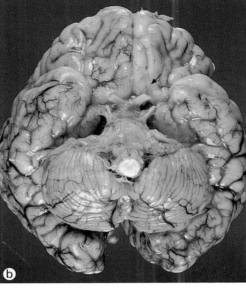

Fig. 3.41 Olfactory aplasia. (a) Bilateral absence of olfactory bulbs and tracts. There is an anomalous orbital convolutional pattern, lacking gyri recti. **(b)** An extremely rare example of right unilateral olfactory aplasia. Compare the abnormal gyral pattern on the right side of the brain with the normal left side, which includes the proximal part of the olfactory tract (arrow).

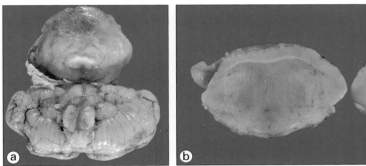
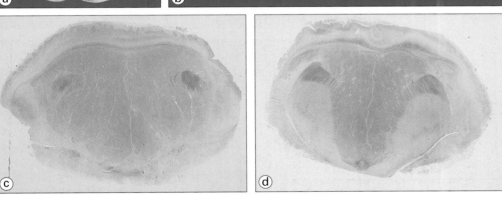
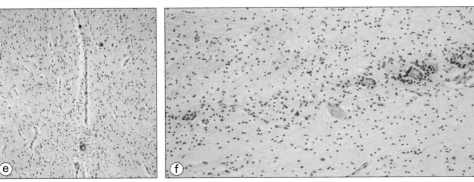
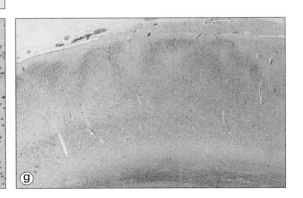

Fig. 3.42 Atelencephaly in a 9-month-old infant. (a) Viewed from below. There is extreme microcephaly (total brain weight 95 g). The tiny uncleaved globular forebrain shows olfactory aplasia, but includes a myelinated optic chiasm. **(b)** When the forebrain is bisected coronally there are few distinguishing features, no visible ventricular cavity, and only a dorsal arch of myelinated fibers. **(c, d)** Histologic sections of the forebrain at low magnification suggest a symmetric organization, confirm the presence of myelinated fibers, and show a thin undulating cortex over the vertex, and a gliomesodermal thickening of the basal leptomeninges. **(e)** Histology also shows a midline raphe containing small calcospherites and tiny ependymal tubules. **(f)** A more laterally placed line of ependymal tubules is seen here, which may represent an abortive attempt to produce a ventricle. **(g)** The looped four-layer cortical ribbon is reminiscent of polymicrogyria.

MACROSCOPIC AND MICROSCOPIC APPEARANCES OF ATELENCEPHALY

The cerebral cortex, basal ganglia, and ventricles are virtually absent, but, unlike anencephaly, there is an intact calvarium sloping sharply to a pointed vertex. There is a tiny globular or multinodular brain remnant rimmed by a thick leptomeningeal gliomesodermal proliferation.

Histologically, atelencephaly is characterized by disorganized gray and white matter with calcifications, ependymal-lined tubules, and a looped polymicrogyric cortex.

MACROSCOPIC AND MICROSCOPIC APPEARANCES OF APROSENCEPHALY

In addition to the features of atelencephaly, aprosencephaly is also characterized by involvement of diencephalic structures, the eyes, optic nerves, mamillary bodies, hypothalamus, and hypophysis. The hindbrain is largely preserved. Facial dysmorphism resembles that found in holoprosencephaly.

AGENESIS OF THE CORPUS CALLOSUM

Agenesis of the corpus callosum may be:
- total or partial (e.g. missing only the splenium)
- isolated or combined with other malformations (e.g. holoprosencephaly)

MACROSCOPIC AND MICROSCOPIC APPEARANCES

If the callosum is deficient, the cingulate gyrus is also deficient. A radiating gyral pattern forms the medial surface of the cerebral hemisphere. The lateral ventricles have a membranous roof with upturned pointed corners, and a large longitudinal myelinated fiber bundle (of Probst) is present laterally. The membranous roof of the (usually distended) third ventricle bulges into the interhemispheric fissure, displacing the fornices laterally from where the widely separated leaves of the septum incline laterally towards the Probst bundles (**Figs 3.43–3.45**). The occipital horns are often markedly dilated. The anterior commissure is variably present, the posterior commissure is always present, and the psalterium is never present.

Callosal anomalies are rarely associated with a midline mass (e.g. cyst, meningioma, hamartoma, lipoma) (**Figs 3.46, 3.47**). There is a high incidence of associated visceral and cerebral anomalies, especially hydrocephalus, and rhinencephalic and migration defects.

ANOMALIES OF THE SEPTUM PELLUCIDUM

Primary agenesis of the septum pellucidum may be an isolated malformation or occur as part of a complex syndrome. Secondary destruction occurs with inflammation, hydrocephalus, or porencephaly, and produces a fenestrated septum or small remaining fragments.

AGENESIS OF THE CORPUS CALLOSUM

- occurs either sporadically or as a familial disorder
- is an important feature of several well-defined syndromes including the X-linked dominant Aicardi syndrome (i.e. infantile spasms, chorioretinopathy and depigmented lacunae, mental retardation, vertebral anomalies, polymicrogyria, and cerebral heterotopias), the autosomal recessive Andermann syndrome (i.e. sensorimotor neuropathy and dysmorphic features), acrocallosal syndrome (i.e. polydactyly, macrocephaly, and mental retardation), Meckel–Gruber syndrome, and hydrolethalus syndrome
- may be entirely asymptomatic or produce subtle perceptual deficits if an isolated anomaly; otherwise clinical signs depend on the associated malformations

ETIOLOGY OF AGENESIS OF THE CORPUS CALLOSUM

- The presence of a longitudinal bundle suggests the involvement of misdirected callosal fibers.
- The importance of a glial sling to guide the growing callosal fibers across the midline has been demonstrated in genetically acallosal mice and by experimentally interfering with the normal embryologic structure.
- The involvement of a mechanical defect is supported by the interposition of hamartomas and lipomas in some cases. The differentiation of these tissue rests may obstruct normal callosal outgrowth.

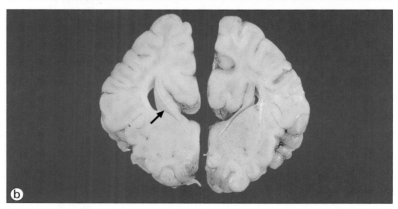

Fig. 3.43 Agenesis of the corpus callosum in a 3-month-old child with maple syrup urine disease. (a) Medial aspect of the hemisphere. The callosum and cingulum are absent, and an irregular arrangement of gyri surrounds the ventricle. **(b)** Frontal coronal sections show the absence of the corpus callosum and anterior commissure. The lateral angles of the lateral ventricles point upwards. There appears to be no septum pellucidum in the midline, but the leaves of the septum are swept laterally to cover the fornices and the bundles of Probst (arrow), which bulge into the medial walls of the frontal horns.

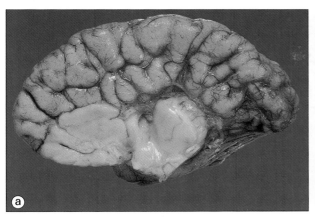

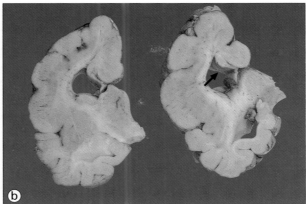

Fig. 3.44 Agenesis of the corpus callosum. (a) Medial aspect of the hemisphere showing replacement of the cingulate gyrus by radiating gyri. **(b)** In coronal sections, the myelinated Probst bundles of misdirected callosal fibers are prominent, and the frontal horn has a characteristic bat-wing appearance.

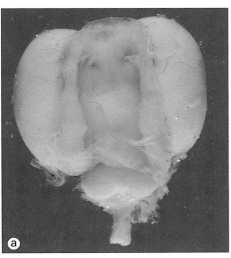

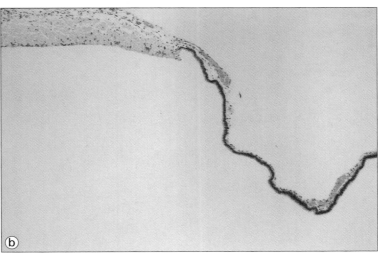

Fig. 3.45 Agenesis of the corpus callosum in a 16-week-old fetus. (a) The delicate membrane roofing the third ventricle balloons upward when placed in water. **(b)** The membrane has two layers: fibrovascular and ependymal.

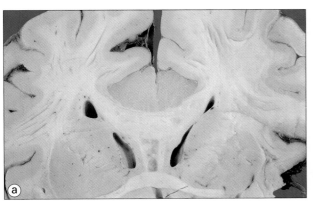

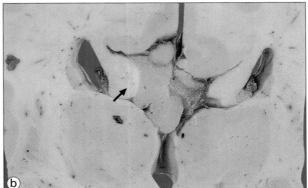

Fig. 3.46 Partial agenesis of the corpus callosum associated with a lipoma. (a) At the level of the anterior commissure the well-formed callosum is covered on its dorsal surface by a yellow lipoma. **(b)** At midthalamic level the callosum is discontinuous, the gap being filled by lipoma. Small longitudinal bundles of Probst can be seen (arrow). (Courtesy of Dr. C. Torre, Rome and Professor F. Scaravilli, Institute of Neurology, London)

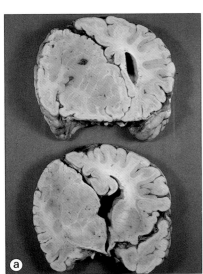

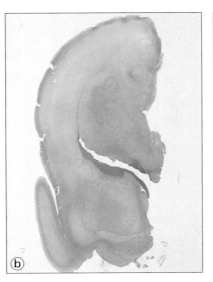

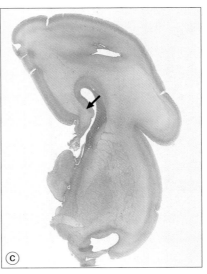

Fig. 3.47 Callosal agenesis associated with a unilateral mass lesion. (a) The left hemisphere is disorganized by massive gray heterotopias so no interhemispheric fibers have formed, while the relatively well-formed right hemisphere has a longitudinal Probst bundle. **(b)** In this 27-week-old fetus a large hamartoma disrupts the left hemisphere. **(c)** The otherwise normal right hemisphere has a Probst bundle (arrow). (Kindly referred by Dr. Jeanne Bell, Edinburgh)

SEPTO-OPTIC DYSPLASIA

Septo-optic dysplasia (**Fig. 3.48**) is the clinical triad of:

- optic hypoplasia
- septal aplasia
- hypopituitarism.

The etiology is unknown, though there is a report of septo-optic dysplasia and semilobar holoprosencephaly following maternal first trimester alcohol abuse. One of the three prime features may occasionally be absent, notably the septal aplasia.

MACROSCOPIC AND MICROSCOPIC APPEARANCES

The main neuropathologic features of septo-optic dysplasia are:

- optic nerve and lateral geniculate hypoplasia

- dysplasia of hypothalamic nuclei
- olfactory aplasia.

Other features that are sometimes seen are posterior pituitary hypoplasia, cerebral heterotopias, polymicrogyia, and cerebellar dysplasias.

CAVUM SEPTI PELLUCIDI AND CAVUM VERGAE

Cavum septi pellucidi (**Fig. 3.49**) and cavum vergae are rostral and caudal cavities, respectively, bounded above by the corpus callosum and laterally by the two leaves of the septum pellucidum and the fornices. They are normally present in fetal life and usually obliterated by term. A cavum septi pellucidi is seen in 20% of brains at necropsy with or without a cavum vergae. Glial tissue lines the cavity, which may contain macrophages.

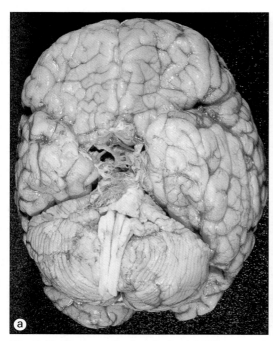
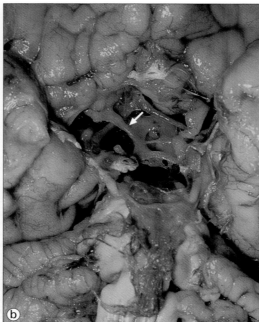
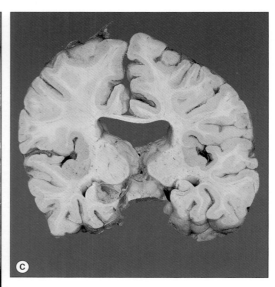

Fig. 3.48 Septo-optic dysplasia. (a) Olfactory aplasia and hypoplastic optic nerves. **(b)** Close-up of the thin gray optic nerves (arrow). **(c)** Coronal section showing absent septum pellucidum and thin callosum with a smooth ventricular surface.

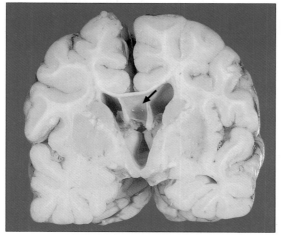

Fig. 3.49 A large cavum septi pellucidi. The cavity (arrow) is enclosed by the corpus callosum above, and the septi pellucidi and fornices on either side.

NEURONAL MIGRATION DEFECTS: CEREBRAL CORTICAL DYSPLASIAS

The classification of these disorders is based on our present rapidly expanding knowledge of the complex development of the cerebral cortex (**Figs 3.50, 3.51**).

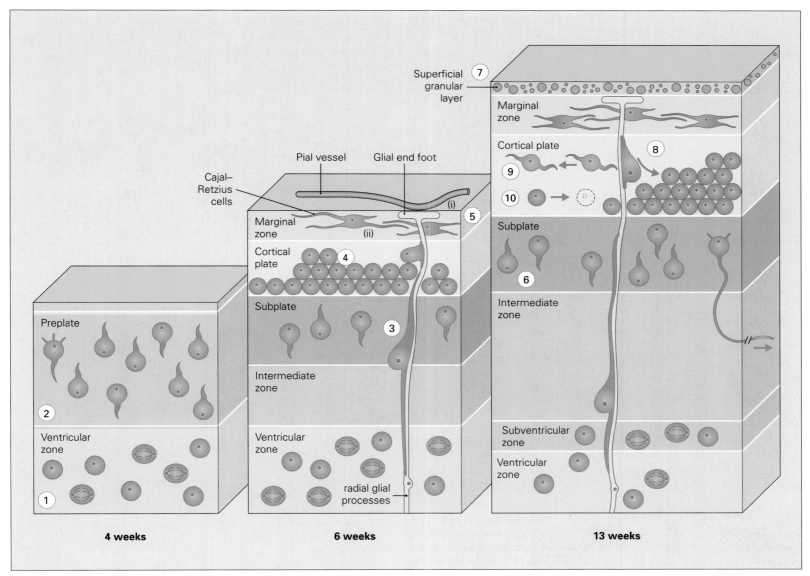

Fig. 3.50 Timing and other aspects of neocortical development. (1) There is initial proliferation of neuronal and glial precursors in the ventricular zone (VZ). **(2)** From 4 weeks' gestation post-mitotic neuroblasts move away from the VZ to form the preplate (PP) under the pia. **(3)** From 6–20 weeks' gestation two major waves of neuroblast migration using radial glial processes (rg) and adhesion molecules to form the cortical plate (CP) in an inside-out manner. The earliest arrivals form the deepest layers. **(4)** The CP splits the PP into an outer marginal zone (MZ) or future molecular layer, and inner subplate (SP). **(5)** Early (at 6 weeks) appearance in the MZ of (i) glia limitans formed from expanded end-feet of rg and basal lamina of pial vessels, and (ii) horizontal processes and synapses of Cajal–Retzius cells (CR), forming a physical barrier to migration. **(6)** SP neurons are transient (most disappear in early postnatal life), have many neuropeptides and growth factor receptors, are important in organizing cortical connections, and act as pioneer corticofugal axons and early temporary targets for thalamic afferents. **(7)** The superficial granular layer (SGL) is transient, lasting from 12–24 weeks' gestation and has an uncertain role. **(8)** Terminal differentiation is a multistep, multifactional process, dependent on birthdate, and therefore laminar position of neuron, environmental events in late S-phase, and switches to initiate and cease migration using adhesion molecules. **(9)** Tangential migration guided by neuronal processes has also been demonstrated. **(10)** Programmed cell death (physiologic pruning of the majority of cells) is critical for achieving correct numbers of cortical neurons. Other aspects of cortical differentiation include synaptic pruning as part of the plasticity of the developing cortex in response to changing patterns of innervation and convolutional folding of the gyri, which may be related to mechanic stresses induced between the various layers within the CP.

A hypothetical scheme of genetic faults responsible for migration defects

Malformation	Possible regulatory gene defects	Result	Other mechanisms
Agyria-pachygyria	Neuroblast proliferation Neuronal size Neuronal type Neuron-glia interaction	Too many or too few neurons Neurons too large or too small Imbalance of neuronal types Malalignment or faulty lamination	
Lissencephaly type II	Neuron-glial interaction	Faulty lamination and overmigration	*Abnormal tangential vascular pattern* *Late disturbance of the cortical plate*
Polymicrogyria	Apoptosis Neuronal size Neuronal type Neuron-glia interaction	Too many or too few neurons Neurons too large or too small Imbalance of neuronal types Malalignment or faulty lamination	
Dysplasia with cytomegaly	Neuron-glia interaction Neuronal size Neuronal type	Malalignment or faulty lamination Abnormal cytomegaly Imbalance of neuronal types	*Abnormal mitotic events* *Glial dysplasia*
Heterotopia	Neuron-glia interaction Neuroblast proliferation Apoptosis Neuronal type	Neurons in ectopic location Excessive neuronal number Failure of expected cell death Imbalance of neuronal types	
Micro-lissencephalies	Neuroblast proliferation Neuronal type Neuronal-glial interaction Neuronal size Apoptosis	Too few neurons Imbalance of neuronal types Faulty lamination and overmigration Neurons too large or too small Excessive neuronal death	*Vascular dysgenesis* *Abnormal mitotic events*

Fig. 3.51 A hypothetical scheme of genetic faults responsible for migration defects.

AGYRIA AND PACHYGYRIA

Agyria and pachygyria refer to an absence of gyri and sulci, or reduced numbers of broadened convolutions, respectively, associated both macroscopically and microscopically with a thickened cortical ribbon (**Figs 3.53, 3.54, 3.56**).

MACROSCOPIC APPEARANCES

The skull vault is small, misshapen, and thickened. Brain weight is usually low, and very occasionally heavy. A markedly thickened cortical ribbon is associated with reduced white matter (see Fig. 3.53). Pachygyria is occasionally combined with polymicrogyria. The claustrum and extreme capsule are absent. Lateral ventricles are dilated and often associated with periventricular nodular heterotopia.

MICROSCOPIC APPEARANCES

The characteristic histological appearance is a four-layer cortex (**Fig. 3.55**):
- molecular layer
- thin, external neuronal layer
- sparsely cellular layer with a tangential myelin fibre plexus
- a thick, inner neuronal layer (**Fig. 3.55c**) which splits in its deeper zone into columns of cells (lissencephaly type I)

Variants may lack lamination or have a more complex horizontal organization.

Associated findings include olivary heterotopia (see Fig. 3.52), and hypoplastic pyramidal tracts. Less common associations are: dentate dysplasia, cerebellar heterotopia and granule cell ectopia.

THE SMOOTH BRAIN

Various synonyms are used in clinical radiologic and pathologic practice when referring to the macroscopic appearances of a smooth brain:
- for almost completely smooth or unconvoluted brains – agyria or lissencephaly
- for reduced numbers of coarse or widened convolutions – macrogyria or pachygyria

Various histologic patterns may be encountered in macroscopically smooth or poorly convoluted cortex:
- agyria or pachygyria with or without four layers (lissencephaly type I)
- cerebro-ocular dysplasia (lissencephaly type II)
- polymicrogyria (unlayered or four-layered)
- cortical dysplasia with cytomegaly – localized, multifocal, or hemimegalencephalic (accurate diagnosis requires microscopic examination)

ETIOLOGY OF AGYRIA AND PACHYGYRIA

- The cell-free third cortical layer suggests a zone of tissue destruction.
- The association with olivary heterotopia implies an initiation time of 11–13 weeks' gestation.
- The considerations above support a mechanism that interferes with the late migration of neuroblasts.

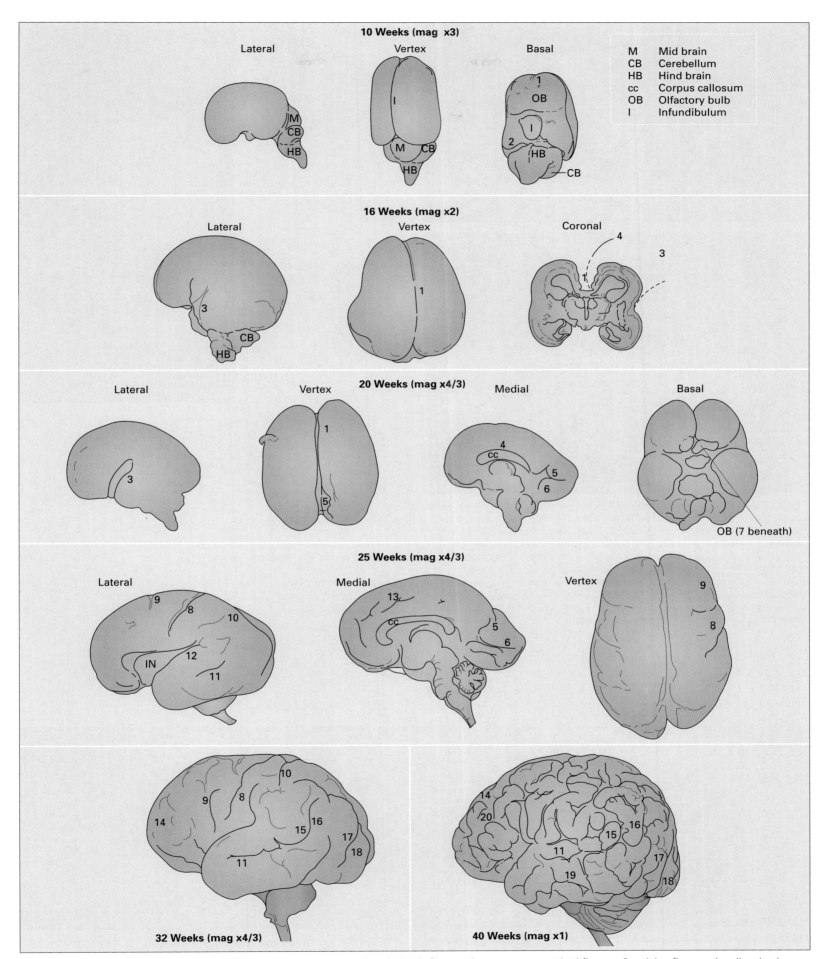

Fig. 3.52 Development of the gyral patterns of the brain. 1, intrahemispheric fissure; 2, transverse cerebral fissure; 3, sylvian fissure; 4, callosal sulcus; 5, parieto-occipital fissure; 6, calcarine sulcus; 7, olfactory sulcus; 8, central sulcus; 9, precentral sulcus; 10, postcentral sulcus; 11, superior temporal sulcus; 12, lateral sulcus; 13, angulate sulcus; 14, superior frontal sulcus; 15, supra-marginal gyrus; 16, angular gyrus; 17, superior occipital gyrus; 18, inferior occipital gyrus; 19, inferior temporal sulcus; 20, inferior frontal sulcus; 21, inter-parietal sulcus.

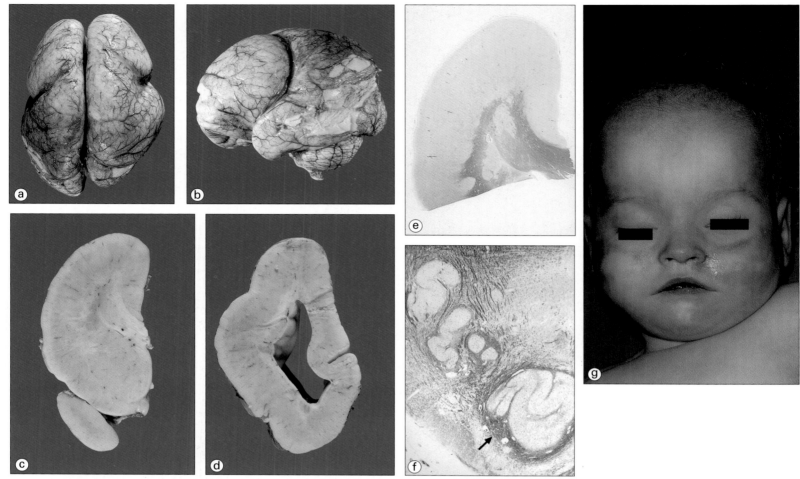

Fig. 3.53 Agyria in a case of Miller–Dieker syndrome. (a) Over the vertex the cortical surface is almost completely smooth. **(b)** Lateral view of the left hemisphere showing a lack of all sulci except the Sylvian fissure. **(c)** Coronal section of the frontal lobe. The cortical surface is smooth and the ribbon is greatly thickened, while the greatly reduced white matter contains a large heterotopia. **(d)** Coronal section of the occipital lobe showing agyria and periventricular gray matter heterotopia. **(e)** Section of the frontal lobe stained with luxol fast blue/cresyl violet. The cortex is extremely thick. Heterotopic gray matter bulges into the ventricular lumen. **(f)** Horizontal section of one side of the medulla showing several islands of heterotopic olivary tissue stranded between the inferior cerebellar peduncle and the dysplastic inferior olivary nucleus (arrow). **(g)** Typical facies with microcephaly, bitemporal hollowing, high forehead, broad nasal bridge and upturned nares, thin upper lip, and micrognathia.

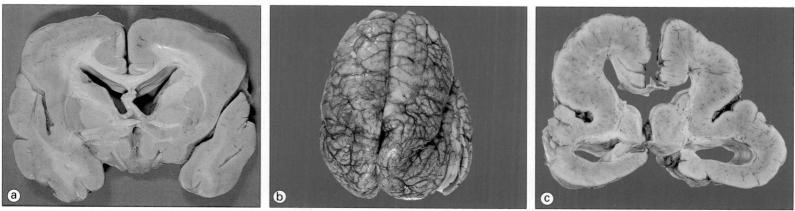

Fig. 3.54 There is a continuous spectrum from agyria to pachygyria. (a) Shallow cingulate and temporal gyri in a 4-year-old microcephalic boy presenting with infantile spasms. **(b)** Marked microcephaly (500 g brain at 8 months). Much of the vertex appears quite smooth. **(c)** In coronal sections of (b) there are cingulate and temporal gyri and a narrow Sylvian fissure, but the insula is poorly formed. Note the very thick cortex, attenuated white matter and corpus callosum, and periventricular heterotopic gray matter.

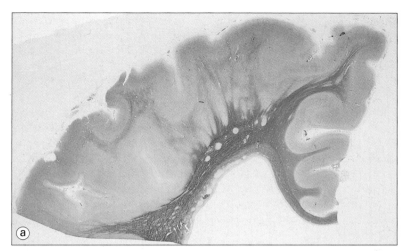

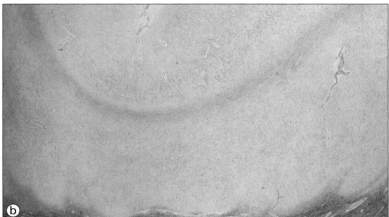

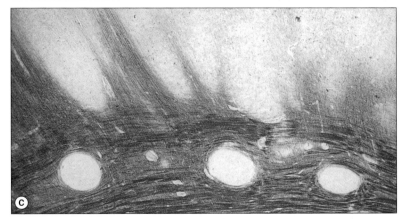

AGYRIA AND PACHYGYRIA

- Agyria and pachygyria are characterized clinically by the lissencephaly sequence of microcephaly, bitemporal hollowing, a small jaw, diminished spontaneous activity, profound mental and motor retardation, feeding problems, early hypotonia, late hypertonia, and epilepsy.
- These malformations occur either sporadically or as familial disorders.
- There are several associated syndromes including Miller–Dieker syndrome (the best known) in which > 90% of patients with the syndrome have a visible or submicroscopic deletion in a critical 350 kb region of chromosome 17p13.3 (LIS-1).
- Other rarer autosomal recessive forms of agyria are characterized by slightly different dysmorphology, severe microcephaly, and a thick cortex with variable lamination.

GENETIC CONTROL OF CORTICAL DEVELOPMENT (EVIDENCE FROM C. ELEGANS AND DROSOPHILA)

Combinations of genes control development at many levels.
- General CNS development, including migration and polarity, is controlled by paired homeobox genes.
- Cell division is regulated by protein kinases.
- Neurogenic genes (such as *notch*) determine cell lineage (i.e. whether cells become epidermal or neuronal).
- Neuroblast production is influenced by prepattern and proneural genes.
- Neuronal differentiation is affected by neuronal precursor selector genes (of the helix-loop-helix family).
- Programmed neuronal death (apoptosis) is controlled by several, sequentially acting genes.

Fig. 3.55 A four-layer cortex in agyria or pachygyria (lissencephaly type I). **(a)** A narrow band of faintly stained myelin fibers indicates the third layer sandwiched between outer and inner gray laminae, the latter sending thick plumes into the thin underlying white matter, which also contains nodular heterotopias. **(b)** Close-up of the four-layer cortex showing the molecular layer, outer neuronal layer, paucicellular layer with myelin, and inner gray layer. **(c)** The deeply placed columns of the innermost layer and heterotopic nodules.

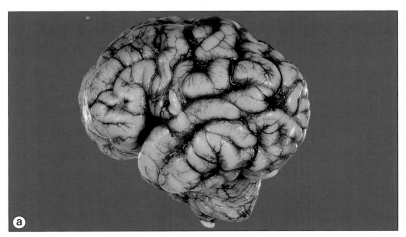

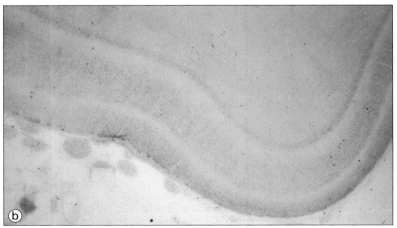

Fig. 3.56 Pachygyria without a four-layer cortex. Not all examples of pachygyria are four layered. **(a)** Marked brachycephaly and simplified broad convolutions in a term neonate. **(b)** Histologically, there are two hypocellular laminae resulting in a remarkable multilayered appearance.

CEREBRO-OCULAR DYSPLASIAS

Cerebro-ocular dysplasias show a distinct histologic form of cerebral cortical thickening and dysplasia (lissencephaly type II). They occur in several rare overlapping autosomal recessive familial syndromes that combine complex cerebral and ocular malformations and muscular dystrophy.

MACROSCOPIC APPEARANCES

An occipital meningocele or encephalocele is common. The cerebral hemispheres are usually enlarged, but occasionally small, and have a smooth surface that lacks convolutions and is covered by adherent thick white leptomeninges (Figs 3.57, 3.58). Fusion of the medial surfaces of the frontal lobes, olfactory aplasia or hypoplasia, thin optic nerves and optic chiasm, small flattened cerebellar hemispheres with a coarsely nodular surface, and a small or absent vermis are sometimes found. A massive hydrocephalus throughout the ventricular system and a thin corpus callosum are evident.

MICROSCOPIC APPEARANCES

Mesodermal proliferation containing prominent glioneuronal heterotopia produces thickened leptomeninges and obliterates the subarachnoid space. A thickened and disorganized cortical ribbon is divided by centripetal fibrovascular septa into irregular neuronal clusters, which sometimes have a wave-like arrangement. The cortical ribbon is separated by a narrow hypocellular zone with thin-walled blood vessels from an inner layer of heterotopic gray matter islands. Cortex on the medial aspects of the hemispheres is often thin and undulating, like polymicrogyria.

Cerebellar cortical dysplasia is associated with numerous heterotopias in the white matter, and dysplastic dentate nuclei. A hypoplastic brain stem is invested with a thick cuirass of fibrous and glial tissue, especially over the midbrain. The pyramidal tracts are absent or misdirected and the inferior olives dysplastic. Dystrophic muscle shows fiber degeneration and regeneration, fibrosis and inflammatory infiltrates.

CEREBRO-OCULAR DYSPLASIA SYNDROMES

- Walker–Warburg or HARD+E (hydrocephalus, agyria, retinal dysplasia plus encephalocele) syndrome is characterized by profound psychomotor retardation, hydrocephalus from birth, ocular anomalies (e.g. central corneal opacity, abnormalities of the iris, cataract, retinal detachment, retinal dysplasia), developmental defects, and death in infancy.
- Cerebro-ocular dysplasia–muscular dystrophy syndrome (COD–MD) produces similar manifestations to Walker–Warburg syndrome, plus electrophysiologic evidence of myopathy, and rising creatine phosphokinase (CPK) concentrations.
- Muscle–eye–brain disease is a further variant with a milder phenotype.
- In Fukuyama congenital muscular dystrophy cerebral malformations are less severe, and comprise microcephaly, extensive unlayered polymicrogyria, and small areas of type II lissencephaly. It is the commonest form of congenital muscular dystrophy in Japan.

PATHOGENESIS OF CEREBRO-OCULAR DYSPLASIA

- The multiplicity of malformations implies a prolonged disruptive process through the second and third trimesters.
- Observations on second trimester abortuses suggest a combination of failure of the pial–glial barrier allowing uncontrolled migration, and disruption of radial migration by the abnormal deep tangential vascular plexus, followed by a late disturbance of surface growth, meningeal proliferation, and fibrovascular invasion of the cortical plate.

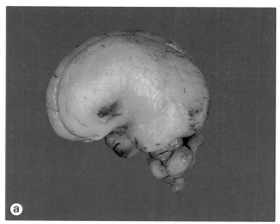

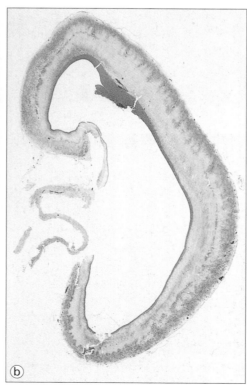

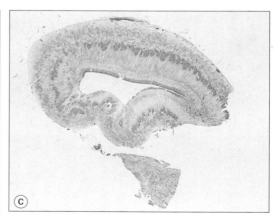

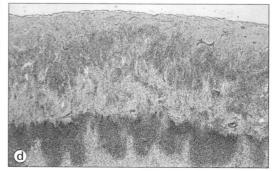

Fig. 3.57 Cerebro-ocular dysplasia in an 18-week-old fetus. (a) Completely smooth lateral surface of the left cerebral hemisphere. **(b)** Microscopy of an occipital coronal section showing massive ventriculomegaly and lissencephalic cortex with deeply placed heterotopias. **(c)** In another fetus of 18 weeks' gestation, extensive deep heterotopias are particularly prominent. **(d)** There is obliteration of the subarachnoid space with gliomesodermal tissue and a thickened patch-like cortex. Parallel with the surface is a linear array of heterotopic nodules.

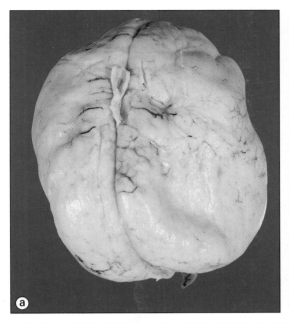

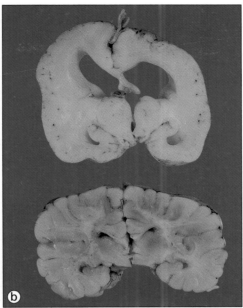

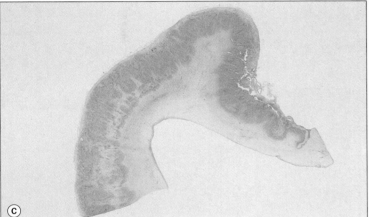

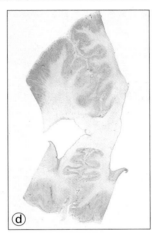

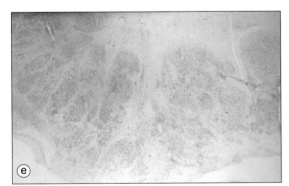

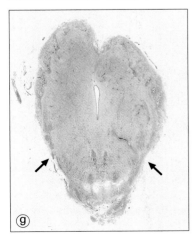

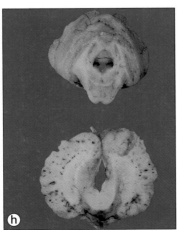

Fig. 3.58 Cerebro-ocular dysplasia (lissencephaly type II; HARD syndrome) in a 6-week-old infant. (a) The vertex of the brain is smooth and white, having no convolutions and very thickened leptomeninges. **(b)** Section at thalamic level compared with an age-matched normal control below, showing ventriculomegaly and a shallow interhemispheric fissure, beneath which the medial surfaces are fused. Although the cortex is abnormally thick, it is pale and difficult to distinguish from white matter. **(c)** Low power microscopy of the frontal lobe shows the irregularly thickened, unlaminated cortex and an archipelago of deeply placed islands of heterotopic gray matter laterally. **(d)** The cortical ribbon on the medial parts of the frontal lobes is thin, undulating, and fused, reminiscent of polymicrogyria. **(e)** The typical histology of lissencephaly type II is of obliterated subarachnoid space and thickened disorganized cortex. **(f)** In places the thickened disorganized cortex is thrown into waves. **(g)** The hypoplastic midbrain, with the tectum above and nigra below, is surrounded by a thick collar of gliomesodermal tissue. There is a rest of neuroblasts dorsal to the aqueduct and the cerebral peduncles appear to be absent, but heterotopic bundles are situated dorsolaterally (arrows). **(h)** Horizontal section of the dysplastic cerebellum and pons below compared with a normal control above. The vermis is absent and normal folial structure is obliterated by extensive cortical dysplasia (see Fig. 3.101a,b).

NEU–LAXOVA SYNDROME

This is a rare lethal autosomal recessive syndrome with a normal karyotype producing severe intrauterine growth retardation, microcephaly, grotesque facies, limb flexion deformities, and skin dysplasia (**Fig. 3.59**).

MACROSCOPIC AND MICROSCOPIC APPEARANCES

The pathology consists of extreme microcephaly, lissencephaly, agenesis of the corpus callosum, and cerebellar hypoplasia. There are preliminary reports of polymicrogyria, growth failure of cortical neurons, and excessive cell death in the ventricular matrix zone.

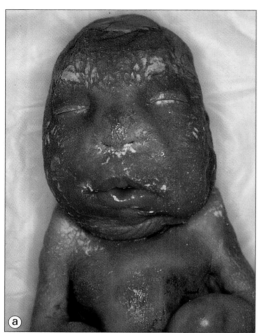

Fig. 3.59 Neu–Laxova syndrome in a 32-week gestation fetus. (a) Note the grotesque facies, microcephaly, prematurely closed fontanelles, hypertelorism, short neck, and protuberant orbits. **(b)** Coronal sections show simplified tiny hemispheres. **(c)** Microscopically, the cortex is thin, immature, and shows status verrucosus. (Courtesy of Dr Antoinette Gelot, Paris, France)

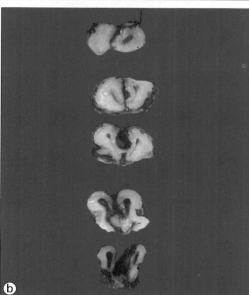

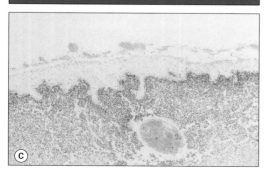

POLYMICROGYRIA

Polymicrogyria is characterized by a hyperconvoluted cortical ribbon of miniature, individually thin gyri, which are often fused together or piled on top of one another.

POLYMICROGYRIA

Polymicrogyria manifests with varying degrees of neurologic disability depending upon the extent of the lesion, and:
- causes profound psychomotor retardation if there are extensive bilateral lesions and microcephaly
- causes spastic diplegia if there is centro-Sylvian involvement resulting in hypoplastic pyramidal tracts
- can cause pseudobulbar palsy, mental retardation, a seizure disorder, or Foix–Chavany–Marie syndrome (facio-pharyngo-glossomasticatory diplegia with voluntary-automatic dissociation) if there is anterior opercular or peri-Sylvian involvement
- may be asymptomatic if it is a focal lesion, particularly if this involves the insula

ETIOLOGY OF POLYMICROGYRIA

Heterogeneous antecedents have been demonstrated.
- Polymicrogyria is acquired in the context of intrauterine ischemia (including encephaloclastic lesions), twinning, or intrauterine infection with cytomegalovirus, varicella–zoster virus, toxoplasmosis, or syphilis.
- Polymicrogyria occurs in rare inherited familial syndromes such as X-linked dominant Aicardi syndrome, and in a few autosomal recessive disorders.
- Polymicrogyria may be associated with metabolic diseases such as Pelizaeus–Merzbacher disease, glutaric acidemia type II, maple syrup urine disease, histidinemia, Leigh's syndrome, and mitochondrial respiratory chain deficiency.
- Polymicrogyria occurs in peroxisomal disorders such as neonatal adrenoleukodystrophy and Zellweger's syndrome.

MACROSCOPIC APPEARANCES

The macrogyric cerebral surface is irregular, and has been likened to cobblestones (**Fig. 3.60**). Sections of the cerebrum reveal heaped up or submerged gyri that widen the cortical ribbon (**Figs 3.61, 3.62**). Polymicrogyria (**Figs 3.63–3.68**) may be:
- widespread in one or both hemispheres
- bilateral and symmetric in a particular arterial territory (usually the middle cerebral artery)
- confined to the opercular region or depths of the insula
- around porencephalic or hydranencephalic defects
- focal in almost any neocortical area except the cingulate or striate cortex.

MICROSCOPIC APPEARANCES

The cortical gray matter is abnormally thin and excessively folded, and there is fusion of adjacent gyri and abnormal cortical lamination. The commonest subtype is unlayered polymicrogyria. A thin unlayered

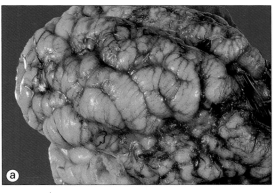
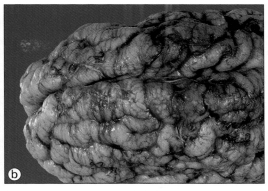

Fig. 3.60 Polymicrogyric cortex has varied external macroscopic appearances. Here are two views of the frontal lobes showing a cobblestone surface.

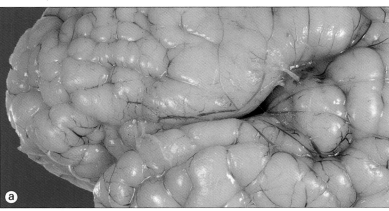
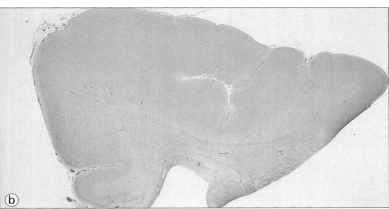

Fig. 3.61   Zellweger syndrome. This typically manifests with a combination of polymicrogyria and pachygyria. **(a)** The surface of the insula and neighboring frontal lobe is coarse and lacks convolutions, while more anteriorly the bumpy surface indicates polymicrogyria. **(b)** Low-power microscopy confirms pachygyria over the vertex and a narrower cortical ribbon with polymicrogyria laterally.

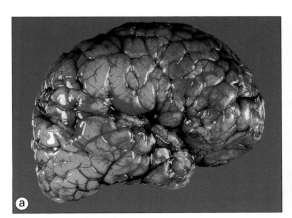
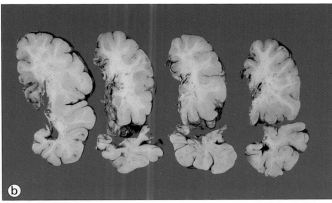

Fig. 3.62 Polymicrogyria in a surgically excised hemispherectomy specimen. **(a)** Lateral view showing broad macrogyric convolutions and a relatively smooth surface. **(b, c)** Coronal slices at frontal and parietal levels showing an irregularly thickened cortical ribbon and buried gray matter. **(d)** Luxol fast blue/cresyl violet-stained section from the left-hand slice in Fig. 3.62c showing that the apparently thick cortex is composed of thin ribbons of fused gray matter and indented by complex branching fingers of the paucicellular molecular layer.

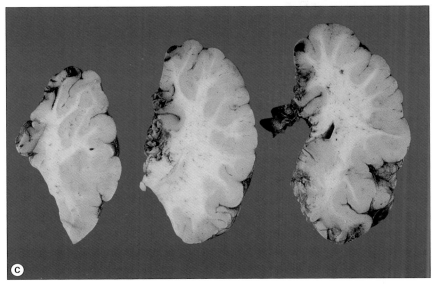
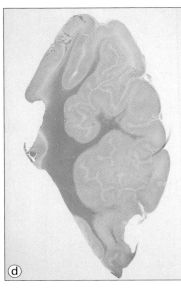

undulating band of gray matter is interrupted by branching 'fingers' of paucicellular tissue that has central blood vessels and radiates out from the overlying molecular layer. A complex pseudoglandular or map-like pattern of irregular neuronal clusters and cell-free zones is produced by the branching and fusing of the molecular layer.

A rarer subtype is four-layer polymicrogyria, which consists of a molecular layer and two layers of neurons sandwiching a paucicellular zone of myelinated fibers. The cortical ribbon is thin and undulating. Both types of polymicrogyria may coexist.

Associated features include glioneuronal leptomeningeal heterotopia and nodular heterotopia. Polymicrogyria is sometimes combined with pachygyria.

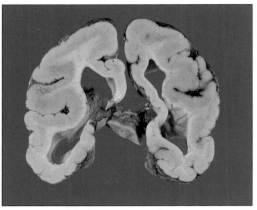

Fig. 3.63 Symmetric polymicrogyria. Polymicrogyria is often symmetric. Here it involves the parietal and insular cortex.

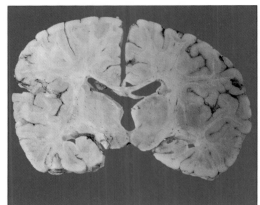

Fig. 3.64 Unifocal polymicrogyria. Polymicrogyria may be unilateral, and if focal can be clinically silent. This shows polymicrogyria limited to the right insula in an 18-month-old child who died following attempted surgical correction of Fallot's tetralogy.

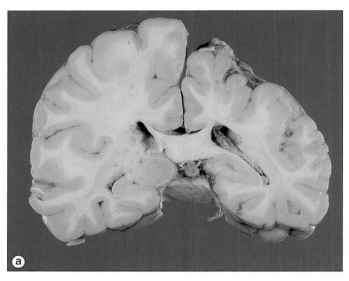

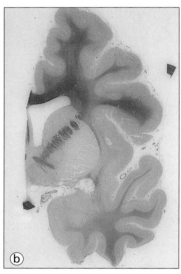

Fig. 3.65 Unilateral polymicrogyria in an asymmetrically small hemisphere. Compare this with Fig. 3.66. **(a)** Coronal section. Compare the smaller hemisphere and abnormal cortical ribbon with the normal left side. (Courtesy of Dr M. Carey, Birmingham) **(b)** Microscopic section showing the branched and fused cortical ribbon and fingers of molecular layer. (Luxol fast blue/cresyl violet)

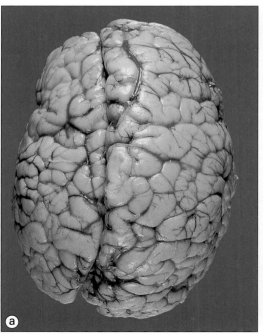

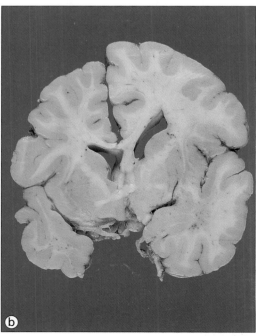

Fig. 3.66 Unilateral polymicrogyria associated with hemimegalencephaly. (a) Viewed from above the enlarged right hemisphere has broad coarse gyri. **(b)** A coronal section emphasizes the abnormality of frontal, insular, and temporal cortices.

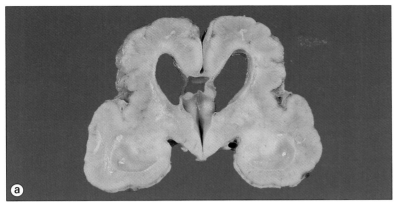

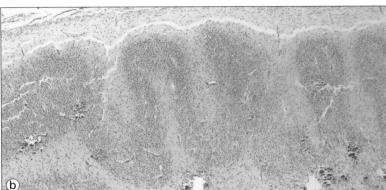

Fig. 3.67 Familial examples of polymicrogyria. These are rare. **(a)** Coronal slice showing microcephaly, macrogyria, white calcific concretions, and ventriculomegaly in one of two affected sisters. **(b)** Microscopy shows a four-layered looped polymicrogyric cortex containing numerous calcifications and covered by glioneuronal heterotopia.

PATHOGENESIS OF POLYMICROGYRIA

- The topography, bilateral symmetry, frequency of middle cerebral artery distribution, juxtaposition to porencephaly, and clinical data suggest a hypoxic–ischemic pathogenesis or transient intrauterine perfusion failure.
- Clinical reports of antecedent catastrophic intrauterine events have led to an estimation that polymicrogyria develops in the fourth to fifth gestational months.
- There are direct observations of the disorder in fetuses of 17–22 weeks' gestation, but ages of deceased co-twins suggest that the onset could be as early as the third to fourth month, implying interference with the later stages of neuronal migration.

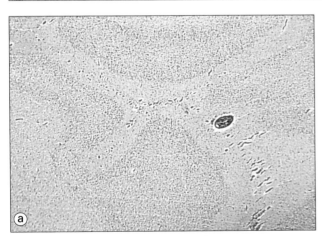

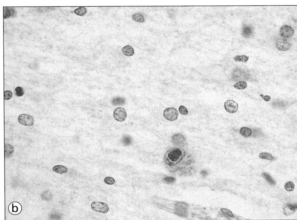

Fig. 3.68 Acquired polymicrogyria. (a) Unlayered polymicrogyria in a case of intra-uterine infection with cytomegalovirus (CMV). Note the centrally placed vessels in the branched cores of the 'fingers' of molecular layer. (Luxol fast blue/cresyl violet) **(b)** CMV immunoreactive inclusion in the white matter. **(c)** Extensive cystic necrosis of the cortex in a case of serologically proven mid-trimester varicella–zoster infection. **(d)** Section from (c) showing four-layer polymicrogyria in the insula. (Cresyl violet)

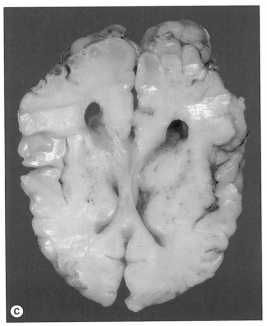

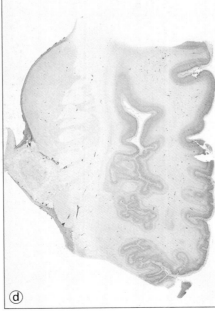

CHONDRODYSPLASIAS

Cortical malformations are prominent features in some chondro-dysplasias:

- In lethal thanatophoric dwarfism (**Fig. 3.69**), abnormally protuberant broad gyri in the temporal lobes show polymicrogyria, leptomeningeal glioneuronal heterotopia, and complete disorganization of Ammon's horns.
- In short-rib polydactyly syndrome (**Fig. 3.70**), there is an extremely bizarre convolutional pattern of deep clefts and disorganized cerebral mantle.

NEURONAL HETEROTOPIAS WITHIN CEREBRAL WHITE MATTER

Heterotopic neurons in the cerebral white matter may be diffusely scattered, clustered into nodules, or grouped in large masses.

NEURONAL HETEROTOPIA

- Neuronal heterotopia may be evident in peroxisomal, mitochondrial, and chromosomal disorders, in certain dysmorphic syndromes, and familial nephrotic syndrome.
- A sub-population of epileptic subjects with normal development and intelligence and an overwhelming female predominance has subependymal nodular heterotopias around the trigones and occipital horns on magnetic resonance imaging (MRI).
- Familial subependymal heterotopia is rare and found only in females, suggesting an X-linked dominant inheritance with prenatal lethality in hemizygous males.

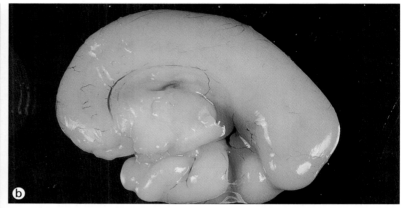

Fig. 3.69 Thanatophoric dwarfism in a 20-week-old fetus. (a) Lateral aspect of the right hemisphere showing an abnormally large and hyperconvoluted temporal lobe. **(b)** Medial aspect of the right hemisphere.

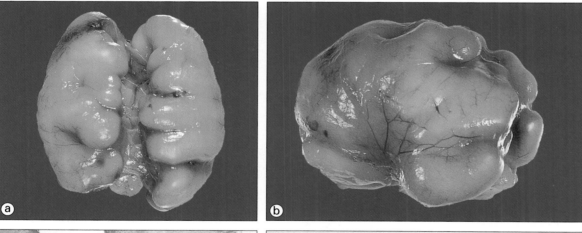

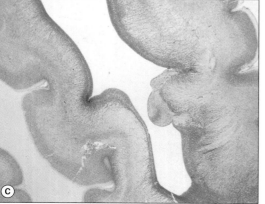

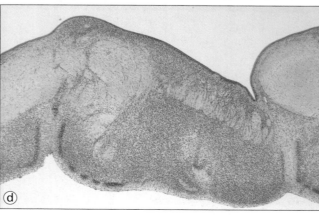

Fig. 3.70 Short-rib polydactyly in an 18-week-old fetus. (a) Superior view of the excessively heavy and precociously convoluted hemispheres. **(b)** Lateral view of the left cerebrum showing irregular deep clefts instead of the smooth outline expected at this age. **(c)** A cresyl violet-stained section of the hemisphere emphasizes the excessive and precocious gyral formation. **(d)** Close-up view of the bizarre cortical dysplasia.

ETIOLOGY OF NEURONAL HETEROTOPIA

- Neuronal heterotopia is reported to follow certain fetal insults such as sustained maternal hyperthermia, methylmercury poisoning, radiation from the atomic bomb, and experimental X-irradiation of rats.
- Heterotopias contain neurons of various types, consistent with differing generation times in the germinal zone and suggesting a fundamental fault in the migratory process or an early focal insult to the germinal zone.

DIFFUSE NEURONAL HETEROTOPIA

Diffuse neuronal heterotopia occurs in some epileptic patients (see microdysgenesis, p. 3.34) and is occasionally a principal finding in early myoclonic epilepsy. It is characterized by the presence of many haphazardly scattered neurons in gyral and central white matter and may be associated with other cerebral malformations (**Fig. 3.71**). Note that occasional neurons are a normal finding in the cerebral white matter, particularly in the anterior temporal region.

NODULAR HETEROTOPIA

Nodules of heterotopic neurons are most often situated in the wall of the lateral ventricle and bulge into its cavity, but are also found in gyral cores and the centrum semiovale. Heterotopias may be single or multiple, varying from small discrete neuronal clusters to large conglomerates, or may occur as irregular serpiginous bands (**Figs 3.72, 3.73**). Nodular heterotopias may be incidental findings, but in necropsy series are often associated with microcephaly or extensive CNS malformations, including megalencephaly.

Histologically, heterotopias vary from simple collections of neurons of random size and orientation to an arrangement resembling cortical lamination.

LAMINAR HETEROTOPIA
MACROSCOPIC APPEARANCES

The brain surface has a normal convolutional pattern, but in coronal slices there are bilateral, symmetric foci of heterotopic gray matter, arranged in extensive bands, wedges, or clustered nodules. These may be situated in most cortical regions except the striate or cingulate cortices, and the fusiform or medial temporal gyri (**Fig. 3.74**).

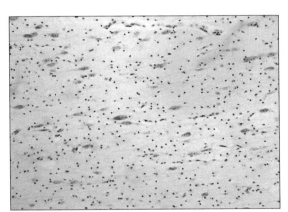

Fig. 3.71 Diffuse gray matter heterotopia. There are shoals of rather fusiform neurons in the white matter of a 4-month-old girl who presented with megalencephaly (brain weight 900 g) and intractable seizures.

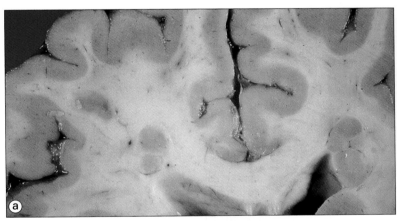

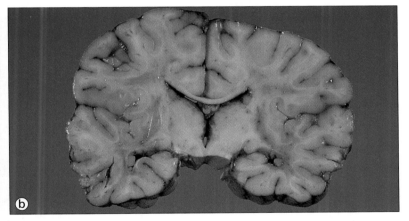

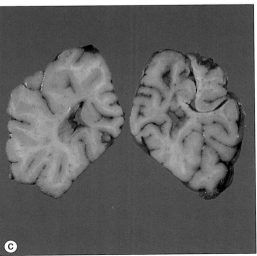

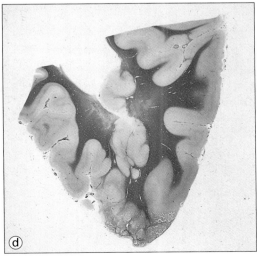

Fig. 3.72 Subependymal nodular gray heterotopia. (a) In a female with longstanding epilepsy, heterotopic gray matter protrudes into the frontal horns. (Courtesy of Professor F. Scaravilli, Institute of Neurology, London) **(b)** Subependymal nodular heterotopia in the temporal horns was an incidental finding in a 5-year-old boy who died of pneumococcal meningitis. **(c)** Occipital lobes in the same case as Fig. 3.72b. Heterotopic gray matter surrounds the occipital horns. **(d)** Histology of the case shown in Fig. 3.89. The inferior part of the temporal lobe shows nodular intracerebral and subependymal heterotopias between the polymicrogyric cortex and ventricle. (Luxol fast blue/cresyl violet)

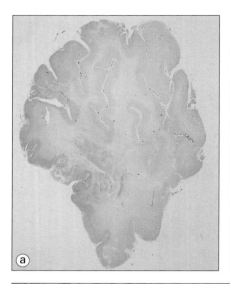

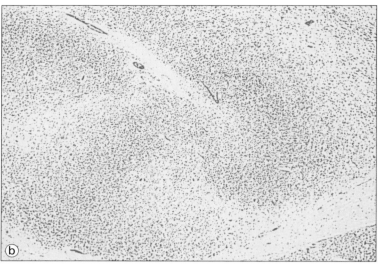

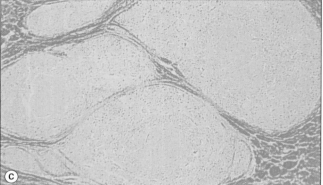

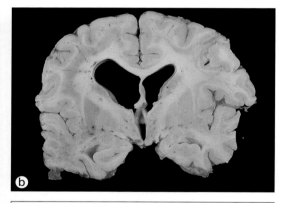

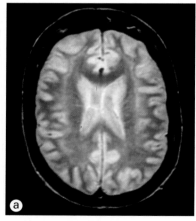

Fig. 3.73 Heterotopias showing elementary organization. (a) Coronal section through the fused frontal lobes of a case of occipital encephalocele and arhinencephaly showing a serpiginous band of heterotopic gray matter. (Luxol fast blue/cresyl violet) **(b)** Close-up view of the folded plate of heterotopic gray matter. **(c)** In these heterotopias a concentric arrangement of neurons around a central cell-poor zone suggests primitive cortical organization. (Luxol fast blue/cresyl violet) **(d)** High-power view of a heterotopic nodule which shows a degree of laminar organization.

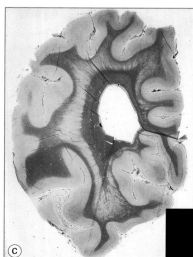

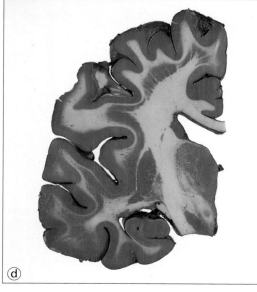

Fig. 3.74 Laminar heterotopia. (a) MRI scan showing extensive gray matter type signal beneath and parallel to the true cortex. (Courtesy of Dr Wendy Taylor, National Hospital for Neurology and Neurosurgery, London) **(b)** In this 37-year-old woman with a 27-year history of epilepsy there are extensive, approximately symmetric, bilateral bands of heterotopic gray matter in subcortical frontal and temporal white matter, clearly separated from the macroscopically normal cortical ribbon by a thin but definite band of white matter. The medial temporal cortex is spared. **(c)** Luxol fast blue/cresyl violet-stained section of the occipital lobe in this case. The heterotopia forms a thick plate laterally and tends to separate into bands or columns in its deeper part. It is a more tenuous structure medially and is absent from the calcarine fissure. (Courtesy of Professor F. Scaravilli, Institute of Neurology, London) **(d)** Laminar heterotopia in another female epileptic. The heterotopic band in the frontal and temporal lobes incorporates the claustrum. (Courtesy of Dr Peter Barber, Birmingham University, UK) (Mulligan's prussian blue)

LAMINAR HETEROTOPIA

- is a very rare non-lethal condition
- usually occurs in females
- can cause mild epilepsy
- is associated with minimal intellectual deterioration
- is associated with family histories of epilepsy

Two families have been described in which mothers and daughters have laminar heterotopia while sons have pachygyria or lissencephaly. These findings suggest differing degrees of the same disorder of neuronal migration and an X-linked dominant inheritance.

Laminar heterotopias are situated just beneath and parallel to the cortex, but separated from it by a narrow layer of white matter. The deep gray nuclei are normal except for the incorporation of the claustrum into the heterotopia.

MICROSCOPIC APPEARANCES

In its outermost part, the heterotopic gray matter shows a haphazard arrangement of neurons and neuropil (**Fig. 3.75**). The intermediate part contains wide columns of cells separated by myelin fiber bundles. The innermost part fragments into islands surrounded by white matter. The cortex overlying the heterotopia has been reported as normal or pachygyric.

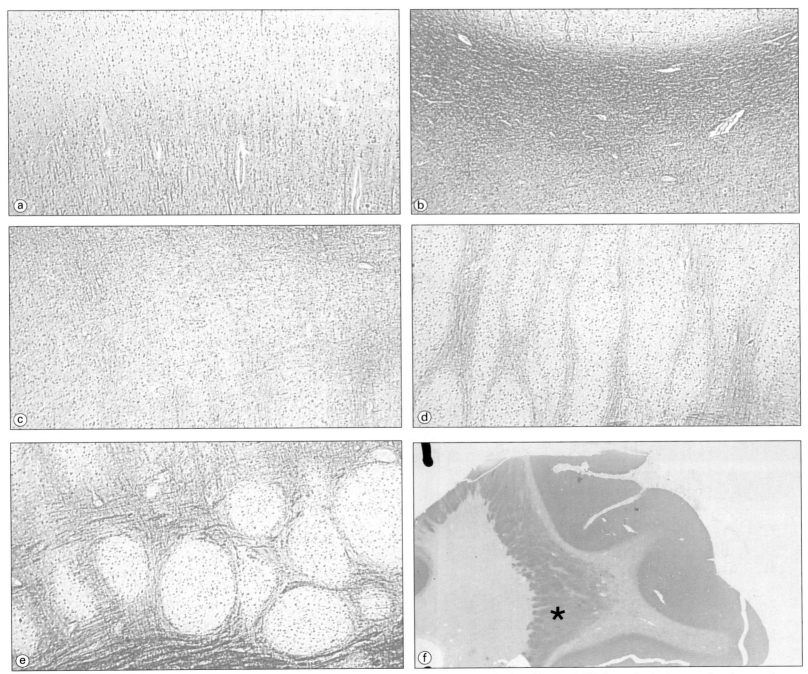

Fig. 3.75 Laminar heterotopia. (a) The cortex overlying the laminar heterotopia in the patient depicted in Fig. 3.73b is qualitatively normal and correctly laminated. (Luxol fast blue/cresyl violet) **(b)** Subcortical white matter clearly separates the cortex from the underlying heterotopia. (Luxol fast blue/cresyl violet) **(c)** The superficial part of the heterotopia is a haphazardly arranged mass of neurons and neuropil. (Luxol fast blue/Nissl method) **(d)** More deeply, the heterotopia begins to break up into columns. (Luxol fast blue/cresyl violet) **(e)** In its deepest part the heterotopia fragments into nodules. (Luxol fast blue/cresyl violet) **(f)** Immunocytochemistry demonstrates similar staining for synaptophysin in both cortex and heterotopia (asterisk).

MICRODYSGENESIS

Some subtle structural abnormalities of cortical architecture have been described in epileptic subjects, notably those with primary generalized epilepsy and Lennox–Gastaut syndrome. These abnormalities consist principally of molecular layer and white matter heterotopias, undulations in layer II, and disorganization of deeper cortical layers.

CORTICAL DYSPLASIA WITH CYTOMEGALY

A characteristic combination of disturbed neuronal migration and abnormal neuronoglial differentiation occurs in the following three distinctive clinicopathologic settings:

- unilateral cortical dysplasia with hemimegalencephaly
- localized cortical dysplasia
- tuberous sclerosis.

CORTICAL DYSPLASIA WITH HEMIMEGALENCEPHALY
MACROSCOPIC APPEARANCES

Total brain weight varies from well below to well above normal. One hemisphere is larger, but this is not always the pathologic one. All or part of the hemisphere shows greatly expanded firm convolutions with a finely pitted surface (**Fig. 3.76**). The cortical ribbon is irregularly thickened and poorly demarcated from underlying white matter. There is usually unilateral enlargement of the centrum semiovale, and occasionally enlargement of one olfactory tract or the basal ganglia.

DIFFERENTIAL DIAGNOSIS OF AN ASYMMETRICALLY ENLARGED HEMISPHERE (HEMIMEGALENCEPHALY)

- pachygyria
- polymicrogyria
- cortical dysplasia with cytomegaly
- tuberous sclerosis

Rarely, hemimegalencephaly is due to an excess of neurons without malformation.

CORTICAL DYSPLASIA WITH HEMIMEGALENCEPHALY

- occurs sporadically if there is no associated hemihypertrophy or viscerocutaneous stigmata of phakomatosis
- causes intractable seizures beginning in infancy
- is associated with a bleak long-term outlook without surgery (i.e. hemispherectomy)

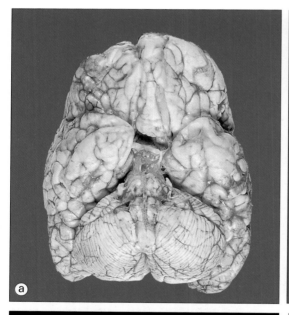

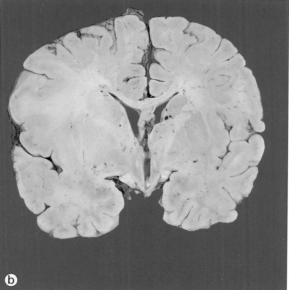

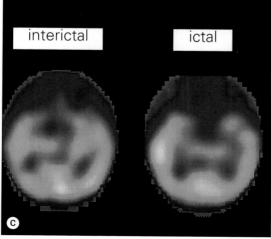

interictal   ictal

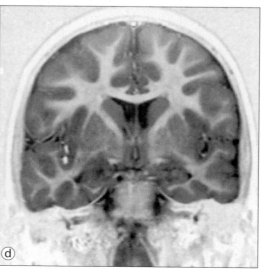

Fig. 3.76 Cortical dysplasia. (a) Cortical dysplasia with hemimegalencephaly. Inferior view shows the asymmetrically enlarged left frontal lobe, olfactory bulb, and tract. **(b)** Cortical dysplasia with hemimegalencephaly. Coronal slice showing widened gyri and loss of gray–white demarcation in the left hemisphere as well as an enlarged corpus striatum with blurred internal markings. **(c)** Localized cortical dysplasia. Functional imaging using single photon emission computerized tomography (SPECT) demonstrates ictal hyperperfusion in the right temporal lobe. **(d)** Localized cortical dysplasia. Same as Fig. 3.75c. Despite the abnormal SPECT, the MRI appearance is normal. (Courtesy of Dr Helen Cross, Great Ormond Street Hospital for Children, London)

MICROSCOPIC APPEARANCES

Architectural anomalies include:

- an abrupt transition from a normal to an abnormal widened cortex with loss of normal lamination (**Fig. 3.77**).
- in some cases, superficial undulations, lissencephaly, or four-layered cortex.
- usually, poor demarcation of the cortex from the white matter.

Cytologic changes include:

- neuronal cytomegaly (**Fig. 3.78**), notably in cortical regions, but also of heterotopic neurons in white matter, and occasionally in the hippo-campus and basal ganglia. Some cells are larger than Betz cells, mis-aligned, and pleomorphic.
- multilobed, vacuolated, or multiple nuclei outlined by a crescentic condensation of Nissl bodies.
- central cytoplasmic clearing of Nissl bodies, abnormal dendritic arborization (as demonstrated by Golgi impregnation), and cyto-skeletal abnormalities (i.e. tangle formation immunopositive for various neurofilament epitopes, tau protein, and ubiquitin).
- astrocytic dysplasia (**Fig. 3.79**), which varies from minimal to massive, evoking the appearance of a neoplasm, and is present in cerebral gray and white matter. Dysplastic cells have swollen glassy cytoplasm and round eccentric nucleolated nuclei. Associated findings are intense astrocytosis and calcification. Rarely Rosenthal fibers and cystic rarefaction in the white matter produce an appearance that may mimic Alexander's disease.

- large globular or 'balloon' cells of indeterminate phenotype, which may show immunohistochemical co-localization of glial fibrillary acidic protein (GFAP) and either vimentin or synaptophysin.

PATHOGENESIS OF HEMIMEGALENCEPHALY

- Dysplastic neurons appear to be deafferented and polyploid.
- Features include faulty migration (extensive neuronal ectopia) and differentiation (neuronal cytoskeletal anomalies and cells of indeterminate phenotype).
- Many of the cytologic findings are similar to those of tuberous sclerosis, and a few cases have been reported to show focal tuberous sclerosis-type genetic abnormalities (see page 3.55).

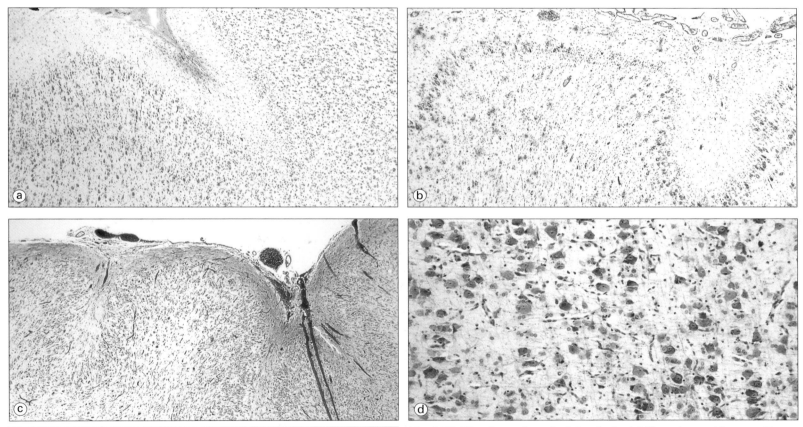

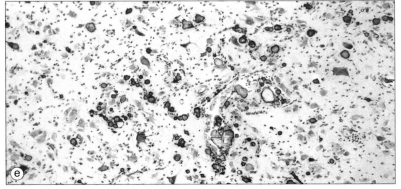

Fig. 3.77 Histology of cortical dysplasia. (a) There is a sudden transition between normally laminated cortex on the right to disordered cortex with very large neurons in a region of localized cortical dysplasia. **(b)** In some examples, as here, superficial undulation of cortical layers is associated with small indenting fingers of molecular layer. This is from a case of hemimegalencephaly. **(c)** Looped abnormal cortex and excessive superficial myelination in another example of cortical dysplasia with hemimegalencephaly. **(d)** Columns of very large neurons in a case of localized cortical dysplasia. **(e)** Completely disorganized cortex, multiple calcifications, prominent astrocytes, and abnormal neurons in a case of cortical dysplasia with hemimegalencephaly. (Luxol fast blue/cresyl violet)

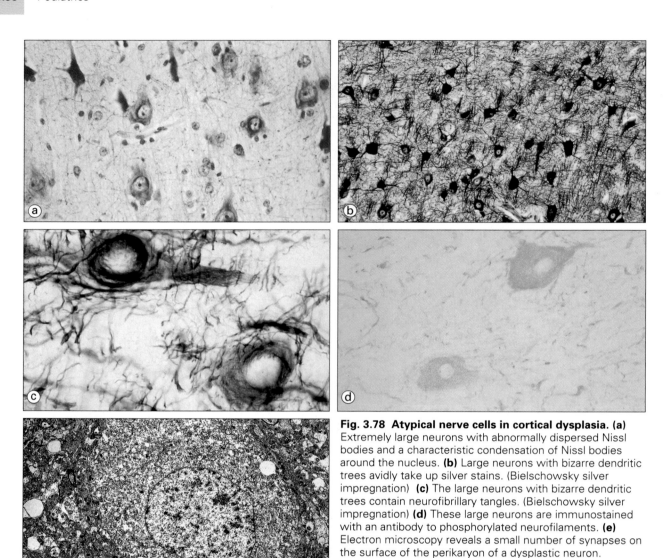

Fig. 3.78 Atypical nerve cells in cortical dysplasia. (a) Extremely large neurons with abnormally dispersed Nissl bodies and a characteristic condensation of Nissl bodies around the nucleus. **(b)** Large neurons with bizarre dendritic trees avidly take up silver stains. (Bielschowsky silver impregnation) **(c)** The large neurons with bizarre dendritic trees contain neurofibrillary tangles. (Bielschowsky silver impregnation) **(d)** These large neurons are immunostained with an antibody to phosphorylated neurofilaments. **(e)** Electron microscopy reveals a small number of synapses on the surface of the perikaryon of a dysplastic neuron.

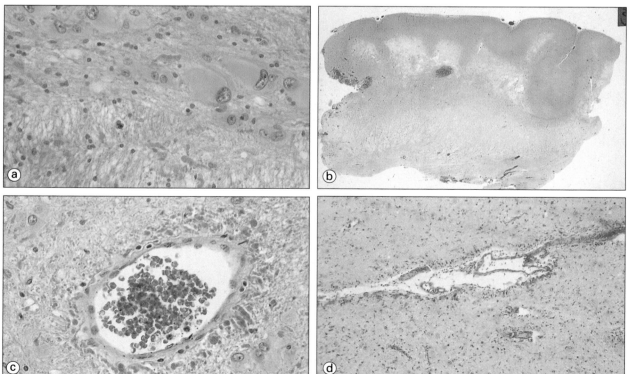

Fig. 3.79 Cytologic changes of cortical dysplasia.
(a) Atypical astrocytes with bloated glassy cytoplasm, and scattered eosinophilic Rosenthal fibers. **(b)** Section from a surgical hemispherectomy showing almost complete destruction of the white matter. (Luxol fast blue/cresyl violet)
(c) Perivascular clustering of Rosenthal fibers may be so profuse that the appearance mimics that of Alexander's disease. **(d)** Subpial rows of Rosenthal fibers simulate Alexander's disease.

LOCALIZED CORTICAL DYSPLASIA

This is usually encountered in circumcribed surgical resections carried out for focal epilepsy and commonly affects only a small part of one gyrus, which may be enlarged.

The principal cytologic changes are neuronal cytomegaly and dysplasia with a variable presence of astrocytic dysplasia and balloon cells. A tangential myelin fiber plexus covering the cortex, loss of lamination, and blurring of the gray-white junction may be evident.

Quantitative functional neuroimaging studies have shown that the dysplastic abnormalities are usually much more extensive than is evident by conventional imaging.

LEPTOMENINGEAL GLIONEURONAL HETEROTOPIA

This is characterized by islands of neuropil, neurons, and glia ectopically situated within the leptomeninges or focal protrusions from the cortical surface into the meninges (**Fig. 3.80**). It is common in malformed brains, especially those with holoprosencephaly and migration defects, and is particularly extensive in cerebro-ocular dysplasias and atelencephaly. Disruption of the pial–glial barrier is the most likely mechanism.

NODULAR CORTICAL DYSPLASIA

Nodular cortical dysplasia (**Fig. 3.81**) is the presence of superficial cortical nodules (brain warts) in otherwise normal cortex or occasionally in microcephalic brains with polymicrogyria. Nodules of 1–5 mm in diameter are scattered over the cortical surface, most often the frontal lobe or near the operculum, on the crown of a gyrus, or in the bank of a sulcus. Histologically, cortical layers II and III protrude through a thin or absent molecular layer. Neurons of various sizes are grouped around a radial bundle of myelinated fibers and a central blood vessel.

STATUS VERRUCOSUS SIMPLEX OR STATUS PSEUDOVERRUCOSUS

This is a microscopic finding in the brains of fetuses from 10–28 weeks' gestation (**Fig. 3.82**). The second cortical layer makes irregular protrusions into the molecular layer, while the external surface is smooth. Although considered by some to be a transient stage of normal development, its presence in some macerated brains and occasional association with polymicrogyria suggest that it may be a true malformation.

HIPPOCAMPAL ANOMALIES

A variety of hippocampal malformations is described including:
- hypoplasia with a dysplastic dentate gyrus (associated with trisomy 18)
- disorganization of the medial temporal lobe with hypoplasia or aplasia of the dentate fascia (thanatophoric dysplasia)
- dispersion or a bilaminar arrangement of the granular layer of the dentate gyrus (seen in patients with temporal lobe epilepsy following febrile convulsions early in life).

Duplication or dispersion of the dentate gyrus can also occur in cases of dysembryoplastic neuroepithelial tumor in the temporal lobe, microdysgenesis, and Sturge–Weber syndrome. In a personal case bilateral duplication of the dentate gyrus was associated with other migration defects and seizures from 6 months of age (**Fig. 3.83**).

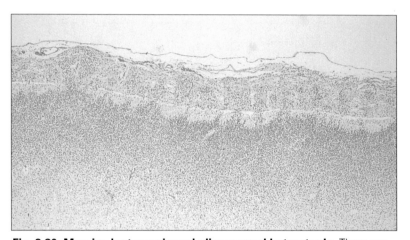

Fig. 3.80 Massive leptomeningeal glioneuronal heterotopia. There are multiple breaches in the pial–glial barrier. 16-week-old fetus: therapeutic termination for hydrocephalus.

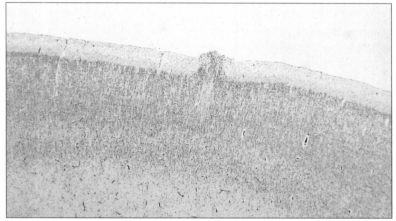

Fig. 3.81 Nodular cortical dysplasia. There is a superficial nodular herniation of layers II and III through the molecular layer. (Luxol fast blue/cresyl violet)

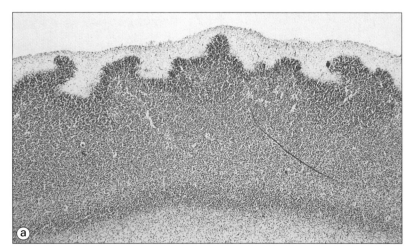

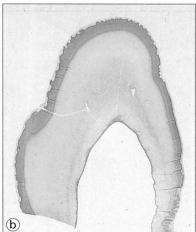

Fig. 3.82 Status verrucosus in a 24-week-old fetus. (a) Layer II protrudes irregularly into the molecular layer, the surface of which remains relatively smooth. **(b)** Status verrucosus extends over the vertex, but polymicrogyria is seen on the medial wall of the hemisphere. (Luxol fast blue/cresyl violet)

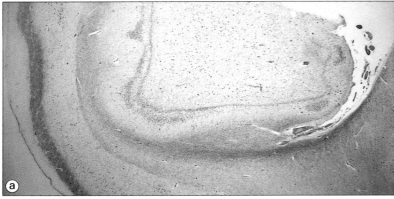

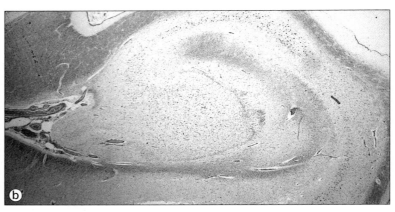

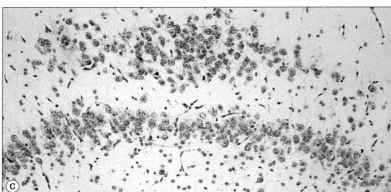

Fig. 3.83 Bilaminar dentate fascia. Bitemporal duplication of the dentate fascia in a 2-year-old boy with a history of developmental delay and seizures from 6 months. Other findings included bilateral hippocampal sclerosis, nodular heterotopias in the temporal and insular white matter, cerebellar heterotopia, brain stem tract anomalies, and unilateral olfactory hypoplasia. **(a)** Left hippocampus. **(b)** Right hippocampus. **(c)** Bilaminar dentate fascia in a surgical specimen from a patient with Sturge–Weber syndrome.

MICROCEPHALY

Microcephaly is a purely descriptive term for a small head, but is also in general use for a small brain, for which the term microencephaly is more appropriate. Brain weights two standard deviations below the mean are considered abnormal. By this definition microcephaly is common, but not invariable in malformed brains. Microcephaly plus associated malformations (**Fig. 3.84**) may be:
• associated with chromosomal or single gene defects

• due to environmental causes
• of unknown etiology (including rare familial examples).
Microcephaly without associated malformations (**Fig. 3.85**) may be:
• primary, in association with proven or possible genetic transmission
• secondary to inborn errors of metabolism
• due to environmental causes, notably intrauterine infection
• of unknown etiology.

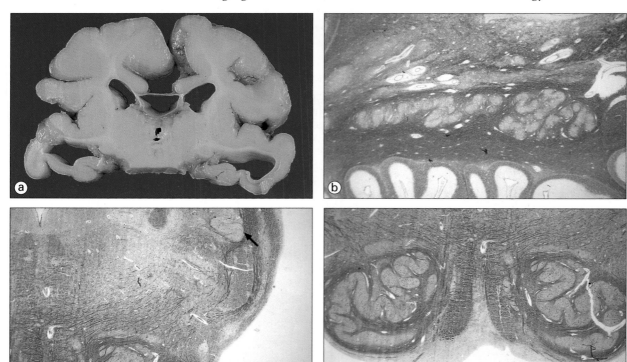

Fig. 3.84 Microcephaly with malformations in a 5-month-old infant with cerebral lactic acidosis due to pyruvate dehydrogenase deficiency. (a) The brain shows microcephaly (brain weight 260 g), a simplified convolutional pattern, and ventriculomegaly. **(b)** There is also dysplasia of the cerebellar dentate nucleus. **(c)** Heterotopic olivary tissue is present within the inferior cerebellar peduncle (arrow). The heterotopic tissue is folded like the normal inferior olivary nucleus. **(d)** Medullary pyramids are absent.

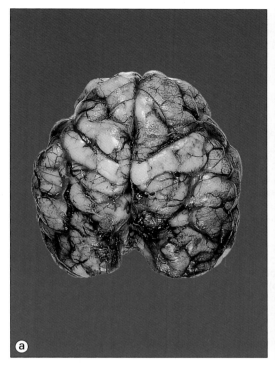

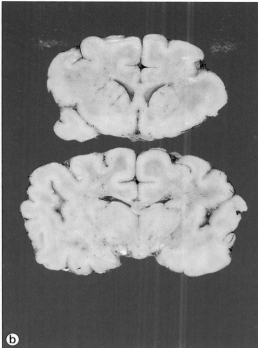

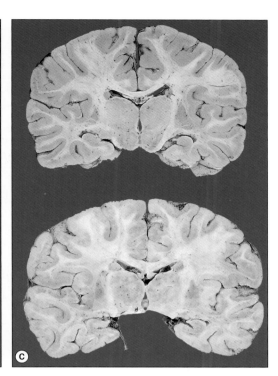

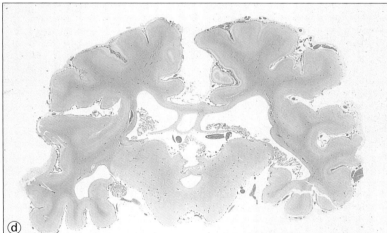

CHROMOSOMAL AND SINGLE GENE DEFECTS

The full range of chromosomal and single gene defects that are associated with CNS malformations is listed in **Figs 3.86, 3.87**.

Trisomy 21 (Down's syndrome)

Brain weights are usually about 1000 g. The cerebrum is brachycephalic and abnormally round and short with an almost vertical occipital contour. Other features include some reduction in secondary sulci, exposure of the insula, and a narrow superior temporal gyrus. The cerebellum and brain stem are small.

ETIOLOGY OF DOWN'S SYNDROME

- Down's syndrome is caused by trisomy of chromosome 21:
  - 95% of cases have three free copies of chromosome 21
  - in 5% of cases, one copy of chromosome 21 is translocated to another acrocentric chromosome (usually chromosome 14 or chromosome 21)
  - some patients have trisomy of only part of chromosome 21 (the 21q22.3 region seems to be particularly important in the genesis of the dysmorphic features)
  - occasionally, patients are mosaics of normal and trisomic cells
- The overall population frequency is 1/650–1000 live births.
- The incidence of trisomy 21 increases with advancing maternal age.
- Familial cases are usually due to translocations.
- Increased levels of the free radical scavenging enzyme Cu/Zn superoxide dismutase are evident in cell lines from both trisomy 21 patients and patients with Alzheimer's disease.
- Down's syndrome cells also show a reduced ability to repair the effects of X-ray damage. Defective DNA repair may contribute to the increased risk of acute leukemias in Down's syndrome.

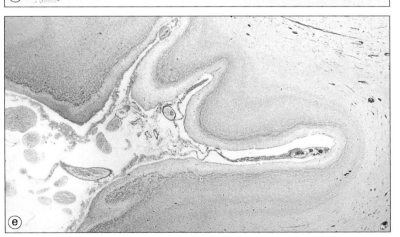

Fig. 3.85 Microcephaly without malformations. (a) 190 g brain from a term infant with a simplified gyral pattern. **(b)** Coronal slices from this case compared with an age-matched control below. **(c)** Coronal sections from a microcephalic infant (brain weight 700 g at 15 months of age) whose mother suffered from phenylketonuria, compared with an age-matched control below. **(d)** Coronal stained section of a tiny 95 g brain with a relatively preserved gyral pattern from a case of familial microcephaly (three sisters died shortly after delivery close to term). (Courtesy of Dr Kari Skulerrud, Oslo) **(e)** Microscopically, the narrowed cortical ribbon has a striking rippled appearance.

Single gene disorders and other syndromes involving CNS malformations

Disorder	CNS malformations	Gene name	Function of gene product	Chromosome location	McKusick number[1]
Aicardi syndrome	Callosal agenesis, polymicrogyria, cerebral heterotopias	ND[2]	ND[2]	Xp22	304050
Angelman syndrome	Microcephaly	ND	ND	15q11	105830
Aniridia/Wilms' association	Cerebral heterotopias in homozygote	PAX6	Nuclear transcription factor	11p13	106210
Apert syndrome	Cerebellar anomalies, agenesis of corpus callosum, limbic defects	Fibroblast growth factor receptor- 2	Cell surface growth factor receptor	10q25-26	101200
Holoprosencephaly 1	Alobar holoprosencephaly	ND	ND	18pter-q11	236100
Holoprosencephaly 2	Alobar or semilobar holoprosencephaly	ND	ND	2p21	157170
Holoprosencephaly 3	Holoprosencephaly	ND	ND	7q36	142945
Kallman syndrome	Agenesis of olfactory lobes	KAL	Secreted protein with similarity to cell adhesion molecules	Xp22.3	308700
Meckel–Gruber syndrome	Occipital encephalocoele, microcephaly, cerebral and cerebellar hypoplasia	ND	ND	ND	249000
Miller–Dieker syndrome	Lissencephaly, cerebral heterotopias, olivary heterotopia	LIS1; Brain platelet-activating factor present in deleted region	Not known	17p13.3	247200
Neu–Laxova syndrome	Microcephaly, lissencephaly, agenesis of corpus callosum, cerebral, cerebellar and pontine atrophy, absence of olfactory bulbs	ND	ND	ND	256520
Pallister–Hall syndrome	Hypothalamic hamartoblastoma	ND	ND	ND	146510
Pettigrew syndrome	Dandy-Walker malformation, basal ganglia anomalies	ND	ND	Xq25-27	304340
Prader–Willi syndrome	Microcephaly	ND	ND	15q11	176270
Sacral agenesis (Currarino triad)	Meningocele	ND	ND	7q36	
Tuberous sclerosis	Hamartomas of CNS and other tissues	TSC1	ND	9q34	191100
		TSC2, Tuberin	Similarity to GTPase binding protein	16p13.3	191092
Waardenburg syndrome type I	Myelomeningocele in homozygous individuals	PAX3	Nuclear transcription factor	2q35	193500
Walker–Warburg syndrome (cerebro-ocular dysplasia; HARD)	Agyria/pachygyria, lissencephaly II, cerebellar vermal hypoplasia cortical dysplasia, occipital encephalocoele, hydrocephaly	ND	ND	ND	236670
X-linked hydrocephalus	Aqueduct stenosis, agenesis of corpus callosum and septum pellucidum, fusion of thalami, absence of pyramids	L1	Cell adhesion molecule, expressed especially on migrating neurons	Xq28	308840
Zellweger syndrome	Pachygyria, polymicrogyria, heterotopia, olivary dysplasia	ND	ND	7q11	214100
		Peroxisomal membrane protein-1	Peroxisome function	1p22-21	170995
		Peroxisomal assembly factor-1	Peroxisome function	8q21.1	170993

1 Catalogue number in McKusick VA. Mendelian Inheritance in Man. A Catalogue of Human Genes and Genetic Disorders. 11th ed. Baltimore: The Johns Hopkins University Press; 1994.

2 Not determined

Fig. 3.86 Single gene disorders and other syndromes involving CNS malformations.

Microscopic anomalies are largely nonspecific. Neuronal density may be increased at birth, but declines markedly from birth onward. Abnormalities in dendritic arborization and decreased numbers of dendritic spines have been detected with Golgi's method in neonates. Delayed myelination is also prominent in infants with congenital heart disease.

Middle-aged patients often develop clinical signs of dementia: their brains show changes of Alzheimer's disease (see chapter 31).

Fragile X syndrome

This is the second most frequent genetic disorder (after Down's syndrome) associated with developmental disability. It has an incidence of 1/1000 liveborn males and is the commonest familial form of mental retardation. The fragile X site at position Xq27 is induced in cells cultured at low folic acid and thymidine concentrations. The defect results from expansion of either of two (FRAXA and FRAXE) specific DNA triplet repeat regions in the FMR1 (Fragile X mental retardation 1) gene. The size of the expansion correlates with the degree of mental retardation.

Trisomy 21 increases the risk of acute lymphoblastic and myeloblastic leukemias by 20-fold and that of acute megakaryocytic leukemia by over 200-fold.

Dysmorphologic features include macro-orchidism, a long face with prominent forehead, and large ears. Neuropathologic findings include microcephaly, neuronal heterotopias, and dendritic spine abnormalities.

ENVIRONMENTAL FACTORS

A list of teratogens that can cause CNS malformations is included in **Fig. 3.88**.

Intrauterine growth retardation

Intrauterine growth retardation may be associated with various malformations, infections, multiple pregnancy, or placental insufficiency from maternal toxemia or renal disease. The small infant has a large brain relative to body weight. The brain is within normal limits for gestational age, and is only very rarely microcephalic.

Phenylketonuria

Children born to a phenylketonuric mother exhibit microcephaly, mental retardation, and low birth weight, which can be prevented if mothers are on a strict diet at the time of conception. Histology of the microcephalic brain is usually nonspecific.

Fetal alcohol syndrome

Microcephaly and many other anomalies have been reported in fetal alcohol syndrome including leptomeningeal glioneuronal heterotopias, agenesis of the corpus callosum, lissencephaly, and other migration disorders.

Chromosomal disorders involving CNS malformations *

Chromosome	Gain	Loss
4	4p+ Microcephaly, agenesis of corpus callosum	4p-(Wolf–Hirschhorn syndrome) Microcephaly
5		5p- (Cri du chat syndrome) Microcephaly
8	8+ Microcephaly, agenesis of corpus callosum	
9	9p+ Macrocephaly, hydrocephaly 9+ Microcephaly, meningocoele	Ms9p Microcephaly
13	13+ (Patau syndrome) Holoprosencephaly, arhinencephaly, agenesis of corpus callosum, hydrocephaly, fusion of basal ganglia, cerebellar heterotopia, cyclopia, myelomeningocoele	13q- Microcephaly, holoprosencephaly
18	18+ (Edwards' syndrome) Microcephaly, gyral anomalies, dysplasias of hippocampus, lateral geniculate nucleus and olive, cerebellar heterotopia	18p- Microcephaly, holoprosencephaly, arhinencephaly 18q- Microcephaly
20	20p+ Hydrocephaly	
21	21+ (Down's syndrome) Microcephaly	
X	XXXY, XXXXY, XXXX, XXXXX, Microcephaly Fragile X	XO (Turner syndrome) Defects of cerebellum, basal ganglia
Triploidy (often mosaic)	Holoprosencephaly, hydrocephaly, Arnold–Chiari malformation, microcephaly, myelomeningocoele	

* Malformations in bold type are present in the majority of cases. Those in normal type are present in a minority of cases.

Fig. 3.87 Chromosomal disorders involving CNS malformations.

Teratogens known or suspected in the production of CNS malformations

Teratogenic agent	Malformations
Alcohol	• Microcephaly, occasional meningomyelocoele and hydrocephaly
Carbamazepine	• Myelomeningocoele
Cytomegalovirus	• Hydrocephalus, microcephaly, polymicrogyria, occasional cerebellar cortical dysplasia
Diabetes mellitus (maternal)	• Neural tube defects, increased incidence
Herpes simplex	• Microcephaly, hydranencephaly
Hyperthermia	• Neuronal heterotopias, microcephaly, ?neural tube defects
Methyl mercury	• Microcephaly, heterotopia
Phenylketonuria (maternal)	• Microcephaly
Phenytoin	• Microcephaly, holoprosencephaly
Retinoids	• Hydrocephaly, microcephaly, neuronal migration defects, cerebellar agenesis/hypoplasia
Rubella	• Microcephaly, occasional hydrocephalus and agenesis of the corpus callosum
Toxoplasmosis	• Necrotising meningoencephalitis, hydrocephalus and calcification, occasional polymicrogyria and hydranencephaly
Valproic acid	• Myelomeningocele
Varicella–zoster	• Necrotizing encephalitis with polymicrogyria
Warfarin	• Microcephaly, hydrocephalus, Dandy–Walker cyst, agenesis of corpus callosum
X-irradiation	• Microcephaly, pachygyria, cerebellar cortical dysplasia, heterotopia

Fig. 3.88 Teratogens known or suspected in the production of CNS malformations.

Irradiation

Pelvic X-ray therapy in the first trimester has been associated with microcephaly and anomalies of the eye, and there have also been reports of cerebellar cortical dysplasia and pachygyria. There was a relatively high incidence of microcephaly and mental retardation among children exposed *in utero* to the atomic explosions at Hiroshima and Nagasaki, but no specific malformations, except for one report of periventricular heterotopia.

Maternal infection (see also Chapter 12)

Rubella: CNS malformations are relatively common (affecting 10–20% of cases) following rubella infection during the first trimester and include chronic meningoencephalitis, microcephaly, and retarded myelination and cytoarchitectonic development. Better known associated malformations are ocular defects (cataract, pigmentary retinopathy, microphthalmos) and sensorineural deafness.

Cytomegalovirus: More than 5% of neonates infected with cytomegalovirus have a rapidly fatal systemic disorder, with brain involvement reported in 10–80% of cases. Clinical features are microcephaly, mental retardation, epilepsy, diplegia, chorioretinitis, and intracerebral calcification. Neuropathologic findings include:
- microcephaly
- hydrocephalus
- necrotizing lesions in ependyma and periventricular tissue.

Other findings that are sometimes seen are porencephaly or hydra-nencephaly, polymicrogyria and cerebellar cortical dysplasia, and perivascular calcifications (see Fig. 3.67a).

Typical viral inclusions are often sparse (see **Fig.** 3.67b); the virus is more readily identified by immunocytochemistry or *in situ* hybridization.

Other viruses: Herpes simplex infection can cause chorioretinitis, microcephaly, hydranencephaly, and microphthalmia.

Varicella–zoster infection in the first or second trimester rarely causes a characteristic embryopathy involving the skin, muscle, eye, and brain. Some necropsy studies report necrotizing encephalitis, and polymicrogyria (see Fig. 3.67c,d).

Other organisms: Intrauterine toxoplasmosis produces necrotizing meningoencephalitis, hydrocephalus, and widespread calcification, sometimes with polymicrogyria and hydranencephaly (see also chapter 18).

MEGALENCEPHALY

Megalencephaly is defined as a brain weight at least 2.5 standard deviations above the mean for age and sex (**Fig. 3.89**). Primary megalencephaly may be:
- an isolated finding
- associated with achondroplasia and endocrine disorders
- familial.

There is a male:female ratio of 2:1, and most patients are mentally retarded and have some sort of neurologic disorder. One-third has cytoarchitectonic or neuronal abnormalities and one-third has macroscopic malformations (**Fig. 3.90**). Megalencephaly with olivary heterotopia is occasionally observed in autistic subjects. Secondary megalencephaly is associated with:
- inborn errors of metabolism such as sphingolipidoses, mucopolysaccharidoses, and certain leukodystrophies (including Alexander's disease and Canavan's disease)
- neurocutaneous syndromes.

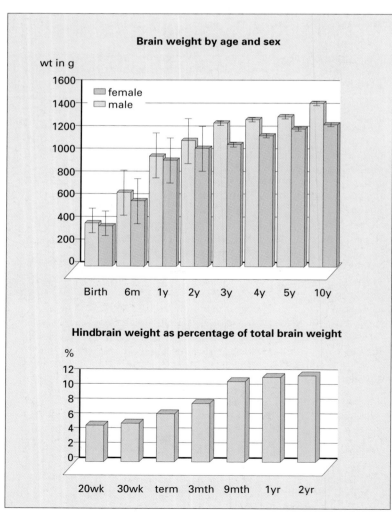

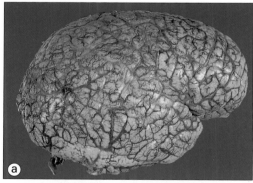
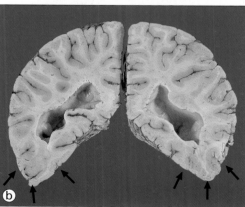

Fig. 3.90 Primary megalencephaly in a 13-year-old boy with a brain weight of 1645 g. (a) Much of the hemispheric surface shows excessive gyration or polygyria as a consequence of early hydrocephalus, which had been successfully shunted in infancy. The inferior surfaces of the temporal and occipital lobes are smoother and delineate an area of polymicrogyria. **(b)** Section showing symmetric polymicrogyria (arrows) associated with subependymal nodular heterotopias (see Fig. 3.72d).

Fig. 3.89 A guide to the weight of the brain during development. The vertical bars indicate ±1SD.

MALFORMATIONS OF THE CEREBELLUM

The classification of cerebellar malformations follows developmental principles (**Fig. 3.91**).

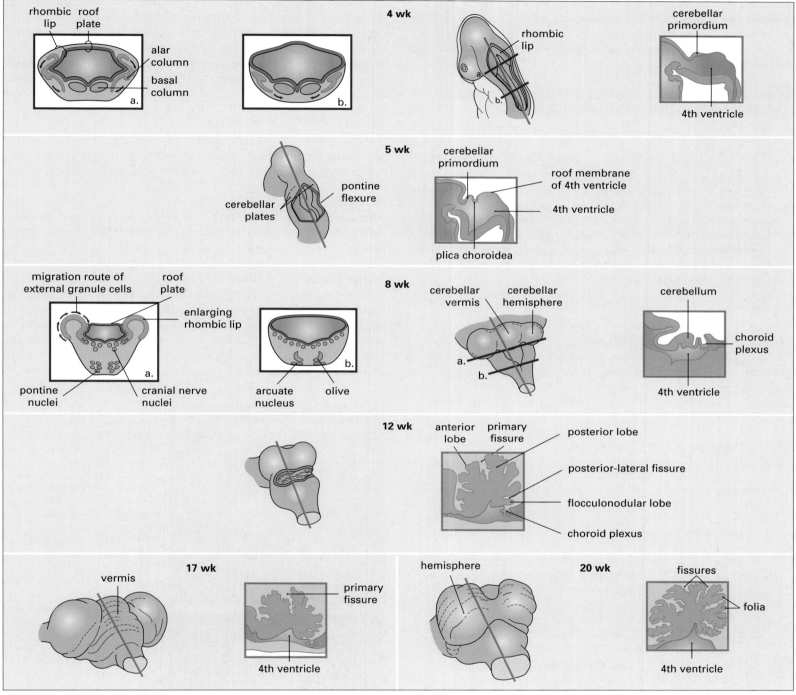

Fig. 3.91 Development of the hind brain. In the fourth week of gestation, the neural tube closes and segments, so that the rhombencephalon becomes temporarily the largest part of the brain. Differential growth in the rhombencephalon during the fifth week results in formation of the pontine flexure, widening the neural tube at this point and thinning its roof which becomes transversely creased as the plica choroidea, which gives rise to the choroid plexus. The pouch-like evagination caudal to it forms a membranous roof to the fourth ventricle which perforates forming the foramen of Magendie by 12 weeks. The roof rostral to the plica is later incorporated into the developing vermis. Also anterior to the plica, the lateral parts of the alar plates undergo intense neuroblastic proliferation, enlarging into the rhombic lips, the paired primordia of the cerebellum which gradually extend dorsomedially to meet the roof of the fourth ventricle and then fuse together in the midline during the third month. Cerebellar growth which has been intraventricular now becomes extraventricular and various subdivisions appear: first the posterolateral or flocculonodular fissure at 9 weeks demarcating the vestibular or archicerebellum from the rest, then at 12 weeks the primary fissure separating anterior from posterior lobes, the spino- or paleo-cerebellum from the ponto- or neo-cerebellum. This last, phylogenetically youngest, part of the cerebellum predominant in mammals, forms its various fissures 4–8 weeks after those of the vermis and flocculonodular lobes. The neurons of the cerebellar cortex and deep nuclei as well as the pontine and arcuate nuclei and inferior olivary nuclei all derive from the alar plates: ventral migrations into the pontine grey and olivary ribbons, and lateral migration into the rhombic lips. The latter has two divergent pathways, inwards through the cerebellar plate for Purkinje cells and deep nuclei, and outwards guided over the surface of the developing cerebellum by pial basal lamina to form the external granular layer (EGL). The rapidly proliferating EGL first appears in week 9, covers the whole cerebellar surface by 14 weeks, and persists until the third postnatal month, disappearing by the end of the first year. From the EGL arise the neurons and glia of the molecular layer, and by inward growth across the molecular layer the internal granule cells.

CEREBELLAR AGENESIS

Total absence of the cerebellum is rare, as the flocculus or nodulus often remains. The nuclei pontis and inferior olives are hypoplastic or dysplastic in association with the cerebellar agenesis.

Partial or total cerebellar agenesis is a feature of large occipital encephaloceles.

Cerebellar agenesis may be unsuspected in life or associated with mental handicap.

DIFFERENTIAL DIAGNOSIS OF PALEOCEREBELLAR MALFORMATIONS INVOLVING THE VERMIS

- Dandy–Walker syndrome
- Joubert syndrome
- tectocerebellar dysraphia with occipital encephalocele in which partial or total vermal agenesis, a severe deformation of the midbrain tectum, and a cerebello-encephalocele coexist
- rhomboencephalosynapsis, a cerebellar hypoplasia consisting of fused hemispheres and dentate nuclei, absent vermis and paleocerebellar roof nuclei, dysplastic olives, and other midline anomalies
- Walker–Warburg syndrome

DANDY–WALKER SYNDROME

This is a combination of vermal agenesis, a cystically dilated fourth ventricle, and an enlarged posterior fossa, and is usually accompanied by hydrocephalus (**Figs 3.92–3.94**). Many systemic and CNS malformations are associated with Dandy–Walker syndrome (**Fig. 3.95**).

DANDY–WALKER SYNDROME

- may present early in life with hydrocephalus, poor head control, motor retardation, spasticity, or respiratory failure
- may present later in childhood with symptoms and signs of a posterior fossa mass
- may be an incidental finding
- can be demonstrated on skull radiography and computerized tomography (CT) by the presence of elevated venous sinuses and torcular, high tentorial attachment, and an enlarged cystic posterior fossa

PATHOGENESIS OF DANDY–WALKER SYNDROME

- The cause of Dandy–Walker syndrome is unknown, but it is occasionally familial.
- The most convincing pathogenetic theory is a developmental arrest of the hindbrain before the third month. This would account for the atretic foramina, associated brain stem anomalies, occasional involvement of the cerebellar hemispheres, and the widespread evidence of arrested CNS development.

MACROSCOPIC APPEARANCES

Although the vermis is sometimes absent, its superior part usually remains. This is anteriorly rotated and blends inferiorly into the membranous roof of the cystic fourth ventricle, which herniates through the tentorial hiatus towards the splenium and attaches laterally to the cerebellar hemispheres and caudally to the medulla. The lateral walls of the cyst are the inner aspects of the cerebellar hemispheres (i.e. white matter covered by ependyma); the floor of the cyst is the dorsum of the brain stem. The outlet foramina of the fourth ventricle are sometimes atretic, but usually patent.

MICROSCOPIC APPEARANCES

The cyst membrane has two layers:
- an outer fibrous leptomeningeal layer
- an inner glio-ependymal layer sometimes including cerebellar remnants.

JOUBERT SYNDROME

This is a familial syndrome of episodic hyperpnea, abnormal eye movements, ataxia, and mental retardation, associated with agenesis of the vermis.

MACROSCOPIC AND MICROSCOPIC APPEARANCES

Rare pathologic reports indicate almost complete absence of the vermis, numerous heterotopias in the cerebellar white matter, a dysplastic segmented dentate nucleus, absent roof nuclei, C-shaped dysplasia of the olives, and anomalies of the pyramidal tracts, cranial nerve nuclei, and midbrain tegmentum. Occipital meningocele, cystic kidneys, and retinal dysplasia are also reported.

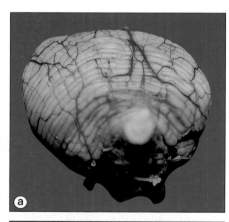

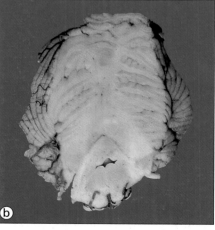

Fig. 3.92 Rhomboencephalosynapsis. **(a)** The hindbrain has a small globular cerebellum unsegmented into hemispheres and vermis. **(b)** Horizontal section through the hindbrain showing folia that are continuous across the midline, there is no recognizable vermis, and the dentate nuclei form a continuous undulating ribbon.

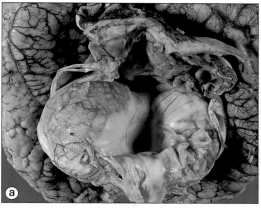
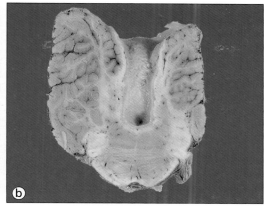
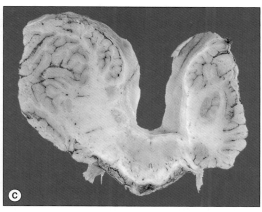
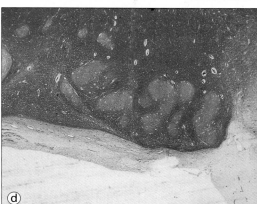

Fig. 3.93 Dandy–Walker malformation. This is the same case as in Fig. 3.89. **(a)** The vermis is absent and there is a widely dilated fourth ventricle with smooth white lateral walls and a roof membrane reinforced by thickened meninges. **(b, c)** Horizontal slices through the brain stem and cerebellum show the remaining superior part of the vermis, the ridged surface of the ventricle with granular ependymal lining, and asymmetry of the cerebellar hemispheres and dentate nuclei. **(d)** The right dentate nucleus is fragmented in the smaller right hemisphere. (Luxol fast blue/cresyl violet)

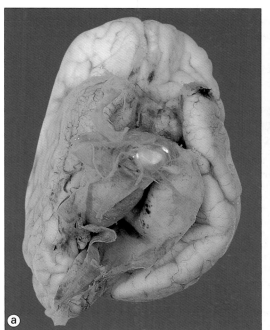
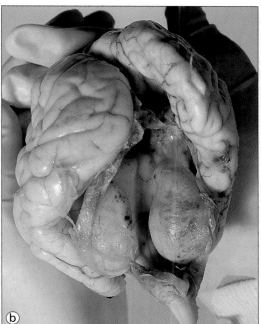
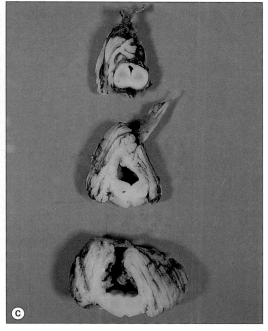
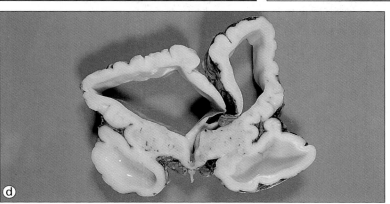

Fig. 3.94 Dandy–Walker malformation. (a) The cystic fourth ventricle has a delicate membranous roof, which is well demonstrated by floating the brain in water. **(b)** The vermis is absent and the lateral walls of the fourth ventricle are cerebellar white matter. **(c)** Horizontal sections of the hindbrain in another case where the superior part of the vermis remains and there is marked hydrocephalus. **(d)** Hydrocephalic cerebral hemispheres. Same case as in (c).

Malformations associated with Dandy-Walker syndrome
CNS

• microcephaly
• callosal agenesis
• polymicrogyria and pachygyria
• aqueduct stenosis
• infundibular hamartomata
• occipital meningocele
• hindbrain abnormalities:
  cerebellar hypoplasia
  cerebellar heterotopias
  cerebellar cortical dysplasia
  dentate dysplasia
  olivary dysplasia and heterotopia
  anomalies of pyramidal tract decussation

Systemic
• Klippel–Feil syndrome • Cornelia de Lange syndrome • cleft palate • polycystic kidneys • spina bifida • polydactyly and syndactyly

Fig. 3.95 Malformations associated with Dandy–Walker syndrome.

PONTONEOCEREBELLAR HYPOPLASIA (PNCH)

PNCH is a severe neocerebellar hypoplasia with relatively well-preserved paleocerebellum, and a peculiar segmentation of the dentate nucleus (**Figs 3.96, 3.97**).

PONTONEOCEREBELLAR HYPOPLASIA

- presents at birth with microcephaly, severe psychomotor retardation, feeding difficulties, choreiform and other abnormal movements, myoclonic jerks, and convulsions
- is usually fatal before the age of 2 years, though survival is possible through the first decade
- is usually sporadic, but familial examples are described

MACROSCOPIC APPEARANCES

There is often severe microcephaly, but the hindbrain is disproportionately small and is usually 3% or less of total brain weight. The extremely small cerebellar hemispheres are virtually smooth or reduced to a few coarse convolutions (see Figs 3.96, 3.97), while the vermis and flocculonodular lobes are almost normal in size. The pons is narrow and the olivary bulges are poorly defined.

MICROSCOPIC APPEARANCES

The hypoplastic cerebellar hemispheres (see Figs 3.96, 3.97) may show normal zones interposed with others where Purkinje and granule cells are completely lacking and replaced by tenuous gliotic tissue. There is only minimal, poorly myelinated, central white matter. The dentate nuclei are disorganized, lacking an undulating ribbon, hilum or amiculum (i.e. a surrounding sheath of myelinated fibers), and the reduced neuronal population is clustered into small neuropil islands embedded in a meshwork of myelin fibers. The vermis, archicerebellum, and roof nuclei are normal.

The superior and middle cerebellar peduncles are thin and poorly myelinated, but the inferior peduncles are preserved. The shallow basis pontis has few transverse fibers and markedly hypoplastic nuclei pontis, the inferior olives are hypoplastic or dysplastic, and the arcuate nuclei are absent.

PATHOGENESIS OF PONTONEOCEREBELLAR HYPOPLASIA

- The disparity in formation of the neocerebellar and paleocerebellar cortices suggests a developmental disturbance at the end of the third month.
- The dentate fragmentation has been ascribed to a developmental arrest or primary malformation, but dentate and brain stem changes could also be secondary anterograde and retrograde atrophy following initial interference with neocerebellar cortical development.

CEREBELLAR HYPOPLASIA IN OTHER CONTEXTS

Various combinations of neocerebellar and paleocerebellar hypoplasia, rudimentary segmented dentate nucleus, large heterotopias in cerebellar white matter, and olivary dysplasia have been reported (**Fig. 3.98a**).

Cerebellar hypoplasia may accompany anterior horn cell degeneration resembling Werdnig–Hoffmann disease (**Fig. 3.98b**). The hemispheres and vermis are equally involved and associated with severe secondary cortical atrophy in the inferior parts of the hemispheres and dentate and olivary dysplasia. Most cases are sporadic, but autosomal recessive inheritance has been recorded.

GRANULE CELL APLASIA

This is a developmental disorder affecting mainly the cerebellar granule cells.

MACROSCOPIC AND MICROSCOPIC APPEARANCES

The brain is usually small, but its convolutional pattern and histology are normal. The brain stem looks relatively normal, but the cerebellum is very small. The cerebellum retains individual folia, but they are shrunken and sclerotic (**Fig. 3.99**).

Microscopically, the folia are short and show a narrow molecular layer above a crowded row of Purkinje cells. The internal granular layer is absent. Purkinje cells are often misplaced into the molecular layer. An abnormal dendritic arborization and spiked expansions of terminal dendrites are common. There are no distinct pericellular baskets, but there are numerous Purkinje torpedo axonal swellings.

Ectopic granule cell somata can be found at any level within the molecular layer. Fibrillary gliosis extends through the cortex and white matter. Dentate and olivary neurons are preserved within a gliotic neuropil.

CEREBELLAR HETEROTOPIAS

Heterotopic gray matter within the cerebellar white matter is quite frequent and often an incidental finding in infants (perhaps present in over 50%). It is more common in the hemispheres, varying from a few cells to large islands of gray matter in which there are clusters of large cells surrounded by neuropil or islands of heterotopic cortex (**Fig. 3.100**).

Heterotopias are notably associated with trisomy 13, cerebellar hypoplasias, brain stem dysplasias, and other migration disorders.

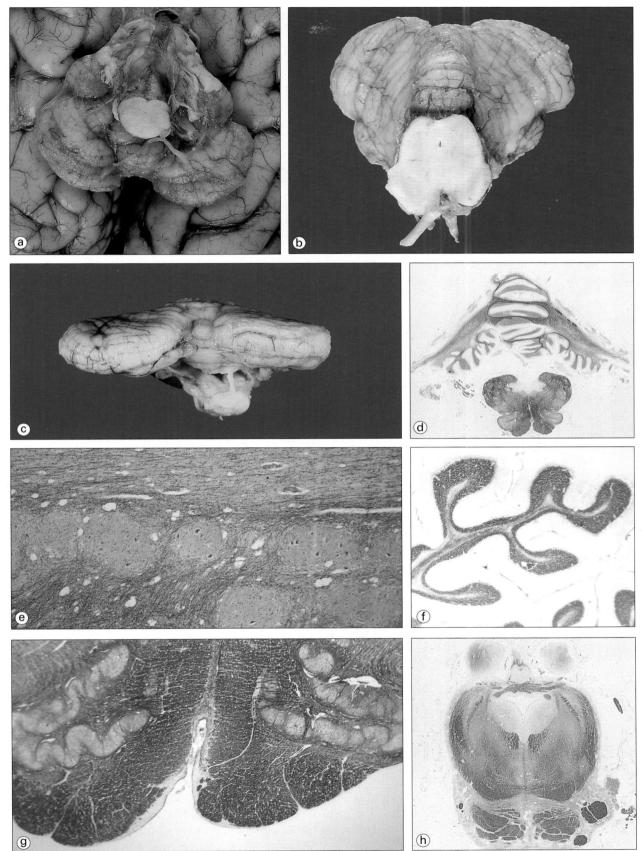

Fig. 3.96 PNCH occurring in two siblings. (a) Inferior view of the brain stem and cerebellum which together accounted for only 2.7% of the total brain weight (normal 12%) in a 9-year-old girl. **(b)** Superior surface of the brain stem and cerebellum shown in (a). The cerebellar hemispheres are reduced to thin plates with clear folial markings, while the preserved vermis and flocculonodular lobes appear unduly prominent. **(c)** The cerebellum seen from behind in the 5-year-old brother is similarly small and flat. **(d)** Horizontal section through the girl's hindbrain showing hypoplastic cerebellar hemispheres and a relatively preserved vermis, dysplastic inferior olives, and fragmented dentate nuclei. **(e)** The dentate nucleus in the boy's cerebellum consists of discrete islands that have been likened to a string of pearls. **(f)** The stubby hypoplastic cerebellar folia can be variably populated by Purkinje and granule cells. **(g)** Olivary dysplasia and absence of the arcuate nucleus in the boy. **(h)** Section through the pons in the girl shows an extremely shallow base due to a lack of transverse pontine fibers and middle cerebellar peduncles, and hypoplastic pontine nuclei.

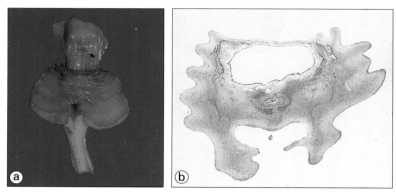

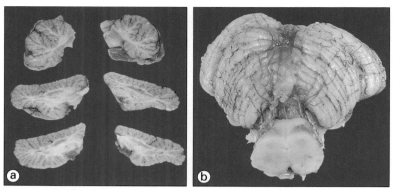

Fig. 3.97 Sporadic case of PNCH in a 5-week-old infant. (a) The tiny cerebellum and brain stem weighed only 3 g (1% of total brain weight) and the cerebellar folia are barely visible. **(b)** There is extreme hypoplasia and the hemispheric folia are virtually devoid of nerve cells. (Luxol fast blue/cresyl violet)

Fig. 3.98 Cerebellar hypoplasia. (a) Combined neocerebellar and paleocerebellar hypoplasia. The folia are short and poorly branching throughout the cerebellum while the dentate is small and accompanied by large heterotopias. **(b)** Cerebellar hypoplasia in a patient with anterior horn cell degeneration, which represents a variant of Werdnig–Hoffmann disease.

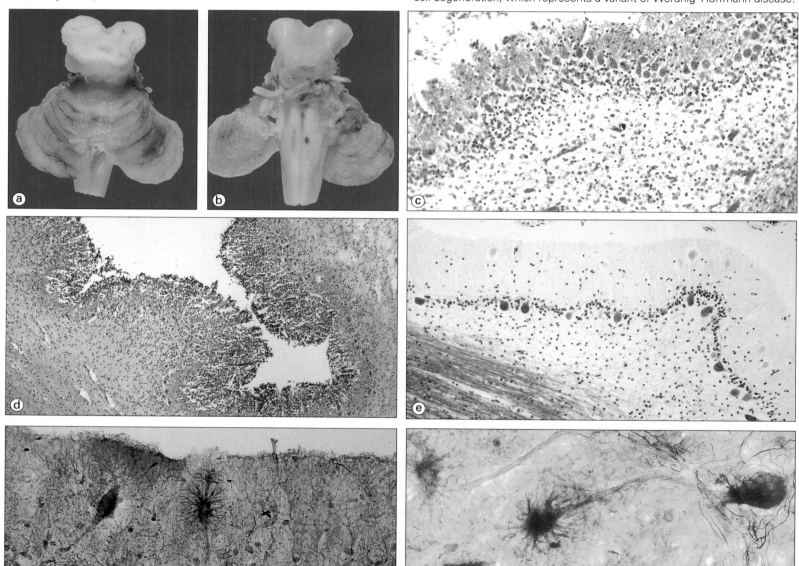

Fig. 3.99 Granule cell aplasia. (a) Superior view of the rudimentary cerebellum and small brain stem (combined weight less than 1% of total brain weight). **(b)** Inferior view of the hindbrain specimen in (a). **(c)** Cerebellar cortex showing absence of the internal granular layer. Purkinje cells form a closely packed row, but some are displaced into the molecular layer. **(d)** In the case shown in (a) and (b) granule cells fill the molecular layer, and there is no internal granular layer. **(e)** In this case of granule cell aplasia, cortical loss is very severe but some Purkinje cells remain. **(f)** Strange starburst-like dendritic protrusions may be demonstrated with silver impregnations. (da Fano's modification of Bielschowsky's method). **(g)** The dendritic asteroid body is in continuity with a Purkinje cell, which retains its associated basket plexus.

CEREBELLAR CORTICAL DYSPLASIA

Small foci of dysplastic cerebellar cortex in the flocculonodular lobes and tonsils and adjacent to the cerebellar peduncles are found in a minority of normal infants. In other parts of the cerebellum, cortical disorganization can be considered to be abnormal (**Fig. 3.101**). It occurs either alone or with many other malformations, but in the cerebro-ocular dysplasias it is particularly extensive and replaces most of the normal cerebellar cortex. Macroscopically, the branched folia are replaced by a smooth or irregularly fissured surface.

Microscopically, the folia are scrambled together with an apparent fusing of apposed molecular layers. However, the cortical layers remain in correct order.

PATHOGENESIS OF CEREBELLAR CORTICAL DYSPLASIA

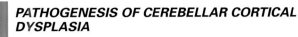

- A relatively late interference with the developing external granular layer is the suggested pathogenesis.
- Selective destruction of cerebellar meningeal cells in rats by 6-hydroxydopamine disrupts the glial scaffold and produces cerebellar cortical dysplasia.

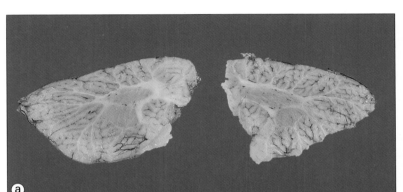

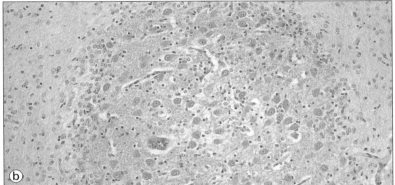

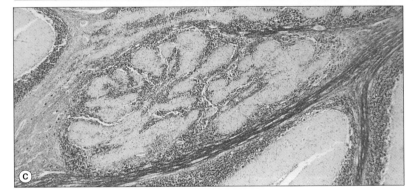

Fig. 3.100 Cerebellar heterotopia. (a) Large bilateral heterotopic gray masses within the central cerebellar white matter. Note also the dysplastic dentate nuclei. **(b)** Most cerebellar heterotopias consist of haphazardly arranged neurons and glia and associated neuropil. **(c)** Heterotopia situated within the folial core of the vermis and consisting of scrambled cerebellar cortex. (Luxol fast blue/cresyl violet)

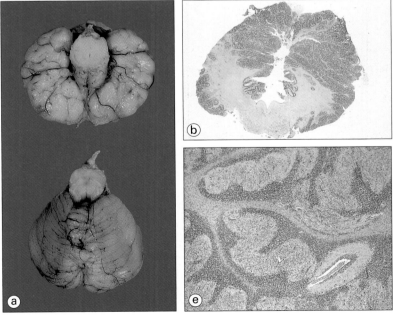

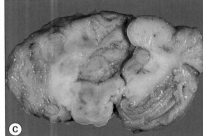

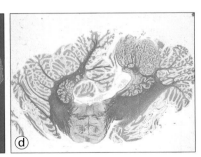

Fig. 3.101 Cerebellar cortical dysplasia. (a) In association with cerebro-ocular dysplasia (lissencephaly type II), the whole of the external surface of the cerebellum is bumpy and lacks folia. Compare with the normal control below. **(b)** Microscopically, the dysplastic cerebellar cortex comprises extensively fused cortical ribbons. This is the same case as shown in Fig. 3.58h. **(c)** A more restricted example of cerebellar cortical dysplasia limited to part of the superior surface in one hemisphere. **(d)** Low magnification cresyl violet-stained section of the specimen shown in (c). **(e)** Histologically, the cortical layers are fused, but their normal relationships to each other are maintained.

BRAIN STEM MALFORMATIONS

OLIVARY HETEROTOPIA

One or more heterotopic fragments of inferior olivary nucleus can be found anywhere along the migration route taken before the end of the third gestational month by their neuroblastic precursors from the rhombic lip to the ventral medulla:

- laterally, near the inferior cerebellar peduncle
- medially, near the rootlets of the hypoglossal nucleus.

These small groups of typical olivary neurons and neuropil can be folded and ensheathed by myelinated fibers rather like the normal nucleus, but the residual main nucleus may be dysplastic (**Fig. 3.102**). Associations include:

- agyria and pachygyria
- Dandy–Walker syndrome
- cerebral lactic acidosis due to pyruvate dehydrogenase deficiency
- megalencephaly

OLIVARY AND DENTATE DYSPLASIAS

Malformations of the inferior olive and dentate nucleus are often combined (**Figs 3.103–3.105**), probably because of their common origin from the rhombic lip.

DENTATO-OLIVARY DYSPLASIA

- Dentato-olivary dysplasia is often part of a more extensive complex of anomalies, the clinical features being those of the disorder as a whole.
- A small number of children with intractable tonic seizures from early infancy and severe developmental delay has been found to have a stereotyped dentato-olivary dysplasia in which the inferior olives are hook-shaped, coarse, and lack undulations, while the dentate nuclei form a compact or club-shaped mass of interconnected gray islands irregularly separated by myelin fibers. A familial occurrence suggests autosomal inheritance.

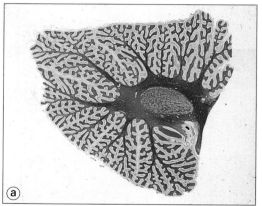
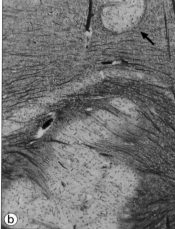

Fig. 3.102 Olivary heterotopia. (a) Small olivary fragments within the inferior cerebellar peduncles. Note the absent pyramids. **(b)** A rare example of a medially placed olivary heterotopia (arrow) near the twelfth nerve in a patient with trisomy 13. Note how the heterotopia mimics the normal folding of the olive, which in this case appears dysplastic. (Courtesy of Dr T. Revesz, Institute of Neurology, London)

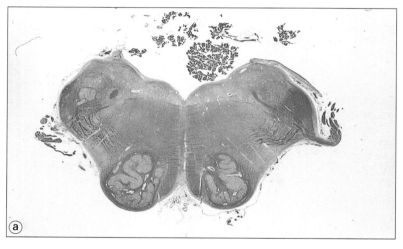
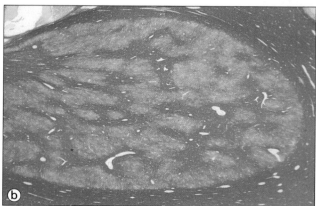

Fig. 3.103 A remarkably stereotyped form of dentato-olivary dysplasia peculiar to a syndrome of intractable, often tonic, seizures that commences in early infancy. Most cases are sporadic, but a familial form has been documented. **(a)** The dentate nucleus is compact and oval, lacking a hilum. **(b)** The dentate nucleus forms a mass of interconnected islands of neuropil and cells. **(c)** The inferior olives are coarse, hook-shaped, and unconvoluted. **(d)** Close-up of the dysplastic unconvoluted olivary ribbon. (Luxol fast blue/cresyl violet)

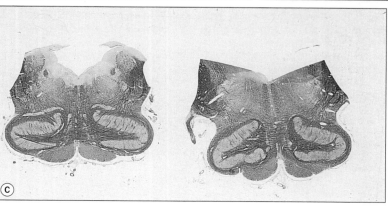
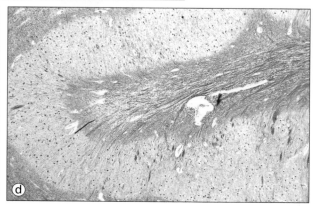

Inferior olivary dysplasia has various forms including:

- excessive folding in thanatophoric dysplasia
- too few convolutions in cerebellar aplasia or hypoplasia
- a simplified C-shaped band lacking folds in Joubert syndrome
- dorsal thickening in trisomy 18
- poverty of convolutions, peripheral margination of neurons, and fragmentation of the cell band, with an overall C shape and dorsal thickening in Zellweger syndrome
- complete disorganization and disruption
- a solid mass of cells
- a horseshoe band resembling an early fetal stage

PATHOGENESIS OF DENTATO-OLIVARY DYSPLASIA

- The pathogenesis of dentato-olivary dysplasia is obscure.
- The precursor neurons have a common ancestry in the rhombic lip, from where they migrate in the third month to form a hook-shaped plate (olive) and diffuse mass of cells (dentate), evolving into their final, folded appearance by about 7 months.

The appearance of dentate dysplasia may be:

- hyperconvoluted in thanatophoric dysplasia
- simplified or broken into islands or segments in cerebellar hypoplasias and in trisomies 13 and 18
- an unfolded thick plate
- interconnected bands and masses of cells
- unrecognizable.

MÖBIUS SYNDROME

Congenital facial diplegia with bilateral abducens palsies produces an expressionless face with internal strabismus in the neonate. The third and fourth cranial nerves and some lower cranial nerves including the twelfth may also be affected. Skeletal abnormalities, absent muscles, and mental retardation are also described, and it may be associated with Poland's anomaly (absent pectoralis muscle and symbrachydactyly). Möbius' syndrome may include:

- aplasia or hypoplasia of cranial nerve nuclei with or without other brain stem malformations
- focal necrosis or calcification of brain stem nuclei (**Fig. 3.106a,b**), possibly secondary to fetal infection or anoxia
- primary peripheral nerve involvement
- myopathy.

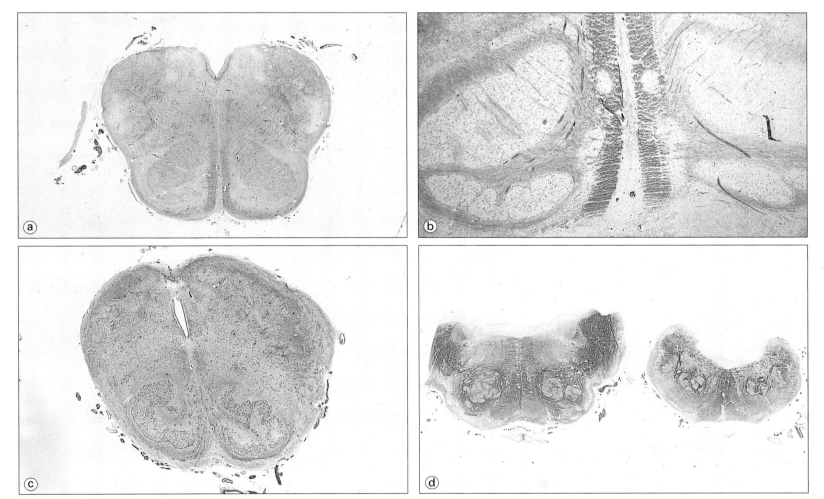

Fig. 3.104 Various types of olivary dysplasia. (a) In trisomy 18 the olive is coarse and C-shaped with thickening of its dorsal part. **(b)** In Zellweger's syndrome the olive is C-shaped with dorsal thickening and also shows fragmentation of the ribbon. **(c)** Disorganized olives in a case of cerebro-ocular dysplasia. **(d)** In a pachygyric brain the olives are broken into a series of convoluted fragments within an abnormally wide medulla. (Luxol fast blue/cresyl violet)

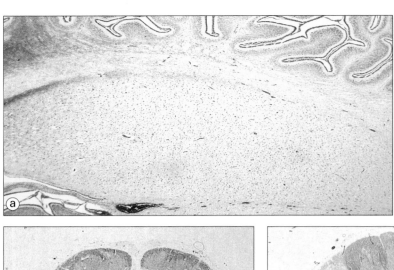

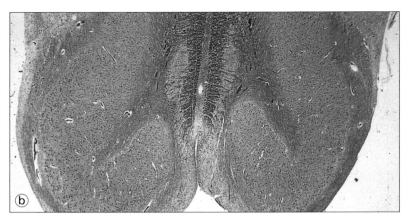

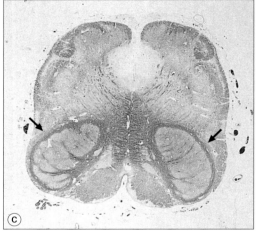

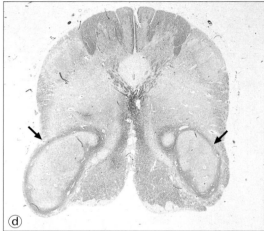

Fig. 3.105 Dentato-olivary dysplasia. (a) and **(b)** A simplified dentate and inferior olive in a neonate with appearances expected in the second trimester. **(c–f)** Specimens from identical twin sisters with identical dentato-olivary dysplasias and identical clinical courses of intractable seizures and death from respiratory infection. The olives (arrows) are lozenge-shaped while the dentate nuclei (arrowheads) are completely disrupted. (c) and (e) are from twin 1. (d) and (f) are from twin 2. (Luxol fast blue/cresyl violet)

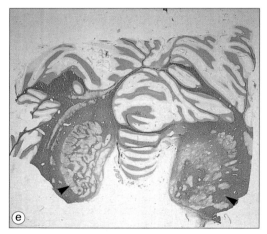

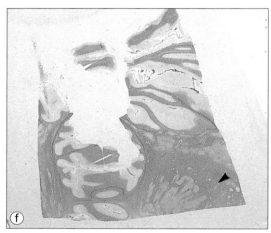

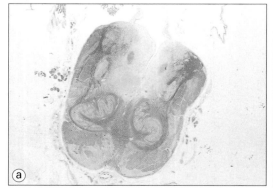

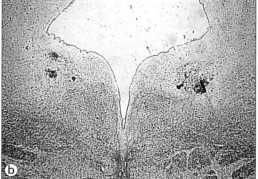

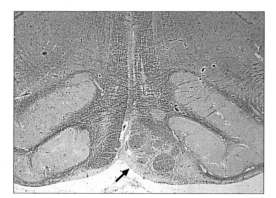

Fig. 3.106 Möbius' syndrome. (a) There are necrosis and calcification within the medullary tegmentum. **(b)** Bilateral calcifications situated close to the ventricle in the pontine tegmentum. (Luxol fast blue/cresyl violet)

Fig. 3.107 Fasciculation of the pyramid. Medulla from a 2-month-old infant showing olivary dysplasia, absent pyramid on one side, and fasciculation of the pyramid (arrow) on the other side.

ABNORMALITIES OF THE PYRAMIDAL TRACTS

Absence of the pyramidal tracts is usual in anencephaly, holoprosencephaly, porencephaly and hydranencephaly, and characteristic of X-linked congenital aqueduct stenosis.

Fasciculation of the pyramids into discrete bundles is an occasional finding in malformed brains (**Fig. 3.107**).

Asymmetric decussation is not uncommon in neonates. Most frequently, the fibers of the left pyramidal tract cross the midline first and pass anteriorly to those of the right. The cord is usually asymmetric.

MALFORMATIONS OF THE SPINAL CORD

Malformations of the spinal cord, principally associated with dysraphic states, are described on p. 3.7. The other principal abnormalities of the spinal cord are syringomyelia and syringobulbia.

SYRINGOMYELIA

Syringomyelia is tubular cavitation of the spinal cord, which may extend over many segments and sometimes occurs in association with hindbrain cavities (i.e. syringobulbia) (**Fig. 3.108a,b**).

SYRINGOMYELIA

- rarely presents in infancy
- usually presents in the second or third decade
- may be slowly progressive or may evolve rapidly before becoming static
- produces wasting and weakness of the hand and forearm muscles, loss of arm reflexes, dissociated or complete anesthesia of the upper limbs, and extensor plantar responses
- causes vasomotor disturbances
- is associated with kyphoscoliosis and Charcot's joints
- is associated with Chiari type I malformation in 90% of patients with idiopathic disease

Syringobulbia

- produces nystagmus, ataxia, facial dissociated sensory loss, and bulbar palsy

MACROSCOPIC APPEARANCES

The cervical cord is often swollen, filling the spinal canal. The syrinx:
- is filled with clear or yellow fluid
- is usually largest in the cervical region, but often absent from the first cervical segment
- extends through the upper thoracic segments for a varying distance
- rarely reaches the lumbosacral enlargement
- typically extends transversely across the cord, passing behind the central canal to involve the more posterior parts of the ventral horns and sometimes the posterior horns
- if bilateral may separate and rejoin at different levels
- at any level may reach the pial surface at the tips of the dorsal horns.

MICROSCOPIC APPEARANCES

Histologically, the walls of the cavity vary greatly along the length of the syrinx. Edematous or densely gliotic neuropil and bundles of peripheral myelinated nerve fibers with Schwann cells are commonly found. A thin layer of collagen covers part of the wall. There may be communication with the central canal, and an ependymal lining may be seen in this region.

SYRINGOBULBIA

Syringobulbia describes the presence of slit-like cavities in the medulla that may be isolated from or associated with syringomyelia (**Fig. 3.108c**).

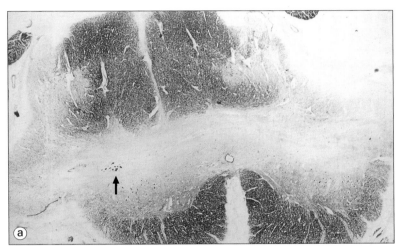

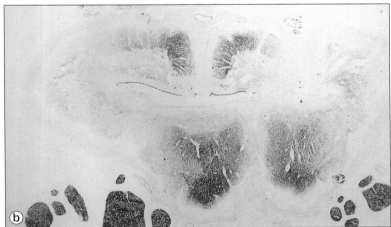

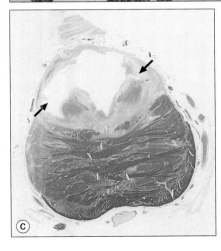

Fig. 3.108 Syringomyelia and syringobulbia. (a) Syringomyelia at lower lumbar level. The slit-like cavity extends right across the cord and into both dorsal horns. It is surrounded by gliotic tissue. Note the tiny bundles of myelinated fibers in the ventral wall of the syrinx on the left side (arrow). **(b)** Syringomyelia at sacral level. The cavity now involves the central canal and is partly lined by ependyma. **(c)** Syringobulbia. An irregular cavity extends out from the fourth ventricle into the tegmentum bilaterally (arrows). (Luxol fast blue/cresyl violet)

MACROSCOPIC APPEARANCES

Features of syringobulbia are variable and can include:

- an anterolateral slit running from the floor of the fourth ventricle to the hypoglossal nucleus in the lower half of the medulla
- an extension of the fourth ventricle along the median raphe, which is usually lined by ependyma
- cavities between the pyramid and the inferior olive that interrupt the emerging fibers of the hypoglossal nerve
- cavities in the pontine tegmentum that destroy fibers in the sixth or seventh cranial nerves or central tegmental tract.

Extensions of the cavity to a higher level such as the midbrain are extremely rare.

ARTHROGRYPOSIS MULTIPLEX CONGENITA

This is a clinical syndrome of multiple congenital contractures and results from the many causes of fetal hypokinesia (**Fig. 3.109**).

Causes of fetal hypokinesia
Neurogenic
Muscle fiber type predominance or disproportion
Dysgenesis of motor nuclei of spinal cord and brain stem
Dysgenesis of central nervous system: abnormal chromosome 18
Arthrogryposis with trisomy 21
Dysgenesis of motor nuclei of brain stem and cord in Pierre–Robin syndrome
Dysgenesis of motor nuclei of brain stem and cord in Möbius syndrome
Dysgenesis of spinal cord and prune belly syndrome
Craniocarpotarsal (Freeman–Sheldon) syndrome
Arhinencephaly, encephalocele; Meckel–Gruber syndrome, dysgenesis of anterior horns
Anencephaly with dysgenesis of anterior horn neurons
Microcephaly alone and with Marden–Walker and Bowen–Conradi syndrome
Arnold–Chiari syndrome
Caudal regression syndrome
Arthrogryposis and Potter sequence
Cerebrohepatorenal (Zellweger) syndrome
X-linked spinal muscular atrophy
Type 1 spinal muscular atrophy
Congenital infection (secondary)
Posterior column and peripheral neuropathy
Myopathic
Congenital muscular dystrophy
Congenital myotonic dystrophy
Central core disease
Nemaline myopathy
Myopathy with increased glycogen
Muscle fibrosis in congenital torticollis
Maternal autoimmune myasthenia gravis
Congenital myasthenic syndrome

Fig. 3.109 Causes of fetal hypokinesia.

ARACHNOID CYSTS

These developmental abnormalities are formed by splitting of the arachnoid membrane, which is reinforced by a thick layer of collagen, to produce a cyst (**Fig. 3.110**). They occur at various sites including the:

- Sylvian fissure (50%)
- cerebellopontine angle
- cisterna magna
- tectal plate
- interhemispheric fissure
- cerebral convexity
- interpenduncular fossa.

Arachnoid cysts may be asymptomatic or form a gradually enlarging space-occupying lesion, which is readily treated by surgery.

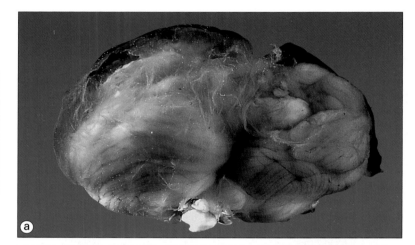

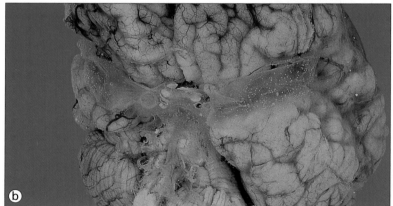

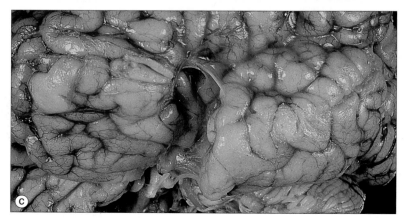

Fig. 3.110 Arachnoid cysts. (a) This cyst covers the basal cistern and was photographed in water. **(b)** Bilateral arachnoid cysts over the Sylvian fissures photographed in water. **(c)** After removal of the cyst an impression produced by pressure within the cyst can be seen in the insula.

DYSGENETIC SYNDROMES

Malformations occur in several dysgenetic syndromes (phakomatoses) including:

- Sturge–Weber syndrome (see below)
- Tuberous sclerosis (see below and also chapter 35)
- Lhermitte–Duclos disease (see chapter 37)
- neurofibromatosis (see chapter 42).

STURGE–WEBER SYNDROME

This syndrome is a neurocutaneous syndrome consisting of:

- a cutaneous vascular nevus in the territory supplied by the sensory branches of the fifth cranial nerve (**Fig. 3.111a**)
- choroidal ocular angioma
- meningeal venous angiomatosis (**Fig. 3.111b**)

The pathogenesis is unknown. Occasional cases are familial

STURGE–WEBER SYNDROME

- This syndrome is characterized clinically by a port wine facial stain, buphthalmos (in 70%), and focal neurologic signs, which may be present at birth.
- Intracranial calcification is present, and can be detected on CT of the brain, even in neonates.
- MRI shows subarachnoid enhancement and cortical atrophy.
- Brain and facial lesions are usually ipsilateral, but can be bilateral.
- Patients present with hemiparesis, hemiplegia, epilepsy, and mental retardation in infancy or early childhood.
- Seizure control may require surgery.

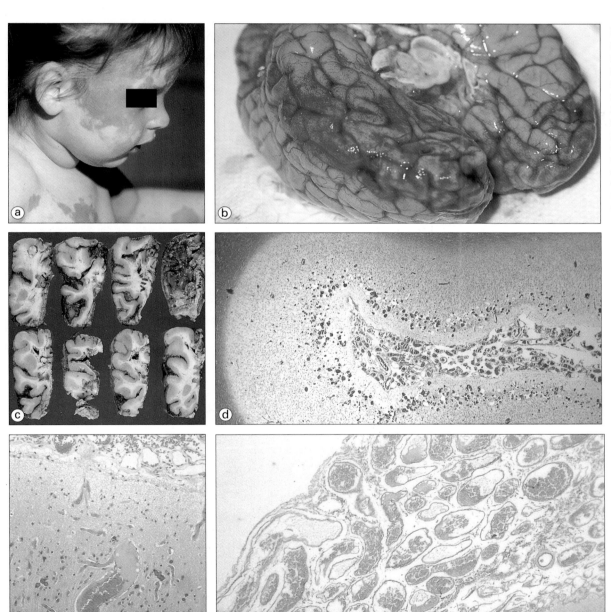

Fig. 3.111 Sturge–Weber syndrome. (a) A typical vascular nevus. **(b)** Bilateral meningeal angiomatosis. **(c)** Coronal slices of a surgical specimen show the narrowed dark granular cortical ribbon. **(d)** Microscopy shows the abnormal leptomeningeal venous plexus and a linear array of superficial calcifications in the thin atrophic cortex. **(e)** Severe astrogliosis with Rosenthal fiber formation and many calcospherites in the superficial cortex. **(f)** The leptomeningeal venous angioma lacks elastic fibers. (Elastic van Gieson)

MACROSCOPIC AND MICROSCOPIC APPEARANCES

The surface of the brain is dark purple due to the excessive vascularity of the meninges. Microscopically, the meningeal vessels and abnormally tortuous veins in the cortex are encrusted with iron and calcium, and foci of dystrophic calcification are scattered in the parenchyma, where there is cortical atrophy and gliosis (**Fig. 3.111c–f**). Polymicrogyria and heterotopias are less common findings.

TUBEROUS SCLEROSIS (BOURNEVILLE'S DISEASE)

Tuberous sclerosis is characterized by CNS malformations, cutaneous lesions, and ocular abnormalities. It causes epilepsy from a few months of age, and mental deficiency (see also chapter 35).

Tuberous sclerosis is inherited as an autosomal dominant trait with high penetrance and a prevalence among children 0–5 years of age of 1:10,000.

MACROSCOPIC APPEARANCES

The cortical tubers are firm, pale, flat or rounded, dimpled nodules projecting from the cortical surface, their diameter varying from a few millimeters to several centimeters (**Fig. 3.112**). Up to forty may be scattered over a single brain. In brain sections, the tubers greatly expand the gyri, blurring the gray–white matter junction.

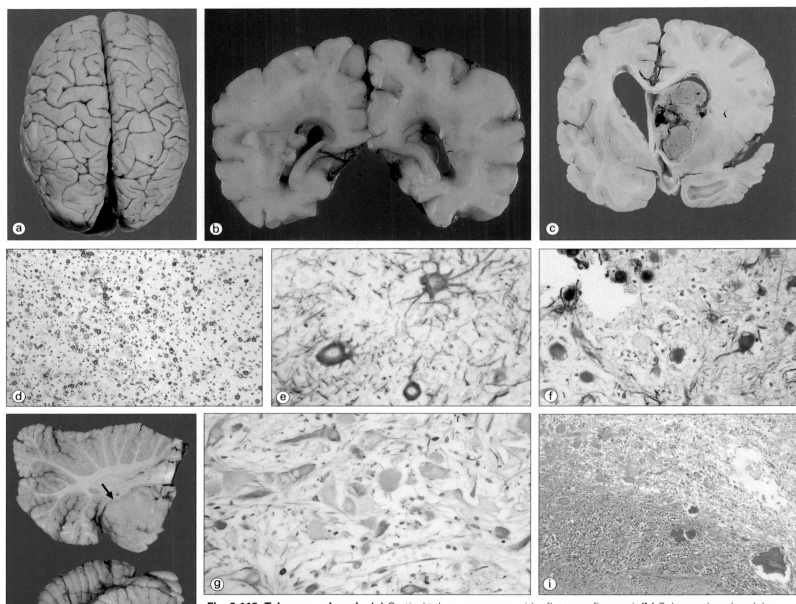

Fig. 3.112 Tuberous sclerosis. (a) Cortical tubers appear as wide, flat, very firm gyri. **(b)** Subependymal nodules and cortical tubers in a neonate. **(c)** Subependymal giant cell astrocytoma blocking the foramen of Monro with resultant hydrocephalus. **(d)** Cortical tuber showing laminar disorganization, large neurons, calcifications, and abnormal astrocytes. **(e)** There is upregulation of expression of phosphorylated neurofilaments within the atypical neurons. **(f)** Variable reactivity for GFAP in the astrocytic population of a tuber. **(g)** Ballooned astrocytes in a subependymal nodule are also variably positive for GFAP. **(h)** A cerebellar tuber (arrow) obliterating the normal folial pattern. **(i)** The cerebellar tuber shown in (h) demonstrates calcification and disorganization of the cortex with atypical astrocytes.

TUBEROUS SCLEROSIS (TSC)

- In the CNS, TSC produces cortical tubers (cerebral and cerebellar), subependymal nodules, and subependymal giant cell astrocytoma.
- Neurologic manifestations include seizures beginning in the first few months, mental retardation, various behavioral problems, and raised intracranial pressure.
- Cutaneous lesions in TSC include hypomelanic macules (seen in 90% of patients), facial angiofibromas or adenoma sebaceum (over the cheeks, nose, lower lip, and chin), - periungual or subungual fibromas (more often on toes than on fingers), shagreen patches or fibrous hamartomas (of dorsal surfaces, forehead, or scalp), poliosis, and leukotrichia.
- TSC involves the eyes in 50% of cases, producing a variety of lesions including retinal giant cell astrocytoma, hypopigmented iris spot, white eyelashes, and eyelid and conjunctival hamartomas.
- TSC commonly involves the heart. Single or multiple cardiac rhabdomyomas may produce fetal hydrops, obstruction to flow, myocardial dysfunction, cardiac arrhythmias, and sudden death.
- TSC causes renal lesions, principally multiple angiomyolipomas and renal cysts.

Subependymal nodules occur singly or in rows (candle gutterings). They are firm or calcified hard protrusions in the wall of the lateral ventricles, particularly near the sulcus terminalis, and less often the third and fourth ventricles or aqueduct. Nodules at the foramen of Monro may obstruct the flow of cerebrospinal fluid, causing hydrocephalus.

ETIOLOGY OF TUBEROUS SCLEROSIS COMPLEX (TSC)

- There is locus heterogeneity with disease-determining genes mapped to chromosome 9q34 (TSC1 gene) and 16p13.3 (TSC2 gene).
- Allele loss (i.e. loss of heterozygosity) for 16p13.3 has been demonstrated in hamartomas, a cortical tuber, and a giant cell astrocytoma from tuberous sclerosis patients. This is consistent with the hypothesis that TSC2 acts as a tumor suppressor gene.

MICROSCOPIC APPEARANCES

Cortical tubers show effacement of the hexalaminar cortex by collections of large bizarre cells with stout processes, peripheral vacuolation, prominent nucleoli, and sometimes multiple nuclei. These cells have a variable immunophenotype that suggests they are atypical astrocytes, atypical neurons, or of indeterminate origin. Clusters of abnormal cells are also found in the deep white matter. Neurofibrillary tangles, argentophilic globules, and granulovacuolar degeneration may also be evident. There is impressive fibrillary gliosis, both beneath the pia and in myelin-depleted gyral cores. Tubers calcify readily. Occasional cerebellar tubers consist of disorganized calcified cortex, abnormal astrocytes, and Purkinje cells.

Subependymal nodules comprise elongated or swollen glial cells and their processes, giant or multinucleated cells, and calcium deposits. Progression to subependymal giant cell astrocytoma (SEGA) is documented. While in clinicopathiological terms the SEGA is neoplastic, not hamartomatous, there is considerable histologic overlap between subependymal nodule and SEGA.

REFERENCES

Harding B and Copp, AJ. (1997) Malformations. In: *Greenfield's Neuropathology*, (6th edition) edited by Graham, D.I. and Lantos, P.L.London:Arnold, p. 397–533.
Friede RL. (1989) *Developmental Neuropathology*, Berlin:Springer-Verlag.

Shaw C.M. and Alvord EC. Jr. (1997) Hydrocephalus. In: *Pediatric Neuropathology*, edited by Duckett S, Malvern. PA:Williams and Wilkins, p. 149–211.
Norman MG, McGillivray BC, Kalousek D., Hill A, and Poskitt KJ. (1995) *Congenital malformations of the brain*, New York:Oxford University Press.

4 Hydrocephalus

Hydrocephalus means an increased volume of cerebrospinal fluid (CSF) in the cranial cavity. The term internal hydrocephalus implies an increased volume of CSF within the ventricular system, but has become interchangeable with hydrocephalus. In childhood, internal hydrocephalus is associated with a huge variety of disorders, which are conveniently subclassified into:

- Those primarily disturbing normal homeostatic control of CSF production and CSF flow or drainage.
- Those principally associated with developmental abnormalities or destructive lesions in the brain (**Fig. 4.1**).

Fig. 4.1 Causes of hydrocephalus in childhood.

Causes of hydrocephalus in childhood	
Pathophysiology	Pathology
Disturbance of CSF homeostasis • Overproduction	• Choroid plexus papilloma
• Failure of absorption Functional changes	• Absence of arachnoid granulations and cilia • Various cranial dysplasias

• Interference with CSF flow
  Reduced propulsion
  Physical block to flow
	• Ciliary dysplasia
	• Neoplasms
	    Intrinsic block, Extrinsic compression
	• Malformation
	    Membranous obstruction of the foramen of Monro
	    Obliteration of the third ventricle
	    Congenital obstruction of the aqueduct of Sylvius
	        Atresia, Stenosis,
	        Vascular anomaly (Vein of Galen, Arteriovenous malformation)
	    Obstruction to foramina of Luschka and Magendie
	        Atresia, Dandy–Walker malformation, Arachnoid cyst
	    Obstruction of foramen magnum
	        Chiari malformation
	    Diffuse obliteration of subarachnoid space
	        Cerebro-ocular dysplasias
	• Infection, hemorrhage, and postinflammatory repair
	    Acute hemorrhage
	        Pre/perinatal germinal matrix hemorrhage
	    Obstruction of foramen of Monro
	    Gliosis in aqueduct
	    Gliosis in fourth ventricular exit foramina
	    Sequestration of fourth ventricle (multiple blocks)
	    Subarachnoid space fibrosis

Developmental anomalies in which ventriculomegaly is an important feature though of uncertain pathogenesis	• Holoprosencephaly, lissencephaly, hemimegalencephaly, hydrolethalus syndrome, Fowler syndrome, congenital lactic acidosis
Following destruction or degeneration of brain tissue	• Hypoxic-ischemic • Degenerative conditions
Combination of disturbance of CSF homeostasis and destruction or degeneration of brain tissue.	

Overproduction of CSF by a choroid plexus papilloma (**Fig. 4.2**), reduced propulsion consequent upon primary ciliary dysplasia, and reduced absorption due to aplasia of arachnoid granulations or raised venous pressure due to bony dysplasia (**Fig. 4.3**) are rare causes of hydrocephalus. More commonly hydrocephalus results from interference with CSF flow at various points in the CSF pathway (**Fig. 4.4**).

Many neoplasms can fill and block the ventricles or subarachnoid spaces, notably those growing close to narrow parts of the ventricular system. For example the foramen of Monro may be blocked by a subependymal giant cell astrocytoma of tuberous sclerosis (**Fig. 4.5**) or a colloid cyst (see chapter 45). Otherwise, obstruction commonly occurs at the aqueduct and the fourth ventricular exit foramina.

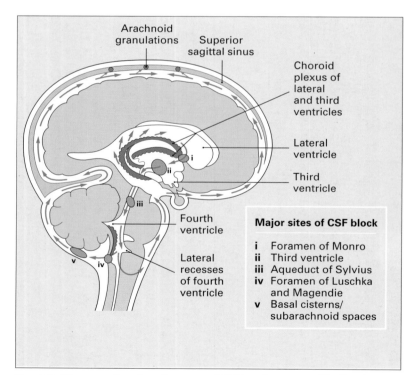

Fig. 4.2 Choroid plexus papilloma. These neoplasms may cause hydrocephalus by obstructing CSF flow or by oversecretion.

Arachnoid granulations   Superior sagittal sinus   Choroid plexus of lateral and third ventricles   Lateral ventricle   Third ventricle   Fourth ventricle   Lateral recesses of fourth ventricle

Major sites of CSF block

i   Foramen of Monro
ii   Third ventricle
iii   Aqueduct of Sylvius
iv   Foramen of Luschka and Magendie
v   Basal cisterns/subarachnoid spaces

Fig. 4.4 Diagram showing the normal CSF pathways and indicating the principal sites of occlusion.

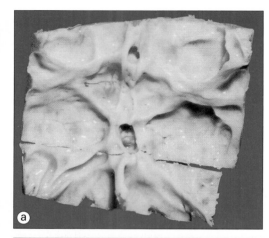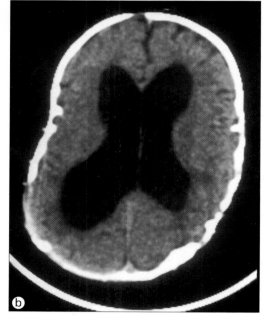

Fig. 4.3 Hydrocephalus associated with bony dysplasia. (a) Part of the skull base from an 8-year-old child who presented with hydrocephalus and chronic tonsillar herniation resulting from craniosynostosis, clover-leaf skull, and Klippel–Feil deformity. The bone is alternately thinned or massively thickened into irregular ridges and contains excessively narrow exit foramina, which compromise venous return and reduce CSF reabsorption, thereby causing hydrocephalus. **(b)** A computerized tomogram of the head of an 18-month-old infant with Crouzon's syndrome shows synostosis, distortion of the skull bones, and hydrocephalus.

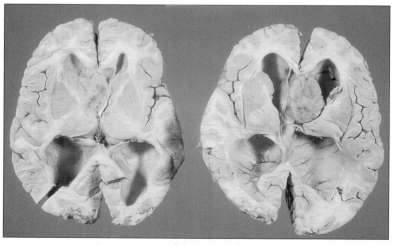

Fig. 4.5 Obstruction of interventricular foramina of Monro by a giant cell astrocytoma in tuberous sclerosis. Horizontal dissection.

OBSTRUCTION OF THE AQUEDUCT OF SYLVIUS

MACROSCOPIC AND MICROSCOPIC APPEARANCES

Stenosis may be sporadic, X-linked, or (rarely) autosomal recessive. It is characterized by a tiny lumen in the usual position, a normal ependymal lining, and an absence of gliosis (**Fig. 4.6**). Experimental and clinical evidence suggests that narrowing can be secondary to compression of the tectal plate by expanding hydrocephalic hemispheres.

In atresia (forking) a normal channel is replaced by groups of ependymal cells, small rosettes, or tiny aqueductules irregularly scattered across the midbrain tegmentum. There is no gliosis (**Fig. 4.7**).

With gliosis, an outline of the aqueduct is still visible. An interrupted ring of ependymal cells, rosettes, and tubules is surrounded and filled by dense fibrillary gliosis, in which there may be one or two small central channels that lack an ependymal lining (**Fig. 4.8**).

OBSTRUCTION OF THE AQUEDUCT OF SYLVIUS

Anatomically, the aqueduct of Sylvius is:
- the narrowest part of the ventricular system
- an irregularly curved tube of variable caliber with two constrictions, above and below a central ampulla
- 0.4–1.5 mm² in its narrowest part in adults
- as small as 0.15 mm² at its narrowest part just cranial to the ampulla in normal children

Obstruction of the aqueduct may result from:
- **Stenosis**, which may be sporadic, X-linked, or (very rarely) autosomal recessive.
- **Atresia**, which may be associated with Arnold–Chiari malformation, hydranencephaly, craniosynostosis, or (possibly) mumps meningoencephalitis, or sporadic.
- **Gliosis**, which is related to previous infection or hemorrhage.
- **A septum.**
- **A vascular malformation**; compression of the tectum by an aneurysm of the great vein of Galen may occlude the aqueduct.
- **X-linked hydrocephalus.**

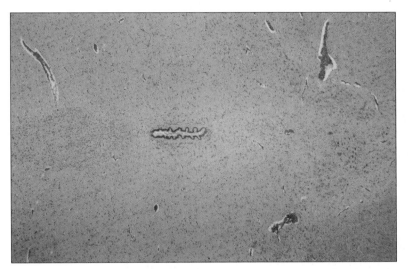

Fig. 4.6 Aqueduct stenosis. This is characterized by a very tiny lumen, intact ependymal lining, and normal surrounding midbrain parenchyma.

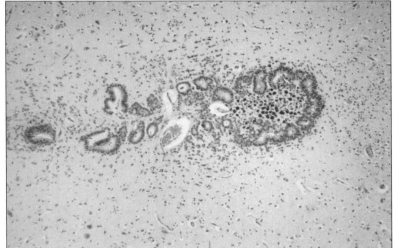

Fig. 4.7 Aqueduct atresia. This is characterized by the presence of many tiny canals or aqueductules scattered through the midbrain tegmentum in the absence of overt gliosis.

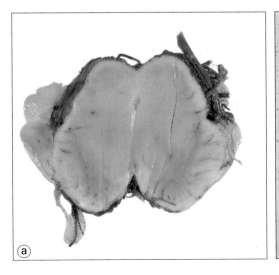

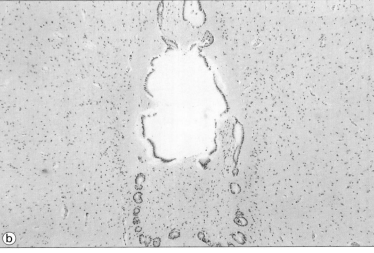

Fig. 4.8 Aqueduct gliosis. (a) Macroscopic view of the midbrain. Although the position of the aqueduct can be seen, it appears blocked. **(b)** Microscopically, the outline of the aqueduct is still visible as an interrupted ring of ependymal canals. Gliotic tissue enmeshes these tubules and fills the aqueductal lumen.

A septum is a rare variant of aqueductal gliosis. A thin translucent glial membrane is surrounded by a ring of ependymal tissue, which interrupts the aqueduct at its caudal end (**Fig. 4.9**).

X-linked hydrocephalus: Ventricular dilatation may be present with or without aqueduct stenosis (**Fig. 4.10**). The cerebrum shows polygyria (excessive gyration with normal histology) (**Fig. 4.11**), which is a common consequence of hydrocephalus in early life. Absence of the medullary pyramids (**Fig.4.12**) is almost invariable. Other findings may be fusion of the thalamic nuclei and agenesis of the corpus callosum.

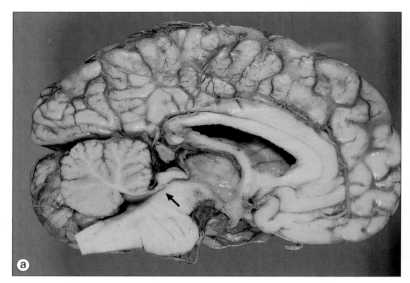
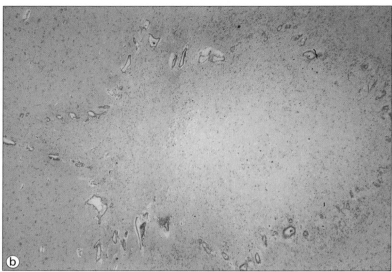

Fig. 4.9 Septum of the aqueduct. (a) A narrow band of white tissue occludes the lower end of the aqueduct (arrow) in this sagittal hemisection of the brain. **(b)** Microscopically the similarity with aqueduct gliosis is striking. A tenuous glial membrane is stretched across the lumen of the Sylvian canal, outlined by a series of ependymal tubules separated and enmeshed by astroglial tissue.

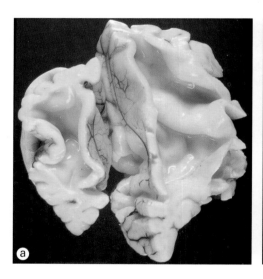
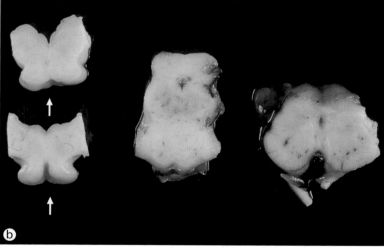

Fig. 4.10 X-linked hydrocephalus. (a) Coronal section through the frontal horns showing marked ventriculomegaly. **(b)** Horizontal section of the hindbrain. The aqueduct is widely patent, but the medullary pyramids are absent (arrows).

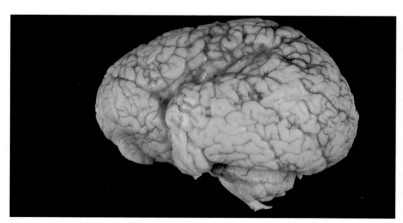
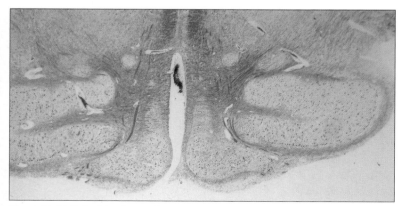

Fig. 4.11 Polygyria. This is evident macroscopically as excessive gyration. It is often associated with congenital hydrocephalus.

Fig. 4.12 X-linked hydrocephalus. An absence of both medullary pyramids is an important association and a useful diagnostic indicator. Note also the dysplastic (simplified) inferior olivary nuclei. (Luxol fast blue/cresyl violet)

X-LINKED HYDROCEPHALUS

- occurs in 1 in 60,000 males
- is characterized by congenital hydrocephalus combined with disproportionately severe mental retardation and spasticity
- usually results in a still birth or death in infancy
- is associated with flexed adducted thumbs in 25% of cases
- has a highly variable clinical expression ranging from thumb spasticity alone through retardation and spasticity without hydrocephalus, to hydrocephalus with or without aqueduct stenosis on neuroimaging

GENETIC ASPECTS OF X-LINKED HYDROCEPHALUS

- Inheritance is X-linked recessive.
- The mutation is located at Xq28.
- The responsible gene, named L1-CAM, codes for a cell adhesion molecule expressed on migrating neurons.
- It appears that X-linked hydrocephalus, X-linked complicated spastic paraplegia, and mental retardation, aphasia, shuffling gait, adducted thumbs (MASA syndrome) can be mapped to the same locus, can occur in the same family, and may represent variable phenotypic expression of the same mutation.

OBSTRUCTION OF THE FOURTH VENTRICULAR EXIT FORAMINA

All three outlets of the fourth ventricle are larger than the aqueduct, so all three must be blocked to compromise CSF flow.

Obstruction may result from Dandy–Walker syndrome, atresia, or arachnoid cysts.

Dandy–Walker syndrome: One or more cerebellar foramina are usually patent. Hydrocephalus is very variable in degree and may be related to the expanding cystic fourth ventricle or the multiplicity of associated malformations.

Atresia: The cerebellar foramina are covered by thin glioependymal membranes (**Fig. 4.13**).

Infratentorial arachnoid cysts can obstruct the exit foramina or compress the aqueduct and fourth ventricle (**Fig. 4.14**).

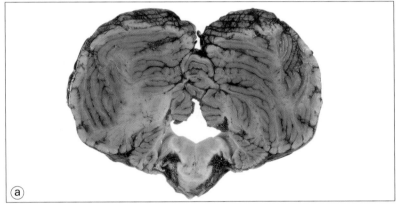
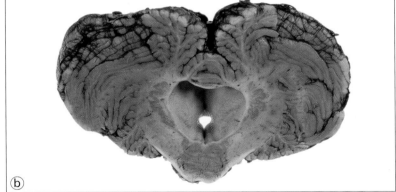

Fig. 4.13 Atresia of the cerebellar exit foramina. (a) At the level of the pontomedullary junction the lateral apertures are dilated and closed over by white membranes. **(b)** At the midpontine level there is marked dilatation of the fourth ventricle and its wall is studded with granular ependymitis.

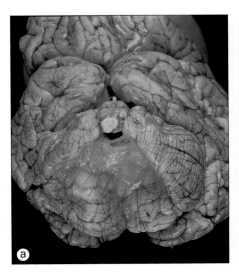
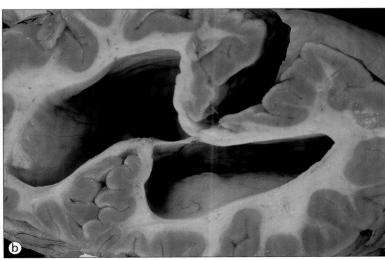

Fig. 4.14 Arachnoid cyst. (a) Infratentorial midline arachnoid cyst. **(b)** Massive ventriculomegaly caused by the cyst in (a).

POST-INFLAMMATORY OR FIBROTIC OBSTRUCTION OF THE CSF PATHWAY

Causes of post-inflammatory or fibrotic obstruction include intrauterine infection, neonatal infection, intraventricular hemorrhage, and mucopolysaccharidosis.

MACROSCOPIC AND MICROSCOPIC APPEARANCES

Intrauterine infection: Congenital toxoplasmosis causes a destructive meningoencephalitis. Progressive ventriculomegaly results from parenchymal destruction, acute aqueduct block (by necrotic debris), ependymitis, and chronic gliosis (**Fig. 4.15**).

Neonatal infection: The exudate of a purulent leptomeningitis caused by Gram-negative enterobacteria, group B streptococci, *Pseudomonas*, or *Candida* may block the foramen of Monro, aqueduct, or fourth ventricular exit foramina. Later organization and scarring lead to gliotic occlusion at one or several of these sites (**Fig. 4.16**). Ventriculitis (**Fig. 4.17**), infarction, and abscess and cavity formation cause ventricular loculations and diverticula which may distend and interfere with CSF flow. Chronic adhesive arachnoiditis may block the basal cisterns.

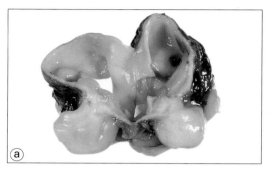
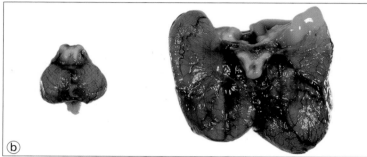

Fig. 4.15 Congenital toxoplasmosis in a 24-week gestation fetus. **(a)** Coronal section showing hydrocephalus, thinning of the pallium, and necrosis of the basal ganglia. **(b)** After detaching the hindbrain, the midbrain appears necrotic and the aqueduct obliterated.

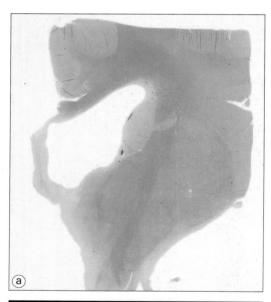
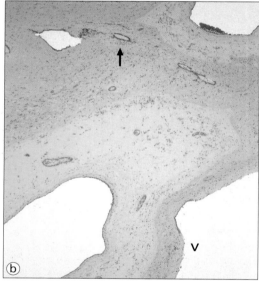

Fig. 4.16 Post-inflammatory scarring resulting in hydrocephalus in an infant who had suffered neonatal meningitis. Post-inflammatory scarring may interfere with CSF circulation at several levels. **(a)** Gliotic occlusion of the foramen of Monro. This low-power histologic section of frontal lobe shows that the foramen of Monro is walled over and the frontal horn is dilated. **(b)** Within the glial tissue occluding the foramen of Monro, ependymal remnants form canals (arrow). Note the interrupted ependymal lining of the ventricle (v). **(c)** Gliotic occlusion of the cerebellar foramina. The foramina of Luschka with choroid plexus are sealed over, and covered by membranous pouches which bulge when the cerebellum is compressed. **(d)** Microscopically, the lateral aperture of (c) is occluded by a delicate sheet of glioependymal tissue, which encloses choroid plexus.

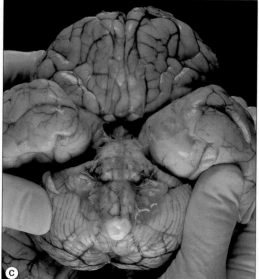
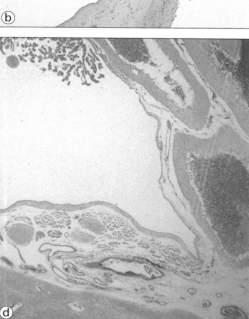

Intraventricular hemorrhage can acutely block the aqueduct, foramen of Monro, and fourth ventricular outlets (**Fig. 4.18**). Later resolution of the hematoma and chronic gliosis may also compromise these foramina, while subarachnoid fibrosis is a common cause of obstructed basal cisterns or fourth ventricular exit foramina (**Fig. 4.19**).

Mucopolysaccharidosis: Hydrocephalus is associated not only with generalized brain atrophy in this condition, but also with blockage of CSF due to leptomeningeal fibrosis (**Fig.4.20**).

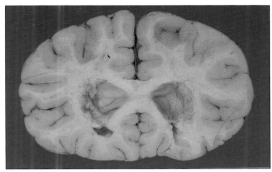

Fig. 4.17 Hydrocephalus complicating haemophilus meningitis. The meningeal exudate has occluded the basal cistern, causing hydrocephalus. Note the ragged ventricular lining due to ventriculitis.

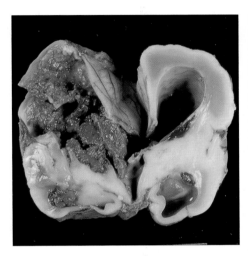

Fig. 4.18 Dilatation of the right frontal horn following blockage of the foramen of Monro by acute hematoma in a premature infant born at 26 weeks' gestation. The acute hematoma resulted from an intraventricular (germinal matrix) hemorrhage and white matter hemorrhagic infarction.

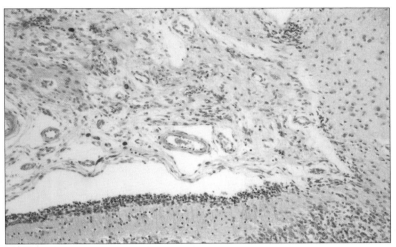

Fig. 4.19 Post-hemorrhagic meningeal fibrosis occluding the cerebellopontine angle. Hemosiderin-laden macrophages are scattered through the tissue.

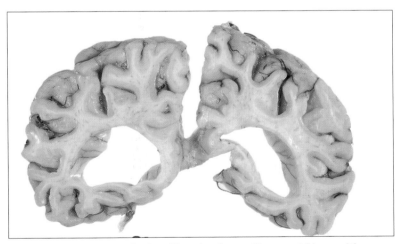

Fig. 4.20 Marked ventricular dilatation in an 11-year-old boy with Sanfillipo A disease (mucopolysaccharidosis type IIIA).

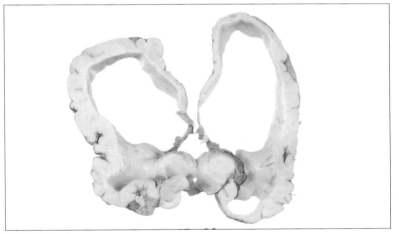

Fig. 4.21 Congenital cerebral lactic acidosis resulting from pyruvate dehydrogenase deficiency. A characteristic combination of malformations, including microcephaly, hydrocephalus, olivary heterotopia, and hypoplastic pyramidal tracts is produced. This is an example of one of the developmental disorders in which hydrocephalus is an essential feature, although its cause remains obscure.

REFERENCES

Friede RL (1989) *Developmental Neuropathology.* pp. 220–246. Berlin: Springer–Verlag.
Russell D (1949) *Observations on the Pathology of Hydrocephalus. MRC Special Report Series* No. 265. London: HMSO.

Weller RO, Kida S, Harding BN (1993) Aetiology and pathology of hydrocephalus. In PH Schurr, CE Polkey (eds) *Hydrocephalus.* pp. 521–538. London: Oxford University Press.

5 *Disorders that primarily affect white matter*

Inherited metabolic disorders that primarily affect white matter are occasionally encountered in children, and even more rarely in adults. A wide range of clinical and morphologic appearances results from the various genetic and biochemical defects that interfere with myelin formation, maintenance, turnover, and catabolism. Some of these conditions, notably those associated with peroxisomal and lysosomal defects, are well characterized and their biochemical defects are sufficiently understood that they are readily diagnosable in life. However, in many cases a definitive diagnosis can be reached only after histologic examination, occasionally following biopsy but more often at autopsy.

The fundamental requirement for the diagnosis of these disorders is the demonstration that there is primary involvement of myelin. The disease process may involve some loss of axons, occasionally manifesting as axonal fragmentation and formation of spheroids, but there is relative preservation of axons.

The leukodystrophies can be distinguished on the basis of their clinical, etiologic, and neuropathologic characteristics (**Figs 5.1–5.4**). This chapter covers the leukodystrophies that are not known to be due to lysosomal or peroxisomal disorders. Those that are caused by lysosomal or peroxisomal disorders are described in more detail in chapter 23.

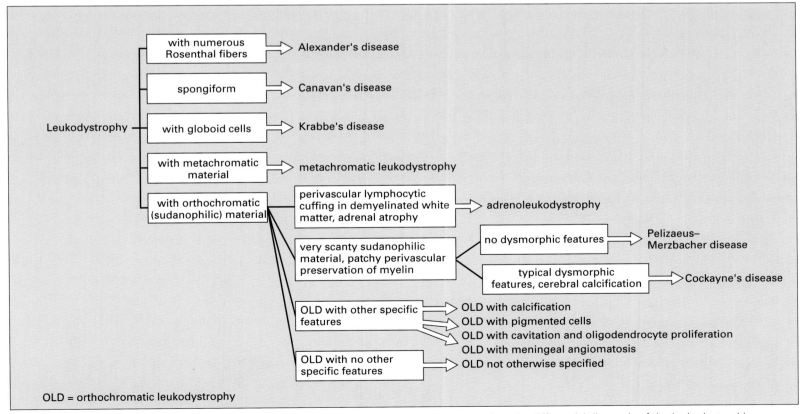

Fig. 5.1 Descriptive classification of leukodystrophies. This provides a morphologic approach to the differential diagnosis of the leukodystrophies.

Clinical features of leukodystrophies

Leukodystrophy	Presentation in infancy	Presentation in childhood	Presentation in adulthood
Krabbe's disease	Irritability, developmental failure, deteriorating motor function, tonic spasms, myoclonic jerks, hyperpyrexia, blindness, bulbar paralysis	Gait disorder, progressive spasticity, peripheral neuropathy, visual disturbance	
Metachromatic leukodystrophy	Progressive motor disability	Behavioral and educational problems, gait disorder	Psychosis, behavioral problems
Adrenoleuko-dystrophy	Hypertonia, seizures, failure to thrive, deafness, retinal degeneration	Loss of skills, educational problems, dementia, problems with hearing and vision, progressive pyramidal, extrapyramidal, or cerebellar disorder	Clumsiness and spasticity, schizophrenia-like syndrome, dementia
Pelizaeus–Merzbacher disease	Rotary nystagmus, stridor, spasticity, ataxia, failure of development, seizures, optic atrophy, either rapidly fatal or with slow progression into third decade		
Canavan's disease	Increased head size which may become less striking later, hypotonia, arrested development, blindness, spasticity, decerebrate posture, myoclonic seizures		
Alexander's disease	Increased head size, progressive loss of skills, seizures, spasticity, brain stem signs	Dementia, psychologic disturbance	

Fig. 5.2 Clinical features of leukodystrophies.

Etiologic classification of leukodystrophies

Type of disorder	Disease	Mechanism	Inheritance
Lysosomal	Krabbe's disease	Galactocerebroside–β –galactosidase deficiency: the gene maps to chromosome 14q31	AR
	Metachromatic leukodystrophy	Aryl sulfatase A deficiency, due to a variety of mutations on chromosome 22, including deletions/splice mutations/substitutions	AR, very rarely AD
Peroxisomal	Adrenoleukodystrophy/adrenomyeloneuropathy	Single peroxisomal enzyme defect of an ATP-binding cassette transporter reduces the capacity to form the coenzyme A derivative of VLCFA: the gene maps to Xq28	X-linked, also in manifesting female carriers
	Neonatal adrenoleukodystrophy	Defective peroxisomal assembly results in absent or severely reduced numbers of peroxisomes and loss of multiple peroxisomal functions. In some patients, disease is due to peroxisome receptor-1 (PXR1) defect which maps to 12p13. Several defects of fatty acid β-oxidation cause similar disease but without loss of peroxisomes	AR
Myelin structural protein	Pelizaeus–Merzbacher disease (PMD)	Deficient or abnormal myelin proteolipid protein, results from mutations/deletions/amplification of Xq21.33-22	X-linked (occasional female cases)
Amino-acidopathy	Canavan's disease	Defective aspartoacylase activity	AR
DNA repair	Cockayne's disease	Defective DNA repair	
Other	Alexander's disease	? astrocytopathy	Usually sporadic, one reported family
	Sudanophil leukodystrophies with various associated features, or with non-specific findings	Unknown	Some are familial

AR: autosomal recessive   AD: autosomal dominant   VLCFA: very long chain fatty acids

Fig. 5.3 Etiologic classification of leukodystrophies.

DIFFERENTIAL DIAGNOSIS OF LEUKODYSTROPHY

- Immunogenic demyelination (see chapters 19 and 20); such as multiple sclerosis and other inflammatory demyelinating diseases: (acute hemorrhagic leukoencephalitis)
- Progressive multifocal leukoencephalopathy (see chapter 13)
- Demyelination associated with systemic disorders; such as central pontine myelinolysis (see chapter 22) and Marchiafava–Bignami syndrome (see chapter 21).

Summary of histologic and histochemical findings in leukodystrophies

	Histology	Histochemistry	Ultrastructure	Other features
Krabbe's disease	Multinucleated macrophages/globoid cells	PAS++ macrophages	Straight or curved tubular inclusions	
Metachromatic leukodystrophy (MLD)	LFB+, PAS+ macrophages in white matter; neuronal storage in basal ganglia, dentate nucleus, and brain stem	Metachromasia (with acidified cresyl violet)	Prismatic inclusions, tuffstone inclusions, zebra-like bodies	Sulfatide stored in kidney tubules, and in urinary sediment
Adrenoleukodystrophy (ALD)	Perivascular inflammation	Sudan++ PAS++ macrophages	Needle-like trilamellar inclusions	Swollen striated adrenocortical cells
Neonatal adrenoleukodystrophy (ALD)	As in ALD, plus cerebral malformation	Sudan± PAS++ macrophages	As in ALD	
Pelizaeus–Merzbacher disease (PMD)	Discontinuous myelin loss, or near total dysmyelination; myelin in peripheral nerves spared	Sudan± macrophages	Segmental demyelination	
Canavan's disease	Spongy white matter, abundant Alzheimer I astrocytes		In cortex, swollen astrocytes contain very long mitochondria with ladder-like cristae	Macrocephaly
Alexander's disease	Cavitation, Rosenthal fibers in glial processes, and small eosinophilic intracytoplasmic bodies		Osmiophilic densities coated with intermediate (glial) filaments	Macrocephaly
Cockayne's disease	Discontinuous myelin loss, calcification, microcephaly	Sudan± macrophages		Dysmorphic, premature aging
Orthochromatic leukodystrophy (OLD) with pigmented glia and macrophages	Pigmented inclusions in glia and macrophages	Sudan+ PAS+ macrophages and glia; also Perls'+ and Masson–Fontana+	Multilamellar inclusions and fingerprint bodies	
OLD with cavitation and oligodendrocyte proliferation	Massive cavities, excessive numbers of oligodendroglia	Sudan+ macrophages		
OLD with meningeal angiomatosis	Meningeal venous angiomatosis	Sudan+ macrophages		
OLD with calcification	Flaky myelin loss, calcifications in white matter and basal ganglia, microcephaly	Sudan+ macrophages		
OLD not otherwise specified	Myelin breakdown	Sudan+ macrophages		

± weak, + moderate, ++ strong, or () variable staining, in frozen sections

Fig. 5.4 Summary of histologic and histochemical findings in leukodystrophies.

PELIZAEUS–MERZBACHER DISEASE
MACROSCOPIC APPEARANCES
These vary in accordance with the clinical phenotype; brains of the connate form with early death are usually normal in weight, but in the classic form prolonged survival may be associated with pronounced atrophy. On slicing the cerebrum, the white matter may look unremarkable in the connate cases, but generally appears gray and firm with a blurred gray–white matter interface (**Fig. 5.5 a, b**). Cerebellar atrophy can be marked. Involvement of brain stem and cord tracts renders them a dull yellow, contrasting with the whiteness of the preserved peripheral myelin in cranial and spinal roots.

MICROSCOPIC APPEARANCES
Myelin staining may be absent (connate variant) or severely reduced but leaving a flaky or tigroid pattern where residual myelin islets have a tendency to hug blood vessels (**Figs 5.5–5.7**). Axons are relatively preserved, though oligodendroglia are reduced and astrocytosis is marked. All central myelin is affected while spinal and cranial nerve roots and peripheral nerves are normal (**Fig. 5.8**). Sudanophilic lipid is sparse and contained in perivascular macrophages. Cerebellar cortical degeneration is quite common (**Fig. 5.9**).

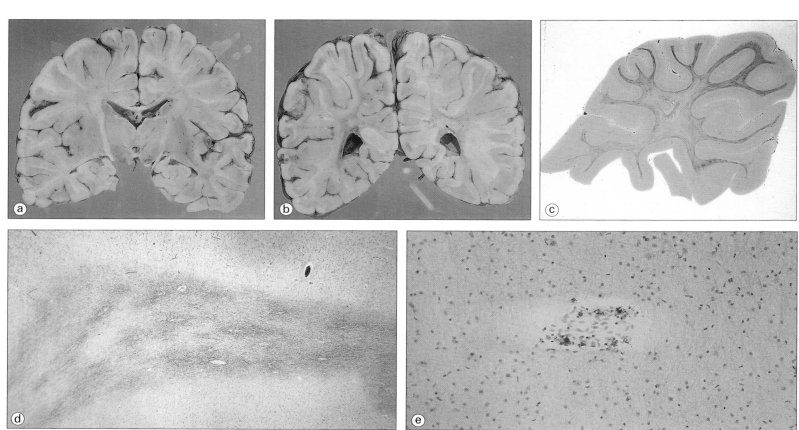

Fig. 5.5 Pelizaeus–Merzbacher disease. (a) and **(b)** Sections of the brain from a 15-year-old male with a typical slowly progressive clinical disorder. Much of the cerebral white matter appears gray and granular, but the U-fibers are relatively spared. The internal capsules and corpus callosum are streaked with gray. **(a)** Coronal section through the basal ganglia **(b)** Coronal section through the parieto-occipital region. **(c)** In the occipital lobe from this patient there is only scant myelin staining. (Luxol fast blue/cresyl violet) **(d)** At higher magnification the white matter takes on a tigroid appearance as islands of residual myelin surround blood vessels. (Luxol fast blue/cresyl violet) **(e)** In this frozen section there is only sparse orthochromatic lipid. (Oil red O)

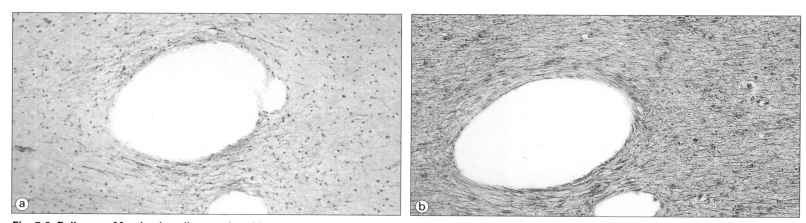

Fig. 5.6 Pelizaeus–Merzbacher disease. As with other leukodystrophies there is a relatively spared population of axons in demyelinated regions. **(a)** Occipital white matter stained for myelin. (Luxol fast blue/cresyl violet) **(b)** An adjacent serial section stained for axons. (Glees)

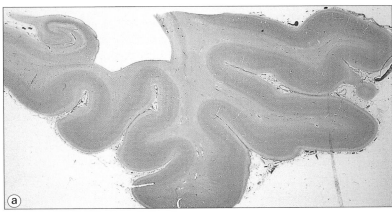

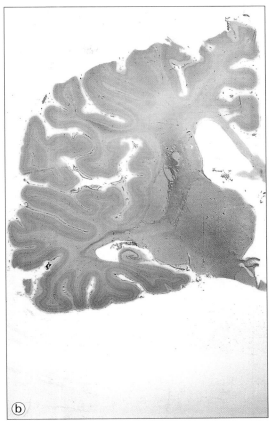

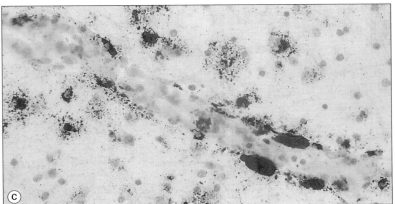

Fig. 5.7 **Myelin and sudanophilic lipid in Pelizaeus–Merzbacher disease. (a)** and **(b)** Coronal sections from a six-month-old child with the connate form of Pelizaeus–Merzbacher disease. Myelin is demonstrable in the internal capsule and optic radiation only. (Luxol fast blue/cresyl violet) **(a)** Temporal lobe. **(b)** Coronal section at mid-thalamic level. **(c)** Moderate amounts of orthochromatic lipid can be demonstrated. (Frozen section, Oil red O)

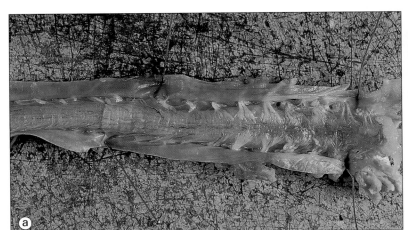

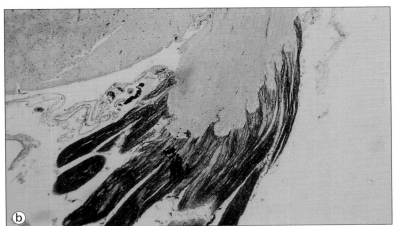

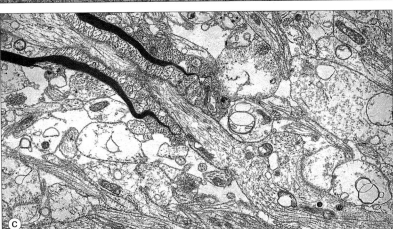

Fig. 5.8 **Sparing of myelin in peripheral nerves in Pelizaeus–Merzbacher disease.** This is a characteristic finding. **(a)** Anterior aspect of the spinal cord showing the marked contrast between the normal white roots and the gray (demyelinated) cord. **(b)** Lateral pons showing the fifth cranial nerve root. Compare the normal peripheral myelin with the umyelinated central structures. (Loyez) **(c)** Ultrastructural examination of the white matter from a cerebral biopsy showing segmental demyelination. The myelin stops abruptly at a heminode, leaving a naked axon continuing through the neuropil.

CANAVAN'S DISEASE
MACROSCOPIC APPEARANCES

Megalencephaly and increased brain weight may occur in the first two years of life, but become less apparent in older patients. At brain cut there is a very poor distinction between cerebral gray and white matter (**Fig. 5.10 a, b**). The soft gelatinous white matter does not cavitate, but the involved subcortical U-fibers may sink below the surface of the brain slices.

MICROSCOPIC APPEARANCES

Extensive vacuolation of the white matter, which is particularly prominent at the deep gray–white matter junction, is associated with diffuse myelin loss(**Fig. 5.10**). Although cortical neurons are normal there are numerous Alzheimer type II astrocytes within the cortex. The vacuoles measure up to 100 μm, and appear empty. There is no sudanophilia and peripheral nerves appear unaffected. Ultrastructural examination reveals swelling of astrocyte processes and splitting of thin myelin lamellae in the white matter. Cortical changes include enlarged pale astrocytes in deeper cortical layers that contain abnormally elongated mitochondria with abnormal ladder-like cristae, unique to Canavan's disease.

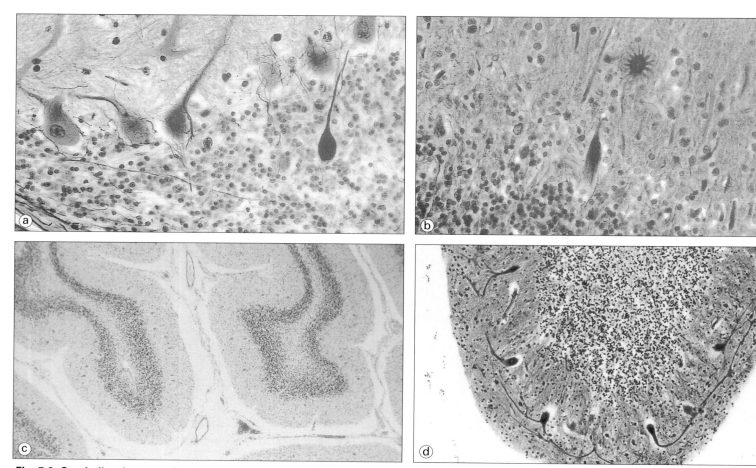

Fig. 5.9 Cerebellar degeneration in Pelizaeus–Merzbacher disease.
Cerebellar degeneration is common in Pelizaeus–Merzbacher disease.
(a) An example of cortical degeneration with loss of Purkinje cells and formation of axonal 'torpedoes'. **(b)** Surviving Purkinje cells have abnormal dendritic swellings — 'asteroid' bodies. (Glees silver impregnation) **(c)** An example of granule cell deficiency and malpositioned Purkinje cells in the molecular layer. **(d)** The ectopic Purkinje cells have 'weeping willow' dendrites. (Glees silver impregnation)

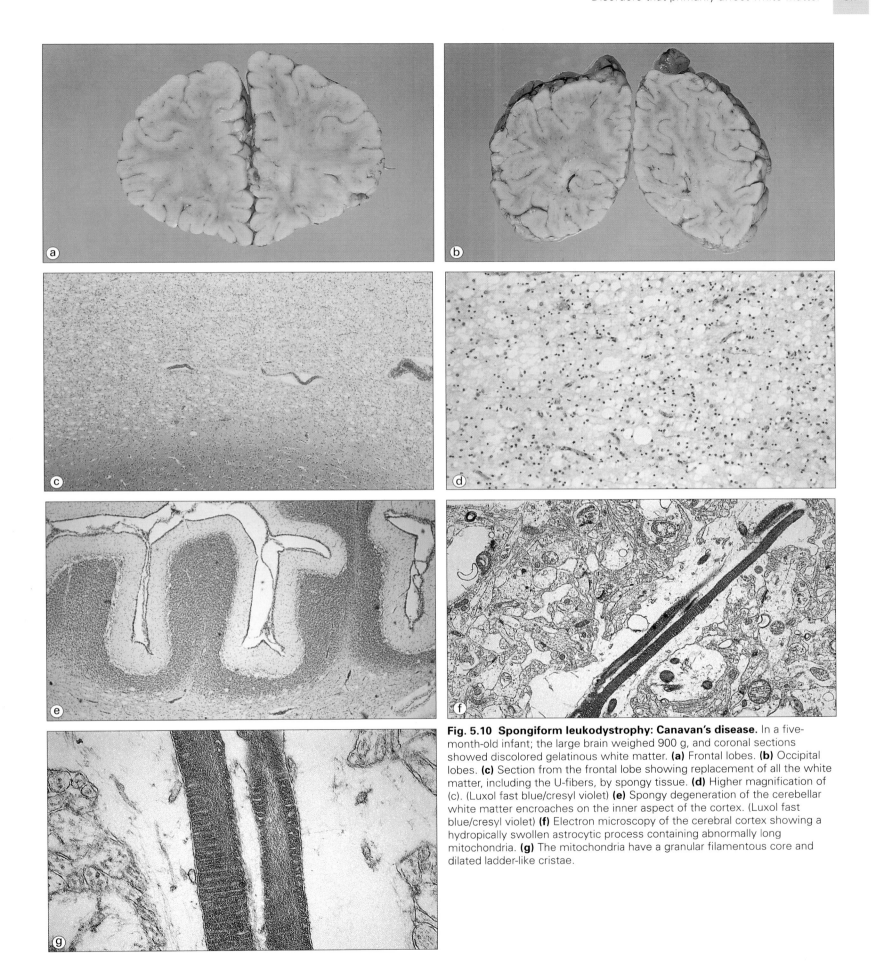

Fig. 5.10 Spongiform leukodystrophy: Canavan's disease. In a five-month-old infant; the large brain weighed 900 g, and coronal sections showed discolored gelatinous white matter. **(a)** Frontal lobes. **(b)** Occipital lobes. **(c)** Section from the frontal lobe showing replacement of all the white matter, including the U-fibers, by spongy tissue. **(d)** Higher magnification of (c). (Luxol fast blue/cresyl violet) **(e)** Spongy degeneration of the cerebellar white matter encroaches on the inner aspect of the cortex. (Luxol fast blue/cresyl violet) **(f)** Electron microscopy of the cerebral cortex showing a hydropically swollen astrocytic process containing abnormally long mitochondria. **(g)** The mitochondria have a granular filamentous core and dilated ladder-like cristae.

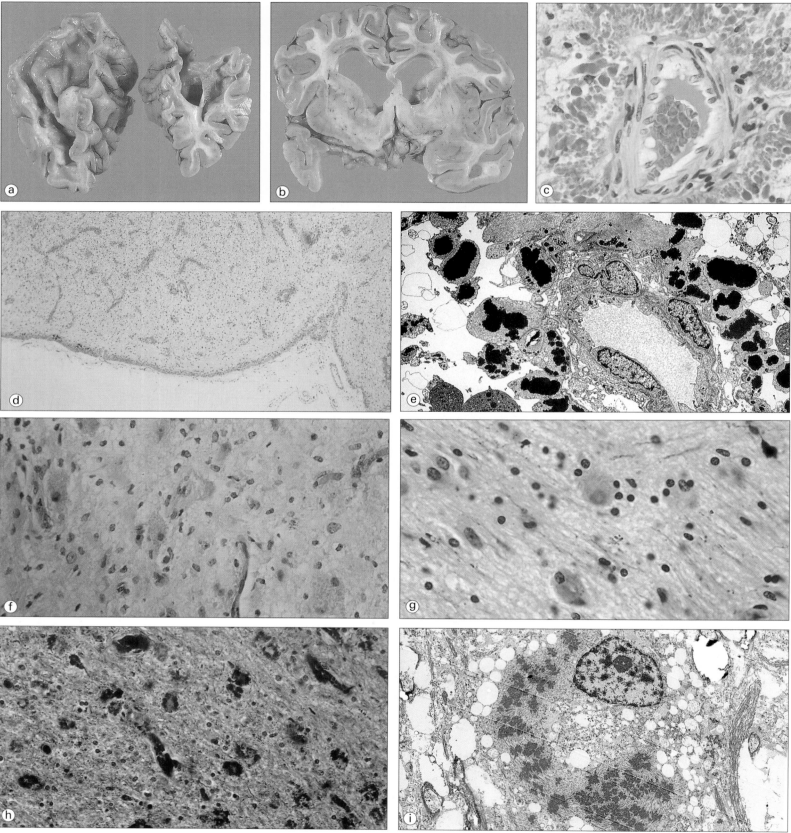

Fig. 5.11 Alexander's disease. (a) and **(b)** Gray gelatinous and collapsed periventricular white matter more posteriorly **(a)**. Coronal sections of the cerebrum. There is cavitation of the white matter anteriorly **(b)**. **(c)** Rosenthal fibers are eosinophilic club-shaped bodies. Typically, they are clustered around blood vessels. **(d)** Rosenthal fibers also accumulate close to the pia. Large numbers are present in this demyelinated pyramid in the ventral medulla. **(e)** Ultrastructurally, the perivascular bodies are composed of astrocytic processes distended by irregular osmiophilic densities covered by glial filaments. **(f)** Astrocyte cell bodies frequently contain small inclusions, which are smaller than typical Rosenthal fibers, but ultrastructurally and tinctorially similar. **(g)** These smaller inclusions stain in a similar fashion to Rosenthal fibers. (Luxol fast blue/cresyl violet) **(h)** Within the astrocyte cell body the small inclusions often have a signet ring appearance. (Phosphotungstic acid/hematoxylin) **(i)** This shape is paralleled by the ultrastructural arrangement of osmiophilic densities.

ALEXANDER'S DISEASE
MACROSCOPIC APPEARANCES

The brain is usually, though not always, enlarged. The cerebral white matter is diffusely discolored, very soft and gelatinous, and often cavitated, especially in the frontal lobes (**Fig 5.11a, b**).

MICROSCOPIC APPEARANCES

Diffuse demyelination leading to rarefaction of CNS white matter, with an abundance of Rosenthal fibers clustered most densely around blood vessels and in subpial and subependymal regions, is the principal feature (**Fig. 5.11**). All white matter is at risk, but the cerebellum is less often affected. As in other pathologic processes the Rosenthal fibers are irreg-

ularly elongated or rounded, hyaline eosinophilic bodies which ultrastructurally take the form of dense round osmiophilic structures coated with thickened glial fibrils within astrocytic processes. Similar but smaller inclusions are also present in the cell bodies of astrocytes, surrounding the nucleus, an appearance apparently restricted to Alexander's disease and therefore of diagnostic utility. Although megalencephaly is a feature up to two years of age with some increase in brain weight, there is a decline to normal weight with longer survival.

OTHER LEUKODYSTROPHIES
MACROSCOPIC AND MICROSCOPIC APPEARANCES

Apart from Cockayne's syndrome, the etiologies of these rare conditions are totally unknown, and so morphologic classification remains paramount (**Figs 5.12–5.15**). Although the tigroid demyelination in Cockayne's syndrome mimics Pelizaeus–Merzbacher there are many differences in this etiologically distinct disorder, notably profound microcephaly and vasocentric calcification in the cerebral cortex and basal ganglia.

Virtually all the other leukodystrophies may be loosely described as sudanophilic as they demonstrate orthochromatic myelin degradation products that are stained with sudan dyes in cryostat sections. All have been reported in families and are presumed to be autosomal recessive. Such is their rarity that their nomenclature is merely a cataloging of their salient morphologic findings. Most readily recognizable is the form with pigmented macrophages which discolor the white matter green. This results from massive lipofuscin deposition in astrocytes and microglia. Also striking microscopically is the association of massive cavitation of the central cerebral white matter with an excessive number of oligodendroglia not just confined to the demyelinated areas or surrounding cavities but also in apparently well-myelinated tracts. Other varieties include cases associated with profuse meningeal angiomatosis and those with no helpful differentiating features.

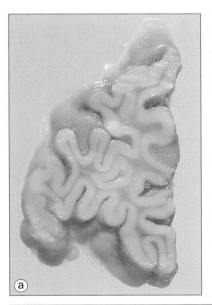
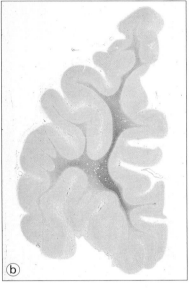

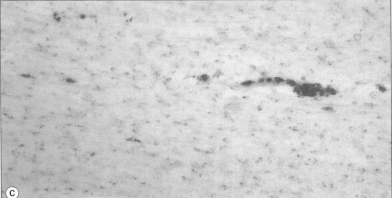

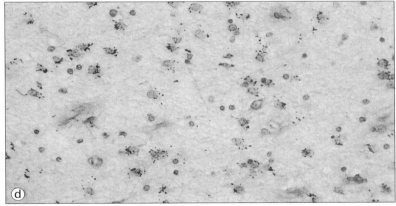

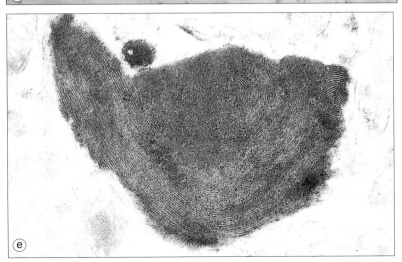

Fig. 5.12 Leukodystrophy with pigmented glia and macrophages (van Bogaert and Nissen disease). **(a)** Coronal section from the frontal pole showing diffuse white matter disease. **(b)** Myelin-stained counterpart of (a). **(c)** Histochemically, there is scanty lipid deposition. (Frozen section, Sharlach-R) **(d)** There is a positive reaction for melanin. (Masson–Fontana) **(e)** Inclusions within the macrophages are multilamellar and include fingerprint profiles.

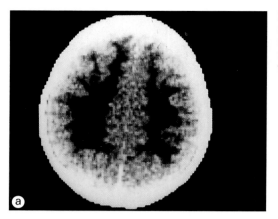

Fig. 5.13 Leukodystrophy with cavitation and oligodendroglial excess (familial example). (a) Computerized tomographic scan indicates massive white matter cavitation in the younger brother. **(b)** Coronal slices from the six-year-old sister's brain show subtotal destruction of the cerebral white matter. **(c)** Histology of the residual white matter around the cavities shows markedly hypercellular tissue made up largely of oligodendrocytes.

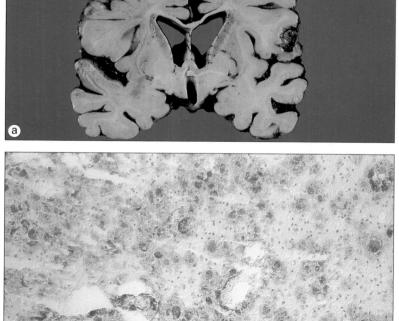

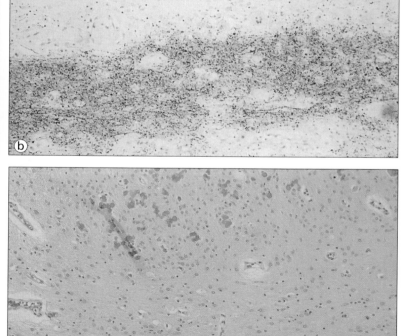

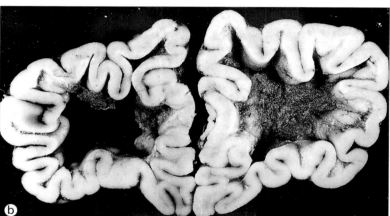

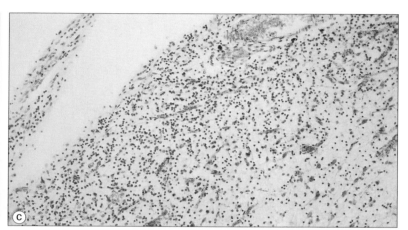

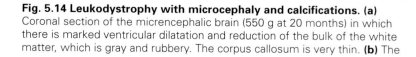

Fig. 5.14 Leukodystrophy with microcephaly and calcifications. (a) Coronal section of the micrencephalic brain (550 g at 20 months) in which there is marked ventricular dilatation and reduction of the bulk of the white matter, which is gray and rubbery. The corpus callosum is very thin. **(b)** The white matter shows poorly stained myelin. (Luxol fast blue/cresyl violet) **(c)** In a frozen section the white matter contains plenty of sudanophilic lipid. **(d)** The white matter also contains scattered calcifications and is markedly gliotic.

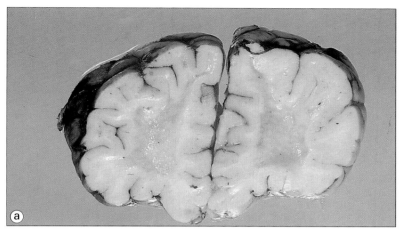

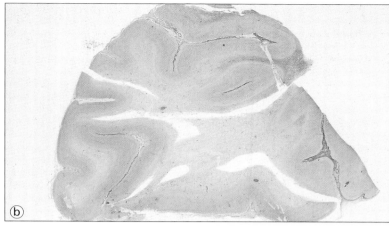

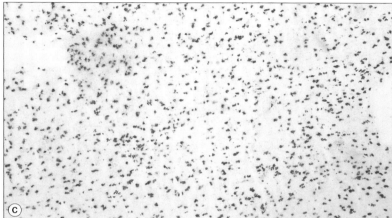

Fig. 5.15 Sudanophilic leukodystrophy with no other specific features (familial example). Despite extensive clinical, biochemical and morphologic examinations, some cases of both familial and sporadic sudanophilic leukodystrophy cannot be classified and remain a major challenge for neuropathologists. **(a)** Coronal section through the frontal lobes of a nine-month-old child showing brown gelatinous white matter. **(b)** Histology reveals a lack of myelin staining. (Luxol fast blue/cresyl violet) **(c)** There are prominent orthochromatic lipid deposits. (Oil red O)

REFERENCES

Lake BD. (1997) Lysosomal and peroxisomal disorders. In *Greenfield's Neuropathology*, (6th ed) Graham DI and Lantos PL (eds) London:Edward Arnold, pp. 658–754.

Friede RL. (1989) *Developmental Neuropathology*, Berlin:Springer-Verlag.

Pridmore CL, Baraitser M, Harding B, Boyd SG, Kendall B and Brett EM. (1993) Alexander's Disease: clues to diagnosis. *J Child Neurol* 35: 727–741.

Harding BN, Malcolm S, Ellis D and Wilson J. (1995) A case of Pelizaeus-Merzbacher disease showing increased dosage of the proteolipid protein gene. *Neuropath and Appl Neurobiol* 21: 111–115.

Gray F *et al.* (1987) Pigmentary type of orthochromatic leukodystrophy (OLD): a new case with ultrastructural and biochemical study. *J Neuropathol Exp Neurol* 46: 585–596.

Graveleau P, Gray F, Plas J, Graveleau J and Brion S. (1985) Cavitary orthochromatic leukodystrophy with oligodendroglial changes. A sporadic adult case. *Rev Neurol Paris.* 141: 713–718.

6 *Neurodegenerative disorders of gray matter in childhood*

A variety of rare neurodegenerative disorders principally affecting gray matter presents in childhood. In most, the precise etiology remains uncertain, but virtually all are presumed to have a metabolic basis. For convenience they are grouped by their most characteristic regional involvement: cerebral cortex, basal ganglia, cerebellum, brainstem, or spinal cord.

CEREBRAL CORTEX

ALPERS–HUTTENLOCHER SYNDROME OR PROGRESSIVE NEURONAL DEGENERATION OF CHILDHOOD (PNDC)

This is a progressive and uniformly fatal disorder of disputed etiology. It primarily involves cerebral cortex and is usually combined with a characteristic hepatopathy.

MACROSCOPIC APPEARANCES

Lesions may be minimal, patchy, or extensive (**Fig. 6.1**). In affected regions the cortical ribbon is thin, granular, and brown, and even dehiscent in some poorly fixed brains. The calcarine cortex is often picked out in a remarkably selective and characteristic way. Rarely, there is softening of the occipital white matter.

MICROSCOPIC APPEARANCES

Histologic abnormalities are more widespread than expected from the macroscopic appearances. The patchy lesions do not conform to vascular territories or watershed zones and show a graded intensification and extension of the degenerative process through the depth of the cortical gray matter. Mild superficial spongiosis gives way to increasing sponginess, neuronal loss, and gliosis extending down through the cortex. In severe lesions, the whole ribbon is replaced by a narrow remnant of hypertrophic astrocytes devoid of nerve cells (**Fig. 6.2**). Neutral fat may be deposited in considerable amounts. Lesions may be symmetric or asymmetric, but there is a striking predilection for the striate cortex. Secondary changes are found in the white matter. Other variable findings include hippocampal sclerosis, cerebellar cortical infarcts, spinal cord tract degeneration, and spongiosis and gliosis in the thalamus (**Fig. 6.3**), amygdala, substantia nigra, and dentate nuclei.

Hepatic pathology

Nearly all patients show characteristic changes in the liver: the hepatocytes undergo severe microvesicular fatty or oncocytic change (**Fig. 6.4**). There are hepatocyte necrosis, diffuse haphazard bile duct proliferation, and bridging fibrosis, with disorganization and regeneration that amount to cirrhosis at one end of the histologic spectrum (**Fig. 6.5**), or end-stage collapse and fibrosis at the other.

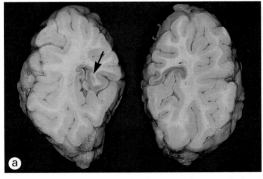
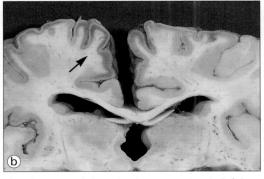
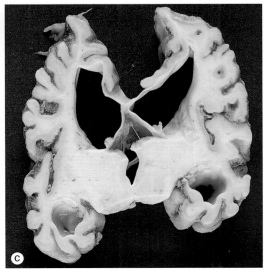

Fig. 6.1 Alpers–Huttenlocher syndrome. Selective involvement of the calcarine cortex is a helpful diagnostic pointer. **(a)** In this child, coronal sections of occipital lobe show the primary visual cortex in both hemispheres delineated by granularity and brown discoloration (arrow). **(b)** Similar discrete areas of cortical thinning and discoloration are present in the posterior frontal cortex at midthalamic level (arrow). **(c)** Although cortical lesions are usually patchy, in extreme cases the whole cortical ribbon may be diffusely and uniformly shrunken. In addition, there is ventricular dilatation, some thalamic atrophy, and marked shrinkage of Ammon's horns.

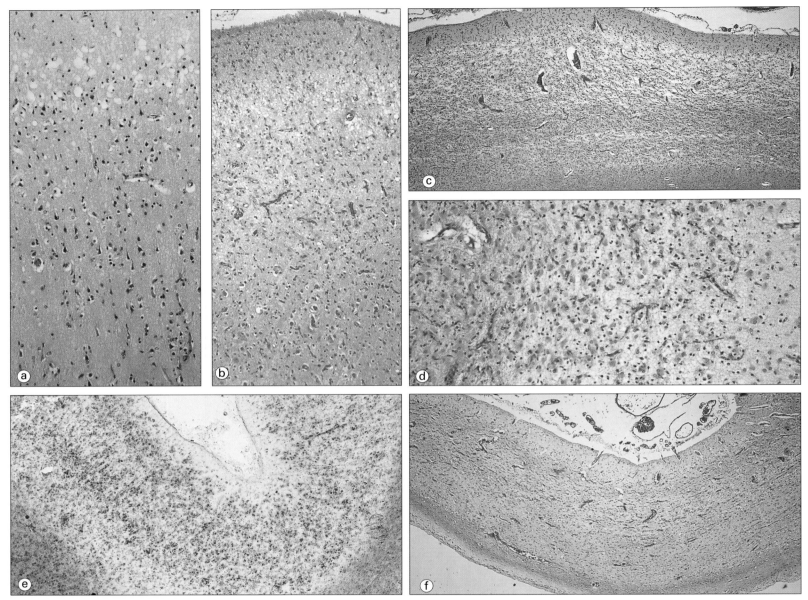

Fig. 6.2 Alpers–Huttenlocher syndrome. (a) The mildest histologic changes consist of a fine spongiosis in the superficial cortical layers. **(b)** Neuronal loss and gliosis gradually extend more deeply through the cortical ribbon. **(c)** Eventually the whole cortex is replaced by hypertrophic astrocytes. This shows the striate cortex, which is especially prone to such severe destruction. **(d)** The neurons and neuropil of the striate cortex are entirely replaced by a cystic meshwork of glial processes emanating from plump hypertrophic astrocytes. **(e)** Massive amounts of neutral fat can be deposited in the degenerating cortex. (Frozen section; Sharlach-R) **(f)** The chronic end stage of this process is a thin poorly cellular gliotic remnant. This shows striate cortex from the same case as in Fig. 6.1c.

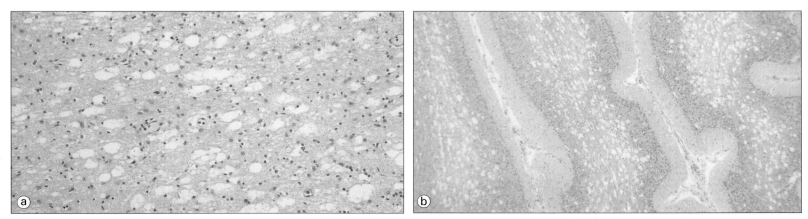

Fig. 6.3 Alpers–Huttenlocher syndrome. (a) There may be prominent neuronal loss and spongy change in the thalamus. **(b)** Occasionally there is marked spongiosis of the cerebellar white matter.

ALPERS–HUTTENLOCHER SYNDROME

Typical course:

- normal birth and neonatal period
- insidious onset of developmental delay in infancy
- failure to thrive
- vomiting
- floppiness
- sudden onset of intractable seizures with protean manifestations, heralding a rapidly progressive downhill course
- variable appearance of clinical liver disorder, sometimes only in terminal stage
- death usually before three years of age

Rare atypical manifestations include:

- prolonged survival to end of second decade
- catastrophic epilepsy without prodrome and very rapid course
- late presentation after four years of age, even in early adulthood

Laboratory investigations:

- computerized tomography: low-density areas in occipital and temporal lobes and progressive cerebral atrophy
- electroencephalogram: characteristic, very slow activity of very high amplitude mixed with low amplitude polyspikes
- electroretinogram: normal while visual evoked potentials become abnormal, usually asymmetrically
- liver function tests: may be significantly deranged, even before seizures commence

DIFFERENTIAL DIAGNOSIS OF ALPERS–HUTTENLOCHER SYNDROME IN THE CONTEXT OF EPILEPSY WITH PROGRESSIVE CEREBRAL ATROPHY

The following discriminating features should be sought:
- **Hypoxic–ischemic encephalopathy**: predilection for vascular boundary zones, relative preservation of gyral crests; striate cortex spared.
- **Hemiatrophy and hemiconvulsions**: unilateral with similar features to hypoxic ischemic encephalopathy.
- **Brain damage post status epilepticus**: ischemic cell change, laminar intensification; striate cortex spared.
- **Hepatic encephalopathy**: involvement of basal ganglia; cavitation of gray–white matter interface.
- **Neuronal storage disorders**: neuronal abnormalities
- **Encephalitis**: inflammatory infiltrate.
- **Rasmussen's disease**: inflammatory infiltrate.

ETIOLOGY OF ALPERS–HUTTENLOCHER SYNDROME

- Prominent spongiosis prompted speculation of a kinship with Creutzfeldt–Jakob disease but one apparently successful animal transmission experiment has not been duplicated.
- A strong familial tendency (the majority of cases occur in siblings) suggests autosomal recessive inheritance.
- There is evidence of mitochondrial dysfunction in some patients.

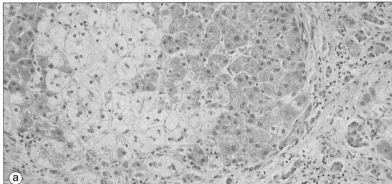

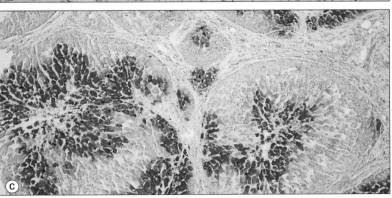

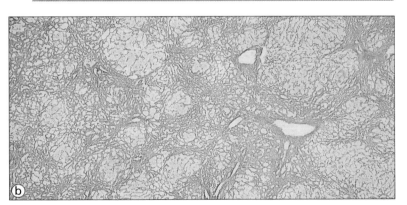

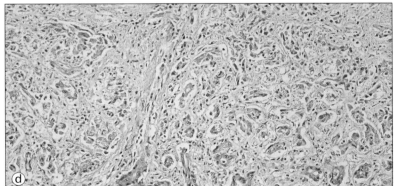

Fig. 6.4 Alpers–Huttenlocher syndrome: liver pathology. Histologic changes in the liver are characteristic and essential for a confident diagnosis. **(a)** The principal features are hepatic steatosis and oncocytic change along with hepatocyte necrosis and a profuse and haphazard proliferation of bile ductules. **(b)** Fibrosis and nodular regeneration often give rise to a cirrhotic pattern. **(c)** Fat may be heavily deposited within the regenerative nodules. (Oil red O, Frozen section) **(d)** In some patients regeneration does not occur and the liver is replaced by dense fibrous tissue and irregular bile ductules. Note the bile retention.

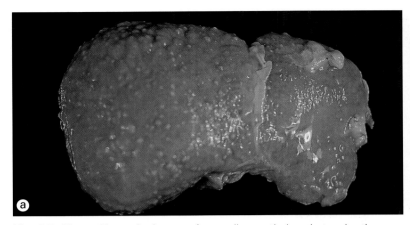

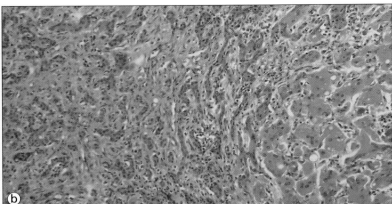

Fig. 6.5 Alpers–Huttenlocher syndrome: liver pathology in two brothers who died from PNDC. One of these brothers received valproate therapy, but both showed typical liver pathology. **(a)** Macroscopic appearance of the finely nodular cirrhotic liver of one brother. **(b)** Liver histology shows the typical changes of PNDC in the other brother. The role of drug therapy and in particular valproate toxicity in the pathogenesis of PNDC is controversial.

BASAL GANGLIA

Progressive disorders primarily affecting the basal ganglia include a number of eponymous neurodegenerative diseases whose morphologic changes overlap to some extent with certain well characterized inborn errors of metabolism.

HOLOTOPISTIC STRIATAL NECROSIS (FAMILIAL STRIATAL DEGENERATION)

This condition causes a clinicopathologic syndrome that resembles Huntington's disease but lacks the relevant genetic defect.

MACROSCOPIC AND MICROSCOPIC APPEARANCES

Two patterns are observed (**Fig. 6.6**):
- Softening and cavitation of the caudate and putamen due to necrosis with macrophage infiltration.

- Atrophy of the corpus striatum and loss of neurons with gliosis. Both patterns may occur in familial cases. Neocortical and cerebellar degeneration may also be found.

HALLERVORDEN–SPATZ DISEASE
MACROSCOPIC AND MICROSCOPIC APPEARANCES

Yellow–brown discoloration of the globus pallidus and substantia nigra are evident (**Fig. 6.7**). Neuronal loss, gliosis, and deposition of iron pigment occur bilaterally in the internal segment of the globus pallidus and the pars reticularis of the substantia nigra. There is also a more widespread distribution of swollen axons (spheroids). Neurochemical studies indicate abnormal cysteine metabolism in the pallidum and it is suggested that cysteine chelates iron, which in turn induces tissue damage mediated by free radicals (see also Neuroaxonal Dystrophy, in chapter 33).

DIFFERENTIAL DIAGNOSIS OF BASAL GANGLIA DISORDERS IN CHILDHOOD

The following discriminating clinicopathological features should be sought.
- **Holotopistic striatal necrosis**: acute necrosis or slow degeneration; recessive inheritance.
- **Hallervorden–Spatz disease**: neuroaxonal spheroids and iron pigment in pallidum and substantia nigra.
- **Leigh's disease**: foci of partial necrosis with vascular proliferation in basal ganglia, brain stem and cord; mitochondrial cytopathy; recessive inheritance.
- **Wilson's disease**: striatal, retinal, and hepatic degeneration.
- **Juvenile Huntington's disease**: striatal degeneration with or without cortical pathology; dominant inheritance; gene abnormality.
- **Juvenile Parkinson's disease**: postencephalitic damage to substantia nigra.
- **Glutaric acidemia**: striatal degeneration; specific biochemical abnormality.
- **Propionic acidemia**: striatal gliosis and/or marbling; specific biochemical abnormality.
- **Methylmalonic acidemia**: infarcts; hemorrhages; specific biochemical abnormality.
- **Urea cycle disorders**: gliosis; neuronal loss with or without cortical atrophy; specific biochemical abnormalities.

HOLOTOPISTIC STRIATAL NECROSIS

- Some cases are familial.
- Onset may be acute (following a febrile illness) or insidious.
- Symptoms include choreoathetosis, abnormal eye movements, seizures, and mental retardation.

HALLEVORDEN–SPATZ DISEASE

- Hallevorden–Spatz disease is a progressive autosomal recessive neurologic disorder that usually presents in the second half of the first decade.
- Pyramidal and extrapyramidal features, principally dystonia, rigidity, spasticity, abnormal speech, and aphonia, are associated with mental deterioration, dementia, and occasionally optic atrophy and pigmentary retinopathy.
- Rarely onset is in adulthood.
- Magnetic resonance imaging may show hypointensity in the pallidum and substantia nigra.
- Survival averages 10 years.

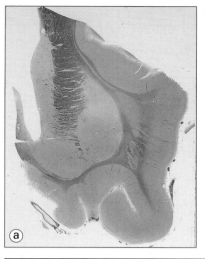

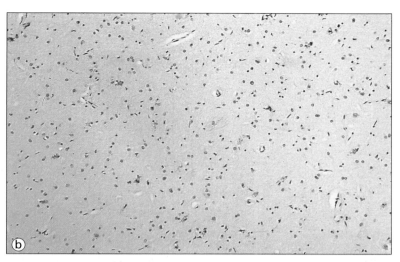

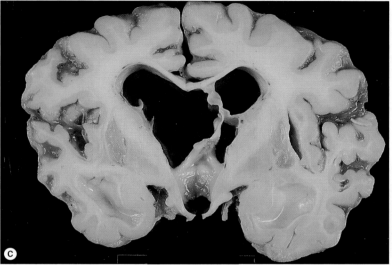

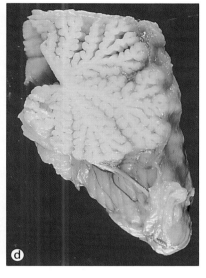

Fig. 6.6 Holotopistic striatal necrosis. (a) Histologic section demonstrating shrinkage and pallor of the dorsal halves of both caudate and putamen. **(b)** Marked neuronal loss and gliosis in the striatum. **(c)** In another patient the caudate nuclei are atrophic brown crescents and the putamina are replaced by cavities outlined by grayish membranes. Ventricular dilatation and cortical atrophy are pronounced. **(d)** In this child there is also cerebellar cortical atrophy, seen here in the vermis.

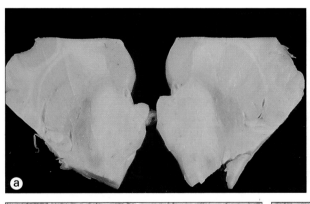

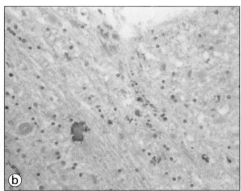

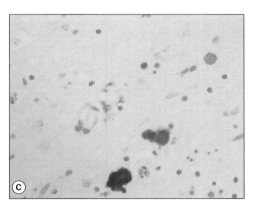

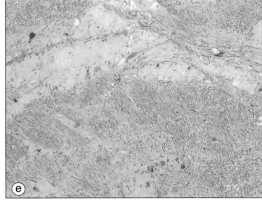

Fig. 6.7 Hallervorden–Spatz disease. (a) Coronal sections at the level of the anterior thalamus demonstrate a remarkable yellow–brown pigmentation in both pallida. **(b)** Microscopically, there are hematoxyphilic mineralizations, eosinophil axonal spheroids, and deposits of brown pigment in the pallidum. **(c)** These deposits stain positively for iron. (Perls' stain) **(d)** Neuroaxonal spheroids demonstrated with antibody to phosphorylated neurofilaments, and mineral concretions (stained blue) within the pallidum. **(e)** Neuroaxonal spheroids, labeled here with an antibody to neurofilament protein, are also plentiful in the gray bridges between caudate and putamen.

CEREBELLUM

MENKES' DISEASE

MENKES' DISEASE

- Seizures commence at 6–8 weeks of age; developmental progress and growth are then slowed, with retardation becoming obvious by the third month.
- Abnormal hair, which looks like steel wool (microscopically twisted, frayed, and nodular with broken ends).
- Progressive deterioration with increasing spasticity, seizures, ataxia, failure to thrive, and frequent infections.
- Death by six years of age despite treatment with parenteral copper.
- Low serum or plasma copper and copper oxidase (ceruloplasmin) concentrations.

MACROSCOPIC AND MICROSCOPIC APPEARANCES

Macroscopic features include marked microcephaly, quite frequent subdural hematomas, and a variable degree of cerebellar atrophy with narrowed folia.

Microscopically there are neuronal loss and myelin deficiency in the temporal cortex and hippocampus. In the cerebellum marked depletion of the granular layer is combined with displacement of Purkinje cells, which show 'torpedoes', dendritic distortions, and somal sprouting (**Fig. 6.8**).

ATAXIA–TELANGIECTASIA

ATAXIA–TELANGIECTASIA

- Normal early development precedes gait and truncal ataxia, which becomes apparent when the child starts to walk.
- Manifestations are titubation, dysarthria, and extrapyramidal features, and rarely choreo-atheosis or dystonia.
- Independent walking is lost by 12 years of age.
- Telangiectasias of conjunctivae are seen after three years of age.
- Skin lesions develop later in sun-exposed areas.
- Increased incidence of respiratory infection is related to abnormal humoral and cellular immunity.
- Increased frequency of neoplasia, particularly T cell leukemia and lymphoma, is evident while malignancy is common in relatives, notably breast carcinoma in mothers.
- Laboratory investigations reveal low IgA, high levels of α-fetoprotein, and enhanced *in vitro* hypersensitivity to ionizing radiation.

MACROSCOPIC AND MICROSCOPIC APPEARANCES

There are cerebellar cortical atrophy with a severe loss of Purkinje and granule cells (**Fig. 6.9**) and posterior column degeneration in the spinal cord. Systemic features include hypoplasia of thymus, lymphoid tissue, and gonads (see also chapter 29).

CARBOHYDRATE-DEFICIENT GLYCOPROTEIN SYNDROME TYPE 1 (CDG 1)

The carbohydrate-deficient glycoprotein syndromes are a recently delineated group of disorders associated with hypoglycosilation of glycoproteins. The principle condition is carbohydrate-deficient glycoprotein syndrome type I, an autosomal recessive multisystem disease with early, severe nervous system involvement, often fatal in early infancy.

CARBOHYDRATE-DEFICIENT GLYCOPROTEIN SYNDROME TYPE 1

- Predominant problems are failure to thrive, hypotonia, growth retardation, and developmental delay.
- Mild facial dysmorphism, inverted nipples, abnormal fat pads over the buttocks, and fatty streaks on the lower limbs are evident on examination.
- Hepatic failure, cardiac failure, and multiple effusions may be present.
- Neurologic signs include axial hypotonia, weakness, and cerebellar ataxia.
- If patients do not die during this infantile phase, they survive into late infancy and childhood showing developmental delay and motor impairment, ataxia, peripheral neuropathy, and epilepsy.
- Diagnosis is best achieved by agarose isoelectric focusing of serum transferrin, which separates bands containing different numbers of sialic acid residues (normal transferrin has 4).

MACROSCOPIC AND MICROSCOPIC APPEARANCES

Brain weight may be normal or slightly reduced, but the hindbrain accounts for 5% or less of the total weight because the cerebellum is globally small with narrow, prominent, and hard folia (**Fig. 6.10**). The pontine base is flattened.

CDG1 is characterized microscopically by a subtotal loss of Purkinje and granule cells, extensive loss of cerebellar white matter, and gliosis, while the dentate nucleus and superior cerebellar peduncles appear well preserved. The pontine nuclei and inferior olives show marked neuronal depletion, and the middle and inferior cerebellar peduncles and transverse pontine fibers are extremely atrophic.

At necropsy, pleural and pericardial effusions and ascites are common. The liver shows macrovesicular fatty infiltration (**Fig. 6.11**), abnormal bile duct plates, and portal fibrosis. The kidneys show pronounced cystic dilation of tubules and collecting ducts.

DIFFERENTIAL DIAGNOSIS OF DISORDERS CHARACTERIZED BY CHILDHOOD INVOLVEMENT OF THE OLIVOPONTOCEREBELLAR AXIS

The following discriminating clinicopathological features should be sought:
- **Menkes' disease**: internal granular cell depletion; abnormal dendrites on Purkinje cells; hair abnormality; X-linked defect of copper metabolism.
- **Ataxia–telangiectasia** : cerebellar and cortical degeneration; telangiectasias of conjunctiva and skin; immunologic disorder.
- **CDG1**: olivopontocerebellar atrophy; renal cysts; hepatopathy; dysmorphic features; specific biochemical abnormalities.
- **Cerebellocortical degeneration (Jervis)**: degenerations of cerebellar cortex, olives and visual system; pons spared; autosomal recessive inheritance.
- **Werdnig–Hoffman variant**: cerebellar cortical degeneration; associated anterior horn cell disease.
- **ADCA II**: olivopontocerebellar atrophy with retinal degeneration; autosomal dominant inheritance.

CHILDHOOD NEURODEGENERATIVE DISORDERS AFFECTING THE CEREBELLUM

Menkes' Disease
- X-linked recessive inheritance
- gene locus Xq12-Xq13
- gene encodes copper-binding ATPase (ATP7A)
- intestinal absorption of copper is impaired

Ataxia–telangiectasia
- recessive inheritance
- gene locus 11q22.3
- abnormal telomeric fusions, particularly in T lymphocytes

Carbohydrate-Deficient Glycoprotein Syndrome Type 1
- recessive inheritance
- complex defects in the terminal carbohydrate residues of various serum glycoproteins (e.g. transferrin)
- CDG1 gene locus in region 16p13.3-16p13.12

Autosomal Dominant Cerebellar Ataxia Type II (ACDA II)
- dominant inheritance with anticipation
- ADCA II gene locus in region 3p12-3p21.1
- an unstable trinucleotide repeat may encode a polyglutamine expansion
- an antibody that recognizes polyglutamine expansion can detect abnormal proteins in ADCA II

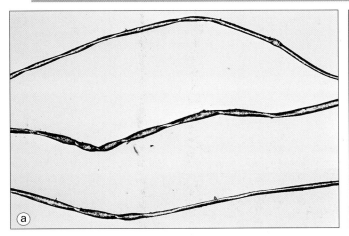

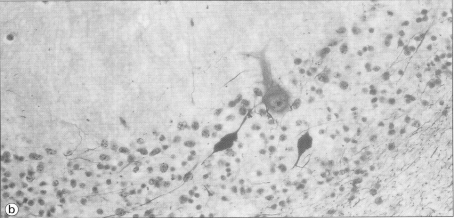

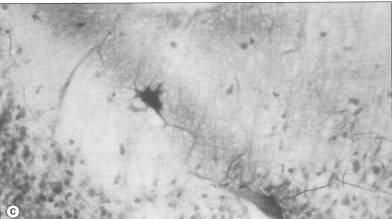

Fig. 6.8 Menkes' disease. (a) Abnormal twisted hairs. **(b)** Cerebellar cortical degeneration with Purkinje cell loss and formation of axonal torpedoes. (Bielschowsky silver impregnation) **(c)** Some Purkinje cells have abnormal dendritic swellings. (Bielschowsky silver impregnation)

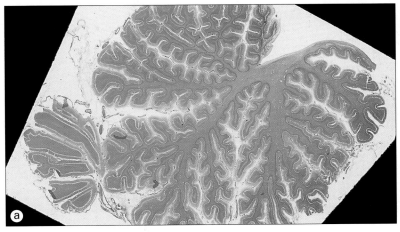

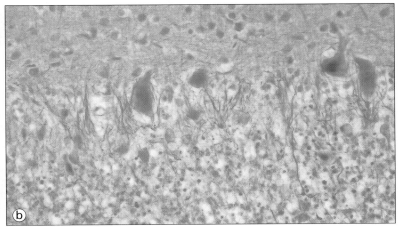

Fig. 6.9 Ataxia–telangiectasia. (a) Atrophy of the cerebellar cortex. **(b)** Cerebellar cortical degeneration with depletion of granule and Purkinje cells and collapsed empty skeins of basket fibers. (Holmes silver impregnation)

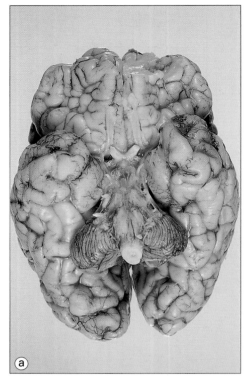

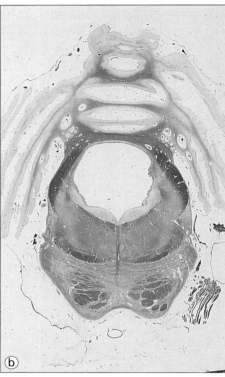

Fig. 6.10 CDG1. (a) Seen from below, the cerebral hemispheres of this infant (one of two affected brothers) are quite normal, but the cerebellum is extremely shrunken, the narrow folia standing out. The base of the pons appears excavated. **(b)** Horizontal section through the hindbrain. The cerebellar folia are reduced to thin unmyelinated plates. The pontine base is shallow and concave in outline; the descending tracts are prominent, but nuclei pontis and transverse fibers are lacking. Compared with the minuscule middle cerebellar peduncles, the superior cerebellar peduncles are well preserved. (Luxol fast blue/cresyl violet) **(c)** Histologic detail of the cerebellar folia. There is extreme atrophy leaving gliotic slivers of tissue devoid of all cortical neurons. **(d)** Occasional axonal 'torpedoes' are encountered in the atrophic cortex. (Glees silver impregnation) **(e)** Horizontal section through the medulla showing moderate fall-out of olivary neurons and loss of hilar and olivocerebellar fibers. (Luxol fast blue/cresyl violet) **(f)** By comparison the dentate neurons are well preserved along with their hilar output to the superior cerebellar peduncles, although the amiculum is quite pale. (Luxol fast blue/cresyl violet)

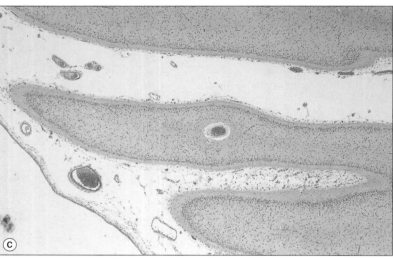

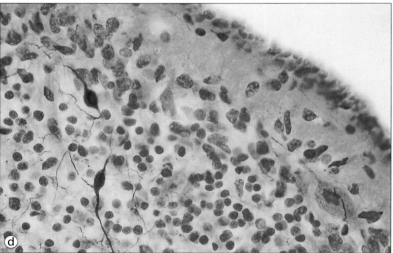

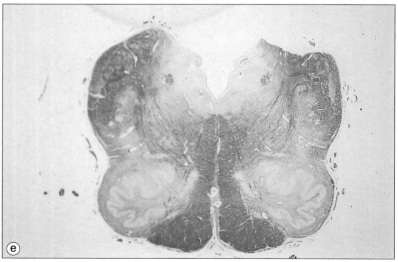

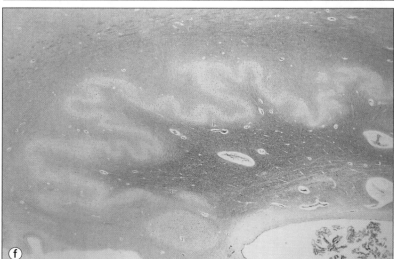

CEREBELLOCORTICAL DEGENERATION (JERVIS)

Sporadic or familial (usually autosomal recessive) examples of cerebellar cortical degeneration are occasionally encountered in children, and were first reported by Jervis. Severe developmental delay and microcephaly from late infancy, epilepsy, and ataxia are the main clinical features, with symptomatic or electrophysiologic evidence of visual failure. Death occurred between 9 months and 16 years of age. These cases may have diverse etiology (see chapter 29 for a discussion of the modern nosology of cerebellar degenerations).

MACROSCOPIC AND MICROSCOPIC APPEARANCES

Microcephaly and marked cerebellar atrophy are seen macroscopically (**Fig. 6.12**). Histologic features are cerebellar cortical degeneration, severe Purkinje cell loss accompanied by 'torpedo' axonal swellings, asteroid dendritic expansions, and variable granule cell involvement. The inferior olivary nuclei are always involved, but the pontine nuclei are spared. Atrophy of the optic nerves, superior colliculi, lateral geniculate nuclei, and visual cortex can also occur.

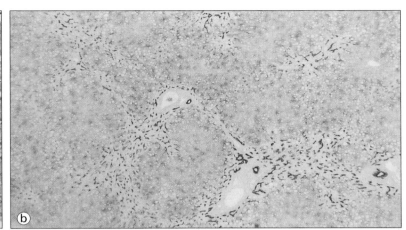

Fig. 6.11 Liver changes in CDG1. (a) Microscopy of the liver shows marked fatty change and prominent bile ducts. **(b)** The abnormal interface between dental plate and surrounding lobule is highlighted in this section immunostained for cytokeratins.

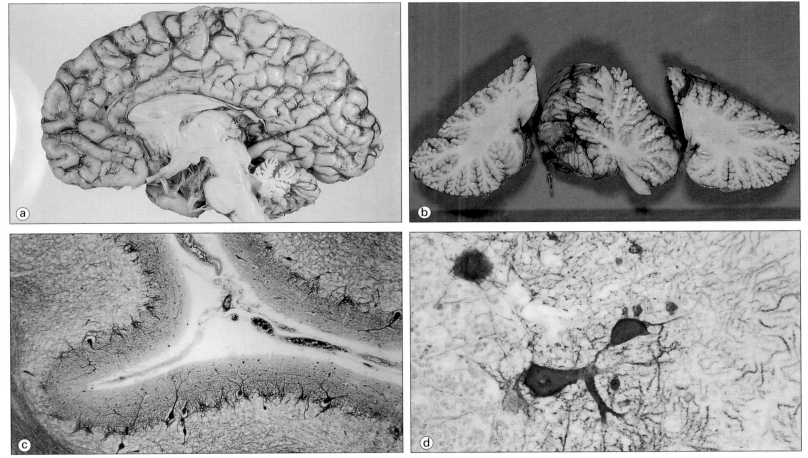

Fig. 6.12 Cerebellocortical degeneration. (a) Mesial view of the hemisected brain. There is severe cerebellar atrophy as well as shrinkage of the optic nerve. **(b)** In another patient there is global cerebellar cortical atrophy. **(c)** Glees silver impregnation shows many empty baskets and some 'torpedo' swellings associated with surviving Purkinje cells. **(d)** Another feature of this type of cerebellar degeneration that is demonstrated here with antineurofilament antibodies is the presence of abnormal dendritic swellings on Purkinje cells.

AUTOSOMAL DOMINANT CEREBELLAR ATAXIA TYPE II (ADCA II)

This form of autosomal dominant ataxia is distinguished by the occurrence of visual failure. Pedigrees can include affected children, with notably a severe infantile presentation.

MACROSCOPIC AND MICROSCOPIC APPEARANCES

Microcephaly, cerebellar atrophy, a shallow pons, and flat inferior olives are accompanied by a subtotal loss of Purkinje cells, lesser depletion of granule cells, Bergmann cell gliosis, severe olivary atrophy, and variable depletion of the nuclei pontis (**Fig. 6.13**).

AUTOSOMAL DOMINANT CEREBELLAR ATAXIA TYPE II

- Presentation is from 6 months to 60 years of age with ataxia and visual failure.
- Neurologic features include pyramidal tract signs and supranuclear ophthalmoplegia.
- The rapidly progressive and fatal infantile form presents before 2 years of age with wasting, weakness, hypotonia, ataxia, regression, and dementia.

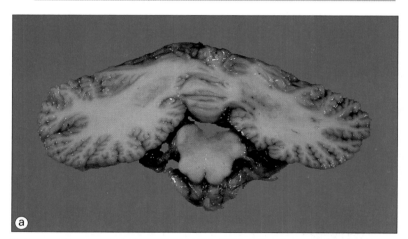

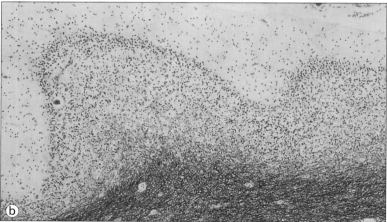

Fig. 6.13 ADCA II. (a) Horizontal section showing prominent folial atrophy throughout the cerebellum. **(b)** Histology shows global devastation of the cerebellar cortex. An occasional Purkinje cell remains among Bergmann's glia. (Luxol fast blue/cresyl violet)

BRAIN STEM

HEREDITARY MOTOR NEUROPATHY

Progressive bulbar palsy presenting in the first two decades of life is associated with two very rare and partially overlapping eponymous disorders:
- Brown–Vialetto–van Laere syndrome.
- Fazio–Londe disease.

MACROSCOPIC AND MICROSCOPIC APPEARANCES

In both Brown–Vialetto–van Laere syndrome and Fazio–Londe disease the main histologic findings are degeneration of:
- motor cranial nerve nuclei, including oculomotor nerve nuclei, in the brain stem
- anterior horn cells in the spinal cord (**Fig. 6.14**) with consequent widespread neurogenic atrophy of muscles, including the tongue

Additionally in Brown–Vialetto–van Laere syndrome there is degeneration of the sensory cochleovestibular nerves and ventral cochlear nuclei.

HEREDITARY BULBAR PALSIES

Bulbar hereditary motor neuropathy type I (Brown–Vialetto–van Laere syndrome)
- Recessive inheritance.
- Presents at 1–30 years of age with an abrupt onset of bilateral nerve deafness concurrently with, or soon followed by, other lower cranial nerve palsies.
- Irregularly progressive with some fatalities.
- EMG shows denervation of limbs and bulbar muscles.

Bulbar hereditary motor neuropathy type II (Fazio–Londe disease)
- There are three clinical subtypes:
  1. Dominant inheritance; presents at 4–20 years of age with dysphagia and dysarthria; progressive and fatal.
  2. Recessive inheritance; presents <5 years of age with respiratory symptoms and stridor; fatal within two years.
  3. Recessive inheritance; onset >5 years of age with dysphagia, dysarthria, and facial weakness; survival for many years.
- EMG shows a neurogenic process in bulbar muscles that may also be seen in limb muscles.

INFANTILE NEURO-AXONAL DYSTROPHY (INAD)

Dystrophic axons containing spheroids can occur in a variety of situations, for example in normal aging, children affected by mucoviscidosis, metabolic disorders, experimental toxicology, and certain inherited disorders (see also chapter 33). The main examples of the latter are:

- Hallervorden–Spatz disease (see p.6.4)
- infantile neuro-axonal dystrophy (INAD)

MACROSCOPIC AND MICROSCOPIC APPEARANCES

Apart from cerebellar atrophy, macroscopic abnormality in INAD is minimal. Axonal spheroids are widely distributed throughout the CNS (Fig. 6.15), but are most easily found in the cerebellum, brain stem, and spinal cord, notably among the long sensory tracts. They are also present in cerebellar and cerebral white matter, basal ganglia, thalamus, and in the cerebral cortex where their small size makes detection difficult with conventional histology.

The axonal spheroids have the appearance of eosinophilic ovoids that sometimes show a cleft. They are irregularly argyrophilic, and immunoreactive with neurofilament antibodies. The nonspecific esterase technique in frozen sections is particularly effective for detecting spheroids in cortical biopsies.

Myelin pallor or degeneration may be widespread in cerebral and cerebellar white matter. Other findings include cerebellar cortical degeneration, neurofibrillary tangles, and Lewy bodies.

Ultrastructurally, the axonal swellings are packed with tubulovesicular membranous material, often surrounding a central cleft.

INFANTILE NEURO-AXONAL DYSTROPHY (INAD)

- The typical presentation is at 9–18 months of age with progressive motor and mental deterioration, bilateral pyramidal signs, hypotonia, and visual disturbance.
- Other patients have shown nonspecific features after minor surgery or febrile illness. These include toe-walking, ataxia, weakness, and severe constipation.
- By 3 years of age the EMG shows signs of denervation (anterior horn cell type) and characteristic fast activity is seen on the EEG. There is progessive abnormality in VEPs.
- Although skin, conjunctiva, muscle, and peripheral nerve biopsies have all been used for diagnosis, failure to find spheroids may not exclude the diagnosis, necessitating brain biopsy or necropsy for ultimate diagnosis.
- Neuroaxonal dystrophy was the main finding in a biopsy from a child with Schindler's disease, (α-N-acetylgalactosaminidase deficiency), but other patients with INAD have not demonstrated this recessive lysosomal disorder.

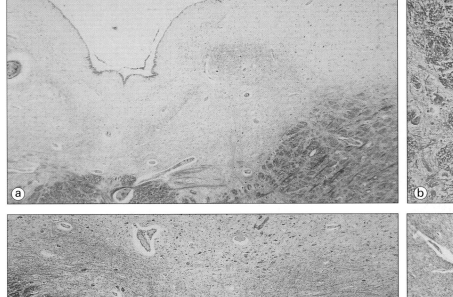

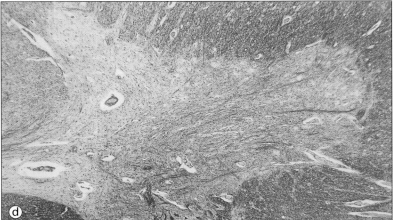

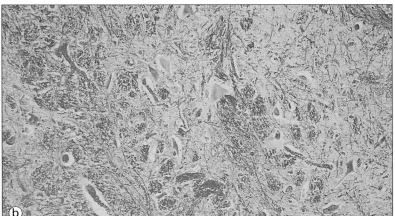

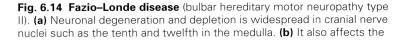

Fig. 6.14 Fazio–Londe disease (bulbar hereditary motor neuropathy type II). **(a)** Neuronal degeneration and depletion is widespread in cranial nerve nuclei such as the tenth and twelfth in the medulla. **(b)** It also affects the motor fifth in the pons. **(c)** The oculomotor nuclei in the midbrain are involved. **(d)** There is anterior horn cell loss in the cord. (Luxol fast blue/cresyl violet)

LEIGH'S DISEASE (SUBACUTE NECROTIZING ENCEPHALOMYELOPATHY)

The pathologic diagnosis of Leigh's disease is based upon the occurrence of a peculiar type of vasculonecrotic lesion in a particular topographic distribution within the CNS. These lesions are the common end result of a variety of metabolic defects of mitochondrial origin.

MACROSCOPIC APPEARANCES

There are characteristic symmetric circumscribed brown patches or gray lesions, which are sometimes cavitated (**Fig. 6.16**). These lesions are present in the striatum, subthalamic nucleus, substantia nigra, inferior olives, and hindbrain tegmentum, and often run in a linear fashion below the ventricle.

MICROSCOPIC APPEARANCES

In typical cases there are many vasculonecrotic lesions distributed symmetrically through the CNS. These lesions take three histologic forms (**Fig. 6.17**), which probably reflect varying chronicity, but the different appearances are often contiguous, suggesting repetitive damage to the area. The oldest lesions are fibrous or cavitated gliotic scars,

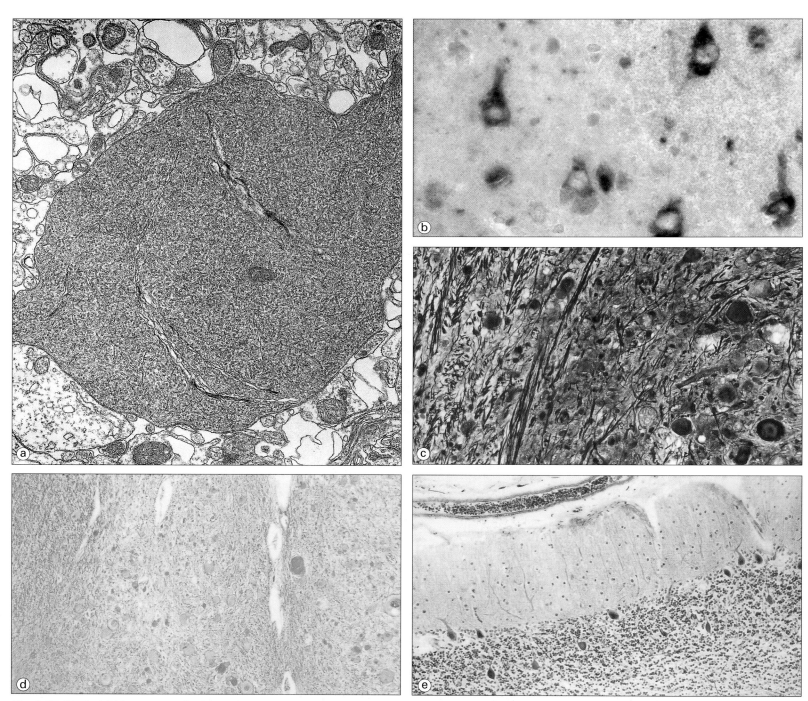

Fig. 6.15 INAD. (a) Ultrastructurally the axonal spheroids contain closely packed tubulovesicular membranes interrupted by narrow clefts. **(b)** The nonspecific esterase technique is a useful method for detecting spheroids, particularly in the cerebral cortex where they are relatively small. Note that the small spheroid to the left of this micrograph contains a curved cleft. Surrounding neurons are also positive with this method. **(c)** Axonal spheroids are particularly common in the dorsal medulla. Silver impregnation gives a variable and irregular result. (Glees and Marsland) **(d)** Spheroids are usually numerous in the dorsal funiculi, but note the variable immunoreactivity with neurofilament antibody. **(e)** Cerebellar cortical degeneration is often associated with INAD and is characterized by marked Purkinje cell fallout and torpedo swellings of proximal axons, which are visualized here with an antibody to neurofilament protein.

LEIGH'S DISEASE

- Initial presentation is usually in the first 2 years, but older patients and rare adult cases are recognized.
- Prenatal onset is occasionally suggested by microcephaly and a few rapidly fatal cases of neonatal disease.
- Most cases are associated with an insidious onset of weight loss, weakness, psychomotor retardation, vomiting, and anorexia in the first year of life. Unexplained fever associated with seizures or other neurologic symptoms may also occur.
- Presentation after the first year is more variable, consisting mainly of movement disorder, ataxia, mental regression, and epilepsy.
- Disturbances of respiration, from dyspnea to Cheyne–Stokes repiration, and abnormal eye movements with or without optic atrophy are common.
- Neurologic signs are more prominent in the later stages of the disease and include hypotonia, reduced reflexes, and a demyelinating type of peripheral neuropathy.
- Although the usual course is chronic and relentlessly progressive, stepwise exacerbations are characteristic. The majority of patients live less than one year from the onset of symptoms, but survival for 15 years and an acute fulminating illness of a few days are also reported.

equivalent to old infarcts. The youngest and least frequent lesions are composed of poorly cellular edematous neuropil with activated macrophages and eosinophilic neurons. The most typical lesion is characterized by numerous foamy macrophages and variable astrocytosis, prominent congested and hypertrophic capillaries, and collapse of the neuropil, within which there are often some normal neurons. This recent lesion (probably several weeks old) resembles the lesions of Wernicke's encephalopathy, but there is never any hemosiderin deposition.

Symmetric lesions, often confined to the same part of a nucleus, are found in many gray areas (**Fig. 6.18**). Lesions are nearly always present in the substantia nigra, but in only about 50% of patients in the striatum and inferior olives, notably in those patients dying after the first year.

Other features include spongy vacuolation or severe myelin loss in the optic nerves and tracts, spinal cord, centrum semiovale, and cerebellar white matter, and patchy loss of Purkinje cells associated with 'torpedo' formation.

LEIGH'S DISEASE

- Autosomal inheritance is suggested in about 50% of patients.
- The other 50% show X-linked mutations of the E1 subunit of pyruvate dehydrogenase complex (PDHC), maternal mitochondrial DNA point mutations, or sporadic inheritance of mitochondrial DNA deletions.
- Biochemical defects include deficiencies of PDHC, respiratory chain complex 1, respiratory chain complex 4, or cytochrome c oxidase.

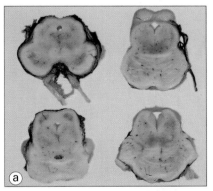
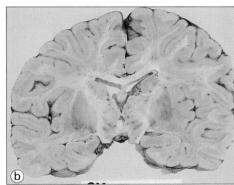
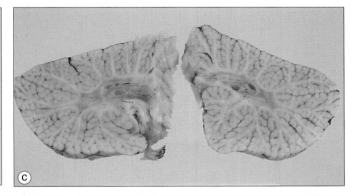
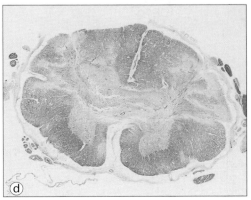
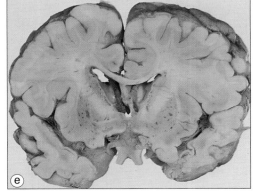
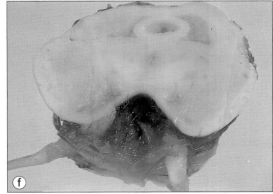

Fig. 6.16 Leigh's disease. (a) The lesions are usually bilateral and are most easy to recognize in the brain stem as brown patches or linear streaks in the tegmentum, inferior colliculi, and substantia nigra. In this eight-month-old child the nigra should not be pigmented! **(b)** Other lesions can be found in the corpus striatum. **(c)** Lesions can also be found surrounding the cerebellar dentate nuclei. **(d)** An extensive lesion may completely transect the spinal cord. (Luxol fast blue/cresyl violet) **(e)** Older lesions become cavitated, as in this example within the striatum. **(f)** Bilateral cavitated lesions in the midbrain within the periaqueductal gray matter and substantia nigra.

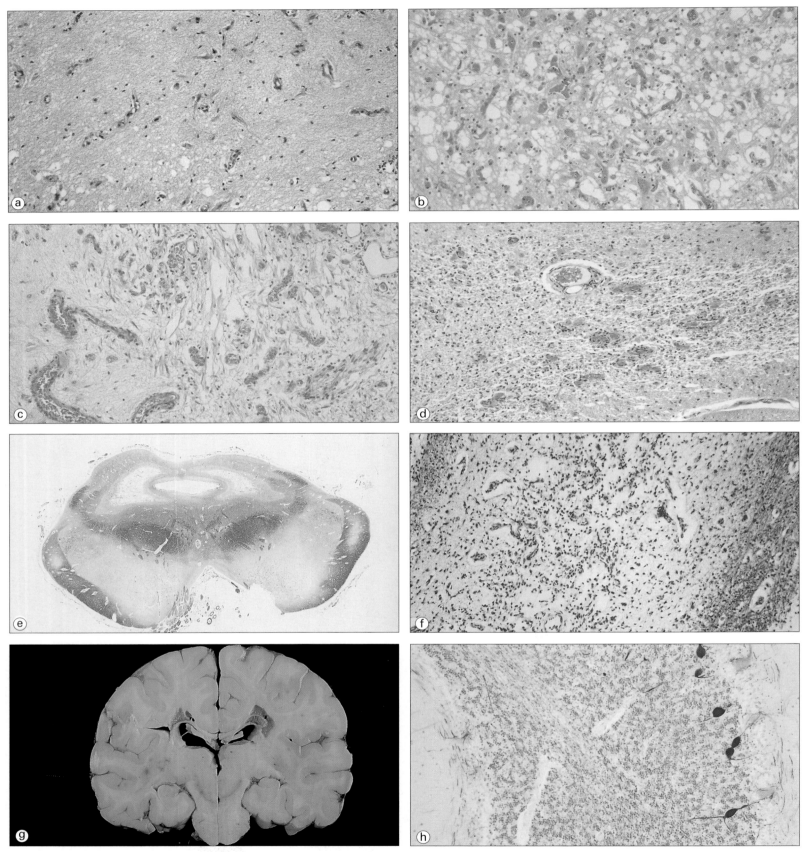

Fig. 6.17 Leigh's disease. (a) In the youngest lesions subtle histologic changes include tissue edema and neuronal necrosis. **(b,c,d)** The more characteristic changes are a variable mixture of tissue necrosis, macrophage infiltration, hypertrophy of astrocytes, and a prominent vascularity. Characteristically, some neurons are intact within the areas of partial necrosis. (Luxol fast blue/cresyl violet) **(e)** The oldest lesions are merely glial-lined cavities. Histologic section of the midbrain shown in Fig. 6.16f.

(f) Degeneration of the central white matter of the optic nerves. (Luxol fast blue/cresyl violet) **(g)** Lesions may also involve the periventricular white matter, here showing very ancient cavities. **(h)** Cerebellar degeneration is quite common. In this example, loss of Purkinje cells is accompanied by profuse 'torpedo' formation, shown by neurofilament protein immunohistochemistry.

SPINAL CORD

SPINAL MUSCULAR ATROPHY (SMA)

The group of disorders known as spinal muscular atrophy is characterized by degeneration of anterior horn cells in the spinal cord. These disorders form the second most common lethal autosomal recessive disorder after cystic fibrosis. The internationally agreed classification divides them into three categories:

- Type I: acute infantile SMA; Werdnig–Hoffman disease.
- Type II: intermediate SMA.
- Type III: chronic SMA; Kugelberg–Welander syndrome.

MACROSCOPIC AND MICROSCOPIC APPEARANCES

At necropsy, there is a striking atrophy of anterior spinal nerve roots and motor nerves (**Fig. 6.19**). There is usually a profound loss of anterior horn cells and gliosis at many levels of the spinal cord. In the early stages there are acute degenerative changes such as chromatolysis and microglial nodules. The degenerative process may also extend to the bulbar cranial nerve nuclei and sometimes to the dorsal root sensory ganglion cells.

Muscle biopsy at first shows atrophy of all fiber types, and then compensatory hypertrophy due to collateral sprouting of residual intact nerve fibers, which produces grouping of large and small fibers. Groups of hypertrophic type I fibers are particularly common in SMA.

Secondary myopathic changes, including endomysial fibrosis, may be prominent in chronic forms of SMA.

SMA variants

There are several similar clinical entities of diverse genetic background that cause anterior horn cell degeneration and these should be differentiated from the typical acute form of SMA. **Fig. 6.20** places them in context alongside SMA and the progressive bulbar palsies of childhood.

GENETIC ASPECTS OF SMA

- The SMA critical region is located on chromosome 5q13.1.
- Two contiguous presumptive SMA genes have been identified: SMN (survival motor neuron gene) and NAIP (neuronal apoptosis inhibitory protein gene).
- Large deletions involving both genes are found in SMA type I patients, but patients with milder phenotypes show deletions involving SMN only.
- So-called SMA variants such as SMA with cerebellar hypoplasia and diaphragmatic SMA are not linked to chromosome 5q.

Frequency of gray matter lesions in Leigh's disease	
Affected region	Approximate frequency
Caudate nucleus	50%
Putamen	50%
Globus pallidus	25%
Substantia nigra	95%
Thalamus	33%
Periaqueductal grey	60%
Mammillary bodies	rare
Subthalamic nucleus	40%
Red nucleus	33%
Superior colliculus	25%
Inferior colliculus	80%
Pontine tegmentum	60%
Cerebellar nuclei	60%
Inferior olivary nucleus	50%
Medullary tegmentum	80%
Spinal grey matter	75%

Fig. 6.18 Frequency of gray matter lesions in Leigh's disease.

SPINAL MUSCULAR ATROPHY

Type I: acute infantile SMA, Werdnig–Hoffman disease

- Onset prenatal to 6 months of age.
- Survival not beyond 3 years of age.
- Manifests with reduced fetal movement, orthopedic deformity at birth, floppy baby, abnormal cry, early feeding difficulty, absent tendon reflexes, and fasciculations.
- Course is characterized by profound hypotonia, delayed motor milestones, intercostal paralysis, and death from respiratory embarrassment and aspiration.

Type II: intermediate SMA

- Onset at 3–15 months.
- Survival beyond 4 years, even to adolescence.
- Manifests with severe weakness, failure to achieve crawling or walking, developing spinal deformity, variable hypotonia, areflexia, and fasciculation.
- Course is characterized by progressive kyphoscoliosis and vulnerability to infection, but speed of progression of weakness is very variable.

Type III: chronic SMA, Kugelberg–Welander syndrome

- Onset from two years of age to adulthood.
- Manifests with slowly progressive limb weakness, waddling gait, asymmetric muscle involvement, and tongue fasciculation, but the face is spared.
- Course is characterized by very slow progression that mimics limb–girdle muscular dystrophy.

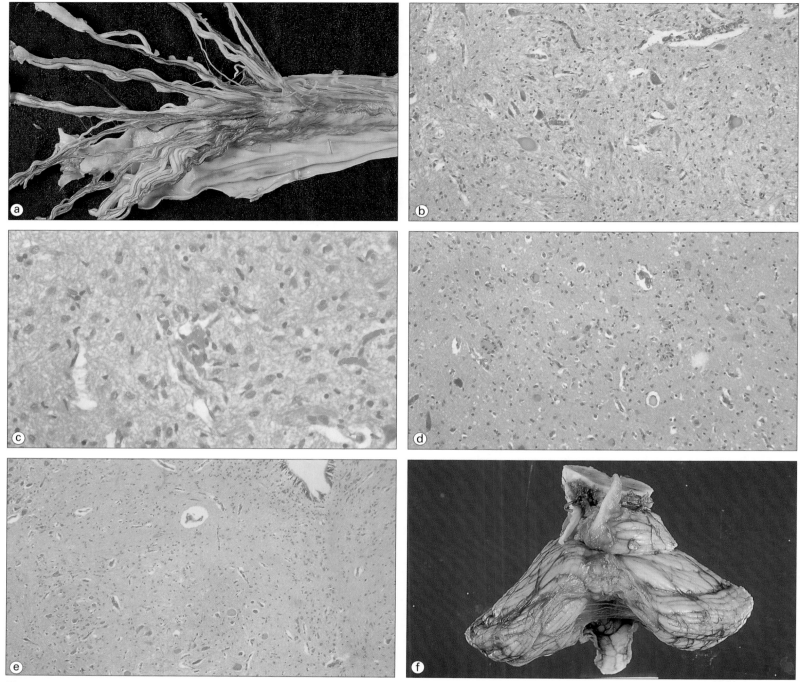

Fig. 16.19 Spinal muscular atrophy. (a) Dissection of the lower cord. Compare the gray atrophic anterior roots with the white well myelinated posterior roots. The cardinal histologic changes are loss of motor neurons from the anterior horn **(b)** the process of degeneration being one of ballooning and chromatolysis, with microglial activation and neuronophagia **(c)**. Usually a similar neuronal degeneration occurs in the thalamus **(d)** and occasionally in brainstem motor nuclei such as the 12th nucleus **(e)**. **(f)** In one variant of SMA there is an associated severe cerebellar degeneration. Here the atrophic cerebellum is viewed from behind.

A comparison of the acute motor neuron degenerations of infancy

	Presentation	Typical duration	Pathology	
			Usual	Occasional
SMA	Early hypotonia	2yr	C, B, T	Dg
Distal infantile SMA with diaphragmatic paralysis	Early diaphragmatic weakness	1yr	C, B, T	
SMA with cerebellar hypoplasia	Hypotonia at birth, mental retardation	2yr	C, B, Cbh	T
SMA with cerebellar atrophy ('infantile neuronal degeneration')	Hypotonia at birth	1yr	C, B, Cba	Bg
Fazio-Londe disease	Bulbar weakness	1-5yr	C, B	Cba, T, Bg

C   = loss of anterior horn cells in spinal cord
B   = loss of cells in bulbar nuclei
T   = loss of cells in thalamus
Cba = cerebellar atrophy
Cbh = cerebellar hypoplasia
Bg = degeneration of basal ganglia cells
Dg = degeneration of dorsal root ganglion cells

Fig. 6.20 A comparison of the acute motor neuron degenerations of infancy.

REFERENCES

Cavanagh JB and Harding BN. (1994) Pathogenic factors underlying the lesions in Leigh's Disease: Tissue responses to cellular energy deprivation and their clinico-pathological consequences. *Brain* **117**:1357–1376.

Ramaekers VT *et al*. (1987) Diagnostic difficulties in infantile neuroaxonal dystrophy: a clinicopathological study of eight cases. *Neuropediatrics* **18**:170–175.

Harding BN. (1990) Progressive Neuronal Degeneration of Childhood with liver disease (Alpers-Huttenlocher syndrome) - a personal review. *Journal of Child Neurology* **5**:273–287.

Horslen SP, Clayton PT, Harding BN, Hall NA, Keir G, and Winchester B. (1991) Neonatal onset olivopontocerebellar atrophy and disialotransferrin deficiency syndrome. *Archives of Disease in Childhood* **66**:1027–1032.

Hagberg BA, Blennow G, Kristriansson B, and Stibbler H. (1993) Carbohydrate-deficient Glycoprotein Syndromes: Peculiar group of new disorders. *Pediatric Neurology* **9**:255–262.

McShane MA, Boyd S, Harding B, Brett EM, and Wilson J. (1992) Progressive bulbar paralysis of childhood: a reappraisal of Fazio-Londe disease. *Brain* **115**:1889–1900.

Lowe J, Lennox G, and Leigh PN. (1997) Disorders of movement and system degenerations. In: *Greenfield's Neuropathology*, (6th edition), vol. 2 edited by Graham, D.I. and Lantos, P.L.London:Arnold, p. 281–366.

Friede RL. (1989) *Developmental Neuropathology*, Berlin:Springer-Verlag.

7 *Miscellaneous pediatric disorders*

VASCULAR DISEASES

Central nervous system vascular pathology is uncommon in children, but there are rare forms of vasculopathy unique to this age group, as well as presentations in childhood of some disorders that are more commonly seen in older individuals (**Fig. 7.1**).

PROLIFERATIVE VASCULOPATHY AND HYDRANENCEPHALY–HYDROCEPHALY (FOWLER'S SYNDROME)

This is a hereditary disorder characterized by hydramnios and hydranencephaly, which can be detected on ultrasound scan as early as 13 weeks' gestation. The disorder is fatal by term.

MACROSCOPIC APPEARANCES

Arthrogryposis, pterygia, muscular hypoplasia, and pulmonary hypoplasia are found at necropsy (**Fig. 7.2a**). Bubble-like hemispheres that are macroscopically indistinguishable from those seen in encephaloclastic hydranencephaly have a diaphenous pallium studded with calcifications (**Fig. 7.2b**).

MICROSCOPIC APPEARANCES

The thin, disorganized pallium has a narrow immature cortical plate.

Glomeruloid endothelial vasculopathy, which is unique to this disorder, is prominent throughout the CNS (**Fig. 7.3**). Endothelial cells in the glomeruloid structures have PAS-positive intracytoplasmic inclusions, which appear on electron microscopy as homogeneous granular material surrounded by rough endoplasmic reticulum (**Fig. 7.4**).

MENINGOCEREBRAL ANGIODYSPLASIA AND RENAL AGENESIS

This sporadic disorder causes stillbirth or premature delivery with minimal survival.

MACROSCOPIC APPEARANCES

Potter's facies, contraction deformities of the limbs, pulmonary hypoplasia, and bilateral renal agenesis are found at necropsy, but there are no cutaneous vascular nevi.

The leptomeninges are extremely vascular, and in some cases there is subarachnoid hemorrhage. The circle of Willis is normal. The brain is small and gyral atrophy is evident. In the cerebrum, there is cortical and white matter necrosis, with or without hemorrhage and calcification.

MICROSCOPIC APPEARANCES

There is diffuse angiodysplasia, consisting of ectatic capillaries and veins. These are present in the leptomeninges, cerebral cortex, cerebellum, and brain stem. The angiodysplasia is complicated by thrombosis, infarction, hemorrhage, hemosiderin-laden macrophages, gliosis and calcification in the cerebral cortex and white matter (**Fig. 7.5**).

Fig. 7.1 Vasculopathy in childhood

Vasculopathy in childhood		
	Fetal presentation	Postnatal onset
Vascular malformation	Proliferative vasculopathy and hydranencephaly–hydrocephaly	Aneurysm of great vein of Galen (see Fig. 7.6)
	Meningocerebral angiodysplasia and renal agenesis	Arteriovenous malformation Cavernous angioma
Aneurysm		Saccular Fusiform (basilar) Infectious (mycotic) Dissecting
Vasculitis		Kawasaki disease Takayasu's arteritis
Coagulopathy		Hemolytic–uremic syndrome Hemorrhagic shock and encephalopathy syndrome

Fig. 7.1 Vasculopathy in childhood.

PATHOGENESIS OF FOWLER'S SYNDROME

The etiology of this disorder is unknown; but hypotheses include:
- congenital infection: against, no microbiologic evidence, familial occurrence, including only one of dizygotic twins
- neuroectodermal failure, occurring before the 7th week (presence of pterygia suggests <12 weeks)
- central role for the glomeruloid vasculopathy which possibly interferes with vascular invasion of the cerebral mantle at the time of neuroblastic migration in the first trimester. Autosomal recessive inheritance is likely.

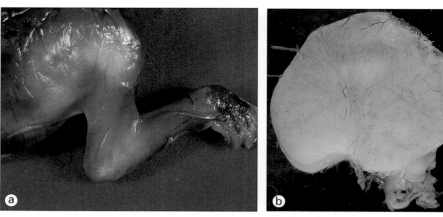

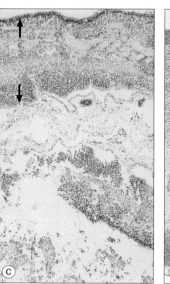

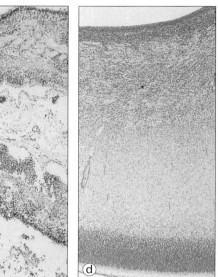

Fig. 7.2 Proliferative vasculopathy and hydranencephaly–hydrocephaly in a 17-week fetus. **(a)** Arthrogryposis and webbing of the elbow joint. **(b)** Lateral aspect of the cystic cerebral hemisphere demonstrated under water. **(c)** The extremely thin pallium (between arrows) is barely one-third of the normal. **(d)** Normal age-matched control for comparison with (c).

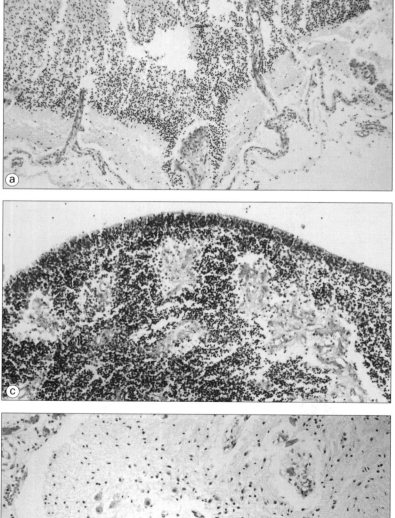

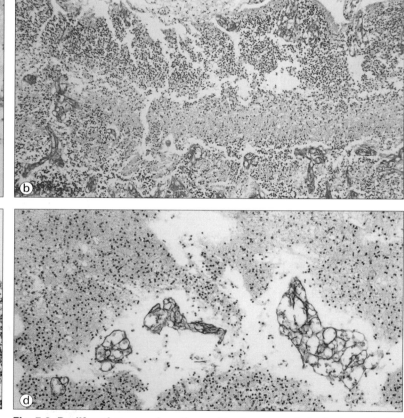

Fig. 7.3 Proliferative vasculopathy and hydranencephaly–hydrocephaly in a fetus. Glomeruloid vascular structures are widespread in the brain and spinal cord. **(a)** Glomeruloid vasculopathy in the marginal zone and cortical plate. **(b)** Prominent vascular expansion involving the intermediate and subventricular zones. (PAS) **(c)** Vasculopathy is also visible in the germinal eminence. **(d)** Glomeruloid structure in the cerebellum (reticulin). **(e)** Glomeruloid vascular expansion in the anterior horn of the spinal cord.

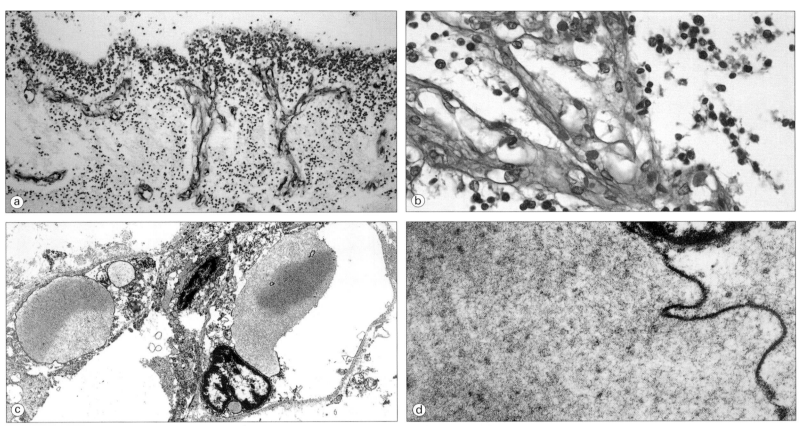

Fig. 7.4 Proliferative vasculopathy and hydranencephaly–hydrocephaly. **(a)** The glomeruloid vascular structures have many small lumina lined by endothelial cells, as demonstrated by immunohistochemistry for *Ulex europaeus* lectin. **(b)** Some endothelial cells contain PAS-positive intracytoplasmic inclusions. **(c)** Electron microscopy reveals endothelial inclusions of very varied size comprising moderately electron-dense granular material surrounded by rough endoplasmic reticulum. **(d)** Close-up of the surrounding rough endoplasmic reticulum.

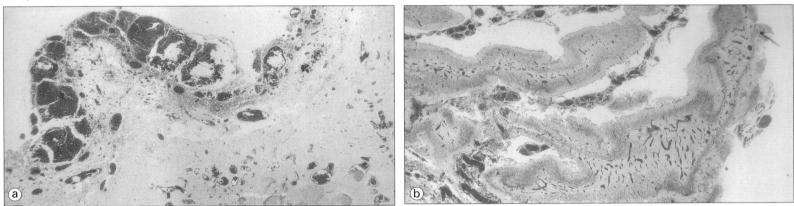

Fig. 7.5 Meningocerebral angiodysplasia and renal agenesis. (a) Engorged and markedly ectatic thin-walled vessels are seen within the pia–arachnoid and also in the underlying partially necrotic cerebral parenchyma. Note also the vascular thrombosis and focal calcification. **(b)** A similar process also affects the cerebellum.

Fig. 7.6 Vein of Galen aneurysm (arteriovenous fistula). (a) and **(b)** The patient is a 15-month-old child who died secondary to extensive encephalomalacia produced by a 'steal' of blood from normal brain through the shunt.

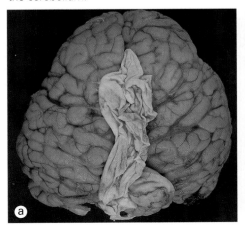

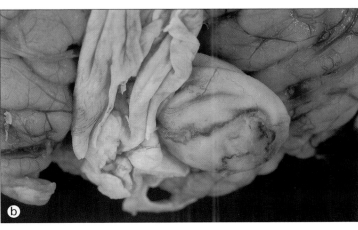

TAKAYASU'S ARTERITIS

This granulomatous angiitis of the aortic arch and its main arterial trunks is an inflammatory vasculopathy of uncertain origin and is a rare cause of stroke in infancy, but more usually affects girls aged 15–20 years.

MACROSCOPIC AND MICROSCOPIC APPEARANCES

Lymphocytic infiltration of the media and destruction of the elastica of affected vessels are associated with giant cells and followed by fibrosis and thickening. The blood vessels are further narrowed by superimposed intimal proliferation and atheroma. Thromboembolic disease leads to cerebral ischemia. Only rarely does the arteritic process directly involve cerebral vessels (**Fig. 7.7**).

KAWASAKI DISEASE (SYNONYM: MUCOCUTANEOUS LYMPH NODE SYNDROME)

This vasculitis of uncertain etiology occurs in epidemics and is particularly frequent in Japan. The suggested pathogenesis is an abnormal immunologic response to certain bacterial infections.

MACROSCOPIC AND MICROSCOPIC APPEARANCES

In fatal cases, there is coronary arteritis with thrombosis and aneurysm formation, interstitial myocarditis, and myocardial infarction. Various medium-sized arteries can be involved, including cerebral vessels (**Fig. 7.8**).

HEMOLYTIC–UREMIC SYNDROME

The childhood form of thrombotic thrombocytopenic purpura is characterized by acute renal failure, hemolytic anemia, thrombocytopenia, and microangiopathy, and is associated with verotoxin-producing *Escherichia coli*.

MACROSCOPIC AND MICROSCOPIC APPEARANCES

Hyaline eosinophilic platelet thrombi occlude small arteries and arterioles, which also show striking endothelial swelling. Multiple microinfarcts are present in cerebral and cerebellar gray matter (**Fig. 7.9**).

CLINICAL ASPECTS OF TAKAYASU'S ARTERITIS

- Cerebral involvement occurs in 5–10% of patients, usually producing acute hemiplegia.
- Absent radial pulses, and radiologic evidence of aortic dilatation suggest the diagnosis.

CLINICAL ASPECTS OF KAWASAKI DISEASE

- Injected conjunctivae, reddening and swelling of hands and feet, lymphadenopathy and ulceration of the oropharynx are associated with fever and striking desquamation of the skin of the digital extremities in the second and third weeks of the illness.
- Most patients recover spontaneously, but coronary artery involvement occurs in 30–40%; if not treated with immunoglobulin and aspirin coronary artery aneurym occurs, with the risk of sudden death from myocardial infarction.
- Other symptoms include arthritis, hepatitis, and aseptic meningitis, which produces irritability and lethargy.

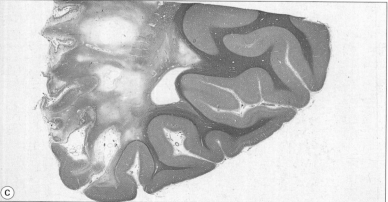

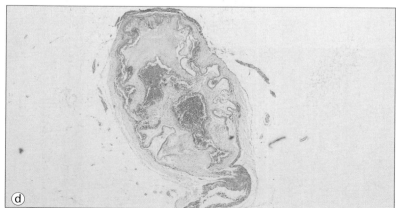

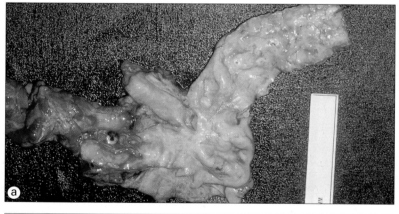

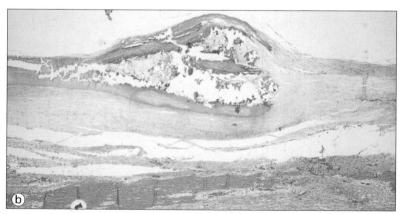

Fig. 7.7 Takayasu's arteritis in a 14-year-old girl. (a) Severe complicated atheroma in the aorta. **(b)** Histologically, the atheroma consists of calcified and atheromatous thickening of the intima and a mononuclear infiltrate disrupting the media. **(c)** Old infarction centered on the parieto-occipital vascular boundary zone. **(d)** All the vessels of the circle of Willis were affected by a chronic arteritic process with intimal thickening, elastic fragmentation, medial atrophy and mononuclear infiltration. The middle cerebral arteries were occluded and recanalized.

HEMORRHAGIC SHOCK AND ENCEPHALOPATHY SYNDROME

This acute disorder of infancy is frequently fatal.

MACROSCOPIC AND MICROSCOPIC APPEARANCES

Cerebral edema is common, and the consequences of profound cerebral hypoperfusion, particularly boundary zone infarction, are sometimes seen (Fig. 7.10).

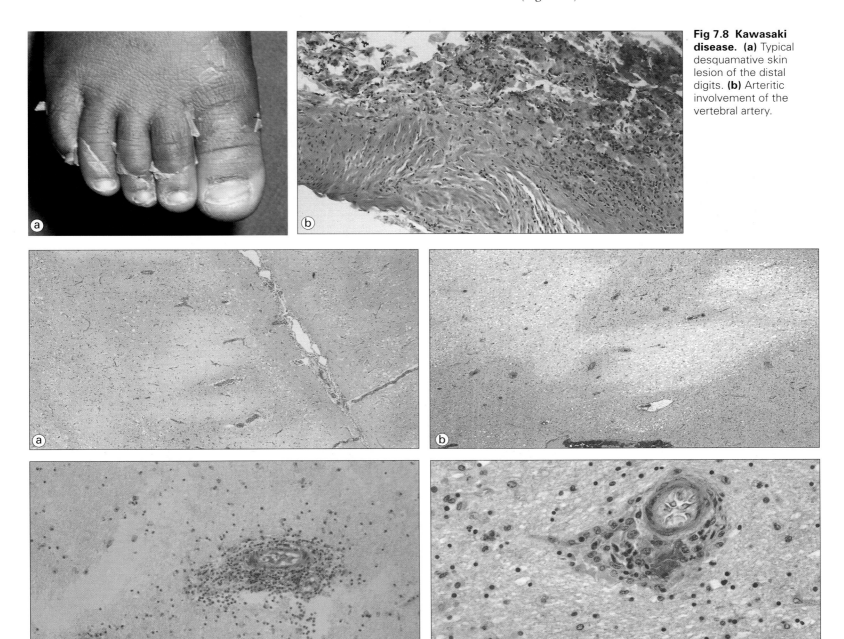

Fig 7.8 Kawasaki disease. (a) Typical desquamative skin lesion of the distal digits. **(b)** Arteritic involvement of the vertebral artery.

Fig. 7.9 Hemolytic–uremic syndrome. (a) Focal cerebral cortical infarction. **(b)** Focal cerebellar white matter infarct.
(c) Occlusive fibrin thrombus in a small arteriole. **(d)** Swollen endothelial cells bulging into the lumen of a small vessel.

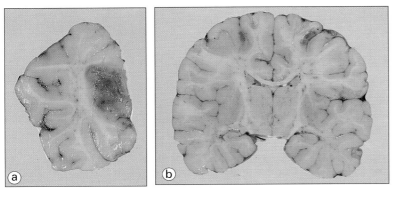

Fig. 7.10 Hemorrhagic shock and encephalopathy syndrome. (a) Subacute infarction in the occipital lobe. **(b)** Bilateral frontal boundary zone infarction (arrows).

EPILEPSY IN CHILDHOOD

Generalized epileptic seizures in childhood may be precipitated by many infective, metabolic, or toxic disorders, and by space-occupying lesions such as a hematoma or neoplasm. In addition, there is an array (**Fig. 7.11**) of more restricted structural lesions associated with focal or unilateral seizures, which are now amenable to surgical treatment. The aim of such treatment is to resect the seizure focus, or, if removal is impossible, to disconnect the focus from the rest of the brain. Most of these disorders are considered elsewhere.

RASMUSSEN'S ENCEPHALITIS

This is a progressive subacute unilateral and intractable seizure disorder with histologic features reminiscent of a chronic viral encephalitis.

MACROSCOPIC AND MICROSCOPIC APPEARANCES

Macroscopic changes may be minimal, but in longstanding cases there is severe and extensive unilateral atrophy with ventricular dilatation. Histologic changes (**Fig. 7.12**) are usually much more widespread than suspected macroscopically and include patchy chronic leptomeningitis and chronic inflammatory changes in the neocortex and hippocampus, subjacent white matter, and sometimes the basal ganglia. The principal features are:

- cuffs of lymphocytes around blood vessels
- lymphocytes, and microglial cells, either scattered across the parenchyma or in clusters ('microglial nodules')
- neuronophagia

In nearly all cases these changes are unilateral. Progressive neuronal loss can lead to an end-stage appearance of a spongy gliotic cortical remnant devoid of nerve cells.

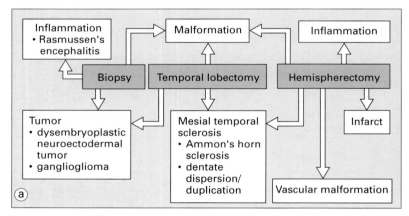

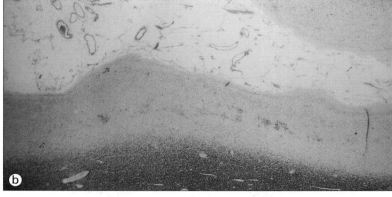

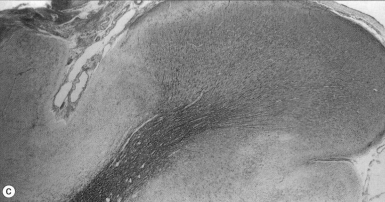

Fig. 7.11 Epilepsy in childhood. (a) A diagrammatic outline of the types of specimen and range of pathology encountered following surgery for pediatric epilepsy. Hypoxic–ischemic lesions around the time of birth can leave a large scar, commonly in the territory of the middle cerebral artery, which becomes a focus for seizure activity. **(b)** This resection contains areas of completely destroyed cortex, with a thin gliotic or cystic remnant including mineralized debris. **(c)** In some places the tips of the gyri are preserved, giving a ulegyric appearance. **(d)** At the edge of the infarcted area there is aberrant myelination, *état fibromyélinique*.

HEMICONVULSIONS–HEMIPLEGIA–EPILEPSY (HHE) SYNDROME, OR ACUTE POSTCONVULSIVE HEMIPLEGIA

Delay in treating febrile convulsions or prolonged status epilepticus in childhood can lead to an acute postconvulsive hemiplegia, which is flaccid at first with notable facial involvement, but is later spastic. Imaging shows unilateral hemispheric edema followed by widespread atrophy. Recovery can be complete, but the usual prognosis is dismal with residual epilepsy, mental retardation, and persistent weakness. Better acute treatment for epilepsy has made the syndrome a rather rare event, but occasional hemispherectomy specimens show the classic features of extensive neocortical neuronal loss, amounting in places to full-thickness destruction with residual cysts (**Fig. 7.13**).

PROGRESSIVE MYOCLONIC EPILEPSIES

These are mostly familial disorders, characterized by severe epilepsy with prominent myoclonus and progressive neurologic deterioration. Progressive myoclonic epilepsies can be subdivided into:

Disorders in which progressive myoclonic epilepsy is the principal manifestation
There are two well-defined conditions in this group:
- Lafora body disease
- Unverricht–Lundborg disease (Baltic myoclonus)

Disorders with other neurologic features but in which progressive myoclonic epilepsy is a consistent, and often the principal, manifestation
- myoclonic epilepsy with ragged red fibers (MERRF) (see chapter 24)
- dentatorubropallidoluysial atrophy (DRPLA) (see chapter 29)

These two disorders may, in some cases, be clinically indistinguishable from Unverricht–Lundborg disease.

Disorders in which progressive myoclonic epilepsy is a frequent, but not the principal, manifestation
These are many and varied, and include:
- many lysosomal storage diseases (see chapter 23)
- several other pediatric degenerative diseases of gray and white matter, such as Alpers disease, Canavan's disease, and Alexander's disease (see chapters 5 and 6)
- some chronic/subacute viral infections of the CNS, particularly subacute sclerosing panencephalitis (see chapter 13)
- Creutzfeldt–Jakob disease (see chapter 32)
- dementia with Lewy bodies
- the late stages of most other neurodegenerative dementing diseases (see chapter 31)

Other causes of myoclonus, with or without progressive neurologic deterioration, are considered in chapter 30.

Ramsay Hunt syndrome

Ramsay Hunt syndrome, of cerebellar ataxia, intention tremor and myoclonus, often associated with tonic-clonic seizures, can be caused by a heterogeneous group of disorders, including Unverricht–Lundborg disease, MERRF, DRPLA, and secondary causes of progressive myoclonic epilepsy.

Lafora body disease

This is an autosomal recessive, rapidly progressive form of myoclonic epilepsy, characterized by the accumulation of Lafora bodies within the brain and several other tissues.

MACROSCOPIC AND MICROSCOPIC APPEARANCES

The brain usually appears macroscopically normal. Histology reveals numerous Lafora bodies in the cytoplasm of neurons and astrocytes in the cerebral cortex (**Fig. 7.14**), basal ganglia (especially the globus pallidus), thalamus, substantia nigra, cerebellar cortex, and dentate nucleus. Fewer inclusions are present in the brain stem and they are sparse in the spinal cord.

The Lafora bodies are composed of polyglucosans (polymers of sulphated polysaccharides) and are similar to corpora amylacea in composition and staining characteristics. The inclusions are round, measuring up to about 30 μm in diameter. They stain strongly with hematoxylin, and with PAS, and metachromatically with methyl violet. Most Lafora bodies contain a deeply hematoxyphilic, PAS-positive central core with a spiculated outline and a surrounding zone of less intensely staining material. The polyglucosans are resistant to diastase digestion. Ultrastructurally, Lafora bodies comprise of aggregates of 6–7 nm filaments. The aggregates are not membrane bound and are admixed with amorphous granular material.

There is usually mild to moderate gliosis and neuronal loss in those regions of the CNS that contain the most numerous Lafora bodies.

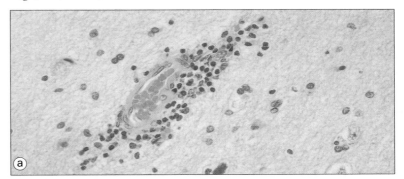

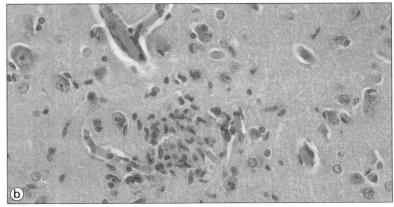

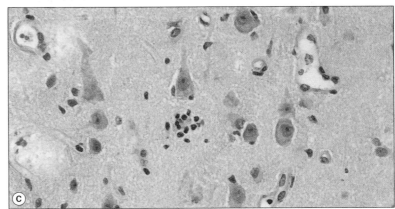

Fig. 7.12 Rasmussen's encephalitis. The typical lesions resemble an indolent viral encephalitis and include the following. **(a)** Mononuclear perivascular cuffs in the cerebral cortex. **(b)** Clusters of lymphocytes and microglial cells in the cortex. **(c)** Neuronophagia.

These changes are most pronounced in the dentate nucleus.

Lafora bodies are present in liver, skeletal and cardiac muscle. An axillary biopsy is useful for confirmation of the diagnosis in life since Lafora bodies occur in myoepithelial cells of the apocrine glands, and in the cells that form the eccrine sweat ducts.

LAFORA BODY DISEASE AND UNVERRICHT–LUNDBORG DISEASE

Lafora body disease
- autosomal recessive inheritance
- age of onset ~15 years
- duration 5–10 years
- clinical manifestations include:
  - generalized seizures
  - myoclonus
  - visual deterioration
  - psychoses
  - rapid intellectual decline with the development of dementia

Unverricht–Lundborg disease (Baltic myoclonus)
- autosomal recessive inheritance
- age of onset 6–13 years
- duration 10–20 years
- clinical manifestations include:
  - generalized seizures
  - violent myoclonus of the proximal limb muscles
  - photosensitive or other forms of stimulus-sensitive myoclonus
  - emotional lability
  - cerebellar ataxia, especially in late stages
  - slow intellectual decline

Unverricht–Lundborg disease (Baltic myoclonus)

This is an autosomal recessive form of progressive myoclonic epilepsy that is most prevalent in the Baltic region of Estonia, eastern Sweden, and Finland. Several affected families in the USA have been reported. The onset of symptoms is usually earlier than in Lafora body disease but the progression is less rapid.

MACROSCOPIC AND MICROSCOPIC APPEARANCES

The brain usually appears macroscopically normal. Histology reveals swelling, vacuolation and severe loss of Purkinje cells, with associated Bergmann cell astrocytosis. The most consistently observed additional histologic abnormalities are neuronal loss and gliosis in the medial thalamic nuclei.

Systemic examination is largely non-contributory but clear membranbe-bound vacuoles have recently been reported to be present in the eccrine sweat gland cells of some patients.

ETIOLOGY OF LAFORA BODY DISEASE AND UNVERRICHT-LUNDBORG DISEASE

Lafora body disease
Gene locus: 6q23-q25
Gene: not known
Genetic defect: not known

Unverricht–Lundborg disease (Baltic myoclonus)
Gene locus: 21q22.3
Gene: encodes cystatin B (stefin B), a cysteine protease inhibitor
Genetic defect: most cases are due to a 15– to 20– base minisatellite repeat expansion in the putative cystatin B gene promoter region. Other mutations have also been reported.

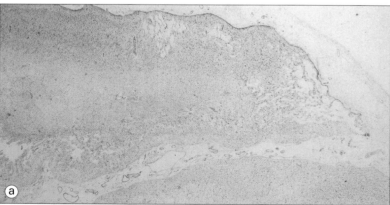

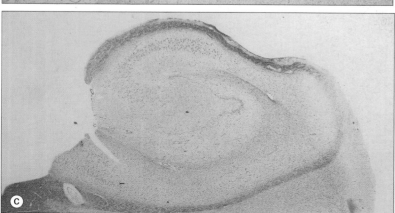

Fig. 7.13 Hemiconvulsions–hemiplegia–epilepsy (HHE) syndrome.
(a) In the hemispherectomy specimen, there are large areas of devastated cystic cortex and subjacent gliotic white matter.
(b) Other areas of remaining cortex show severe neuronal fallout.
(c) The hippocampus shows typical Ammon's horn sclerosis.

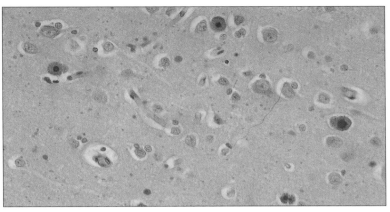

Fig. 7.14 Lafora body disease. Lafora bodies ranging from 1–2 μm to about 25 μm in diameter are visible within neurons and astrocytes in the cerebral cortex. The section has been stained with PAS reagent, with which the Lafora bodies react strongly. The Lafora bodies have a central deeply stained core with a spiculated outline, and a surrounding zone of less intensely stained material.

AN APPROACH TO THE NEUROPATHOLOGY OF FATAL PEDIATRIC TRAUMA

In its widest sense, trauma can include:
- accidental injury resulting from a variety of incidents (road traffic accident, fall, or drowning)
- intoxication (suicidal or as a consequence of drug abuse)
- homicide from poisoning or child abuse (so called non-accidental injury)

Thorough investigation of the past medical history, the social circumstances of the child, and the particular medical circumstances surrounding their sudden or unexpected death helps the pathologist to interpret the necropsy findings and assess the possibility, however remote, that the cause of death was non-accidental as well as unnatural.

INDICATORS OF NON-ACCIDENTAL INJURY

- Consider non-accidental injury particularly if there are multiple injuries of varied chronicity or if a child aged <1 year has a cranial injury.
- Radiologic features include metaphyseal fragmentation, periosteal thickening and calcification, transverse and spiral fractures of the shafts of long bones, multiple rib fractures, and skull fracture.
- At autopsy, external features include external or internal bruising or laceration of the lips, injuries to the gums, tearing of the frenulum, vitreous or retinal hemorrhage, lens opacity, displacement of the lens, skin bruising, especially of the pinnae, discoid bruises around large joints and around the throat, injuries to the chest, abdomen, buttocks, and thighs, linear marks from beating, burns, scalds, and bite marks.

- Internal features include head and abdominal injuries, which are the commonest causes of death.
- CNS injuries include skull fracture(s), subdural hemorrhage, cerebral edema, contusions and lacerations, hemorrhagic tears in cerebral white matter (especially in the orbitofrontal region or temporal lobes), and diffuse axonal injury (not in infant brain stem) (**Figs 7.15, 7.16**).
- Non-CNS injuries include ruptured liver, intestinal laceration, pancreatitis, retroperitoneal and perirenal hematomas, rib fracture, lung laceration, subcutaneous hematoma, poor nutrition or hygiene, and animal bites.

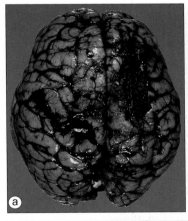
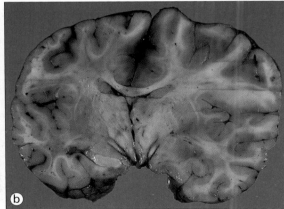
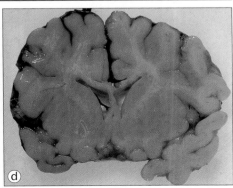

Fig. 7.15 Traumatic cranial injuries. The child's brain is exquisitely sensitive to injury, hypoxia, or surgical manipulation, and may swell very rapidly. **(a)** In this patient subdural hemorrhage followed a road traffic accident. **(b)** This led very rapidly to unilateral brain swelling and midline shift. **(c)** It also led very rapidly to transtentorial herniation, coning, and Duret hemorrhages. **(d)** Hemorrhagic tears are a characteristic finding in young children suffering closed head injury. These so-called contusional tears are especially common in orbitofrontal or temporal white matter.

REQUIREMENTS FOR AN ADEQUATE NECROPSY EXAMINATION OF THE TRAUMATIZED CHILD

- On-site availability of photography and radiology.
- Toxicologic, microbiologic, histochemical and biochemical services.
- Retention of the eyes and whole brain for examination after fixation.
- Full examination of the spinal cord: a posterior approach may be necessary to examine the surrounding soft tissues properly, and in the event of vertebral injury it is preferable to remove part or all the column together with the cord for adequate anatomic correlation of bony and spinal lesions.

- Photographs of external abnormalities and any visceral and intracranial lesions.
- Photographs of the sectioned fixed brain.
- A full radiological skeletal survey is the essential minimum.

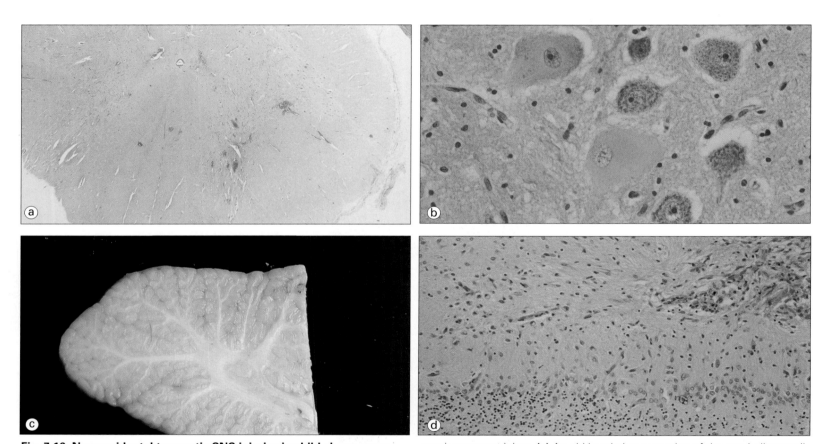

Fig. 7.16 Non-accidental traumatic CNS injuries in child abuse cases. Multiple traumatic incidents are the rule. **(a)** In this baby the necropsy disclosed an acute cord hemorrhage presumably related to the fatal injury. **(b)** There was also chromatolysis in anterior horn cells, which suggests previous recent injury. **(c)** An old herniation contusion of the cerebellar tonsil (similar to that seen in a boxing injury) was also evident. **(d)** Microscopically the tonsillar lesion contained hemosiderin-laden macrophages.

REFERENCES

Brett EM and Neville BGR. (1997) Epilepsy and convulsions; the surgical treatment of epilepsy in childhood. In: *Paediatric Neurology*, (3rd edition) Brett, E.M (ed.) New York:Churchill Livingstone pp. 333–406.

Buchhalter JR. (1994) Inherited epilepsies of childhood. *J Child Neurol* 9 (Suppl 1): S12–9

Delgado-Escueta AV, *et al.* (1994) Progress in mapping human epilepsy genes. *Epilepsia* 35 (Suppl 1): S29–40.

Harding BN, Ramani P, and Thurley P. (1995) The familial syndrome of proliferative vasculopathy and hydranencephaly-hydrocephaly: immunocytochemical and ultrastructural evidence for endothelial proliferation. *Neuropathology and Applied Neurobiology* 21:61–67.

Honavar M and Meldrum BS. (1997) Epilepsy. In: *Greenfield's Neuropathology* (6th edition) Graham DI and Lantos PL (eds) London:Arnold, pp. 931-991.

Kalimo H, Kaste M, and Haltia M. (1997) Vascular diseases. In: *Greenfield's Neuropathology*, edited by Graham, D.I. and Lantos, P.L. London:Arnold pp. 315–396.

Leestma J. (1995) Forensic Neuropathology. In: *Pediatric Neuropathology* Duckett S and Malvern PA. (eds) Williams and Wilkins, pp. 243-283.

Levin M. and Walters S. (1997) Infections of the nervous system. In: *Paediatric Neurology*, 3rd edition, Brett EM (ed). New York:Churchill Livingstone pp. 621-690.

Serratosa JM *et al.* (1995) The gene for progressive myoclonus epilepsy of the Lafora type maps to chromosome 6q. *Hum Mol Genet* 4: 1657–1663.

Valdivieso EMB and Scholtz CL. (1986) Diffuse meningocerebral angiodysplasia. *Pediatric Pathology* 6:119–126.

Virtaneva K *et al.* (1997) Unstable minisatalite satellite expansion causing recessively inherited myoclonus epilepsy, EPM1. *Nature Genet.* 15:393-396

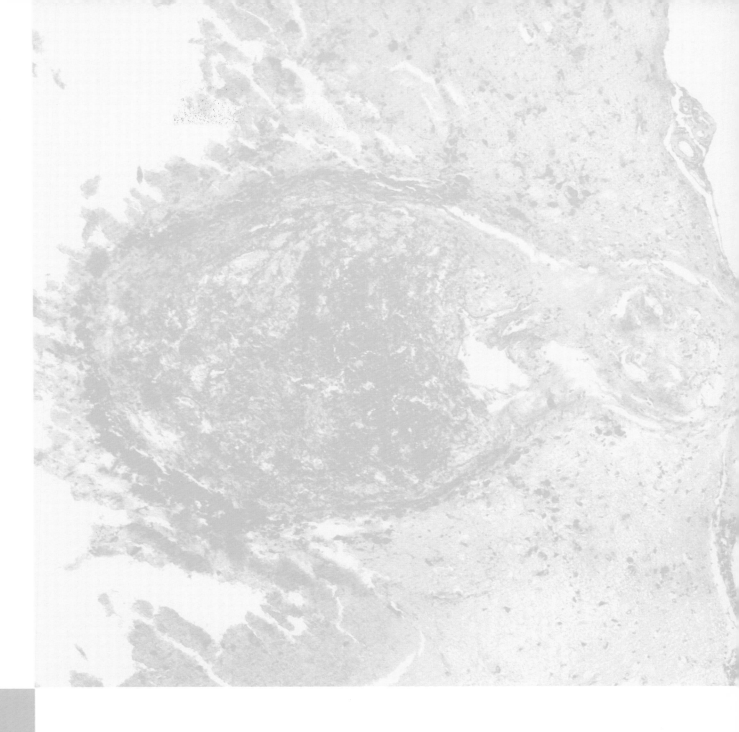

3 Vascular Disorders

8 Adult hypoxic and ischemic lesions

TERMINOLOGY

Although the terms 'hypoxia' and 'ischemia' are often used interchangeably, these conditions have different pathophysiology and CNS sequelae:

- Local brain ischemia is usually due to arterial stenosis or occlusion, and any resulting infarction is within the perfusion territory of the affected artery.
- Global brain ischemia is due to a fall in cerebral perfusion pressure below the threshold for autoregulation (see below), i.e. when systemic blood pressure falls very low (e.g. due to cardiac tamponade, heroin overdose), or intracranial pressure rises to a level that compromises perfusion of the brain (e.g. after severe head injury). The resulting brain damage or infarction is accentuated in the watershed regions — the boundaries between the perfusion territories of the major cerebral or cerebellar arteries — particularly in the depths of sulci.
- In hypoxia, the blood flow to the CNS may be entirely normal or even increased. Damage is greatest in certain populations of neurons that are particularly vulnerable to hypoxia (see box on next page).

In practice, many causes of hypoxemic hypoxia (such as respiratory arrest or carbon monoxide poisoning — see box on next page) also depress cardiac output and so produce a combination of hypoxic and global ischemic brain injury.

Brain respiration is dependent on glucose, and the neuropathologic findings in hypoglycemic brain injury are similar to those caused by hypoxia, although not identical (see chapter 22, page 22.1)

HYPOXIC–ISCHEMIC BRAIN DAMAGE

- Hypoxic–ischemic encephalopathy has a very variable clinical presentation.
- Clinical recovery is generally better after hypoxemic hypoxia than after global brain ischemia.
- The severity and duration of hypoxic-ischemic encephalopathy after transient cerebral hypoxia or ischemia depend upon the duration of the insult, the completeness of the insult, the blood glucose level (high levels lead to a poorer outcome), and the CNS temperature (a lower temperature is protective).
- Long-term sequelae after transient cerebral ischemia may be difficult to predict. Assessment requires careful patient observation over days or weeks.

Adult and developing (especially infant) brains react differently to hypoxia and ischemia (see chapter 2). In general, infants are more resistant to hypoxia than adults, and hypoxic-ischemic lesions have a different distribution in infants and adults (**Fig. 8.1**).

Hypoxic-ischemic encephalopathy and head trauma are the commonest causes of persistent vegetative state.

PATHOLOGY

Despite the relatively straightforward clinical stratification of syndromes, the macroscopic and microscopic features of hypoxic-ischemic lesions are extremely variable. Lesions can be considered as either acute/subacute or chronic.

CEREBRAL BLOOD FLOW (CBF)

$$\frac{\text{cerebral perfusion}}{\text{pressure}} = \frac{\text{systemic arterial}}{\text{blood pressure}} - \frac{\text{intracranial}}{\text{pressure}}$$

- So long as the mean cerebral perfusion pressure remains above about 5.3kPa (~40 mmHg), the tone of the smooth muscle of intracranial arteries and arterioles (and hence the cerebrovascular resistance) adjusts in response to changes in the perfusion pressure, to maintain CBF at a constant value of approximately 50 ml/100g/min in adults (the value is higher in children). This phenomenon is known as autoregulation.
- Although overall CBF remains constant while cerebral perfusion pressure remains above the threshold for autoregulation, the blood flow does vary somewhat locally, according to demand for O_2 and glucose (ie. according to brain activity), a process of 'local autoregulation'.
- The density of capillaries is greater in gray matter than in white matter, reflecting the difference in their metabolic requirements and resulting in a corresponding difference in blood flow:
  - 80–100 ml/100 g/min in gray matter.
  - 20–25 ml/100 g/min in white matter.
- If the mean cerebral perfusion pressure falls below about 5.3kPa, autoregulation fails and CBF falls dramatically.
- The threshold CBF for infarction in primate brain is approximately 10–12 ml/100g/min.

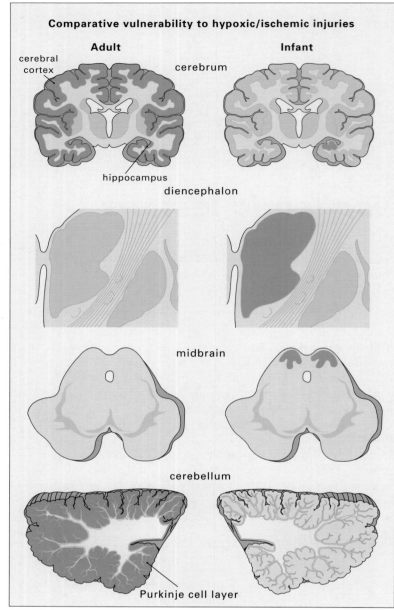

Comparative vulnerability to hypoxic/ischemic injuries

Adult | **Infant**

cerebral cortex — cerebrum

hippocampus

diencephalon

midbrain

cerebellum

Purkinje cell layer

Fig. 8.1 Regions of selective vulnerability to hypoxic–ischaemic damage are different in the adult and infant brain. Those regions most susceptible to such an insult are colored in the above diagram, though individual cases may show much variation.

PRINCIPAL CAUSES OF HYPOXIA

Hypoxemic hypoxia (low O_2 content in blood)
- Carbon monoxide poisoning (mechanisms include displacement of O_2 from hemoglobin and direct binding to heme-containing proteins in the brain)
- Near drowning
- Respiratory arrest (drug-induced, status asthmaticus, aspiration)
- Prolonged status epilepticus

Stagnant hypoxia (inadequate supply of oxygenated blood i.e. ischemia)
- Cardiac arrest with prolonged asystole, or hypotension due to myocardial infarction, cardiac tamponade, or major cardiac dysrhythmia.
- Intraoperative hypotensive episode(s), particularly if there is a sustained and profound drop in blood pressure or if there is extensive underlying vascular disease (e.g. atherosclerosis in the carotid or vertebral arteries).
  There is evidence that microemboli released into the circulation during such surgery may also contribute to the subsequent encephalopathy.
- Severe increases in intracranial pressure, when intracranial pressure reaches mean arterial blood pressure, brain perfusion ceases.
- Cessation of brain perfusion has usually been prolonged in patients coming to autopsy after having been maintained for a long period on a respirator. The (imprecise) term 'respirator' brain is sometimes used to describe such brains.

Histotoxic hypoxia (inability of tissues to utilize O_2)
- Cyanide and sulfide exposure (due to inhibition of mitochondrial enzymes involved in oxidative respiration).

SELECTIVE VULNERABILITY AND EXCITOTOXICITY

Selective vulnerability refers to the differential susceptibility of CNS regions to an hypoxic–ischemic event. The following regions are listed in roughly decreasing order of vulnerability to hypoxia in adults: hippocampus, cerebral neocortex, cerebellum, thalamus, basal ganglia, brain stem, hypothalamus and spinal cord.
- Within the hippocampus, the CA1 field (Sommer sector) is most vulnerable and the CA2 field least so.
- Within the cerebral neocortex, the most vulnerable neurons are in laminae 3 and 5.
- Within the cerebellum, the Purkinje cells are most susceptible to hypoxic injury.
- In premature and term infants, the pattern of neuronal susceptibility to hypoxic-ischemic injury differs from that in adults (see chapter 2).

Determinants of selective vulnerability to neuronal necrosis are complex, but include:
- Variable O_2 and energy requirements of different neurons and neuronal populations.
- Glutamate receptor densities. Glutamate acts as an excitotoxic neurotransmitter acting upon various receptor subtypes, including NMDA, kainate, AMPA (α-amino-3-hydroxy-5-methyl-4-isoxazole propionic acid), and metabotropic.
- Activation of immediate early genes (e.g. heat shock protein, c-fos) by ischemia-induced free radicals, and the vasodilatory activity of nitric oxide.

MACROSCOPIC APPEARANCES

Acute/subacute lesions include the following abnormalities:

- precursors of cystic infarcts (especially in watershed territories, see chapter 9)
- cortical laminar necrosis (if very severe)
- patchy gray discoloration of the cortex with blurring of the junction between the gray and white matter (i.e. appearance resembling subacute infarction)
- bright pink discoloration and edema in the acute stages following carbon monoxide poisoning
- generalized dusky discoloration and softening — the appearance of a nonperfused brain ('respirator' brain) (**Fig. 8.2**).

There may be no macroscopic abnormality.

Chronic: Changes that evolve from the acute/subacute lesions often become more obvious, for example:

- Watershed infarcts (**Fig. 8.3**).
- Cortical laminar necrosis (**Fig. 8.4**).
- Characteristic cystic necrosis in carbon monoxide poisoning. This is usually symmetrical and affects the globus pallidus. Occasionally this pattern is seen without well-documented carbon monoxide exposure (**Fig. 8.5**), and can occur as a result of cyanide poisoning, heroin overdose or other causes of global cerebral hypoxia and ischemia.
- Hypoxic-ischemic leukoencephalopathy (see Fig. 8.11).
- Hippocampal atrophy due to 'sclerosis' (see page 8.7).

In some cases no macroscopic abnormality is evident. However, most patients who have been in a persistent coma or vegetative state due to hypoxic-ischemic injury will show macroscopic abnormalities.

MICROSCOPIC APPEARANCES

Acute/subacute: Ischemic neurons have pyknotic nuclei and bright pink cytoplasm in sections stained with hematoxylin and eosin. At later times, as the chromatin is degraded, the nuclei become more eosinophilic and appear to blend in with the surrounding cytoplasm. These changes are first discernible histologically after several hours' survival, last for about 2 weeks, and are particularly likely to be seen in neurons that are sensitive to hypoxia (e.g. hippocampal neurons in the CA1 field, pyramidal neurons in the cerebral necortex, cerebellar Purkinje cells) (**Figs 8.6, 8.7**). The neuropil may show slight vacuolation or be normal. Normal neurons may be seen adjacent to severely affected cells. Hypoxic-ischemic neuronal change is sometimes dramatically demonstrated in smear/squash preparations of affected brain region(s) (**Fig. 8.8**).

Ultrastructurally, ischemia in animal models produces changes of cellular necrosis, with breaks in nuclear and cell membranes and flocculent densities in mitochondria. Mitochondrial swelling is an early feature but in the absence of further changes is thought to be reversible.

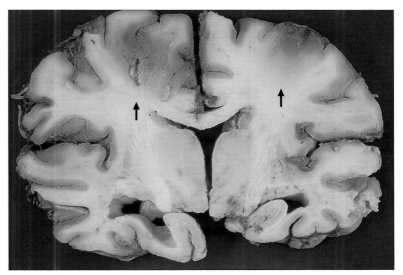

Fig. 8.2 Coronal section through a nonperfused ('respirator') brain. This shows an edematous brain with patchy gray-brown discoloration throughout the cortex and extending into the subcortical white matter, most notably in the watershed regions (arrows) between the perfusion territories of the middle and anterior cerebral arteries.

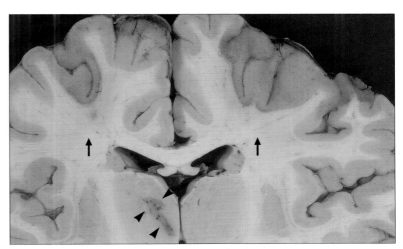

Fig. 8.3 Relatively recent bihemispheric watershed infarcts in anterior cerebral artery/middle cerebral artery border zones. Note the dusky gray-brown discoloration of the cortex in these regions (arrows), which is accentuated at the junction between the gray and white matter. There is also a region of necrosis in the left thalamus (arrowheads). The patient was a 2-year-old child with double outlet right ventricle who underwent the Fontan procedure. Intraoperative and postoperative complications led to death 15 days later.

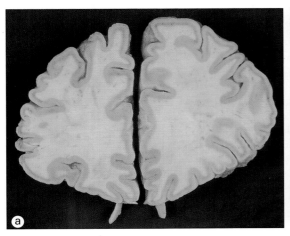

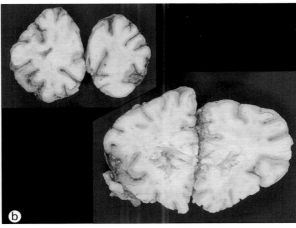

Fig. 8.4 Cortical laminar necrosis. (a) Coronal section through the brain of a 53-year-old man who underwent an orthotopic liver transplant and became severely obtunded approximately 1 month before death. Note the variably dense line in the cortical ribbon just above the junction between gray and white matter. This is indicative of laminar necrosis. **(b)** Sections through the brain of a 41-year-old man who experienced numerous cardiorespiratory arrests after complicated bowel surgery and died 1 month later. Note the severe cortical necrosis with virtual separation of the cortical ribbon from underlying white matter.

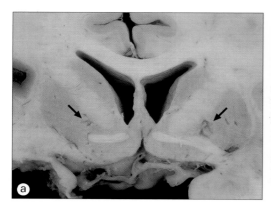

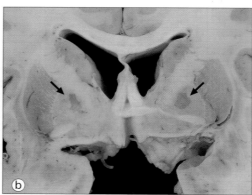

Fig. 8.5 Bilateral pallidal cystic necrosis. (a) Pallidal necrosis in a patient who died after surgery for a malignant glioma in the left temporal lobe. The hemorrhagic surgical bed is seen at the lower left. He had previously attempted suicide by carbon monoxide poisoning several months before his death. Note the bilateral pallidal cystic necrosis (arrows), which is more extreme on the right than on the left. **(b)** Comparable section from the brain of a 75-year-old woman with severe toxic epidermal necrolysis syndrome and no history of carbon monoxide poisoning. Recent bihemispheric parieto-occipital infarcts (not shown) and bilateral partial necrosis of globus pallidus (arrows) were noted at necropsy.

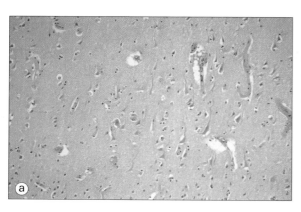

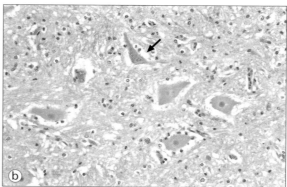

Fig. 8.6 Acute hypoxic neuronal change. (a) Neocortical neurons with eosinophilic cytoplasm and smudged or pyknotic nuclei. **(b)** Pronounced cytoplasmic eosinophilia, loss of definition of cell membranes, and pyknotic nuclei in several anterior horn cells. Anterior horn cells of the spinal cord are rarely affected by hypoxia-ischemia except when an hypoxic-ischemic episode is severe or prolonged. A single neuron (arrow) has preserved Nissl substance and a relatively intact appearance.

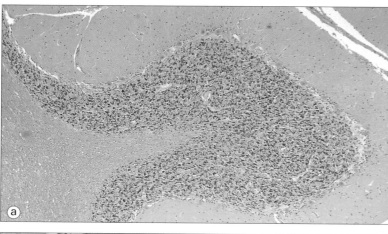

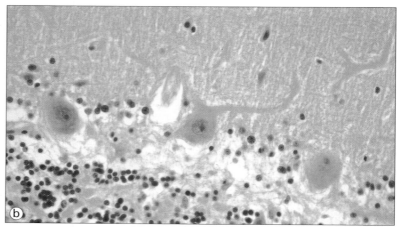

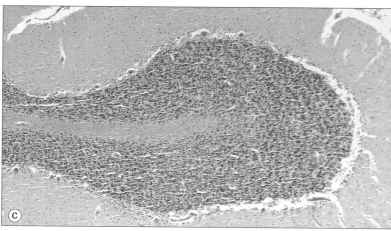

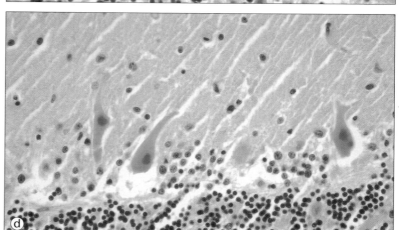

Fig. 8.7 Hypoxic change in cerebellar Purkinje cells. The cerebellum is especially vulnerable to hypoxic-ischemic lesions. **(a)** Low-power view of normal cerebellum. **(b)** High-power view of normal cerebellum. **(c)** Low-power view of cerebellar cortex from a 74-year-old patient who died shortly after complicated open heart surgery. At low magnification there is little obvious difference between this specimen and that in (a). **(d)** High-power view of (c) showing eosinophilic Purkinje cells with smudged and pyknotic nuclei, which contrast with the normal Purkinje cells that have plump large vesicular nuclei and prominent nucleoli (b).

'Delayed neuronal death' describes a loss of neurons hours to days after a global ischemic insult and is well documented in the hippocampus.

Nonperfused 'respirator' brain shows autolysis and anterior pituitary necrosis but no inflammatory and macrophage infiltrate. The tissue remains soft even after fixation, and stains poorly in histologic sections. If the brain swelling has been severe, fragments of disrupted cerebellum may be identified in the subarachnoid space around the spinal cord.

Chronic: Laminar necrosis usually affects the middle cortical layers, especially laminae 3 and 5. In extreme instances, there may be full-thickness (rather than laminar) cortical necrosis (**Fig. 8.9**). The necrosis is

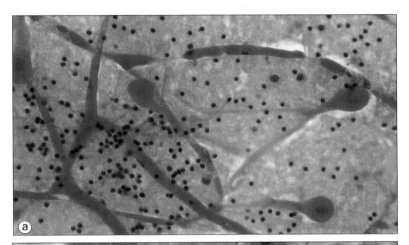

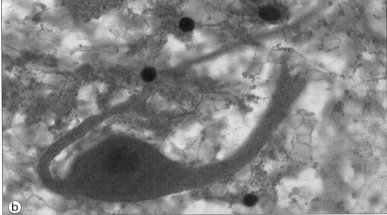

Fig. 8.8 Hypoxic change. This is often clearly demonstrated in smear/squash preparations. **(a)** Cerebellum. **(b)** Cerebral cortex.

PERSISTENT VEGETATIVE STATE (PVS)

Definitions*

The *vegetative state* is a clinical condition of complete unawareness of the self and the environment, accompanied by sleep-wake cycles, with either complete or partial preservation of hypothalamic and brainstem autonomic functions. In addition, patients in a vegetative state show no evidence of sustained, reproducible, purposeful, or voluntary behavioral responses to visual, auditory, tactile, or noxious stimuli; show no evidence of language comprehension or expression; have bowel and bladder incontinence; and have variably preserved cranial nerve and spinal reflexes.

Persistent vegetative state is defined as a vegetative state present 1 month after acute traumatic or non-traumatic brain injury or lasting for at least 1 month in patients with degenerative or metabolic disorders or developmental malformations.

The neuropathologic findings vary according to the underlying etiology but usually include one or more of the following:

- **Diffuse cortical injury**
  This is usually hypoxic-ischemic, metabolic (e.g. as a result of hypoglycemic injury, or lysosomal storage disease), or degenerative (e.g. in late-stage Alzheimer's disease) in etiology.
- **Bilateral thalamic injury**
  This is almost always due to hypoxia/ischemia
- **Diffuse white matter damage**
  The commonest cause is diffuse axonal injury due to head trauma (see chapter 11). PVS due to diffuse white matter damage rarely complicates hypoxia-ischemia (see Fig. 8.11), and may also result from leukodystrophies associated with lysosomal or peroxisomal enzyme defects.
- **Major developmental malformations**, such as holoprosencephaly, hydraencephaly etc.

Secondary changes, caused for example by seizures, effects of medication, and infections, are often present.

*Multi-Society Task Force on PVS. (1994) Medical aspects of the persistent vegetative state. N Engl J Med; **330**:1499–508.*

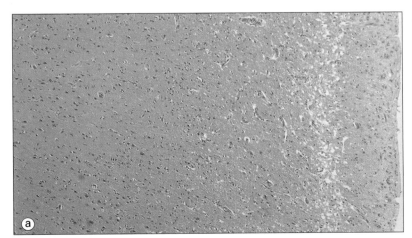

Fig. 8.9 Hypoxic-ischemic cortical injury in two patients. (a) 80-year-old patient who underwent pituitary surgery 1 month before death. At necropsy there were minimal macroscopic abnormalities of the brain, but microscopically there was widespread hypoxic neuronal change, vacuolation of the superficial cortex, subtle microvascular proliferation, and gliosis.

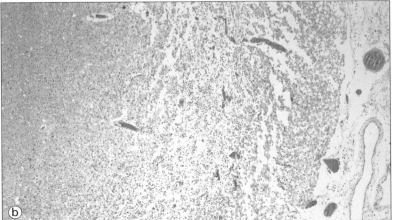

(b) Severe cortical necrosis. This is from the brain shown in Fig. 8.4b. It shows severe pancortical necrosis tantamount to infarction. The cellular infiltrate replacing the neuronal layers comprises a mixture of astrocytes and macrophages.

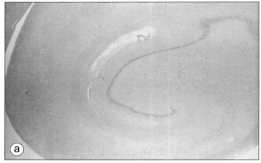
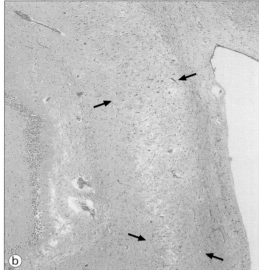
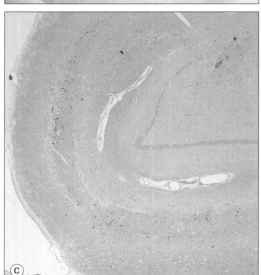
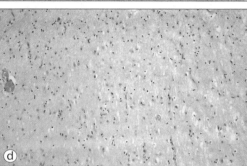

Fig. 8.10 Selective vulnerability to hypoxic-ischemic change in the hippocampus. (a) Normal hippocampus at low magnification. The figure includes part of the granule cell layer and part of the pyramidal cell layer as far as the prosubiculum/CA1 junction. **(b)** Segmental loss of neurons and slight neuropil vacuolation within the CA1 field or sector. Note the abrupt transitions (arrows) between intact neurons in the pyramidal cell layer and the region of neuron loss and gliosis (sclerosis). **(c)** There is an infarct involving virtually the entire CA1 field or sector and extending into the prosubiculum. Neuron loss and spongy change seen in the affected neuropil. The endplate (CA3/4) region is also involved, but note the preservation of the CA2 field or sector and the granule cell layer (dentate fascia). **(d)** Magnified view of the pyramidal cell layer in an elderly patient who had severe intra- and perioperative hypotension and hypoxia years before death, resulting in an amnestic syndrome. This shows sparse surviving neurons and severe astrocytic gliosis.

usually accentuated in watershed zones. Watershed infarcts are described in chapter 9.

In many regions long-term hypoxic-ischemic change may appear simply as a focal loss of neurons with reactive gliosis. This is particularly dramatic in the hippocampus where the CA1 sector is very vulnerable to hypoxia whereas the CA2 sector is relatively resistant (**Fig. 8.10**). A distinction is often made between 'selective neuronal loss and gliosis' in which neurons disappear with attendant gliosis, and 'infarction' in which all cellular elements die and macrophages infiltrate to remove the cellular debris. In practice, the two processes may be difficult to differentiate months or years after the insult has occurred, though cystic change and encephalomalacia are more pronounced after infarction.

A leukoencephalopathy may coexist with hypoxic-ischemic gray matter damage (**Fig. 8.11**), and exceptionally may be the predominant finding after prolonged hypoxia in association with hypotension. It has been associated with carbon monoxide poisoning, but can occur in other settings, such as drug overdose. Histologically, there may be necrosis with abundant macrophages, or loss of myelin in association with relative sparing of axons, reactive astrocytosis, and activation of microglia.

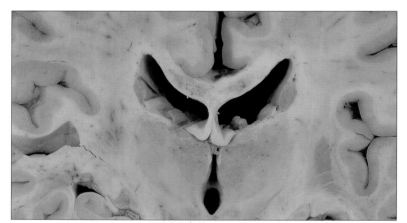

Fig. 8.11 Hypoxic-ischemic leukoencephalopathy. Note the white matter discoloration and the necrosis of the central part of the corpus callosum. This was seen at necropsy of a 69-year-old patient who underwent complicated aortic surgery and developed 'mental status changes' and spinal cord paralysis secondary to a cord infarct one month before death. There were also widespread necrotic lesions in the cortex and subcortical white matter. Histologic changes included dense collections of histiocytes.

REFERENCES

Adams JH, Brierley JB, Connor RCR, Treip CS (1966) The effects of systemic hypotension upon the human brain. Clinical and neuropathological observations in 11 cases. *Brain* **89**: 235–268.

Auer RN, Benveniste H (1996) Hypoxia and related conditions. In Graham DI and Lantos PL (eds) *Greenfield's Neuropathology. Sixth edition.* pp. 263–314. London: Arnold.

Auer RN, Siesjö BK (1988) Biological differences between ischemia, hypoglycemia, and epilepsy. *Ann Neurol* **24**: 699–707.

Ginsberg MD, Hedley-Whyte ET, Richardson EP Jr (1976) Hypoxic-ischemic leukoencephalopathy in man. *Arch Neurol* **33**: 5–14.

Kinney HC, Samuels MA (1994) Neuropathology of the persistent vegetative state. A review. *J Neuropathol Exp Neurol* **53**: 548–558.

Levy DE, Caronna JJ, Singer BH, Lapinski RH, Frydman H, Plum F (1985) Predicting outcome after hypoxic-ischemic coma. *JAMA* **253**: 1420–1426.

Moody DM, Bell MA, Challa VR, Johnston WE, Prough DS (1990) Brain microemboli during cardiac surgery or aortography. *Ann Neurol* **28**: 477–486.

Siesjö BK (1988) Hypoglycemia, brain metabolism, and brain damage. *Diab Metab Rev* **4**: 113–144.

Wass CT, Lanier WL (1996) Glucose modulation of ischemic brain injury: review and clinical recommendations. *Mayo Clin Proc* **71**: 801–812.

Whetsell WO Jr (1996) Current concepts of excitotoxicity. *J Neuropathol Exp Neurol* **55**: 1–13.

9 *Vascular disease and infarcts*

Infarcts are to be distinguished from focal or generalized hypoxic–ischemic change, which primarily affects neurons (see chapter 8), and intracranial hemorrhage (see chapter 10). An infarct is defined as a region of brain tissue in which all cellular elements undergo necrosis (cell death), usually as the result of a cessation of flow of oxygenated blood to the region. Infarcts can become secondarily hemorrhagic and may mimic primary hemorrhage.

The clinical term 'stroke' describes a syndrome of rapidly evolving or sudden onset, non-epileptic, neurologic deficit that lasts more than 24 hours. By convention, stroke has come to mean either brain infarction or hemorrhage. A transient ischemic attack (TIA) lasts less than 24 hours. Infarcts can be caused by:
- large vessel or macrovascular (arterial) disease
- small vessel or microvascular (arterial) disease
- emboli
- venous thrombosis

The first part of this chapter covers the various types of vascular disease that cause infarcts of the CNS, and the latter part covers the pathology of CNS infarcts *per se*.

EPIDEMIOLOGIC ASPECTS OF STROKE

- In the USA there are approximately 0.5 million new 'strokes' annually and almost 3 million 'survivors' of a stroke. Stroke is the third most common cause of mortality causing 150,000 deaths each year, although this figure has been declining.
- Incidence of stroke increases with age, being 100/100,000 for people aged 45–54 years and increasing to over 1800/100,000 for those over 85 years of age.
- The major, largely modifiable, risk factors for stroke are hypertension, cardiac disease, cigarette smoking, hyperlipidemia and diabetes mellitus.
- Other risk factors for stroke include oral contraceptive use, hematologic diseases (e.g. sickle cell disease, polycythemia), some inherited coagulation disorders, and various cardiac and vascular diseases.
- In most US series, brain infarction is approximately ten times more common than brain hemorrhage. The ratio is lower in some European and virtually all Japanese studies; some studies from the Orient have found hemorrhage to be almost as common as infarction.

LARGE VESSEL DISEASE

ATHEROSCLEROSIS

Atherosclerosis is by far the leading systemic vasculopathy that produces brain infarcts, especially in older patients. It can affect both intracranial and extracranial large arteries.

RISK FACTORS FOR ATHEROSCLEROSIS

Major risk factors for atherosclerosis include:
- age
- family history
- diabetes mellitus
- cigarette smoking
- hypertension
- abnormalities of lipid metabolism
- truncal obesity

ATHEROSCLEROSIS AND STROKE

- Atherosclerotic stroke is usually associated with documented risk factors for or a family history of atherosclerosis and patients may have coronary artery disease or peripheral vascular disease.
- TIA is a common presentation. This is a focal neurologic deficit resolving within 24 hours and referable to the vessel involved by severe atheroma, for example a right carotid artery atheromatous plaque may produce transient or episodic right monocular blindness (amaurosis fugax) and left hemiparesis. Platelet–fibrin emboli can sometimes be visualized on fundoscopic examination.
- A patient who suffers a TIA has a high risk of developing a completed stroke.
- Atherosclerotic strokes result from dislodgement and embolization of platelet–fibrin material, or occlusive thrombosis of the atherosclerotic artery.
- The thrombosis often originates extracranially, at the bifurcation of the carotid artery or within the intraosseous part of the vertebral artery, although the thrombus may propagate to involve intracranial arteries.
- Less often an atherosclerotic intracranial artery is the site of primary thrombosis.

MACROSCOPIC APPEARANCES

The severity of atherosclerosis can vary significantly in different vessels. The degree and extent of aortic or coronary artery atherosclerosis do not predict involvement of the cerebral vasculature. Atherosclerosis is often most severe at the origins of the vertebral arteries and carotid bifurcation (**Figs. 9.1, 9.2**). Intracranial atherosclerosis is most severe in the major branches of the circle of Willis and vertebrobasilar system (**Fig.**

9.3a). Atheroma in distal arterial branches is more common in Asian and African–American patients. The extent and topography of atherosclerosis in the basal vessels are often best documented by removing the circle of Willis (**Fig. 9.3b**). Carotid endarterectomy specimens from patients with TIAs or threatened stroke may be submitted for histology and the extent and severity of atheroma should be assessed (see **Fig. 9.2**)

THE AUTOPSY OF A STROKE PATIENT

- The emphasis of the postmortem investigations varies acccording to whether the 'stroke' was ischemic or hemorrhagic (or a combination of these).
- Clinical history and imaging studies assist this assessment.

Especially important for infarction:

- Assess patency of major arteries (carotid and vertebral) in the neck:
  - Inject water at their origins and monitor 'through-flow' in the cranial cavity after the brain has been removed
  - If any vessel is obstructed, prosector should attempt to establish:
    - site(s) of occlusion/severe stenosis, and
    - cause(s) of occlusion (e.g. atherosclerosis, embolus, dissection)
  - Vessels should be dissected until significant lesions are documented; this sometimes requires removal of entire carotid or vertebral artery.
  - Dissection of the intraosseous part of the vertebral arteries is facilitated by prior removal of the cervical vertebral bodies. This is achieved from an anterior approach by making a parasagittal saw cut through the medial part of the vertebral pedicles (a laterally placed cut will damage the arteries).
- Carefully inspect the heart paying particular attention to:
  - possible endocarditis (infectious or non-infectious); culture/histology of any valvular lesions may be helpful
  - any possible cause of a right-to-left shunt (e.g. septal defect, patent foramen ovale)
  - abnormalities of the valves, especially on the left side of heart (e.g. myxomatous degeneration/prolapse of mitral valve, calcific aortic sclerosis)

- Look for infarcts in other organs.
- If there is little evidence of macro/microvascular disease, and cardiac examination is normal, consider: hematologic disorders (e.g. antiphospholipid syndrome, or abnormalities of coagulation, platelets, erythrocytes); these need to be sought in non-neuropathologic components of the autopsy, and antemortem laboratory values.

Especially important for hemorrhage (see chapter 10):

- In the medical history and general autopsy, seek evidence of disease that may be of etiologic significance:
  - Hypertension - cardiomegaly with left ventricular hypertrophy, nephrosclerosis
  - Dementia – especially in elderly patients dementia may point to cerebral amyloid angiopathy in association with Alzheimer's disease
  - Neoplasia – hemorrhage in association with metastasis
  - History suggesting drug abuse
- When a hematoma is documented at time of brain removal, establish:
  - in which compartment it exists (e.g. subdural, subarachnoid, combined subarachnoid/intraparenchymal or intraventricular)
  - its approximate volume
  - in a young patient, by dissecting the circle of Willis and its major branches, whether a ruptured cerebral aneurysm has caused subarachnoid (or intracerebral) hemorrhage.
- When a hematoma is first discovered when the fixed brain is cut:
  - sample surrounding tissues generously to document microvascular disease or remnants of hemangioma/neoplasm.

HYPERHOMOCYSTEINEMIA, ATHEROMA AND BRAIN INFARCTS

- Hyperhomocysteinemia occurs in a range of inherited disorders, including homocystinuria (due to cystathionine β-synthase deficiency), and several rare disorders of vitamin B_{12} or folate metabolism (see chapter 21).
- Elevated levels of homocysteine in the blood increase the risk of atheroma and of arterial and venous thomboses in several organs, including the brain.

- Several mechanisms are probably involved. Homocysteine promotes the proliferation of vascular smooth muscle cells. It also inhibits the proliferation of endothelial cells ands increases their release of thrombogenic factors.
- There is strong epidemiologic evidence that acquired mild hyperhomocysteinemia, in most cases probably due to subclinical folate deficiency, is a risk factor for the development of atheroma and of brain infarcts.

MICROSCOPIC APPEARANCES

The histologic features of atheroma are best demonstrated with:

- stains that differentiate elastica, fibrous tissue, and smooth muscle (e.g. elastica van Gieson, Movat pentachrome)
- immunohistochemistry using primary antibodies to vascular smooth muscle actin

Fibromuscular intimal hyperplasia with an intact endothelium and variable attenuation of the vascular lumen is noted in 'early' and asymptomatic vascular lesions, and often discovered incidentally at necropsy (**Fig. 9.4**).

Complicated plaques show cholesterol clefts, prominent macrophages, and evidence of old hemorrhage (hemosiderin and hematoidin), and may be calcified. There is usually significant narrowing of the vessel lumen, often in association with ulceration and overlying mural or occlusive thrombus (**Fig. 9.5**).

The distal circulation (i.e. parenchymal and meningeal arteries) may show atherosclerotic changes or platelet–fibrin or atheromatous emboli (**Fig. 9.6**).

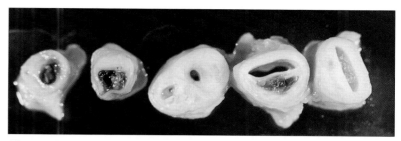

Fig. 9.1 Atheroma of carotid artery. Sections of common carotid (right) and internal carotid arteries removed at necropsy from a patient with severe atherosclerotic cerebrovascular disease. Note the severe stenosis of the lumina and eccentric intimal thickening of the internal carotid artery.

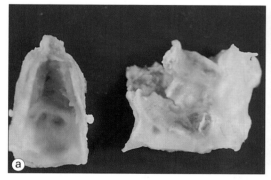
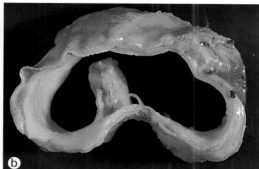

Fig. 9.2 Carotid endarterectomy specimens from two patients. (a) A specimen cut open to reveal grumous fractured eggshell-like atheromatous material and superimposed mural thrombus. **(b)** Another specimen cut in cross section showing atheroma at the carotid bifurcation. (Courtesy of Dr Sophia Apple, Dept of Pathology and Lab Medicine, UCLA Medical Center, U.S.A.)

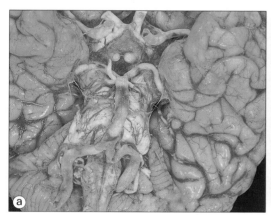
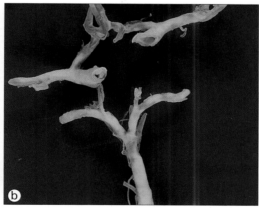

Fig. 9.3 Severe atherosclerosis of the circle of Willis and its major branches. (a) Patchy yellow discoloration of the arterial branches indicates underlying atheroma. **(b)** Severe atheroma involving the basal arteries of the brain of an 82-year-old patient.

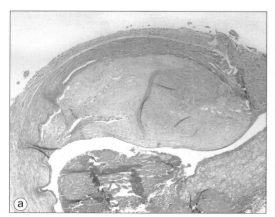
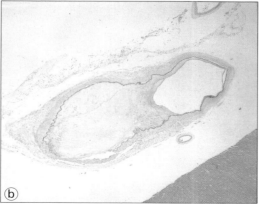
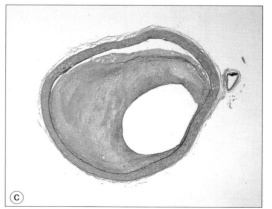

Fig. 9.4 Atherosclerosis with fibromuscular intimal hyperplasia. Eccentric atheroma is prominent in these arteries, but is largely composed of smooth muscle cells and 'ground substance' (glycosaminoglycans), though scattered cholesterol clefts are also present. Note the intact endothelium in all instances. The single elastic lamina (as is the case in intracerebral arteries) is also largely intact. **(a)** Middle cerebral artery. **(b)** An intracerebral (meningeal) artery, a branch of the posterior cerebral artery. **(c)** Posterior cerebral artery. (Elastic van Gieson)

FIBROMUSCULAR DYSPLASIA (FMD)

FMD is an idiopathic systemic vascular disease characterized by non-atherosclerotic abnormalities of smooth muscle and fibrous and elastic tissues in small and medium-sized arteries. It is much less common than atherosclerosis.

The pathogenesis is unknown, but some studies have suggested a relationship to segmental arterial mediolysis (a disorder in which smooth muscle cells in the outer part of the tunica media undergo vacuolation and lysis). This occurs mainly in coronary and splanchnic arteries and is thought to be due to vasospasm of undetermined etiology.

FMD of the renal arteries is estimated to occur in one in every 100 necropsies. The cephalic arteries are affected in 25% of reported cases and are the second most commonly involved arteries after the renal arteries. The carotid artery is much more often involved than the vertebral artery; carotid artery involvement is bilateral in over 50% of patients. Vessel wall involvement is medial in over 90% of cases, intimal in 5% of cases, or very rarely, adventitial. Intracranial arteries very rarely contain FMD.

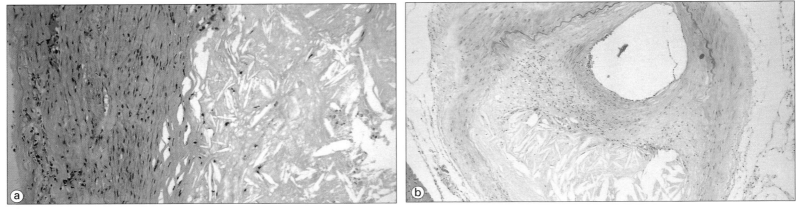

Fig. 9.5 Complicated atherosclerosis. (a) Severe atherosclerosis in a carotid endarterectomy specimen. Note the cholesterol clefts adjacent to a region of smooth muscle cell hyperplasia.
(b) Prominent eccentric atheroma with smooth muscle cell hyperplasia and cholesterol clefts in an intracranial meningeal artery. The atheroma has produced significant stenosis.

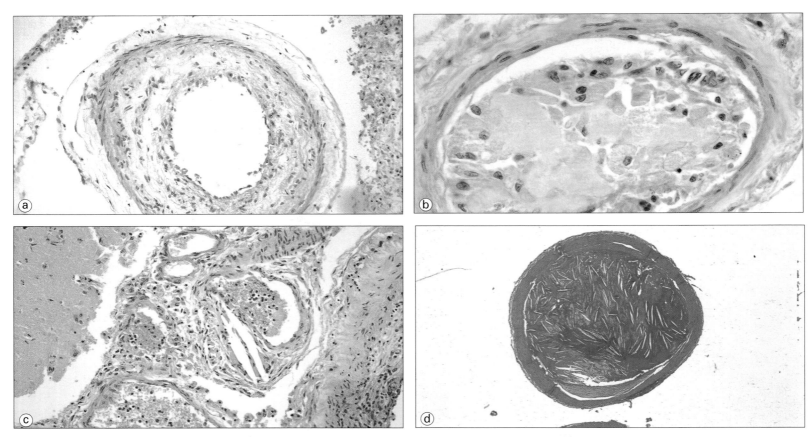

Fig. 9.6 Cerebral atherosclerosis and complications of atheroma. (a) Atherosclerosis in a small artery (external diameter approximately 500 μm) manifests as fibromuscular intimal hyperplasia. **(b)** Intraluminal macrophages and histiocytes related to embolic material from fragmented atheromatous plaques in a 58-year-old hypertensive woman with multiple cerebral and cerebellar infarcts in both watershed and non-watershed territories. **(c)** Cholesterol clefts related to emboli from fragmented atheromatous plaques in the same case as (b). **(d)** Larger artery in another patient showing occlusive thrombus composed primarily of atheromatous material ('athero-embolus') with residual cholesterol clefts. An 'embolic' origin of the atheromatous material is suggested by the relative absence of intrinsic atherosclerosis in the artery itself.

MACROSCOPIC AND MICROSCOPIC APPEARANCES

FMD is easily distinguished from atherosclerosis by:

- the absence of features of complicated atherosclerosis (see above)
- the presence of smooth muscle cell hyperplasia or thinning, destruction of elastica, fibrosis, and general disorganization of arterial wall components (Fig. 9.7)
- negligible inflammatory infiltrate

MOYAMOYA DISEASE

Moyamoya disease is a rare idiopathic condition that presents with progressive stenosis and eventual occlusion of basal intracerebral arteries. Compensatory dilatation of lenticulostriate arteries produces a characteristic 'puff of smoke' appearance on angiography.

Thrombotic lesions in the circle of Willis implicate abnormal thrombogenesis in the pathogenesis of this disorder, and regions of intimal thickening may represent organizing thrombi.

Moyamoya disease was initially thought to occur only in Japan, but is now well documented among many other populations, including Caucasians, African Americans, and Native Americans.

FIBROMUSCULAR DYSPLASIA

- FMD shows female predominance.
- FMD usually becomes symptomatic in the fourth or fifth decade.
- Connective tissue disorders and α1-antitrypsin deficiency are associated with FMD.
- Ischemic infarcts secondary to vascular stenosis or occlusion may occur.
- As many as 10–20% of patients with carotid dissections show angiographic features of FMD.
- FMD is rarely associated with the formation of aneurysms on intra- or extracranial arteries.

MOYAMOYA DISEASE

- Moyamoya disease presents with subarachnoid or intraparenchymal hemorrhage (35% of cases), cerebral infarction (20% of cases), TIA (20% of cases), seizures (10% of cases), or a combination of these.
- An upper respiratory tract infection often procedes initial symptoms.
- Cerebral angiography, which shows dilated lenticulostriate arteries and other collaterals is usually diagnostic.
- The prognosis is poor if both anterior and posterior branches of the circle of Willis are involved.

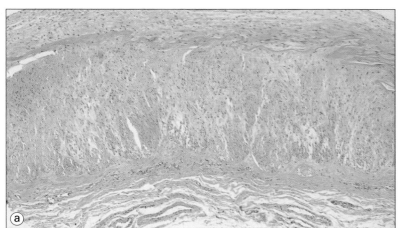

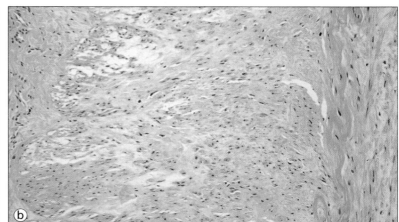

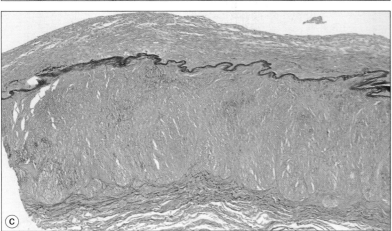

Fig. 9.7 FMD of extracranial internal carotid artery (ICA) associated with aneurysm formation. (a) The tunica media shows disorganization and loss of smooth muscle cells. **(b)** The loss of smooth muscle cells, and abnormal orientation of many that remain, is more obvious at higher magnification. **(c)** The internal elastic lamina may appear irregular or disrupted. (Elastic van Gieson). (Courtesy of M. Miyauchi and S. Shionoya)

MACROSCOPIC AND MICROSCOPIC APPEARANCES

Arteries of the circle of Willis show thrombotic lesions in over 50% of patients. The most commonly involved vessels are the internal carotid arteries, posterior communicating arteries, and posterior cerebral arteries. Severely stenotic non-complicated atherosclerosis with intimal fibromuscular hyperplasia but negligible lipid, inflammation, and disruption of the elastica are the histologic features (**Fig. 9.8**). Platelet–fibrin thrombi are often seen at the intimal surface.

ARTERIAL DISSECTION

Arterial dissection is rare and tends to affect young and middle-aged adults. The dissection is usually spontaneous but can be initiated by blunt trauma, often mild (e.g. chiropractic manipulations of the neck). Rarely other etiologic factors are involved (see box). The dissection may involve the extracranial or intracranial part of the vertebral artery (more common in women) or carotid artery (more common in men). An intimal tear leads to a medial or subendothelial hematoma. The expanding hematoma occludes the vessel lumen, producing infarction. Dissection of intracranial arteries may rarely extend to involve the adventitia, producing subarachnoid hemorrhage.

MACROSCOPIC AND MICROSCOPIC APPEARANCES

A subarachnoid hemorrhage or ischemic infarct with cerebral edema is evident macroscopically. Demonstration of the point of origin of the dissection usually necessitates complete examination of the intracranial and extracranial parts of the affected carotid or vertebral artery. A subendothelial or intramural hematoma is found within the vessel wall (**Fig. 9.9**).

HUMAN IMMUNODEFICIENCY VIRUS (HIV)-ASSOCIATED ARTERIOPATHIES

When a stroke occurs in a patient with HIV infection, it may be difficult to determine its precise cause. Many of the opportunistic infections frequently seen in such patients may cause, mimic, or contribute to cerebrovascular disease, especially cytomegalovirus (CMV) and varicella–zoster virus (VZV) infections, toxoplasmosis, aspergillosis, and tuberculosis.

One study found evidence of cerebrovascular disease in 5–10% of necropsies carried out on patients with AIDS. Non-bacterial thrombotic endocarditis (marantic endocarditis) should be considered and sought at necropsy in any patient with AIDS who develops an acute arterial occlusion. Chronic basal meningitis and angiitis (including granulomatous angiitis) occasionally cause cerebral ischemia.

As many as 20–25% of children with AIDS have evidence of cerebral hemorrhage or infarction (in roughly equal proportions).

> ### POSSIBLE ETIOLOGIC FACTORS IN ARTERIAL DISSECTION
>
> *Most cases are spontaneous. Possible etiologic factors in some patients include:*
> - Fibromuscular dysplasia
> - Moyamoya disease
> - Migraine
> - Hypertension
> - Cystic medial necrosis
> - Atherosclerosis

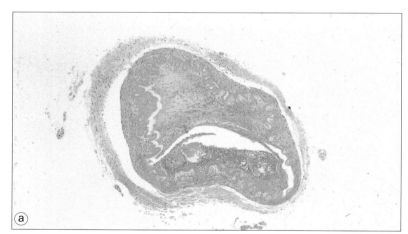

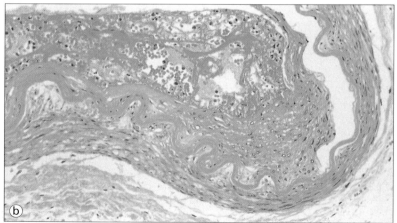

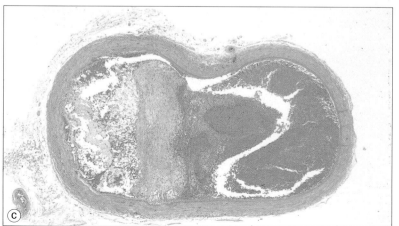

Fig. 9.8 Moyamoya disease. (a and b) Sections of the internal carotid artery from a 15-year-old boy with Moyamoya disease. There is marked intimal thickening with platelet fibrin thrombi on the intimal surface. **(c)** Posterior cerebral artery from a 52-year-old woman with Moyamoya disease. The artery contains mural thrombus composed of red blood cells and fibrin. (Courtesy of Professor E. Ikeda and Professor Y. Hosoda, Tokyo, Japan)

MACROSCOPIC AND MICROSCOPIC APPEARANCES

An HIV-associated arteriopathy is characterized by intimal fibromuscular hyperplasia and aneurysmal dilatation of vessel walls in association with fragmentation of the internal elastic lamina, consistent with 'healed arteritis' (**Fig. 9.10**).

HIV-1 has been demonstrated immunohistochemically in affected vessel walls (probably within the cytoplasm of macrophages), but its pathogenetic role is unclear.

CEREBROVASCULAR DISEASE ASSOCIATED WITH ANTIPHOSPHOLIPID ANTIBODIES

Antibodies that bind phospholipids (APLAs) are associated with various thromboembolic syndromes including recurrent venous and arterial thrombosis (see box). Nearly 20% of APLA-related thromboses affect the cerebral circulation. Anticardiolipin antibodies are an independent risk factor for initial ischemic stroke. These antibodies are detected by enzyme-linked immunosorbent assay (ELISA) using cardiolipin as the antigen or by demonstrating lupus anticoagulant activity.

MACROSCOPIC AND MICROSCOPIC APPEARANCES

There are no distinctive features in occluded vessels to suggest vasculitis or vasculopathy. The cerebral vessels are occluded by bland thrombus. The pial branches of vessels undergo occlusion to produce infarcts.

ANGIITIS AND VASCULITIS AFFECTING LARGE ARTERIES

Most forms of angiitis involving the CNS affect the microvasculature. The only two types affecting major arteries feeding the CNS are:
- giant cell arteritis (also known as temporal arteritis)
- Takayasu's arteritis (also known as aortic arch syndrome)

GIANT CELL ARTERITIS

Giant cell arteritis (GCA) involves large- and medium-sized arteries including the carotid and vertebral arteries and their major branches. Most significant clinical effects involve the eye or brain. The etiology of GCA is unknown, but it may be an anomalous granulomatous response to the elastic component of arterial walls. GCA responds well to treatment with steroids.

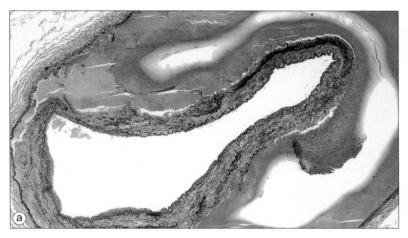
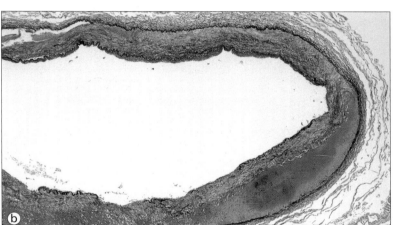
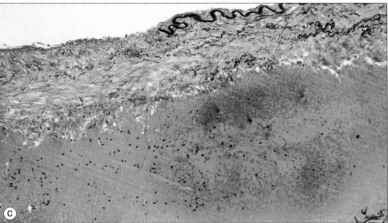
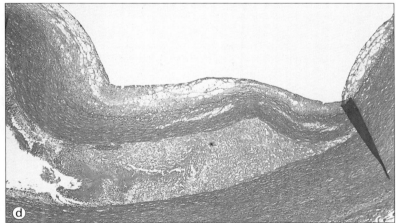

Fig. 9.9 Vertebral artery dissection following chiropractic neck manipulation. (a) There is almost circumferential dissection of blood between the internal and external elastic laminae. (Elastic van Gieson) **(b)** This shows only a thin 'strip' of blood between the internal and external elastic laminae. (Elastic van Gieson) **(c)** This shows a breach of the internal elastic lamina (possibly related to the entry point for the dissection). (Material studied by courtesy of Professor Michael A. Farrell, Dublin) (Elastic van Gieson) **(d)** Intracranial basilar artery dissection in another patient. A subintimal 'wedge' of blood extends into the media.

GIANT CELL ARTERITIS (GCA)

- has an incidence of 15–20/100,000 among those over 50 years of age.
- occurs almost exclusively in elderly patients.
- is a systemic illness that produces fever, malaise, weakness, and limb pain.
- is associated with polymyalgia rheumatica.
- produces headache and visual symptoms if the temporal artery is involved.
- can cause blindness.
- is diagnosed by temporal artery biopsy, but the presence of 'skip' lesions means that a negative result does not exclude the disease. Multiple sections should be taken from the tissue block.
- is accompanied by a normal erythrocyte sedimentation rate (ESR) in 5% of cases.

ANTIPHOSPHOLIPID ANTIBODY SYNDROME

- The antiphospholipid antibodies (APLAs) of most clinical importance are those to a complex of cardiolipin and β2-glycoprotein, and the lupus anticoagulants.
- Low levels of APLAs are a relatively common, usually transient, finding, particularly during or after viral infection (including that due to HIV), or in patients taking chlorpromazine, and probably do not carry an increased risk of thrombotic disease.
- 30-50% of patients with SLE and some patients with other autoimmune diseases have high levels of APLAs and are at risk of thrombotic disease including recurrent strokes in early adulthood from arterial or venous thrombosis.
- Other manifestations of hypercoagulability in patients with APLAs can include optic atrophy, systemic (e.g. myocardial) infarcts, recurrent fetal loss (associated with placental microthrombi), and livedo reticularis.
- Most patients whose SLE is complicated by thrombotic cerebrovascular disease have high titers of APLAs.
- The mainstay of treatment is warfarin but other forms of anticoagulation are also used.

APLA syndrome

- This is defined as the combination of APLA and one or more of the following: venous or arterial thrombosis, thrombocytopenia, or recurrent miscarriages.
- As noted above, APLA syndrome may be a complication of SLE, but can also occur outside of this context, in which case it is known as primary APLA syndrome.
- Unlike SLE (which is predominantly a disease of women), primary APLA syndrome is more common in men. The usual presentation is recurrent small vessel strokes in middle age. These may progress to vascular dementia (see chapter 31)

Sneddon's syndrome

This describes the association of livedo reticularis and strokes, and is associated with APLAs.

MACROSCOPIC AND MICROSCOPIC APPEARANCES

GCA is characterized by widespread granulomatous inflammation of the arterial walls and can cause cerebral infarction. The aorta and coronary, carotid, and vertebral arteries, and their major branches (**Fig. 9.11**) are particularly affected. Multinucleated giant cells are usually evident, and their cytoplasm may contain fragments of elastic lamina.

TAKAYASU'S ARTERITIS

Takayasu's arteritis is a rare disease of the aorta and its branches that sometimes affects the carotid arteries in the neck. It is characterized by granulomatous inflammation (panarteritis) with resultant scarring and destruction.

INHERITED DISORDERS OF COAGULATION THAT INCREASE THE RISK OF DEVELOPING BRAIN INFARCTS

These disorders are relatively uncommon, but should be considered in children and young adults with brain infarcts, particularly if there is a history of previous venous or arterial thrombotic disease involving tissues outside of the CNS. The principal inherited coagulation disorders that have been linked to brain infarcts are:

- Protein C deficiency. This increases the risk of arterial and venous brain infarcts, especially if associated with use of oral contraceptives or with other thrombogenic conditions (e.g. protein S deficiency).
- Factor V Leiden mutation (Arg 506 Gln). This mutation prevents the inactivation of factor V by protein C (and is also known as activated protein C resistance). The main risk is of developing systemic venous thromboses but rarely factor V Leiden mutation is found in children with brain infarcts.
- Protein S deficiency. This is an occasional finding in children and young adults with brain infarcts.
- Antithrombin III abnormalities. Deficient or defective antithrombin III is predominantly associated with venous thombosis and is a rare cause of brain infarcts.
- Carbohydrate-deficient glycoprotein synthase type I. This rare enzyme deficiency affects the synthesis of multiple coagulation factors and their inhibitors and substantially increases the risk of venous thrombosis and brain infarcts.

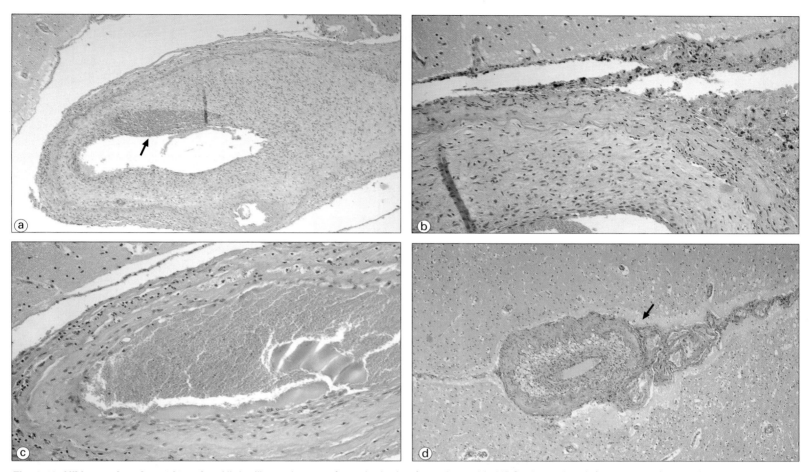

Fig. 9.10 HIV-associated arteriopathy. All the illustrations are from the brain of a patient with AIDS who had multifocal areas of necrosis and hemorrhage at necropsy. **(a)** There are eccentric intimal fibromuscular hyperplasia with focal attenuation of the elastic lamina and a small organizing mural thrombus (arrow) **(b)** This shows another artery with a relatively intact elastic lamina and superimposed intimal hyperplasia, including some macrophage-like cells. **(c)** and **(d)** Two arteries showing intimal hyperplasia with variable numbers of foamy histiocytes in the 'plaque'.

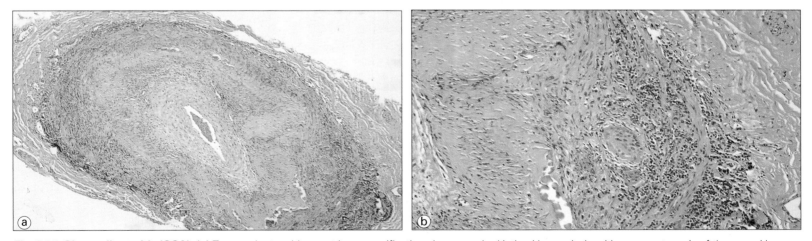

Fig. 9.11 Giant cell arteritis (GCA). (a) Temporal artery biopsy at low magnification shows marked intimal hyperplasia with severe stenosis of the vessel lumen, transmural (but especially prominent adventitial) chronic inflammation, and sparse multinucleated giant cells. **(b)** This shows a rare multinucleated giant cell more clearly. Also note the focal calcification adjacent to and probably involving the internal elastic lamina.

SMALL VESSEL DISEASE (MICROANGIOPATHY)

This is arbitrarily defined as disease affecting arteries with a cross-sectional diameter of 250 µm or less. There are significant exceptions to this rule when considering angiitis, which is, however, most conveniently categorized with this group of conditions. The three most common cerebral microvasculopathies or microangiopathies are:

- arteriosclerosis or arteriolosclerosis
- lipohyalinosis, which is closely linked to arteriosclerosis
- cerebral amyloid angiopathy (CAA)

These conditions commonly produce intraparenchymal hemorrhage (see chapter 10). Arteriosclerosis and lipohyalinosis are also associated with cerebral infarcts, especially small lacunar infarcts, whereas the association between CAA and ischemic lesions is less clear-cut.

ANGIITIS AND VASCULITIS

Patients who have an ischemic infarct or a cerebral hemorrhage as a result of vasculitis usually have systemic as well as cerebrovascular symptoms so presentation is often different from non-vasculitic stroke. CNS abnormalities may be just one facet of multi-organ disease. The investigation of these patients focuses on hematologic and immunologic tests as well as imaging studies of the CNS.

Angiitis and vasculitis may be due to:

- disease that involves the CNS exclusively, for example primary angiitis of the CNS (PACNS), which shows a male predominance and tends to occur in the elderly.
- disease that involves the CNS as part of a systemic disorder, for example miscellaneous vasculitides, which may present with encephalopathy, epilepsy, focal neurologic deficits, cranial neuropathies, meningism, and subarachnoid or intracranial hemorrhage.

PRIMARY ANGIITIS OF THE CNS (PACNS)

PACNS is probably multifactorial in origin. It may be an unusual response to autoantigens or viral infection and varicella-zoster virus has been implicated in some cases.

Macroscopic and microscopic features of PACNS are similar to those of systemic giant cell arteritis, with widespread granulomatous inflammation of leptomeningeal and parenchymal blood vessels including branches of the circle of Willis; it is therefore not exclusively a microangiopathy. Giant cells may be present in the granulomas and fibrinoid necrosis is common (**Fig. 9.12**). Rare examples of severe granulomatous inflammation have recently been described in association with extensive CAA.

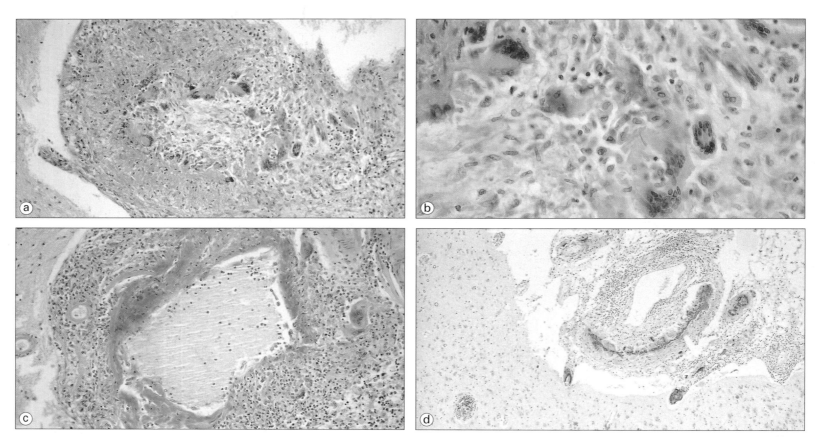

Fig. 9.12 Primary angiitis of the CNS (PACNS), (with a major giant cell component) associated with amyloid angiopathy (CAA). (a) Severe transmural inflammation with occlusion of the arterial lumen and numerous multinucleated giant cells in the vessel wall. **(b)** Detail of the giant cells shown in (a). **(c)** Fibrinoid necrosis of another artery from the same patient. **(d)** Anti-Aβ immunostained section from another patient. Note the prominently immunoreactive Aß amyloid in the walls of meningeal and cortical arteries.

ANGIITIS DUE TO MISCELLANEOUS VASCULITIDES
MACROSCOPIC AND MICROSCOPIC APPEARANCES

These vary as follows:

- Polyarteritis nodosa is a multifocal panarteritis with destruction of the elastica affecting small and medium-sized arteries. The acute phase is characterized by polymorph neutrophil infiltration and fibrinoid necrosis. The chronic and healing phase is characterized by vascular fibrosis. End-organ damage results from thrombosis, ischemia, and infarction.
- Allergic angiitis and granulomatosis (Churg–Strauss syndrome) is an allergic diathesis with consistent lung involvement and eosinophilia and produces fibrinoid necrosis and an eosinophilic granulomatous inflammation in small and medium-sized arteries, capillaries, and venules.
- Wegener's granulomatosis is characterized by a granulomatous vasculitis of the respiratory tract with or without glomerulonephritis. It results in fibrinoid necrosis, the presence of inflammatory cells in small arteries and veins, and granulomas containing prominent giant cells.
- Lymphomatoid granulomatosis is characterized by an angiodestructive lesion of cerebral (intraparenchymal) arteries and arterioles, and a polymorphous transmural infiltrate of atypical leukocytes which is often combined with fibrinoid necrosis. It may be a variant of primary CNS lymphoma (angiocentric T cell lymphoma) (**Fig. 9.13**).

MICROVASCULOPATHY ASSOCIATED WITH DEMENTIA

Two distinct entities need to be considered:

- Binswanger's subcortical arteriosclerotic leukoencephalopathy (BSL).
- Cerebral autosomal dominant arteriopathy with subcortical infarcts and leukoencephalopathy (CADASIL).

However, note that CAA (see chapter 10) is a common microangiopathy and is one of the microscopic lesions of Alzheimer's disease.

MISCELLANEOUS VASCULITIDES

Polyarteritis nodosa

- affects all organs except lung and spleen.
- involves the CNS in 20–40% of patients.
- involves the peripheral nervous system in over 50% of patients.
- commonly causes hypertension.
- in the USA, is associated with hepatitis B antigenemia in about 30% of patients (the figure is lower in most UK and European series).
- is an immune complex vasculitis.

Wegener's granulomatosis

- involves the CNS in 20–40% of patients.
- is associated with anti-neutrophil cytoplasmic autoantibodies

Lymphomatoid granulomatosis

- is a controversial entity that appears to link vasculitis with primary CNS lymphoma.
- involves the CNS in 10–15% of patients.

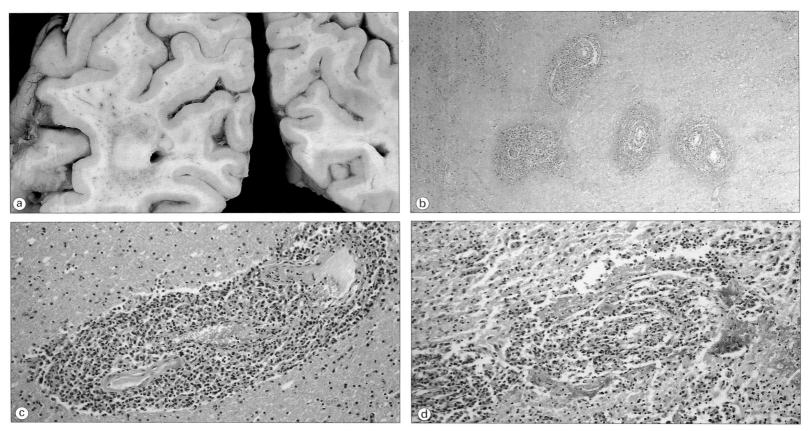

Fig. 9.13 Lymphomatoid granulomatosis in a patient with AIDS. (a) Section of brain showing a focus of necrosis adjacent to the left lateral ventricle. **(b)** Section from a necrotic region that includes small vessels with transmural and adventitial inflammatory infiltrates. **(c)** A non-necrotic focus showing a polymorphous inflammatory infiltrate, primarily in the vascular adventitia. **(d)** A severely inflamed vessel wall with patchy fibrinoid necrosis.

in microvascular thrombosis and end-organ (including cerebral) ischemia (**Fig. 9.20**).

In siderocalcinosis and ferruginization of microvessels, arteries and arterioles, particularly those in the basal ganglia or dentate fascia of the hippocampus, become encrusted with iron and calcium. This is associated with variable collagenous thickening of the intima and narrowing (or obliteration) of the lumen (**Fig. 9.21**). In a few elderly people, a proportion of whom have hypoparathyroidism (see Fahr's disease, chapter 22) many small and medium-sized blood vessels in the basal ganglia and cerebellum become calcified.

EMBOLIC DISEASES

An 'embolic' stroke may result when any solid material:
- forms within the arterial circulation.
- is introduced into the arterial circulation.
- forms in the venous circulation and has a conduit to the arterial circulation (e.g. via a right-to-left shunt in the heart).

The resultant infarct is usually:
- clinically abrupt in onset due to sudden cessation of flow.
- hemorrhagic, possibly because of dissolution of the embolus with re-establishment of flow into necrotic tissue (**Fig. 9.22**).

The differential diagnosis of embolic stroke includes:
- ischemic infarct from any other cause
- cerebral hemorrhage.

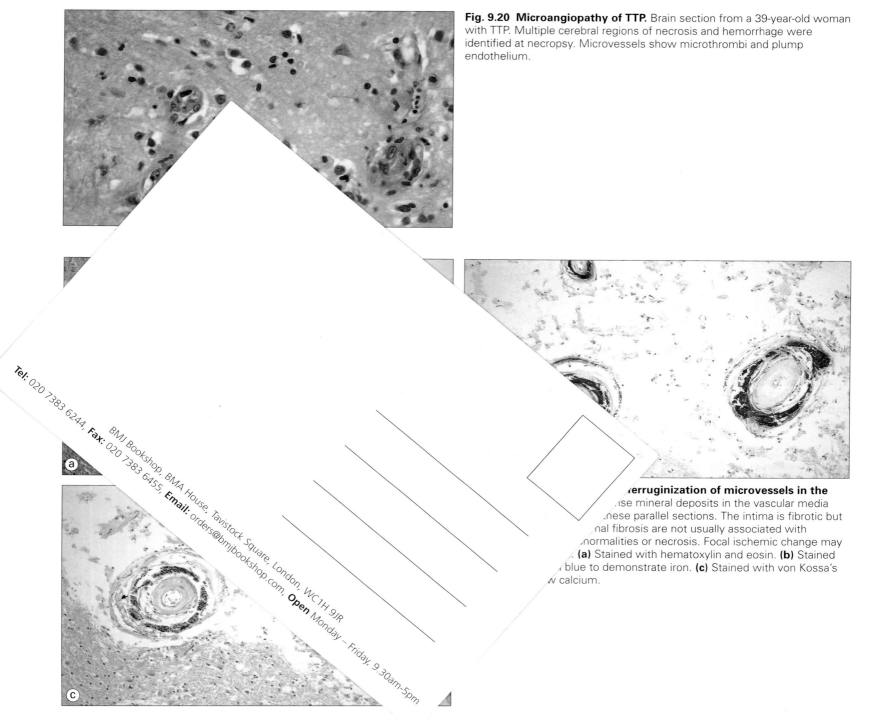

Fig. 9.20 Microangiopathy of TTP. Brain section from a 39-year-old woman with TTP. Multiple cerebral regions of necrosis and hemorrhage were identified at necropsy. Microvessels show microthrombi and plump endothelium.

...ferruginization of microvessels in the ...se mineral deposits in the vascular media ...nese parallel sections. The intima is fibrotic but ...nal fibrosis are not usually associated with ...normalities or necrosis. Focal ischemic change may ... **(a)** Stained with hematoxylin and eosin. **(b)** Stained ...blue to demonstrate iron. **(c)** Stained with von Kossa's ...calcium.

ANGIITIS DUE TO MISCELLANEOUS VASCULITIDES
MACROSCOPIC AND MICROSCOPIC APPEARANCES
These vary as follows:

- Polyarteritis nodosa is a multifocal panarteritis with destruction of the elastica affecting small and medium-sized arteries. The acute phase is characterized by polymorph neutrophil infiltration and fibrinoid necrosis. The chronic and healing phase is characterized by vascular fibrosis. End-organ damage results from thrombosis, ischemia, and infarction.
- Allergic angiitis and granulomatosis (Churg–Strauss syndrome) is an allergic diathesis with consistent lung involvement and eosinophilia and produces fibrinoid necrosis and an eosinophilic granulomatous inflammation in small and medium-sized arteries, capillaries, and venules.
- Wegener's granulomatosis is characterized by a granulomatous vasculitis of the respiratory tract with or without glomerulonephritis. It results in fibrinoid necrosis, the presence of inflammatory cells in small arteries and veins, and granulomas containing prominent giant cells.
- Lymphomatoid granulomatosis is characterized by an angiodestructive lesion of cerebral (intraparenchymal) arteries and arterioles, and a polymorphous transmural infiltrate of atypical leukocytes which is often combined with fibrinoid necrosis. It may be a variant of primary CNS lymphoma (angiocentric T cell lymphoma) (**Fig. 9.13**).

MICROVASCULOPATHY ASSOCIATED WITH DEMENTIA
Two distinct entities need to be considered:

- Binswanger's subcortical arteriosclerotic leukoencephalopathy (BSL).
- Cerebral autosomal dominant arteriopathy with subcortical infarcts and leukoencephalopathy (CADASIL).

However, note that CAA (see chapter 10) is a common microangiopathy and is one of the microscopic lesions of Alzheimer's disease.

MISCELLANEOUS VASCULITIDES

Polyarteritis nodosa

- affects all organs except lung and spleen.
- involves the CNS in 20–40% of patients.
- involves the peripheral nervous system in over 50% of patients.
- commonly causes hypertension.
- in the USA, is associated with hepatitis B antigenemia in about 30% of patients (the figure is lower in most UK and European series).
- is an immune complex vasculitis.

Wegener's granulomatosis

- involves the CNS in 20–40% of patients.
- is associated with anti-neutrophil cytoplasmic autoantibodies

Lymphomatoid granulomatosis

- is a controversial entity that appears to link vasculitis with primary CNS lymphoma.
- involves the CNS in 10–15% of patients.

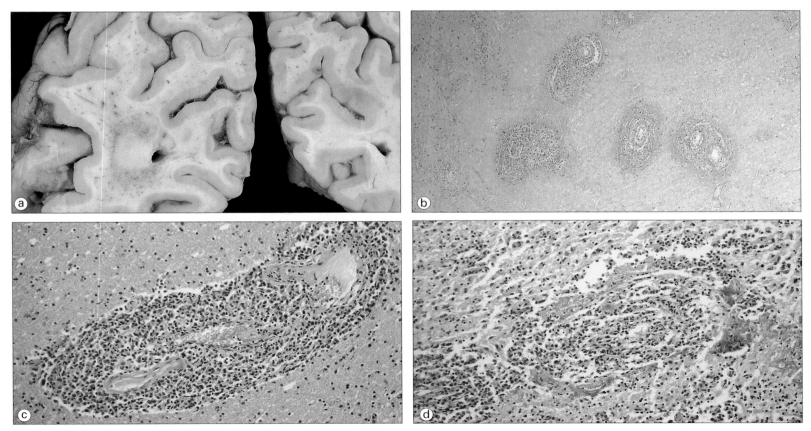

Fig. 9.13 Lymphomatoid granulomatosis in a patient with AIDS. (a) Section of brain showing a focus of necrosis adjacent to the left lateral ventricle. **(b)** Section from a necrotic region that includes small vessels with transmural and adventitial inflammatory infiltrates. **(c)** A non-necrotic focus showing a polymorphous inflammatory infiltrate, primarily in the vascular adventitia. **(d)** A severely inflamed vessel wall with patchy fibrinoid necrosis.

Binswanger's Subcortical Arteriosclerotic Leukoencephalopathy (BSL)

BSL is an entity of controversial nosology. It is a disease of elderly hypertensive patients and is characterized by a leukoencephalopathy, which may be associated with hypertensive microvascular changes. Implicated pathogenetic factors include ischemia, hypoxia, infarction in watershed zones, and hydrocephalus.

MACROSCOPIC AND MICROSCOPIC APPEARANCES

There is diffuse myelin pallor with or without well-defined large or small subcortical infarcts. (**Fig. 9.14**). Microscopic sections confirm infarction with reactive change (**Fig. 9.15**). Microvascular changes are usually those of arteriosclerosis and, lipohyalinosis (see chapter 10).

CADASIL

CADASIL has some similarities with BSL, but is distinguished by its familial tendency and the deposition of abnormal material in vessel walls. Individuals with CADASIL have missense mutations of the *Notch 3* gene on chromosome 19p. The onset is usually in the fifth or sixth decade and the presentation that of systemic vasculopathy with predominant CNS features.

MACROSCOPIC AND MICROSCOPIC APPEARANCES

These include cortical and subcortical atrophy with myelin loss, astrocytosis, and 'lacunes' in the subcortical white matter (**Fig. 9.16**). Small arteries show fibrosis and replacement of the media by eosinophilic, periodic acid–Schiff-positive, Congo red-negative granular material (**Fig. 9.17**). Ultrastructural studies reveal compact electron-dense granular material around myocytes (**Fig. 9.18**).

BINSWANGER'S SUBCORTICAL ARTERIOSCLEROTIC LEUKOENCEPHALOPATHY

- is a slowly progressive condition, typically showing stepwise deterioration and episodes of partial recovery that are characteristic of multiple infarcts.
- usually starts in the sixth or seventh decade.
- causes prominent disorders of memory, mood, and cognition.
- also causes focal motor signs and less commonly a pseudobulbar syndrome in association with deterioration of gait and loss of sphincter control.

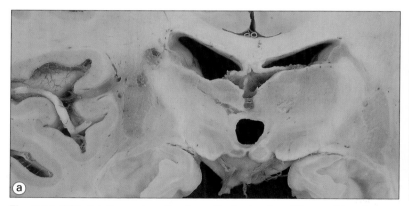

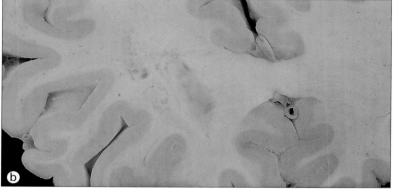

Fig. 9.14 BSL. (a) Coronal section from the brain of an 87-year-old patient with a longstanding 'confusional state.' Note the lacunar infarcts in the left internal capsule and deep gray matter; adjacent white matter shows an irregular 'pitted' appearance with gray discoloration. **(b)** Section of brain of an 86-year-old female with a four-year history of dementia. Note the diffuse leukomalacia in the left frontal lobe.

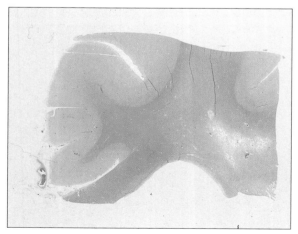

Fig. 9.15 BSL. Low-power histologic section showing a lacunar infarct typical of BSL in white matter adjacent to cingulate cortex. This was one of many noted throughout the cerebral white matter in this demented patient.

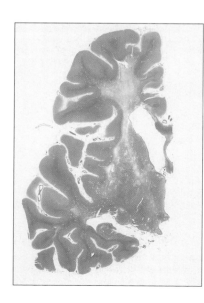

Fig. 9.16 CADASIL. Coronal section through left cerebral hemisphere showing lacunar infarcts and diffuse myelin pallor of the deep white matter with sparing of subcortical U-fibers. (Courtesy of Professor Françoise Gray, Paris)

MISCELLANEOUS MICROANGIOPATHIES

These include systemic lupus erythematosus (SLE), thrombotic thrombocytopenic purpura (TTP), and siderocalcinosis and ferruginization of microvessels.

MACROSCOPIC AND MICROSCOPIC APPEARANCES

SLE is more commonly associated with infarction than hemorrhage and may cause stroke as a result of emboli associated with Libman–Sacks endocarditis or hypertension associated with renal disease. It is often associated with the presence of microinfarcts and hemorrhages in the postmortem brain, but vasculitis is rarely observed. Hyaline change in the walls of thickened small arteries is sometimes associated with perivascular lymphocytes (**Fig. 9.19**).

TTP preferentially involves gray matter. An interaction of platelets with platelet-aggregating factor or unusual multimers of factor VIII:von Willebrand's factor may cause abnormal platelet agglutination resulting

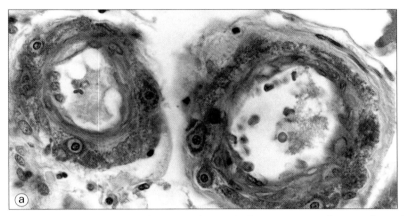
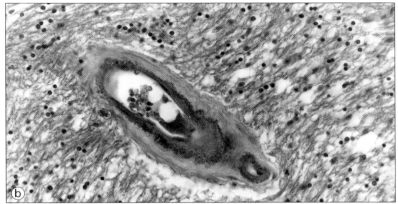

Fig. 9.17 These sections illustrate the typical appearance of parenchymal microvessels in CADASIL.
Note the concentric thickening of arterial wall with intimal hyperplasia, granular deposits surrounding swollen myocytes in the media, and adventitial fibrosis. (Courtesy of Professor Françoise Gray)

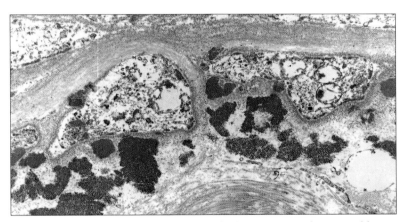

Fig. 9.18 Ultrastructural appearance of white matter microvessel in CADASIL. Swollen myocytes are surrounded by compact electron-dense granular material. (Courtesy of Professor Françoise Gray, Paris)

MISCELLANEOUS MICROANGIOPATHIES

SLE

- This is predominantly a disease of young adult women.
- Neuropsychiatric symptoms affect up to 75% of patients in some series.
- Brain infarcts occur in about 5% of patients.
- SLE is commonly associated with APLAs.

TTP

- This is predominantly a disease of children but can also affect young adults.
- The incidence is less than 1:1,000,000.
- CNS symptoms are associated with a variety of systemic manifestations including hemolytic anemia, thrombocytopenia, renal insufficiency and a purpuric rash over the trunk and limbs.

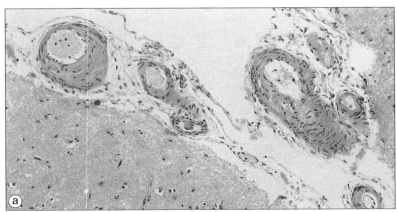
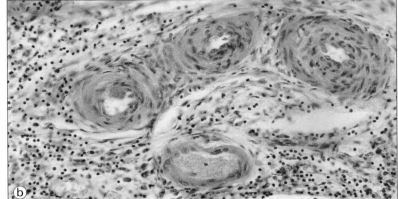

Fig. 9.19 Microangiopathy associated with SLE. (a) This patient with SLE died of non-neurologic disease, but had scattered microinfarcts throughout the CNS. Thickened hyalinized walls are seen in microvessels. **(b)** Perivascular lymphocytes are observed in some cases.

in microvascular thrombosis and end-organ (including cerebral) ischemia (**Fig. 9.20**).

In siderocalcinosis and ferruginization of microvessels, arteries and arterioles, particularly those in the basal ganglia or dentate fascia of the hippocampus, become encrusted with iron and calcium. This is associated with variable collagenous thickening of the intima and narrowing (or obliteration) of the lumen (**Fig. 9.21**). In a few elderly people, a proportion of whom have hypoparathyroidism (see Fahr's disease, chapter 22) many small and medium-sized blood vessels in the basal ganglia and cerebellum become calcified.

EMBOLIC DISEASES

An 'embolic' stroke may result when any solid material:
- forms within the arterial circulation.
- is introduced into the arterial circulation.
- forms in the venous circulation and has a conduit to the arterial circulation (e.g. via a right-to-left shunt in the heart).

The resultant infarct is usually:
- clinically abrupt in onset due to sudden cessation of flow.
- hemorrhagic, possibly because of dissolution of the embolus with re-establishment of flow into necrotic tissue (**Fig. 9.22**).

The differential diagnosis of embolic stroke includes:
- ischemic infarct from any other cause
- cerebral hemorrhage.

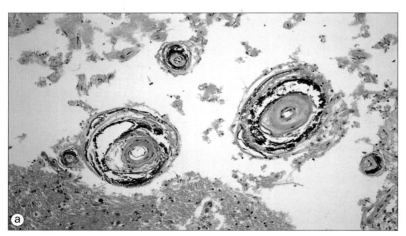

Fig. 9.20 Microangiopathy of TTP. Brain section from a 39-year-old woman with TTP. Multiple cerebral regions of necrosis and hemorrhage were identified at necropsy. Microvessels show microthrombi and plump endothelium.

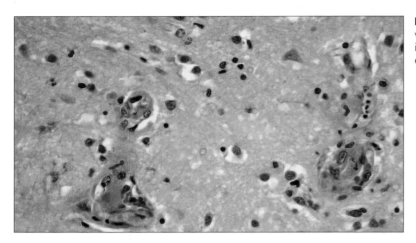

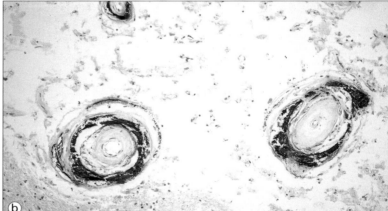

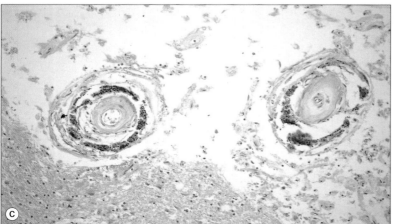

Fig. 9.21 Siderocalcinosis and ferruginization of microvessels in the globus pallidus. There are dense mineral deposits in the vascular media and adventitia, as shown in these parallel sections. The intima is fibrotic but the mineralization and intimal fibrosis are not usually associated with specific parenchymal abnormalities or necrosis. Focal ischemic change may occur in severe cases. **(a)** Stained with hematoxylin and eosin. **(b)** Stained with Perls' Prussian blue to demonstrate iron. **(c)** Stained with von Kossa's technique to show calcium.

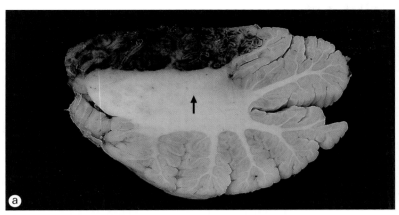

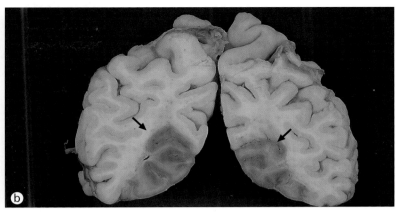

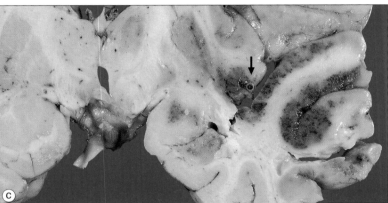

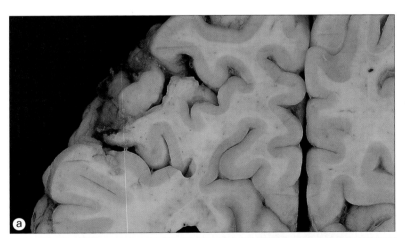

Fig. 9.22 Hemorrhagic embolic infarction. (a) and **(b)** Embolic infarcts are typically hemorrhagic. Acute and organizing hemorrhagic infarcts, respectively, in the cerebellum (arrow) (a) and medial inferior parieto-occipital regions (arrows) (b) in sections of brain from two elderly patients with basilar artery atherosclerosis and distal artery-to-artery emboli of atheromatous material. **(c)** Recent hemorrhagic infarct involving the superior part of the temporal lobe, the insula and inferior part of the frontal lobe, the insula and inferior part of the frontal lobe, and resulting from an embolus which is macroscopically visible in the middle cerebral artery (arrow).

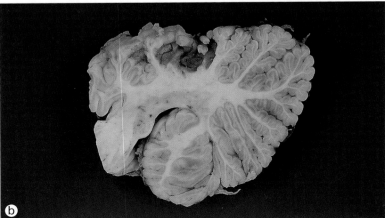

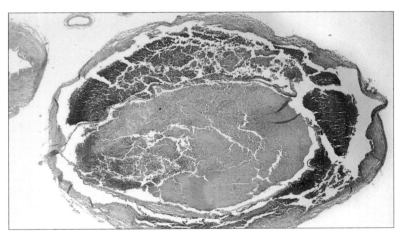

Fig. 9.24 Embolism due to bacterial endocarditis. Section of MCA from a man with HIV who developed *Streptococcus viridans* sepsis and bacterial endocarditis of the mitral valve. Note the large thrombus surrounded by masses of inflammatory cells and the red blood cells outside the internal elastic lamina. If the patient had survived, an infectious or mycotic aneurysm may have developed (see also chapter 10).

Fig. 9.23 Emboli of cardiac origin. A 54-year-old African–American male with a four-year history of idiopathic cardiomyopathy and multiple embolic strokes. At necropsy, multiple regions of remote encephalomalacia were identified in the brain. **(a)** Left parieto-occiptal region. **(b)** Cerebellum.

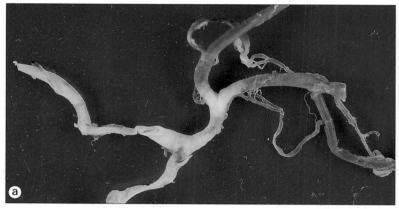

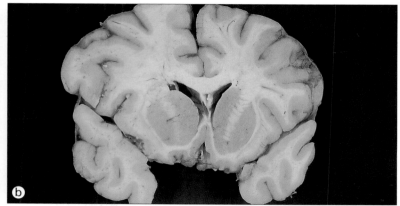

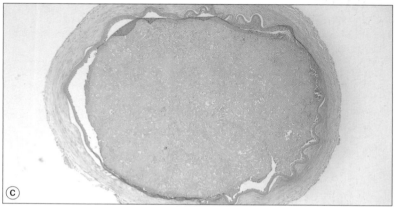

Fig. 9.25 The cerebrovascular consequences of non-bacterial thrombotic endocarditis. (a) There is a solid yellowish-white 'saddle embolus' at the bifurcation of the middle cerebral artery (MCA). **(b)** Large left hemispheric subacute infarct, with early midline shift in a 44-year-old woman with widely metastatic breast carcinoma. **(c)** Infarction in (b) was due to a left MCA embolus. **(d)** The embolus in (c) arose from a mitral valve vegetation, illustrated here. The MCA embolus shows a comparable degree of organization to that seen in the mitral valve vegetation.

SOURCES OF BRAIN AND SPINAL CORD EMBOLI

Atheroma

- Plaques of complicated atherosclerosis in the aorta and its branches serve as a nidus for material that can embolize to produce infarction.

Cardiogenic

Emboli associated with cardiac pathology are an important cause of ischemic stroke in young people who are relatively free of atherosclerosis.

Principal sources of cardiac emboli are:

- Thrombus in a non-contractile left atrium in a patient with atrial fibrillation.
- Mural thrombi from the endocardial surface of a hypokinetic left ventricular wall in association with cardiomyopathy, myocardial infarction, or ventricular aneurysm. (**Fig. 9.23**).
- Endocarditis, either bacterial in association with a prosthetic valve or after rheumatic fever, or non-bacterial thrombotic endocarditis. The resultant emboli may be either septic (**Fig. 9.24**) or platelet–fibrin (**Fig. 9.25**).
- Platelet–fibrin emboli from miscellaneous valve lesions such as rheumatic valve disease, mitral valve prolapse, and calcific aortic sclerosis (**Fig. 9.26**).
- Paradoxic embolus in association with a right-to-left shunt.
- Cardiac neoplasms, especially as a trial myxoma.

Fat

- Symptomatic fat embolism is usually associated with fractures of long bones or the pelvis but rarely complicates soft tissue trauma, or open-chest cardiac surgery
- The postmortem brain shows petechial hemorrhages within gray and white matter (although usually more prominent in the latter).
- Fat emboli can be conclusively demonstrated in appropriately stained frozen sections (**Fig. 9.27**).

Neoplasms and parasites

- Very rarely solid neoplasms fragment and embolize to the CNS (**Fig. 9.28**).
- Rarely parasites or parasitic ova embolize to the brain.

Iatrogenic causes

- Iatrogenic emboli may result from a variety of materials introduced into the arterial circulation during vascular surgery or angiography. Cotton fiber is the most common of these and has a characteristic appearance on polarization (**Fig. 9.29**).
- Treatment of brain vascular malformations includes intentional iatrogenic embolization or 'embolotherapy'.

Miscellaneous

- Embolization of intervertebral disc material to the spinal cord has rarely been reported (**Fig. 9.30**).
- Air embolism occurs in decompression sickness and cardiac bypass surgery. Bubbles cause microinfarcts, particularly in the spinal cord in decompression sickness.

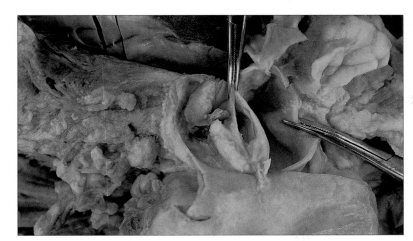

Fig. 9.26 Calcific sclerosis of a bicuspid aortic valve. This pathology is occasionally a source of emboli to the brain.

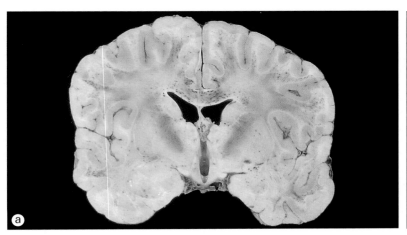

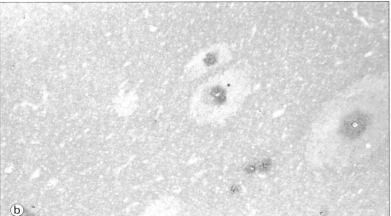

Fig. 9.27 Cerebral fat emboli. (a) Multiple petechial hemorrhages in the cerebral white matter. **(b)** Frozen section of brain tissue stained for lipid. (Oil red-o) (Courtesy of Dr Cynthia T. Welsh)

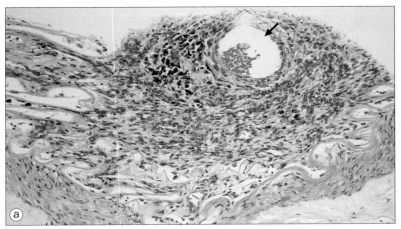

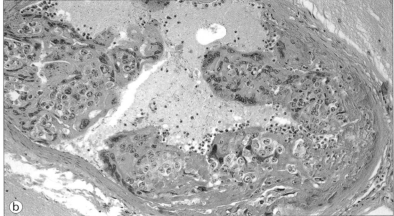

Fig. 9.28 Neoplastic emboli in the brain. (a) Neoplastic embolus in a patient who had widely disseminated sarcoma and an old cerebral infarct underlying the occluded vessel. Note the small recanalized lumen (arrow).

(b) Embolic choriocarcinoma in the meningeal artery with focal invasion of the vessel wall and early aneurysm formation. The patient died of multiple cerebral hemorrhages (see chapter 10).

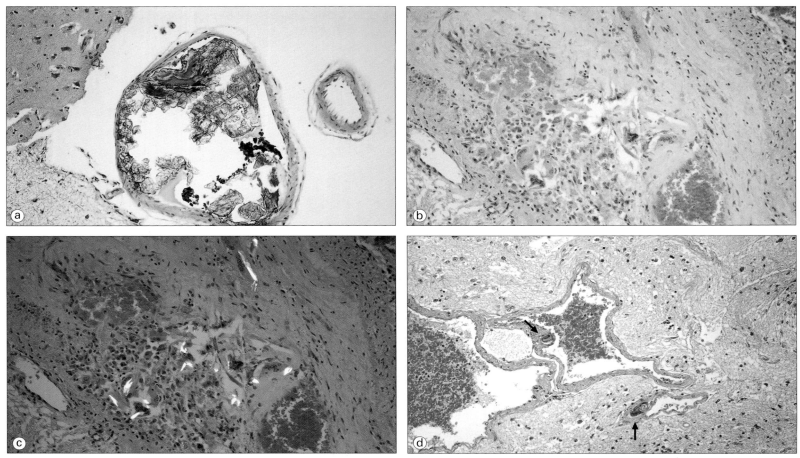

Fig. 9.29 Iatrogenic emboli take many forms, and may be intentional or accidental. (a) Particulate material found in a meningeal artery from a patient who underwent a complicated cardiothoracic surgical procedure. (Courtesy of Dr Virginia M. Walley) **(b)** Longstanding mesencephalic arteriovenous malformation (AVM) in a patient who had undergone multiple therapeutic embolizations. Foreign body giant cell reaction is noted in the depths of the AVM. **(c)** The same section as (b) viewed after polarization demonstrates acellular refractile particles, which probably represent cotton fiber introduced during an interventional procedure or angiography. **(d)** An AVM that had not undergone therapeutic embolization shows small basophilic particles surrounded by foreign body giant cells and 'embedded' within the vessel walls (arrows). Such 'foreign' materials are particularly likely to lodge in AVMs because of their high and turbulent blood flow which is associated with the arteriovenous shunting.

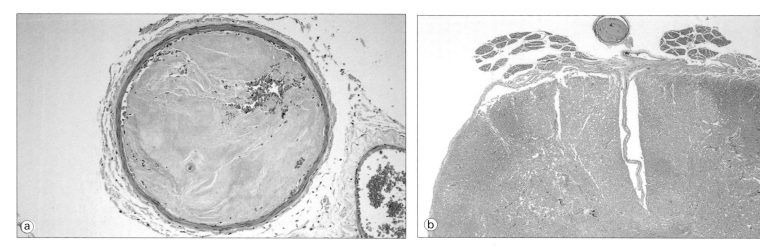

Fig. 9.30 Embolism of intervertebral disc material. (a) Embolus of intervertebral disc material to the anterior spinal artery, has resulted in this extensive spinal cord infarct **(b)**. (Courtesy of Professor Michael A. Farrell, Dublin)

CEREBRAL VENOUS THROMBOSIS (CVT)

CVT is a much less common cause of stroke than arterial disease, though necropsy series probably underestimate its true incidence. Infection is becoming a relatively less important causal factor. Cavernous sinus thrombosis is the most common example of septic venous thrombosis.

MACROSCOPIC AND MICROSCOPIC APPEARANCES

The macroscopic findings depend on the interval between CVT and death. The most consistent feature is severe and extensive hemorrhagic necrosis in the brain, often with evolution into parenchymal hematomas (**Fig. 9.31**). The thrombosed sinus is usually engorged, and the thrombus is palpable (**Fig. 9.32**).

Histology shows hemorrhagic necrosis (**Fig. 9.33**). If there is a septic component, microorganisms can be demonstrated and inflammatory cells are more abundant.

CEREBRAL VEIN THROMBOSIS (CVT)

- Patients manifest a wide variety of signs and symptoms: the most common are headache, papilledema, sensorimotor deficit, and epilepsy.
- The clinical presentations have been subclassified as: isolated intracranial hypertension, focal neurologic deficit, syndrome of cavernous sinus thrombosis, or (unusual) miscellaneous presentations.
- The superior sagittal and lateral sinuses are most often involved.

ETIOLOGY OF CVT

- Local etiologic factors include infections, either intracranial or in adjacent facial and bony structures, head injury, neurosurgical procedures, and neoplasms.
- General risk factors include pregnancy and the puerperium, oral contraceptive use, cyanotic congenital heart disease, hematologic abnormalities (e.g. polycythemia, sickle cell disease, coagulation disorders), severe dehydration, malignancy, and inflammatory and connective tissue disorders (e.g. Behçet's syndrome).

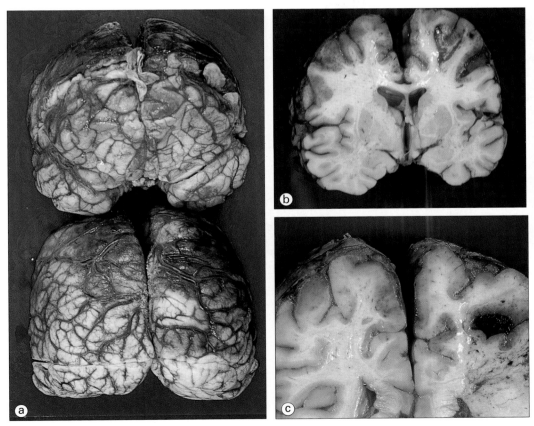

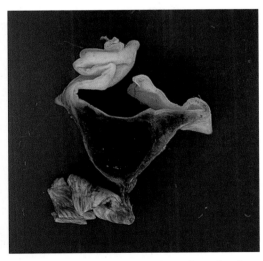

Fig. 9.32 Superior sagittal sinus thrombosis. Coronal section through the superior sagittal sinus showing recent thrombus.

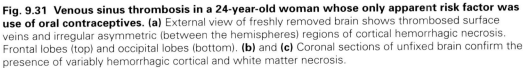

Fig. 9.31 Venous sinus thrombosis in a 24-year-old woman whose only apparent risk factor was use of oral contraceptives. (a) External view of freshly removed brain shows thrombosed surface veins and irregular asymmetric (between the hemispheres) regions of cortical hemorrhagic necrosis. Frontal lobes (top) and occipital lobes (bottom). **(b)** and **(c)** Coronal sections of unfixed brain confirm the presence of variably hemorrhagic cortical and white matter necrosis.

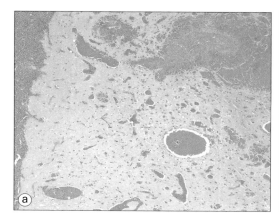
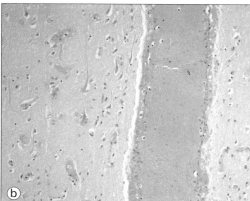

Fig. 9.33 Venous infarction. Cortex showing extensive subacute hemorrhagic necrosis. **(a)** There is extravasation of red blood cells into brain parenchyma. **(b)** This is accompanied by eosinophilic hypoxic–ischemic neuronal change.

CNS INFARCTION

MACROSCOPIC APPEARANCES

The macroscopic appearances of a brain or spinal cord infarct at necropsy depend on the interval between the stroke and death. The evolution of these appearances corresponds to a sequence of microscopic abnormalities. The dating of infarcts using macroscopic and microscopic criteria is, however, relatively imprecise.

Acute infarction

An infarct that has occurred 5–8 hours before a patient's death is almost always undetectable macroscopically and even microscopic abnormalities will be minimal.

Changes that develop within 12–36 hours include slight blurring of the gray/white matter interface, dusky discoloration of gray matter and slight softening of the tissue. These changes may be relatively easy to detect, especially if confined to the territory of a major cerebral artery (**Fig. 9.34**).

Subacute infarction

Infarction with an antemortem interval of 2–4 days appears as softening, with blurring of the gray/white matter junction and dusky gray discoloration of brain tissue. At this stage, the most telling abnormality is cerebral edema (**Fig. 9.35**).

Chronic infarction

Stage I: As the edema subsides, the region of infarction starts to undergo liquefactive necrosis, eventually leading to cavitation (**Fig. 9.36**).

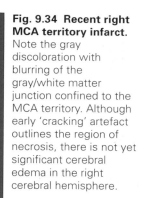

Fig. 9.34 Recent right MCA territory infarct. Note the gray discoloration with blurring of the gray/white matter junction confined to the MCA territory. Although early 'cracking' artefact outlines the region of necrosis, there is not yet significant cerebral edema in the right cerebral hemisphere.

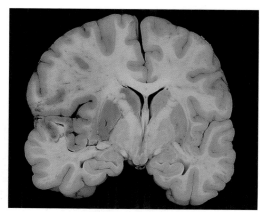

Fig. 9.35 Left MCA territory infarct consistent with survival of 2–4 days. The macroscopic appearance is similar to that noted in Fig. 9.34 except that there is significant left to right shift of midline structures.

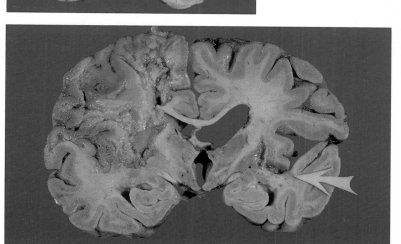

Fig. 9.36 Liquefactive necrosis in a left MCA territory infarct that occurred a few days before death. Much of the the edema has subsided. The arrow in the right cerebral hemisphere indicates older foci of cystic encephalomalacia in the right putamen and adjacent insular cortex.

Stage II: an old infarct (older than several months) will appear as a cystic cavity within the brain substance and is surrounded by atrophic brain tissue (**Fig. 9.37**). In some cases a well-defined cavity does not form. Instead, there is a 'moth-eaten' appearance to the area of encephalomalacia.

MICROSCOPIC APPEARANCES

Acute infarction

This produces neuronal eosinophilia with pyknosis, as in anoxic–ischemic encephalopathy (see chapter 8), and is associated with vacuolation of the surrounding neuropil (**Fig. 9.38**).

Subacute infarction

Neuronal eosinophilia persists at this stage. Variable degrees of polymorph neutrophil infiltration are evident, often adjacent to necrotic microvessels. Early microglial activation and the formation of foamy histiocytes are responses to the tissue damage (**Fig. 9.39**). Endothelial proliferation and neovascularization are found at 5–12 days, but are variable in extent and timing.

Chronic infarction

Foamy macrophages, often containing hemosiderin, sometimes persist over many months. Thin-walled blood vessels pass through the cystic cavity. Abundant reactive astrocytes encircle the infarct. In large cerebral cortical infarcts, there is a characteristic pattern of relative preservation of the molecular layer (lamina 1), which contains abundant reactive astrocytes (**Fig. 9.40**). Residual neurons and axons in and around the infarct may become encrusted with iron and calcium (i.e. ferruginization and siderocalcinosis) (**Fig. 9.41**). Rarely there are thrombosed vessels adjacent to the infarct (**Fig. 9.42**). The cellular events in the evolution of an infarct are shown in **Fig. 9.43**.

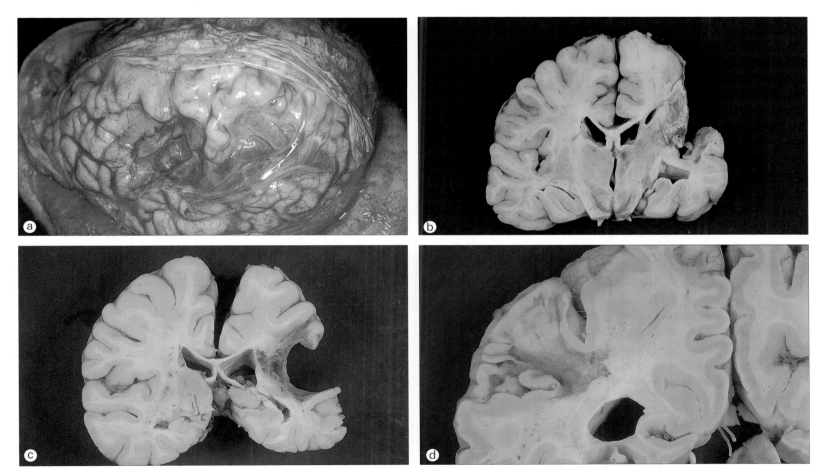

Fig. 9.37 Old cystic infarcts in MCA territory in different patients. (a) Appearance of brain before removal shows collapse of brain substance (left fronto-parietal region) with apparent opacification and hypervascularity of overlying leptomeninges. **(b)** There is an old cystic infarct in the right MCA territory. The surrounding scars are partly the result of subsequent infection of the necrotic tissue in this patient, a distinctly unusual complication of a cerebral infarct. **(c)** Chronic cortical and white matter infarction. **(d)** A predominantly subcortical infarct in left parietal lobe.

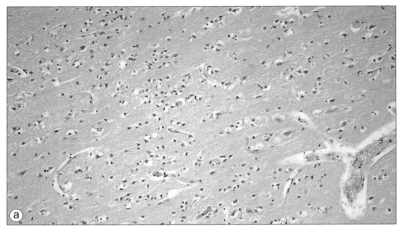

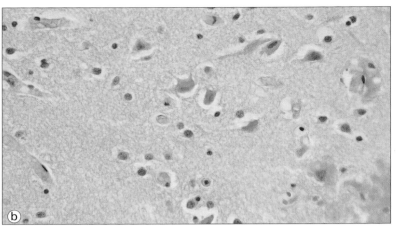

Fig. 9.38 Histology of acute cerebral infarct. The appearances are consistent with an 8–12-hour interval between stroke and death. **(a)** Note the neuronal eosinophilia, which is best appreciated at higher magnification in **(b)**, and vacuolation of the neuropil. **(c)** The interface between the pale infarct and the more deeply stained 'preserved' tissue is often most easily appreciated at low magnification in a routine section as here. Vacuolation tends to be most pronounced at the edge of the infarct.

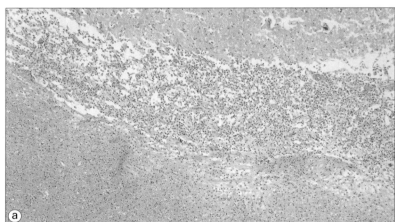

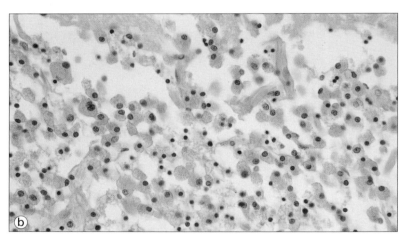

Fig. 9.39 Histology of subacute cerebral infarct. (a) Edge of infarct (top) with early macrophage infiltration. **(b)** The infiltrating macrophages have a characteristic round shape, eccentric nucleus, and foamy or granular cytoplasm, which in some instances contains altered blood pigment. **(c)** Vascular endothelial proliferation is often seen at the edge of an infarct after 1–2 weeks.

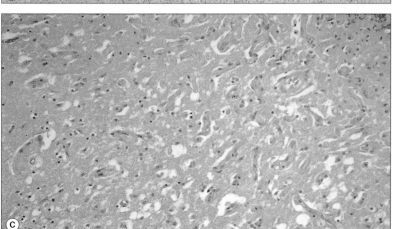

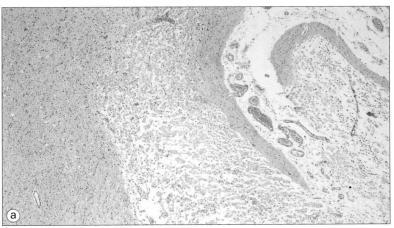

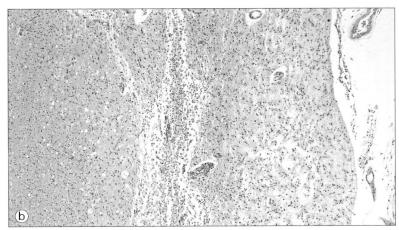

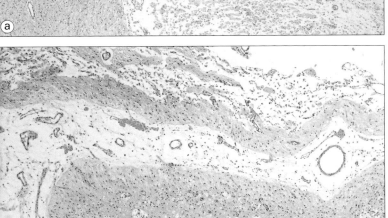

Fig. 9.40 Histologic features of an old infarct. After a few weeks, the precise 'age' of an infarct becomes increasingly difficult to judge. **(a)** Here the meninges are on the right and a thin rim of preserved subpial tissue overlies a zone of cortex in which necrotic debris is identified, and large numbers of macrophages are present. **(b)** A subpial rim of gliotic tissue is seen above a large collection of histiocytes in a region of cortical collapse. The meninges are on the right. **(c)** With time, macrophages and histiocytes partly or completely resorb the damaged tissue, leaving a cystic cavity surrounded by a dense rim of reactive astrocytes.

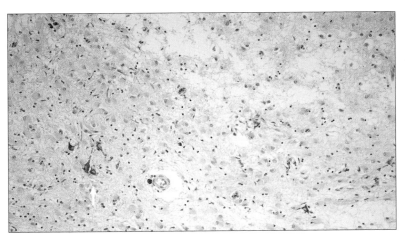

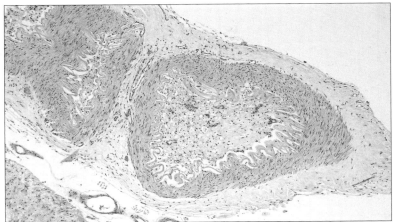

Fig. 9.41 Ferruginization. Reactive astrocytes are seen adjacent to neurons and axons that have become encrusted with basophilic material composed of calcium and iron (arrow) in neuroglial tissue surrounding an old infarct.

Fig. 9.42 Old thrombosis. Occasionally, a meningeal or parenchymal artery showing old thrombosis will be noted adjacent to an infarct. Such a finding is, however, exceptional.

INFARCTS CAUSED BY OCCUSION OF LARGE ARTERIES

The territories supplied by the major cerebral arteries are illustrated in **Fig. 9.44**. If a destructive lesion fits within one of these discrete regions, its etiology is likely to be ischemic (**Figs 9.45–9.49**). If an encephalomalacic lesion appears *between* two major territories of supply, it is likely to represent a watershed/border zone infarct (**Fig. 9.53** and also chapter 8).

SPINAL CORD INFARCTION

Infarction in the spinal cord is much less frequent than infarction in the brain. Atherosclerosis of the spinal arteries does not occur, and atherosclerotic plaques in the aorta tend not to occlude the ostia of arteries that supply the cord.

Spinal cord infarction is caused by:
- embolization of:
  - material from complicated plaques of atherosclerosis in the aorta (postmortem studies indicate that this can be asymptomatic)
  - fibrocartilaginous material, usually following trauma to the back
- severe hypotension

- decompression sickness
- pathology in the aorta:
  - dissection, in association with hypertension, Marfan's syndrome, or arterial cannulation
  - coarctation
  - clamping of the aorta during abdominal surgery
- venous occlusion, in association with septicaemia or metastatic carcinoma which predisposes to thrombosis
- Foix-Alajouanine syndrome

In addition, infarction may be part of the pathophysiology of spinal cord damage following trauma.

MICROSCOPIC APPEARANCES

The histology of spinal cord infarction appears and evolves identically to brain infarction (see above). Infarction in the distribution of the anterior spinal artery is most common and affects the anterior gray matter (**Fig. 9.50, 9.51**) and the medial anterior tracts. Infarction secondary to hypotension preferentially affects the anterior zones and in mild cases may affect anterior horn motor neurons preferentially, resulting in their loss and associated gliosis. The most vulnerable watershed zone is around the level of T_4.

Foix-Alajouanine syndrome

This rare vascular malformation of the spinal cord usually presents in middle-aged men with a progressive myelopathy characterized by an areflexic paraparesis, sensory disturbances, and bladder, bowel, and sexual dysfunction.

MACROSCOPIC AND MICROSCOPIC APPEARANCES

The surfaces of the caudal, and to a lesser degree, the rostral spinal cord are covered by dilated blood vessels which also course through the cord itself. The cord may show focal atrophy. Histologically, zones of necrotic cord are surrounded by thick-walled tortuous blood vessels (**Fig. 9.52**). Areas of necrosis contain lipid-laden macrophages and are surrounded by gliosis. The structure of the abnormal vessels does not permit their characterization as arterioles or venules. Perivascular lymphocytes may occasionally be seen.

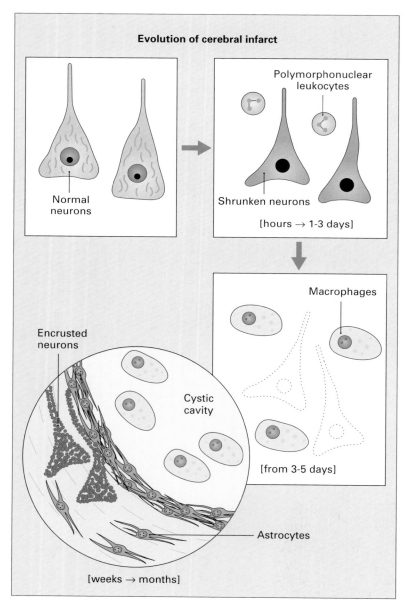

Evolution of cerebral infarct

Normal neurons

Polymorphonuclear leukocytes

Shrunken neurons

[hours → 1-3 days]

Encrusted neurons

Macrophages

Cystic cavity

[from 3-5 days]

Astrocytes

[weeks → months]

Fig. 9.43 The sequence of microscopic changes in the evolution of a cerebral infarct.

> ### CORTICAL DYSFUNCTION DUE TO MAJOR CEREBRAL ARTERIAL TERRITORY INFARCTION
>
> *Listed below are some of the clinical features associated with specific cerebral arterial territory infarcts.*
> - MCA: hemiparesis (face and arm, possibly leg), aphasia (dominant hemisphere), and hemisensory disturbance.
> - ACA: hemiparesis (leg, possibly face and arm), transcortical motor aphasia, and abulia.
> - PCA: thalamic syndrome, hemianopia (cortical blindness if bilateral), and alexia (dominant hemisphere).

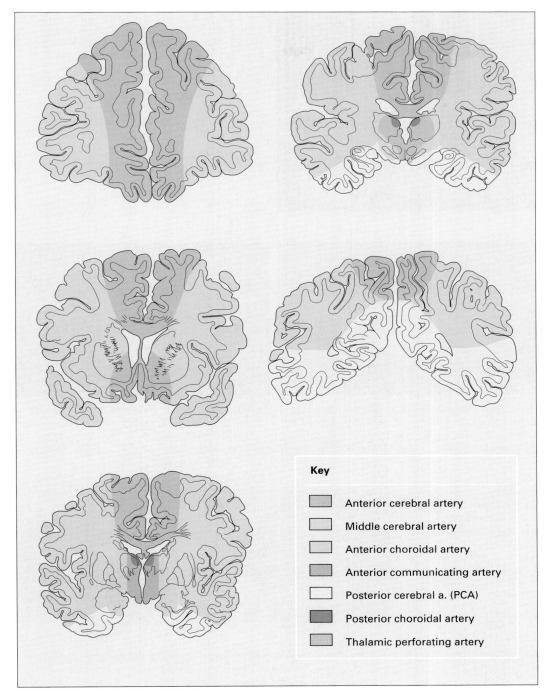

Fig. 9.44 The territories supplied by the major cerebral arteries.

Key

- Anterior cerebral artery
- Middle cerebral artery
- Anterior choroidal artery
- Anterior communicating artery
- Posterior cerebral a. (PCA)
- Posterior choroidal artery
- Thalamic perforating artery

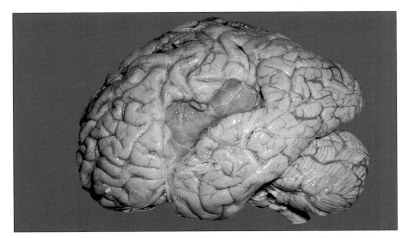

Fig. 9.45 Lateral view of old left MCA territory infarct in fixed brain.

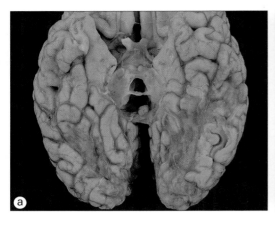
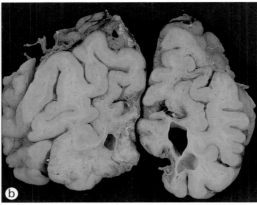

Fig. 9.46 PCA territory infarcts. (a) View of the undersurface of the brain. **(b)** Coronal slice through the same specimen as in (a). Note that atherosclerosis unusually extends even into leptomeningeal arteries.

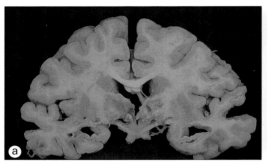
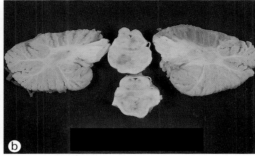
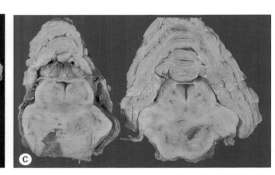

Fig. 9.47 Basilar artery thrombosis. (a) Infarction had occurred several days before death in this 79-year-old diabetic with severe vertebrobasilar atherosclerosis. Note the multifocal necrosis in the thalami and inferior temporal lobes. **(b)** There is also multifocal necrosis in the brain stem and cerebellum. The mechanism for some of the infarcts was almost certainly that of 'artery-to-artery' emboli (e.g. basilar artery to right superior cerebellar artery). **(c)** Sections of brain stem from another patient showing regions of old cystic encephalomalacia in the basis pontis.

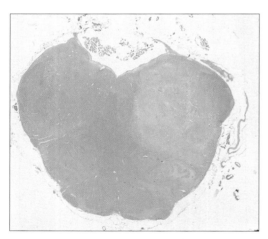

Fig. 9.48 Vertebral artery thrombosis. Lateral medullary syndrome in a 77-year-old woman who had a vertebral artery thrombosis 3–5 days before death.

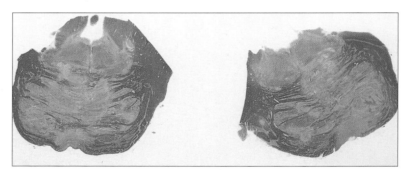
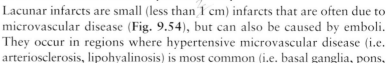

Fig. 9.49 Basilar artery thrombosis. Sections of pons stained for myelin showing geographic areas of recent necrosis, primarily in the basis pontis, but extending focally into the tegmentum.

WATERSHED OR BORDER ZONE INFARCTS

Watershed infarcts usually occur in elderly people with significant atherosclerosis who experience a prolonged episode of hypotension and reduced cerebral blood flow (e.g. intraoperatively or after cardiac arrest). They are also a common complication of severely raised intracranial pressure, especially after head injury (see chapters 8 and 11). The infarct is usually wedge-shaped, with its base at the pial surface. Infarction may be symmetric within cerebral hemispheres and usually at least partly hemorrhagic (an appearance attributed to reflow into necrotic tissue) (**Fig. 9.53**).

LACUNAR INFARCTS (LACUNES)

Lacunar infarcts are small (less than 1 cm) infarcts that are often due to microvascular disease (**Fig. 9.54**), but can also be caused by emboli. They occur in regions where hypertensive microvascular disease (i.e. arteriosclerosis, lipohyalinosis) is most common (i.e. basal ganglia, pons, internal capsule).

Lacunar infarcts may be an incidental finding at necropsy but can produce a range of focal neurologic deficits, which depend on the region in which the infarct occurs, for example:

- pure motor hemiparesis due to a capsular lesion.
- dysarthria–clumsy hand syndrome due to a lacune in upper paramedian basis pontis near the medial lemniscus).

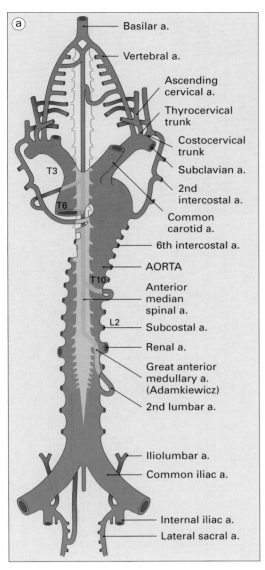

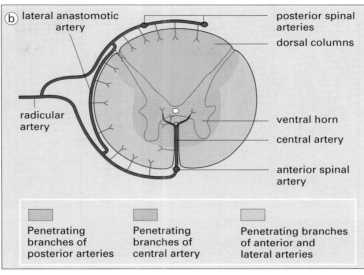

Fig. 9.50 **Blood supply of the spinal cord. (a)** The major arterial branches to the spinal cord. **(b)** The regions supplied by the arteries of the spinal cord.

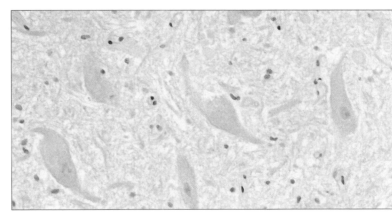

Fig. 9.51 **Spinal cord infarction.** Eosinophilic neurons in the ventral horn of the spinal cord following a severe episode of hypoxia–ischemia.

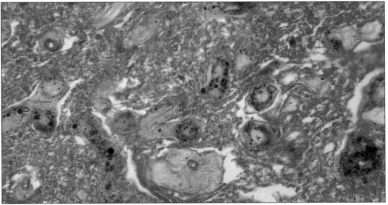

Fig. 9.52 **Foix–Alajouanine syndrome.** Zones of necrotic cord surrounded by thick walled and tortuous blood vessels.

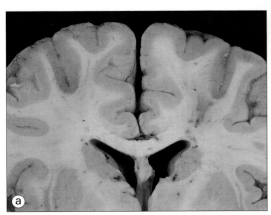
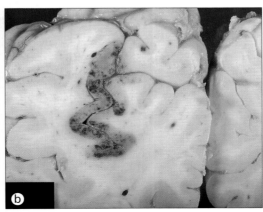

Fig. 9.53 **Watershed infarcts in slices of brain from two patients. (a)** Asymmetric anterior/middle cerebral artery (ACA/MCA) watershed zone infarcts, more prominent on the right. Note the dusky gray discoloration of the cortex, which contrasts with the surrounding pale cortical ribbon, with necrosis extending into subcortical white matter on the right side. **(b)** Section from parieto-occipital region showing a hemorrhagic ACA/MCA watershed infarct in another patient.

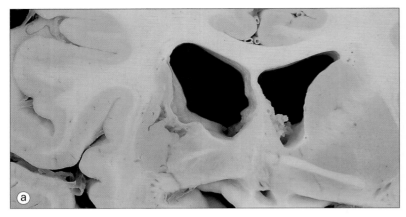

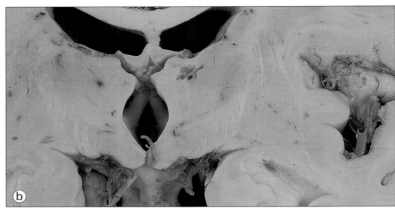

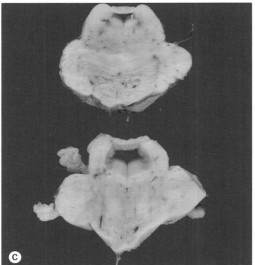

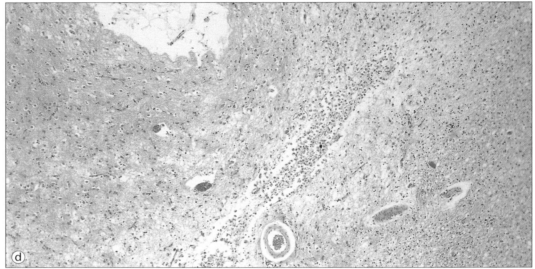

Fig. 9.54 Lacunar infarcts in the deep central gray matter. (a) Lacunar infarcts in left caudate, putamen, and internal capsule. They are so extensive that there is enlargement of the overlying left lateral ventricle. **(b)** Lacunar infarcts in the right diencephalon and thalamus at the coronal level of the mamillary bodies. **(c)** Lacunar infarcts in the basis pontis imparting a 'moth-eaten' appearance to this structure. **(d)** On histologic section, lacunar infarcts share microscopic features with larger infarcts. There are collections of macrophages and histiocytes surrounded by reactive astrocytes.

REFERENCES

Barnett HJM, Mohr JP, Stein BM, Yatsu FM. (eds) (1992) *Stroke. Pathophysiology, Diagnosis. and Management. Second edition.* 1270 pp. New York: Churchill Livingstone.

Beal MF, Williams RS, Richardson EP Jr, Miller Fisher C. (1981) Cholesterol embolism as a cause of transient ischemic attacks and cerebral infarction. *Neurology* 31: 860–865.

Berger JR, Harris JO, Gregorios J, Norenberg M. (1990) Cerebrovascular disease in AIDS: a case-control study. *AIDS* 4: 239–244.

Bogousslavsky J, Barnett HJM, Fox AJ, Hachinski VC, Taylor W for the EC/IC Bypass Study Group. (1986) Atherosclerotic disease of the middle cerebral artery. *Stroke* 17: 1112–1120.

Bogousslavsky J, Van Melle G, Regli F. (1988) The Lausanne Stroke Registry: Analysis of 1,000 consecutive patients with first stroke. *Stroke* 19: 1083–1092.

Castaigne P *et al.* (1973) Arterial occlusions in the vertebro–basilar system A study of 44 patients with post-mortem data. *Brain* 96: 133–154.

DiNubile MJ. (1988) Septic thrombosis of the cavernous sinuses. *Arch Neurol* 45: 567–572

Farrell MA, Gilbert JJ, Kaufmann JCE. (1985) Fatal intracranial arterial dissection: clinical pathological correlation. *J Neurol Neurosurg Psych* 48: 111–121.

Fisher CM. (1989) Binswanger's encephalopathy: a review. *J Neurol* 236: 65–79.

Fisher CM, Gore I, Okabe N, White PD. (1965) Atherosclerosis of the carotid and vertebral arteries—extracranial and intracranial. *J Neuropathol Exp Neurol* 24: 455–476.

Fisher M. (1994) *Clinical Atlas of Cerebrovascular Disorders.* London: Mosby–Wolfe.

Gacs G, Fox AJ, Barnett HJM, Vinuela F. (1983) Occurrence and mechanisms of occlusion of the anterior cerebral artery. *Stroke* 14: 952–959.

Gray F, Robert R, Labrecque R, Chretien F, Baudrimont M, Fallet–Bianco C, Mikol J, Vinters HV. (1994) Autosomal dominant arteriopathic leukoencephalopathy and Alzheimer's disease. *Neuropathol Appl Neurobiol* 20: 22–30.

Hachinski V, Norris JW. (1985) The Acute Stroke. 286 pp. Philadelphia: FA Davis.

Hart RG. (1988) Vertebral artery dissection. *Neurology* 38: 987–989.

Ikeda E, Hosoda Y. (1993) Distribution of thrombotic lesions in the cerebral arteries in spontaneous occlusion of the circle of Willis: cerebrovascular Moyamoya disease. *Clin Neuropathol* 12: 44–48.

Kubik CS, Adams RD. (1946) Occlusion of the basilar artery—a clinical and pathological study. *Brain* 69: 73–121.

Levie SR, Brey RL, Sawaya KL, *et al* (1995) Recurrent stroke and thrombo-occlusive events in the antiphospholipid syndrome. *Annals of Neurology* 38:119–124.

Mettinger KL (1982) Fibromuscular dysplasia and the brain. II. Current concept of the disease. *Stroke* 13: 53–58.

Mizusawa H, Hirano A, Llena JF, Shintaku M. (1988) Cerebrovascular lesions in acquired immune deficiency syndrome (AIDS). Acta Neuropathol 76: 451–457.

Mohr JP. (1982) Lacunes. *Stroke* 13: 3–11.

Moore PM, Fauci AS. (1981) Neurologic manifestations of systemic vasculitis. *Am J Med* 71:517–524.

Pessin MS, Adelman LS, Barbas NR. (1989) Spontaneous intracranial carotid artery dissection. *Stroke* 20: 1100–1103.

Rhodes RH, Madelaire NC, Petrelli M, Cole M, Karaman BA. (1995) Primary angiitis and angiopathy of the central nervous system and their relationship to systemic giant cell arteritis. *Arch Pathol Lab Med* 119: 334–349.

Ross R. (1993) The pathogenesis of atherosclerosis: a perspective for the 1990s. *Nature* 362: 801–809.

Save–Soderbergh J, Malmvall B–E, Andersson R, Bengtsson B–A. (1986) Giant cell arteritis as a cause of death. *JAMA* 255: 493–496.

Torvik A. (1984) The pathogenesis of watershed infarcts in the brain. *Stroke* 15: 221–223.

Torvik A, Jorgensen L. (1964) Thrombotic and embolic occlusions of the carotid arteries in an autopsy material. Part 1. Prevalence, location and associated diseases. *J Neurol Sci* 1: 24–39.

Toubi E, Khamashta MA, Panarra *et al*, (1995) Association of antiphospholipid antibodies with central nervous system disease in systemic lupus erythematosus. *American Journal of Medicine* 99:397-401.

Vinters HV. (1991) Interactions between the heart and brain. In Silver MD (ed.) *Cardiovascular Pathology. Second edition.* pp. 1029–1071. New York: Churchill Livingstone.

Walley VM, Stinson WA, Upton C, Santerre JP, Mussivand T, Masters RG, Ghadially FN. (1993) Foreign materials found in the cardiovascular system after instrumentation or surgery (including a guide to their light microscopic identification). *Cardiovasc Pathol* 2:157–185.

Welch KMA. (ed.) (1993) Cerebrovascular diseases: Eighteenth Princeton conference. *Stroke* 24(Suppl I).

10 Hemorrhage

The term 'intracranial hemorrhage' describes extravasation of blood into brain substance, regions defined and enclosed by the meninges and skull, or the ventricular cavities. Intracranial hemorrhage can be classified on anatomic grounds as:
- extradural (epidural) hemorrhage
- subdural hemorrhage
- subarachnoid hemorrhage
- encephalic or brain hemorrhage (which can be further subdivided into cerebral, cerebellar, or brain stem hemorrhage).

The term 'cerebral hemorrhage' should be used only for bleeding into the parenchyma of the cerebral hemispheres, though it is sometimes incorrectly applied to bleeding into any part of the brain parenchyma, including the brain stem and cerebellum.

EXTRADURAL HEMORRHAGE (EDH)

EDH is also considered in chapter 11, in relation to craniocerebral trauma, with which it is almost invariably associated.

MACROSCOPIC AND MICROSCOPIC APPEARANCES

EDH is easily diagnosed at necropsy as a biconvex hematoma that is readily seen on removing the calvarium but before breaching the dura (**Fig. 10.1**). As patients who have died of EDH are often the subject of a forensic investigation, the size and site of any (causal) skull fracture and the volume of hematoma should be measured. Hematomas of 75–100 ml are usually fatal. The maximum volume that is likely to accumulate is approximately 300 ml. The neuropathologist should also document the effects of the EDH (e.g. distortion or herniation of brain substance), and the presence of any other traumatic lesions.

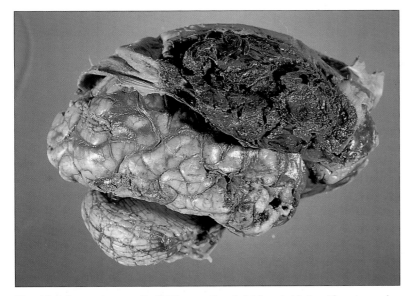

Fig. 10.1 Large traumatic EDH over the right frontal lobe. (Courtesy of Professor Michael A. Farrell, Dublin, Ireland)

EXTRADURAL HEMORRAGE

- EDH is much less common than SDH (see p 10.2) in large clinicopathologic series incorporating necropsy data from patients who have died from head injury. EDH and SDH often occur together.
- EDH occurs in 5–15% of fatal non-missile head injuries.
- The hemorrhage usually results from a skull fracture that produces tearing of a dural artery (most often the middle meningeal artery). This mechanism accounts for over 90% of cases. Much less frequently, EDH results from tearing of the sagittal or lateral venous sinus.
- EDH is most common in the temporal fossa in adults.
- EDH is most common in the posterior fossa in children.
- EDH is less common in children than adults.
- EDH may be associated with a lucid interval lasting hours to days after the head injury. Injury to the underlying brain may be minimal.

SUBDURAL HEMORRAGE (SDH)

Compared with EDH, SDH has a more diverse clinical presentation and etiology, and is not invariably associated with (documented) head trauma.

The acute and chronic forms of SDH have distinctive clinical and pathologic features. However, both types result from rupture of 'bridging' veins between the brain and the dura.

MACROSCOPIC AND MICROSCOPIC APPEARANCES

As with EDH, the extent of an acute SDH should be carefully documented at necropsy, along with its effects on the underlying brain (**Figs 10.2–10.4**). Associated skull fractures (if any) and contusions (with acute SDH) should be noted when the brain is removed and subsequently sectioned. If the SDH is chronic or subacute, histologic sections of hematoma will show vascular and variably fibrotic granulation tissue with an admixture of blood breakdown products (**Fig. 10.5**). As dural neoplasms and hemangiomas are, rarely, associated with SDH, surgically removed hematoma submitted for pathologic evaluation should be examined with these possibilities in mind.

PATHOGENESIS OF SUBDURAL HEMATOMAS

- Acute SDH usually results from trauma in which the head is subjected to rapid acceleration or deceleration. Because of the inertia of the brain, its movement lags behind that of the skull. This causes traction on, and tearing of, the bridging veins between brain and dura mater, since the latter is adherent to the inside of the skull.
- Chronic SDH starts with rupture of bridging veins and is followed by cycles of organization and rebleeding, due to the formation of densely vascular granulation tissue (pseudomembrane) around the hematoma. Large caliber thin-walled blood vessels in this tissue tend to bleed spontaneously and perpetuate the pathologic process. Osmotic forces may also lead to enlargement of the hematoma.
- SDH may occur in association with dural neoplasms (e.g. meningiomas and metastases) and dural hemangiomas.
- Patients with abnormal hemostasis are at risk of developing spontaneous acute or chronic SDH.

CHRONIC SUBDURAL HEMORRHAGE

- This mainly affects patients over 50 years of age.
- The precipitating head injury may be trivial or unrecognized.
- The frequency in men and women is roughly equal.
- Progression of symptoms and signs may be slow and stepwise, including stroke-like episodes and, in elderly patients, may include dementia.
- Chronic SDH is particularly common in elderly patients with cerebral atrophy due to aging or Alzheimer's disease. It can be difficult to differentiate dementia secondary to parenchymal disease from that associated with chronic SDH.

ACUTE SUBDURAL HEMORRHAGE

- SDH should be suspected in any patient of any age who has experienced significant head trauma. Its existence can be verified by appropriate imaging studies (i.e. CT or MRI).
- It causes predominantly non-localizing symptoms and signs (e.g. headache, drowsiness) rather than a focal deficit.
- SDH can be bilateral.
- SDH is recorded at necropsy in 25–50% of patients with fatal non-missile head injuries.
- Compared with EDH, SDH carries a worse prognosis because it is more often associated with underlying contusional brain injury, which can itself be a major cause of mortality and morbidity.
- The mortality rate in patients under 10 years of age is approximately 50% of that in patients over 60 years of age.

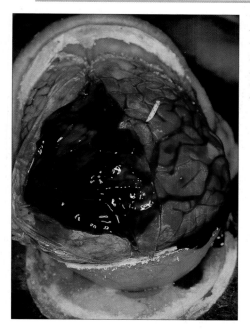

Fig. 10.2 Acute SDH over the left hemisphere. This was seen at necropsy of a 30-year-old woman with acute leukemia and disseminated intravascular coagulation.

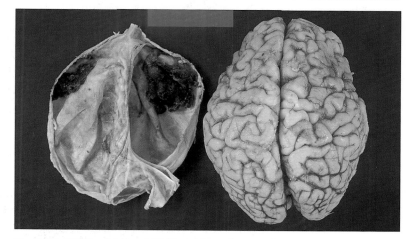

Fig. 10.3 Bilateral frontal SDHs with early organization. The dura has been reflected from the convexities of the fixed brain of a 47-year-old woman with SDHs due to antiphospholipid syndrome.

SUBARACHNOID HEMORRHAGE (SAH)

SAH describes an acute extravasation of blood into the space between the arachnoid membrane and pia mater. Spontaneous SAH should be distinguished from that associated with brain trauma (see chapter 11). Spontaneous SAH occurs when a weakened vessel in the subarachnoid space ruptures. Such weakening results from a focal abnormality due to either a pathologic process or a congenital malformation:

- berry (saccular) aneurysms, which are the commonest cause of spontaneous SAH
- infectious (mycotic) aneurysms (IAs)
- fusiform aneurysms
- arteriovenous malformations (see p 10.17–10.18)
- cerebral amyloid angiopathy (see p 10.13)

Because the last two of these more often cause brain hemorrhage than SAH, they are considered together with other causes of brain hemorrhage (from p 10.9). Traumatic SAH is covered in chapter 11.

BERRY (SACCULAR) ANEURYSMS

Berry aneurysms are an incidental finding in up to 3% of unselected necropsies, and usually there is no history and there are no pathologic

features to suggest previous hemorrhage. Unlike the incidences of strokes due to brain hemorrhage or infarction, which have declined over recent decades, the incidence of SAH due to berry aneurysm has remained constant.

SAH DUE TO RUPTURE OF BERRY ANEURYSMS

- Aneurysmal SAH has an annual incidence of approximately 10–12/100,000.
- The incidence increases with age up to the fifth or sixth decade. Some studies have shown a decline in the incidence of SAH in subsequent decades.
- SAH due to a ruptured berry aneurysm is fatal or disabling in over two-thirds of patients: one-third die from the initial hemorrhage within 72 hours, and a further third die or become significantly disabled due to the complications of SAH (i.e. vasospasm with brain ischemia, re-bleeding, acute or chronic hydrocephalus, and complications of surgical intervention).
- Major SAH is preceded by warning symptoms in over 50% of patients. The symptoms are usually related to a 'sentinel leak' from the lesion 2–3 weeks before the overt SAH.
- The clinical manifestations of SAH due to a ruptured aneurysm are determined by the location of the aneurysm (e.g. an aneurysm of the posterior communicating artery can compress the third cranial nerve), the size of the hemorrhage, and the regions into which the hemorrhage extends (e.g. brain parenchyma, ventricular system).
- Massive SAH can lead to coma and death within minutes.
- Less extensive SAH often produces prominent localizing signs and symptoms (e.g. hemiparesis, akinetic mutism, or lower limb paresis due to a ruptured anterior communicating artery aneurysm).
- If treated successfully (by surgical 'clipping') an aneurysm will not usually cause further symptoms or affect lifespan.
- Berry aneurysms that rupture are usually smaller than 1 cm in diameter. Approximately 10–15% are smaller than 5 mm. Giant aneurysms (i.e. larger than 2–2.5 cm in diameter) bleed less frequently and more commonly behave as a mass lesion within the CNS.

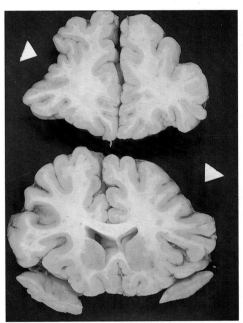

Fig. 10.4 Indentation and displacement of brain parenchyma by SDHs. The arrows show the location of bilateral frontal SDHs during life. Coronal sections of the brain illustrated in Fig. 10.3.

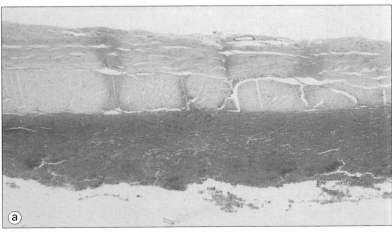
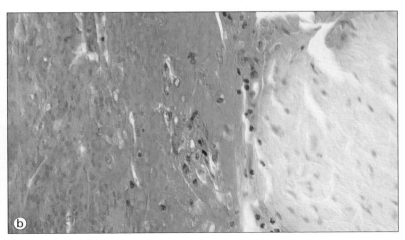

Fig. 10.5 Organizing pseudomembrane in SDH. (a) At low magnification, a thin pseudomembrane composed of early granulation tissue is seen immediately beneath the fibrous dura. **(b)** Magnified view shows evidence of blood breakdown (hemosiderin), and capillary buds and fibroblasts that have infiltrated the hematoma.

MACROSCOPIC APPEARANCES

Abundant SAH is obvious at necropsy. However, when the ruptured dome of an aneurysm is embedded in brain parenchyma, a purely intraparenchymal bleed will result, with negligible SAH. This should be borne in mind when someone, especially a young person, dies from a brain hemorrhage of occult origin (**Figs 10.6–10.9**). Massive SAH in a young or middle-aged patient (**Fig. 10.10a**) from a clinically unproven source of bleeding strongly suggests a berry aneurysm. Blood at the base of the brain should be dissected away gently until the aneurysm is discovered (**Fig. 10.10b, c**). This dissection should not be deferred until the brain has been fixed because hematoma is then difficult to dissect, making the source of bleeding much more difficult to locate. The possibility that there is more than one aneurysm, or a combination of vascular abnormalities (berry aneurysm and an AVM), should always be considered. A 'ruptured' aneurysm is usually identified by the proximity of abundant hematoma and the 'tear' in the aneurysm wall (see below). Anterior circulation aneurysms occur at major branch points on the circle of Willis (**Fig. 10.11**), most commonly:

- the middle cerebral artery trifurcation in the Sylvian fissure
- the internal carotid artery/posterior communicating artery junction
- the anterior cerebral artery/anterior communicating artery junction

'Posterior circulation' aneurysms constitute 10–30% of cases, and most arise at the basilar artery bifurcation (basilar 'tip') (**Fig. 10.11**).

For patients who survive an SAH for days to weeks, the pathologist should note:

- the degree and extent of meningeal discoloration and fibrosis
- the severity of hydrocephalus, if present
- ischemic lesions within the CNS that may have resulted from vasospasm
- the location and status of any aneurysm clips placed by the neurosurgeon (**Figs 10.12, 10.13**)

Incidental berry aneurysms are found in up to 3% of non-selected adult autopsies. An incidental aneurysm can be quite large, and in elderly patients there may be superimposed atherosclerotic change within its walls.

PATHOGENESIS OF BERRY ANEURYSMS

Although berry aneurysms are said to be 'congenital', they are very seldom present in infants and children. Certain segments of the vascular tunica media (especially at arterial branch points, where blood flow is most turbulent) are prone to develop aneurysms in later life. The risk is increased in association with:

- *hypertension*
- *cerebral arteriovenous malformations (AVMs): up to 10% are associated with coexisting berry aneurysm(s) involving arteries hemodynamically affected by the increased flow of blood through the AVM*
- *some systemic vascular diseases (e.g. fibromuscular dysplasia)*
- *defective vascular collagen, smooth muscle, and elastic tissue (e.g. Ehlers–Danlos syndrome, acid maltase deficiency)*
- *polycystic kidney disease and coarctation of the aorta, probably because these conditions produce hypertension*
- *Moya-Moya disease*

Hypertension is not only a risk factor for the development of berry aneurysms but also increases the likelihood of their rupturing. Rupture of berry aneurysms may be precipitated by abuse of cocaine, presumably due to the associated hypertensive surge.

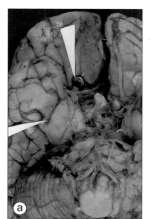
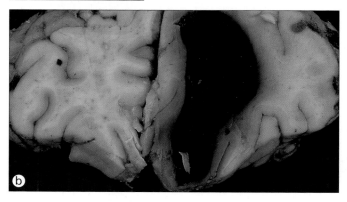

Fig. 10.6 Right carotid–ophthalmic artery aneurysm treated by balloon embolization. (a) Basal view showing severe right mesial temporal herniation (lower arrow) and balloon occlusion of the aneurysm adjacent to dusky discoloration on the undersurface of right frontal lobe in cortex overlying the hematoma (upper arrow). **(b)** Coronal section showing that the dome of the aneurysm had ruptured into the frontal lobe to produce a well-demarcated intracerebral hematoma.

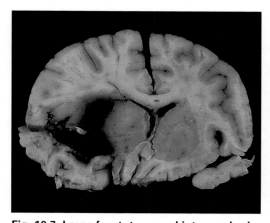

Fig. 10.7 Large frontotemporal intracerebral hematoma adjacent to the left basal ganglia. The patient was a young man who presented with severe rapid-onset headache and died within 72 hours.

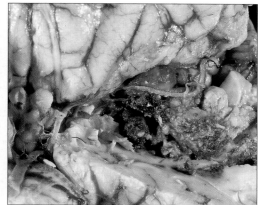

Fig. 10.8 Large left middle cerebral artery bifurcation berry aneurysm that has bled directly into the brain substance rather than the subarachnoid space. This is from the same patient as shown in Fig. 10.7. The left temporal tip has been cut away.

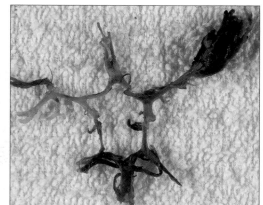

Fig. 10.9 Large left middle cerebral artery trifurcation berry aneurysm. This circle of Willis is from the brain of the patient shown in Figs 10.7 and 10.8.

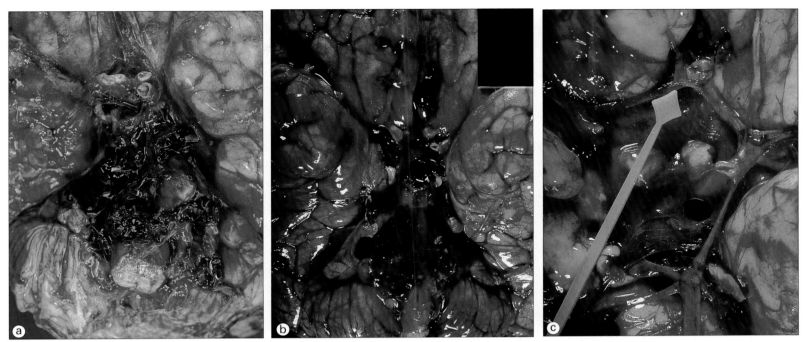

Fig. 10.10 Massive spontaneous SAH. (a) Basal view of freshly removed brain. A berry aneurysm on the circle of Willis should be suspected in all cases of spontaneous SAH. **(b)** Closer view of similar brain from another patient.

(c) Dissection of blood from (b) at the time of necropsy revealed a ruptured left anterior cerebral artery/anterior communicating artery aneurysm (arrow).

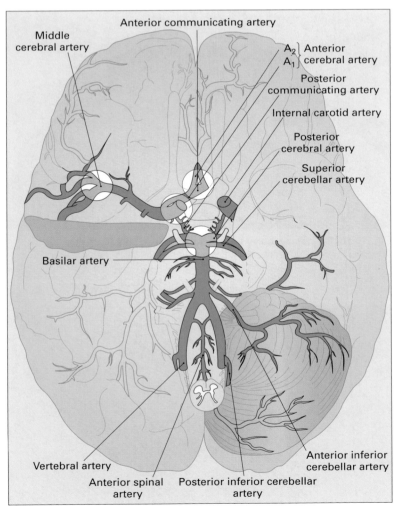

Fig. 10.11 Schematic illustration of the circle of Willis showing the most common locations for berry aneurysms at major arterial bifurcation points. Approximately 30% of patients in whom an aneurysm is identified will have one or more aneurysms elsewhere in the circle of Willis.

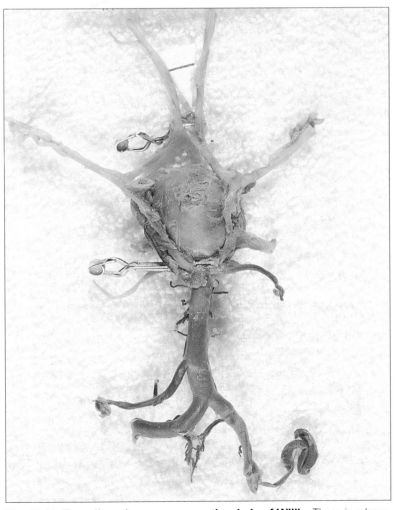

Fig. 10.12 Two clipped aneurysms on the circle of Willis. There is a large basilar tip aneurysm with a clip at its base and a smaller anterior cerebral artery/anterior communicating artery aneurysm.

MICROSCOPIC APPEARANCES

The histologic features of a berry aneurysm, either ruptured or intact, are optimally demonstrated by an elastic stain (e.g. elastic/van Gieson, Movat pentachrome). The aneurysm may be unilobular or multilobular (**Fig. 10.14**), and characteristic features include attenuation and focal loss of elastic tissue and muscularis, generally most marked close to the site of rupture. There is variable fibrosis of the aneurysm wall and foci of atherosclerosis may be evident (**Figs 10.15, 10.16**). Blood breakdown products in the vicinity may reflect earlier bleeds. Giant berry aneurysms (usually greater than 1.5–2 cm in diameter) often show mural calcification, and thrombosis with or without recanalization (**Figs 10.17, 10.18**).

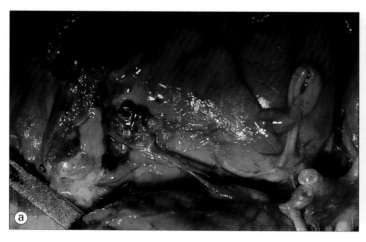
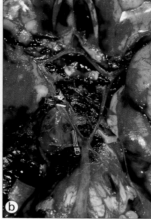

Fig. 10.13 Berry aneurysms. (a) Middle cerebral artery trifurcation aneurysm in the Sylvian fissure. For orientation, the optic chiasm and cut section of the internal carotid artery are seen at the right of the illustration. The brain around the aneurysm shows yellow-orange discoloration that is probably related to previous hemorrhage. The patient died of disease unrelated to the aneurysm, which shows no evidence of acute hemorrhage. **(b)** Large berry aneurysm in the vicinity of the right posterior cerebral artery/posterior communicating artery junction. Note the two aneurysm clips. There is abundant acute hemorrhage. The patient also had a large AVM in the right temporal lobe.

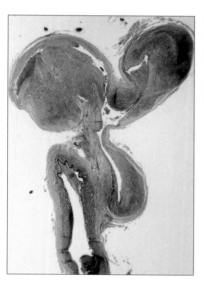

Fig. 10.14 Microscopic section of a berry aneurysm. A Movat pentachrome stain has been used to highlight the vascular components. The aneurysm wall shows variable thinning and fibromuscular intimal hyperplasia.

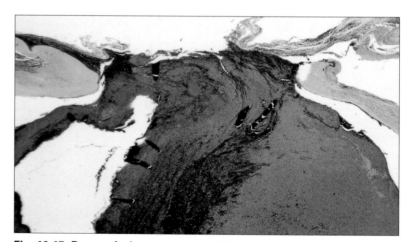

Fig. 10.15 Dome of a berry aneurysm. Thinning and attenuation of the aneurysm wall and local absence of elastic tissue are seen near the site of rupture. (Elastic/van Gieson)

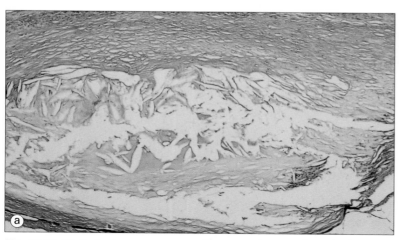
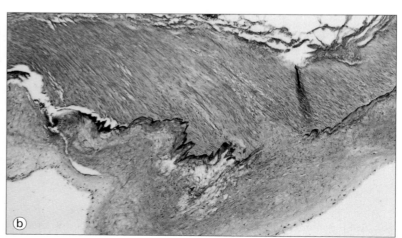

Fig. 10.16 Wall of a berry aneurysm. These sections are from the berry aneurysm shown in Fig. 10.15. **(a)** Fibrosis and focal atherosclerotic change with cholesterol clefts, and an absence of elastic tissue. **(b)** A region of wall remote from the rupture site, with focal loss of the internal elastic lamina, and intimal fibromuscular hyperplasia.

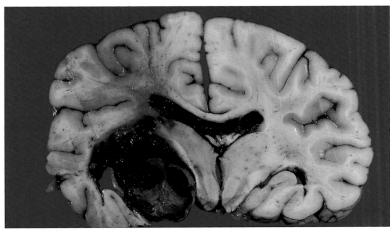

Fig. 10.17 Giant aneurysm in the left temporal lobe. Note the mass effect caused by this large aneurysm which has displaced and distorted adjacent temporal lobe and thalamic structures. The lumen of the aneurysm contains laminated thrombus and there are only small residual patent lumina. The cause of death was rupture of the aneurysm into the brain with intraventricular extension of hemorrhage.

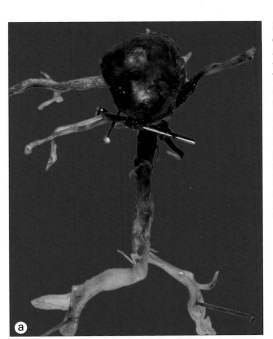

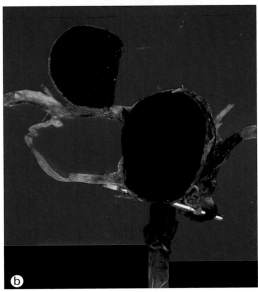

Fig. 10.18 Giant clipped basilar tip aneurysm. (a) In-situ view on the circle of Willis. **(b)** Section demonstrating recent thrombus. Nearby regions of brain stem and cerebellum showed ischemic necrosis, probably secondary to thrombus propagation into the superior cerebellar artery. (Courtesy of Dr MA Verity, UCLA, U.S.A.)

INFECTIVE ANEURYSMS (IAS)
MACROSCOPIC AND MICROSCOPIC APPEARANCES
Diagnosis of IAs depends on the pathologist's having a high index of suspicion in a patient with a predisposing medical condition who has a subarachnoid or parenchymal brain hemorrhage. IAs are usually situated distal to the circle of Willis and may be impossible to identify macroscopically. In this case, sections incorporating small arteries from the edge of a hematoma are likely to reveal an IA. Elastic stains demonstrate breaches in the elastic tissue of the vessel, while stains for fungi and bacteria are likely to show the causal organism in the vessel wall (Figs 10.19, 10.20).

INFECTIVE ANEURYSMS

- account for 5–6% of all intracranial aneurysms.
- present with SAH, brain hemorrhage, infarction, or headache.
- are often asymptomatic until the time of hemorrhage, but there may be symptoms of the predisposing condition (usually endocarditis).
- have a mortality rate of approximately 30% if bacterial, and of approximately 90% if fungal.

PATHOGENESIS OF IAs

- IAs result from bacterial or fungal colonization of the vessel wall.
- As bacterial infection is the most common cause, the term 'mycotic' aneurysm is best avoided since mycotic implies the presence of a fungal infection.
- Infection-induced inflammation weakens the vessel wall, resulting in ectasia and an IA.
- The colonizing microorganisms may be of hematogenous origin (e.g. associated with subacute endocarditis) or from a local infection (e.g. meningitis, osteomyelitis).
- As many as 3% of patients with infectious endocarditis develop IAs.
- IAs often involve the distal branches of cerebral blood vessels, particularly in cases due to bacterial infection. Bacterial colonization may be facilitated by the absence of vasa vasorum in the branches of these vessels. Inflammation and destruction of the vessel appear to proceed from the adventitia inwards.

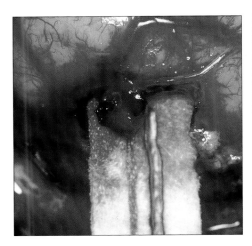

Fig. 10.19 IA in a young intravenous drug abuser. Intraoperative photograph showing the aneurysm involving a small leptomeningeal artery. (Courtesy of Dr NA Martin, UCLA, U.S.A.)

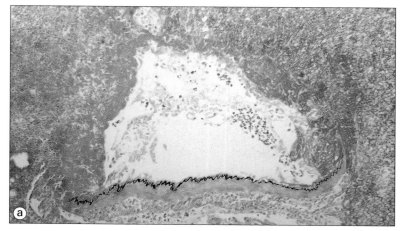

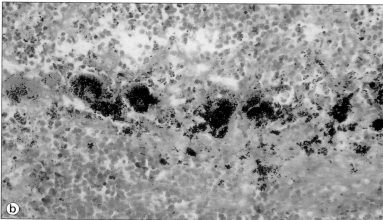

Fig. 10.20 **IA in a young intravenous drug abuser. Sections of the aneurysm shown in Fig. 10.19. (a)** The elastic tissue is intact along part of the vessel wall (bottom of the illustration) but ends abruptly in a mass of fibrin and inflammatory cells. (Elastic/van Gieson) **(b)** Part of the aneurysm wall stained to show the presence of Gram-positive cocci, which had colonized the vessel wall and produced the aneurysmal dilatation.

FUSIFORM ANEURYSMS

These rare aneurysms are formed from ectatic, often tortuous, basal arteries. Most involve the vertebrobasilar system. Fusiform aneurysms may be several centimeters in diameter.

Most patients are elderly. They may present with:

- brain stem and cranial nerve compression secondary to a basilar aneurysm
- ischemia secondary to thrombosis
- hemorrhage

MACROSCOPIC AND MICROSCOPIC APPEARANCES

Fusiform aneurysms usually affect the basilar artery, especially the middle segment of the artery (**Fig. 10.21**), but may extend inferiorly to involve the upper part of one of the vertebral arteries. There is usually marked atherosclerosis in the affected vessel wall. The histologic features are those of severe complicated atherosclerosis and include foamy histiocytes, evidence of old intraplaque hemorrhage, calcification, thrombosis (either mural or occlusive), and variable degrees of inflammation.

OTHER CAUSES OF SAH

SAH is rarely caused by neoplastic aneurysms, especially those originating in occlusive emboli from cardiac myxoma or choriocarcinoma, which invade multiple foci in the distal vasculature to produce ectasia and focal rupture.

The cause of SAH remains 'occult' in approximately 15–20% of patients (**Fig. 10.22**).

Possible causes of bleeding in some patients include:

- a ruptured small aneurysm that has sealed off or thrombosed
- rupture of a small, angiographically undetectable vascular malformation
- an undiscovered bleeding diathesis

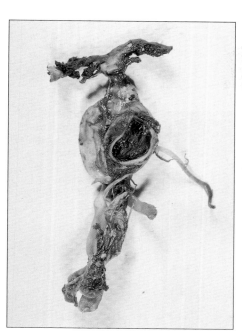

Fig. 10.21 **Fusiform atherosclerotic aneurysm of the basilar artery.** The vessel has been dissected away from the brain stem. The vertebral arteries are at the bottom of the illustration, the basilar bifurcation at the top. Note the severe atherosclerosis. There is a large region of ectasia, with rupture near the bifurcation (tip) of the basilar artery.

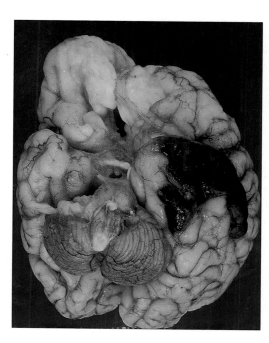

Fig. 10.22 **Acute idiopathic SAH over the left temporal lobe.** The patient was a 1-month-old child with severe respiratory distress secondary to a viral infection.

ENCEPHALIC OR BRAIN HEMORRAGE (BH)

The term BH encompasses cerebral, cerebellar and brain stem parenchymal hemorrhages. These commonly extend into ventricles, leptomeninges, and basal cisterns, producing secondary intraventricular hemorrhage and SAH. Conditions associated with BH are:

- hypertension
- trauma (see chapter 11)
- cerebral amyloid (congophilic) angiopathy (CAA)
- berry (saccular) aneurysm (see p 10.3)
- vascular malformations
- bleeding diathesis, due to systemic disease or anticoagulant therapy
- vasculitis
- illicit drug use
- neoplasms
- infection (including infective aneurysm)

HYPERTENSIVE BH

Hypertension is a major risk factor for BH. Although the incidence of hypertensive BH in the USA declined by approximately 50% between 1945–60 and 1977–87, hypertension continues to account for about 40–50% of BHs.

PATHOGENESIS OF HYPERTENSIVE BH

Hypertensive BH results from rupture of parenchymal arterioles that have become less compliant, and weakened, due to:

- replacement of smooth muscle by fibrocollagenous tissue
- fragmentation of elastic tissue
- in some cases, focal dilatation, with formation of a Charcot–Bouchard microaneurysms (**Fig. 10.31**) – these have been reported to be 5–10 times more frequent in the basal ganglia and pons of brains with hypertensive BH than in controls.

HYPERTENSIVE BH

- Hypertensive BH may be associated with a documented history of hypertension and related visceral complications (e.g. left ventricular hypertrophy and nephrosclerosis).
- Cardiac, renal and other visceral complications of hypertension may be discovered only at the time of BH.
- Symptoms and signs depend on the site of BH, but usually include a severe headache. Localizing syndromes associated with BH include:
  - hemiparesis, hemisensory loss, and visual field deficit (**putamen**),
  - hemiparesis, hemisensory loss, gaze abnormalities, and vomiting (**thalamus**)
  - vomiting, headache, truncal or limb ataxia, cranial nerve abnormalities, and coma if there is significant brain stem compression (**cerebellum**)
  - coma, quadriparesis or quadriplegia, and small reactive pupils (**large pontine hemorrhage**)
  - gaze paresis, ataxia, and contralateral sensorimotor deficit (**small pontine hemorrhage**)
- BH is 5–10 times less common than cerebral infarction.

MACROSCOPIC APPEARANCES

Hypertensive BH most commonly originates in the putamen, thalamus, cerebellum, or pons. Smaller hemorrhages may occur in the subcortical white matter. The acute hematoma appears as a soft red mass distinct from brain parenchyma (**Figs 10.23–10.25**); the hematoma hardens during formalin fixation and may fall away from the brain slice when the fixed brain is cut. The hemorrhage may extend into the ventricular system (**Fig. 10.26**), but very rarely dissects directly into the subarachnoid space, though may reach it after passing through the exit foramina of the fourth ventricle. There is usually significant brain swelling and herniation.

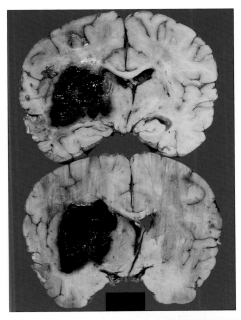

Fig. 10.23 Massive hypertensive (lateral ganglionic) BH. Coronal sections through the cerebral hemispheres of a man of about 30 with intractable hypertension. The hematoma has produced severe left-to-right shift of the midline structures.

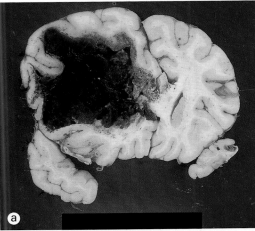

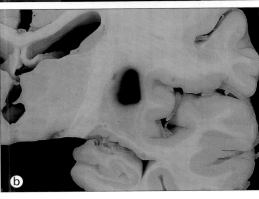

Fig. 10.24 Hypertensive BH. (a) There is massive left-to-right shift. Note the characteristic petechial hemorrhages at the margins of the hematoma. The patient was a 76-year-old woman and the BH probably originated in the left basal ganglia and extended into the left centrum semiovale. **(b)** A much smaller hematoma in the posterior part of the putamen in another patient.

Older hematomas may resorb, leaving a cystic cavity lined by orange–brown altered blood pigment (Figs 10.27, 10.28). Old BH can usually be distinguished from an infarct or encephalomalacia by:

- its location, as the location of the hematoma cavity does not usually correspond to a particular vascular territory
- the amount of altered blood pigment that remains in the wall of the cavity, as this is usually larger after BH than after infarction

If a BH in the region of the basal ganglia has been sufficiently large and longstanding, Wallerian degeneration is usually evident in descending long tracts in the brain stem and spinal cord (**Fig. 10.28c**).

MICROSCOPIC APPEARANCES

Sections of an acute hypertensive BH reveal fresh blood where it has dissected through the tissue planes and along tracts. After 2–3 days, inflammatory cells accumulate including neutrophils initially and, later macrophages. Hemosiderin- and lipid-laden macrophages, hematoidin, and cytoid bodies, remain visible for months or years within the cavity and adjacent gliotic margins of older hematomas(10.29).

The microvascular pathology usually affects arterioles of 50–200 μm diameter. Onion-skin type thickening (arteriosclerosis and arteriolosclerosis) is evident in many vessels, but is particularly prominent where

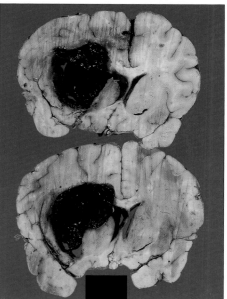

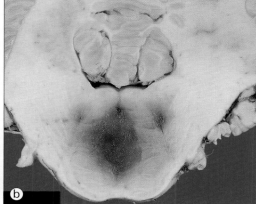

Fig. 10.25 Hypertensive pontine hemorrhage (a) and **(b).** This occurred several days before the patient's death. The hemorrhage extends to the edge of the fourth ventricle (a) and shows early signs of organization.

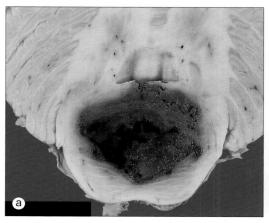

Fig. 10.26 Intraventricular extension of hypertensive BH. This is from the same patient as shown in Fig. 10.23. Note the significant left hemisphere swelling with left-to-right shift, and extension of the hematoma into the lateral ventricles.

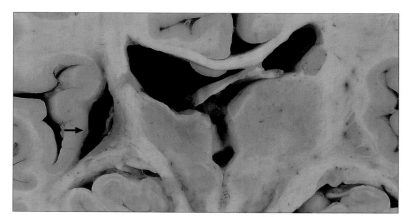

Fig. 10.27 Old resorbed hypertensive hematoma. Note the collapse of surrounding tissue and the smooth surface and orange-yellow discoloration of the hematoma cavity wall. The location of the cavity and the prominent discoloration by blood breakdown products distinguish this from an old infarct.

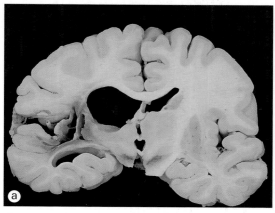
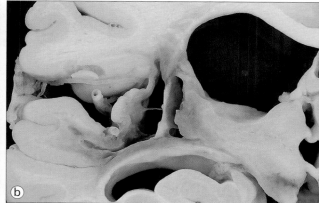
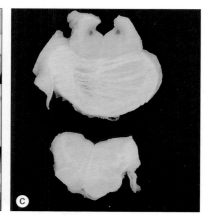

Fig. 10.28 Brain section from a 67-year-old man who had had a 'stroke' 13 years before death. (a) Note the large area of encephalomalacia in the left basal ganglia which extends into the adjacent insular region, and subcortical white matter of the left temporal lobe. **(b)** Magnified view. Note the compensatory dilatation of the left lateral ventricle and the degeneration of the ipsilateral corticospinal tract **(c).**

hypertensive BHs are common (see p 10.9) (**Fig. 10.30**). Lipohyalinosis describes thickening of the vessel wall by hyaline (non-amyloid) material and lipid-bearing macrophages, resulting in narrowing or obliteration of the lumen (**Fig. 10.31a, b**). Charcot–Bouchard microaneurysms may be seen as ectatic outpouchings in an abnormal vessel wall (**Fig.**

10.31c, d). Their lumina may be partly or entirely obliterated and surrounded by recent hemorrhage or altered blood pigment. They are believed to be of pathogenetic importance, although they are observed relatively infrequently in histologic sections and may occur in association with other forms of microangiopathy (e.g. CAA, see p 10.13).

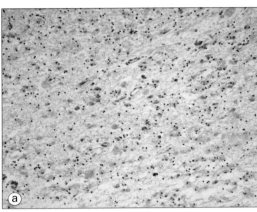
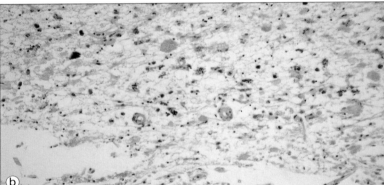

Fig. 10.29 Brain parenchyma around an old hematoma. (a) and (b) These show cystic microcavitation, hemosiderin, eosinophilic (granular) cytoid bodies, sparse histiocytes, and reactive astrocytes.

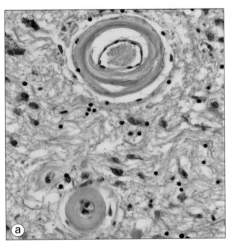
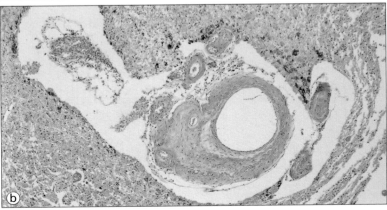

Fig.10.30 Arteriosclerotic change and lipohyalinosis. (a) In smaller arterioles. (b) In larger arterioles.

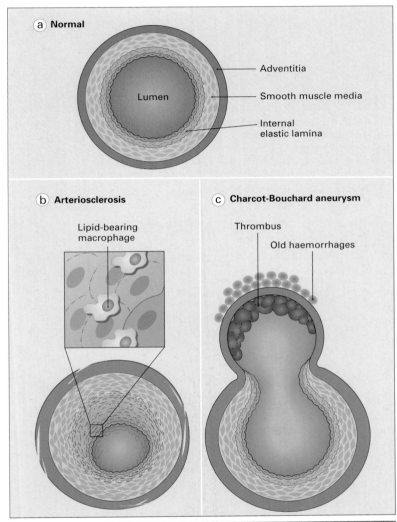
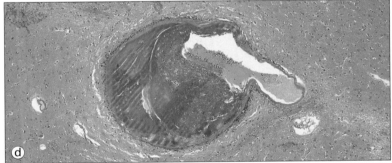

Fig. 10.31 Diagram showing normal arterioles, and arteriosclerotic change. (a) Normal brain intraparenchymal arteriole structure. (b) Arteriosclerotic change, which is usually associated with prolonged hypertension. There is thickening of the media, adventitial fibrosis, fragmentation and reduplication of elastic tissue, and intimal thickening, sometimes with accumulation of macrophages and histiocytes (i.e. lipohyalinosis). (c) Sometimes there is Charcot–Bouchard microaneurysm formation with a focal loss of elastic tissue and ballooning of the vessel wall. These aneurysms can contain mural thrombi and are not specific for hypertensive arteriosclerotic microvascular disease as they are also seen in severe CAA (see p 10.13). (d) Charcot–Bouchard microaneurysm in the putamen. This patient had systemic changes of longstanding hypertension. The microaneurysm is largely filled with thrombus.

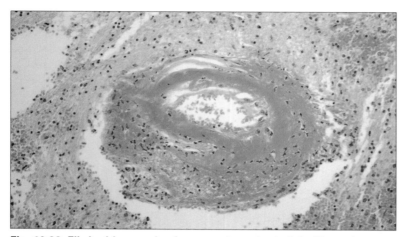

Fig. 10.32 Fibrinoid necrosis of a parenchymal arteriole. The patient was a 97-year-old woman with severe arteriosclerotic disease, Alzheimer's disease, and severe CAA (see below), who had a terminal BH. Note effacement of the normal arteriolar structures (see Fig. 10.31). The vessel wall has been replaced by deeply eosinophilic hyaline material and is surrounded by acute hemorrhage.

Arterioles adjacent to foci of hemorrhage may show changes of fibrinoid necrosis (**Fig. 10.32**).

Attempting to define the microvessel(s) from which a BH originated can be frustrating and non-productive. The point of origin of the hemorrhage is often obliterated by the hemorrhage itself.

ASSOCIATED WITH MALIGNANT (ACCELERATED) HYPERTENSION

A rapid rise in blood pressure to levels in excess of 200/150mm Hg can produce an encephalopathy, the manifestations of which include severe headache, vomiting, visual disturbances, seizures, focal neurologic deficits, stupor, and coma. The commonest predisposing conditions are glomerulonephritis, toxemia of pregnancy, systemic vasculitis, scleroderma, pheochromocytoma, and benign essential hypertension (especially after sudden withdrawal of some antihypertensive drugs, such as clonidine).

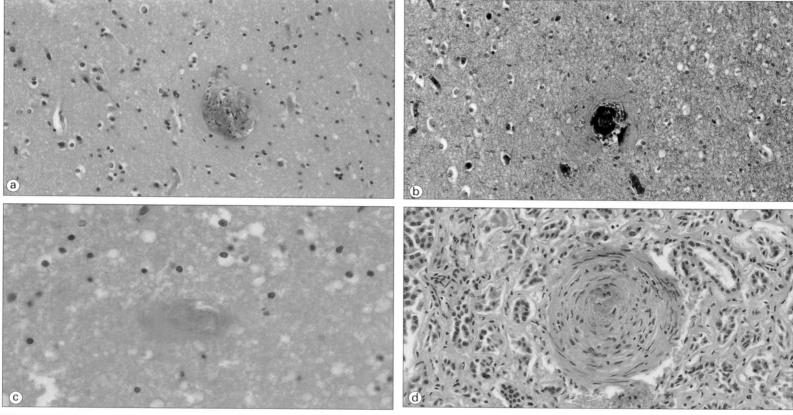

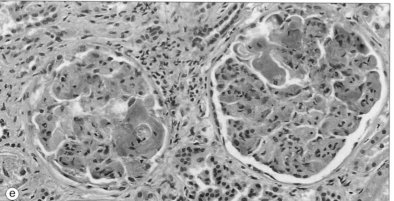

Fig. 10.33 Vascular abnormalities in hypertensive encephalopathy of malignant hypertension complicating scleroderma. (a) Fragmented nuclei and fibrinoid exudate in the wall of a small blood vessel **(b)** Small blood vessels containg fibrin thrombi. (Phosphotungstic acid/hematoxylin) **(c)** Necrosis of small blood vessel, with complete loss of nuclear staining. A proteinaceous exudate surrounds the blood vessel. The adjacent white matter is severely edematous. **(d)** 'Onion skin' appearance of a small renal artery, and **(e)** Fibrinoid necrosis of afferent glomerular arterioles in a kidney of the patient whose cerebral vascular changes are shown in 10.33a, b and c.

MACROSCOPIC AND MICROSCOPIC APPEARANCES

The brain appears swollen and may contain circumscribed clusters of petechial hemorrhages, or one or more large hemorrhages. Histology shows perivascular or parenchymal hemorrhages, acute microinfarcts (especially in the pons and basal ganglia), and characteristic changes in small parenchymal arteries and arterioles. There is fragmentation or loss of nuclei in the walls of affected blood vessels (**Fig. 10.33**). Some contain fibrin thrombi, others are surrounded by a proteinaceous exudate or admixed fibrin and hemorrhage. Typical histologic changes of malignant hypertension are evident in other organs, especially the kidneys (see Fig. 10.33 d, e).

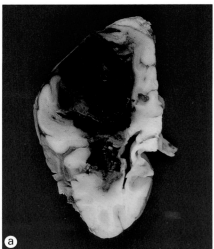
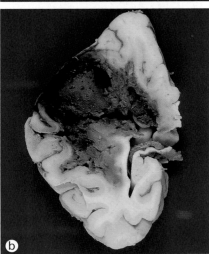
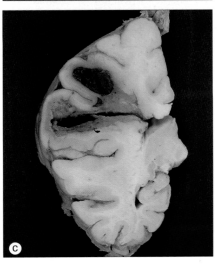

Fig. 10.34 BH secondary to CAA. Serial coronal slices of fixed brain from an elderly patient with Alzheimer's disease and CAA. **(a)** and **(b)** There is a large left parietal hematoma, which clearly extends into the subarachnoid space and the lateral ventricle. **(c)** Two smaller foci of hemorrhage at the coronal level of the lateral geniculate nucleus. The lower hematoma appears to be undergoing resorption.

CEREBRAL AMYLOID ANGIOPATHY (CAA)

In many series CAA is the second most frequent cause of primary non-traumatic BH, accounting for as many as 10–15% of all cases. The most common form of CAA is strongly associated with Alzheimer's disease (including the Alzheimer's disease pathology seen in the context of Down syndrome) and with aging. In CAA the media of parenchymal microvessels (mainly arterioles) is replaced by skeins of microfilaments, which are 7–10 nm thick and show (by light microscopy) the tinctorial properties of amyloid (e.g. affinity for Congo red and yellow–green birefringence when subsequently viewed by polarized light). CAA also involves meningeal arteries, though amyloid deposition in these arteries is usually more adventitial than medial.

MACROSCOPIC APPEARANCES

CAA-related BH is almost always cerebral (**Figs 10.34–10.36**). The smaller CAA-related hematomas are usually superficial, in the cortex or just near to it. The superficial origin of larger CAA-related hematomas may not be apparent. In both cases the hematomas tend to rupture into the subarachnoid space (unlike hypertensive BHs, which are more likely to rupture into the ventricles). As with hypertensive BH, the macroscopic features of CAA-related BH depend on its duration:

- Recent lesions are evident as fresh cortical or superficial subcortical hematomas in the brain.
- Old hematomas may resorb, leaving a cavity with surrounding brown dicoloration (**Fig. 10.37**).

MOLECULAR GENETICS OF CAA

The common (Alzheimer's disease-, Down syndrome-, and age-associated) forms of CAA result from deposition of the Aβ peptide within the vessel wall. This 4 kD peptide is derived from a much larger precursor protein, amyloid precursor protein (APP). In Alzheimer's disease brains, deposits of Aβ within the neuropil form plaques, and in vessel walls produce CAA.
Two much rarer, regional familial forms of CAA are:

Icelandic CAA or hereditary cystatin C amyloid angiopathy (HCCAA)

Previously known as hereditary cerebral hemorrhage with amyloidosis–Icelandic (HCHWA–I). This is:
- *inherited as an autosomal dominant trait*
- *associated with BH in young adult or middle-aged patients*
- *biochemically distinct from Aβ CAA*

HCCAA is characterized by vascular deposition of a mutant form of cystatin C/gamma trace (a cysteine proteinase inhibitor), in which glutamine is replaced by leucine as a result of a single nucleotide substitution in codon 68.

Dutch CAA or hereditary cerebral hemorrhage with amyloidosis–Dutch (HCHWA–D).

- This is inherited as an autosomal dominant trait.
- Amyloid deposition in arteriole walls in the brain leads to BH in middle-aged and elderly patients.
- Amyloid and preamyloid are also deposited in the neuropil, but less extensively than in Alzheimer's disease.
- The vascular amyloid is related to Aβ protein; the condition results from a mutation at codon 693 of APP.

A Flemish form of BH secondary to CAA (with AD changes) results from an APP codon 692 mutation.

MICROSCOPIC APPEARANCES

Reactive changes in the brain surrounding the hematoma are as described for hypertensive BH. Rarely, severe CAA is seen in regions of encephalomalacia, though it is more often associated with hemorrhagic than ischemic lesions (**Fig. 10.38**).

All biochemical types of CAA can be demonstrated by Congo red or thioflavin staining, though the appearances of affected blood vessels in hematoxylin and eosin-stained sections may be strongly suggestive of this diagnosis (**Fig. 10.39**). Specific CAA subtypes may be suggested by demographic associations. The diagnosis of Alzheimer's disease-related CAA or HCHWA–D can be confirmed by anti-Aβ immunohisto-chemistry, while a diagnosis of HCCAA can be confirmed with anti-cystatin C antibodies (**Fig. 10.40**).

CAA-associated microangiopathies are characterized by the presence of microaneurysms indistinguishable in hematoxylin–eosin sections from hypertension associated Charcot–Bouchard aneurysms, hyalinosis, variable degrees of inflammation, fibrinoid necrosis, and, rarely, thrombosis (**Fig. 10.41**). CAA is rarely associated with the development of a granulomatous angiitis (**Fig. 10.41c**)

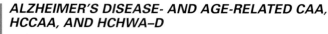

ALZHEIMER'S DISEASE- AND AGE-RELATED CAA, HCCAA, AND HCHWA–D

- Although Alzheimer's disease is common, CAA-related BH is not, especially in view of the large number of people with Alzheimer's disease.
- Lobar BH in an elderly person with the clinical features of an Alzheimer's disease-type dementia is likely to be due to CAA.
- CAA-related hematomas may be multiple, occurring simultaneously or over a period of months or years.
- BH associated with HCCAA or HCHWA–D resembles that associated with Alzheimer's disease-related CAA, but HCCAA and HCHWA–D are distinguished by their genetic and geographic context, and by the biochemical/immunohistochemical features of the amyloid protein.
- Patients with HCCAA have abnormally low concentrations of cystatin C in the cerebrospinal fluid.
- Patients at risk of HCHWA–D can be screened for the appropriate APP mutation.

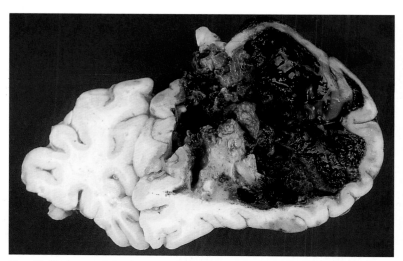

Fig. 10.35 Large right frontal BH in a 97-year-old woman with severe arteriosclerotic disease, Alzheimer's disease, and CAA. The hematoma has dissected into the subarachnoid space and has produced massive right-to-left shift of the midline structures.

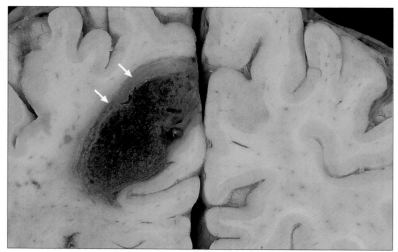

Fig. 10.36 Relatively small CAA-associated BH in the medial part of the left parietal lobe. Unlike the hematoma shown in Fig. 10.34, which was probably the immediate cause of death, this was one of many BHs that had occurred in the brain over several years. The hematoma communicates medially with the subarachnoid space. Note that there is evidence of early organization at its edges (arrows).

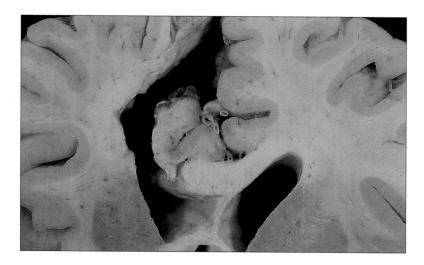

Fig. 10.37 Old CAA-related hematoma. A cystic cavity is seen in the left frontal lobe after resorption of a hematoma that resulted from CAA. Note the rust-orange color of the cavity wall, signifying previous hemorrhage.

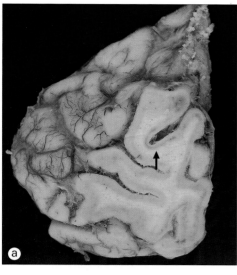

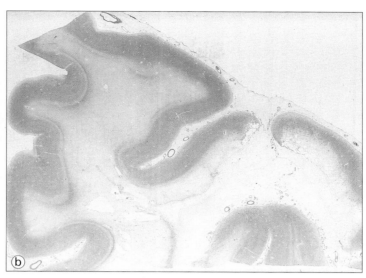

Fig. 10.38 CAA-related ischemic brain lesions. CAA is associated with ischemic brain lesions less consistently than with BH. **(a)** Occipital region of brain of an elderly woman who died after long-term care in a nursing home with presumed Alzheimer's disease. Some regions of the cortex show a picture resembling laminar necrosis (arrow). Microscopic sections showed only severe CAA with stenosis of microvessels (some of which were occluded) in this area and in other areas throughout the brain. **(b)** Section from another patient with severe neocortical CAA showing cystic encephalomalacia of the underlying white matter.

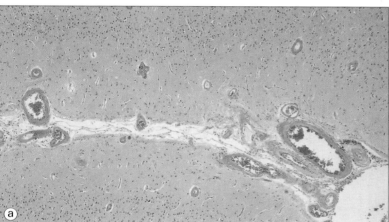

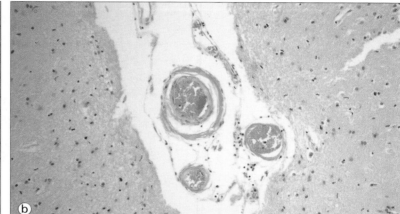

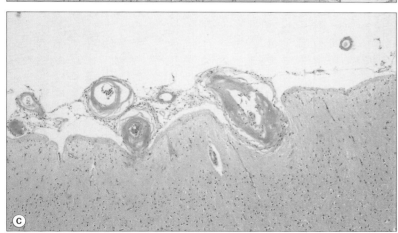

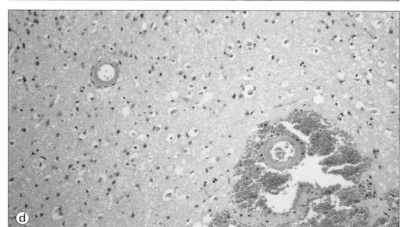

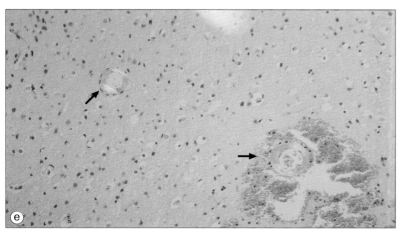

Fig. 10.39 Routine histology of CAA. (a) In routine hematoxylin and eosin-stained sections, the cellular components of the arteriolar wall are replaced by hyaline material. **(b)** Meningeal arteries and arterioles often show a 'lumen within a lumen' appearance, the outer wall having the characteristic staining properties of amyloid. **(c)** Affected vessels often show medial thickening and fibrosis in addition to amyloid deposition. **(d)** Congo red-stained biopsy tissue from brain adjacent to a large hematoma viewed without polarized light. **(e)** Same section as in (d) viewed with polarized light. Note the yellow–green birefringence of CAA-affected arterioles (arrows).

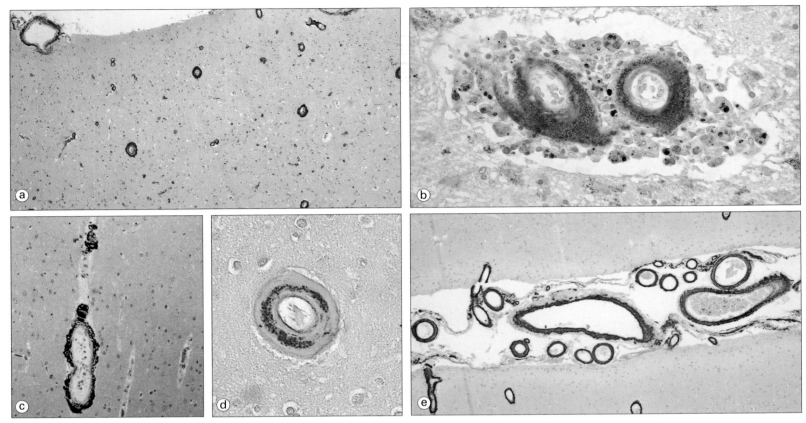

Fig. 10.40 CAA immunohistochemistry. (a) Severe CAA demonstrated using an anti-Aβ polyclonal antibody. Note that Aβ deposition is almost exclusively microvascular. **(b)** Brain section from another patient with a CAA-related BH showing extensive Aβ immunoreactive material in the vascular media and adventitia. **(c)** 1 μm thick plastic section stained with a silver-enhanced immunogold technique showing Aβ peptide around smooth muscle cells in the arteriolar wall (preparation by Diana Lenard Secor). **(d)** HCHWA–D can also be highlighted with anti-Aβ antibodies. **(e)** HCCAA affecting meningeal and parenchymal arteries and arterioles is demonstrated with anti-cystatin C antibodies and an immunoperoxidase technique.

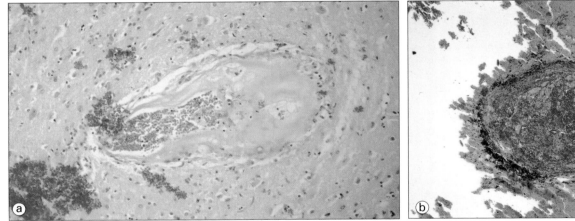

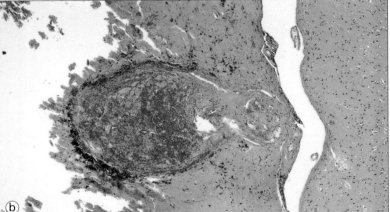

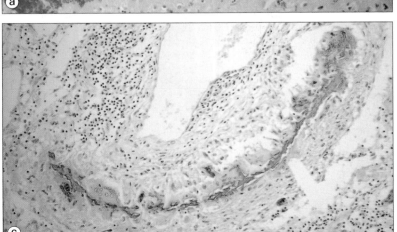

Fig. 10.41 Arteries and arterioles affected by CAA. (a) There can be marked fibrosis of arterial and arteriolar walls with histiocytic infiltration and ectasia with focal thinning. **(b)** CAA-related Charcot–Bouchard microaneurysm formation. Note the mural thrombus, adjacent old blood pigment, and acute hemorrhage. **(c)** Rarely there is a giant cell arteritis and angiitis. Here anti-Aβ immunohistochemistry shows severe CAA of a leptomeningeal artery with vasculitis and multinucleated giant cells. (Courtesy of Dr Mario Kornfeld, Albuquerque, New Mexico, U.S.A.)

VASCULAR MALFORMATIONS

Vascular malformations (**Fig. 10.42**) including arteriovenous malformation (AVM), cavernous hemangioma, venous angioma, telangiectasia, arteriovenous fistula, and berry aneurysm may present with BH or may be an incidental finding at necropsy. Their pathogenesis is unknown, but as a group they account for about 5% of BH. Of the vascular malformations, only AVMs are a significant cause of SAH (see p 10.3).

arteriovenous malformation (avm)

AVM is the vascular malformation that most commonly produces BH and is the second most common cause of SAH (after berry aneurysms, see p 10.3).

ARTERIOVENOUS MALFORMATIONS (AVMs)

AVMs occur at any age but are most common in the third and fourth decades. They are slightly more common in men than women. AVMs:

- can present with BH, SAH, or focal ischemia. Ischemia may be secondary to a 'steal' phenomenon resulting from an arteriovenous shunt
- are rarely familial
- are rarely multiple, but are associated with a berry aneurysm on a feeding artery in up to 10% of cases
- are defined angiographically as having a nidus, 'feeding' artery or arteries, and draining veins
- are the most common form of vascular malformation encountered in surgical specimens

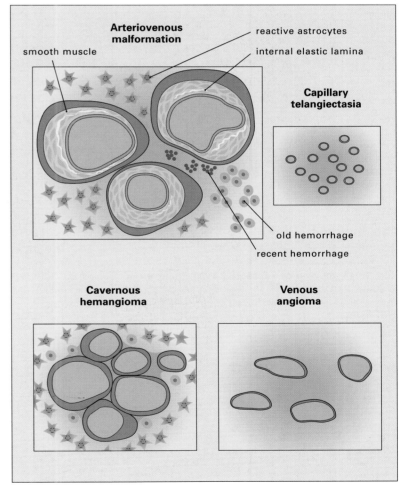

Fig. 10.42 Types of CNS vascular malformation.

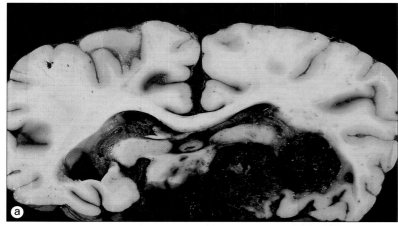
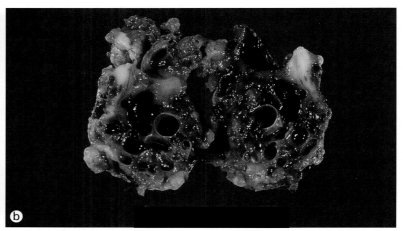

Fig. 10.43 AVMs. (a) Large right medial temporal and hippocampal AVM
extending from the ventricular lining to the subarachnoid space. It ruptured into both compartments.
(b) A resected AVM showing the characteristic appearance of vascular channels of variable caliber
and wall thickness, embedded in disorganized hemorrhagic brain parenchyma.

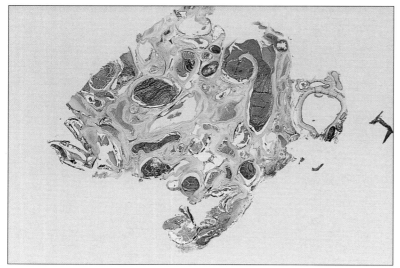
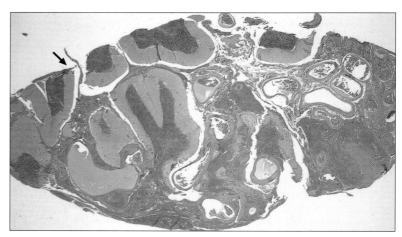

Fig. 10.45 Cerebellar AVM. This is at a slightly higher magnification than
that shown in Fig. 10.44. Note the similar features, though the cerebellar
architecture is still recognizable (arrow). The AVM extends from the brain
parenchyma into the subarachnoid space. The AVM includes very thin and
attenuated vessel walls, which are presumably the sites of AVM rupture. In
practice the exact point of rupture is found much less commonly than is the
case for berry aneurysms.

Fig. 10.44 Section of a resected AVM. There are tortuous and
disorganized vascular channels of varying diameter and wall thickness,
some containing laminated thrombus. (Trichrome stain)

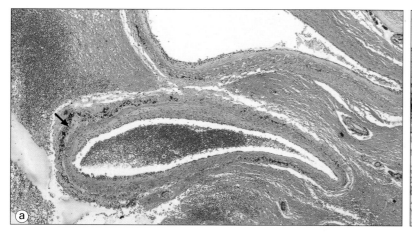
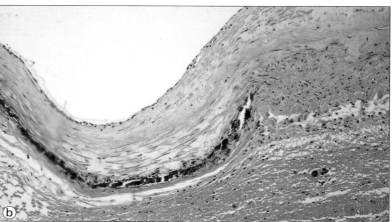

Fig. 10.46 AVM calcification. This is common within both parenchymal and vascular components of an
AVM. **(a)** Punctate calcification (arrow) immediately exterior to the fragmented elastic tissue. **(b)** Linear
calcification on the intimal aspect of the internal elastic lamina.

MACROSCOPIC AND MICROSCOPIC APPEARANCES

AVMs often extend from brain parenchyma into the subarachnoid space. They contain arteries, veins, and abnormal vessels with thin walls and a prominent internal elastic lamina, or thick walls and no elastic tissue (**Figs 10.43–10.45**). The caliber and wall thickness of vessels in an AVM vary markedly, and there are often varying degrees of calcification in the vessel walls and surrounding brain (**Fig. 10.46**). Intimal 'cushions'

caused by fibromuscular hyperplasia and hyalinization are prominent features, but 'complicated' atheroma (with foamy histiocytes, cholesterol clefts and plaque ulceration) is rare (**Fig. 10.47**). The surrounding brain shows reactive changes, including gliosis, old hemorrhage, cytoid bodies, and Rosenthal fibers (**Figs 10.48, 10.49**). Brain parenchyma is seen between the abnormal vessels.

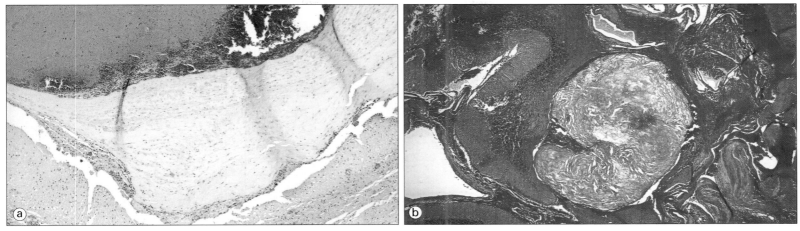

Fig. 10.47 Intimal hyperplasia and hyaline change in AVMs. (a) Intimal hyperplasia is frequently encountered in segments of vessels from an AVM, as in this example. These regions can protrude into the vascular lumen. **(b)** Hyaline change within the vessels can be extensive and can occlude the vascular lumen, as shown here.

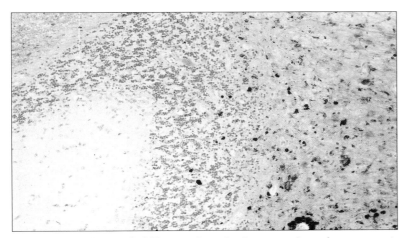

Fig. 10.48 Evidence of old hemorrhage in the parenchymal component of an AVM. This is often seen and is shown here in the cerebellum of a patient with an adjacent AVM. (Perls' stain)

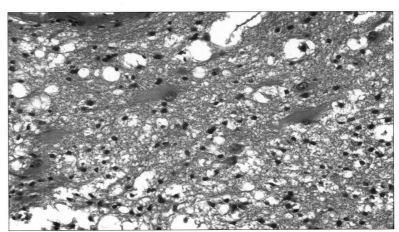

Fig. 10.49 Parenchymal gliosis. Gliosis is common in the disorganized brain parenchymal component of an AVM.

AVMs are commonly treated by embolization with various thrombus-inducing substances (**Fig. 10.50**), which can lead to a pronounced inflammatory and foreign body giant cell reaction in the vessel lumina and walls.

Cavernous hemangioma (cavernoma)

Cavernous hemangioma often occurs as a familial disorder, in which case the hemangiomas may be multiple. The presentation is with hemorrhage, focal neurologic deficits, or seizures.

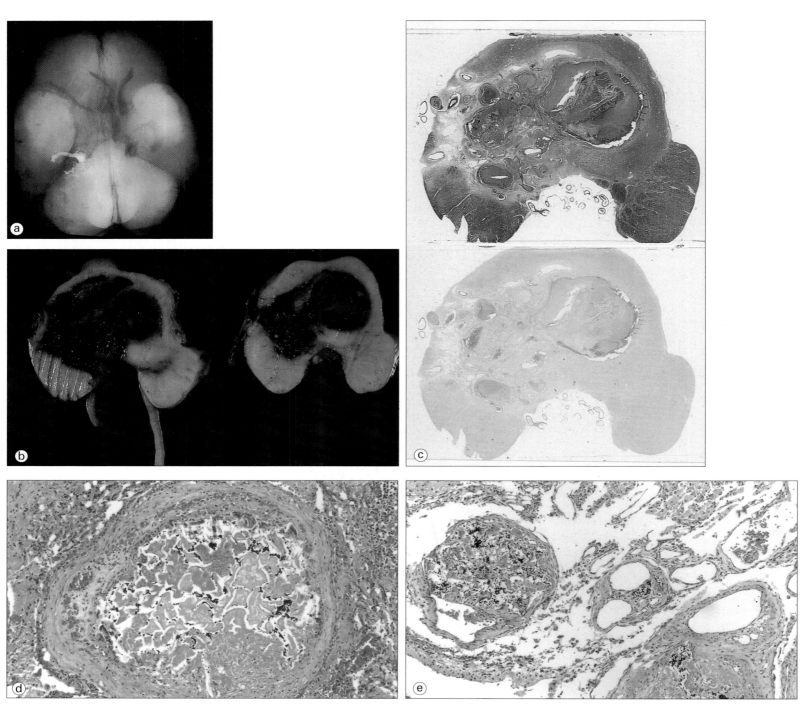

Fig. 10.50 Therapeutic embolization of AVMs. (a) Soft tissue autopsy radiograph of the brain of a patient with an AVM that had been treated with embolization. A 'cast' of radio-opaque material is seen in the right temporal lobe. Also note the shift of midline structures from right to left. The patient had a BH after embolization. **(b)** Mesencephalon with a large inoperable AVM that had been treated repeatedly with embolization therapy. **(c)** Whole mount sections of the lesion shown in (b) stained with hematoxylin and eosin (bottom) and an elastic tissue stain (top). **(d)** Embolization with a mixture of cyanoacrylate–tantalum produces cleft-like spaces in the lumen which represent sites where cyanoacrylate has been dissolved by tissue processing. The black particulate material is tantalum powder, which is added as a radio-opaque marker. Cyanoacrylate causes a foreign body giant cell reaction. **(e)** Over weeks or months, cyanoacrylate–tantalum occluded vessels can recanalize, leaving the 'iatrogenically' introduced material in the vessel wall and recognizable as a black particulate substance (residual tantalum).

MACROSCOPIC AND MICROSCOPIC APPEARANCES

Macroscopically the cavernous hemangioma resembles a small hematoma within the brain parenchyma (**Fig. 10.51a,b**). Microscopically, there is a tightly packed collection of hyalinized vessels lacking intervening brain parenchyma. The hemangioma is often surrounded by abundant old hemorrhage and reactive gliosis (**Fig. 10.51c–e**).

Venous angioma

Venous angiomas rarely bleed except when they occur in the cerebellum. They are probably the most common type of vascular malformation encountered at necropsy.

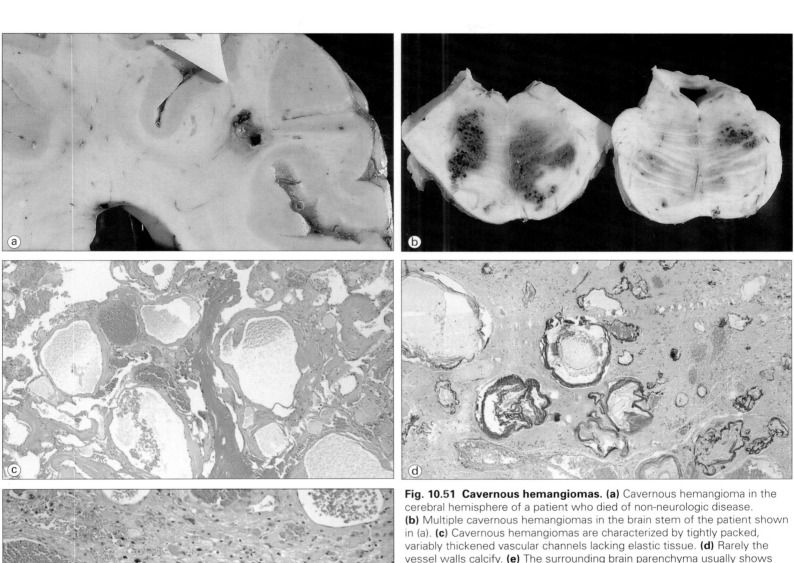

Fig. 10.51 Cavernous hemangiomas. (a) Cavernous hemangioma in the cerebral hemisphere of a patient who died of non-neurologic disease. **(b)** Multiple cavernous hemangiomas in the brain stem of the patient shown in (a). **(c)** Cavernous hemangiomas are characterized by tightly packed, variably thickened vascular channels lacking elastic tissue. **(d)** Rarely the vessel walls calcify. **(e)** The surrounding brain parenchyma usually shows extensive old hemorrhage and reactive changes, even more consistently than around an AVM.

MACROSCOPIC AND MICROSCOPIC APPEARANCES

Venous angiomas are found in the subcortical white matter of the cerebral hemispheres (Fig. 10.52a, b). Macroscopically, they resemble petechial hemorrhages. These angiomas are composed of thin-walled, dilated vascular channels lying within otherwise normal brain parenchyma (Fig. 10.52c).

Capillary telangiectasia

This malformation is almost always an incidental necropsy finding. It is usually found in the pons, and is virtually never hemorrhagic.

MACROSCOPIC AND MICROSCOPIC APPEARANCES

Telangiectasia appears as a collection of small-caliber, very thin-walled channels surrounded and separated by normal brain (**Fig. 10.53**).

Arteriovenous fistula

As strictly defined, an arteriovenous fistula is not a vascular malformation. It usually results from rupture of an aneurysm into a venous sinus (e.g. carotid–cavernous fistula). The vein of Galen aneurysm (see chapter 7) is an arteriovenous fistula in infants and children.

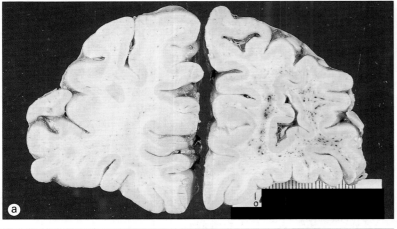

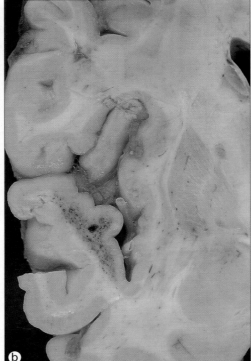

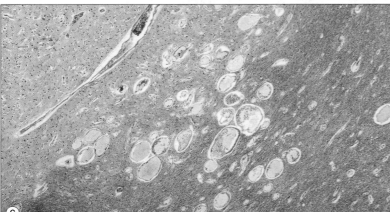

Fig. 10.52 Venous angiomas. (a) and **(b)** Examples encountered as incidental findings at necropsy. They may be mistaken for petechial hemorrhages, except that they are seen only focally rather than diffusely throughout white matter. **(c)** The microscopic appearance is usually of thin-walled, somewhat dilated venous channels, that have little effect on the surrounding brain. (Masson trichrome stain)

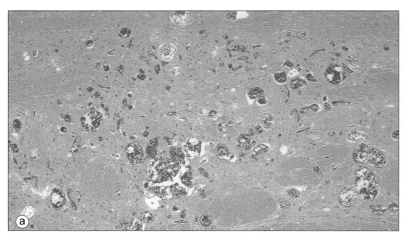

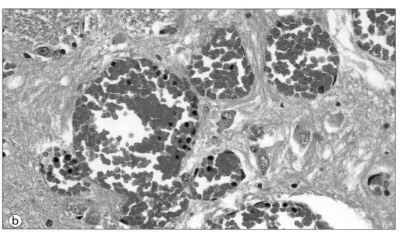

Fig. 10.53 Capillary telangiectasia. This is usually an incidental finding at necropsy, often in the pons, as in this patient. The lesion consists of thin-walled, small-caliber vascular channels and there is no surrounding reactive change, tissue disorganization, or old hemorrhage. **(a)** Low magnification. **(b)** High magnification.

BH SECONDARY TO SYSTEMIC DISEASE OR MEDICAL THERAPY

This group includes conditions of diverse etiology and may be the commonest cause of BH in tertiary medical centers. The most frequent causes of BH in this group are leukemia, coagulopathy, and the administration of thrombolytic agents.

MACROSCOPIC AND MICROSCOPIC APPEARANCES

The hematomas are often multiple, but can have a similar distribution to those associated with hypertension or CAA. However, microscopic examination fails to yield any evidence of the type of microangiopathy seen with hypertension or CAA.

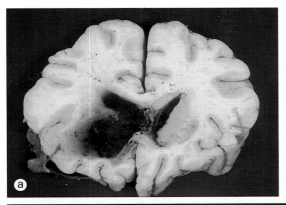

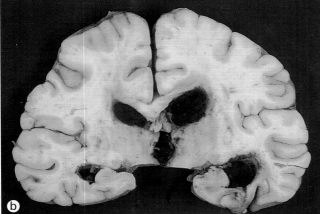

Fig. 10.54 BH due to pancytopenia. Sections of brain from a 59-year-old man with acute myelogenous leukemia who was treated with an allogeneic bone marrow transplant 2 months before death, but then developed pancytopenia and BH. **(a)** Left basal ganglia hematoma, the site and appearance of which mimic hypertensive BH. **(b)** The BH has ruptured into the ventricles, forming a blood cast in the posterior ventricular system. Green discoloration around the hematomas is due to jaundice, and bilirubin leakage into regions of brain with a disrupted blood–brain barrier.

BH DUE TO SYTEMIC DISEASE OR MEDICAL THERAPY

Leukemia

BH may be due to:
- thrombocytopenia secondary to either bone marrow involvement or treatment or both, or very high peripheral white blood counts
- pancytopenia before therapeutic bone marrow transplantation (**Figs 10.54–10.55**)

Coagulopathy

Coagulopathy causing BH may be:
- induced by iatrogenic anticoagulation (the overall frequency of BH in anticoagulated patients is of the order of 1%).
- secondary to hepatic disease (**Fig. 10.57**).

Administration of thrombolytic agents

Streptokinase, urokinase, and tissue plasminogen activator predispose to BH and can aggravate the tendency to BH with CAA.

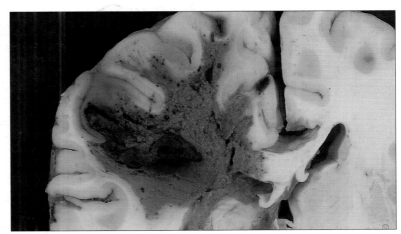

Fig. 10.55 BH due to bone marrow hypoplasia with pancytopenia. Section of brain from a 10-year-old boy who had had acute lymphoblastic leukemia for 6 years and developed testicular and CNS relapses. Two months before death he had a bone marrow transplant. Five weeks later he developed a large left parietal hemorrhage secondary to bone marrow hypoplasia. The photograph shows a large organizing hematoma extending into the corpus callosum and the left lateral ventricle with peripheral 'satellite' hemorrhages in the subcortical white matter.

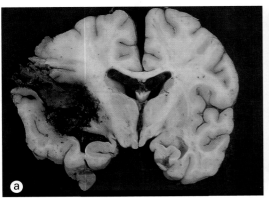

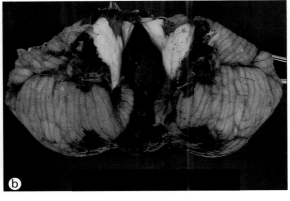

Fig. 10.56 BH due to pancytopenia. A 47-year-old male with refractory anemia who had a bone marrow transplant and subsequently developed pancytopenia and a BH. **(a)** Massive left parietotemporal BH extending into the ventricular system. **(b)** View of the cerebellum after the brain stem had been removed by cutting through the cerebellar peduncles. A cast of blood is present in the fourth ventricle, and there is extensive SAH.

BH SECONDARY TO ILLICIT DRUG USE

Drugs with which BH is commonly associated include cocaine (especially 'crack'), amphetamine, phencyclidine, and phenyl-propanolamine. The neuropathologic substrate and the pathogenesis of BH secondary to illicit drug use are unclear. BH may be related to:
* sudden rises in blood pressure
* drug-associated vasculitis. This has been diagnosed on the basis of a suggestive (though not specific) 'beaded' appearance on angiography, but has rarely been documented pathologically.

MACROSCOPIC AND MICROSCOPIC APPEARANCES

The macroscopic and microscopic features of drug-related BH are not unique. Many features resemble those of classic hypertensive bleeds. The diagnosis depends on knowledge of the clinical context in which the hemorrhage occurs.

BH SECONDARY TO NONVASCULAR PATHOLOGIES

All that bleeds in the brain is not vascular and both neoplasms and specific infections can present with BH. These include:
* oligodendrogliomas, glioblastomas, metastatic melanomas, and choriocarcinomas (**Fig. 10.58**). A metastatic neoplasm may present as BH before the primary neoplasm is evident.
* disseminated angioinvasive fungal infection (**Fig. 10.59**)

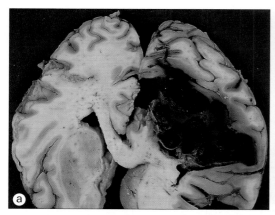

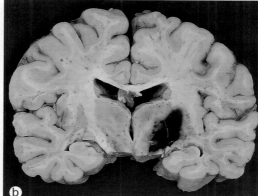

Fig. 10.57 BH associated with hepatic dysfunction. (a) Horizontal slice of fixed brain of a 42-year-old male with coagulopathy secondary to hepatitis C and after two orthotopic liver transplants. A large multiloculated BH fills the right parietal white matter and extends into the subarachnoid space. **(b)** Brain of a 59-year-old man with a history of macronodular cirrhosis, hepatocellular carcinoma, and hepatic necrosis after therapeutic hepatic embolization. A large hematoma extends into the right internal capsule, thalamus, and basal ganglia.

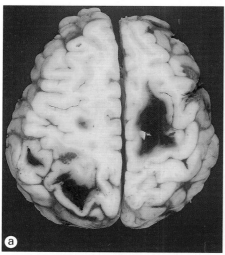

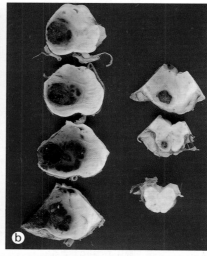

Fig. 10.58 Neoplasms 'masquerading' as BH.
(a) Horizontal sections through the brain of a patient with metastatic choriocarcinoma. The mechanism of hemorrhage was probably neoplastic emboli to the parenchymal and meningeal arteries with 'pseudoaneurysm' formation and rupture, though fragments of neoplasm were noted within the hematomas on microscopic section. **(b)** Large mesencephalic and pontine hematoma secondary to metastatic, clinically unsuspected, pulmonary carcinoma. The clinical diagnosis was of a brain stem vascular malformation. Only tiny fragments of neoplasm were present in serial blocks through the lesion. **(c)** Magnified view of one section in (b). Note the similarity to the hypertensive brain stem hematoma shown in Fig. 10.25. **(d)** Neoplasm in the pons that extends into the middle cerebellar peduncle in a patient who developed primary CNS B cell lymphoma after orthotopic liver transplant. The appearance resembles an organizing BH.

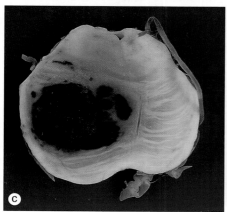

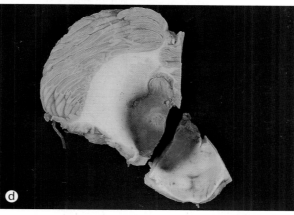

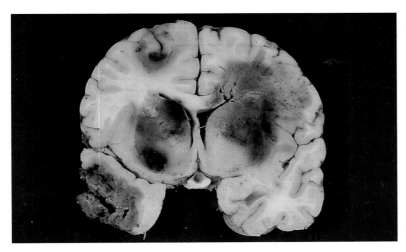

Fig. 10.59 Aspergillosis-induced BH. Coronal section of brain showing multiple intensely hemorrhagic regions of necrosis secondary to *Aspergillus* infection in a 12-year-old boy with acute lymphoblastic leukemia after a therapeutic bone marrow transplant. The surrounding brain substance shows green bile discoloration because the patient had hepatic veno-occlusive disease associated with graft-versus-host disease.

REFERENCES

Barnett HJM, Mohr JP, Stein BM, Yatsu FM (eds) (1992) *Stroke. Pathophysiology, Diagnosis, and Management. Second edition.* 1270 pp. New York: Churchill Livingstone.

Bennett M, O'Brien DP, Phillips JP, Farrell MA (1995) Clinicopathologic observations in 100 consecutive patients with fatal head injury admitted to a neurosurgical unit. *Irish Med J* **88**(2): 60–62.

Challa VR, Moody DM, Brown WR (1995) Vascular malformations of the central nervous system. *J Neuropathol Exp Neurol* **54**: 609–621.

Cole FM, Yates PO (1968) Comparative incidence of cerebrovascular lesions in normotensive and hypertensive patients. *Neurology* **18**: 255–259.

Crooks DA (1991) Pathogenesis and biomechanics of traumatic intracranial haemorrhages. *Virchows Archiv A Pathol Anat* **418**: 479–483.

Drapkin AJ (1991) Chronic subdural hematoma: pathophysiological basis for treatment. *Brit J Neurosurgery* **5**: 467–473.

Fisher CM (1971) Pathological observations in hypertensive cerebral hemorrhage. *J Neuropathol Exp Neurol* **30**: 536–550.

Fisher M (1994) *Clinical Atlas of Cerebrovascular Disorders.* London: Mosby–Wolfe.

Freytag E (1968) Fatal hypertensive intracerebral haematomas: a survey of the pathological anatomy of 393 cases. *J Neurol Neurosurg Psych* **31**: 616–620.

Hachinski V, Norris JW (1985) *The Acute Stroke.* 286 pp. Philadelphia: FA Davis.

Kassell NF, Sasaki T, Colohan ART, Nazar G (1985) Cerebral vasospasm following aneurysmal subarachnoid hemorrhage. *Stroke* **16**: 562–572.

Omae T, Ueda K, Ogata J, Yamaguchi T (1989) Parenchymatous hemorrhage: etiology, pathology and clinical aspects. In JF Toole (ed) *Handbook of Clinical Neurology, Vol. 10 (54): Vascular Diseases Part II.* pp. 287–331. New York: Elsevier.

Rinkel GJE, van Gijn J, Wijdicks EFM (1993) Subarachnoid hemorrhage without detectable aneurysm. A review of the causes. *Stroke* **24**: 1403–1409.

Shokunbi MT, Vinters HV, Kaufmann JCE (1988) Fusiform intracranial aneurysms. Clinicopathologic features. *Surg Neurol* **29**: 263–270.

Ueda K, Hasuo Y, Kiyohara Y, Wada J, Kawano H, Kato I *et al.* (1988) Intracerebral hemorrhage in a Japanese community, Hisayama: Incidence, changing pattern during long-term follow-up, and related factors. *Stroke* **19**: 48–52.

Vinters HV (1987) Cerebral amyloid angiopathy. A critical review. *Stroke* **18**: 311–324.

Vinters HV, Lundie MJ, Kaufmann JCE (1986) Long-term pathological follow-up of cerebral arteriovenous malformations treated by embolization with bucrylate. *N Engl J Med* **314**: 477–483.

Vinters HV, Wang ZZ, Secor DL (1996) Brain parenchymal and microvascular amyloid in Alzheimer's disease. *Brain Pathology* **6**: 179–195.

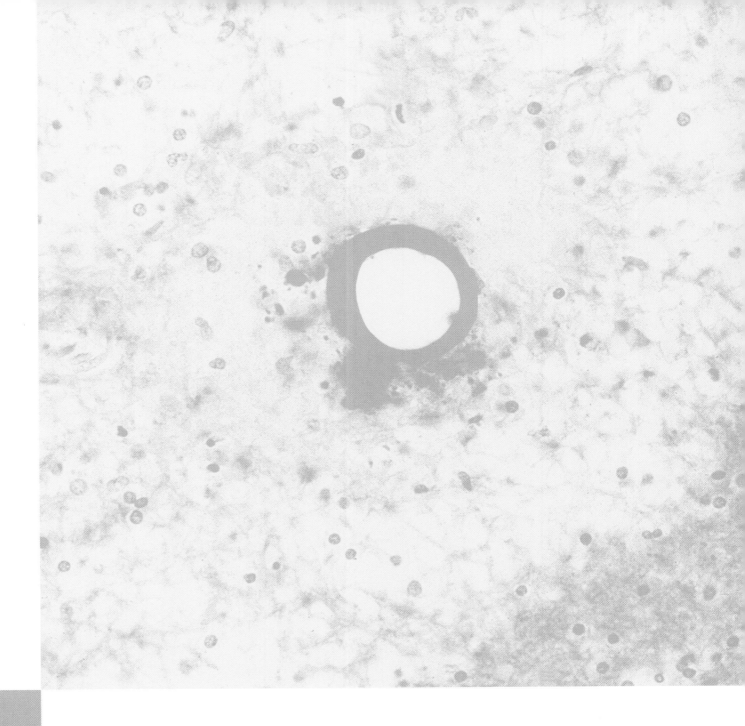

4 Trauma

11 Head and spinal injuries

HEAD INJURY

Head injury, whether accidental, criminal, or suicidal, is the leading cause of death in people under 45 years of age in developed countries. It accounts for 1% of all deaths, 30% of deaths from trauma, and 50% of deaths due to road traffic accidents.

The severity of head injury is often assessed using the Glasgow coma scale. This yields scores of 3 (the worst score) to 15 (the best score) based on an assessment of eye, verbal, and motor responses (**Fig. 11.1**).

In the USA, an estimated 700,000 individuals each year sustain severe head injury, and 150/100,000 of the population have a persisting handicap resulting from trauma-induced brain damage (i.e. approximately 450,000 individuals). Improvements in the acute management of trauma have led to an increase in the number of disabled survivors.

NATURE OF LESIONS IN HEAD INJURY
Type of head injury:
- Non-missile or blunt head injury, associated with acceleration or deceleration forces to the head that cause brain movement within the skull. This is the commonest pattern of head trauma seen clinically.
- Missile head injury results from penetration of the skull or brain by an external object such as a bullet.

Distribution of lesions:
The lesions can be subdivided according to their distribution as:
- Focal.
- Diffuse (**Fig. 11.2**)

Time course:
Brain damage following trauma can be viewed as occurring in two phases (**Fig 11.3**):
- Primary damage resulting from the immediate physical stresses involved (see next page).
- Secondary damage, initiated by the process of injury, but presenting later and mainly involving physiologic responses to trauma, hypoxia, and ischemia.

Progressive neurologic deterioration over many years has been noted in 15% of patients who have suffered severe head trauma (see p. 11.20).

Glasgow coma scale	
Best eye response (maximum = 4)	
1. No eye opening.	3. Eye opening to verbal command.
2. Eye opening to pain.	4. Eyes open spontaneously.
Best verbal response (maximum = 5)	
1. No verbal response.	4. Confused.
2. Incomprehensible sounds.	5. Oriented.
3. Inappropriate words.	
Best motor response (maximum = 6)	
1. No motor response.	4. Withdrawal from pain.
2. Extension to pain.	5. Localizing to pain.
3. Flexion to pain.	6. Obeys commands.

Coma Score	Clinical correlate
13 or above	Mild brain injury
9 - 12	Moderate injury
8 or less	Severe brain injury

Teasdale G., Jennett B., Lancet (ii) 81–83, 1974.

Fig. 11.1 The Glasgow coma scale.

HEAD INJURY

- May result in loss of consciousness (varying from momentary dazing to prolonged coma), mental confusion, amnesia, and a wide range of focal deficits.
- In general the longer the period of unconsciousness and the deeper the level of coma, the greater the likelihood that the patient has suffered brain damage and will have neurologic and neuropsychiatric sequelae.
- Most patients (60%) make a good recovery and have no residual deficits. The remainder suffer from a range of chronic problems ranging from brief periods of amnesia to personality changes, severe disabilities, a chronic degenerative disease process, or a vegetative state.
- Outcome surveys in the UK, USA, and the Netherlands indicate that for every 100 head injury survivors up to 5 remain in a vegetative state, up to 15 are still severely disabled 6 months after injury, 20 have minor psychiatric or psychologic problems, and 60 make a good recovery.

NON-MISSILE HEAD INJURY

MECHANISMS OF PRIMARY DAMAGE IN NON-MISSILE HEAD INJURY

Contact damage

Focal injuries may be sustained at or just deep to the point of impact of the head against an object or surface.

Acceleration or deceleration damage

Applying force to the head causes the skull to accelerate in a linear or rotational fashion. Due to inertia, the movement of the brain lags behind that of the skull and damage may result from the following mechanisms:

- Contact of the inner surface of the moving skull with the stationary brain may produce contusions, particularly in places where the skull protrudes internally. When the moving head is abruptly halted, the brain continues briefly to move due to its inertia. Impact of the moving brain against the stationary skull may again produce contusions.
- Traction on the bridging veins may cause them to tear, resulting in subdural hemorrhage.
- Differential movement and distortion of different parts of the brain produces shearing, traction, and compressive stresses, which may damage small parenchymal blood vessels, and cause diffuse injury to axons.

FOCAL DAMAGE

Focal lesions of the scalp

Laceration or bruising of the scalp is a common form of focal injury and a good indicator of the site of the trauma (**Fig. 11.4**).

Focal lesions of the skull

The presence of a skull fracture indicates that the head has been subjected to localized trauma of considerable force. It is very important that the dura is stripped as a routine procedure at necropsy examination after head injury otherwise fractures are easily missed. The type of fracture is partly dictated by the nature of the object that has made traumatic contact with the skull:

- Contact with a flat surface tends to produce closed fissure fractures, which often extend into the base of the skull.
- Contact with angled or pointed objects tends to produce localized fractures, which are often open and depressed (i.e. displaced inwards by at least the thickness of the skull).
- Contrecoup fractures (i.e. fractures located at a distance from the point of injury that are not direct extensions of the fracture originating at the point of injury) occur principally in the roofs of the orbits, and the ethmoid plates, following falls or other blunt impact involving the back of the skull.

The risk of intracranial hematoma is significantly increased in patients with skull fractures.

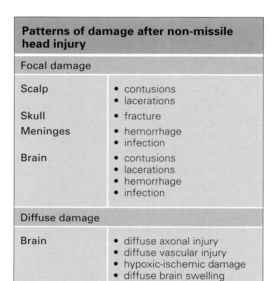

Patterns of damage after non-missile head injury	
Focal damage	
Scalp	• contusions • lacerations
Skull	• fracture
Meninges	• hemorrhage • infection
Brain	• contusions • lacerations • hemorrhage • infection
Diffuse damage	
Brain	• diffuse axonal injury • diffuse vascular injury • hypoxic-ischemic damage • diffuse brain swelling

Fig. 11.2 Patterns of damage after non-missile head injury.

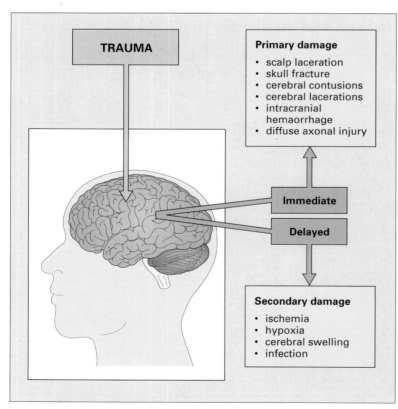

Fig. 11.3 Primary and secondary damage related to non-missile head injury.

TRAUMA

Primary damage
- scalp laceration
- skull fracture
- cerebral contusions
- cerebral lacerations
- intracranial hemaorrhage
- diffuse axonal injury

Immediate

Delayed

Secondary damage
- ischemia
- hypoxia
- cerebral swelling
- infection

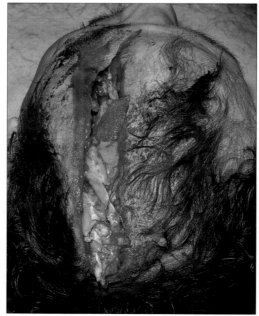

Fig. 11.4 Focal lesion to scalp. Deep scalp laceration associated with fracture of the skull and laceration of the brain in a patient who was struck on the head by a falling object. Lacerations can bleed copiously and are often the site, or route of entry, of subsequent infections.

Fractures of the base of the skull predispose to:

- Infection, as they often pass through the petrous temporal bone or the anterior cranial fossa and cause leakage of cerebrospinal fluid (CSF) through the ear, nose, or nasopharynx. These breaks in the integrity of the skull are also routes for the spread of infection.
- Aeroceles (trapping of air in the cranial cavity), which occur in up to 30% of patients with leakages of CSF and can cause raised intracranial pressure and displacement of the brain.

Depressed fractures may tear the dura and associated blood vessels leading to intracranial hemorrhage (see p. 11.4).

Focal lesions of the brain

Contusions and lacerations

Contusions are superficial bruises of the brain. Cerebral and, to a lesser extent, cerebellar contusions are frequent but not inevitable after head injury.

MACROSCOPIC APPEARANCES

Acutely, contusions appear as superficial hemorrhagic areas associated with some hemorrhage into the overlying leptomeninges and variable brain swelling (Figs 11.5, 11.6). Over subsequent days and weeks their color changes to brown or orange and as necrotic tissue is resorbed the involved gyri become indented or superficially cavitated. In brain slices, old contusions often have a triangular shape, with the point in the depths of the cortex or underlying white matter and a wide base at the surface of the crest of the gyrus (Fig. 11.7, see also Fig. 11.25). Contusions can be distinguished from foci of old ischemic damage, which are almost invariably more severe within the depths of sulci.

Contusions may occur in the region of impact (a form of contact damage), particularly if this causes fracturing, but also occur elsewhere over the brain in a stereotyped distribution that is much the same whatever the site of the original injury. The contusions occur on the crests of gyri that come into contact with protuberances within the skull

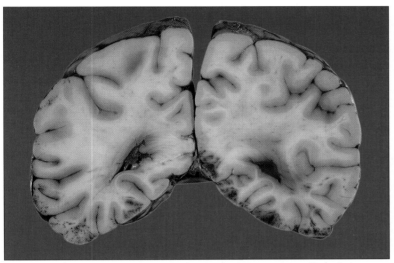

Fig. 11.5 Superficial contusions on the underside of the occipital lobes. The contusions in the left occipital lobe are superficial whereas those on the right are more hemorrhagic and involve the full thickness of the cortex.

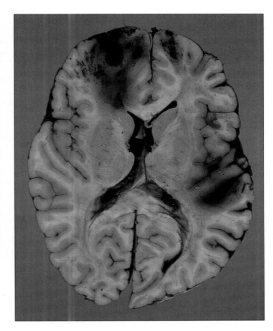

Fig. 11.6 Severe cerebral contusions. Severe frontal and temporal lobe contusions associated with extensive hemorrhage into the overlying subarachnoid space.

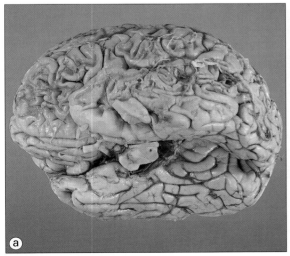
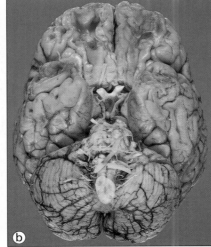
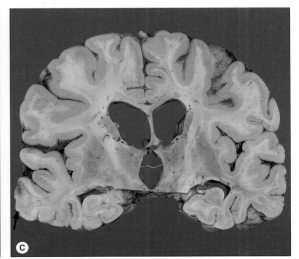

(a)   (b)   (c)

Fig. 11.7 Old cerebral contusions. (a) Old contusions over the lateral aspect of frontal, temporal and parietal lobes. These appear as as brown or orange-stained indentations on the crests of gyri. **(b)** Old contusions on inferior aspect of frontal lobes **(c)** Old wedge-shaped contusion of the left inferior temporal gyrus (arrow). There is also evidence of old diffuse axonal injury: the ventricles are dilated, the corpus callosum thinned and yellow, and the temporal and right parasagittal frontal white matter show gray discoloration.

(**Figs 11.8, 11.9**). Contusions are therefore located in the following regions:

- frontal poles
- orbital surface of the frontal lobes
- temporal poles
- lateral and inferior surfaces of the temporal lobes
- cortex adjacent to the sylvian fissures

Contusions may also occur in the cerebellar hemispheres (**Fig. 11.9e,f**).

Lacerations develop when the severity of trauma has been sufficient to cause tearing of the pia. This may occur in association with a depressed skull fracture. The most severe pattern of cerebral laceration is embraced by the term 'burst lobe'. This is often associated with a skull fracture and most commonly involves the frontal and temporal lobes, which show confluent intracerebral and subarachnoid bleeding associated with massive disruption of the affected lobe (**Fig. 11.10**).

MICROSCOPIC APPEARANCES

The appearance of contusions evolves with time through several stages:

- Initially the contusion is visible as microscopic regions of perivascular hemorrhage (**Fig. 11.11a**) following the track of small vessels in the cortex and usually running perpendicular to the cortical surface. The hemorrhage occurs within seconds or minutes of the injury.
- Over several hours blood continues to seep into the adjacent cortex, which shows local swelling and confluent hemorrhage. If the contu-

sion is severe there is extension into the underlying white matter. During this phase, neurons in the immediate vicinity begin to degenerate (**Fig. 11.11b,c**).

- If there is survival, the damaged area undergoes progressive organization characterized by activation and proliferation of astrocytes and microglia, infiltration of blood-derived phagocytes, and removal of necrotic material.
- What remains eventually is a superficial, roughly wedge-shaped, region of neuronal loss and glial scarring (**Fig. 11.12**). Hemosiderin pigment is found in scattered residual macrophages and astrocytes. The remaining neurons may become mineralized. The subjacent white matter is rarefied and gliotic.

Intracranial hemorrhages

Bleeding in and around the brain is a common feature of head injury. Intracranial hematomas may evolve over a period of time after the impact. The resulting brain swelling or compression is one of the most important forms of secondary brain damage and the commonest reason for deterioration and death in patients who are initially well after their injury.

Extradural hematoma occurs in approximately 10% of severe head injuries and up to 15% of fatal head injuries. It results from torn vessels in the meninges and is usually associated with a skull fracture in adults, but may occur without an associated skull fracture in children. The bleeding vessel is often the middle meningeal artery, which is torn as a result of a fracture of the squamous temporal bone.

Extradural hematomas are relatively localized and may accumulate slowly over a period of hours because of the adherence between the dura and the inner aspect of the calvaria. They are evident macroscopically on removal of the calvaria as a biconvex accumulation of clotted blood lying between the skull and the dura (**Fig. 11.13**).

Death due to an extradural hematoma is usually the result of cerebral compression and transtentorial herniation.

Subdural hematoma usually results from tearing of bridging veins that cross the subdural space, especially those related to the superior sagittal sinus. Blood from the ruptured vessels spreads freely through the subdural space and can envelope the entire hemisphere (**Fig. 11.14**).

Acute subdural hematomas generally consist of soft, recently clotted blood. With time, the firm blood clot of less acute subdural hematomas is broken down, so that only a few foci remain after about a month. A serous fluid tinged with blood pigments is characteristic of chronic hematomas, but repeated small, acute hemorrhages may produce a mixed picture.

Chronic subdural hematomas become surrounded by a 'membrane' of organizing granulation tissue. This is usually evident on the dural aspect of the hematoma within about 1 week, and later on its deep surface. Progressive enlargement of the hematoma may occur, mainly due to recurrent bleeding from friable blood vessels in the granulation tissue, although an osmotic effect of blood breakdown products may also contribute. Attempted dating of subdural hematomas by histologic examination of the 'membranes' has proven unreliable.

Traumatic subarachnoid hemorrhage There are several possible sources of subarachnoid bleeding after head injury:

- Subarachnoid blood may derive from severe contusions and lacerations (**Fig. 11.15**, see also Figs 11.6, 11.10).
- Fractures of the skull base can rupture large vessels at the base of the brain.
- Blood from intraventricular hemorrhage enters the subarachnoid

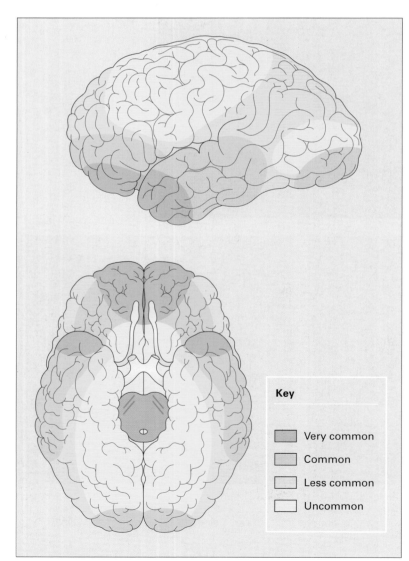

Key

■ Very common

■ Common

□ Less common

□ Uncommon

Fig. 11.8 Sites of predilection for cerebral contusions.

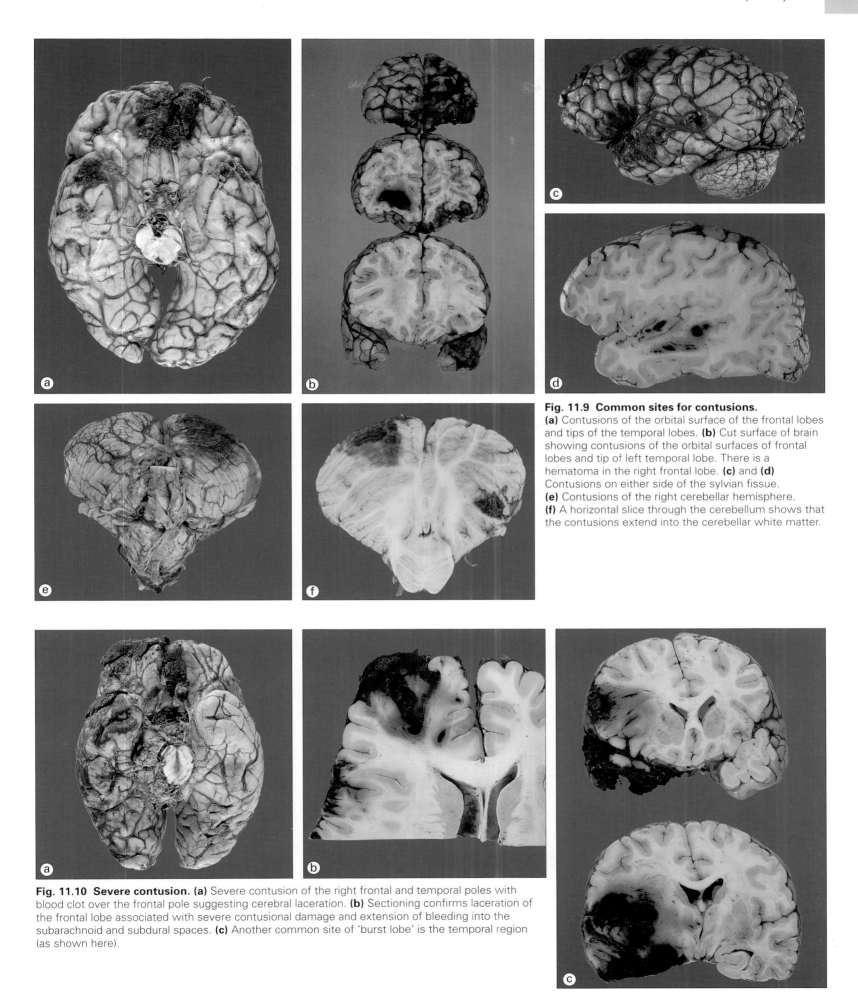

Fig. 11.9 Common sites for contusions.
(a) Contusions of the orbital surface of the frontal lobes and tips of the temporal lobes. **(b)** Cut surface of brain showing contusions of the orbital surfaces of frontal lobes and tip of left temporal lobe. There is a hematoma in the right frontal lobe. **(c)** and **(d)** Contusions on either side of the sylvian fissue.
(e) Contusions of the right cerebellar hemisphere.
(f) A horizontal slice through the cerebellum shows that the contusions extend into the cerebellar white matter.

Fig. 11.10 Severe contusion. (a) Severe contusion of the right frontal and temporal poles with blood clot over the frontal pole suggesting cerebral laceration. **(b)** Sectioning confirms laceration of the frontal lobe associated with severe contusional damage and extension of bleeding into the subarachnoid and subdural spaces. **(c)** Another common site of 'burst lobe' is the temporal region (as shown here).

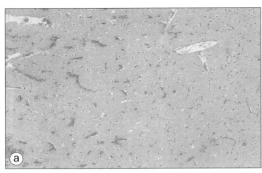 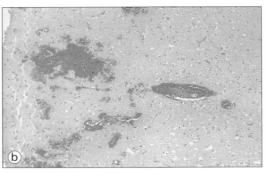 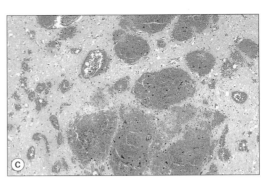

Fig. 11.11 Microscopic appearance of early contusions. (a) Early contusions showing small perivascular hemorrhages. **(b)** Early contusions showing extravasation of blood into the cortex associated with acute degeneration of the surrounding neurons. **(c)** Later evolution leads to more extensive perivascular hemorrhages in the cortex and superficial white matter.

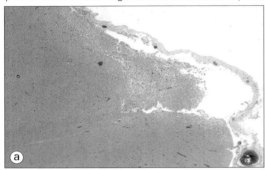 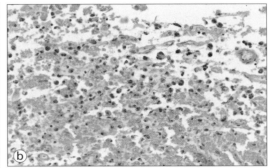

Fig. 11.12 Resolution of contusions. (a) At low magnification resolving contusions are seen as wedge-shaped superficial lesions. **(b)** Higher magnification shows the resolving contusion to contain numerous hemosiderin-laden macrophages.

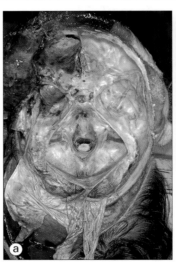 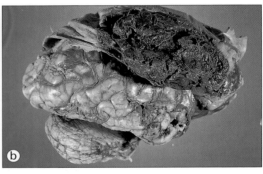

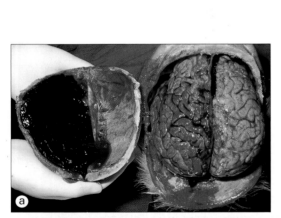

Fig. 11.13 Extradural hematoma. (a) Fracture of the left squamous temporal bone with an associated extradural hematoma. Extradural blood is visible through the dura in the left middle and anterior cranial fossae. **(b)** Extradural hematoma overlying right fronto-parietal dura. (Courtesy of Professor Michael A. Farrell, Dublin, Ireland)

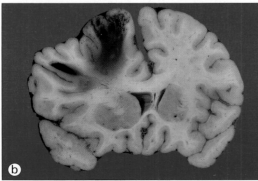 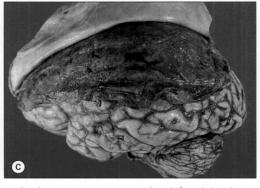 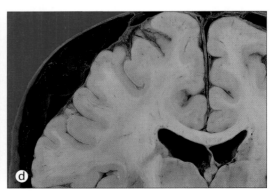

Fig. 11.14 Subdural hematoma. (a) Removal of the calvarium at necropsy reveals a left subdural hematoma that has compressed the underlying brain. The arachnoid surface of the left cerebral hemisphere is blood-stained and the gyri are flattened. **(b)** Indentation of the left cerebral hemisphere due to a subdural hematoma. Note the contusion, hemorrhage, and focal infarction in the underlying brain tissue. **(c)** Chronic subdural hematoma enclosed in a thin 'membrane' of granulation tissue. Although the hematoma was known to be more than 2 weeks old, it consisted of clotted blood. **(d)** Subdural hematoma showing compression of brain.

space through the exit foramina of the fourth ventricle.
In trauma associated with subarachnoid bleeding a careful search should be made for cerebral arterial aneurysms since these may have important medicolegal implications.

A late consequence of traumatic subarachnoid hemorrhage is the development of hydrocephalus due to obstruction of CSF drainage pathways.

Cerebral and cerebellar hematomas   Superficial lobar hematomas are generally related to overlying contusional damage and are mainly seen in the frontal and temporal lobes (**Fig. 11.16**). They also occur in association with contusions in the cerebellum (**Fig. 11.17**). Deep hematomas tend to be related to the basal ganglia and thalamus (**Fig. 11.18**, see also Fig. 11.24a) and are often associated with coexisting diffuse axonal injury.

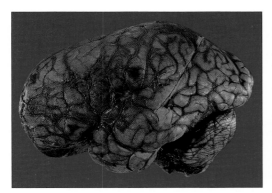

Fig. 11.15 Traumatic subarachnoid hemorrhage. Blood is present over the cerebral convexity and in the sylvian fissure.

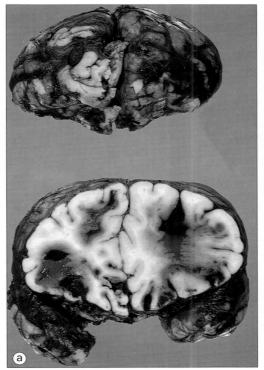

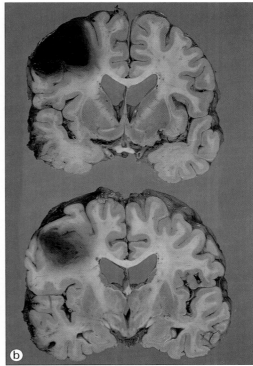

Fig. 11.16 Cerebral hematomas. (a) Hematomas in the white matter of the frontal lobe associated with severe contusions. **(b)** Superficial lobar hematoma in the posterior frontal region. The hematoma was related to a cortical laceration associated with a depressed skull fracture.

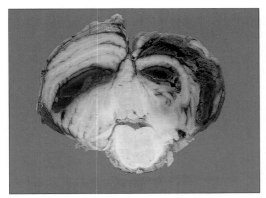

Fig. 11.17 Cerebellar hematoma. Hematomas in the cerebellum are usually associated with severe contusional damage to the cerebellar hemispheres, which is often related to a skull fracture in the posterior fossa.

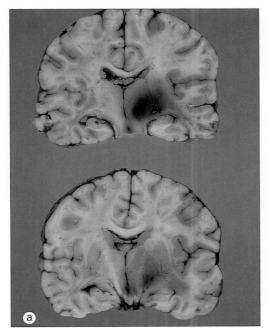

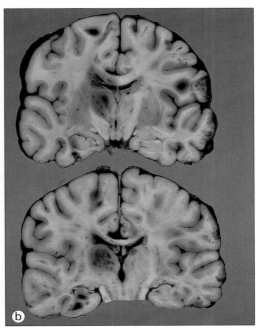

Fig. 11.18 Hematomas of the basal ganglia and thalamus. (a) Traumatic hematoma in the right basal ganglia associated with mass effect and compression of the ventricular system. The appearance resembles that of a primary intracerebral bleed. Histologic examination revealed diffuse axonal injury in a wide distribution. **(b)** A cluster of hematomas in the left thalamus caused by head injury. There is other damage in the form of cortical contusions, and a small hematoma in the hippocampus. A hemorrhagic lesion in the corpus callosum is indicative of diffuse axonal injury.

Traumatic hematomas may develop several days after the injury. In some cases, a parenchymal hematoma develops following evacuation of an extradural or subdural hematoma, and probably reflects reperfusion of brain tissue that has sustained ischemic injury as a result of the compression.

DISTINGUISHING PRIMARY AND TRAUMATIC INTRACEREBRAL HEMATOMAS

- Distinguishing a primary intracerebral hematoma from one secondary to head injury is occasionally of medicolegal importance, usually in relation to motor vehicle collisions.
- It is often impossible to resolve whether a deep hematoma in the basal ganglia is a primary event leading to an accident or developed as a result of the accident.
- Assessment of the extent of diffuse axonal injury and associated vascular pathology may be helpful. If there is evidence of associated diffuse axonal damage in the brain and an absence of other vascular pathology it is likely that the deep hematoma is caused by trauma. If there is hyaline arteriolosclerosis in the basal ganglia regions and an absence of features of diffuse axonal injury, it is likely that the deep hematoma is a primary event.

Uncommon types of focal brain damage

Uncommon types of focal brain damage include:
- Ischemic brain damage due to traumatic dissection and thrombosis resulting from stretching of the vertebral or carotid arteries by hyperextension of the neck (**Fig. 11.19**).
- Infarction of the pituitary gland due to traumatic transection of the pituitary stalk.
- A pontomedullary rent resulting from severe injury associated with hyperextension of the neck (**Fig. 11.20**).

- Cranial nerve avulsion (most commonly the olfactory nerve fibres, the optic nerve, the facial nerve, and the auditory nerve).

INFECTION

Infection is predominantly a complication of skull fractures:
- Fractures of the calvarium or skull base can provide a route for bacteria to pass from the major air sinuses into the subarachnoid space and cause meningitis. Such fractures are often associated with a leakage of CSF or the formation of an aerocele.
- Open head injuries predispose to the development of brain abscesses, particularly if the brain is lacerated or sustains a missile injury.

The incidence of brain abscesses is, however, increased even after closed head injuries, presumably because the devitalized tissues are prone to colonization in the event of a transient bacteremia (see chapter 15).

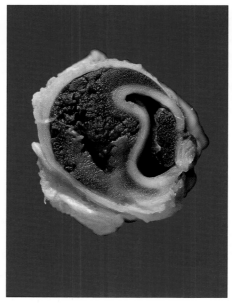

Fig. 11.19 Traumatic arterial dissection. Traumatic dissection and associated thrombosis of the vertebral artery in a patient who developed brain stem infarction after head injury.

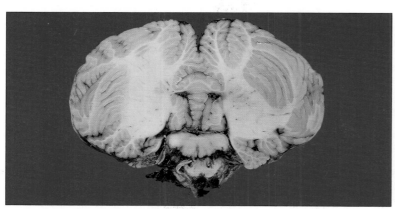

Fig. 11.20 A pontomedullary rent. Tearing of the brain stem at the junction between the upper medulla and lower pons has produced a hemorrhagic lesion termed a pontomedullary rent. In this case the injury resulted from a high-speed motor cycle collision in which the patient suffered a hyperextension injury to the neck. At necropsy there was a large quantity of subarachnoid blood in the posterior fossa, but no clear site of origin of the hemorrhage. Once the brain had been fixed and sliced it became clear that the site of bleeding had been this injury to the brain stem.

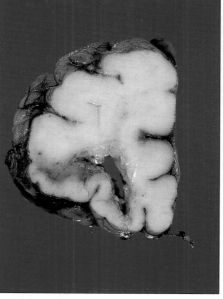

Fig. 11.21 Contusional tear in the frontal lobe of an infant aged 2 months who had a sustained non-accidental shaking injury. This distinctive pattern of damage is due to differential movement of the cerebral cortex and white matter and may be related to the poor myelination of the white matter at this age. Non-hemorrhagic contusional tears are difficult to see and may be misinterpreted as artefacts produced during removal of the brain. Histologic examination is needed to resolve this: a vital reaction is seen even in recent contusional tears and is characterized by swelling of astrocytes and, later, infiltration by macrophages.

NON-ACCIDENTAL INJURIES IN CHILDREN

- Non-accidental injuries in children are associated with distinct patterns of head injury.
- There may be impact damage, with focal lesions of the scalp and skull.
- Even in the absence of impact damage, vigorous shaking of the child can cause:
  - subdural hematomas, which are often bilateral.
  - cerebral contusions
  - retinal hemorrhage
  - diffuse axonal injury
  - intracerebral hemorrhage
  - diffuse brain swelling with secondary ischemic injury

In early childhood shaking or impact damage can produce a characteristic lesion called a **contusional tear**, which is characterized by separation of the cortex from the underlying white matter forming a small slit-like tear (**Fig. 11.21**). This may become hemorrhagic or be associated with localized swelling. Non-hemorrhagic lesions are very hard to see macroscopically, but can be found on histologic examination, which reveals the axonal tearing and local glial reaction.

DIFFUSE DAMAGE

DIFFUSE AXONAL INJURY (DAI)

DAI is the term given to the widespread damage to axons within the CNS that results from severe acceleration or deceleration of the head. Patients who have sustained severe DAI are typically unconscious from the moment of impact, do not experience a lucid interval, and remain unconscious, vegetative, or at least severely disabled until death. Lesser degrees of DAI are compatible with recovery of consciousness, with persisting neurologic deficits of varying severity.

MACROSCOPIC APPEARANCES

DAI can be diagnosed only by histologic examination, but there are macroscopic abnormalities from which the presence of DAI can be inferred including:

- Focal lesions in the corpus callosum, which appear as clusters of petechial hemorrhages or soft hemorrhagic foci (**Fig. 11.22**). The lesions may disrupt the interventricular septum, in which case there is often associated intraventricular hemorrhage.
- Focal lesions in the dorsolateral quadrants of the rostral brain stem. Small lesions appear as discrete foci of petechial hemorrhage in and adjacent to the superior cerebellar peduncles. More severe damage results in hemorrhagic softening of the dorsal part of the midbrain and rostral pons (**Fig. 11.23**).

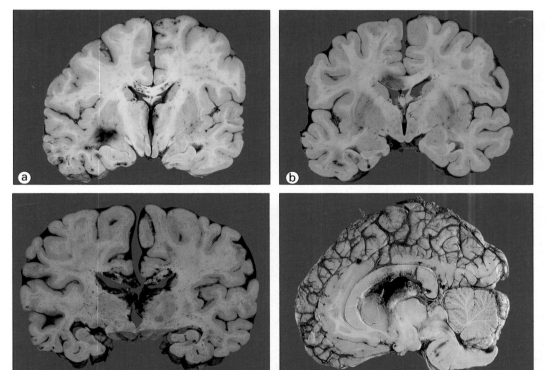

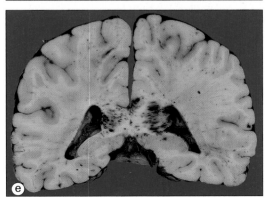

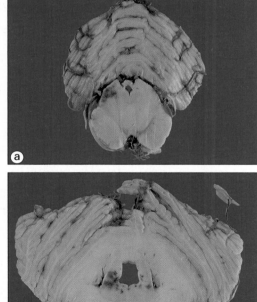

Fig. 11.22 Lesions in the corpus callosum in DAI. These may vary from small petechiae to larger foci of hemorrhagic discoloration and softening and extensive hemorrhagic disruption. **(a)** Small petechiae. **(b)** Larger focus of hemorrhagic discoloration and softening. **(c)** Extensive hemorrhagic disruption. **(d)** In the sagittal plane lesions typically involve the corpus callosum for several centimetres along its length. **(e)** The lesions may occur anywhere along the corpus callosum, but there is a tendency for them to be concentrated in the splenium

Fig. 11.23 Brain stem lesions associated with DAI. These consist of clusters of petechial hemorrhages or foci of hemorrhagic softening in the dorsolateral part of the midbrain and dorsolateral part of the rostral pons. **(a)** The right dorsolateral part of the midbrain contains petechiae. **(b)** The dorsolateral part of the rostral pons shows petechiae bilaterally.

• 'Gliding contusions,' which are hemorrhagic lesions affecting the parasagittal white matter in the superior part of the cerebral hemispheres. Small lesions occur close to the junction between the white matter and the overlying cortex, but larger lesions curve downwards through the parasagittal white matter towards the corpus callosum (**Fig. 11.24**). Gliding contusions are often bilateral, but typically are not symmetric.

The brains of long-term survivors of DAI typically show moderate to marked cerebral atrophy with dilatation of the lateral and third ventricles, thinning of the corpus callosum (sometimes marked), ill-defined gray discoloration of the cerebral white matter, and, in some cases, atrophy of the cerebral peduncles, base of the pons, and medullary pyramids (**Fig. 11.25**). In the absence of other injuries such as cerebral contusions the cortical ribbon usually appears normal.

MICROSCOPIC APPEARANCES

Histology is needed to substantiate the diffuse damage to axons. The main regions affected are:

• superior parasagittal cerebral white matter
• corpus callosum

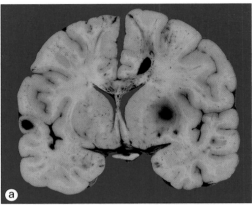
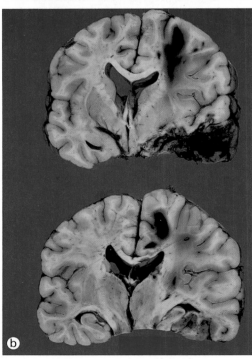

Fig. 11.24 Gliding contusions.
(a) Bilateral gliding contusions in the parasagittal white matter. The one on the left is no more than a perivascular streak of hemorrhagic white matter discoloration. The one on the right includes several hemorrhagic foci and a larger hematoma. There are also typical DAI-related lesions in the corpus callosum, contusions over both unci, and several other hematomas, including one in the right putamen. **(b)** Large lesions extending through the parasagittal white matter towards the corpus callosum. In this case there is also severe contusion of the temporal lobe and petechial hemorrhages are present in the corpus callosum in the lower slice.

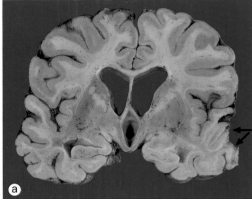
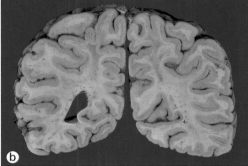
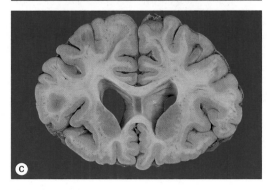

Fig. 11.25 Long-term effects of DAI.
(a) Old trauma with contusions of the right middle and superior temporal gyri (arrows) and ventricular dilatation. Note the ill-defined gray discoloration of the white matter due to DAI. This is most marked in the temporal lobes (including the non-contused left temporal lobe), but also involves the corpus callosum and internal capsule.
(b) Gray discoloration of the parasagittal white matter in the posterior part of the parietal lobes. **(c)** The gray-brown streaks in the parasagittal white matter in this brain are due to previous gliding contusions.

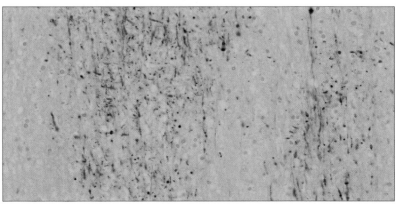

Fig. 11.26 Clusters of axons with abnormal accumulation of APP early after head injury. A few axons show focal swelling, but this is still mild and many of the axons appear to be intact.

- subcortical fiber tracts (fornix, internal and external capsules)
- superior cerebellar peduncles
- brain stem (corticospinal tracts, medial lemnisci, medial longitudinal bundles, central tegmental tracts)

The time course of histologic changes is as follows:

- Within 4–5 hours there are focal axonal accumulations of β-amyloid precursor protein (APP) and other anterogradely transported proteins. These can be identified immunohistochemically at a time when conventional tinctorial stains do not show definite abnormalities (**Fig. 11.26**).

- By 12–24 hours axonal varicosities may be evident on conventional histologic examination (**Fig. 11.27**).
- From 24 hours to 2 months after the injury conventional histology reveals axonal swellings. These are eosinophilic (**Fig. 11. 28a,c**), but are best demonstrated by silver impregnation techniques (**Fig. 11.28b,d**). Axonal swellings can also be detected by immunohistochemistry for ubiquitin, APP, or neurofilament protein, but these are less sensitive at later times.

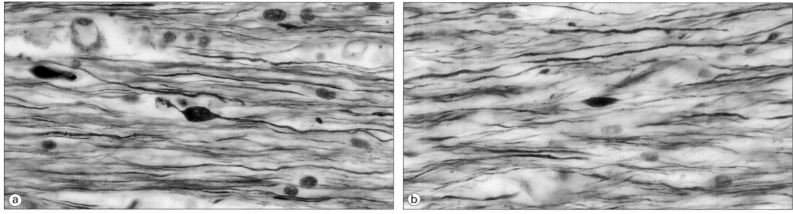

Fig. 11.27 Microscopic changes 12–24 hours after head injury with DAI. (a) and **(b)** Silver impregnation may reveal axonal varicosities, as shown in these illustrations.

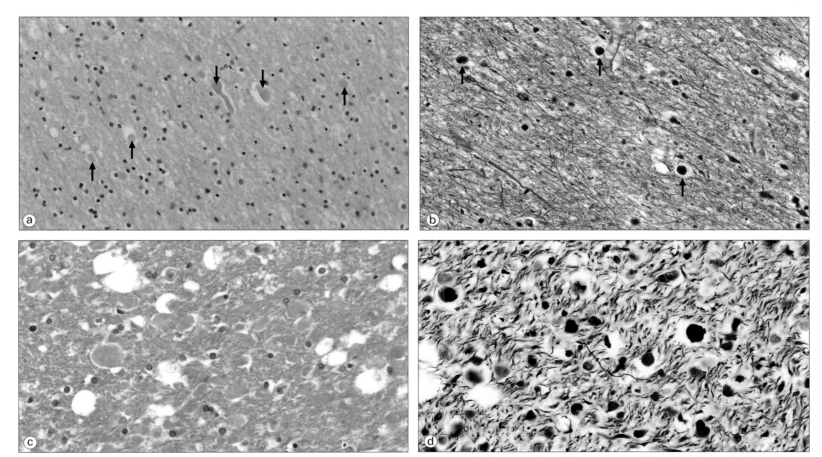

Fig. 11.28 Microscopic changes after head injury with DAI. In sections stained with hematoxylin and eosin, the axonal swellings are generally small and inconspicuous, but they are well visualized by silver impregnation. **(a)** Hematoxylin and eosin section. The axonal swellings (arrows) are small and inconspicuous. **(b)** Silver impregnation highlights the axonal swellings (arrows). **(c)** The axonal swellings may be obvious in a hematoxylin and eosin section in severe DAI, particularly if the patient survives for several days as here. **(d)** Palmgren silver impregnation of section adjacent to (c) showing large axonal swellings.

- Two weeks to 5 months after the injury clusters of microglia are seen in the affected regions (**Fig. 11.29**).

- From 2 months to years after the injury wallerian degeneration leads to loss of myelinated fibers (**Fig. 11.30**).
  Grading of DAI is shown in **Fig. 11.31**.

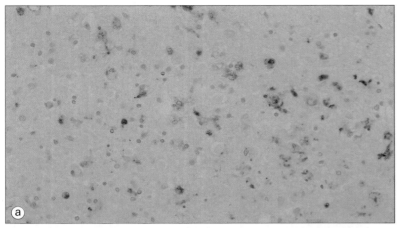

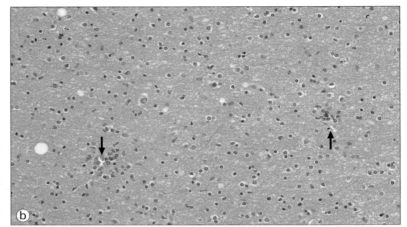

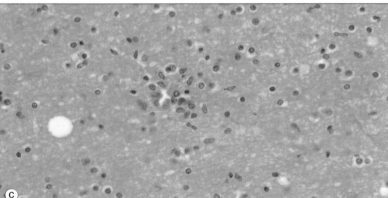

Fig. 11.29 Clustering of microglial cells after head injury with DAI. From about 2 weeks after the injury and persisting for many months, the white matter contains numerous clusters of microglial cells. **(a)** Macrophages can be identified within regions of DAI within 3 or 4 days. (CD68 immunostain) **(b)** Clustering of cells, seen at low magnification (arrows). This is particularly well demonstrated in thick sections cut at 20 μm, as here. **(c)** At higher magnification, the clusters are seen to consist of microglia.

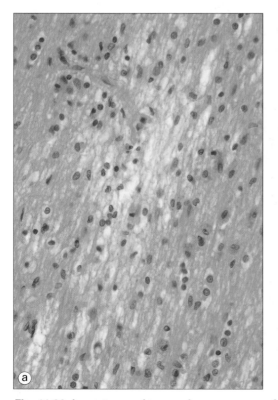
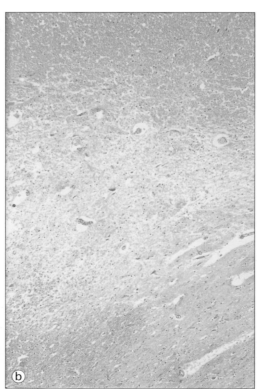
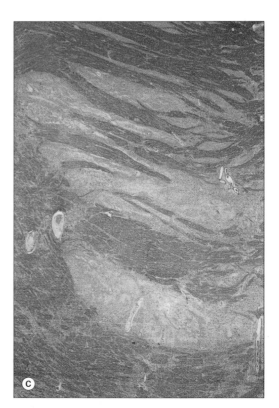

Fig. 11.30 Long-term microscopic appearance of head injury with DAI. (a) Focal glial scarring in a long-term survivor of head injury with DAI. **(b)** Focal rarefaction of the white matter in a long-term survivor of head injury with DAI. **(c)** Patchy depletion of corticospinal fibers in the pons of a patient who survived several months with severe DAI. (Solochrome cyanin)

PATHOGENESIS OF DAI

- Clinical and experimental studies suggest that there are two mechanisms of diffuse axonal injury (**Fig. 11.32**): primary axotomy, which is is almost immediate and secondary axotomy, which occurs over a period of hours after the injury.
- The importance of the concept of secondary axotomy as a mechanism of diffuse axonal damage is that it implies that strategies for neuroprotection and preventing secondary ischemic damage may lead to improved survival of axons.

Primary axotomy

- Large axolemmal tears allow an influx of calcium, activation of calcium-activated proteases, severe cytoskeletal disruption at the site of the tear, and rapid disconnection of the distal axon.
- Axoplasmic transport results in an accumulation of material proximal to the discontinuity and ballooning of the truncated axon.

Secondary axotomy

- Calcium-activated proteases focally damage the axonal cytoskeleton, but immediate axonal disconnection does not ensue, possibly because the resulting small membrane tears are resealed.
- Failure of cellular repair mechanisms or secondary neuronal damage, possibly ischemic, results in disconnection of the distal axonal segment.
- Axoplasmic transport continues and results in accumulation of material proximal to the damaged segment with localized axonal swelling.

Grading of DAI

	Axonal damage	Lesions in corpus callosum	Lesions in brain stem
Grade 1	Present	Absent	Absent
Grade 2	Present	Present	Absent
Grade 3	Present	Present	Present

Fig. 11.31 Grading of DAI. (Adams JH *et al.* (1989) Diffuse axonal injury in head injury: definitions, diagnosis and grading. *Histopathology* **15**: 49–59.

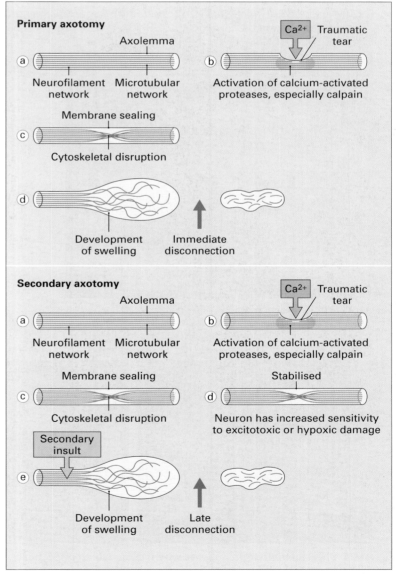

Fig. 11.32 Pathogenesis of DAI. See basic science box above for explanation.

DIFFUSE VASCULAR INJURY

In a small proportion of patients who die within minutes after head injury, the only discernible structural abnormalities are petechial hemorrhages in the white matter of the frontal and temporal lobes, thalamus, and brain stem (**Fig. 11.33**). This diffuse vascular damage probably results from traction and shearing of parenchymal blood vessels due to differential movement and distortion of different parts of the brain during severe acceleration or deceleration of the head. All parts of the vascular system seem to be affected and hemorrhages may occur around arteries, veins, and capillaries.

DIFFUSE VASCULAR INJURY AND FAT EMBOLISM

- Diffuse vascular injury should be distinguished from CNS fat embolism, which is probably underdiagnosed in patients with head injury and usually manifests clinically with dyspnea, hypoxia and confusion only 2–3 days after trauma, but can present earlier if severe.
- Most patients with fat embolism will have sustained multiple injuries, including long bone fractures, and will have radiologic and pathologic evidence of pulmonary fat emboli (which can be demonstrated in touch preparations of fresh lung tissue), although fat embolism can also occur in other clinical contexts (see Chapter 10).

Macroscopic features of fat embolism

- If death occurs within two days the brain may appear macroscopically normal.
- After survival of three or four days the brain contains numerous petechial hemorrhages and small perivascular foci of gray discoloration (**Fig. 11.34**). At later periods, these appear as scattered small foci of necrosis. The lesions are most prominent in the cerebral white matter, but may also involve the cerebral and cerebellar cortex, deep gray nuclei, and brain stem.

Microscopic features of fat embolism

- Histology reveals scattered capillaries surrounded by small ring or ball hemorrhages (**Fig. 11.35**).
- Some of the capillaries show fibrinoid necrosis.
- The brain tissue immediately adjacent to the affected capillaries is usually edematous with fragmented axons, or frankly infarcted.
- Lipid globules are demonstrable within the necrotic capillaries by appropriate staining of frozen sections. The lipid persists for several days.
- Later there is infiltration by macrophages and glial scarring.

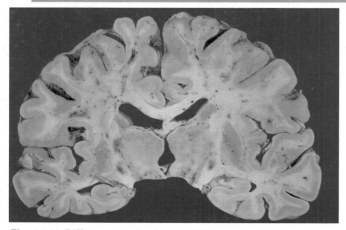

Fig. 11.33 Diffuse vascular injury. Diffuse vascular injury has produced numerous petechial hemorrhages in this brain from a patient who died within minutes after severe head injury.

BRAIN SWELLING AND RAISED INTRACRANIAL PRESSURE

Brain swelling and herniation are common forms of secondary brain damage after head injury. Brain swelling occurs in about 75% of patients and is a major factor (along with hemorrhages) contributing to an increase in intracranial pressure. It is thought to result from:

- cerebral vasodilatation and an increase in cerebral blood volume (i.e. congestive brain swelling)
- damage to blood vessels and extravasation of edema fluid through the defective blood–brain barrier (i.e. vasogenic edema)
- an increase in the water content of neurons and glia (i.e. cytotoxic cerebral edema)

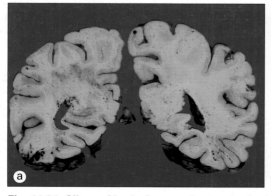
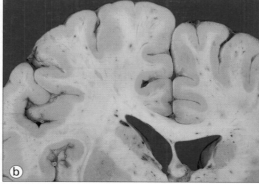
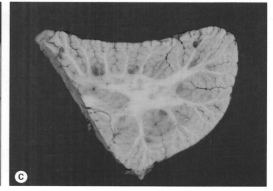

Fig. 11.34 Slices of brain from patients who had sustained direct head injury but also developed fat embolism. The lesions may appear as petechial hemorrhages or small perivascular foci of grey discoloration. Both gray and white matter are usually involved, although lesions in the white matter are easier to see on macroscopic examination. **(a)** Petechial hemorrhages and foci of gray discoloration in the white matter of the occipital lobes. **(b)** Perivascular foci of gray discoloration in the frontal lobe. **(c)** Petechial hemorrhages and foci of gray discoloration in the cortex and white matter of the cerebellum.

Three patterns of brain swelling are encountered in patients who have sustained a head injury:

- Swelling adjacent to contusions. Physical disruption of blood vessels in the surrounding brain tissue results in increased capillary permeability and a loss of normal blood flow regulation at the arteriolar level.
- Diffuse swelling of one cerebral hemisphere. This is especially common after evacuation of an ipsilateral subdural hematoma (**Fig. 11.36**),

which may also be followed by delayed intracerebral hemorrhage, probably due to reperfusion of infarcted tissue.

- Diffuse swelling of both cerebral hemispheres. This is seen mainly in children and adolescents (**Fig. 11.37**) and is thought to result from a global increase in brain blood volume. It is associated with epileptic activity and status epilepticus.

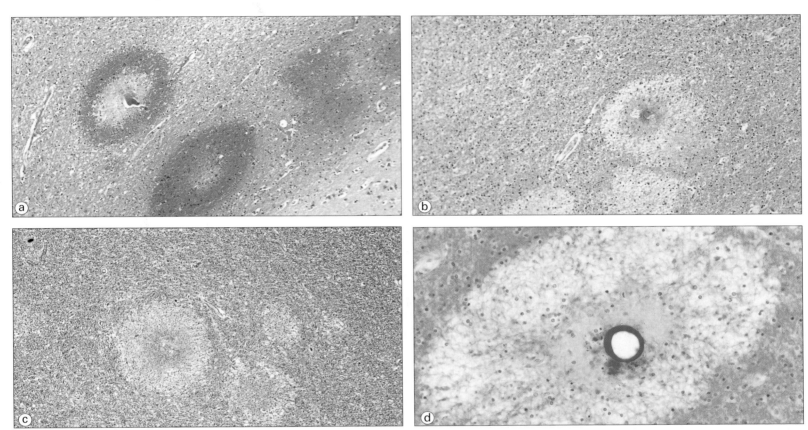

Fig. 11.35 Microscopic features of fat embolism. (a) Hemorrhagic lesions due to fat embolism, some of which are obviously centered on capillaries showing fibrinoid necrosis. **(b)** Non-hemorrhagic lesions, some of which are also centered on capillaries showing fibrinoid necrosis. **(c)** Silver impregnation reveals fragmentation of axons immediately adjacent to the necrotic capillaries. **(d)** In a frozen section lipid globules can be demonstrated in and around the necrotic foci by oil red O staining.

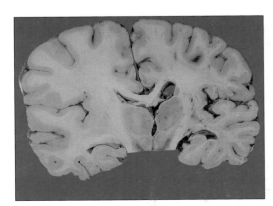
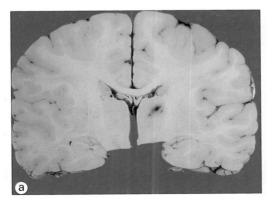
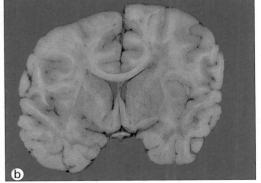

Fig. 11.36 Diffuse swelling of one cerebral hemisphere. Swelling of the left cerebral hemisphere after evacuation of an ipsilateral subdural hematoma.

Fig. 11.37 Diffuse brain swelling. (a) Diffuse brain swelling after head injury. There is a small hematoma in the thalamus. **(b)** Diffuse brain swelling in a child due to non-accidental head injury.

Herniation

The cranial cavity is subdivided by the relatively rigid tentorium and falx cerebri into three compartments with limited capacity to accommodate accumulations of blood or swelling due to edema without an increase in pressure. Differences in pressure between two adjacent intracranial compartments, or between an intracranial compartment and the spinal canal cause displacement of the soft substance of the brain into the lower pressure compartment (i.e. internal herniation). There are three sites where this tends to occur, resulting in subfalcine, tentorial, or tonsillar herniation (**Figs 11.38–11.41**). Raized intracranial pressure can also lead to external herniation of brain tissue through a skull fracture or craniotomy.

Internal herniation may result in compression or stretching of blood vessels, leading to secondary ischemic damage (**Figs 11.42, 11.43**). It is important to recognize the secondary nature of these lesions and not attribute the bleeding to primary pontine hemorrhage. Compression of the oculomotor nerves by downwards displacement of the posterior cerebral arteries can cause focal nerve contusion.

Focal contusion or hemorrhagic infarction of the hippocampus or parahippocampal gyrus may result from compression of these structures against the edge of the tentorium during trans-tentorial herniation (**Figs**

RAISED INTRACRANIAL PRESSURE

Brain damage may occur when the pressure begins to exceed the upper range of normal for minutes at a time.
- Mild increases to 15–22 mm Hg are reasonably well tolerated.
- Moderate increases to 30 mm Hg require intervention.
- Severe increases above 37.5 mm Hg are associated with ischemic brain damage.
- Pressures over 60 mm Hg often indicate a terminal state.
- If intracranial pressure equals arterial pressure, cerebral blood flow and all neurologic function cease.

11.39, 11.40). Similar damage may result from subfalcine herniation of the cingulate gyrus (see Fig. 11.40). Trans-tentorial herniation also produces distortion of the midbrain and compression of the cerebral peduncles (**Fig. 11.44**). In many cases this causes necrosis of the contralateral cerebral peduncle due to its compression against the edge of the tentorium or of the ipsilateral cerebral peduncle due to its compression by the herniated uncus.

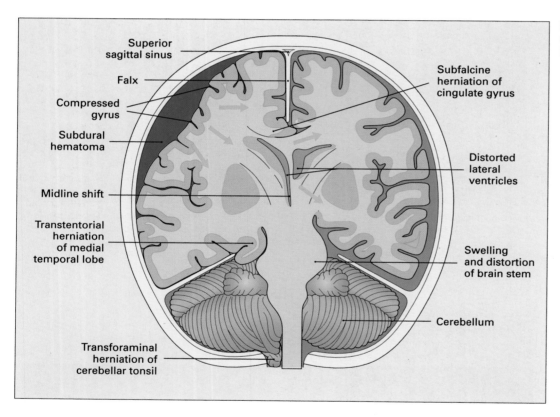

Fig. 11.38 Internal brain herniation. Space occupancy by an expanding lesion causes herniation at several sites.

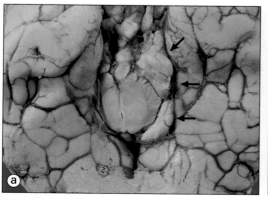
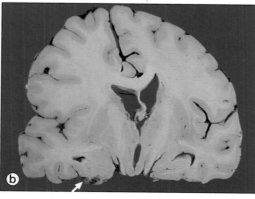

Fig. 11.39 Trans-tentorial herniation. (a) Herniation of the parahippocampal gyrus through the tentorial hiatus. The free edge of the tentorium cerebelli has indented the cerebrum (arrows) along the margin of the herniated brain tissue. **(b)** Herniation contusions (arrow) may be visible where the uncus or parahippocampal gyrus has been pressed against the edge of the tentorium, in this case by a subdural hematoma (not visible in figure). Histologic examination of the contusions reveals focal necrosis and small hemorrhages. The subdural hematoma has also displaced midline structures and caused subfalcine herniation of the cingulate gyrus (arrowhead).

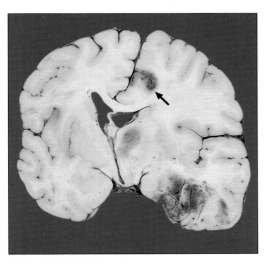

Fig. 11.40 Cerebral herniation. In this case contusional damage and hemispheric swelling have caused subfalcine herniation of the right cingulate gyrus. This has resulted in adjacent hemorrhagic infarction (arrow). Note also the shift of midline structures and herniation of the uncus.

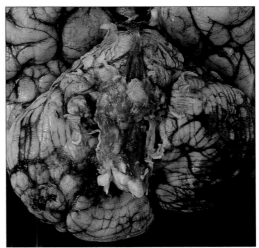

Fig. 11.41 Tonsillar herniation and necrosis. In this case head injury has resulted in severe tonsillar herniation and necrosis. The medulla is partly ensheathed by the necrotic tonsillar tissue.

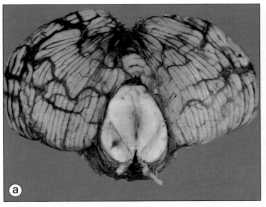

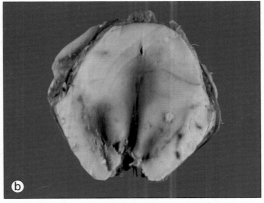

Fig. 11.42 Effects of internal herniation. With severe persisting herniation there is downwards displacement of diencephalic structures and descent of the pons, resulting in anteroposterior kinking or buckling of the brain stem with traction on the extramedullary segments of penetrating arteries and compression of their intramedullary segments. This results in foci of necrosis, and hemorrhages termed Duret hemorrhages, in the midbrain and upper pons. **(a)** Small Duret hemorrhage appearing as a linear area of midline hemorrhage. **(b)** A more severe lesion associated with hemorrhage in the midline and substantia nigra. **(c)** Duret hemorrhages appearing as extensive foci of hemorrhagic necrosis. **(d)** Marked hemorrhage and necrosis in the pons. **(e)** and **(f)** Sagittal sections, which demonstrate the buckling of the upper brain stem and the distribution of hemorrhagic lesions. (e) Early Duret hemorrhages. (f) Later, more extensive Duret hemorrhages. **(g)** Although internal herniation and brain stem hemorrhage are usually terminal events, rarely survival is long term, in which case the lesions in the midbrain and pons undergo organisation and appear as soft cystic areas of cavitation.

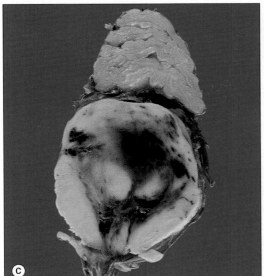

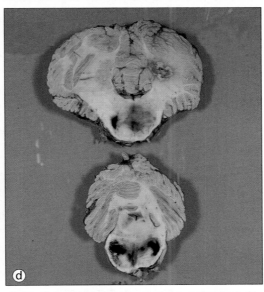

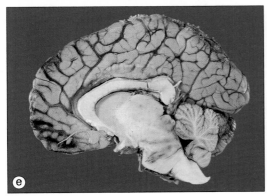

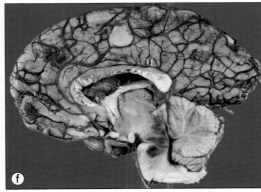

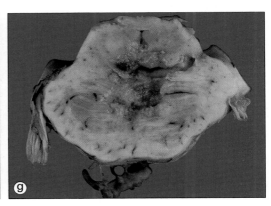

ISCHEMIC DAMAGE

Infarction and widespread hypoxic–ischemic brain damage are common after head trauma. Hypoxic–ischemic damage is likely in patients who have had:

- clinically evident hypoxia
- hypotension with a systolic blood pressure less than 80 mm Hg for at least 15 minutes
- episodes of raised intracranial pressure (i.e. over 30 mm Hg)

Evidence of hypoxic–ischemic damage may be confined to the hippocampus (**Fig. 11.45**) or associated with more widespread changes in the cerebral cortex (**Fig. 11.46**) and deep gray matter. Cortical damage is often accentuated in the border zones between the major cerebral arterial territories, particularly between the anterior and middle cerebral arteries (**Fig. 11.47**), but may be diffuse. The damage is bilateral in most cases. Infarction may be restricted to the territory supplied by a single artery, but this is comparatively rare.

Internal herniation may be complicated by secondary infarction, especially of the occipital lobes (see Fig. 11.43) and upper brain stem (see Fig. 11.42).

MISSILE HEAD INJURY

Missile injuries are caused by objects that fall or are propelled through the air. The resulting damage is generally focal. As the head is not significantly accelerated or decelerated, diffuse damage is not a characteristic feature, except in very high velocity missile injury, in which the shock wave can cause widespread brain damage. The extent and depth of a missile injury is a function of the shape and speed of the missile, and the location of impact. The injury may be classified as depressed, penetrating, or perforating.

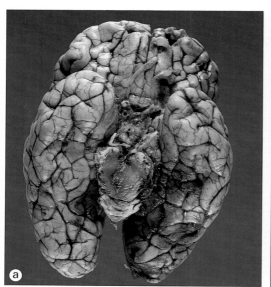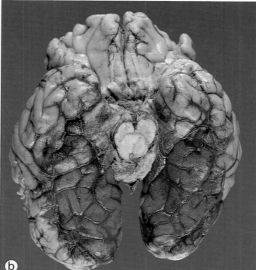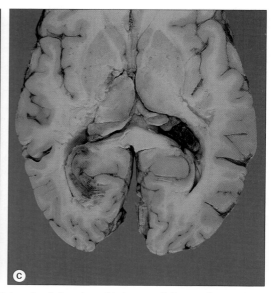

Fig. 11.43 Posterior cerebral infarction due to herniation of the parahippocampal gyrus. During herniation of the parahippocampal gyrus the posterior cerebral artery is compressed against the free edge of the tentorium. This can cause occipital lobe infarction, in some cases largely confined to the primary visual cortex in the calcarine fissure, but much more extensive in others. **(a)** Extensive infarction of inferomedial part of the left occipital lobe and a small region of the right occipital lobe. **(b)** Bilateral inferomedial occipital and adjacent temporal infarction. **(c)** Cut surface of brain showing medial occipital infarction.

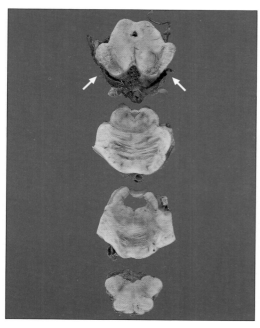

Fig. 11.44 Long term damage to brain stem after trans-tentorial herniation. Sections through the brain stem of a patient who survived several months after head injury with bilateral uncal herniation. There is bilateral necrosis of the cerebral peduncles (arrow), and associated gray discoloration and focal cavitation of the descending fiber tracts in the base of the pons and medullary pyramids.

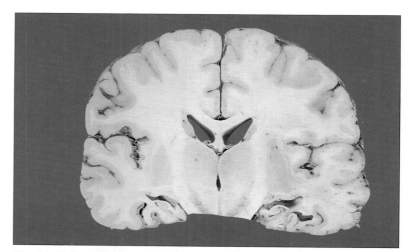

Fig. 11.45 Hypoxic brain damage. Bilateral hippocampal necrosis caused by hypoxic damage resulting from head injury.

In **depressed injuries** the object does not penetrate the skull, but can cause a depressed fracture and focal contusions. Consciousness is rarely lost.

In **penetrating injuries** the object enters the skull. Small sharp objects (e.g. a spike) can cause minimal injury and damage may be overlooked if the missile is no longer embedded in the skull. The brain damage is focal. There is often no loss of consciousness. Penetrating head injuries carry a high risk of infection (e.g. abscess, meningitis) and of causing post-traumatic epilepsy, which occurs in approximately 40% of cases.

In **perforating injuries**, the missile (usually a bullet) enters and exits the skull, in most cases passing through the brain (**Figs 11.48–11.50**).

- Low-velocity missiles are more likely to fragment or ricochet within the skull, producing a penetrating rather than a perforating injury, and to drive fragments of cloth, bone, and scalp into the brain.
- High-velocity bullets can pass through the skull without knocking the victim down or causing an immediate loss of consciousness. However, the brain damage is often severe. Exit wounds are generally larger than entry wounds. The shock wave produced by high-velocity missiles tends to cause severe brain injury that extends well away from the missile track and includes remote contusions of the frontal and temporal poles and the undersurface of the cerebellum, and contrecoup fractures of the orbital plates.

Typically, approximately 10% of patients shot in the head survive for more than 24 hours and only approximately 5% for more than 7 days.

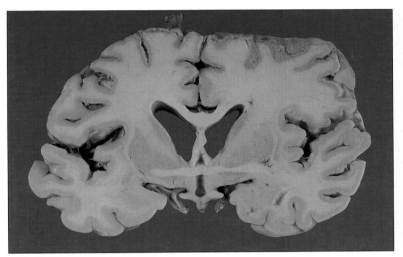

Fig. 11.46 Hypoxic–ischemic damage caused by head injury. Appearance of bilateral cortical necrosis in the perfusion territories of the middle cerebral arteries after survival of several weeks.

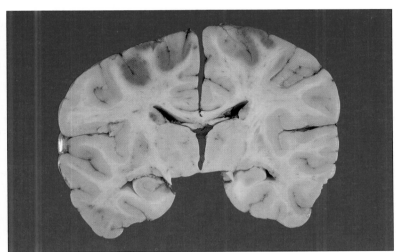

Fig. 11.47 Hypoxic–ischemic damage caused by head injury. Acute boundary zone infarction in the watershed between the anterior and middle cerebral arterial territories bilaterally.

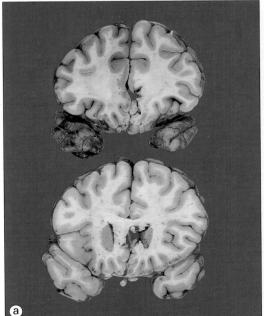
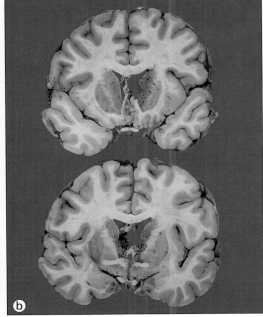
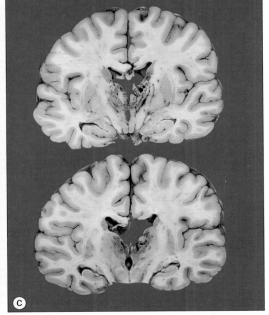

(a) **(b)** **(c)**

Fig. 11.48 Penetrating injury due to bullet from a small-bore handgun. Note that the slices are viewed from the front. The entry wound was in the forehead in the midline. The exit wound was in the occipital region of the skull. **(a)** The missile has passed through the corpus callosum and head of caudate nucleus on the left. **(b)** There is hemorrhagic disruption of the caudate nucleus and interventricular septum. **(c)** There is also bilateral thalamic damage.

PROGRESSIVE NEURODEGENERATION

Progressive decline over an extended period of time of 10–15 years has been noted in approximately 15% of people who have suffered severe head trauma. The pathophysiologic mechanisms responsible for this process are not known. Case studies have documented Alzheimer-type pathologic changes in the brains of some patients.

Punch-drunk syndrome (dementia pugilistica)

Exposure of the head to large numbers of concussive or subconcussive blows tends to produce minor brain damage. Regions of cerebral hypoperfusion have been demonstrated in amateur boxers by single photon emission computed tomography (SPECT) imaging. Computerized tomography (CT) and magnetic resonance imaging (MRI) studies of professional fighters have shown focal abnormalities, ventricular enlargement, and cortical atrophy.

MACROSCOPIC AND MICROSCOPIC APPEARANCES

The brains of patients with punch-drunk syndrome show a characteristic pattern of brain damage, the principal features of which are (**Fig. 11.51**):

- fenestrated septum pellucidum
- degeneration of the substantia nigra with neuronal loss
- neuronal loss from the cortex and cerebellum
- neurofibrillary tangle formation in the cerebral cortex
- diffuse Aβ plaques in the cerebral cortex

PUNCH-DRUNK SYNDROME

- becomes clinically obvious years after the last fight.
- progresses through three stages:
  - stage 1 – affective disorder and mild incoordination
  - stage 2 – dysphasia, apraxia, agnosia, apathy, and blunting of affect
  - stage 3 – global cognitive decline and parkinsonism
- is present in about 20% of older professional boxers over 50 years of age.
- is more likely to develop in boxers with long careers who have been dazed or knocked out on many occasions.

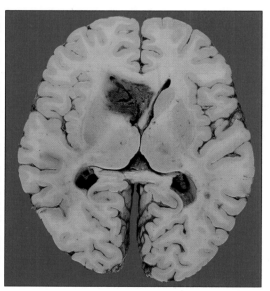

Fig. 11.49 Suicide resulting from discharge of a small-bore handgun in the mouth. The bullet passed through the nasopharynx and base of skull and produced a hemorrhagic lesion in the caudate nucleus and corpus callosum.

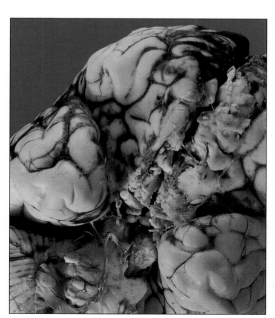

Fig. 11.50 Penetrating injury due to bullet from a small-bore handgun. The entry wound was in the forehead in the midline. The missile has passed along the floor of the anterior cranial fossa, lacerating the orbital surface of the left frontal lobe, and through the left side of the upper midbrain, destroying a large part of the left cerebral peduncle.

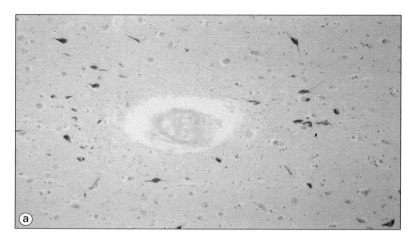

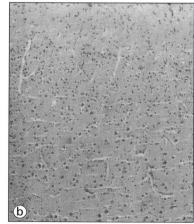
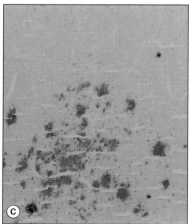

Fig. 11.51 Punch-drunk syndrome. (a) Neurofibrillary tangles in the cerebral cortex of a 23-year-old boxer. The tangles were most numerous in the vicinity of cortical blood vessels and were immunoreactive for tau protein, as shown here. In older boxers tangles may be present in larger numbers in the cerebral cortex and brain stem, and do not show this relationship to blood vessels. (Courtesy of Dr J. Geddes, Royal London Hospital) **(b)** and **(c)** Diffuse Aβ plaques in the cerebral cortex of a professional boxer. The plaques can be demonstrated in sections of cerebral cortex that have been treated with formic acid before immunohistochemistry. An untreated section is shown on the left (b), while an adjacent section that was treated with formic acid is shown on the right (c). Both were immunostained for Aβ peptide.

SPINAL INJURY

Included in this chapter are injuries to the spinal cord resulting from trauma and degenerative disease of the spinal column (**Fig. 11.52**). Neoplastic, ischemic, infectious, toxic, and metabolic disorders that may affect the spinal cord are considered in the appropriate chapters elsewhere in this book.

TRAUMATIC SPINAL CORD INJURY

Trauma to the spinal cord is a major cause of disability after motor vehicle, horse riding, and diving accidents, other sport-related injuries, falls, and knife and firearms assaults. Cervical cord and cervicomedullary injuries are also a feature of non-accidental whiplash injuries resulting from violent shaking of infants.

Nature of lesions

Types of injury
- Indirect (usually closed) injury, results from focal compression, flexion, or extension of the cord by fracture or fracture–dislocation of the spinal column.
- Direct open injury, results from penetration of the cord by an external object such as a knife or bullet.

Distribution
The nature and site of injury varies according to the underlying etiology:
- 60–70% involve the cervical cord, but this proportion is higher in diving and other sport-related injuries.
- Approximately 25% involve the thoracic cord.
- 5–15% involve the lumbar cord.
In descending order of frequency vertebral fractures involve C1/C2, C4–C7, T11–L2, and then other vertebrae.

Time course
Cord damage after trauma can be viewed as occurring in two phases:
- Primary damage resulting from cord compression, contusion, laceration, and hemorrhage.
- Secondary damage initiated by the trauma, but developing over several hours or even days and mainly involving physiologic responses to trauma, hypoxia, and ischemia. Systemic hypotension, loss of autoregulation of blood flow in the injured cord, local edema, generation of free radicals, and release of excitotoxic neurotransmitters may all be contributory factors.

Delayed neurologic deterioration months or years after injury may result from progressive cavitation of the cord (post-traumatic syringomyelia), continued cord compression, or progressive meningeal fibrosis and atrophy of the cord.

CLINICAL FEATURES OF SPINAL CORD INJURY

- There is usually pain at the level of injury and, depending on the extent of the cord damage, variable loss of motor and sensory function below.
- Severe cord injury is generally followed by a 2 to 3 week period of spinal shock and flaccidity, followed by the development of spasticity and hyperreflexia that includes autonomic overactivity.
- Delayed neurologic deterioration may occur months or years after spinal cord injury. The causes may include post-traumatic syringomyelia, continued cord compression, or progressive meningeal fibrosis and atrophy of the cord.

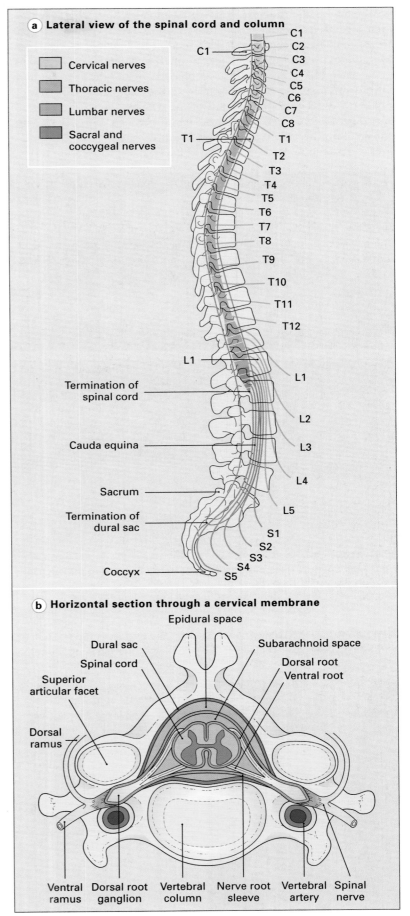

a Lateral view of the spinal cord and column

Cervical nerves
Thoracic nerves
Lumbar nerves
Sacral and coccygeal nerves

C1, C2, C3, C4, C5, C6, C7, C8
T1, T2, T3, T4, T5, T6, T7, T8, T9, T10, T11, T12
L1, L2, L3, L4, L5
S1, S2, S3, S4, S5

Termination of spinal cord
Cauda equina
Sacrum
Termination of dural sac
Coccyx

b Horizontal section through a cervical membrane

Epidural space
Dural sac
Spinal cord
Superior articular facet
Subarachnoid space
Dorsal root
Ventral root
Dorsal ramus
Ventral ramus
Dorsal root ganglion
Vertebral column
Nerve root sleeve
Vertebral artery
Spinal nerve

Fig. 11.52 Spinal anatomy.

MACROSCOPIC APPEARANCES

In most cases the soft tissues around the vertebral column are hemorrhagic and the fracture or fracture–dislocation is visible or at least palpable on external examination of the column. The site of the fracture is obvious on dividing the column (**Figs 11.53, 11.54**). Blood is usually visible in the extradural space and may also be present in the subarachnoid space around the cord. The macroscopic damage to the adjacent cord varies from mild focal indentation to severe hemorrhagic disruption that may extend several segments above and below the level of the fracture (**Fig. 11.55**). Even in the absence of obvious hemorrhage, the injured cord is usually swollen and congested.

In long-term survivors, the meninges at the site of injury are thickened and fibrotic, and the cord may be atrophic. Slit-like cavitation of the cord may be visible at and above the level of injury.

ASSESSMENT OF THE SPINAL CORD AFTER VERTEBROSPINAL TRAUMA OR OTHER COMPRESSIVE CORD LESIONS

- Adequate assessment of the anatomic relationships between the spinal cord and vertebral column often necessitates the removal of all or part of the spinal column at necropsy and fixation of the intact column with the enclosed cord before dissection.
- After fixation, the spinal cord can be exposed by sawing through the vertebral laminae or pedicles. The cord should be dissected gently away from the vertebral column, carefully avoiding excessive traction or angulation. Inexpert removal of the cord can produce artefactual lesions that simulate central cord necrosis or post-traumatic syringomyelia.
- Lesions of the vertebral bodies and disc spaces are usually best demonstrated by sawing midsagittally through the anterior part of the column.

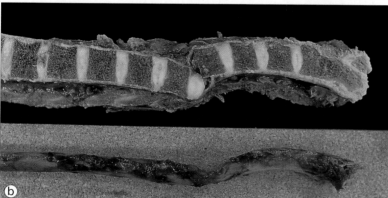

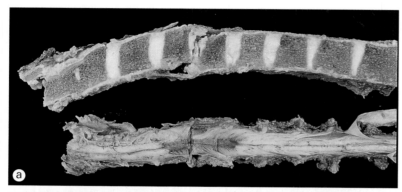

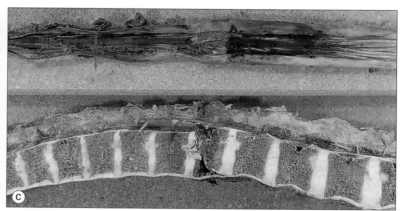

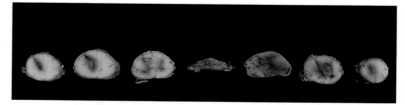

Fig. 11.53 Fracture–dislocations demonstrated by sawing midsagittally through the vertebral bodies. (a) Fracture–dislocation of the cervical column. The anterior longitudinal ligament is torn, but despite the displacement, the posterior longitudinal ligament is still intact and there is only scanty hemorrhage into the soft tissues around the spinal column or extradural space. The cervical cord is swollen and contused. The horizontal slice through the cord was made in the course of examination.

(b) Fracture–dislocation of the cervical column. The marked displacement has caused severe compression of the cord and is associated with more marked soft tissue and extradural hemorrhage than in (a). (Courtesy of Dr. T Moss, Frenchay Hospital, Bristol). **(c)** Fracture–dislocation of the lumbar column. The fractured vertebral body has compressed and lacerated the cord and is associated with extensive extradural and subarachnoid hamorrhage. (Courtesy of Dr. T Moss, Frenchay Hospital, Bristol)

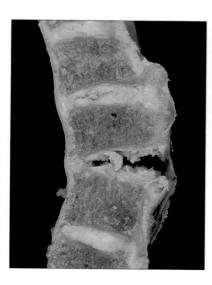

Fig. 11.54 Hyperextension injury of the cervical cord. In this case, the patient had degenerative spinal disease with anterior osteophytes. As a result of a fall, he sustained a cervical hyperextension injury causing cord compression. There has been tearing of the anterior longitudinal ligament and intervertebral disc space, but the posterior longitudinal ligament is intact and there is no horizontal displacement of the column.

Fig. 11.55 Hemorrhagic cord lesion. Hemorrhagic disruption extending several segments above and below the level of cord compression at the site of vertebral fracture–dislocation. The rostral and caudal ends of the hemorrhagic lesion have a typical tapering spindle shape. (Courtesy of Dr. T Moss, Frenchay Hospital, Bristol)

MICROSCOPIC APPEARANCES

During the acute phase after spinal injury, histology reveals variable combinations of edema, disruption of long tracts with prominent axonal swellings, hemorrhage, and foci of infarction (**Figs 11.56–11.58**). Over the next few weeks there is infiltration by macrophages, and gradual removal of myelin and neuronal debris (**Figs 11.59, 11.60**). Rostral and caudal segments of cord show degeneration of the ascending and descending long tracts that were damaged at the level of cord injury. The gray matter at the level of injury may become necrotic and, later, cavitated (**Fig. 11.61**) and often shows prominent proliferation and later hyaline thickening of small blood vessels. With time there is often infiltration by fibroblasts and associated collagenous fibrosis. Frequently, cavitation also involves the anterior part of the posterior columns. Such cavitation is usually maximal at the level of gray matter injury, but can extend several segments above and below (post-traumatic syringomyelia). The cavitation may continue to extend rostrally and caudally within the cord over many years.

Peripherally myelinated nerve fibers, usually of posterior root origin may grow into the damaged cord along blood vessels and into the collagenous scar tissue.

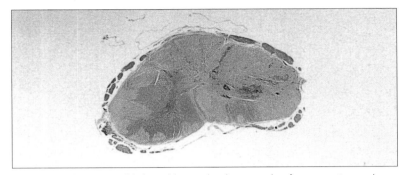

Fig. 11.56 Acute cord injury. Hemorrhagic necrosis of gray matter and disruption and extensive infarction of white matter in the compressed cord at the level of a cervical fracture–dislocation. (Solochrome cyanin)

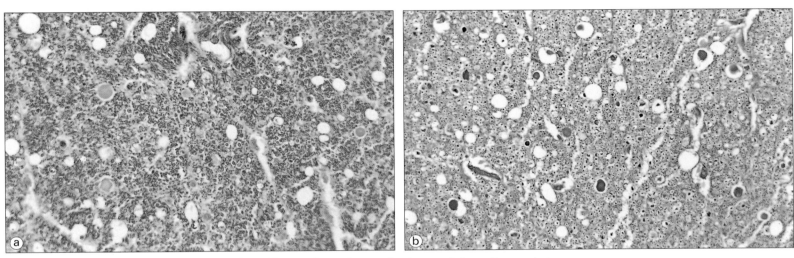

Fig. 11.57 Microscopic appearance of spinal cord in a patient who survived several days after cord injury. (a) There are scattered axonal spheroids in the lateral columns. (Solochrome cyanin). **(b)** The axonal spheroids are well demonstrated by Palmgren silver impregnation.

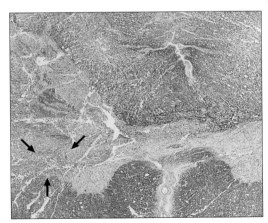

Fig. 11.58 Microscopic appearance of spinal cord 1 week after cord injury. At the level of injury the cervical cord is disrupted and there are foci of gray matter necrosis with infiltration by macrophages (arrows).

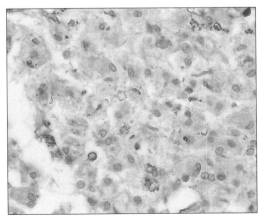

Fig. 11.59 Infiltration of injured cord by macrophages. Removal of myelin debris from the posterior columns of an injured cord by infiltrating macrophages. (Solochrome cyanin)

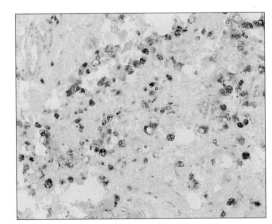

Fig. 11.60 Infiltration of injured cord by macrophages. CD68-immunoreactive macrophages in an injured spinal cord.

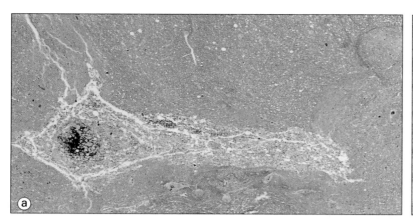

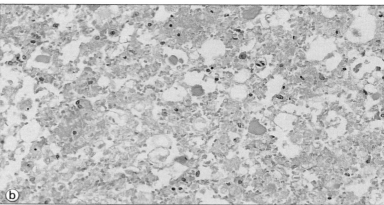

Fig. 11.61 Necrosis of cord after trauma. (a) Necrosis of central gray matter and immediately adjacent part of the posterior columns above the level of a spinal fracture. (Solochrome cyanin) **(b)** Higher magnification of a hematoxylin and eosin-stained section reveals necrotic hemorrhagic tissue, scattered macrophages, and a few axonal spheroids.

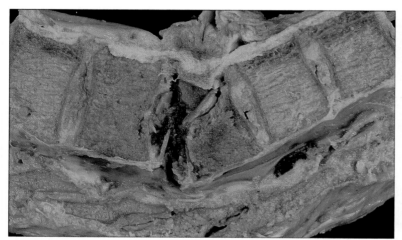

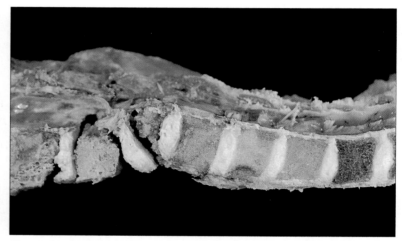

Fig. 11.62 Osteoporotic vertebral collapse. Little remains of the collapsed, wedge-shaped vertebra. In some patients with osteoporotic vertebral collapse, symptoms and signs of cord compression are delayed several weeks as the fragments of bone are gradually extuded posteriorly.

Fig. 11.63 Osteonecrotic vertebral collapse. Verterbal collapse due to osteonecrosis complicating radiotherapy for spinal Hodgkin's disease.

NON-TRAUMATIC SPINAL CORD INJURY

In most cases the spinal white and gray matter are damaged by a combination of direct compression injury and ischemia due to vascular compression. The white matter damage results in ascending and descending fiber tract degeneration above and below the level of injury.

NON-TRAUMATIC CAUSES OF CORD COMPRESSION

Atlantoaxial deformities or subluxation

- Odontoid hypolasia or dysplasia and resulting atlantoaxial instability causing compression due to atlantoaxial subluxation or associated thickening of the dura mater in the craniocervical region: Down syndrome; Morquio's syndrome (mucopolysaccharidosis type IVA); rarely other mucopolysaccharidoses or mucolipidoses; primary bone dysplasias; achondroplasia.
- Basilar invagination or posterior inclination of the odontoid: congenital (in some cases associated with Klippel–Feil syndrome or occipitalized atlas); acquired as a result of rheumatoid arthritis (see below), rickets, or osteomalacia.
- Atlantoaxial arthritis causing subluxation, especially in rheumatoid arthritis (see below), less commonly in ankylosing spondylitis, and rarely in other arthritides.

Severe kyphosis with or without scoliosis

- Idiopathic (e.g. Scheuermann's disease).
- Due to vertebral collapse (see below).
- Due to chronic neurogenic or myopathic weakness involving muscles of the vertebral column.

Vertebral expansion or collapse

- Tumors: primary; secondary.
- Osteomyelitis.
- Osteoporosis (**Fig. 11.62**). In some cases, the onset of neurologic signs and symptoms may be delayed by weeks or months after an osteoporotic fracture as fragments of bone are slowly displaced posteriorly.
- Osteonecrosis: usually associated with corticosteroid administration or radiotherapy (**Fig. 11.63**).
- Metabolic disorders involving bone: Paget's disease; hyperparathyroidism causing osteitis fibrosa cystica ('brown tumor') of vertebrae; Gaucher's disease; severe rickets or osteomalacia (e.g. due to familial hypophosphatemic rickets).

Developmental or idiopathic spinal stenosis

Connective tissue, intervertebral disc, and joint disease

- Rheumatoid arthritis (rarely ankylosing spondylitis or psoriatic arthritis) can cause C1/C2 (atlantoaxial), C2/C3 (subaxial), or much less commonly, C3/C4 subluxation (**Fig. 11.64**).
- Acute disc prolapse (**Fig. 11.65**).
- Spondylosis (**Fig. 11.66**). The changes in the spinal cord are due to several factors: the direct effects of compression and indentation; ischemic injury caused by vascular compression; root damage due to entrapment; and possibly injury caused by traction of the denticulate ligament. There is often associated fibrous thickening of the leptomeninges and of the walls of blood vessels within the cord. Occasionally the cord is invaded by peripheral nerve fibers as in other forms of chronic cord injury.
- Ossification of the posterior longitudinal ligament (OPLL) or, rarely, of the ligamentum flavum. The risk of OPLL is increased in ankylosing spondylitis.
- Amyloidosis, particularly due to β2-microglobulin deposition in patients on chronic hemodialysis (**Fig. 11.67**). This can cause an arthropathy as well as thickening of the posterior longitudinal ligament and ligamentum flavum.
- Tophaceous gout and rarely chondrocalcinosis (pseudogout).

Epidural space-occupying lesions (see also chapters 16, 17, 18, 46, 47)

- Tumors: primary including lipoma and angiolipoma; secondary, especially lymphoma.
- Epidural abscess (tuberculous or pyogenic).
- Epidural cyst.
- Hemorrhage (**Fig. 11.68**): spontaneous or due to a bleeding diathesis, most commonly after the administration of streptokinase or tissue plasminogen activator for treatment of a myocardial infarct.
- Extramedullary hemopoiesis, especially in thalassemia or myelofibrosis.

Subdural and subarachnoid space-occupying lesions (see also chapters 16, 17, 18, 46, 47)

- Infections: pyogenic (e.g. subdural empyema); tuberculosis, very rarely syphilis; fungal (e.g. coccidioidomycosis, paracoccidioidomycosis, cryptococcosis); parasitic (e.g. cysticercosis, hydatid disease, schistosomiasis).
- Tumors: primary nerve sheath or meningeal tumors or intrinsic CNS tumors including those that have metastasized within the subarachnoid space; secondary tumors.
- Cysts: arachnoid; enterogenous; epidermoid or dermoid; perineurial.

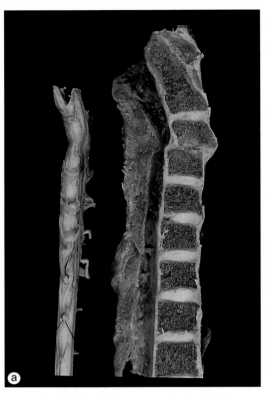

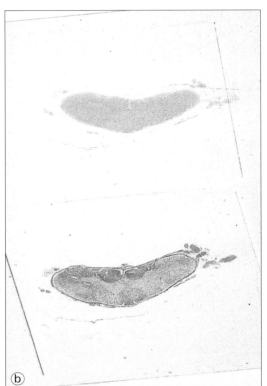

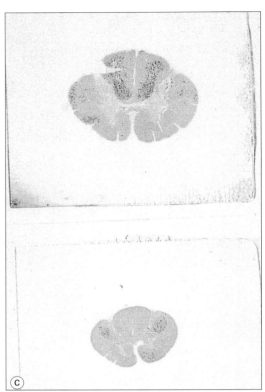

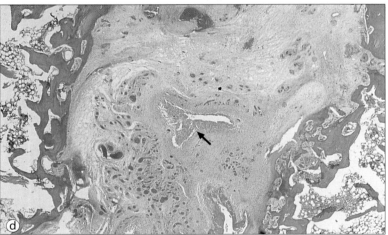

Fig. 11.64 Cord damage due to rheumatoid arthritis. (a) C3/C4 subluxation due to rheumatoid arthritis with resulting cord compression. **(b)** There is extensive white matter damage at the level of cord compression. (Top section: hematoxylin and eosin. Bottom section: luxol fast blue/cresyl violet.) **(c)** Marchi preparations reveal symmetric posterior column degeneration at the C2 level (top section) and pyramidal tract degeneration in the thoracic cord (bottom section). **(d)** The affected intervertebral disc space is replaced by vascular fibrous connective tissue with occasional foci of fibrinoid necrosis (arrow). (Hematoxylin/van Gieson) **(e)** Higher magnification through a focus of fibrinoid necrosis shows peripheral pallisading by fibroblasts and macrophages.

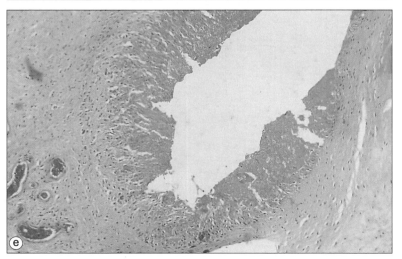

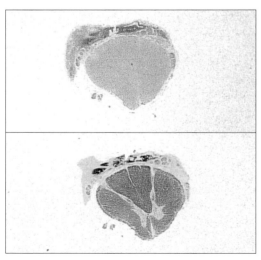

Fig. 11.65 Acute disc prolapse. Indentation of the thoracic cord due to acute anterolateral disc prolapse. (Top section: hematoxylin and eosin. Bottom section: luxol fast blue/cresyl violet.)

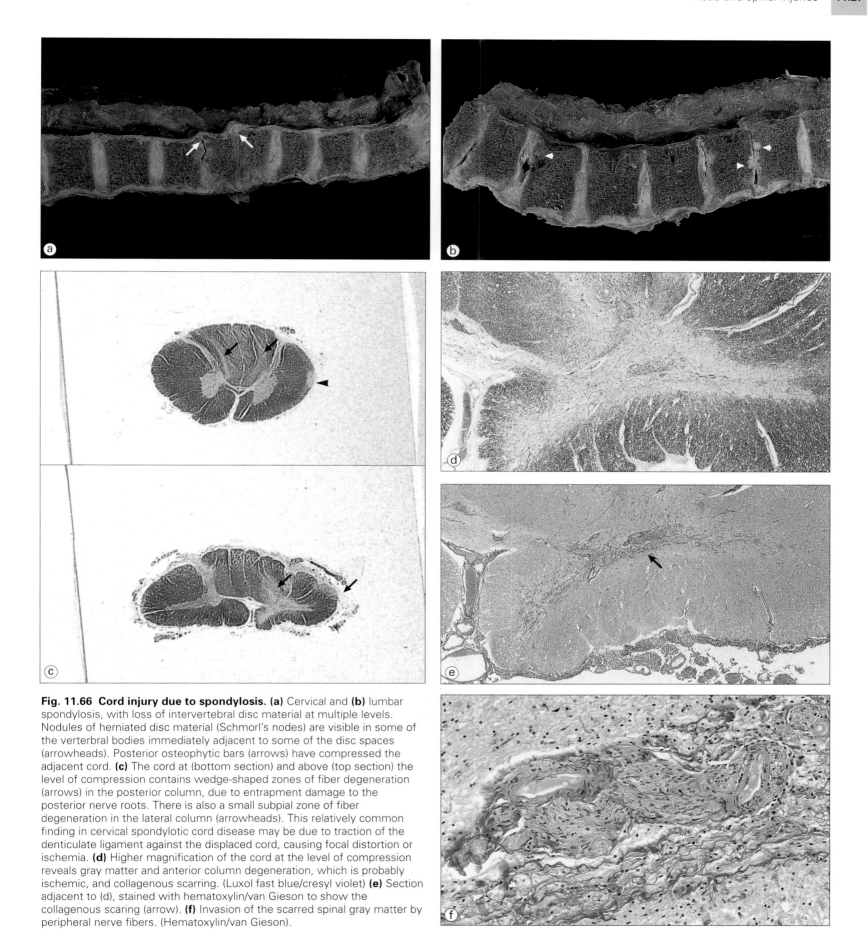

Fig. 11.66 Cord injury due to spondylosis. (a) Cervical and **(b)** lumbar spondylosis, with loss of intervertebral disc material at multiple levels. Nodules of herniated disc material (Schmorl's nodes) are visible in some of the verterbral bodies immediately adjacent to some of the disc spaces (arrowheads). Posterior osteophytic bars (arrows) have compressed the adjacent cord. **(c)** The cord at (bottom section) and above (top section) the level of compression contains wedge-shaped zones of fiber degeneration (arrows) in the posterior column, due to entrapment damage to the posterior nerve roots. There is also a small subpial zone of fiber degeneration in the lateral column (arrowheads). This relatively common finding in cervical spondylotic cord disease may be due to traction of the denticulate ligament against the displaced cord, causing focal distortion or ischemia. **(d)** Higher magnification of the cord at the level of compression reveals gray matter and anterior column degeneration, which is probably ischemic, and collagenous scarring. (Luxol fast blue/cresyl violet) **(e)** Section adjacent to (d), stained with hematoxylin/van Gieson to show the collagenous scaring (arrow). **(f)** Invasion of the scarred spinal gray matter by peripheral nerve fibers. (Hematoxylin/van Gieson).

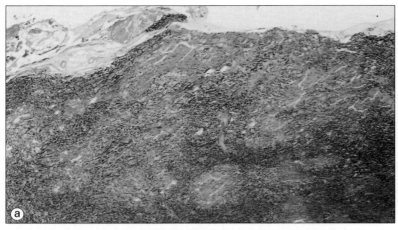

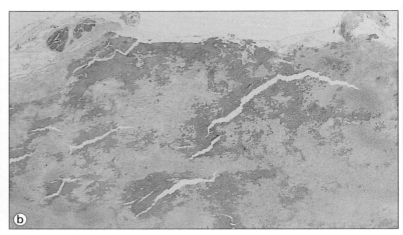

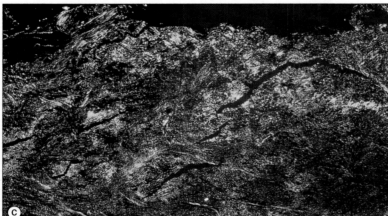

Fig. 11.67 Cord compression due to amyloid. Adjacent sections showing deposits of β_2-microglobulin amyloid in and adjacent to the ligamentum flavum in a patient on chronic hemodialysis. **(a)** Van Gieson/Weigert's elastic stain. **(b)** Sirius red viewed with unpolarized light. **(c)** Sirius red viewed with polarized light.

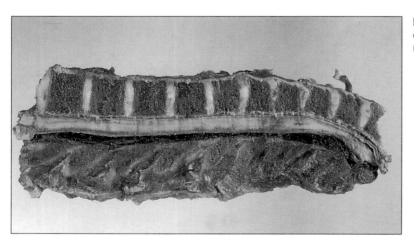

Fig. 11.68 Spinal epidural hematoma. Posterior compression of the spinal cord by an epidural (extradural) hematoma in a patient who had been receiving streptokinase for treatment of a myocardial infarct.

REFERENCES

Davis RL and Roberston DM (eds).(1997) *Textbook of Neuropathology* (3rd edition) Baltimore: William & Wilkins.

Graham DI, Adams JH, Nicoll JAR, Maxwell WL, Gennarelli TAT. (1995) The nature, distribution and causes of traumatic brain injury. *Brain Pathology* 5: 397–406.

Graham DI and Lantos PL (eds). (1997) Greenfield's Neuropathology, (6th edition) London: Edward Arnold, vol 1 pp. 658–754.

Jennett B. (1996) Epidemiology of head injury. *J Neurol Neurosurg and Psych* 60: 362–369.

Nicoll, JAR, Roberts GW, Graham DI. (1995) Apolipoprotein E epsilon4 allele is associated with deposition of amyloid beta- protein following head injury. *Nature Medicine* 1: 135–137.

Povlishock JT, Jenkins LW. (1995) Are the pathobiological changes evoked by traumatic brain injury immediate and irreversible? *Brain Pathology* 5: 415–426.

Tator, CH (1995) Update on the pathophysiology and pathology of acute spinal cord injury *Brain Pathology* 5: 407–413.

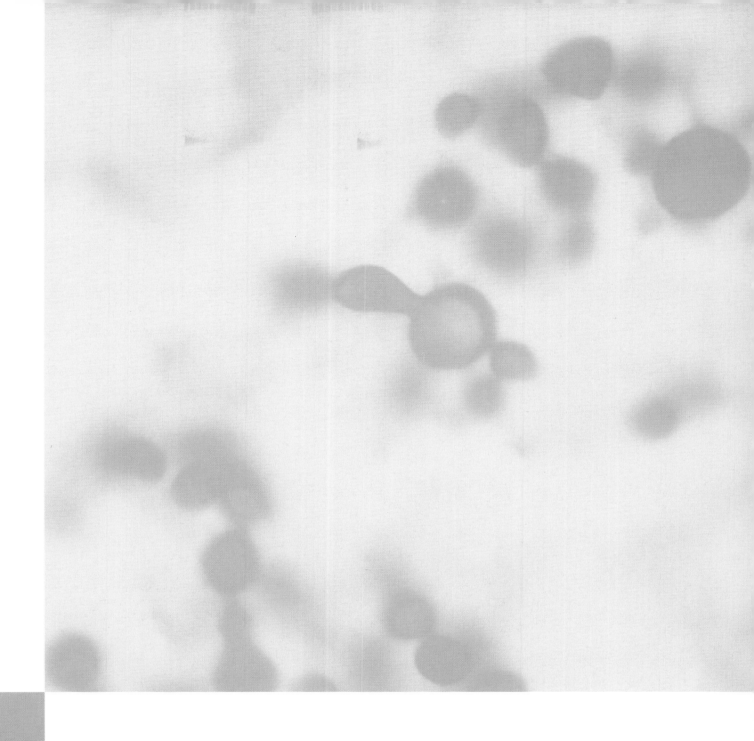

5 | **Infectious Diseases**

12 *Acute viral infections*

Classifications of viral infections of the CNS such as those shown in **Fig. 12.1** are of help in making an accurate diagnosis. In practice, a combination of approaches is generally used to classify and diagnose these disorders.

ASEPTIC MENINGITIS

This is a benign, usually short-lived, syndrome of meningeal inflammation that is not attributable to any of the common bacterial pathogens. A wide range of viruses can produce aseptic meningitis (**Fig. 12.2**); much less commonly it can be produced by some bacteria (for example, syphilis and Lyme disease) or other microorganisms, and some noninfectious disorders (for example, Behçet's disease). One form of recurrent aseptic meningitis (Mollaret's meningitis) that was previously regarded as noninfective in nature has been linked to infection with herpes simplex virus especially herpes simplex virus type 2.

The causes of aseptic meningitis show considerable geographic and seasonal variation. The peak incidence of cases due to enteroviral infection, which is the commonest overall cause of this syndrome, is during late summer and fall.

MACROSCOPIC AND MICROSCOPIC APPEARANCES
Since aseptic meningitis is by definition benign, reports of the neuropathologic findings are uncommon. Occasionally, patients with aseptic meningitis die as a result of a concurrent systemic illness (e.g. viral myocarditis). Histologic examination of the CNS then reveals a scanty infiltrate of lymphocytes in the meninges, in the perivascular space surrounding some of the superficial cortical blood vessels (**Fig. 12.3**), and in the choroid plexus.

Viral infections of the central nervous system	
These may be classified according to:	
Course of disease	**Patient age group**
acute	intrauterine
subacute or chronic	neonatal
Target tissue	child
meningitis	adult
poliomyelitis, polioencephalomyelitis	**Patient immune status**
viral leukoencephalopathy	**Etiologic agent**
panencephalitis	

Fig. 12.1 Viral infections of the central nervous system.

POLIOMYELITIS

This disorder is characterized by lytic infection of motor neurons. The destructive effects may be confined to the spinal cord or may also involve neurons within the brain (polioencephalomyelitis).

MACROSCOPIC APPEARANCES: ACUTE PHASE
It is unusual to see macroscopic lesions. In severe cases, vascular congestion, petechial hemorrhages, and focal necrosis may be evident in the spinal gray matter.

POLIOMYELITIS

- Polioviruses are small RNA viruses of the genus Enterovirus (along with group A and B coxsackieviruses, echoviruses, and enteroviruses). Spread of the virus is feco-oral, and is facilitated by crowding and poor sanitation.
- There are three antigenic types of poliovirus: types 1, 2, and 3. Until the development and widespread use of poliovirus vaccines, these viruses were responsible for almost all cases of poliomyelitis, including the epidemics of paralytic poliomyelitis in Europe and North America in the latter half of the nineteenth century.
- The introduction of the Salk vaccine containing inactivated virus in the 1950s, and of the Sabin vaccine comprising live attenuated poliovirus in the early 1960s, caused a sharp decline in the incidence of poliomyelitis.
- Outbreaks of paralytic infection by wild-type (i.e. unmodified) poliovirus do still occur in developing parts of the world and in communities that refuse vaccination (e.g. for religious reasons). However, in vaccinated populations poliomyelitis is usually caused either by the rare reversion to neurovirulence of attenuated vaccine-related strains of poliovirus or by other enteroviruses, especially group A coxsackieviruses and enterovirus 71.
- CNS infection by poliovirus and other enteroviruses is hematogenous. After initial intestinal infection and viral replication, there is a primary viremia with spread to the reticuloendothelial system where further replication leads to a secondary viremia, during which the virus enters the CNS.

MICROSCOPIC APPEARANCES: ACUTE PHASE

The extent of histologic involvement almost always exceeds that predicted by the clinical manifestations. The distribution of lesions is variable. The spinal gray matter is usually involved, particularly the anterior horn cells. The disease also shows a predilection for the motor nuclei in the pons and medulla, the reticular formation, and deep cerebellar nuclei (**Fig. 12.4**). Apart from the precentral gyrus, the cerebral cortex is usually spared.

There is intense inflammation in the leptomeninges and affected gray matter (**Fig. 12.5**). Neutrophils are found initially, but lymphocytes soon predominate. Lymphocytic cuffing of blood vessels is a conspicuous feature.

The histologic hallmark of the viral infection of neurons is neuronophagia (aggregation of microglia and macrophages around dead neurons, **Fig. 12.6**). Clusters of microglia (microglial nodules) mark the sites of destroyed neurons for several weeks after their resorption.

There is often congestion of small blood vessels in the areas of inflammation. This may be associated with perivascular hemorrhage and, occasionally, focal necrosis.

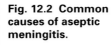

Common causes of aseptic meningitis
• echovirus
• coxsackie B
• coxsackie A
• herpes simplex virus (HSV)-2
• mumps
• measles
• adenovirus

Fig. 12.2 Common causes of aseptic meningitis.

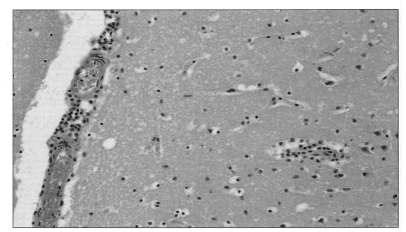

Fig. 12.3 Aseptic meningitis. This section shows a meningeal and scanty perivascular infiltrate of lymphocytes in a child who died of coxsackievirus myocarditis. (Courtesy of Dr David Hilton, Derriford Hospital, Plymouth, U.K.)

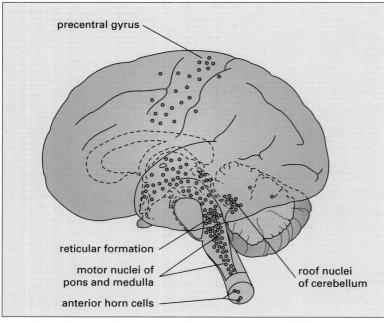

precentral gyrus

reticular formation

motor nuclei of pons and medulla

anterior horn cells

roof nuclei of cerebellum

Fig. 12.4 Schematic illustration of the regions of the CNS that are susceptible to poliomyelitis.

■ POLIOVIRUS INFECTION

- Most patients experience no more than a minor nonspecific illness at the time of the primary viremia, 1–5 days after exposure to the virus. Symptoms include: gastrointestinal upset, mild pyrexia, headache, and general malaise.
- Some days after resolution of the nonspecific illness or approximately 10 days after the initial exposure, a small percentage of patients develop paralytic polioencephalomyelitis. In children, paralytic disease is usually heralded by pyrexia, headache, vomiting, neck stiffness, and irritability. In adults, these prodromal symptoms may be less pronounced.
- Patients may experience muscle pain or stiffness before the development of paralysis.
- The distribution of the paralysis depends on that of the lesions within the CNS. The spinal cord is usually involved. The paralysis is typically asymmetric, the lower limbs being involved more often than the upper limbs or trunk. Bulbar disease manifests with cranial nerve palsies, and involvement of the reticular formation with cardiac arrhythmias and abnormal patterns of breathing.

Post-polio syndrome

- This is a syndrome of increasing weakness or muscular atrophy developing many years later in survivors of poliomyelitis who do not have any other neuromuscular disease. The cause is not known.

MACROSCOPIC AND MICROSCOPIC APPEARANCES: CHRONIC PHASE

In patients coming to necropsy several years after the acute illness, there is wasting of the affected muscles, and thinning and gray discoloration of the corresponding anterior nerve roots.

Examination of the affected regions shows an obvious loss of motor neurons (**Fig. 12.7**) and atrophy and fibrosis of anterior nerve roots. There is no residual inflammation and, apart from these changes, the parenchyma of the affected spinal cord or brain stem is usually remarkably well preserved.

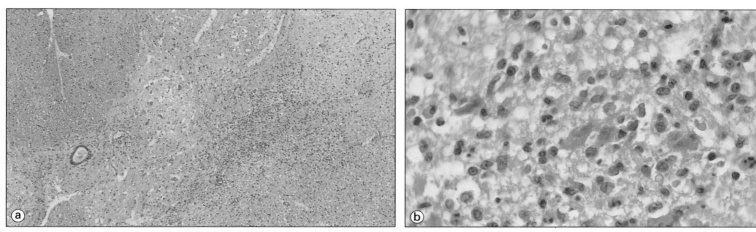

Fig. 12.5 Poliomyelitis. (a) and **(b)** show mixed inflammatory infiltrate in the spinal gray matter in coxsackievirus poliomyelitis. (Courtesy of Dr David Hilton, Derriford Hospital, Plymouth, U.K.)

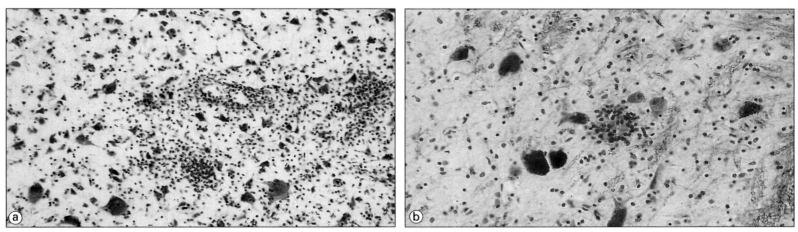

Fig. 12.6 Neuronophagia and microglial nodule formation in poliovirus infection. (a) Florid brain stem inflammation and neuronophagia in poliovirus poliomyelitis. (Cresyl violet) **(b)** Microglial nodule in the brain stem in coxsackievirus polioencephalomyelitis.

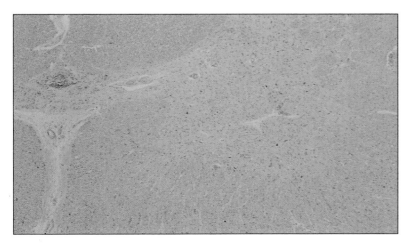

Fig. 12.7 Chronic phase of poliomyelitis. Marked depletion of anterior horn cells from the spinal cord of a long-term survivor of poliomyelitis. (Cresyl violet)

HERPESVIRUS INFECTIONS

The herpesviruses are relatively large, enveloped, double-stranded DNA viruses. The group includes several that are human pathogens and can cause CNS disease (**Fig. 12.8**), including herpes simplex virus type 1, herpes simplex virus type 2, Epstein–Barr virus, cytomegalovirus, and human herpesvirus 6. The simian herpesvirus, B virus, can also infect humans and cause CNS disease. When these viruses invade the CNS they tend to cause necrotizing destruction of both gray and white matter (i.e. panencephalitis or panmyelitis).

HERPES SIMPLEX VIRUS INFECTION
Classical herpes simplex encephalitis (HSE)
This is one of the commonest forms of acute necrotizing encephalitis. Approximately 50 cases are reported in the United Kingdom each year, but there are undoubtedly more cases that are not recognized and therefore not reported.

MACROSCOPIC APPEARANCES: ACUTE PHASE
Most cases show obvious congestion and hemorrhagic necrosis involving the temporal lobes (**Figs 12.10, 12.11**) and, to a greater or lesser extent, the insulae, cingulate gyri, and posterior orbital frontal cortex (see Fig. 12.11). The lesions are often asymmetric. The brain is usually swollen, particularly the hemorrhagic regions, but in patients dying some weeks after the onset of disease the liquefactive necrosis in these regions will have progressed to cavitation and atrophy.

HERPES SIMPLEX ENCEPHALITIS

- Patients present with a combination of:
  - nonspecific features of encephalitis (e.g. headache, pyrexia, neck stiffness, drowsiness, coma)
  - focal neurologic signs (e.g. dysphasia, hemiparesis, focal seizures).
- Without treatment, the disease progresses rapidly over the course of a few days and is usually fatal.
- Some patients do survive, with behavioral abnormalities, memory disturbances, and other neurologic deficits of varying severity.
- Since the introduction of vidarabine and later acyclovir, the mortality and morbidity rates have fallen substantially, although 25–50% of patients still die despite treatment, the risk being greatest in the elderly and in those whose level of consciousness is severely depressed when treatment is started.

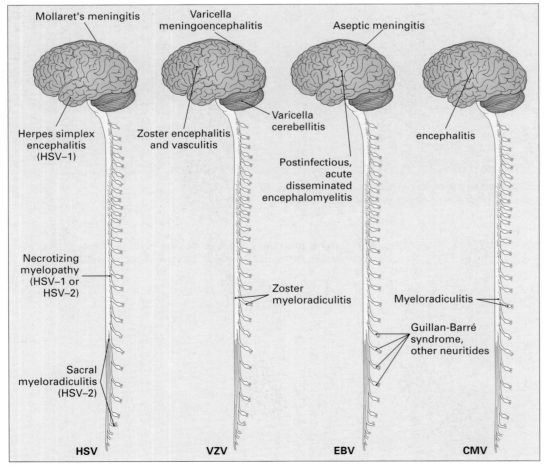

Fig. 12.8 Patterns of herpesvirus infections in children and adults.

HERPES SIMPLEX ENCEPHALITIS

Classical herpes simplex encephalitis (HSE) is caused by herpes simplex virus type 1 (HSV-1), which is spread by direct contact with infected secretions, usually from orolabial vesicles ('cold sores').

Primary mucocutaneous infection

In most patients, initial infection by HSV-1 involves the mucocutaneous border of the lips or the oropharyngeal mucosa.

Establishment of latency in the trigeminal ganglion

*After local replication the virus is conveyed by retrograde axonal transport along sensory fibers to the trigeminal ganglion, where, after further replication, latent infection is established (**Fig. 12.9**). (In contrast, HSV-2 causes genital herpes infection and establishes latency in the sacral dorsal root ganglia.) HSV-1 genome and latency-associated transcripts (the only viral mRNAs produced during latent infection) can be detected in the trigeminal ganglia in 50–75% of adults.*

Reactivation of virus

Reactivation of the virus within the trigeminal ganglia results in its anterograde axonal transport to the skin or mucosa and the development of cold sores. Reactivation may occur spontaneously, or be precipitated by local mucocutaneous trauma or ultraviolet irradiation, or by systemic factors such as pyrexia, emotional stress, physiologic fluctuations in estrogen and progesterone concentrations during the menstrual cycle, and immunosuppression.

Involvement of the olfactory pathway

HSV-1 DNA has been detected in the olfactory bulbs in approximately 15% of adults, suggesting that retrograde transport of the virus along the olfactory nerve fibers may occur after primary nasopharyngeal infection. It is not known whether the virus in the olfactory bulbs is susceptible to reactivation. In experimental studies, attempts at reactivation from central nervous tissue have been unsuccessful.

Entry of HSV-1 into the CNS

The mechanism of entry of HSV-1 into the CNS to cause HSE has been much debated. Proposals include:

- Spread along olfactory nerve fibers and tracts either during primary nasopharyngeal infection or after reactivation of latent virus in the olfactory bulbs. This route would explain the predilection of the disease for the posterior orbital, frontal, and limbic regions.
- Reactivation of latent virus in the trigeminal ganglia and axonal spread along either centrally projecting fibers into the brain stem or peripheral trigeminal sensory fibers innervating the dura. This route would not account for the restricted distribution of lesions in herpes encephalitis, the lack of correlation between the development of herpes labialis and herpes encephalitis, or the occasional difference in the strain of virus isolated from cold sores and the brain.
- Reactivation of virus that has previously established latent infection within the temporal lobes or other parts of the CNS affected by herpes encephalitis. This is the most speculative proposal, although there are reports that tiny amounts of HSV DNA have been detected in the brains of adults without neurologic disease.

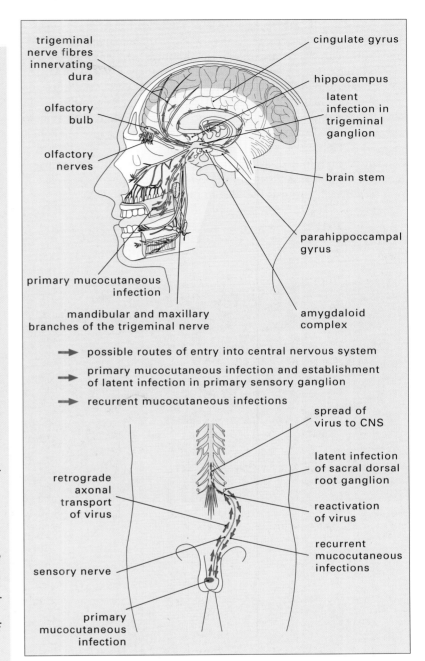

Fig. 12.9 Spread of HSV-1, and possible routes of entry of virus into the CNS

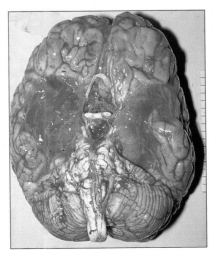

Fig. 12.10 Macroscopic appearance of a brain in HSE. Undersurface of unfixed brain from a patient with HSE showing hemorrhagic necrosis of the temporal lobes.

MICROSCOPIC APPEARANCES: ACUTE PHASE

The earliest lesions contain relatively scanty parenchymal inflammation, although there are moderate numbers of lymphocytes and macrophages in the overlying leptomeninges (**Figs 12.12, 12.13**). The lesions extend from the pial surface through the cerebral cortex and into the white matter. The affected neurons, glia, and endothelial cells tend to have slightly hypereosinophilic cytoplasm. Many of the nuclei are pyknotic or disintegrating; others contain homogeneous eosinophilic inclusions (**Fig. 12.13, 12.14**), some surrounded by an irregular rim of condensed marginated chromatin. Clumps of eosinophilic inclusion material may also be visible in the cytoplasm. Inclusions are usually best seen in cells towards the edge of the lesions.

Most lesions are usually at a more advanced stage, containing sheets of necrotic cells, foci of hemorrhage, and an intense perivascular and interstitial infiltrate of lymphocytes and macrophages (**Fig. 12.15**). There may be neuronophagia and, later, microglial nodules. Nuclear inclusions are sparse at this stage.

Herpesvirus nucleocapsid particles are approximately 100 nm in diameter and may be seen within the nuclei of infected cells by electron microscopy (**Fig. 12.16**). Viral antigen is readily demonstrable by immunohistochemistry (**Fig. 12.17**) for up to approximately 3 weeks after the onset of encephalitis, and viral DNA can be detected in frozen or paraffin sections by in-situ hybridization (**Fig. 12.18**) or polymerase chain reaction (PCR) amplification with suitable primers.

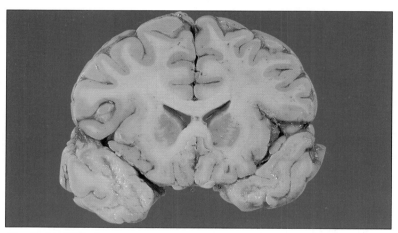

Fig. 12.11 HSE. Coronal slice through the fixed brain, showing temporal, orbital frontal, and focal insular necrosis.

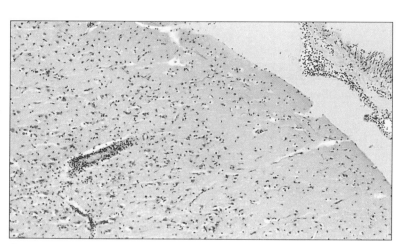

Fig. 12.12 Early HSE. Meningeal, perivascular, and scanty parenchymal inflammation. (Luxol fast blue/cresyl violet)

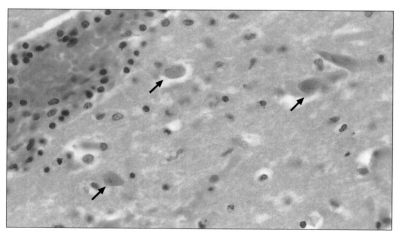

Fig. 12.13 Early herpes encephalitis. This section shows scanty perivascular inflammation and scattered cells containing viral inclusions (arrows).

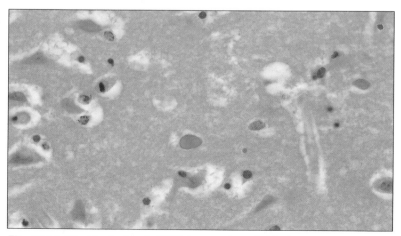

Fig. 12.14 Viral inclusion in HSE. Intranuclear viral inclusion is seen in this section, towards the edge of the affected region of the temporal lobe in HSE.

MACROSCOPIC AND MICROSCOPIC APPEARANCES: CHRONIC PHASE

In long-term survivors of untreated or unsuccessfully treated herpes encephalitis, the affected parts of the brain are shrunken and cavitated and show yellow-brown discoloration (**Fig. 12.19**).

The normal gray and white matter is replaced by cavitated glial scar tissue (**Fig. 12.20**). Occasional clusters of lymphocytes are still seen in the meninges and brain parenchyma (**Fig. 12.21**).

Although virus is no longer demonstrable by culture, electron microscopy, or immunohistochemistry, in most cases viral DNA is readily detectable, even in paraffin-embedded material, by PCR. It should be noted, however, that on using highly sensitive nested PCR techniques, very small amounts of herpesvirus DNA have been detected in apparently normal brain tissue.

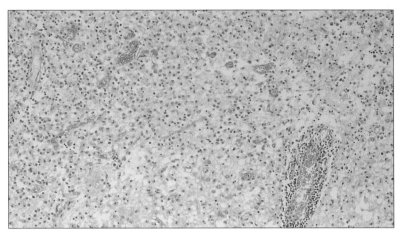

Fig. 12.15 Necrotizing inflammation in HSE. Sheets of foamy macrophages and perivascular cuffing by lymphocytes in a case of HSE.

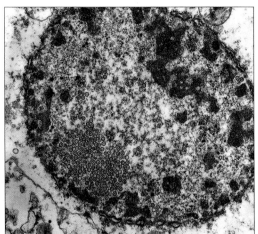

Fig. 12.16 Ultrastructural appearance of HSV. Electron micrograph showing intranuclear herpesvirus nucleocapsid particles.

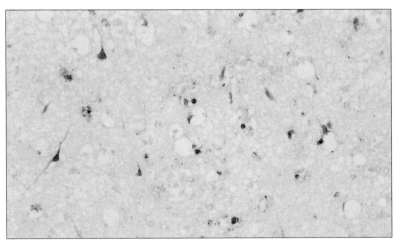

Fig. 12.17 Immunohistochemical demonstration of HSV antigen.

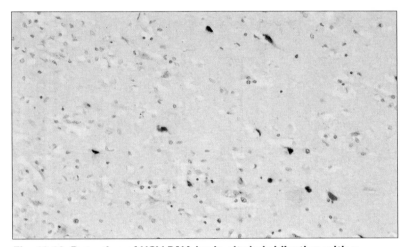

Fig. 12.18 Detection of HSV DNA by *in-situ* hybridization with a biotinylated probe.

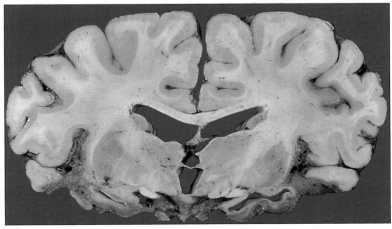

Fig. 12.19 Long-term survivor of herpes encephalitis. Marked atrophy and yellow-brown discoloration affect the temporal lobes and insulae.

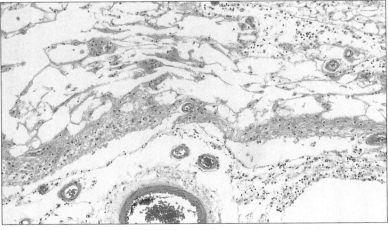

Fig. 12.20 Long-term survivor of HSE. Cavitated temporal lobe in a case of 'burnt out' HSE.

ATYPICAL HERPES SIMPLEX ENCEPHALITIS

In occasional patients, HSE predominantly involves the brain stem or follows a more subacute clinical course than usual (**Fig. 12.22**). Although the likelihood of developing HSE is probably not increased by immunosuppression, anecdotal reports suggest that immunosuppression may predispose to atypical forms of the disease.

NECROTIZING MYELOPATHY

Both HSV-1 and HSV-2 can cause this rare disorder. Histology shows extensive necrosis and inflammation involving the spinal gray and white matter (**Fig. 12.23**). Herpesvirus is usually demonstrable within the cord by immunohistochemistry (**Fig. 12.24**).

NEONATAL HSV ENCEPHALITIS

Neonatal HSE differs in its pathogenesis and clinical and pathologic manifestations from the adult disease.

PATHOGENESIS OF NEONATAL HSV ENCEPHALITIS

- Most cases of neonatal HSV infection are due to HSV-2 and are acquired during delivery from contact between the fetus and infected maternal genital lesions. The disease can, however, be acquired from the mother *in utero*, even during early gestation, or by contact with infected secretions from the mother or another source during the postnatal period.
- Primary maternal HSV-2 infection during pregnancy and prolonged rupture of the membranes in a woman with active genital infection are particular risk factors for fetal infection.
- Approximately 15–20% of neonatal HSV infections are due to HSV-1 and these are predominantly acquired postnatally.

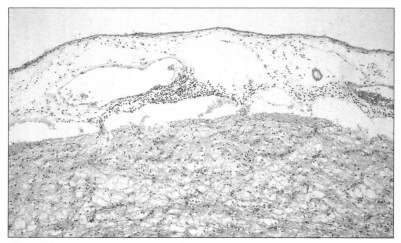

Fig. 12.21 Long-term survivor of HSE. Scattered aggregates of lymphocytes persist in the meninges or brain parenchyma for many years.

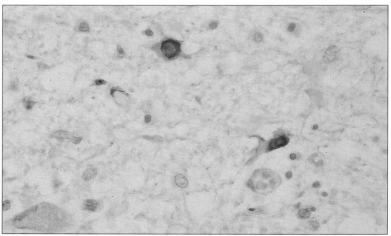

Fig. 12.22 Atypical HSE. Immunohistochemical demonstration of atypical non-necrotizing HSV-1 infection of the brain stem in a patient with AIDS.

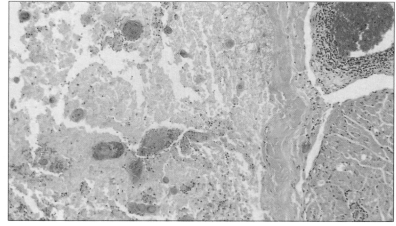

Fig. 12.23 Necrotizing myelopathy due to HSV-1 infection. There is extensive necrosis within the spinal cord and perivascular inflammation in the leptomeninges. (Courtesy of Professor Clayton Wiley, University of Pittsburgh.)

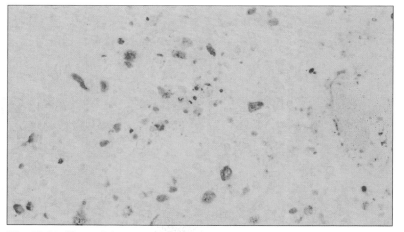

Fig. 12.24 Necrotizing myelopathy due to HSV-1 infection. Immunohistochemical demonstration of HSV-1 in the necrotic spinal cord. (Courtesy of Professor Clayton Wiley, University of Pittsburgh.)

NEONATAL HSV INFECTION

- In approximately one-third of neonates with HSV infection the disease is confined to the skin, eyes, and mouth.
- In one-third there is also (or only) encephalitis.
- Approximately one-third show evidence of widely disseminated disease, usually involving the brain, liver, and adrenals, and, less consistently, other internal organs.
- Vesicular skin lesions and keratoconjunctivitis are usually but not always present.
- CNS involvement usually manifests nonspecifically, with poor feeding, irritability, lethargy, and seizures.
- Treatment with acyclovir has reduced the mortality of localized neonatal HSE to approximately 15% and nearly 50% of survivors develop normally.
- The mortality of disseminated infection is much higher (approximately 50%), but approximately 85% of the survivors develop normally.

MACROSCOPIC APPEARANCES

The brains of neonates or infants dying of disease acquired intrapartum or postnatally are usually swollen, with generalized softening and variable congestion and hemorrhage. Intrauterine infection may produce severe cystic encephalomalacia.

MICROSCOPIC APPEARANCES

The lesions of HSE in neonates do not show a predilection for any particular part of the brain and can involve gray and white matter in the cerebrum, cerebellum, and brain stem (**Fig. 12.25**). As in adults, the features are of a necrotizing encephalitis, associated with meningeal and parenchymal infiltration by lymphocytes and macrophages (**Fig. 12.25a**). Nuclear inclusions (**Fig. 12.25c**), viral antigen (**Fig. 12.25b, d**), and DNA (**Fig. 12.25e**) are usually demonstrable in abundance, particularly during the first few days of infection.

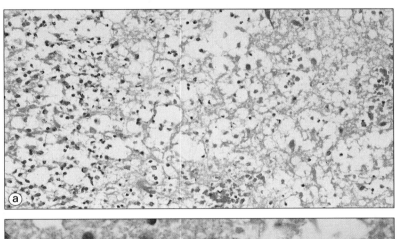

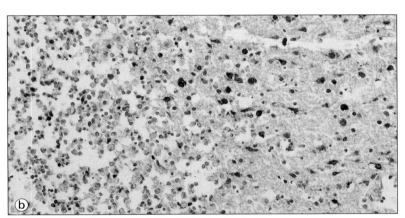

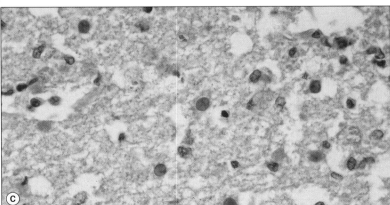

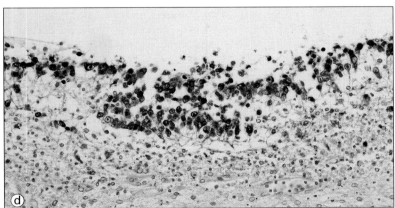

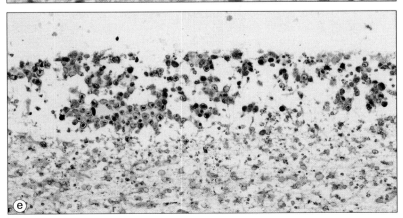

Fig. 12.25 Neonatal HSV-1 encephalitis. (a) There is a mixed inflammatory infiltrate towards the edge of a zone of necrosis within the cerebral cortex. **(b)** Immunohistochemistry reveals abundant HSV-1 antigen within the necrotic tissue. **(c)** There are typical herpesvirus intranuclear inclusions in this case of neonatal HSE. **(d)** Immunohistochemical demonstration of periventricular HSV-1 infection. **(e)** Section adjacent to that in (d) showing *in-situ* hybridization of a biotinylated probe for HSV DNA.

VARICELLA-ZOSTER VIRUS (VZV) INFECTION

VZV is the cause of varicella (chickenpox) and herpes zoster (shingles).

VARICELLA-ZOSTER VIRUS

- After presumed upper respiratory infection, primary viremic spread to the reticuloendothelial system, and secondary viremia, the virus spreads throughout the body, including to the skin, to cause the typical manifestations of chickenpox.
- Latent infection is subsequently established in the dorsal root or trigeminal ganglia or both, probably after retrograde axonal transport of virus from the periphery.
- Reactivation of latent virus usually manifests as shingles, which may involve the head and neck (the ophthalmic division of the trigeminal nerve is commonly involved), trunk, or extremities.
- Reactivation often occurs without an obvious precipitating event, but there are recognized risk factors, including cancer, lymphoma (especially Hodgkin's disease), ionizing radiation, and immunosuppression.
- The CNS may be involved during the primary infection (varicella) or the recrudescent disease (herpes zoster) (**Fig. 12.26,** and see Fig. 12.7).

Varicella cerebellitis

This complicates approximately 1 in 4000 cases of chickenpox and is usually a benign short-lived illness manifesting with meningism and ataxia. Viral antigen and DNA have been identified in the cerebrospinal fluid (CSF), which shows mild to moderate lymphocytosis.

Varicella meningoencephalitis

Less commonly, varicella is complicated by an encephalitic illness in which seizures and impaired consciousness are often prominent features. The onset of the encephalitis may precede or follow the development of the skin rash. There are conflicting reports concerning its pathology and probable pathogenesis. Some describe only scanty lymphocytic cuffing and edema; others record changes resembling those of acute disseminated encephalomyelitis. In most reports, virus has not been identified within the CNS, suggesting that the neurologic damage is immunologically mediated. Although most patients make a good recovery, a small percentage die during the acute illness or suffer permanent neurologic disability.

CNS manifestations of the VZV infection in children and adults	
Condition	CNS manifestation
Varicella	• cerebellitis • meningoencephalitis
Zoster	• encephalitis • myeloradiculitis • vasculopathy and vasculitis

Fig. 12.26 CNS manifestations of VZV infection in children and adults.

Zoster encephalitis and myeloradiculitis

These conditions usually occur in patients who are immunosuppressed. Many of the descriptions of zoster encephalitis and myeloradiculitis in the scientific literature relate to patients with AIDS.

ZOSTER ENCEPHALITIS AND MYELORADICULITIS

- A zosteriform skin rash usually (although not always) occurs 1–2 weeks before the development of the encephalitis or myeloradiculitis.
- Encephalitis presents nonspecifically with altered mentation, seizures, and variable neurologic deficits. Depending on the pattern of infection (see text), visual or bulbar symptoms may predominate.
- In myeloradiculitis, the presenting neurologic symptoms are usually ipsilateral to the rash. Paralysis is more prominent than sensory loss.

MACROSCOPIC AND MICROSCOPIC APPEARANCES

Several patterns are described, including:
- multifocal lesions predominantly involving the cerebral white matter
- ventriculitis
- encephalitis involving the visual system
- brain stem encephalitis
- myeloradiculitis

The first two patterns of infection are probably caused respectively by hematogenous and ventricular spread of virus, the third by spread from conjunctival and corneal lesions of ophthalmic zoster, and the last two by direct spread from the trigeminal or dorsal root ganglia. In all cases, the infection is typically necrotizing and associated with perivascular and interstitial infiltration by lymphocytes and macrophages. Intranuclear viral inclusions may be seen, and viral antigen and DNA are usually demonstrable. Neuronophagia and microglial nodules tend to be prominent features of brain stem zoster encephalitis. Parenchymal infection may be associated with a necrotizing or granulomatous vasculitis involving small or large intracranial blood vessels and causing infarcts or hemorrhages. These manifestations of VZV infection have been largely confined to patients with AIDS.

Zoster intracranial vasculopathy and vasculitis

Vasculitis may be a feature of VZV infections of the CNS. However, VZV may be associated with a CNS vasculopathy in the absence of parenchymal infection. Viral particles and antigen have been demonstrated in the walls of intracranial blood vessels in some cases and it has been postulated that an autoimmune process accounts for others.

A well-recognized, albeit rare complication of ophthalmic zoster is the development of contralateral hemiplegia. Angiography may demonstrate cerebral infarction due to inflammation (which may be granulomatous), focal necrosis, and thrombosis of the ipsilateral internal carotid artery or a major parenchymal artery (**Fig. 12.27**). In other patients the infarction is due to vasculitis involving smaller intracerebral arteries (**Fig. 12.28**).

Intrauterine VZV infection

Intrauterine VZV infection can cause varicella embryopathy, which is a syndrome of limb hypoplasia, CNS abnormalities (cerebral cortical atrophy, microcephaly, or hydrocephalus), cicatricial skin lesions, and ocular defects (chorioretinitis, cataracts, microphthalmia, optic atrophy). The risk is highest if maternal varicella occurs during the first 20 weeks of pregnancy. Although fetal infection occurs in approximately 25% of cases of maternal chickenpox, the risk of varicella embryopathy is much lower (approximately 2%).

MACROSCOPIC AND MICROSCOPIC APPEARANCES

In addition to the features described above, neuropathologic examination usually reveals foci of cystic degeneration, glial scarring, and microcalcification, but no viral inclusions or antigen. There may be inflammatory infiltrates. Very rarely, there is evidence of active necrotizing infection with viral inclusions and antigen (**Fig. 12.29**).

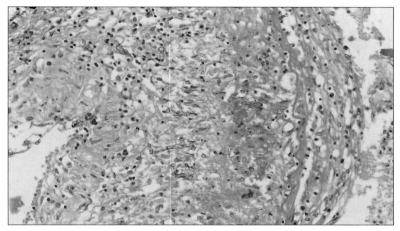

Fig. 12.27 Zoster vasculitis. Fibrinoid necrosis in the wall of the posterior cerebral artery in VZV infection. This is associated with an infiltrate of lymphocytes, macrophages, and multinucleated cells.

Neonatal VZV infection

Neonatal VZV infection complicates up to 35% of cases of maternal varicella during the late part of the third trimester or the postpartum period. Although a severe infection with multiple organ involvement may ensue, CNS lesions are uncommon.

EPSTEIN–BARR VIRUS (EBV) INFECTION

EBV is the etiologic agent of infectious mononucleosis. It is also associated with Burkitt's lymphoma and nasopharyngeal and other poorly differentiated or lymphoepithelioma-like carcinomas of the stomach, salivary gland, lung, and thymus. EBV probably contributes to the development of a range of B cell lymphoproliferative disorders, particularly in immunosuppressed patients, in whom it also causes oral hairy leukoplakia, and may play a role in the development of smooth muscle neoplasms.

EBV is present in the saliva during infectious mononucleosis and is usually spread in droplets and by direct contact. It establishes latent infection in B cells and causes their immortalization *in vitro*. Latent virus has also been detected in EBV-associated carcinomas and at necropsy in a wide range of tissues without EBV-related disease.

EBV may be associated with several peripheral nervous system disorders, including Guillain–Barré syndrome, mononeuritis, and polyneuritis (see Fig. 12.7). CNS complications of EBV infection are much less common and include aseptic meningitis (see p. 12.1), acute disseminated encephalomyelitis, and an acute cerebellitis resembling that associated with VZV (see p. 12.10). Rarely, the virus causes an encephalitis or myelitis, which may be combined with peripheral neurologic manifestations of infection. Most patients make a good recovery.

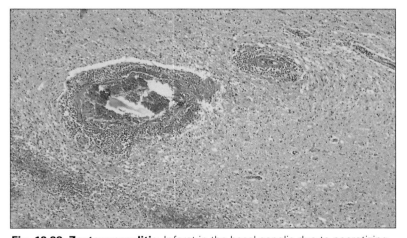

Fig. 12.28 Zoster vasculitis. Infarct in the basal ganglia due to necrotizing vasculitis in a patient with ophthalmic zoster.

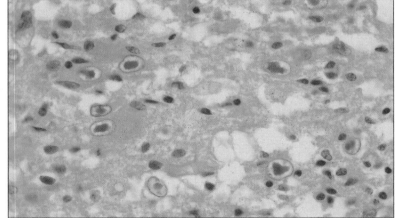

Fig. 12.29 Congenital VZV infection. Many of the nuclei in the cerebral cortex, deep gray matter, and brain stem contained viral inclusions. This unusual case complicated maternal chickenpox at 12 weeks' gestation. (Courtesy of Dr L.R. Bridges, University of Leeds.)

CYTOMEGALOVIRUS (CMV) INFECTION

In immunocompetent children and adults, CMV infection causes an infectious mononucleosis-like syndrome. The virus may be spread through saliva, urine, sexual contact, or blood transfusion. Spread is facilitated by crowded living conditions and, as a result, infection tends to occur at an earlier age in lower socioeconomic groups. Latent infection is probably established in peripheral blood lymphocytes and monocytes.

CMV encephalitis and myeloradiculitis

Although CMV may cause encephalitis and myeloradiculitis, these complications of infection are uncommon in patients with normal immune function. Much of the literature on CMV encephalitis and myeloradiculitis concerns patients with AIDS (see chapter 13), in whom several patterns of infection may occur (see below). The majority (approximately 90%) of patients with AIDS and CMV encephalitis also have CMV retinitis; conversely, approximately 40% of those with CMV retinitis also have CMV encephalitis. Although CMV retinitis usually responds well to ganciclovir or foscarnet, these agents do not prevent the development of CMV encephalitis. The development of symptoms of CMV encephalitis (i.e. impaired mentation, confusion, disorientation, and, in some patients, nystagmus and cranial nerve palsies) carries a poor prognosis in patients with AIDS.

MACROSCOPIC AND MICROSCOPIC APPEARANCES

Several patterns are described, including:
- low-grade encephalitis, with cytomegalic inclusion cells, usually but not always within microglial nodules
- necrotizing encephalitis, with large cystic foci resembling old infarcts
- ventriculoencephalitis, with hemorrhagic necrosis of periventricular brain tissue
- lumbosacral myeloradiculitis

These are discussed and illustrated under HIV infection (see chapter 13).

Congenital CMV infection

This is the commonest of the known intrauterine viral infections, affecting 0.2–2.2% of live births.

MACROSCOPIC AND MICROSCOPIC APPEARANCES

During the acute infection, the neuropathologic features are of a necrotizing encephalitis or ventriculoencephalitis with infiltration by lymphocytes and macrophages, microglial nodules, and typical cytomegalic inclusion cells (**Fig. 12.31**). Neurons, glia, and endothelial cells may be infected. Immunohistochemistry or in-situ hybridization reveals that many more cells are infected by virus than those showing cytomegalic change.

Residual lesions in those surviving the acute neonatal illness include microcephaly, microgyria, porencephalic cysts, hydrocephalus, and periventricular calcification.

HUMAN HERPESVIRUS 6

Human herpesvirus 6 is the cause of exanthem subitum (roseola infantum), a benign disease of infants and children characterized by a high fever and, as the fever subsides, a faint maculopapular rash. The pre-eruptive stage of the disease may be complicated by febrile seizures or, rarely, an encephalitic illness. Viral DNA has been detected in the CSF of some patients. Most make a good recovery.

B VIRUS

This herpesvirus is indigenous to Old World monkeys, but can cause human infection. Transmission to humans is usually by monkey bite, but rare cases of monkey-to-human spread are presumed to have been mediated by infected respiratory droplets and human-to-human transmission has occurred. In humans, B virus tends to cause a rapidly progressive necrotizing infection of the CNS (i.e. ascending myelitis leading to widespread panencephalitis).

CONGENITAL CMV INFECTION

- In most cases, congenital CMV infection is due to transplacental spread of virus from an infected mother.
- The risk of fetal transmission is approximately 40% during primary maternal infection, but less than 2% during recrudescent maternal disease.
- As women in lower socioeconomic groups living in crowded conditions are more likely to have been exposed to CMV in childhood, only approximately 10% of these women are susceptible to primary infection during pregnancy compared with up to 50% of women from higher socioeconomic groups in developed countries.
- The risk of fetal complications is related to the gestational age at the time of infection, and is highest when infection occurs during the first trimester.
- Neonatal infection is occasionally acquired postnatally by contact with infected genital secretions, saliva, or breast milk.

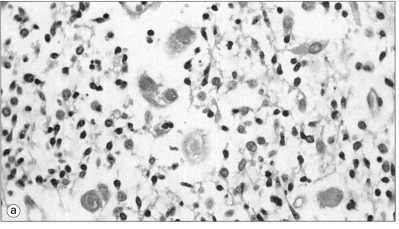
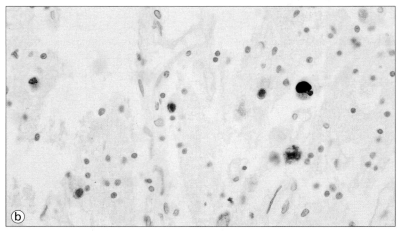

Fig. 12.30 Congenital CMV encephalitis. (a) Scattered cytomegalic inclusion cells are seen within the germinal matrix. **(b)** Immunohistochemical demonstration of CMV in scattered cells in the disrupted basal ganglia. Not all of the virus-containing cells have a cytomegalic appearance.

MANIFESTATIONS OF CONGENITAL CMV INFECTION

- Only 10–15% of infected neonates develop symptomatic infection although careful examintion of 'asymptomatic' cases often discloses minor neurologic impairment, particularly sensorineural hearing loss.
- The manifestations of symptomatic neonatal infection include hepatosplenomegaly with liver dysfunction and consumptive coagulopathy, microcephaly with intracranial calcifications, and chorioretinitis.
- Up to 30% of infants die during the acute illness.
- Most survivors have residual neurologic defects, including mental retardation, microcephaly, learning difficulties, seizures, sensorineural hearing loss, chorioretinitis, and optic atrophy.

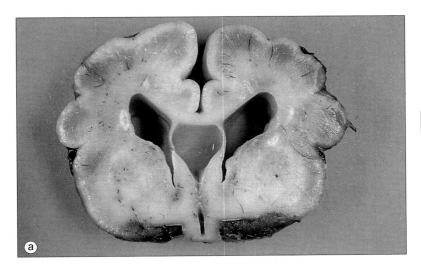

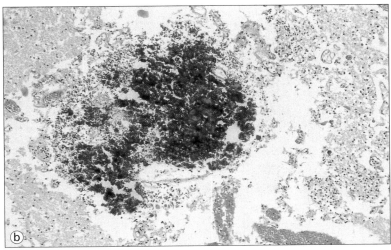

Fig. 12.31 Congenital CMV encephalitis. (a) Note the ventricular dilation and periventricular calcification. (Courtesy of Dr. Helen Porter, Bristol Children's Hospital, U.K.) **(b)** Large focus of periventricular calcification due to CMV encephalitis.

RUBELLA ENCEPHALITIS

ETIOLOGY AND PATHOGENESIS OF RUBELLA

- Rubella virus is a small enveloped RNA virus and is the only member of the genus Rubivirus in the Togavirus family.
- In children and adults, this virus causes German measles, which is a benign exanthematous disease complicated in some cases by arthritis, and rarely, by postinfectious acute disseminated encephalomyelitis.
- It is, however, the fetus that is most at risk from rubella virus.
  - Most cases of fetal infection are associated with symptomatic maternal infection during pregnancy, but in approximately 35% of cases the maternal infection is subclinical.
  - The risk of teratogenic fetal damage declines from approximately 50% during the first month of pregnancy to 5% by the fourth month.
  - Congenital rubella is now rarely seen in countries with vaccination programs for female children, but remains a health problem in developing regions.

RUBELLA INFECTION

- The classic rubella syndrome of cardiac and vascular malformations, cataracts, mental retardation, microcephaly, and deafness occurs only after first trimester infections.
- In second trimester infections, fetal damage, when it occurs, is usually limited to mental retardation and deafness.
- Neonates may manifest an 'expanded' syndrome of continuing rubella infection, which includes pneumonitis and hepatosplenomegaly with severe thrombocytopenia. This syndrome may persist for several months after birth. Occasionally, it develops after an initial period of apparent quiescence.
- Very rarely, congenital or postnatal rubella infection manifests up to a decade or more later as a slowly progressive panencephalitis.

MACROSCOPIC AND MICROSCOPIC APPEARANCES

Macroscopic abnormalities are usually a consequence of first-trimester infection. The commonest are microcephaly, hydrocephalus, and foci of cavitation in the cerebral white matter.

Microscopically, the 'expanded' rubella syndrome may be associated with active meningoencephalitis. Much more commonly, histology reveals only chronic lesions, consisting of vascular and parenchymal mineralization, particularly in the basal ganglia and thalamus (**Fig. 12.32**).

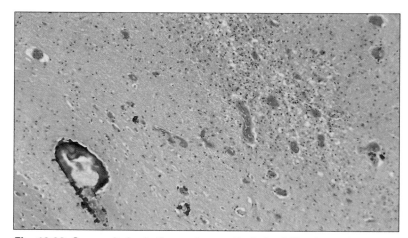

Fig. 12.32 Congenital rubella syndrome. Foci of calcification and necrosis in the basal ganglia of an infant with first trimester infection, who also had cardiac malformations and cataracts.

RABIES

ETIOLOGY AND PATHOGENESIS OF RABIES

Rabies virus is an RNA virus of the genus Lyssavirus in the Rhabdovirus family (Fig. 12.33).

Etiology

- The disease is endemic in animals in the Americas, large parts of Europe, Africa, and Central Asia. Rabies-free countries include the United Kingdom, Sweden, Portugal, Japan, Australia, and New Zealand.
- Rabies is usually transmitted by the bite of a rabid animal. Dogs are still an important source of human rabies in many parts of the world.
- In most developed countries, however, vaccination programs have limited or eradicated rabies in domestic dogs; as a result, wild animals are usually responsible for transmitting the disease. These include foxes (particularly in Europe, but also in North America), skunks, raccoons, and lynx (in North America), vampire bats (particularly in South America), wolves (in Asia and parts of Europe), jackals (in Africa), and mongooses (in Africa and parts of Asia).
- The disease may also be spread by nonimmune domestic cats.
- Aerosol transmission is a recognized but rare consequence of visiting caves populated by infected bats.

Pathogenesis

- In most cases, rabies virus replicates within skeletal muscle at the site of inoculation before being taken up by axons and transported centripetally to the CNS. At this stage, the virus replicates and spreads within the CNS through the spinal cord and brain stem to the cerebrum and cerebellum.
- Virus is also transported centrifugally within nerve fibers to peripheral tissues, including the salivary and lacrimal glands, from which virus is shed in saliva and tears. Transmission has occurred by corneal transplantation.

MACROSCOPIC AND MICROSCOPIC APPEARANCES

The brain and spinal cord may appear swollen, but are usually macroscopically normal.

Microscopically, the appearances are of a widespread polioencephalomyelitis. The classic histologic feature is the presence of Negri bodies, which are sharply delineated, round or oval, eosinophilic inclusions in the neuronal cytoplasm (**Fig. 12.34**). Some neurons contain less well-defined (although ultrastructurally similar) eosinophilic inclusions, termed lyssa bodies. There may occasionally be coarse vacuolation of the cytoplasm of infected neurons. The inclusions can occur in most parts of the CNS, but tend to be easiest to find in Purkinje cells, hippocampal pyramidal cells, and brain stem nuclei.

Although there are usually leptomeningeal and perivascular

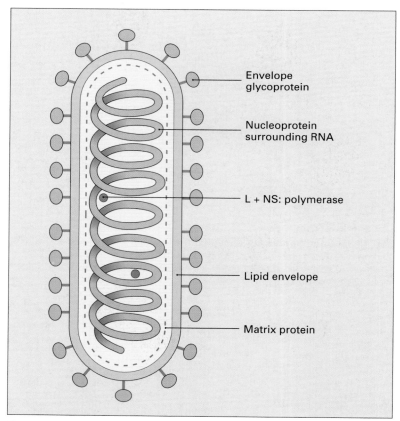

Fig. 12.33 Schematic illustration of rabies virus.

Envelope glycoprotein

Nucleoprotein surrounding RNA

L + NS: polymerase

Lipid envelope

Matrix protein

lymphocytic infiltrates and neuronophagia, there may be a striking disparity between the abundance of virus and the limited degree of inflammation. The clusters of microglia that remain after neuronal destruction are known as Babès' nodules (**Fig. 12.35**).

Paralytic rabies is characterized by striking neuronal destruction and inflammation involving the brain stem, gray matter of the spinal cord, and dorsal root ganglia, with relatively scanty inclusion bodies in these regions, although Negri bodies can usually be found in the Purkinje cells and hippocampus.

Immunostaining of virus usually shows it to be much more abundant than is evident on conventional microscopy (**Fig. 12.36**). Virus can be identified by immunofluorescence in corneal cells and in cutaneous nerve fibers. The disease can therefore be confirmed by examining corneal impressions or nuchal skin biopsies.

RABIES INFECTION

Incubation period

The incubation period ranges from as little as 10 days to as long as 1 year, or, very rarely, longer. The incubation period is shorter in children than adults and also varies according to the proximity of the site of inoculation to the CNS, the onset of symptoms being most rapid after bites on the head.

Prodrome

The onset of CNS disease is heralded by a 2–10-day period of flu-like symptoms (i.e. headache, fever, malaise) and occasionally pain or paresthesia at the site of the bite.

Acute neurologic disease

The acute neurologic disease lasts 2–7 days. This takes one of two forms, which may overlap:
- 'Furious' rabies is the commoner form and is characterized by agitation, insomnia, aggressive behavior (which may include biting), hallucinations, hydrophobia, and brain stem dysfunction (including dysphagia, dysarthria, nystagmus, and cardiorespiratory disturbances).
- 'Dumb' rabies, the other form, is characterized by paralysis of one or more limbs and sometimes ascending paralysis simulating Guillain–Barré syndrome, sensory loss, and incontinence.

Terminal stage

- The acute neurologic disease progresses to stupor, coma, and death. Complications that may occur during this terminal stage include inappropriate ADH secretion, diabetes insipidus, cardiac and respiratory failure.

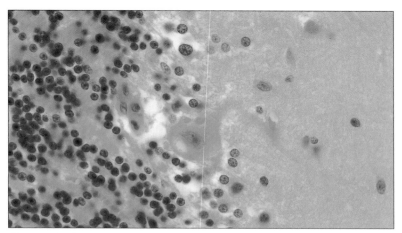

Fig. 12.34 Negri bodies. This section from a case of rabies encephalitis shows a Purkinje cell containing two Negri bodies (arrows). Note the absence of inflammation.

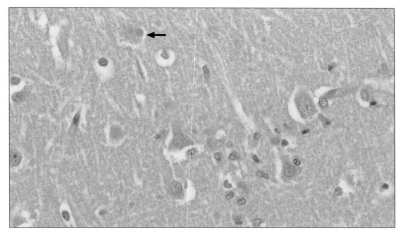

Fig. 12.35 Rabies encephalitis. Cluster of microglia (arrowheads) in the parahippocampal gyrus. One of the remaining neurons contains a Negri body (arrow). (Courtesy of Professor Francoise Gray, Hôpital Raymond Poincare, Paris)

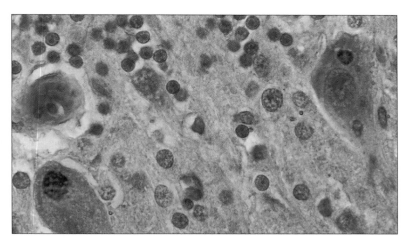

Fig. 12.36 Rabies encephalitis. The red immunolabeling product highlights the abundant rabies virus antigen in infected Purkinje cells. (Courtesy of Professor Francoise Gray, Hôpital Raymond Poincare, Paris)

ARBOVIRUS INFECTIONS

Arboviruses are small enveloped RNA viruses transmitted predominantly by arthropod vectors (i.e. arthropod-borne viruses). Most arbovirus infections are asymptomatic or produce only a mild febrile illness. Although some arboviruses are capable of causing hemorrhagic fever or encephalitis, these occur in only a small proportion of infections. Arbovirus encephalitis is rarely encountered in neuropathology practice. Four virus families harbor arboviruses: Togaviridae, Flaviviridae, Bunyaviridae, and Reoviridae. Only those arboviruses that are capable of causing encephalitis are considered here.

PATHOGENESIS OF ARBOVIRUS INFECTIONS

- The virus enters the vector (usually a mosquito or tick) while it is feeding on the blood of an infected host. It is then transmitted to further hosts in the salivary secretions of the vector as it feeds. The natural hosts of most arboviruses are birds or small mammals such as rodents: Humans (and horses, in the case of the equine encephalitides) are dead-end hosts.
- The virus replicates at the site of host inoculation and then spreads to regional lymph nodes and other lymphoreticular tissues (primary viremia) where it proliferates before disseminating hematogenously (secondary viremia) to systemic tissues, including, in some cases, the CNS.

ETIOLOGY OF ARBOVIRUS INFECTIONS

Togaviridae
- Genomes comprise positive-sense, single-stranded, polyadenylated, non-segmented RNA.
- Only the genus Alphavirus includes arboviruses, three of which are important causes of mosquito-borne encephalitis: Eastern equine encephalitis, Western equine encephalitis, and Venezuelan equine encephalitis (VEE); the related VEE II Everglades virus is readily spread in aerosol form.
- The genus Rubivirus is also in the Togavirus family and includes rubella virus, which is not an arbovirus and is considered on p.12.13.

Flaviviridae
- Genomes comprise positive-sense, single-stranded, non-polyadenylated, non-segmented RNA.
- Causes of mosquito-borne encephalitis in this family include: St Louis encephalitis, Japanese encephalitis, Murray Valley encephalitis.
- This family also includes a group of closely related tick-borne encephalitis-causing viruses such as the viruses that cause Powassan encephalitis and Russian spring–summer encephalitis.

Bunyaviridae
- Genomes comprise segmented, single-stranded, non-polyadenylated RNA that is negative-sense (apart from the genus Phlebovirus, which contains ambisense RNA, the 5′-end being positive-stranded and the 3′-end negative-stranded).
- Two genera in this family (i.e. Bunyavirus and Phlebovirus) include arboviruses that cause mosquito-borne human encephalitis.
  - Bunyavirus encephalitides include those caused by California serogroup viruses (especially La Crosse virus), Tahyna virus, and Jamestown Canyon virus.
  - The Phlebovirus most often associated with human encephalitis is Rift Valley fever virus, which can be spread in aerosol form.

Reoviridae
- Genomes comprise double-stranded RNA.
- Colorado tick fever virus in the genus Orbivirus is the only significant cause of human tick-borne encephalitis in this family.

EPIDEMIOLOGY OF ARBOVIRUS INFECTION

- The geographic distribution of different arboviruses reflects that of the natural hosts and insect vectors (**Fig. 12.37**).
- There is marked seasonal variation in the incidence of most arbovirus infections corresponding to the fluctuation in quantity of insect vectors. Infections are most numerous in the summer and early fall months. The number of cases also varies considerably from year to year.
- Some types of infection have a predilection for the young: Western equine encephalitis usually infects children less than 1 year of age; Eastern equine encephalitis infects children and the elderly; La Crosse virus encephalitis is the commonest pediatric arbovirus encephalitis in the U.S.A.

The geographic distribution of different arboviruses	
Virus	Geographic distribution
Eastern equine encephalitis	• Eastern and Gulf coast states of USA, Caribbean, and South America, and rarely further inland
Western equine encephalitis	• Predominantly western and midwestern USA
VEE	• South and Central America, Florida, and southwestern USA
St Louis encephalitis virus	• Endemic throughout the Americas
Japanese encephalitis	• Southeast Asia
Murray valley encephalitis	• Southwestern Australia, New Guinea
Powassan encephalitis	• Canada, northern USA, and Russia
Russian spring–summer encephalitis	• Russia, east Asia
La Crosse virus	• Mainly midwestern USA
Tahyna virus	• Czech Republic, Slovakia
Jamestown Canyon virus	• Northern central USA

Fig. 12.37 The geographic distribution of different arboviruses.

MACROSCOPIC APPEARANCES

The brain tends to be moderately congested and swollen (**Fig. 12.39**). There may be petechial hemorrhages. The most severely affected parts of the brain are the basal ganglia, thalamus, and brain stem in Western or Eastern equine encephalitis, and the midbrain and thalamus in St Louis encephalitis. In Japanese encephalitis the lesions may be widely distributed throughout the brain and spinal cord (see Fig. 12.41).

ARBOVIRUS INFECTION

- The incubation period is usually <1 week but can be up to 3 weeks.
- Patients present acutely with fever (sometimes marked), malaise and myalgias.
- Manifestations of neurologic disease are relatively nonspecific and include:
  - headache and vomiting
  - an altered level of consciousness, disorientation
  - flaccid or spastic paralysis
  - seizures.
- Progression to coma may occur rapidly.
- In some cases the neurological features are solely of aseptic meningitis.
- The precise viral etiology is usually determined by serologic tests or by isolation of virus or specific viral RNA from the CSF.
- The mortality and morbidity of the encephalitis caused by different arboviruses vary considerably (**Fig 12.38**).

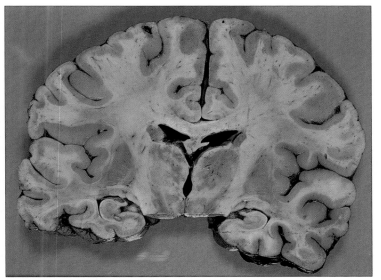

Fig. 12.39 Coronal slice through the brain in a case of Japanese encephalitis. The brain is congested and there is mottled dusky discoloration of the thalamus and upper part of the midbrain. (Courtesy of Professor Francesco Scaravilli, Institute of Neurology, Queen Square, London)

Mortality and morbidity of arbovirus encephalitis		
Causative virus	Mortality	Morbidity
Eastern equine encephalitis	50–75%	90% of survivors have persistent neurologic disability
Western equine encephalitis and VEE	Less than 5%	
St Louis encephalitis	Less than 5%	Persistent neurologic disability in approximately 25% of survivors
Japanese encephalitis	Up to 50%	Persistent neurologic disability in a high proportion of survivors
LaCrosse virus	Less than 1%	
Tick-borne encephalitides	Varies from less than 1% to over 10%	A small proportion of patients with Russian spring–summer encephalitis who recover from the acute illness later develop a chronic encephalitis with intractable epilepsy and progressive paralysis

Fig. 12.38 Mortality and morbidity of arbovirus encephalitis.

MICROSCOPIC APPEARANCES

Histology reveals leptomeningeal, perivascular, and parenchymal infiltration, predominantly by lymphocytes and microglia or macrophages (**Fig. 12.40, 12.41**). Affected gray matter regions contain perivascular cuffs of mononuclear inflammatory cells, especially lymphocytes, perivascular hemorrhages, and microglial nodules, often surrounding degenerating neuronal cell bodies (neuronophagia) (**Fig. 12.42**). The perivascular inflammation in the white matter is associated with focal

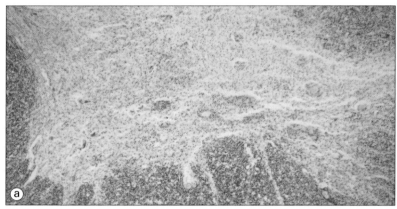

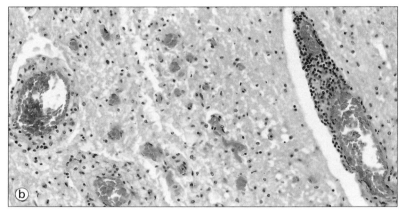

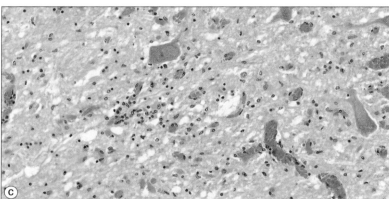

Fig. 12.40 Inflammatory lesions in the cervical cord in Japanese encephalitis. (a) There is extensive destruction of anterior horn cells and infiltration of the gray matter by mononuclear inflammatory cells. (Luxol fast blue/cresyl violet) **(b)** Higher magnification of a section stained with hematoxylin and eosin shows accumulation of foamy macrophages and perivascular cuffing by lymphocytes. **(c)** Cluster of lymphocytes and macrophages within the gray matter in a better-preserved part of the spinal cord. (Courtesy of Professor Francesco Scaravilli, Institute of Neurology, London)

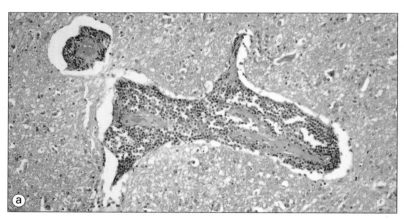

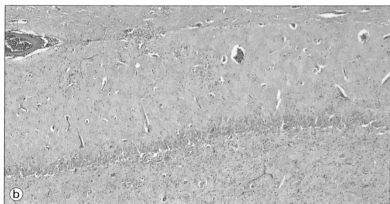

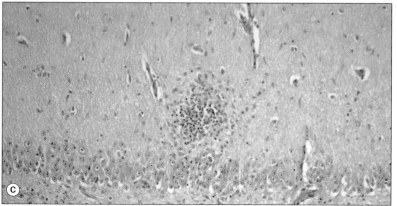

Fig. 12.41 Eastern equine encephalitis in a horse. (a) There is prominent cuffing of blood vessels by mononuclear inflammatory cells with vacuolation of the surrounding gray matter. **(b)** The hippocampus contains parenchymal infiltrates of inflammatory cells. **(c)** The hippocampus also contains compact microglial nodules similar to those seen in other forms of viral encephalitis. (Prepared from material provided by Dr R.V. Jones and Bruce H. Williams, Armed Forces Institute of Pathology, Washington D.C., U.S.A.)

necrosis of myelinated fibers. Other features include thrombosed small blood vessels and, rarely, large regions of necrosis.

These viruses do not produce distinctive nuclear or cytoplasmic inclusions. If viral infection is suspected at necropsy or biopsy, material should be taken for electron microscopy and viral culture.

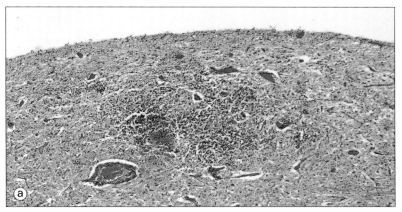

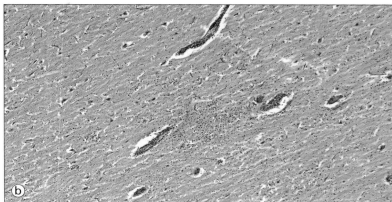

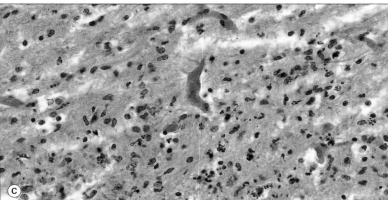

Fig. 12.42 Deep gray matter in a horse with Venezuelan equine encephalitis. (a) There is dense inflammation and focal hemorrhage in the subependymal region. The ependyma itself has sloughed. **(b)** There are perivascular and parenchymal infiltrates of inflammatory cells in the gray matter. **(c)** Higher magnification reveals parenchymal hemorrhage, neuronal necrosis, and surrounding acute and chronic inflammation. Prepared from material provided by Dr R.V. Jones and Bruce H. Williams, Armed Forces Institute of Pathology, Washington D.C., U.S.A.

REFERENCES

Amlielefond C, KleinschmidtDeMasters BK, Mahalingam R, Davis LE, Gilden DH (1995) The vasculopathy of varicella-zoster virus encephalitis. *Ann Neurol* **37**: 784–790.

Anonymous (1992) Arboviral diseases—United States, 1992. *Morbid Mortal Weekly Rep* **42**: 467–468.

Ansari MZ, Shope RE (1994) Epidemiology of arboviral infections. *Publ Health Rev* **22**: 1–26.

Bodian D (1949) Poliomyelitis: pathologic anatomy. In *Poliomyelitis: Papers and Discussions Presented at the First International Poliomyelitis Conference*. pp. 62–84. Philadelphia: Lippincott.

Calisher CH (1994) Medically important arboviruses of the United States and Canada. *Clin Microbiol Rev* **7**: 89–116.

Freij BJ, Sever JL (1992) Congenital viral infections. *Curr Opin Infect Dis* **5**: 558–568.

Gray F *et al.* (1994) Varicella-zoster virus infection of the central nervous system in the acquired immune deficiency syndrome. *Brain* **117**: 987–989.

Griffin DE (1995) Arboviruses and the central nervous system. *Springer Semin Immunopathol* **17**: 121–132.

Liedtke W, Opalka B, Zimmermann CW, Lignitz E (1993) Age distribution of latent herpes simplex virus-1 and varicella-zoster virus genome in human nervous tissue. *J Neurol Sci* **116**: 6–11.

Mackenzie JS, Lindsay MD, Coelen RD, Broom AK, Hall RA, Smith DW (1994) Arboviruses causing human disease in the Australian zoogeographic region. *Arch Virol* **136**: 447–467.

Miller E, Cradock Watson JE, Pollock TM (1982) Consequences of confirmed maternal rubella at successive stages of pregnancy. *Lancet* **2**: 781–784.

Mrak RE, Young L (1994) Rabies encephalitis in humans—pathology, pathogenesis and pathophysiology. *J Neuropathol Exp Neurol* **53**: 1–10.

Nicoll JAR, Maitland NJ, Love S (1991) Necropsy neuropathological findings in 'burnt out' herpes simplex encephalitis and use of the polymerase chain reaction to detect viral DNA. *Neuropathol Appl Neurobiol* **17**: 375–382.

Pastuszak AL *et al.* (1994) Outcome after maternal varicella infection in the first 20 weeks of pregnancy. *N Engl J Med* **330**: 901–905.

Picard FJ, Poland SD, Rice GPA (1993) New developments with herpesviruses and the nervous system. *Curr Opin Neurol Neurosurg* **6**: 169–175.

Rotbart HA (1995) Enteroviral infections of the CNS. *Clin Infect Dis* **20**: 971–981.

Sever JL (1979) Congenital rubella. *Clin Perinatal* **6**: 347–352.

Sloots TP, Mackay IM, Pope JH (1995) Diagnosis of human herpesvirus-6 infection in 2 patients with central nervous system complications. *Clin Diag Virol* **3**: 333–341.

Suga S *et al.* (1993) Clinical and virological analyses of 21 infants with exanthem subitum (roseola infantum) and central nervous system complications. *Ann Neurol* **33**: 597–603.

Vinters HV *et al.* (1989) Cytomegalovirus in the nervous system of patients with the acquired immune deficiency syndrome. *Brain* **112**: 245–268.

Wattre P, Dewilde A, Lobert PE (1995) Actualités sur la pathologie du cytomegalovirus humain. *Rev Med Intern* **16**: 354–367.

Whitley R *et al.* The National Institute of Allergy and Infectious Diseases Collaborative Antiviral Study Group (1991) Predictors of morbidity and mortality in neonates with herpes simplex virus infections. *N Engl J Med* **324**: 450–454.

Whitley RJ (1991) Arthropod-borne encephalitides. In Scheld WM, Whitley RJ, Durack DT (eds) *Infections of the Central Nervous System*. pp. 87–111. New York: Raven Press.

Whitley RJ, Middlebrooks M (1991) Rabies. In Scheld WM, Whitley RJ, Durack DT (eds) *Infections of the Central Nervous System*. pp. 127–144. New York: Raven Press.

Whitley RJ, Schlitt M (1991) Encephalitis caused by herpesviruses, including B virus. In Scheld WM, Whitley RJ, Durack DT (eds) *Infections of the Central Nervous System*. pp. 41–86. New York: Raven Press.

Whitley RJ, Stagno S (1991) Perinatal viral infections. In Scheld WM, Whitley RJ, Durack DT (eds) *Infections of the Central Nervous System*. pp. 167–200. New York: Raven Press.

Chronic and subacute viral infections of the CNS

Chronic/subacute viral infections of the central nervous system (CNS) tend to progress over months or years rather than days or weeks. The incubation period is usually considerably longer than that of acute viral infections. In the past, classifications of chronic (slow) virus infections have included Creutzfeldt–Jakob disease and other spongiform encephalopathies, but according to current understanding of the pathogenesis of these diseases this designation is inappropriate. The spongiform encephalopathies are considered in chapter 32.

SUBACUTE MEASLES ENCEPHALITIDES

MEASLES INCLUSION BODY ENCEPHALITIS

MACROSCOPIC AND MICROSCOPIC APPEARANCES

Macroscopically, the brain usually appears normal, although there may be foci of softening and discoloration. Histology reveals occasional or numerous foci of hypercellularity (**Fig. 13.1**), within which many neurons and some astrocytes and oligodendrocytes contain eosinophilic inclusion bodies (**Fig. 13.2**). Most of these are intranuclear, largely filling the nucleus, apart from a few pyknotic clumps of marginated chromatin. Less well-defined eosinophilic inclusions may be visible in the cytoplasm (see Fig. 13.2). The lesions also contain reactive astrocytes and microglia (**Fig. 13.3**), and occasional multinucleated cells may be seen (**Fig. 13.4**). The lesions occur in any part of the brain. The inclusions are readily seen in hematoxylin–eosin preparations and can also be demonstrated immunohistochemically (**Fig. 13.5**) or by electron microscopy (**Fig. 13.6**).

MEASLES

Measles virus is an enveloped virus of the Morbillivirus genus in the Paramyxovirus family. It contains single-stranded, negative-sense RNA and six proteins (NP, L, P, H, F, and M), of which one, the M (matrix) protein, is required for virus particle assembly. The virus is highly contagious and is acquired by inhalation of infected fomites. It usually causes a short-lived febrile disease and a characteristic maculopapular rash.
CNS involvement commonly produces an aseptic meningitis (see p 12.1) or, acute disseminated encephalomyelitis, which is a postinfectious inflammatory disorder. Much less commonly, measles causes a subacute or chronic infective encephalitis, of which there are two forms:
- Measles inclusion body encephalitis, which develops within months of the initial systemic infection in patients with impaired cell-mediated immunity.
- Subacute sclerosing panencephalitis (SSPE), which is a more delayed manifestation of the initial infection and occurs in patients without any immunologic impairment. Its pathogenesis remains uncertain, but involves defective expression of M protein despite the presence of an intact coding sequence. The disease is characterized serologically by high levels of circulating antibodies to most measles antigens apart from M protein.

MEASLES INCLUSION BODY ENCEPHALITIS

- Measles inclusion body encephalitis is a rare disorder, developing within several months of exposure to, or apparent recovery from, measles.
- Most patients have depressed cell-mediated immunity.
- Presenting symptoms and signs include seizures, confusion, and a variety of focal neurologic deficits, and later coma.
- It is usually fatal within a few weeks of onset.

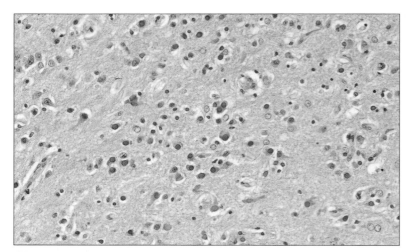

Fig. 13.1 Measles inclusion body encephalitis. There is a focal region of hypercellularity in the cerebral cortex.

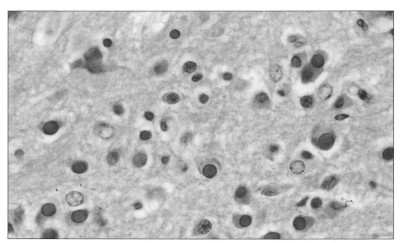

Fig. 13.2 Inclusion bodies in measles inclusion body encephalitis. These fill the nuclei of neurons and glia. Eosinophilic inclusions are also visible in the cytoplasm of some of the cells.

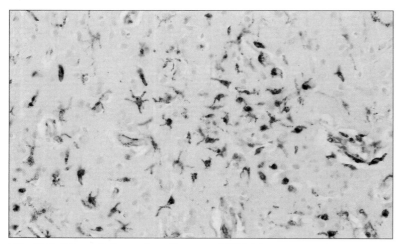

Fig. 13.3 Microglial reaction. Clusters of CD68–immunoreactive microglia are present within the foci of hypercellularity in measles inclusion body encephalitis.

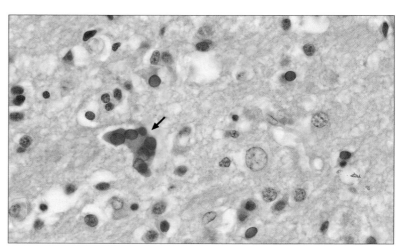

Fig. 13.4 Measles inclusion body encephalitis. Multinucleated cell (arrow) with nuclear inclusion bodies.

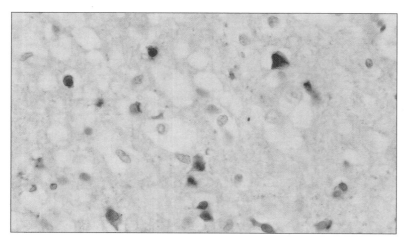

Fig. 13.5 Immunohistochemical demonstration of measles virus antigen. In contrast to the paucity of viral antigen in SSPE, in measles inclusion body encephalitis antigen is abundant.

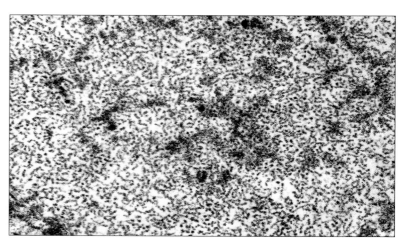

Fig. 13.6 Measles virus nucleocapsid particles in the nucleus of an infected neuron.

SUBACUTE SCLEROSING PANENCEPHALITIS (SSPE)

SUBACUTE SCLEROSING PANENCEPHALITIS

SSPE is a chronic progressive encephalitis that follows exposure to the measles virus by several years.
- Age of onset is usually 5–15 years.
- SSPE is more likely if the initial exposure to measles occurs at less than 18 months of age.
- The course of disease is variable. It can result in death within months or progress only intermittently. Survival in excess of 10 years is well documented.

Clinical staging of SSPE
- I. Intellectual impairment and behavioral changes.
- II. Repetitive, symmetric myoclonic jerks every 5–10 seconds.
- III. Increasing mental deterioration, development of various combinations of ataxia, spasticity, choreoathetosis and dystonias, and gradual disappearance of myoclonus.
- IV. Stupor, autonomic disturbances, coma, and eventually death.

MACROSCOPIC APPEARANCES

Often the brain is macroscopically normal. However, in cases of longer duration, there is usually moderate to marked brain atrophy and the white matter may have an abnormally firm texture and a mottled gray appearance.

MICROSCOPIC APPEARANCES

There is a chronic encephalitis, with leptomeningeal, perivascular, and parenchymal infiltration by lymphocytes (predominantly T cells) and microglia (**Fig. 13.7**).

The distribution and severity of lesions are variable, but the cerebral cortex, white matter, basal ganglia, and thalamus are usually involved. The affected gray matter shows inflammation, gliosis (**Fig. 13.8a**), loss of neurons, occasional neuronophagia, and sparse intranuclear inclusions, which are sharply defined eosinophilic bodies with a surrounding clear space ('halo') (**Fig. 13.8b**). In most cases these sparse inclusion bodies can be detected immunohistochemically. Another finding, in some cases of several years' duration, is the presence of Alzheimer-type neurofibrillary tangles (**Fig. 13.9**). These are most often found in the cerebral cortex and hippocampus, and may be numerous.

The affected white matter is severely gliotic and is characterized by a predominantly perivascular inflammation and a patchy loss of myelinated fibers (see Fig. 13.7b, 13.8a).

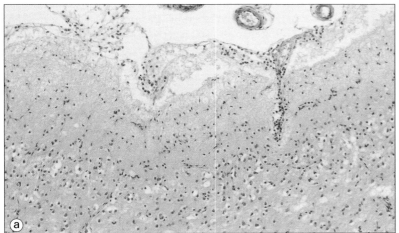

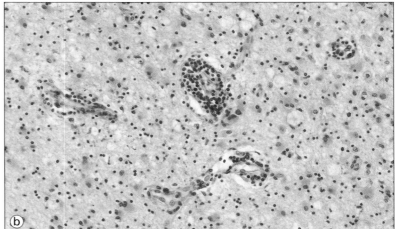

Fig. 13.7 SSPE. Leptomeningeal, perivascular, and parenchymal infiltration of the cerebral cortex **(a)** and white matter **(b)** by mononuclear inflammatory cells in SSPE. Note the marked reactive gliosis.

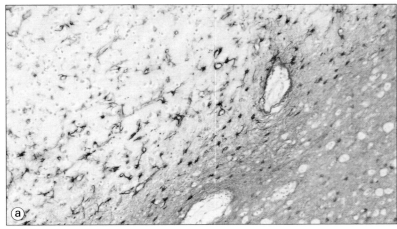

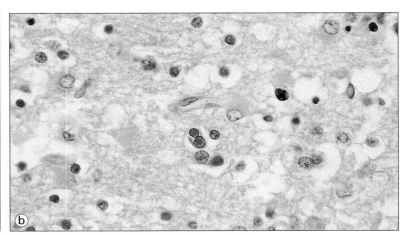

Fig. 13.8 Gliosis and intranuclear inclusions in SSPE. (a) Dense gliosis of the white matter and deep cerebral cortex in SSPE. Immunostained for glial fibrillary acidic protein. **(b)** Intranuclear inclusions. These are sparse in

SSPE and may be absent, particularly if the disease has run a protracted course.

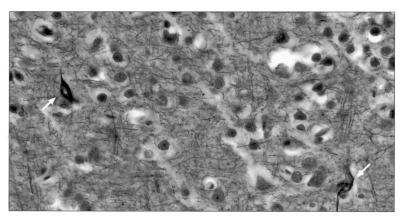

Fig. 13.9 SSPE. Scattered neurofibrillary tangles (arrows) in the cerebral cortex. These are most numerous in cases with illness of long duration. (Palmgren silver impregnation)

PROGRESSIVE RUBELLA PANENCEPHALITIS

This is a very rare, delayed complication of intrauterine or childhood rubella infection, presenting years later with intellectual impairment, ataxia, seizures, spasticity, and choreoathetosis. The disease progresses slowly over several years until the patient becomes decerebrate and eventually dies.

MICROSCOPIC APPEARANCES
Reported findings include widespread neuronal and white matter destruction with leptomeningeal and perivascular infiltration by lymphocytes and macrophages, severe gliosis, fibrinoid necrosis, and mineralization of small blood vessels. No inclusion bodies are seen.

PROGRESSIVE MULTIFOCAL LEUKOENCEPHALOPATHY (PML)

Until two decades ago, this was a rare disease, predominantly affecting small numbers of patients with leukemias, lymphomas, and renal transplants. Since then, the incidence of PML has increased several-fold, mainly because of its relatively frequent occurrence in patients with AIDS.

MACROSCOPIC APPEARANCES
The cut surface of the fixed brain affected by PML appears asymmetrically pitted by small foci of gray discoloration mixed with larger confluent areas of abnormal parenchyma, which may be centrally necrotic (**Figs 13.10, 13.11**). The lesions tend to be most numerous in the cerebral white matter, but also involve the cerebral cortex and deep gray matter (**Figs 13.10, 13.12**). The cerebellum (**Fig. 13.13**), brain stem, and much less commonly the spinal cord, may also be involved.

MICROSCOPIC APPEARANCES
There are multiple foci of demyelination (**Figs 13.14, 13.15**). Some are small and rounded, others confluent and irregular and occasionally centrally necrotic. These lesions contain moderate numbers of foamy macrophages (**Fig. 13.15**), but only scanty perivascular lymphocytes. Lymphocytic infiltrates may be commoner in PML associated with AIDS and may confer a slightly better prognosis.

A striking feature, particularly in older lesions, is the presence of very large astrocytes with bizarre, pleomorphic, hyperchromatic nuclei (**Figs 13.15, 13.16**). These cells resemble the individual astrocytes that can be seen in glioblastomas. Typical reactive astrocytes are also present.

PROGRESSIVE MULTIFOCAL LEUKOENCEPHALOPATHY

- usually presents with focal neurologic deficits including dysarthria, limb weakness, visual disturbances, ataxia, personality changes, and occasionally seizures.
- usually progresses relentlessly over a few months, resulting in increasing neurologic impairment, dementia, and eventually death.

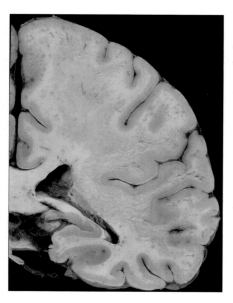

Fig. 13.10 PML. Numerous small and larger confluent foci of gray discoloration in the cerebral cortex and white matter. Some of the foci are partly cavitated.

PROGRESSIVE MULTIFOCAL LEUKOENCEPHALOPATHY

- PML is caused by the JC virus, one of two ubiquitous polyomaviruses, the other being BK virus.
- Infection in humans is generally asymptomatic.
- Latent JC or BK virus is demonstrable in the kidneys of most adults and in the brains of some.
- PML is thought to result from reactivation of latent JC virus residing within the CNS or in peripheral tissues, usually as a result of impaired cell-mediated immunity.
- JC virus can be detected in circulating B lymphocytes in a high proportion of patients with PML, suggesting that these cells may play a role in viral entry into the CNS.

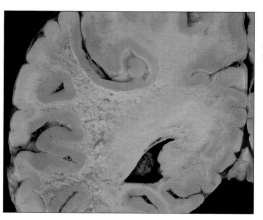

Fig. 13.11 PML. Extensive granularity and cavitation of the white matter.

Mitoses are rare. Those that do occur may appear atypical. However, despite the nuclear pleomorphism, the lesions are easily distinguishable from neoplasm by their relatively low cellularity and the presence of viral inclusions, which are seen towards the periphery of the foci of demyelination in the enlarged nuclei of oligodendrocytes. The homogeneous amphophilic inclusions (see Fig. 13.16) largely fill the nuclei and consist of closely packed polyomavirus particles, which are readily

identifiable on electron microscopy (**Fig. 13.17**). The virus can be detected and specifically identified by in-situ hybridization.

Occasionally, in cases of PML involving the cerebellum, accumulations of cells with large vesicular nuclei and central nucleoli can be seen in the granule cell layer. These probably represent altered granule cells.

Very rarely, astrocytic neoplasms have been reported in PML.

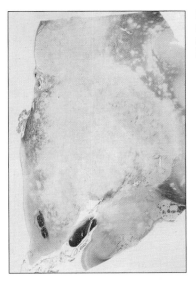

Fig. 13.12 PML. Extensive loss of myelin staining in the basal ganglia and hypothalamus. (Luxol fast blue/cresyl violet)

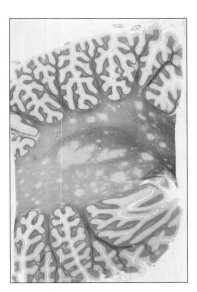

Fig. 13.13 PML. Foci of demyelination in the white matter of the cerebellum. (Luxol fast blue/cresyl violet)

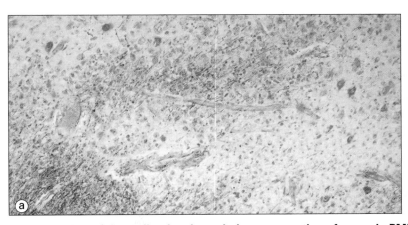
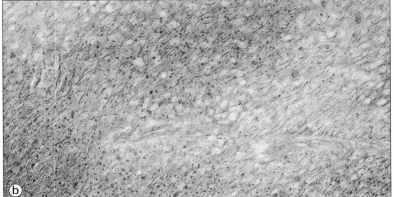

Fig. 13.14 Foci of demyelination, but relative preservation of axons in PML. (a) Section stained for myelin with solochrome cyanin. **(b)** Adjacent section stained for axons (Palmgren silver impregnation). Axons traverse the foci of demyelination. The scattered cells with very large nuclei (seen best in (a)) are atypical astrocytes.

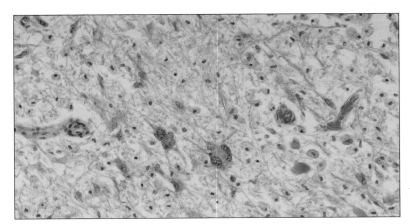

Fig. 13.15 PML. Foamy macrophages, bizarre astrocytes, and very sparse lymphocytes in a region of demyelination.

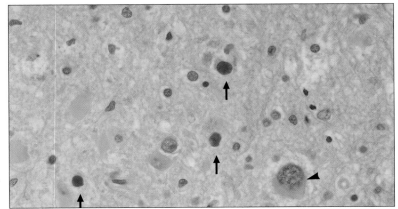

Fig. 13.16 PML. Oligodendrocytes at the edge of a focus of demyelination have enlarged nuclei containing amphophilic viral inclusions (arrows). Note the large atypical astrocyte (arrowhead).

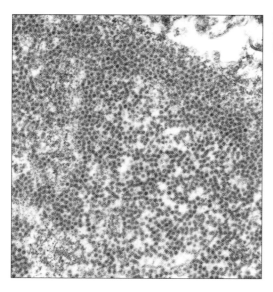

Fig. 13.17 Intranuclear polyomavirus particles in PML.

HUMAN T CELL LEUKEMIA/LYMPHO-TROPIC VIRUS-1 (HTLV-1)-ASSOCIATED MYELOPATHY (HAM) (TROPICAL SPASTIC PARAPARESIS)

MACROSCOPIC APPEARANCES

In longstanding cases of HAM, there may be meningeal thickening (**Fig. 13.18**) and atrophy of the spinal cord, particularly in the lower thoracic region. Lateral funicular degeneration may also be visible.

MICROSCOPIC APPEARANCES

An infiltrate of lymphocytes and macrophages is seen in the leptomeninges and parenchyma of the spinal cord (**Figs 13.19, 13.20**), and is most marked in the lower thoracic region. Hyaline thickening of small blood vessels is a prominent feature (see Fig. 13.18). Intramyelinic vacuolation and demyelination may be evident early in the course of disease, but soon progress to symmetric degeneration and gliosis involving the long tracts in the spinal cord (**Fig. 13.21**). The degeneration tends to be most severe in the lateral columns. The anterior and less commonly the posterior columns may also be involved. The neurons are relatively well preserved (**Figs 13.20, 13.21**). Sparse viral nucleic acids may be detectable within the spinal cord by in-situ hybridization or by the polymerase chain reaction. Adventitial fibrosis and scanty perivascular inflammation have been observed in the cerebral white matter and less commonly in the cerebellum and brain stem.

HUMAN T CELL LEUKEMIA/LYMPHOTROPHIC VIRUS-1 (HTLV-1)-ASSOCIATED MYELOPATHY (HAM)

- HAM is caused by HTLV-1, which was the first human retrovirus to be identified. As the name suggests, it can also cause adult T cell leukemia.
- HTLV-I is endemic in the Caribbean, South America, parts of Africa, southern Japan, the Seychelles, and probably parts of India. HAM is therefore most common in these parts of the world, with prevalence figures ranging from 5–130/100,000 inhabitants.
- HTLV-1 infection is transmitted by sexual contact, breast feeding, or blood transfusion. The incubation period varies from one year to as long as 25 years, and may depend to some extent on the route of infection; in several reported cases of transfusion-related infection, the incubation period has been less than two years.
- The extent of inflammation and paucity of virus within the spinal cord, and the presence of high titers of HTLV-I-specific antibodies in the serum and cerebrospinal fluid has been interpreted as suggesting that the cord injury is immunologically mediated.

HUMAN T CELL LEUKEMIA/LYMPHOTROPHIC VIRUS-1 (HTLV-1)-ASSOCIATED MYELOPATHY

- Age of onset is usually 25–60 years.
- HAM causes progressive spastic paraparesis and sphincter disturbance, and most patients are chairbound within 10 years.
- Backache is common.
- HAM can cause sensory disturbances in the legs.
- A history of other sexually transmitted disease(s) is often elicited.

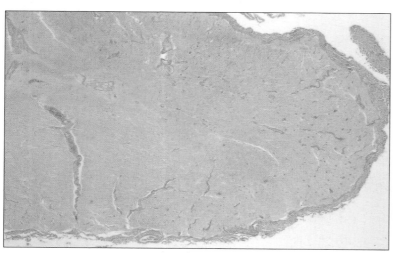

Fig. 13.18 HAM. Collagenous thickening of the spinal leptomeninges and the walls of parenchymal blood vessels. (Hematoxylin/van Gieson)

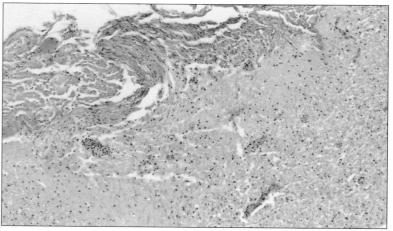

Fig. 13.19 HAM. Higher magnification view showing thickened leptomeninges and patchy infiltration by lymphocytes in the dorsal root entry zone. (Hematoxylin/van Gieson)

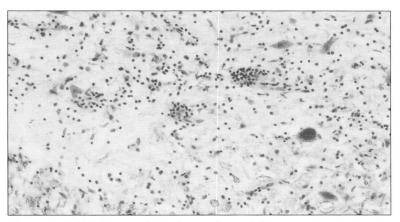

Fig. 13.20 HAM. Perivascular and parenchymal infiltrates of lymphocytes in the spinal gray matter in HAM. (Luxol fast blue/cresyl violet)

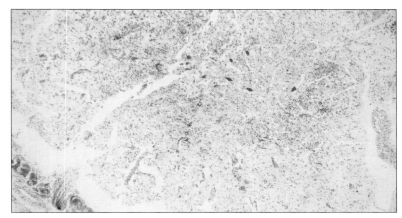

Fig. 13.21 HAM. Degeneration of myelinated fibers in the anterior and lateral funiculi of the spinal cord with relative preservation of anterior horn cells. (Luxol fast blue/cresyl violet)

HUMAN IMMUNODEFICIENCY VIRUS (HIV) INFECTION

HIV was first recognized as a cause of human disease in the early 1980s. Although other subtypes exist, most human disease results from infection with HIV-1 (referred to below simply as HIV), which is the major cause of acquired immunodeficiency syndrome (AIDS). HIV infection is pandemic, although the prevalence varies worldwide.

Definition of AIDS
AIDS is a clinical syndrome associated with HIV infection and defined since 1 January 1993 by the Centers for Disease Control, Atlanta, in very specific terms as follows:

A patient with AIDS is an HIV-infected person with CD4-positive T lymphocytes totalling less than $200/\mu l$, or accounting for less than 14% of all T lymphocytes, who also has one of 23 specific (AIDS-associated or AIDS-defining) illnesses (e.g. cryptosporidiosis, Kaposi's sarcoma, various fungal and viral infections, HIV encephalopathy or dementia, wasting syndrome, pulmonary tuberculosis, recurrent pneumonia, or invasive cervical cancer).

HIV infection is detected by serology or by polymerase chain reaction (PCR) assay for HIV nucleic acids.

Factors that lead to progression from 'simple' HIV infection to AIDS are not yet fully understood, and the time interval between the two may be many years. Neurologic disease in people infected with HIV may result from:
- direct HIV infection of the CNS
- immunosuppression caused by HIV infection, leading to opportunistic infections and neoplasms, especially lymphoma
- systemic factors and miscellaneous conditions related to an illness that causes cachexia, metabolic derangement, hypoxia, and other diverse abnormalities
- treatment.

HUMAN IMMUNODEFICIENCY VIRUS

HIV is a retrovirus of the Lentivirus subfamily. Like other retroviruses it is an enveloped positive-strand RNA virus (Fig. 13.22).
Transmission of infection occurs by:
- Vaginal or anal intercourse in 70–80% of cases.
- Intravenous drug injection in 5–10% of cases.
- Infected mother to child transmission in 5–10% of cases.
- Blood transfusion in 3–5% of cases (this transmission rate is declining as blood supplies are monitored more carefully).
- Health care or occupational exposure in 0.01% of cases.

Viral entry into T lymphocytes or macrophages is mediated by binding of the Env envelope glycoprotein to CD4 receptors on the cell surface. DNA provirus is synthesized from the RNA genome by the viral enzyme reverse transcriptase, which is packaged within the core particle of the virus and released on its entry into the cell. The provirus enters the nucleus and integrates at random sites in the cellular genome.
Once a patient is infected, 'clearance' does not occur except in very rare circumstances.

EPIDEMIOLOGIC ASPECTS OF HIV INFECTION

- By the early 1990s over 11 million people worldwide were infected by HIV-1 and there were an estimated 1.5 million or more cases of AIDS.
- The number of people infected with HIV in different geographic areas are as follows: >1 million in the United States; >1 million in Latin America; >7 million in Africa; >1 million in Southeast Asia.
- In some populations (e.g. Southern California) AIDS is the leading cause of death among men aged 25–44 years, and almost 25% of deaths in this age group result from AIDS.

DIRECT HIV INFECTION OF THE CNS
MACROSCOPIC APPEARANCES
The brain may appear normal or show diffuse atrophy with ventriculomegaly (**Fig. 13.23**) and ill-defined gray discoloration of the centrum semiovale.

MICROSCOPIC APPEARANCES
Histology reveals the following abnormalities in various combinations:
* Widespread low-grade inflammation with microglial nodules and perivascular lymphocyte cuffing (**Fig. 13.24**). MGNE (microglial nodule encephalitis) is also a feature of some opportunistic infections including CMV, toxoplasmosis, and certain fungal infections.
* Leukoencephalopathy with patchy demyelination and white matter gliosis (**Fig. 13.25**).
* Multinucleated cells, usually pericapillary, with scanty cytoplasm (morulae) or abundant cytoplasm (true giant cells) (**Fig. 13.26**) in which HIV antigen can be demonstrated with antibody to gp41 or p24 (**Fig. 13.27**). Even without immunohistochemistry, the multinucleated cells are sufficiently characteristic to allow a diagnosis of HIV encephalitis provided that other causes of granulomatous inflammation with giant cell formation are ruled out.

DEMENTIA DUE TO HIV INFECTION OF THE BRAIN

A dementing illness with memory and personality changes may be a presenting feature of AIDS and is also one of the 'AIDS-defining' illnesses (see above). This has received various descriptive names including AIDS–dementia complex, HIV-related cognitive–motor deficit, subacute encephalitis of AIDS, HIV encephalitis, and AIDS/HIV-related encephalopathy.
The reported frequency is extremely variable and
* exceeds 50% of patients in some series.
* has become less common since the widespread use of antiviral agents, particularly zidovudine, which was also known as azidothymidine (AZT).
* may be altered by combination therapy including protease inhibitors but this remains to be evaluated fully.

PATHOGENESIS OF DIRECT HIV INFECTION OF THE CNS

In the CNS, HIV infects mainly microglial cells or macrophages.
This results in the secretion of:
* Cytokines such as tumor necrosis factor (TNF) and interleukins (e.g. IL-1, IL-6).
* Other potentially damaging chemicals such as nitric oxide, superoxide anion, hydroxyl radical, peroxides, and quinolinate.
The pathologic substrate of the resulting encephalopathy has been extensively studied.
* Initial attention focused on a leukoencephalopathy or leukoencephalitis as the cause of neurologic deterioration.
* More recently the emphasis has been on neocortical abnormalities such as neuron, synapse, and dendrite loss.
* There has been much debate as to whether HIV encephalopathy and dementia are related to the viral burden within the CNS or the secretion of cytokines and other damaging substances by relatively few infected cells.
Direct HIV infection of brain is a relatively more common cause of neurologic deterioration in HIV-positive infants and children than in adults with HIV, in whom opportunistic infections and other miscellaneous conditions are more often responsible.

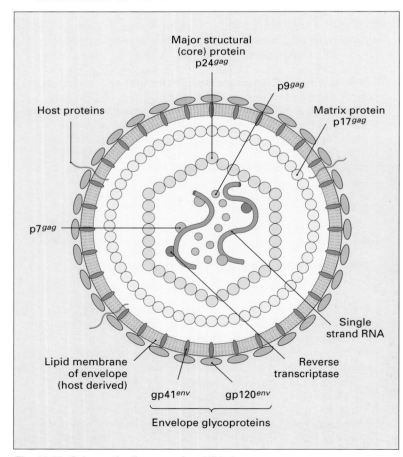

Fig. 13.22 Schematic diagram of an HIV virus.

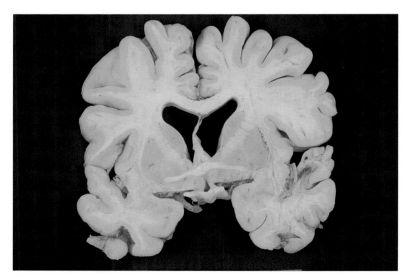

Fig. 13.23 Macroscopic appearance of brain in AIDS dementia. This occurred in a 39-year-old man with multiple complications of HIV infection including widespread microglial nodule encephalitis and vacuolar myelopathy. Note the mild diffuse cortical atrophy and ventricular enlargement with blunting of the angles of the lateral ventricles.

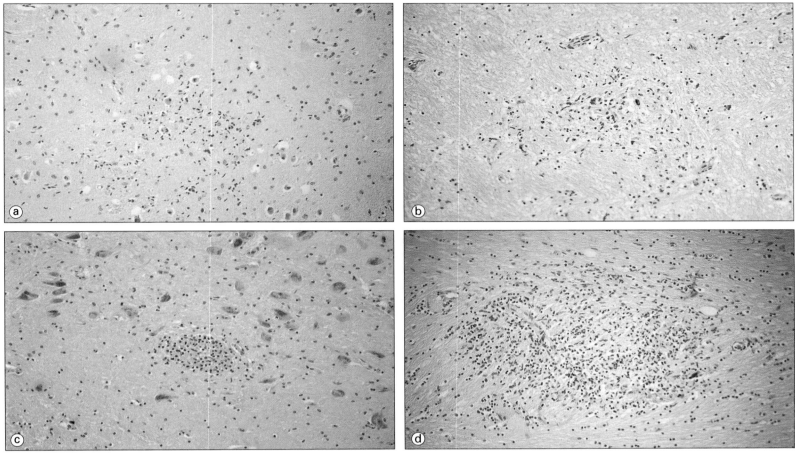

Fig. 13.24 Microglial nodule encephalitis. This is a characteristic finding in the brains of people with HIV and may be due to an identified agent (e.g. HIV, CMV, toxoplasmosis), but occasionally no causal microorganism is found. Inflammatory foci contain varying numbers of microglia and some lymphocytes and even astrocytes. **(a)** Poorly defined region of microglial activation. **(b,c)** Compact collections of microglia. **(d)** Large aggregates of microglia. The presence of multinucleated cells in **(b)** and **(d)** indicates probable HIV infection of the brain.

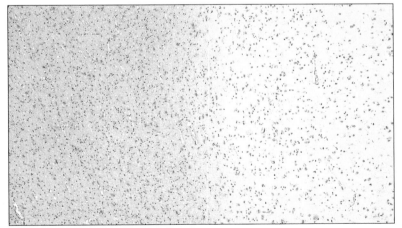

Fig. 13.25 HIV leukoencephalopathy. This is characterized by pallor of myelin staining, and mild to moderate white matter astrocytic gliosis as illustrated here. (GFAP immunohistochemistry)

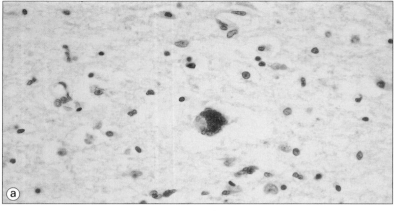

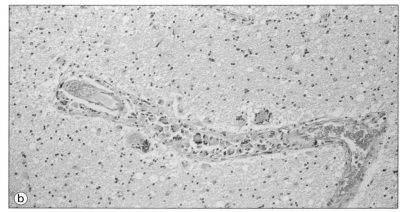

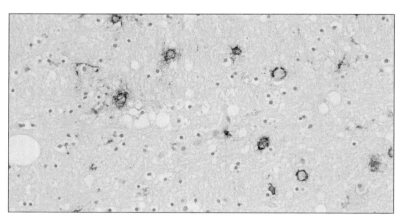

Fig. 13.26 Multinucleated cells in HIV infection of brain. (a) The cells may have a morular appearance. **(b)** Alternatively, the cells may contain relatively abundant eosinophilic or foamy cytoplasm, which may be central or peripheral to the multiple nuclei within the cell. HIV-type multinucleated cells have the immunophenotype of microglia or macrophages and tend to aggregate around blood vessels (especially capillaries). **(c)** HIV-type multinucleated cells adjacent to a CNS lymphoma.

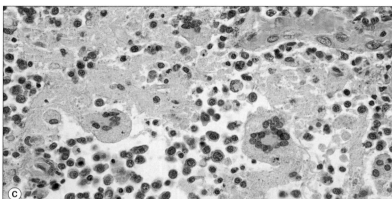

Fig. 13.27 HIV brain infection. Immunohistochemical demonstration of HIV p24 antigen in scattered microglia/macrophages and mutinucleated cells.

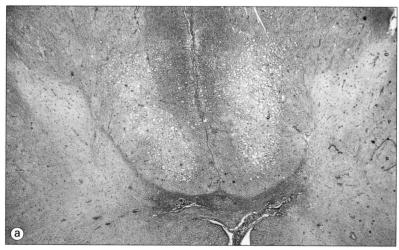

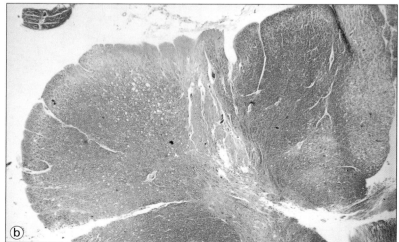

Fig. 13.28 The vacuolar myelopathy of AIDS. This resembles subacute combined degeneration of the spinal cord. **(a)** Note the vacuolar change in the posterior columns (Luxol fast blue/cresyl violet).
(b) There may also be vacuolar change in the lateral corticospinal tract, but usually to a lesser extent.

Vacuolar myelopathy
MACROSCOPIC AND MICROSCOPIC APPEARANCES

The vacuolar myelopathy resembles subacute combined degeneration of the spinal cord (**Fig. 13.28**) (see chapter 21). There is vacuolation of the spinal white matter in the posterior columns and lateral corticospinal tracts, most pronounced in the thoracic segments. Breakdown of myelin, and later axons, is accompanied by an accumulation of macrophages containing debris.

VACUOLAR MYELOPATHY

- Vacuolar myelopathy affects up to 25% of people with AIDS and causes spastic paraparesis, ataxia, and incontinence.
- The cause is unclear. It may result from direct infection of macrophages within the spinal cord or an indirect mechanism not associated with productive HIV infection.

Necrotizing leucoencephalopathy

Rarely, HIV infection of the CNS produces a severe necrotizing leuko-encephalopathy (**Fig. 13.29**).

HIV infection of the brain in children

Children with AIDS are less prone to opportunistic infections and brain neoplasms than adults with AIDS, but often develop HIV-associated progressive encephalopathy of childhood. This is characterized by progressive mental deterioration associated with immunosuppression, which is usually severe. Brain imaging reveals severe atrophy and calcification, particularly involving the basal ganglia.

MACROSCOPIC AND MICROSCOPIC APPEARANCES

The neuropathologic findings are of HIV encephalitis, but with particularly prominent perivascular chronic inflammatory infiltrates and dystrophic parenchymal and angiocentric calcification (**Fig. 13.30**).

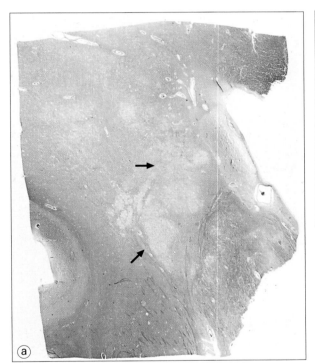

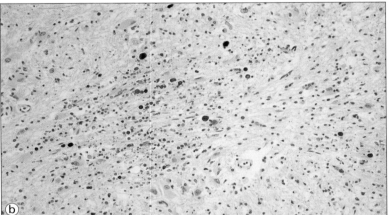

Fig. 13.29 Necrotizing leucoencephalopathy associated with HIV infection. (a) Patchy necrosis (arrows) of the internal capsule.
(b) Dystrophic calcification and reactive (gemistocytic) astrocytes in a focus of white matter necrosis.

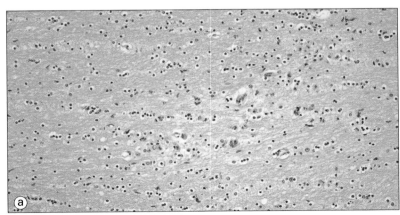

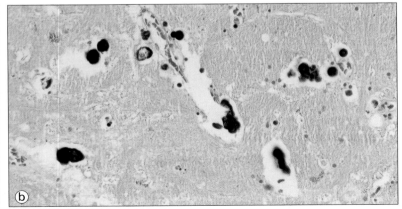

Fig. 13.30 Pediatric HIV encephalopathy. (a) Subtle giant cell encephalitis in a 6-year-old child with congenital HIV infection. **(b)** Cerebral calcification is a common finding in AIDS, but especially in children. (von Kossa)

HIV-ASSOCIATED IMMUNOSUPPRESSION AND NEUROLOGIC DISEASE

Deficient cell-mediated immunity due to HIV infection may lead to:

- fungal infection (see also chapter 17)
- viral infection (see also chapter 13)
- parasitic infection (see also chapter 18)
- bacterial infection (see also chapter 16)
- neoplastic changes (see also chapter 42).

Fungal infections of the CNS in AIDS

Cryptococcus neoformans infection (see p 17.6): In most series, *C. neoformans* is the commonest fungal opportunistic infection of the CNS in AIDS, affecting up to 5–10% of patients. It presents as a meningitis, which is often low grade. The brain usually has a glistening sheen on external examination and a cribriform appearance (**Fig. 13.31**) on sectioning as a result of fungal proliferation in the perivascular spaces. Rarely, there is a necrotic abscess. The inflammatory response may be virtually nonexistent, mild, or rarely of severe granulomatous type (**Fig. 13.32**).

Aspergillus fumigatus infection (see p 17.2): *A. fumigatus* infection causes abscesses that present as space-occupying lesions. CNS involvement is usually associated with widely disseminated infection and the brain contains multiple necrotic, often hemorrhagic, lesions (**Fig. 13.33**). Histology reveals angioinvasive fungal hyphae, vascular thrombosis and infarction, and variable inflammation. Mycotic aneurysms are common (see chapter 10).

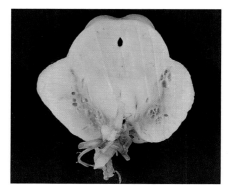

Fig. 13.31 Section through the midbrain of an AIDS patient with cryptococcal infection. Distension of the perivascular spaces by proliferating fungi gives the affected parts of the brain (in this case, the substantia nigra) a cribriform appearance. The gray matter is more vascular and usually more severely affected than the white matter.

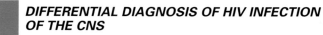

DIFFERENTIAL DIAGNOSIS OF HIV INFECTION OF THE CNS

- The precise cause of a dementing condition in an HIV-infected patient is often not determined until necropsy.
- A wide range of HIV-related infections and neoplasms may be responsible or the encephalopathy may be multifactorial (e.g. due to HIV brain infection combined with PML, primary CNS lymphoma, or hypoxia).
- The possibility of a non-HIV-related dementia should be kept in mind, though most of these are rare in young people, who constitute the majority of patients with AIDS.
- Causes of myelopathy in patients with AIDS, other than vacuolar myelopathy of AIDS, include herpesvirus (CMV, VZV, or herpes simplex virus) myelitis, other opportunistic infections, lymphoma within the spinal cord, and cord compression related to opportunistic infection or lymphoma.

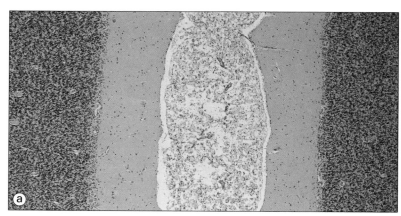

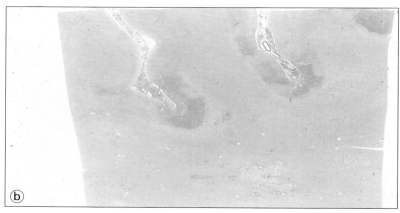

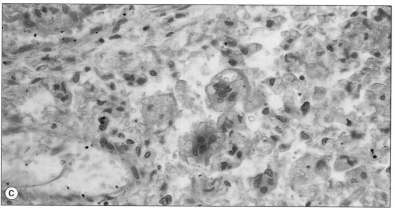

Fig. 13.32 Variable inflammatory response to cryptococcal infection in AIDS. (a) This shows fungal yeasts expanding the subarachnoid space surrounding the cerebellum, with virtually no associated inflammation. **(b)** Severe granulomatous inflammation in the subarachnoid space, with necrosis of the underlying cortex and white matter. (Periodic acid–Schiff) **(c)** Higher magnification of the granulomatous inflammatory infiltrate revealing cryptococcal yeasts in the cytoplasm of multinucleated giant cells.

Coccidioides immitis infection (see p 17.11): This is an important AIDS-related infection in areas where the fungus is common in dusty soil (e.g. southwestern United States, especially the San Joaquin Valley of central California). Macroscopic examination of the brain reveals meningitis and abscesses (**Fig. 13.34**). Histology reveals large spherules with enclosed endospores, often engulfed by multinucleated giant cells (**Fig. 13.35**) and associated with acute or chronic granulomatous, inflammation. Fibrinoid necrosis of small vessels and endarteritis obliterans are common.

Other fungal infections: Many other fungal infections have been described in the CNS of patients with AIDS, including histoplasmosis, candidiasis, and mucormycosis (see chapter 17).

Viral encephalitides and myelitides in AIDS

CMV infection (see p 12.13): This is the commonest viral opportunistic infection involving the CNS in AIDS. It is found in as many as 15–20% of necropsies of patients with AIDS. The neuropathologic manifestations are variable and include:

- Low-grade microglial nodule encephalitis (MGNE). Cytomegalic cells occur within microglial nodules (**Fig. 13.36**) or without any associated inflammation.
- Severe necrotizing encephalitis with large regions of cystic encephalomalacia (**Fig. 13.37**) resembling infarcts.

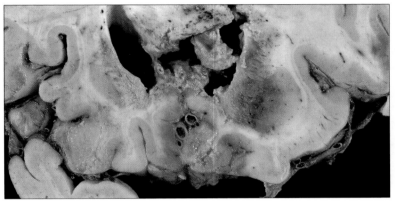

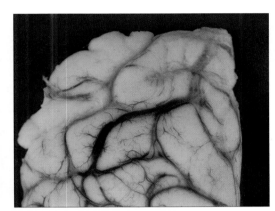

Fig. 13.34 Coccidioidomycosis in a patient with AIDS. Note the thickened white meninges overlying some of the superficial vessels.

Fig. 13.33 *Aspergillus* infection in a patient with AIDS. Multiple foci of hemorrhagic necrosis are typical of CNS aspergillosis.

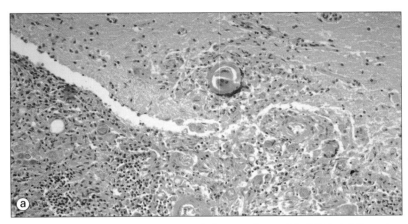

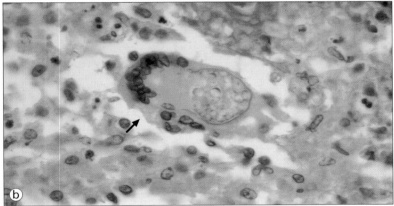

Fig. 13.35 Florid coccidioidomycosis in a patient with AIDS. (a) Granulomatous meningoencephalitis. **(b)** The fungal endospores are encapsulated within spherules, some of which are engulfed by foreign body-type giant cells (arrow). (Courtesy of Dr Paul S. Mischel)

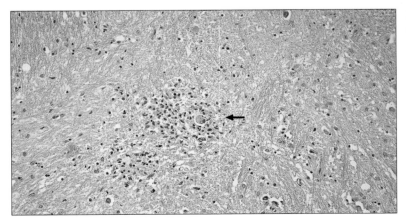

Fig. 13.36 CMV-related MGNE involving the medulla of a patient with AIDS. A cytomegalic cell (arrow) is present within the microglial nodule.

- Ventriculoencephalitis (Figs 13.38, 13.39) visible macroscopically (or on imaging studies) as sugar icing-like material lining the ventricular surfaces with hemorrhagic necrosis of adjacent brain parenchyma.
- Meningoradiculitis and myelitis (Fig. 13.40) with a clinical presentation simulating Guillain–Barré syndrome. This is often due to CMV-associated vasculopathy with microvascular thrombi in and around the nerve roots.
- Rarely, widespread infection of microvascular endothelial cells (Fig.

13.41) that sometimes also involves the peripheral nerve and skeletal muscle.
- Foci of demyelination.

There is evidence of occasional coinfection of single cells by HIV and CMV.

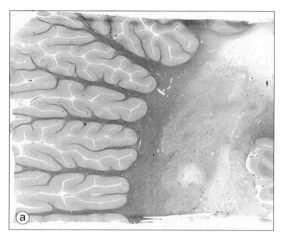
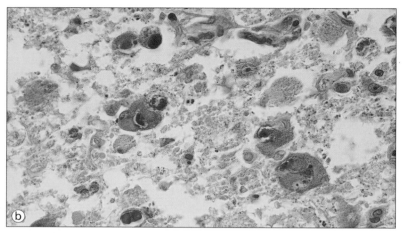

Fig. 13.37 Severe necrotizing CMV encephalitis in a patient with AIDS. (a) Large regions of cystic encephalomalacia resembling infarcts are seen here in the cerebellar white matter. **(b)** Cytomegalic cells with characteristic nuclear and cytoplasmic inclusions at the periphery of the necrotic foci.

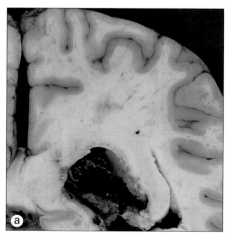
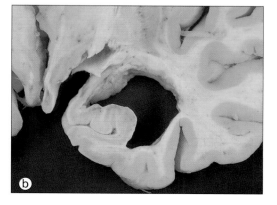

Fig. 13.38 Necrotizing CMV ventriculoencephalitis.
(a) There is congestion and focal hemorrhagic necrosis of the ventricular ependymal lining. This figure also shows hemorrhage into the choroid plexus, which is often infected by CMV. **(b)** The temporal horn of the lateral ventricle, as shown here, is often involved.

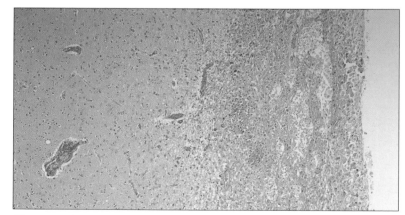

Fig. 13.39 Necrotizing CMV ventriculoencephalitis. The ventricle at right of figure is surrounded by inflamed, partly necrotic, ependymal and subependymal tissue. Cytomegalic cells are prominent, especially near the ventricular cavity. Multinucleated HIV-type giant cells are also present, deeper within the brain parenchyma.

Varicella-zoster virus (VZV) infection (see p 12.11): This is much less common than CMV infection, but also produces heterogeneous neurologic manifestations, including:

- Leukoencephalopathy and leukoencephalitis with sharply demarcated necrotizing lesions.
- Encephalitis involving the visual system.
- Brain stem encephalitis.
- Myeloradiculitis (**Fig. 13.42**; see also Fig. 13.45).

- Ventriculitis.
- Vasculitis or non-inflammatory vasculopathy.

Other herpesviruses infections: Herpes simplex encephalitis (see p 12.6) occurs rarely in patients with AIDS, while Epstein–Barr virus infection is associated with primary CNS lymphoma in AIDS patients (see below and chapter 42). The role of human herpesvirus-6 in the pathogenesis of AIDS-related neurologic syndromes has not yet been

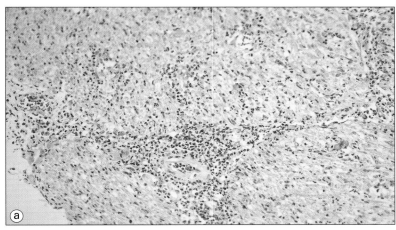

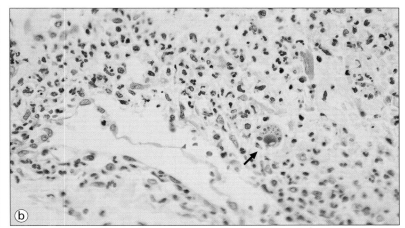

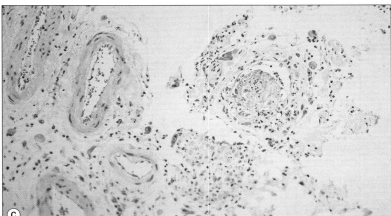

Fig. 13.40 CMV radiculitis in an AIDS patient who presented with a Guillain–Barré-type syndrome. (a) The nerve roots include a chronic inflammatory infiltrate **(b)** within which are typical CMV inclusions (arrow). **(c)** Foci of necrosis are associated with microthrombi in small meningeal arteries harboring CMV in their walls.

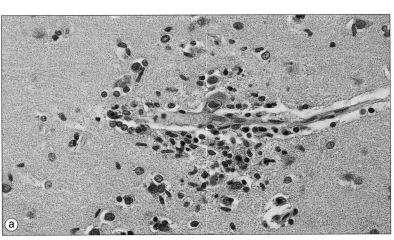

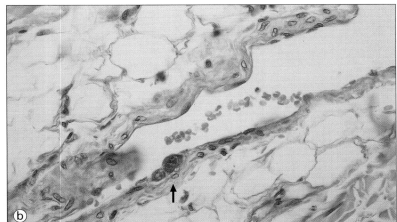

Fig. 13.41 CMV infection of endothelial cells. (a) In the brain. **(b)** In the epineurium (arrow).

defined. A newly recognized herpesvirus, designated human herpesvirus 8 (HHV8) or Kaposi's sarcoma-associated herpesvirus (KSHV), has a role in the pathogenesis of Kaposi's sarcoma and primary effusion (body cavity-based) lymphomas, but not directly in the development of neurologic disease.

The neuropathology of PML is described on p 13.4–13.6.

Other viral infections of the CNS that have rarely been reported in patients with AIDS include adenovirus encephalitis (**Fig. 13.43**) and measles inclusion body encephalitis (see p 13.1).

Diagnosis of the specific viral infection in the histological material can be achieved by:

- Immunohistochemistry for viral antigen(s) (Figs 13.27, 13.42).
- In-situ hybridization to viral DNA and RNA (**Fig. 13.44**).
- PCR amplification of viral DNA and RNA (**Fig. 13.45**).
- In-situ PCR.

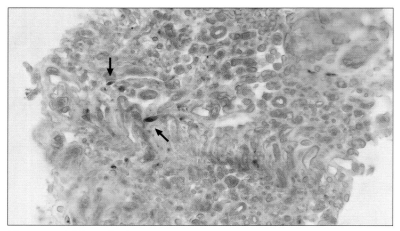

Fig. 13.42 VZV radiculitis. Immunostained VZV-infected cells (arrows) in nerve root. (Courtesy of Professor Françoise Gray, Hôpital Raymond Poincare, Paris, France)

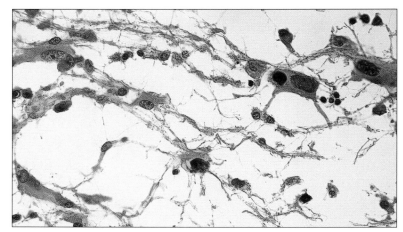

Fig. 13.43 Intranuclear adenovirus inclusions in adenovirus ventriculoencephalitis in a child with AIDS.

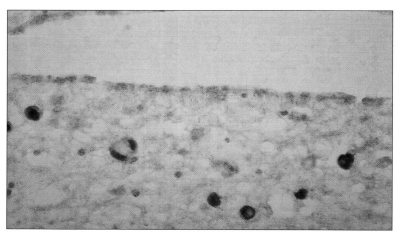

Fig. 13.44 Detection of CMV by in-situ hybridization. (Courtesy of Lorna Cheng, University of California, Los Angeles, U.S.A.)

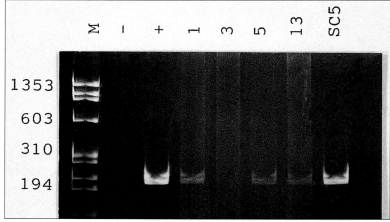

Fig. 13.45 Detection of VZV in paraffin sections by PCR amplification with VZV-specific primers. The PCR products were separated by polyacrylamide gel electrophoresis, stained with ethidium bromide, and transilluminated with ultraviolet light. DNA size markers are in lane 'M'. Negative and positive controls are in lanes labeled '–' and '+' respectively. The remaining lanes contain amplified DNA from different regions of brain with vasculitis, but no VZV inclusions. The most intense band ('SC5') is from sections of spinal cord with extensive myeloradiculitis. PCR results should be interpreted with caution because of the extraordinary sensitivity of the technique. (Courtesy of Jennifer Cheng and Diana Lenard Secor, University of California, Los Angeles, U.S.A)

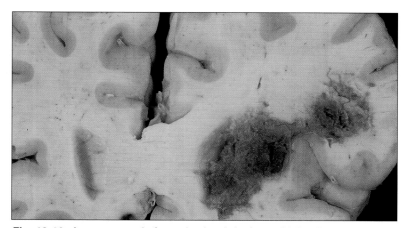

Fig. 13.46   Large necrotic focus in the right frontal lobe due to toxoplasmosis.

Parasitic infections of the CNS in AIDS

The most important parasitic infection of the CNS in AIDS is toxoplasmosis, which usually produces large necrotic abscesses (**Fig. 13.46**). The neuropathology of parasitic infections is discussed in detail in chapter 18.

Bacterial infections of the CNS in AIDS

The commonest bacterial infections in AIDS are due to acid-fast bacilli, including:

- *Mycobacterium avium-intracellulare*, which is found in large numbers in the cytoplasm of infected macrophages within the CNS. This usually produces only mild parenchymal injury, but rarely causes focal necrosis.
- *Mycobacterium tuberculosis* (see chapter 16).

The incidence of neurosyphilis is increased in patients with AIDS.

Neoplasms of the CNS in AIDS

The principal neoplastic CNS complication in patients with AIDS is lymphoma, resulting from either:

- Meningeal spread of a systemic lymphoma, which is a common complication of AIDS.
- Primary CNS lymphoma (PCNSL) (see also chapter 42).

Non-Hodgkin's lymphomas (not just those within the CNS) are 50 to 60 times more common in patients with AIDS than in the general population.

PCNSL in AIDS is usually of high-grade, non-Hodgkin's, B cell-type and associated with Epstein–Barr virus infection. The prognosis is dismal despite aggressive radiotherapy. Neuropathology reveals unifocal or multifocal lesions that may mimic a glioblastoma macroscopically (**Fig. 13.47**) and are often centrally necrotic.

CNS lymphomatoid granulomatosis has been reported in AIDS. Kaposi's sarcoma rarely involves the CNS.

HIV-ASSOCIATED SYSTEMIC FACTORS AND MISCELLANEOUS CONDITIONS CAUSING NEUROLOGIC DISEASE
Cerebrovascular disease in AIDS

Cerebral hemorrhages and infarcts occur in patients with AIDS, but are uncommon and more often seen in children than adults. Related factors include:

- Endocarditis, either bacterial, fungal, or marantic (non-bacterial).
- Thrombocytopenia and coagulopathy.
- HIV-associated vasculopathy of unknown etiology manifesting as intimal thickening mainly of meningeal arteries (**Fig. 13.48**).
- Opportunistic infections.
- PCNSL.

COMMONEST CAUSES OF A CEREBRAL MASS LESION IN A PATIENT WITH HIV

- Toxoplasmosis
- Primary CNS lymphoma (PCNSL)
- Fungal infection (especially *Aspergillus*)
- Tuberculoma
- PML
- Cytomegalovirus (CMV) infection
- A lesion not related to HIV (e.g. glioma, metastatic cancer)

Diagnosing the cause of the cerebral mass

- A stereotactic biopsy usually suffices for diagnosis and planning treatment.
- Smear or squash preparations performed for rapid diagnosis or perioperative consultation allow neoplasia to be distinguished from infection; often a precise etiologic diagnosis is possible.

The possibility of mixed or multiple lesions should be borne in mind.

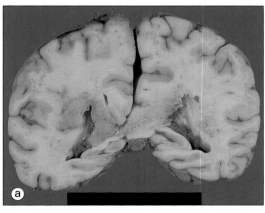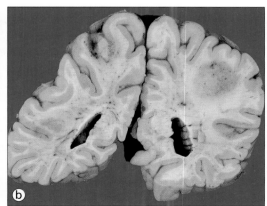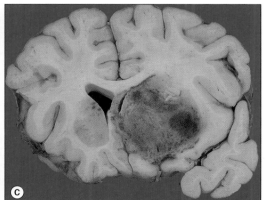

Fig. 13.47 PCNSL in AIDS. (a) PCNSL mimicking a glioblastoma. **(b)** Multifocal PCNSL. **(c)** Hemorrhage and necrosis in AIDS-related PCNSL.

Metabolic and nutritional abnormalities in AIDS

Hypoxic encephalopathy may occur, as expected in patients who often develop respiratory failure due to overwhelming pneumonia (e.g. caused by *Pneumocystis carinii* or CMV). Wernicke's encephalopathy (secondary to thiamine deficiency) is rarely observed, but has been documented (**Fig. 13.49**). Alzheimer type II astrocytosis is usually associated with liver failure and hepatic encephalopathy (see chapter 22), but is often observed in patients with AIDS in the absence of liver failure.

Central pontine myelinolysis is seen occasionally in association with AIDS and not always after rapid correction of hyponatremia (see chapter 22). It should be distinguished from multifocal necrotizing leuko-encephalopathy, which may also complicate AIDS (see chapter 22).

COMPLICATIONS OF HIV TREATMENT THAT CAUSE NEUROLOGIC DISEASE

These tend not to affect the CNS directly. The best documented is zidovudine (AZT) myopathy: zidovudine interferes with the replication of mitochondrial DNA and causes a mitochondrial myopathy.

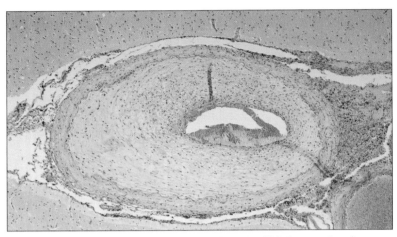

Fig. 13.48 Intimal thickening in HIV arteriopathy. This is an entity of unclear etiology, but is observed in a small number of patients with AIDS and may be associated with 'stroke' syndromes (see chapters 9 and 10).

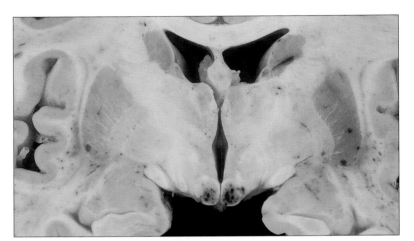

Fig. 13.49 Typical mammillary body lesions of Wernicke's encephalopathy in an AIDS patient. These developed shortly after starting zidovudine therapy.

RASMUSSEN'S ENCEPHALITIS

This is a rare syndrome characterized by:
- slowly progressive neurologic deterioration over months or years
- lateralized brain destruction and atrophy
- pathologic features of chronic encephalitis.

ETIOLOGY AND PATHOGENESIS OF RASMUSSEN'S ENCEPHALITIS

- Many patients have a history of a 'flu-like illness before the onset of seizures.
- No viral pathogen has been consistently identified in studies with molecular and immunohistochemical probes for herpesviruses and other viruses.
- It has been suggested that vascular immune complex deposition may play a role.
- A Rasmussen's encephalitis-like picture has been seen in rabbits immunized with a glutamate receptor (GluR3) fusion protein.

RASMUSSEN'S ENCEPHALITIS

- Rasmussen's encephalitis causes epilepsy that almost always starts before 15 years of age.
- Patients experience various types of seizure including simple partial and generalized tonic–clonic convulsions, and status epilepticus.
- Rasmussen's encephalitis is usually associated with the development of epilepsia partialis continua.
- Abnormalities are exclusively or predominantly confined to one cerebral hemisphere on neuroimaging.

MACROSCOPIC AND MICROSCOPIC APPEARANCES

The affected cerebral hemisphere shows variable focal atrophy and, in some cases, cavitation.

Microscopically, the cortex is consistently affected by multifocal patchy inflammation, astrocytosis, and spongy cavitation. These changes are often seen in the white matter also (**Figs 13.50–13.54**). The inflammation is characterized by:

- Microglial activation (**Fig. 13.55**).
- Microglial nodules (Fig. 13.52), which may surround pyknotic neurons.

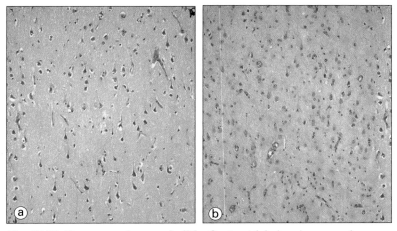

Fig. 13.50 Rasmussen's encephalitis. Contrast (**a**) showing normal neuropil and complement of neurons with (**b**) from a patient with Rasmussen's encephalitis in which there is neuronal loss, marked gliosis, and a suggestion of hypervascularity.

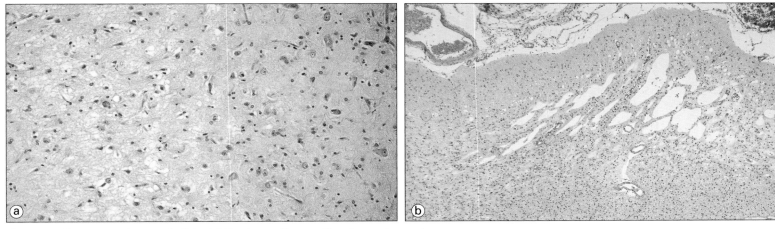

Fig. 13.51 Rasmussen's encephalitis. (a) Patchy capillary proliferation and spongiosus. **(b)** Cystic cavitation of the affected cortex.

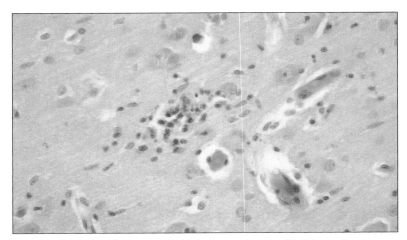

Fig. 13.52 Microglial nodule in Rasmussen's encephalitis.

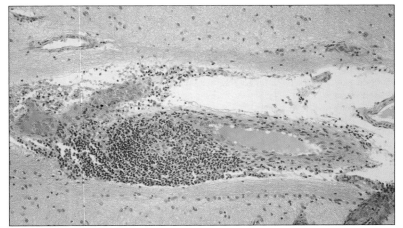

Fig. 13.53 Ramussen's encephalitis. Focal inflammation involving a meningeal vein.

- Perivascular and parenchymal lymphocytic infiltrates composed mainly of T cells (**Fig. 13.56**).
- Focal meningitis with lymphocytic cuffing and even infiltration of meningeal veins (Fig. 13.52).

The affected parenchyma may appear hypervascular with evidence of capillary proliferation (Fig. 13.50b). The abnormalities can be remarkably well-demarcated producing a sharp transition from normal to affected areas.

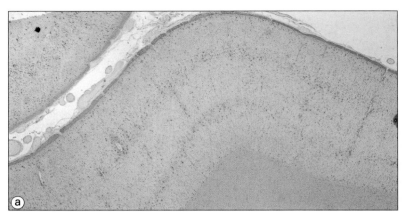
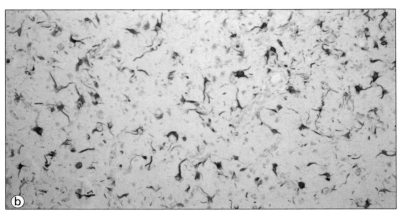

Fig. 13.54 Rasmussen's encephalitis. (a) Laminar gliosis. (GFAP immunostain) **(b)** Diffuse gliosis. (GFAP immunostain)

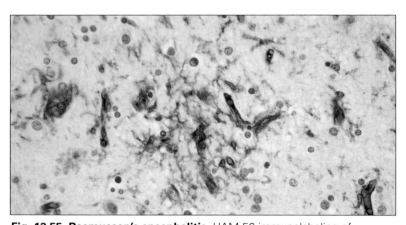
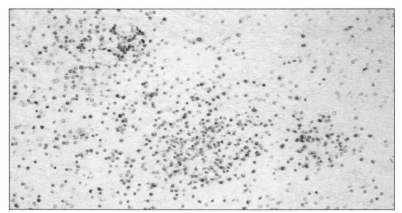

Fig. 13.55 Rasmussen's encephalitis. HAM-56 immunolabeling of endothelial cells, microglia, and macrophages within the brain parenchyma.

Fig. 13.56 Rasmussen's encephalitis. Immunohistochemical demonstration of perivascular and parenchymal T cells.

REFERENCES

Andermann F. (ed.) (1991) *Chronic Encephalitis and Epilepsy.* Boston/London: Butterworth–Heinemann.

Brew BJ, Rosenblum M, Cronin K, Price RW. (1995) AIDS dementia complex and HIV-1 brain infection: Clinical–virological correlations. *Ann Neurol* 38: 563–570.

Budka H *et al.* (1991) HIV-associated disease of the nervous system: Review of nomenclature and proposal for neuropathology-based terminology. *Brain Pathol* 1: 143–152.

Chrétien F, Gray F, Lescs MC, Geny C, Dubreuil-Lemaire ML, Ricolfi F, Baudrimont M, Levy Y, Sobel A, Vinters HV. (1993) Acute varicella-zoster virus ventriculitis and meningo-myelo-radiculitis in acquired immunodeficiency syndrome. *Acta Neuropathol* 86: 659–665.

Cruickshank JK *et al.* (1989) Tropical spastic paraparesis and human T cell lymphotropic virus type 1 in the United Kingdom. *Brain* 112: 1057–1090.

Farrell MA, DeRosa MJ, Curran JG, Secor DL, Cornford ME, Comair YG, Peacock WJ, Shields WD, Vinters HV. (1992) Neuropathologic findings in cortical resections (including hemispherectomies) performed for the treatment of intractable childhood epilepsy. *Acta Neuropathol* 83: 246–259.

Farrell MA, Droogan O, Secor DL, Poukens V, Quinn B, Vinters HV. (1995) Chronic encephalitis associated with epilepsy: immunohistochemical and ultrastructural studies. *Acta Neuropathol* 89: 313–321.

Gessain A, Gout O. (1992) Chronic myelopathy associated with human T-lymphotropic virus type I (HTLV-I). *Ann Int Med* 117: 933–946.

Gray F (ed.). (1993) *Atlas of the Neuropathology of HIV Infection.* Oxford: Oxford University Press.

Ijichi S, Osame M. (1995) Human T lymphotropic virus type I (HTLV-1)-associated myelopathy/tropical spastic paraparesis (HAM/TSP): Recent perspectives. *Int Med* 34: 713–721.

Iwasaki Y. (1990) Pathology of chronic myelopathy associated with HTLV-1 infection (HAM/TSP). *J Neurol Sci* 96: 103–123.

Mangano MF, Plotkin SA. (1991) Viral vaccines that protect the central nervous system. In WM Scheld, RJ Whitley, DT Durack (eds) *Infections of the Central Nervous System.* pp. 233–258. New York: Raven Press.

Mischel PS, HV Vinters. (1995) Coccidioidomycosis of the central nervous system: Neuropathological and vasculopathic manifestations and clinical correlates. *Clin Infect Dis* 20: 400–405.

Montgomery RD. (1989) HTLV-1 and tropical spastic paraparesis. 1. Clinical features, pathology and epidemiology. *Trans R Soc Trop Med Hyg* 83: 724–728.

Mustafa MM, Weitman SD, Winick NJ, Bellini WJ, Timmons CF, Siegel JD. (1993) Subacute measles encephalitis in the young immunocompromised host — report of 2 cases diagnosed by polymerase chain reaction and treated with ribavirin and review of the literature. *Clin Infec Dis* 16: 654–660.

Rogers SW, Andrews PI, Gahring LC, Whisenand T, Cauley K, Crain B, Hughes TE, Heinemann SF, McNamara JO. (1994) Autoantibodies to glutamate receptor GluR3 in Rasmussen's encephalitis. *Science* 265: 648–651.

Sharer LR. (1992) Pathology of HIV-1 infection of the central nervous system. A review. *J Neuropathol Exp Neurol* 51: 3–11.

Townsend JJ *et al.* (1975) Progressive rubella panencephalitis. Late onset after congenital rubella. *N Engl J Med* 292: 990–993.

Vinters HV, Anders KH. (1990) *Neuropathology of AIDS.* Florida: CRC Press Inc.

Vinters HV, Kwok MK, Ho HW, Anders KH, Tomiyasu U, Wolfson WL, Robert F. (1989) Cytomegalovirus in the nervous system of patients with the acquired immune deficiency syndrome. *Brain* 112: 245–268.

Vinters HV, Wang R, Wiley CA. (1993) Herpesviruses in chronic encephalitis associated with intractable childhood epilepsy. *Hum Pathol* 24: 871–879.

Weil ML *et al.* (1975) Chronic progressive panencephalitis due to rubella virus simulating subacute sclerosing panencephalitis. *N Engl J Med* 292: 994–998.

Wiley CA, Achim CL. (1995) Human immunodeficiency virus encephalitis and dementia. *Ann Neurol* 38: 559–560.

14 Rickettsial infections

Although historically an important cause of human infection (epidemic typhus was responsible for over three million deaths in Russia between 1915 and 1925), rickettsiae are rarely encountered in neuropathology practice.

Rickettsiae are obligate intracellular microorganisms measuring 1–2 μm in length and 0.3 μm in diameter. Their appearance and staining characteristics are of gram-negative coccobacilli. They usually infect animals and only infrequently cause human disease.

HUMAN RICKETTSIAL DISEASES

Human rickettsial diseases fall into the following four main groups:

- Spotted fever: Rocky Mountain spotted fever (R. rickettsii), boutonneuse fever (R. conori), North Asian tick typhus (R. sibirica), rickettsialpox (R. akari), Queensland tick typhus (R. australis).
- Typhus: epidemic typhus (R. prowazekii), endemic/murine typhus (R. typhi).
- Scrub typhus/tsutsugamushi fever (R. tsutsugamushi).
- Q fever (Coxiella burnetii).

- The definitive hosts of the first 3 groups are usually rodents. Human disease is acquired from the vectors, which are ticks or mites (spotted fever and scrub typhus), fleas (endemic typhus) or lice (epidemic typhus).
- The definitive hosts of Coxiella burnetii include cattle, sheep, goats, and other mammals. Q fever is transmitted between animals by ticks but humans acquire it by inhalation.

EPIDEMIOLOGY OF RICKETTSIAL INFECTION

- Human rickettsial diseases are relatively rare, even in endemic areas.
- Typhus group infections and Q fever occur worldwide.
- Most of the other rickettsial diseases are mainly concentrated in specific geographic regions: for example, Rocky Mountain spotted fever in North, Central, and South America, and in predominantly southeastern states of the USA; boutonneuse fever in the Mediterranean region, Asia, and Africa; Queensland tick typhus in northern Australia; scrub typhus in southeast Asia and the Pacific region.

PATHOGENESIS OF RICKETTSIAL INFECTIONS

- Rickettsiae apart from C. burnettii are inoculated into the bloodstream by feeding ticks or mites, or when skin onto which infected flea or louse feces have been deposited is scratched.
- The rickettsiae are disseminated hematogenously. From the bloodstream they enter, proliferate within, and cause damage to vascular endothelial and smooth muscle cells.
- Most of the manifestations of human disease (including the spotted fever rash) are a consequence of vasculitis (**Fig. 14.1**).

- C. burnettii is present in the urine, feces, milk, and placentas of infected sheep, cattle, and goats.
- Humans are infected by inhalation of the microorganisms in contaminated aerosols or dust. This results in lung and systemic infection but usually not vasculitis.

MACROSCOPIC AND MICROSCOPIC FEATURES

Most of the scanty published data relate to typhus and Rocky Mountain spotted fever. In fatal cases the brain is swollen and contains petechial hemorrhages (**Fig. 14.2**). Histology reveals angiocentric inflammation, thrombosis, and microinfarcts, in the absence of fibrinoid necrosis. Microglial nodules are usually detected in the gray matter. Rickettsiae can be demonstrated by immunofluoresence or, less consistently, by tinctorial methods (**Fig. 14.3**): Brown and Hopps modified Gram stain is most sensitive. There may be a mononuclear inflammatory infiltrate with a variable amount of hemorrhage in the leptomeninges.

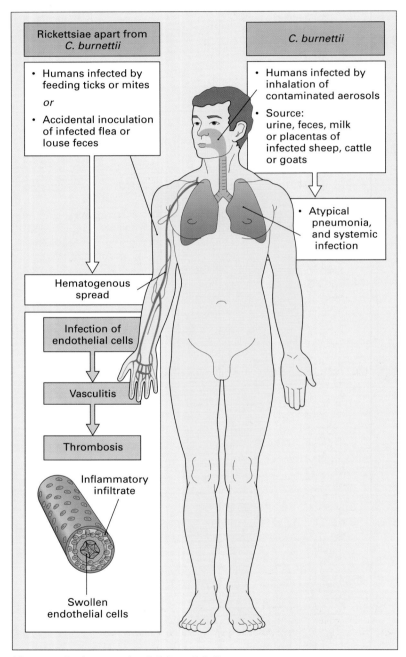

Fig. 14.1 Pathogenesis of rickettsial disease.

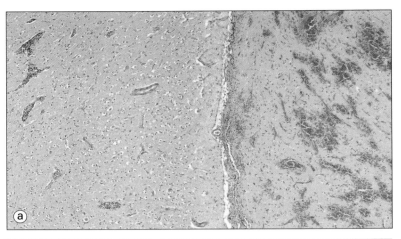

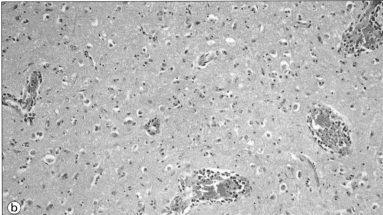

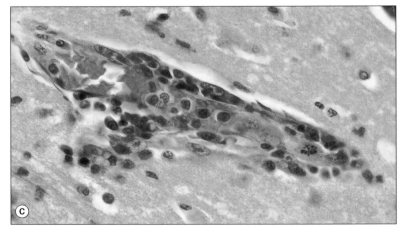

Fig. 14.2 Rocky Mountain spotted fever in a dog. (a) Section through part of 2 adjacent gyri. The gyrus on the right shows hemorrhagic necrosis. There is mild inflammation in the meninges and mononuclear cell cuffing of blood vessels in the cortex of the left gyrus. **(b)** Cuffing of blood vessels by mononuclear inflammatory cells. **(c)** At higher magnification, the inflammatory infiltrate is seen to comprise a mixture of lymphocytes and macrophages. Note the absence of neutrophils or of fibrinoid necrosis. (All prepared from material provided by Bruce H. Williams, MAJ, VC, USA, Department of Veterinary Pathology, Armed Forces Institute of Pathology, Washington DC, USA.)

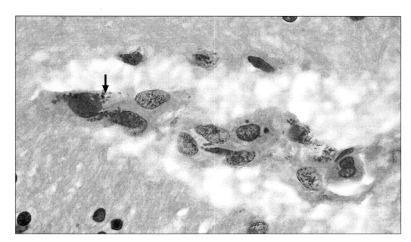

Fig. 14.3 Human Rocky Mountain spotted fever. Inflammation in the brain was minimal. Gram-negative coccobacilli (arrow) are, however, visible at high magnification, in the cytoplasm of endothelial cells. (Brown and Hopps modified Gram stain) (Prepared from material provided by Dr Robert V. Jones, COL, MC, USAR, Department of Pathology, Armed Forces Institute of Pathology, Washington DC, USA.)

REFERENCES

Hackstadt T (1996) The biology of rickettsiae. *Infect Agent Dis* 5: 127–143.

Kim JH, Durack DT (1991) Rickettsiae and the central nervous system. In WM Scheld, RJ Whitley, DT Durack (eds) *Infections of the Central Nervous System.* pp. 411–424. New York: Raven Press.

Silpapojakul K, Ukkachoke C, Krisanapan S, Silpapojakul K (1991) Rickettsial meningitis and encephalitis. *Arch Int Med* 151: 1753–1757.

Walker DH (1995) Rocky mountain spotted fever: A seasonal alert. *Clin Infect Dis* 20: 1111–1117.

15 Acute bacterial infections and bacterial abscesses

PYOGENIC INFECTIONS

NEONATAL BACTERIAL MENINGITIS

*In the United Kingdom, United States, and in many other developed countries, group B streptococci and Escherichia coli account for over 65% of cases of neonatal bacterial meningitis. However, the range of bacteria responsible for meningitis in neonates is wide (**Fig. 15.1**) and varies in different regions and even at different times in the same region.*

- Outbreaks of neonatal meningitis due to group B streptococci or other bacteria may be caused by cross-contamination within hospital wards. Epidemics of listerial meningitis have been traced to contaminated batches of unpasteurized cheese and other uncooked foods.
- Infants of low birth weight are at particular risk. Other risk factors include prolonged rupture of the amniotic membranes and postpartum maternal pyrexia.
- The absence of alveolar macrophages, a relatively small pool of neutrophils, and low levels of secretory IgA and IgG and a limited capacity for their synthesis, all render neonates particularly susceptible to bacterial infection.
- The initial portal of entry is usually oral, from contaminated amniotic fluid, the maternal genital tract, or the hands of the mother or ward staff. The bacteria cross the respiratory or gastrointestinal mucosa, proliferate within the blood, and enter the CNS.

NEONATAL BACTERIAL MENINGITIS

- Initial symptoms are usually nonspecific (e.g. poor feeding, diarrhea, vomiting, irritability).
- Progression to lethargy and coma occurs within a few hours.
- Nuchal rigidity, a bulging fontanelle, and septic shock are poor prognostic features.
- Mortality rate is 30–60%.
- Long-term morbidity (e.g. mental retardation, epilepsy, hydrocephalus, spasticity, deafness, and blindness) affects approximately 35% of survivors.

NEONATAL BACTERIAL MENINGITIS
MACROSCOPIC APPEARANCES

The brain is swollen and congested. Hemorrhagic infarcts are common and may be extensive (**Fig. 15.2**), and a purulent exudate is seen over the cerebral hemispheres or the base of the brain or both (**Fig. 15.3**). The ventricles may appear compressed by the swollen cerebral hemispheres, or distended if the aqueduct has been obstructed by purulent material. There may be coexistent cerebral abscesses, particularly in association with *Citrobacter diversus* or *Proteus mirabilis* meningitis.

Principal bacterial causes of neonatal meningitis
Gram-positive • Group B streptococcus (*Streptococcus agalactiae*) • *Listeria monocytogenes* • *Staphylococcus aureus* **Gram-negative** • *Escherichia coli* • *Citrobacter* species (especially *C. diversus*) • *Klebsiella* and *Enterobacter* species • *Pseudomonas aeruginosa* • *Proteus* species • *Salmonella* species

Fig. 15.1 Principal bacterial causes of neonatal meningitis.

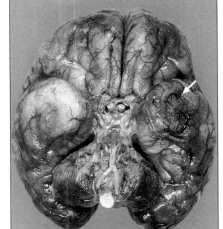

Fig. 15.2 Neonatal meningitis caused by group B streptococcus. There is focal left temporal infarction (arrow) with thrombosis of the overlying meningeal blood vessels. Elsewhere the meninges are markedly congested and there is blood in the subarachnoid space. (Courtesy of Dr Helen Porter, Bristol Children's Hospital, U.K.)

MICROSCOPIC APPEARANCES

The meningeal exudate contains large numbers of neutrophils, scattered macrophages, fibrin, and necrotic cellular debris. The exudate may be particularly prominent over the base of the brain. It extends along perivascular spaces into the brain parenchyma. Bacteria are usually demonstrable within the exudate.

Inflammatory cells tend to infiltrate the walls of leptomeningeal and cortical arteries and veins (**Fig. 15.4**). Intimal accumulations of

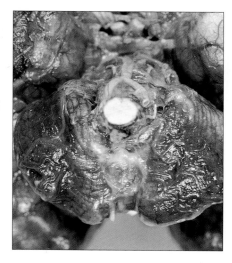

Fig. 15.3 Group B streptococcal meningitis. Purulent exudate over the inferior part of the cerebellum. (Courtesy of Dr Helen Porter, Bristol Children's Hospital, U.K.)

inflammatory cells may be a prominent feature. Venous thrombosis and infarction are often evident (see Figs 15.2, 15.4b) and may be extensive.

Purulent material is usually seen in the choroid plexus and may also adhere to ventricular walls. An acute, predominantly perivascular, inflammatory infiltrate is present in the adjacent tissue.

Complications

Complications of acute meningitis are:
* obstructive (non-communicating) or communicating hydrocephalus (see chapter 5)
* cavitating foci in cerebral gray (**Fig. 15.5**) and white matter.

ACUTE BACTERIAL MENINGITIS IN CHILDREN AND ADULTS
MACROSCOPIC APPEARANCES

The brain is swollen and the leptomeninges are congested. A purulent exudate is seen in the subarachnoid space over the cerebral hemispheres and the base of the brain (**Fig. 15.6**), and accumulating in the basal cisterns and cerebral sulci. The exudate associated with pneumococcal infections may be particularly prominent over the cerebral convexities (**Fig. 15.7**). There may be little or no macroscopically discernible exudate in patients dying very acutely or those who have been partially treated with antibiotics. Sectioning of the brain may reveal edematous white matter and compressed ventricles or ventricular enlargement due to obstructive hydrocephalus. There is usually purulent fluid within the

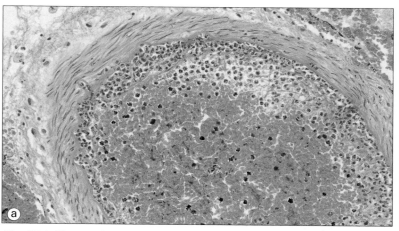

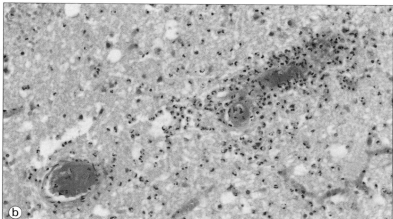

Fig. 15.4 Neonatal bacterial meningitis. (a) Intimal infiltration of meningeal artery by neutrophils. **(b)** Inflammatory cell infiltration and thrombosis of small cortical veins with acute infarction of the surrounding tissue.

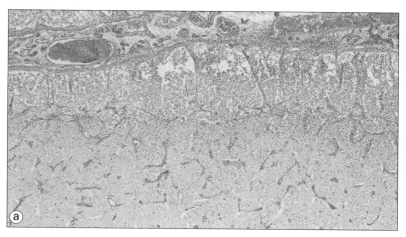

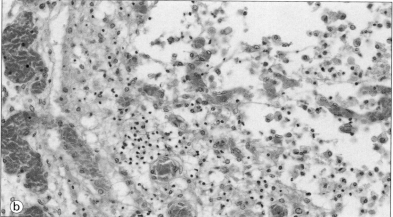

Fig. 15.5 Neonatal bacterial meningitis. (a) Extensive superficial cavitation of cerebral cortex in a case of neonatal group B streptococcal meningitis. **(b)** At higher magnification the cortex is seen to consist of cystic spaces containing newly formed blood vessels, foamy macrophages, and scattered lymphocytes.

ACUTE BACTERIAL MENINGITIS

The responsible organisms vary according to age:

- In children, especially those aged between 1 month and 5 years, *Haemophilus influenzae* type b and *Neisseria meningitidis* (meningococcus) are responsible for approximately 80% of cases. *H. influenzae* is a particularly common cause in children under 2 years of age. *Streptococcus pneumoniae* (pneumococcus) accounts for a further 10–20% of cases.
- In adults, *S. pneumoniae* is the commonest cause of bacterial meningitis, accounting for up to 50% of all cases. People at particular risk are the elderly or debilitated, and those with an immunodeficiency disorder or a dural fistula (usually post-traumatic) or those who have had a splenectomy. A dural fistula may be associated with recurrent bacterial meningitis. *N. meningitidis* meningitis is slightly less common overall and tends to occur in outbreaks, being facilitated by crowded living conditions and poor hygiene.
- The risk of infection with any of the three main pathogens is reduced by the presence of circulating specific anticapsular antibodies and increased by high rates of nasopharyngeal carriage in contacts. The carriage rate tends to be much lower for *H. influenzae* type b than for *N. meningitidis* or *S. pneumoniae*, but is increased for all these bacteria among the contacts of infected patients, in closed populations, and in crowded living conditions. Patients with *H. influenzae* or *S. pneumoniae* meningitis have often experienced a preceding upper respiratory tract infection or otitis media. Up to 50% of patients with pneumococcal meningitis have an associated pneumonia.
- Gram-negative bacilli are responsible for approximately 65% of cases of meningitis complicating neurosurgery, and a smaller but significant proportion occurring after head injury. *Escherischia coli*, *Klebsiella* species, and *Pseudomonas aeruginosa* are most often involved. Gram-negative bacterial meningitis and occasionally meningitis due to *Staphylococcus aureus* may also occur in the context of severe debilitation, diabetes mellitus, or chronic alcoholism.
- Patients with ventricular or lumbar shunts have a risk of developing ventriculitis and meningitis, due particularly to slime-producing strains of *S. epidermidis*. Less commonly, *S. aureus* or gram-negative bacilli are responsible. The infection is usually introduced at the time of surgery, although the manifestations may be delayed for weeks or even months.

BACTERIAL MENINGITIS IN CHILDREN AND ADULTS

- Bacterial meningitis typically presents with pyrexia, headache, vomiting, nuchal rigidity, and photophobia. Patients may develop seizures, cranial nerve palsies, or focal neurologic deficits. These are particularly common in pneumococcal meningitis.
- Initial symptoms and signs may progress rapidly over a few hours to obtundation and coma or, most notably in some children with *Haemophilus influenzae* meningitis, may evolve over several days.
- Bacterial meningitis commonly causes symptoms and signs of raised intracranial pressure. Occasionally, these are due to the development of a subdural effusion (an accumulation of albumin-rich fluid). This is much more frequently seen in infants and children, in whom the effusion sometimes becomes infected, resulting in a subdural empyema (see p. 5.9).
- Over 50% of patients with meningococcal meningitis develop a rash. This is initially maculopapular, but later becomes petechial or purpuric. In a small proportion of children with meningococcal meningitis, overwhelming septicemia results in bilateral adrenal hemorrhage and circulatory collapse (Waterhouse–Friederichsen syndrome).

Lumbar shunt infection

- usually causes the classic signs and symptoms of meningitis
- may have an insidious onset

Ventricular shunt infection

- causes ventriculitis rather than meningitis
- presents with pyrexia, headache, and confusion, without nuchal rigidity or photophobia.
- may be associated with pain and inflammation at the distal end of the shunt in the peritoneal or pleural cavity

Ventriculoatrial shunt infection

- causes bacteremia and, rarely, shunt nephritis

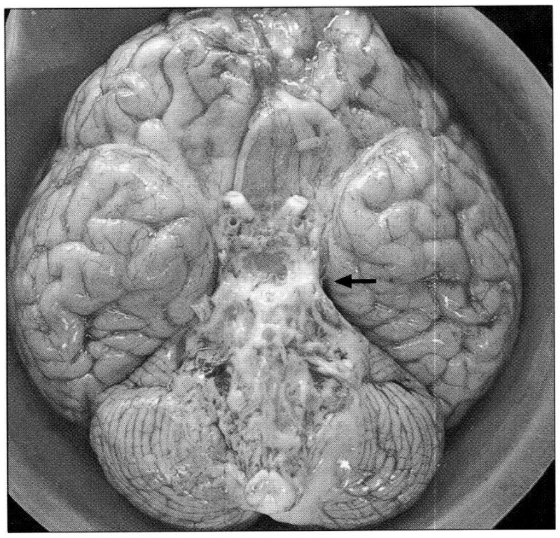

Fig. 15.6 Purulent meningitis with a thick basal exudate (arrow).

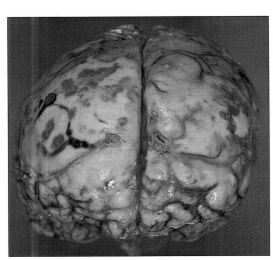

Fig. 15.7 Pneumococcal meningitis. The brain is swollen with a purulent exudate over the cerebral convexities and foci of infarction in the underlying cortex.

ventricles. The ventricular exudate may be pronounced in patients with ventricular shunt infection (**Fig. 15.8**), in whom the leptomeninges appear remarkably clear. Occasionally, the coagulopathy associated with meningococcal septicemia is complicated by ventricular hemorrhage. Small infarcts may result from thrombosis of penetrating arteries (**Fig. 15.9**). Venous thrombosis and hemorrhagic infarcts are less common than in neonatal meningitis.

Subdural effusions are an occasional complication of meningitis in children and appear as accumulations of clear fluid over the cerebral convexities or in the interhemispheric fissure.

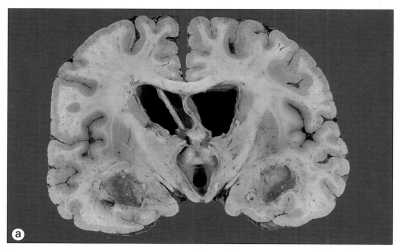
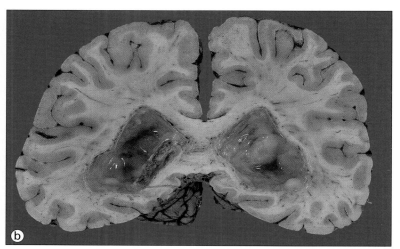

Fig. 15.8 Ventriculitis due to *Staphylococcus aureus* shunt infection. (a) The shunt tubing is visible in one of the lateral ventricles. The ventricles are dilated and their lining markedly congested. **(b)** The purulent exudate is well seen in the occipital horns.

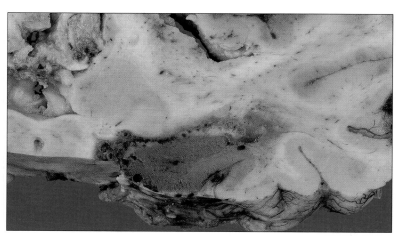

Fig. 15.9 *Proteus* meningitis. There are multiple foci of infarction (one involving the hippocampus) due to arterial thrombosis.

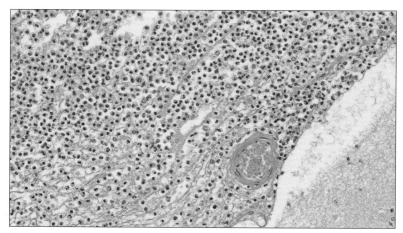

Fig. 15.10 Meningeal exudate in acute purulent meningitis. The exudate includes numerous neutrophils and strands of fibrin.

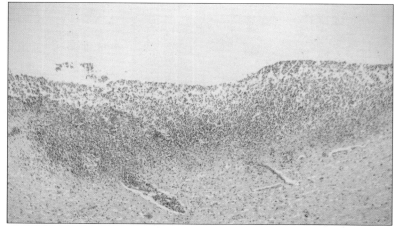

Fig. 15.11 Purulent ventricular exudate. An inflammatory infiltrate is present in the ventricles and the periventricular white matter.

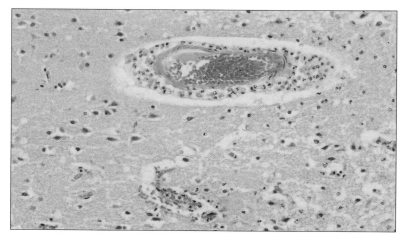

Fig. 15.12 Acute purulent meningitis. Perivascular spread of inflammatory cells in the superficial cerebral cortex is a common finding.

MICROSCOPIC APPEARANCES

During the first few days, the subarachnoid (**Fig. 15.10**) and ventricular (**Fig. 15.11**) exudate contains large numbers of neutrophils and necrotic debris. Intracellular and extracellular bacteria can usually be demonstrated. The exudate extends along perivascular spaces into the cerebral cortex (**Fig. 15.12**), cerebellum, brain stem, and spinal cord. There is usually purulent material in the choroid plexus (**Fig. 15.13**). Perivascular inflammation and fibrinoid necrosis of blood vessels may be seen in the periventricular white matter (**Fig. 15.14, see Fig. 15.11**). With time, the numbers of various mononuclear leukocytes increase, and by the end of the first week these predominate. There is usually some proliferation of fibroblasts.

Inflammatory cells tend to infiltrate the walls of leptomeningeal and cortical arteries and veins and may accumulate in the intima (**Fig. 15.15**). Thrombosis of small meningeal and cortical blood vessels (**Fig. 15.16**) with associated focal infarction is relatively common in cases coming to necropsy (see Figs 15.7, 15.9, 15.16).

Complications

As noted above, the complications include:
- cerebral edema, which may be marked
- arterial and venous infarcts (**Fig. 15.17**)
- obstructive or communicating hydrocephalus
- subdural effusions
- subdural empyema.

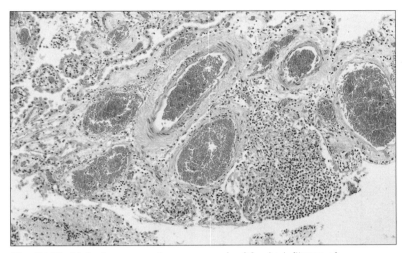

Fig. 15.13 *Listeria monocytogenes* **meningitis.** An infiltrate of inflammatory cells is present in the choroid plexus.

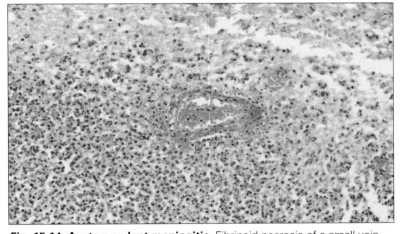

Fig. 15.14 Acute purulent meningitis. Fibrinoid necrosis of a small vein within an acute inflammatory cell infiltrate in the periventricular white matter.

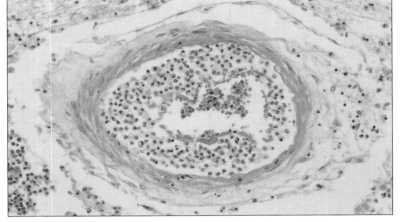

Fig. 15.15 Acute purulent meningitis. Intimal infiltrate of inflammatory cells in a meningeal artery.

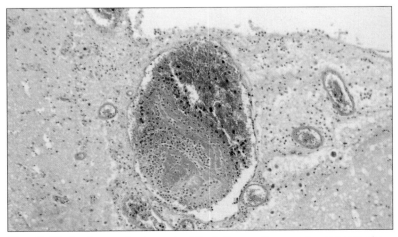

Fig. 15.16 Acute purulent meningitis. Inflammation and thrombosis of a cortical vein with infarction of the adjacent parenchyma.

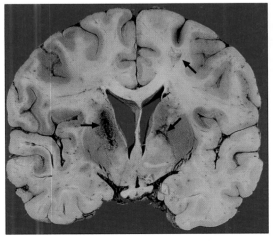

Fig. 15.17 Multiple cerebral infarcts (arrows) complicating pneumococcal meningitis.

BRAIN ABSCESS

BRAIN ABSCESS

Direct spread

- The cause of approximately 50% of brain abscesses is spread of infection from a septic focus in the paranasal sinus, middle ear, or dental root. The proportion of brain abscesses caused by spread from local infection is higher in parts of the world where such infections are neglected until at an advanced stage than in developed countries, where sinusitis and otitis media tend to receive relatively early medical attention.
- *Streptococcus milleri* is the most commonly implicated pathogen, but isolates include both aerobic and anaerobic streptococci, staphylococci, *Bacteroides fragilis*, *Actinomyces israelii* (an anaerobic, filamentous, gram-positive bacterium), and aerobic gram-negative bacilli. Mixed infections are common.

Hematogenous spread

- In approximately 25% of brain abscesses, the infection is of hematogenous origin.
- In children, congenital heart disease with right-to-left shunting is usually responsible. Bypassing of the pulmonary circulation by small septic emboli, cerebral hypoxia, and increased blood viscosity due to polycythemia are probably all contributory factors.
- In adults, the source of hematogenous infection is septic emboli, usually from bronchiectasis, a lung abscess, or subacute endocarditis. *Streptococcus viridans*, and microaerophilic or anaerobic streptococci are the commonest isolates.

Other antecedents of brain abscesses include cranial trauma, neurosurgery, and immunodeficiency, either disease-related (e.g. AIDS, leukemia) or iatrogenic (e.g. after organ or bone marrow transplantation). Even closed head injuries pre-dispose to abscess formation, suggesting that the presence of devitalized brain tissue is an important predisposing factor. This is presumably why cerebral infarcts are, rarely, complicated by abscess formation.
Immunodeficiency is an increasingly important predisposing factor and associated pathogens include:
- *Toxoplasma gondii.*
- *Nocardia asteroides* (an aerobic, filamentous, gram-positive bacterium).
- *Listeria monocytogenes.*
- Gram-negative bacilli.
- Mycobacteria.
- Diverse fungi (see chapter 17).
Abscesses occasionally develop in association with Citrobacter diversus *or* Proteus mirabilis *meningitis in infants.*

BRAIN ABSCESS

- A brain abscess may present with headache, fever, epilepsy, nausea and vomiting, altered sensorium, nuchal rigidity, or localizing neurologic signs.
- Early changes of local cerebritis may be evident on magnetic resonance imaging (MRI) before any abnormality can be seen on computerized tomography (CT).
- Poor prognostic factors include extremes of age (the very young or very old), an altered sensorium at presentation, or concomitant systemic infection.
- Mortality is approximately 20%.
- Approximately 50% of the survivors have persistent epilepsy, intellectual impairment, or focal neurologic signs, or a combination of these complications.

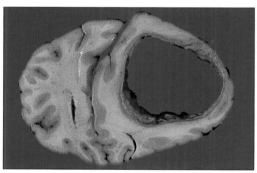

Fig. 15.18 Brain abscess due to direct spread of infection. Frontal abscess complicating chronic frontal sinus infection.

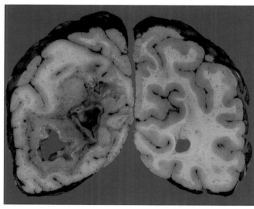

Fig. 15.19 Hematogenous brain abscesses. Multiple abscesses in a patient with a ventriculoseptal defect complicated by pulmonary hypertension and right-to-left shunting (Eisenmenger's syndrome).

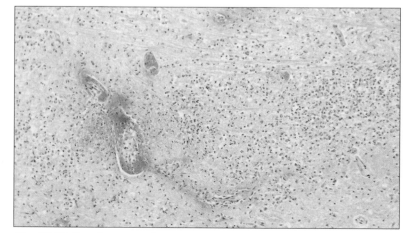

Fig. 15.20 Focal suppurative encephalitis due to *Listeria monocytogenes* infection. Fibrinoid vascular necrosis is a common finding in *Listeria* meningoencephalitis.

MACROSCOPIC APPEARANCES

As would be expected, abscesses caused by direct spread of local infection tend to be located in the frontal (**Fig. 15.18**) or temporal lobes or the anterior parietal region, adjacent to the source of infection. Less commonly, otogenic infection may be complicated by a cerebellar abscess. Abscesses caused by hematogenous spread of infection tend to occur at junctions between gray and white matter and are often multiple (**Fig. 15.19**). They may be situated in any part of the brain, although the perfusion territory of the middle cerebral arteries is usually involved.

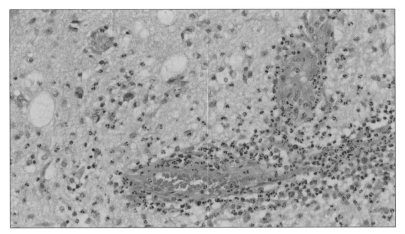

Fig. 15.21 Acute cerebritis. The inflamed brain tissue was adjacent to a focus of middle ear and petrous temporal bone infection.

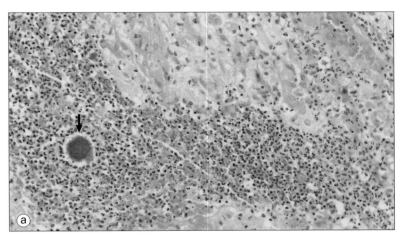

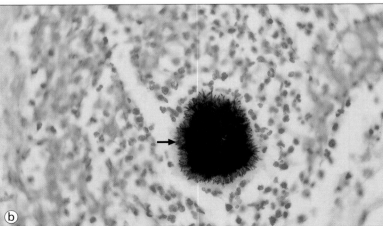

Fig. 15.22 Focal suppurative encephalitis with confluent necrosis due to _Actinomyces israelii_ infection. (a) and **(b)** The characteristic 'sulfur' granules (arrow in **a**) are composed of numerous filamentous gram-positive bacteria (arrow in **b**). Established _Actinomyces_ abscesses tend to be multiloculated.

The earliest stage of focal cerebritis appears macroscopically as an ill-defined region of hyperemia with surrounding white matter edema. It takes about 1–3 weeks for an abscess with a visible capsule and purulent center to become macroscopically discernible. Over weeks and months, the abscess enlarges by expanding into the white matter. The capsule gradually thickens, although this occurs to a greater extent in the subcortical region than in the deep white matter, where the capsule tends to remain relatively thin. Abscesses caused by hematogenous spread of infection tend to be less well encapsulated than those caused by local spread. A large abscess occasionally ruptures into the ventricular system, causing a purulent ventriculitis.

MICROSCOPIC APPEARANCES

The evolution of a cerebral abscess can be subdivided into the following four stages:
- focal suppurative encephalitis (days 1–2)
- focal suppurative encephalitis with confluent central necrosis (days 2–7)
- early encapsulation (days 5–14)
- late encapsulation (from day 14)

Focal suppurative encephalitis lasts 1–2 days and is characterized by swelling of endothelial cells, and perivascular and parenchymal infiltration by neutrophils (**Figs 15.20, 15.21**). Small foci of necrosis develop rapidly. Only occasional mononuclear inflammatory cells are present at this stage.

Focal suppurative encephalitis with confluent central necrosis is characterized by adjacent foci of necrosis, which soon enlarge and become confluent (**Fig. 15.22**). By day 3 or 4, foamy macrophages are much more numerous and the infiltrate includes lymphocytes and some plasma cells.

Early encapsulation is seen by days 5–7: an early granulation tissue response is evident around the margin of the necrotic tissue, with newly formed capillaries and scattered fibroblasts (**Fig. 15.23**). Over the next few days, the fibroblasts proliferate and deposit reticulin (**Fig. 15.24**). The surrounding brain tissue is edematous and contains swollen reactive astrocytes. Parenchymal blood vessels have plump endothelial cells and tend to be surrounded by small aggregates of lymphocytes.

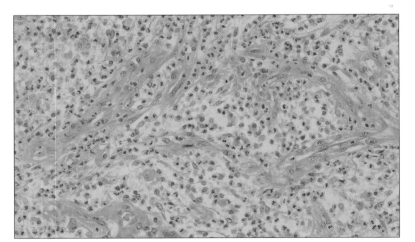

Fig. 15.23 Early encapsulation of a cerebral abscess with newly formed capillaries and scattered fibroblasts. The inflammatory infiltrate includes macrophages and lymphocytes as well as neutrophils.

Late encapsulation is seen from about day 14 when most abscesses have a clearly defined structure consisting of:

- Central necrotic material.
- A surrounding rim of granulation tissue within which are numerous neutrophils, foamy macrophages, and scattered lymphocytes.
- A capsule composed of multiple concentric layers of fibroblasts and collagen (**Fig. 15.25**), and variable numbers of inflammatory cells, mainly lymphocytes and macrophages. The capsule is penetrated by small blood vessels, most of which are radially oriented, in contrast to the fibroblasts and collagen.
- Reactive brain tissue.

Progressive collagen deposition over subsequent weeks thickens the capsule. The thickness varies at different points, tending to be greater on the cortical than on the ventricular aspect (**Fig. 15.26**). Occasionally, the infection in a chronic abscess resolves in the absence of treatment, leaving a dense fibrous capsule lined by sparse macrophages and amorphous material.

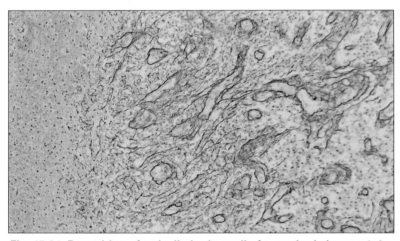

Fig. 15.24 Deposition of reticulin in the wall of a cerebral abscess 1–2 weeks in age.

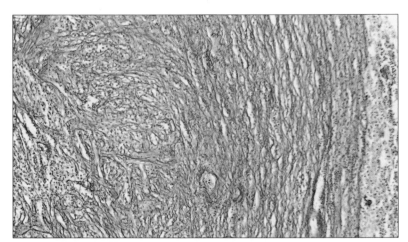

Fig. 15.25 Numerous closely packed layers of circumferentially oriented reticulin in the wall of a chronic cerebral abscess.

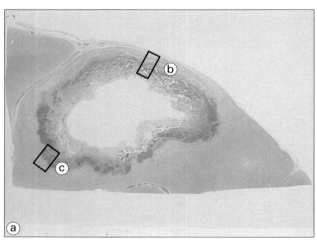

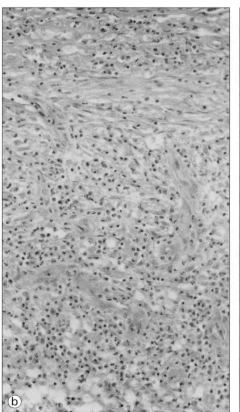

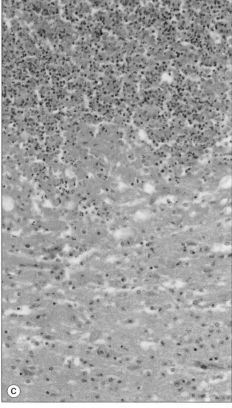

Fig. 15.26 Varying thickness of the wall of an established cerebral abscess. (a) Established cerebral abscess at the junction of cortex and white matter. **(b)** Higher magnification view of the subcortical superficial part of the abscess wall (marked in **a**). A thick zone of granulation tissue is covered by circumferential layers of collagen and fibroblasts. **(c)** On the deep surface of the same abscess (marked in **a**), the wall is poorly defined, with scarcely any separation of the contents of the abscess and the adjacent brain tissue.

SUBDURAL EMPYEMA

SUBDURAL EMPYEMA

- Bacteria usually reach the subdural space by local spread or direct contamination, the commonest antecedents of subdural empyema being sinusitis, otitis media, cranial trauma, and neurosurgery.
- In infants and young children, subdural empyema may complicate meningitis (see p. 15.3).
- Less commonly, the bacteria are of hematogenous origin (e.g. in patients with bronchiectasis, systemic abscesses, or a congenital heart defect with a right-to-left shunt).
- The range of bacteria causing subdural empyemas and cerebral abscesses is similar: *Streptococcus milleri* is most often isolated and mixed infections are common. *S. pneumoniae* or *Haemophilus influenzae* is usually responsible for an empyema complicating meningitis.
- The rare spinal subdural empyemas are usually caused by hematogenous spread of *Staphylococcus aureus*.

SUBDURAL EMPYEMA

- Intracranial subdural empyema presents with worsening headaches, fever, vomiting, depressed consciousness, epilepsy (especially in children), or focal neurologic signs.
- Spinal subdural empyema presents with local pain and tenderness, or symptoms and signs of cord compression.
- Both are usually associated with a pronounced leukocytosis and elevated erythrocyte sedimentation rate and C-reactive protein concentration.

MACROSCOPIC AND MICROSCOPIC FEATURES

In most cases, an empyema is situated above the tentorium (**Fig. 15.27**), occasionally adjacent to the falx cerebri. Empyema occurs less commonly in the posterior fossa (**Fig. 15.28**) or, rarely, in the spinal canal. Subdural empyema consists of pus surrounded by granulation tissue and a mixed inflammatory infiltrate.

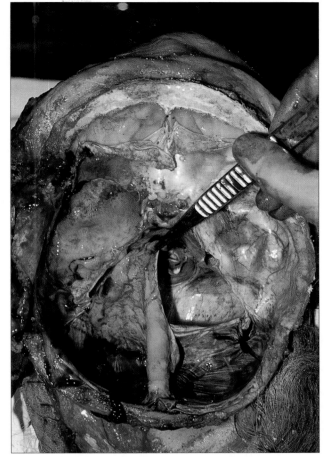

Fig. 15.27 Subdural empyema of hematogenous origin complicating congenital heart defect with a right-to-left shunt. Purulent material covers the left side of the tentorium cerebelli and the dura mater in the left middle cranial fossa.

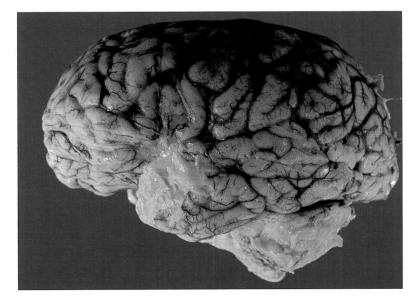

Fig. 15.28 Subdural empyema involving the middle and posterior cranial fossae. *Staphylococcus aureus* was isolated from this empyema and also from a psoas abscess in this patient.

EPIDURAL ABSCESS

EPIDURAL ABSCESS

- Most epidural abscesses occur in the spinal canal. The source of infection may be local (e.g. vertebral osteomyelitis, retropharyngeal abscess, infected dermal sinus tract) or distant (e.g. a furuncle or soft tissue abscess). Infection may also be introduced as a result of trauma or surgical procedures. *Staphylococcus aureus* is the usual infective agent. Gram-negative bacilli are occasionally isolated.
- The pathogenesis of intracranial epidural abscess is similar to that of subdural empyema: both tend to arise from otogenic or sinus infection, local trauma, or surgery. They differ, however, in that epidural abscesses are hardly ever a sequel of childhood meningitis.

EPIDURAL ABSCESS

- Epidural abscess typically manifests clinically with tenderness and local or radicular pain, pyrexia, and neurologic deficits associated with root, cord, or (in the case of an intracranial epidural abscess) brain compression.
- Non-specific associations are an elevated white blood cell count, ESR, and C-reactive protein concentration.
- The abscess can usually be diagnosed by MRI.

MACROSCOPIC AND MICROSCOPIC APPEARANCES

A spinal epidural abscess usually extends over several vertebral levels (**Fig. 15.29**). Intracranial epidural abscesses tend to be biconvex in shape, sharply delimited by the skull and the displaced dura.

Histology reveals extradural purulent material (**Fig. 15.30**) surrounded by inflamed granulation tissue. Osteomyelitis involving the vertebrae adjacent to a spinal epidural abscess may also be evident.

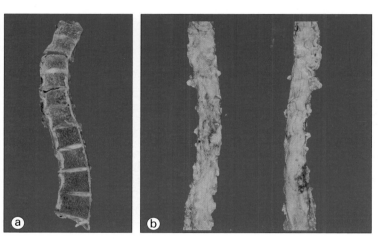

Fig. 15.29 Spinal epidural abscess complicating vertebral osteomyelitis. (a) A midsagittal section through the vertebral column reveals yellow discoloration and softening of several adjacent cervical vertebral bodies and some of the intervening discs. **(b)** There is purulent material on the outer aspect of the dura surrounding the cervical cord.

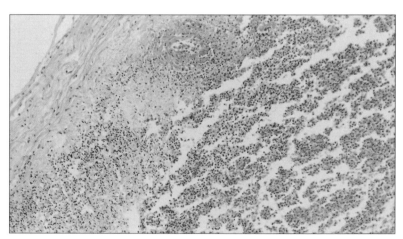

Fig. 15.30 Histologic confirmation of purulent epidural spinal exudate.

REFERENCES

Adams RD, Kubik CS, Bonner FJ (1948) The clinical and pathological aspects of B influenzal meningitis. *Arch Pediatr* 65: 408–411.

Dill SR, Cobbs CG, McDonald CK (1995) Subdural empyema: analysis of 32 cases and review. *Clin Infect Dis* 20: 372–386.

Garvey G (1983) Current concepts of bacterial infections of the central nervous system. Bacterial meningitis and bacterial brain abscess. *J Neurosurg* 59: 735–744.

Gellin BG, Weingarten K, Gamache FW Jr, Hartman BJ (1991) Epidural abscess. In WM Scheld, RJ Whitley, DT Durack (eds) *Infections of the Central Nervous System*. pp. 499–514. New York: Raven Press.

Gray F, Nordmann P (1997) Bacterial infections. In Graham DI, Lantos PL, (eds) *Greenfields Neuropathology*, Sixth edition. London: Arnold. pp113–152.

Helfgott DC, Weingarten K, Hartman BJ (1991) Subdural empyema. Epidural abscess. In WM Scheld, RJ Whitley, DT Durack (eds) *Infections of the Central Nervous System*. pp. 487–498. New York: Raven Press.

Hlavin ML, Kaminski HJ, Fenstermaker RA, White RJ, Horwitz NH, Long DM (1994) Intracranial suppuration: A modern decade of postoperative subdural empyema and epidural abscess. *Neurosurgery* 34: 974–981.

Pfister HW, Borasio GD, Dirnagl U, Bauer M, Einhaupl KM (1992) Cerebrovascular complications of bacterial meningitis in adults. *Neurology* 42: 1497–1504.

Pfister HW, Feiden W, Einhaupl KM (1993) Spectrum of complications during bacterial meningitis in adults. Results of a prospective clinical study. *Arch Neurol* 50: 575–581.

Roos KL, Tunkel AR, Scheld WM (1991) Acute bacterial meningitis in children and adults. In WM Scheld, RJ Whitley, DT Durack (eds) *Infections of the Central Nervous System*. pp. 335–410. New York: Raven Press.

Smith AL, Haas J (1991) Neonatal bacterial meningitis. In WM Scheld, RJ Whitley, DT Durack (eds) *Infections of the Central Nervous System*. pp. 313–334. New York: Raven Press.

Synnott MB, Morse DL, Hall SM (1994) Neonatal meningitis in England and Wales: A review of routine national data. *Arch Dis Child* 71: F75–F80.

Tunkel AR, Scheld WM (1991) Pathogenesis and pathophysiology of bacterial infections of the central nervous system. In WM Scheld, RJ Whitley, DT Durack (eds) *Infections of the Central Nervous System*. pp. 297–312. New York: Raven Press.

Wispelwey B, Dacey RG Jr, Scheld WM (1991) Brain abscess. In WM Scheld, RJ Whitley, DT Durack (eds) *Infections of the Central Nervous System*. pp. 457–486. New York: Raven Press.

Yang SY, Zhao CS (1993) Review of 140 patients with brain abscess. *Surg Neurol* 39: 290–296.

16 *Chronic bacterial infections and neurosarcoidosis*

TUBERCULOSIS

TUBERCULOUS MENINGITIS

- The human tubercle bacillus, *Mycobacterium tuberculosis*, is usually responsible. *M. bovis* only rarely causes meningitis.
- Vaccination of immunosuppressed patients with the attenuated bacille Calmette–Guérin (BCG) strain occasionally produces disseminated disease, including meningitis. Immunosuppressed patients are also susceptible to infection by atypical mycobacteria, including *M. avium-intracellulare*, but the pattern of CNS infection in these patients is usually parenchymal rather than meningeal.

- Tuberculous meningitis may complicate the initial hematogenous dissemination of a primary droplet-acquired pulmonary infection. In some cases, this complication of primary infection occurs in the context of miliary disease.
    - In developing countries, particularly in Asia and Africa, the primary infection usually occurs in infancy or childhood.
    - Exposure to *M. tuberculosis* is much less common in developed countries, as a result of which primary infection, although infrequent, occurs at any age.
    - In some urban communities in developed countries, the incidence of primary tuberculosis is increasing, owing to the rising prevalence of active pulmonary tuberculosis among people with AIDS and indigent inner city inhabitants.
- The growth of mycobacteria after the initial hematogenous dissemination is usually arrested by the development of cell-mediated immunity. However, dormant but viable bacilli may persist within small tubercles in the lungs (as part of the primary complex) or in other tissues. A 'Rich's focus' is a persisting primary tubercle within the CNS.
- Depression of cell-mediated immunity may allow reactivation of infection in primary tubercles. Rupture of a reactivated Rich's focus into the subarachnoid space or ventricles results in tuberculous meningitis. Tuberculous meningitis may also complicate hematogenous dissemination from reactivated infection elsewhere in the body.

MACROSCOPIC APPEARANCES

Tuberculous meningitis is characterized by a gelatinous subarachnoid exudate. This may appear slightly nodular and is usually thickest in the Sylvian fissures, over the base of the brain (**Fig. 16.1a**), and around the spinal cord. Sectioning of the brain usually reveals a similar exudate within the choroid plexus and lining the ventricles. Tubercles may be visible in the meninges, usually adjacent to sulcal veins (see Fig. 16.1a), and in the ventricular lining (**Fig. 16.1b**). Small superficial tuberculomas are quite

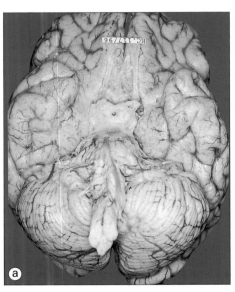

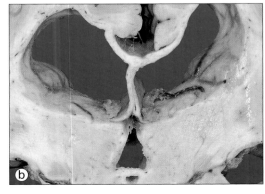

Fig. 16.1 Tuberculous meningitis. (a) Thick pale yellow exudate over the base of the brain, particularly around the optic chiasm. Several tubercles are visible. **(b)** Tubercle granulomas in the lining of the lateral ventricles.

common (**Fig. 16.2**) and may be associated with an overlying meningeal exudate. Large tuberculomas occasionally occur, but are rare in patients with meningitis.

The ventricles are often moderately dilated, owing to the development of obstructive or communicating hydrocephalus. There may be infarcts.

TUBERCULOUS MENINGITIS

- initially presents over 2–3 weeks with a combination of headache, lethargy, nausea, and vomiting
- subsequently causes a variety of neurologic signs including cranial nerve palsies, other focal neurologic deficits, epilepsy, and increasing obtundation
- may cause signs of raised intracranial pressure
- is more commonly associated with a documented history of tuberculosis exposure or infection in children than in adults

Examination of the cerebrospinal fluid (CSF) usually reveals lymphocytosis, a reduced glucose concentration, and an increased protein concentration. M. tuberculosis can be detected in the CSF by use of PCR-based techniques

MICROSCOPIC APPEARANCES

The meningeal and ventricular exudate contains lymphocytes, macrophages, and sparse plasma cells, admixed with necrotic material and fibrin (**Fig. 16.3a**). There may be accumulations of epithelioid cells and fibroblasts, multinucleated giant cells (**Fig. 16.3b**), and well-defined tuberculous granulomas (**Fig. 16.4**) with central caseous necrosis.

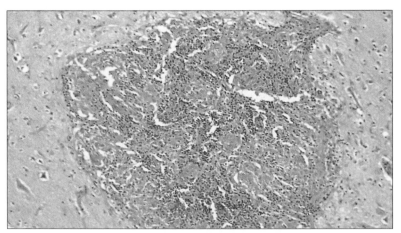

Fig. 16.2 Small cortical tuberculoma in a patient with tuberculous meningitis.

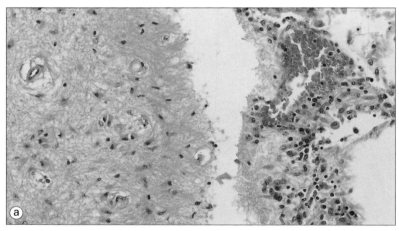

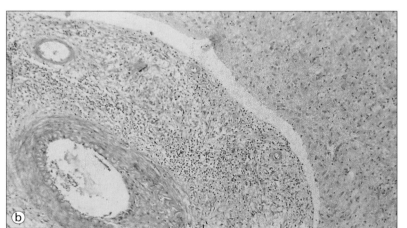

Fig. 16.3 Histology of tuberculous meningitis. (a) There is a meningeal exudate of macrophages, lymphocytes, plasma cells, and fibrin. The superficial cortex is densely gliotic. **(b)** Meningeal artery surrounded by lymphocytes, macrophages, and an occasional multinucleated giant cell. There is mild endarteritis, with proliferation of subintimal fibroblasts.

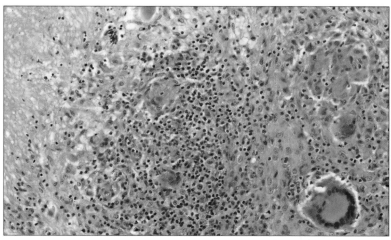

Fig. 16.4 Part of a caseating meningeal granuloma in tuberculous meningitis. There is a characteristic infiltrate of lymphocytes, epithelioid macrophages, and Langhans'-type multinucleated giant cells.

DIFFERENTIAL DIAGNOSIS OF TUBERCULOUS MENINGITIS

- This includes several infectious and non-infectious disorders.
- The principal infectious differential diagnoses are coccidioidomycosis (see chapter 17), particularly in the southwestern United States and Central and South America, and histoplasmosis (see chapter 17). In these, as in tuberculous meningitis, accurate diagnosis depends on identifying the relevant organisms by staining or culture of CSF or brain tissue.
- Granulomatous fungal infections that are less likely to be mistaken for tuberculous meningitis include cryptococcosis, paracoccidioidomycosis and sporotrichosis (see chapter 17). *Non-infectious causes of granulomatous meningitis are considered in detail under neurosarcoidosis on page 16.9.*

Mycobacteria may be readily demonstrable or very sparse. Silver impregnation reveals a loss of reticulin in the caseous material (see Fig. 16.9b). In immunosuppressed patients the mycobacteria are usually numerous and the inflammation less granulomatous and without multinucleated giant cells (**Fig. 16.5**).

The inflammation extends into the subpial and periventricular brain tissue, which shows reactive astrocytosis (see Fig. 16.3) and microglial proliferation. This may cause degeneration of white matter adjacent to the ventricles and in the spinal cord.

The inflammatory cells tend to infiltrate through the adventitia, into the media and even the intima, of blood vessels within the exudate (**Fig. 16.6**, see Fig. 16.3b). Thrombosis occurs in some blood vessels. In others, the inflammation provokes a subintimal intimal fibroblastic reaction that narrows and can occlude the lumen (**Fig. 16.7**, see Fig. 16.3b). Infarcts are therefore common (**Fig. 16.8**), particularly in the superficial cortex and, due to the involvement of perforating branches of the middle cerebral artery, in the basal ganglia.

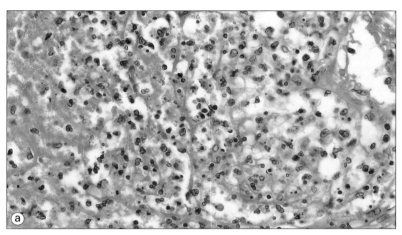
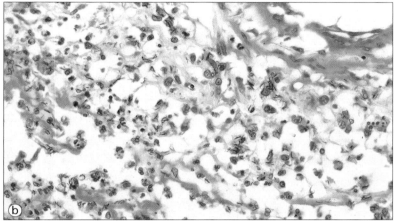

Fig. 16.5 Tuberculous meningitis in an immunosuppressed patient. (a) Inflammation in the leptomeninges of a patient with AIDS. Note the absence of a typical granulomatous tissue reaction. **(b)** Numerous acid-fast bacilli in AIDS-associated tuberculous meningitis.

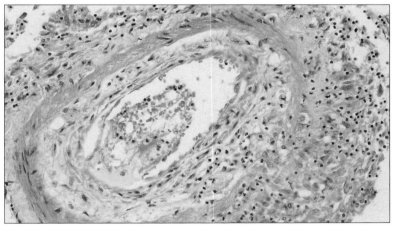

Fig. 16.6 Mild tuberculous endarteritis. Extension of granulomatous inflammation through the adventitia and media of a meningeal artery.

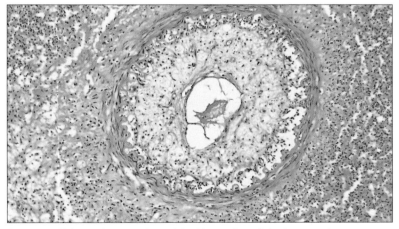

Fig. 16.7 Tuberculous endarteritis. Narrowing of the lumen of an inflamed meningeal artery by proliferation of intimal connective tissue.

Fig. 16.8 Acute infarction of superficial brain parenchyma in tuberculous meningitis. Several arteries in the overlying leptomeninges are occluded or severely stenosed by intimal fibroplasia.

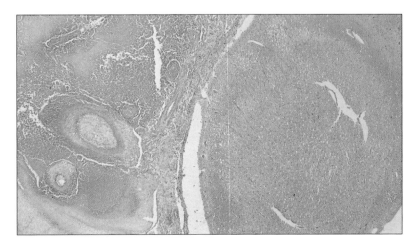

TUBERCULOMAS OF THE CNS

Tuberculomas result from the growth of tubercles, which enlarge within the CNS parenchyma or remain encapsulated within the meninges, rather than rupturing into the CSF to cause meningitis (see above), except in some cases at a late stage.

Patients present with a subacute onset of focal neurologic signs and symptoms, and often with evidence of raised intracranial pressure. The majority have evidence of systemic tuberculosis. Most tuberculomas respond to antibiotic therapy, although this can, very occasionally, cause central liquefaction and formation of a tuberculous abscess, and exacerbate the disease. Rarely, central liquefaction occurs spontaneously.

MACROSCOPIC APPEARANCES

Tuberculomas appear as solitary encapsulated yellow or gray masses or multinodular aggregates of smaller masses. They are most often cerebral or cerebellar, but can occur anywhere within the neuraxis. The central tissue, though necrotic, has a firm consistency when cut.

MICROSCOPIC APPEARANCES

Histology reveals solitary or confluent tuberculous granulomas with central caseous necrosis surrounded by lymphocytes, epithelioid cells, Langhans'-type multinucleated giant cells, and an outer zone of collagen, fibroblasts, lymphocytes, and macrophages (**Fig. 16.9**). Older lesions may calcify. The adjacent parenchyma is usually markedly gliotic.

SPINAL EPIDURAL TUBERCULOSIS

This is caused by extension of tuberculous vertebral osteomyelitis into the epidural space. There is usually a history of backache and general malaise over a period of weeks or months. Compromise of the spinal cord ('Pott's paraplegia') is caused by focal compression, which is often exacerbated by local vertebral collapse and kyphosis and, in some cases, spinal infarction. The thoracic cord is most often involved.

MACROSCOPIC APPEARANCES

There is usually extensive destruction, which may be associated with collapse of the affected vertebral bodies and intervertebral discs . This is associated with variable protrusion of gray multinodular granulomatous tissue into the epidural space (**Fig. 16.10**).

MICROSCOPIC APPEARANCES

The epidural mass shows typical granulomatous tuberculous inflammation with caseation. Changes in the spinal cord reflect a combination of focal compression by epidural inflammatory tissue or vertebral kyphosis, ischemia (see chapter 9), and secondary long tract degeneration. Compression of the anterior spinal artery may produce a typical 'watershed' infarct (see chapter 9) involving the upper and middle parts of the thoracic cord.

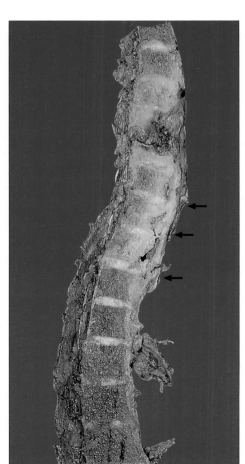

Fig. 16.10 Tuberculous osteomyelitis. The osteomyelitis involves cervical vertebrae and is associated with epidural extension of the granulomatous infiltrate (arrows).

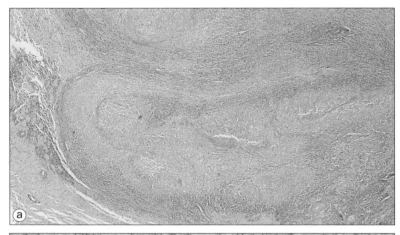

Fig. 16.9 Cerebral tuberculoma. (a) Section through part of a cerebral tuberculoma. (Hematoxylin/Van Gieson) **(b)** Loss of reticulin in the region of caseous necrosis within the tuberculoma.

SYPHILIS

CLASSIFICATION

The different types of CNS involvement in syphilis have been classified as:

- asymptomatic CNS involvement, associated with CSF pleocytosis and increased immunoglobulin concentration, and positive CSF syphilis serology
- syphilitic meningitis
- meningovascular syphilis
- parenchymatous neurosyphilis (general paresis and tabes dorsalis).
- gummatous neurosyphilis

SYPHILITIC MENINGITIS

This complication of syphilis occurs 1–2 years after the initial infection. Although invasion of the leptomeninges during secondary syphilis is relatively common, symptomatic meningitis is rare. In addition to the typical clinical manifestations of meningeal inflammation, patients may develop cranial nerve palsies and acute hydrocephalus. The disease usually resolves, spontaneously or with treatment.

MENINGOVASCULAR SYPHILIS

This is due to a combination of chronic meningitis and multifocal arteritis. The peak incidence is approximately 7 years after the initial infection. Although blood vessels in any part of the CNS may be involved, the middle cerebral arterial tree is most susceptible.

Meningovascular syphilis presents with headache, apathy, irritability, insomnia, and focal neurologic deficits that reflect the distribution of arteritis.

SYPHILIS

Syphilis is caused by the spirochete Treponema pallidum *and is usually acquired by mucous membrane or cutaneous inoculation during venereal contact. The disease is subdivided into three stages (Fig. 16.11).*

- Primary syphilis, due to proliferation of the spirochetes at the site of inoculation. This stage is characterized by the development of a chancre, which heals spontaneously after 2–6 weeks.
- Secondary syphilis, due to subsequent hematogenous dissemination of spirochetes. This occurs after approximately 6 weeks in untreated patients and manifests with generalized lymphadenopathy, a maculopapular rash, condyloma lata, and mucous patches, and lasts for weeks or months after which the 'infection' enters a latent phase. Patients may develop latent syphilis without developing the signs and symptoms of secondary syphilis.
- Months or years after the mucocutaneous lesions of secondary syphilis have resolved, approximately 30–50% of untreated patients with latent syphilis develop tertiary syphilis. There are cardiovascular (much the commonest), ocular, neuroparenchymal, and gummatous forms, which are all associated with a chronic inflammatory process that causes progressive irreversible tissue damage.

There is some evidence that syphilitic involvement of the CNS is commoner in patients with concomitant HIV infection. The fetus becomes susceptible to transplacental spread of spirochetes from approximately 16 weeks' gestation. The risk is greatest during the first few years of maternal infection. The CNS is involved in approximately 35% of cases of congenital syphilis.

MACROSCOPIC APPEARANCES

There is thickening and fibrosis of the leptomeninges, which rarely contain miliary gummas. Sectioning of the brain may reveal infarcts due to syphilitic arteritis and hydrocephalus.

MICROSCOPIC APPEARANCES

The meninges contain scattered lymphocytes and plasma cells. The gummas, if present, resemble tubercles, but the central (gummatous) necrosis differs histologically because the reticulin is preserved. The arteritis can involve large, medium-sized, or small arteries and arterioles. It is characterized histologically by lymphocytic and plasma cell infiltration of the adventitia and media (**Fig. 16.12a,b**) and concentric collagenous thickening of the intima, which eventually occludes the lumen (**Fig.16.12c**).

GENERAL PARESIS (OF THE INSANE)

This is due to chronic meningoencephalitis. The peak incidence is 10–20 years after the initial infection. General paresis is much more common in men than in women. It presents with an insidious impairment of attention and cognition. In the absence of treatment it causes psychiatric disturbances, progressive intellectual decline, seizures, loss of motor control, incontinence, and eventual death.

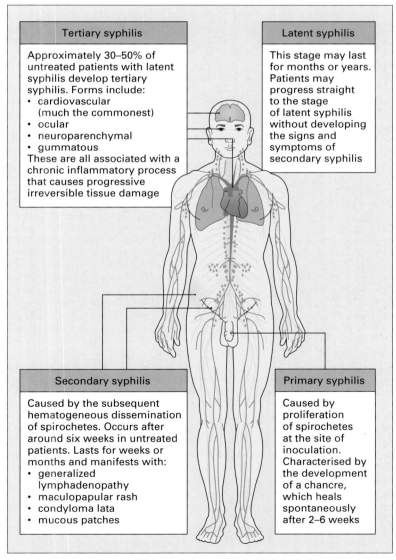

Tertiary syphilis

Approximately 30–50% of untreated patients with latent syphilis develop tertiary syphilis. Forms include:
- cardiovascular (much the commonest)
- ocular
- neuroparenchymal
- gummatous

These are all associated with a chronic inflammatory process that causes progressive irreversible tissue damage

Latent syphilis

This stage may last for months or years. Patients may progress straight to the stage of latent syphilis without developing the signs and symptoms of secondary syphilis

Secondary syphilis

Caused by the subsequent hematogeneous dissemination of spirochetes. Occurs after around six weeks in untreated patients. Lasts for weeks or months and manifests with:
- generalized lymphadenopathy
- maculopapular rash
- condyloma lata
- mucous patches

Primary syphilis

Caused by proliferation of spirochetes at the site of inoculation. Characterised by the development of a chancre, which heals spontaneously after 2–6 weeks

Fig. 16.11 Stages of syphilis

MACROSCOPIC AND MICROSCOPIC APEARANCE

The meninges are thickened and fibrotic and the underlying brain is firm and atrophic. Histology reveals scanty meningeal and perivascular parenchymal aggregates of lymphocytes and plasma cells, moderate loss of neurons from the cerebral cortex, reactive gliosis, and striking proliferation of rod-shaped microglia (**Fig. 16.13**). Spirochetes are demonstrable in the cortex by silver impregnation in a minority of cases.

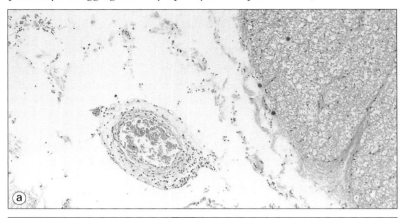

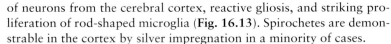

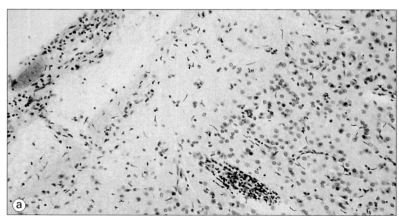

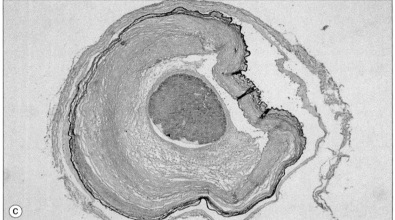

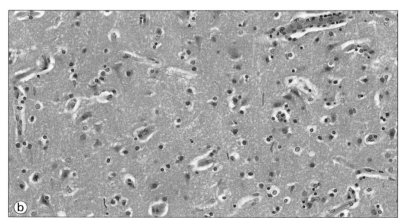

Fig. 16.12 Histology of meningovascular syphilis. A lymphocytic infiltrate is present in the adventitia and media of leptomeningeal **(a)** and parenchymal **(b)** arteries and arterioles. **(c)** Marked collagenous intimal thickening in end-stage syphilitic arteritis involving the middle cerebral artery. (Elastic/Van Gieson).

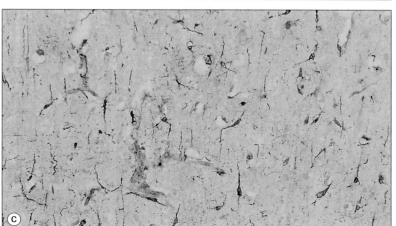

Fig. 16.13 Histology of general paresis. (a) Scanty meningeal and perivascular infiltrate of lymphocytes in syphilitic general paresis. Scattered elongated nuclei or rod-shaped microglia are visible in the cortex. (Hematoxylin/Van Gieson) **(b)** The rod-shaped microglia (arrows) are relatively inconspicuous in conventional histologic preparations. **(c)** The microglia are well demonstrated by silver carbonate impregnation. (Nomenko–Feigin). Figures **(a)** and **(b)** are from material generously provided from the Corsellis collection, Runwell Brain Bank.

TABES DORSALIS

The manifestations of tabes dorsalis are due to chronic inflammatory disease of the dorsal roots and ganglia with associated degeneration of the posterior columns of the spinal cord. The peak incidence is 15–20 years after the initial infection.

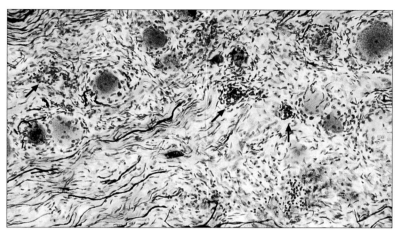

Fig. 16.14 Tabes dorsalis. A lymphocytic infiltrate is present in this dorsal root ganglion. Nodules of Nageotte (arrows) are seen where ganglion cells have degenerated. (Silver/cresyl violet)

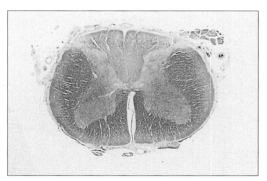

Fig. 16.15 Tabes dorsalis. Loss of myelinated fibers from the posterior columns in the lumbar region of the spinal cord. (Luxol fast blue/cresyl violet)

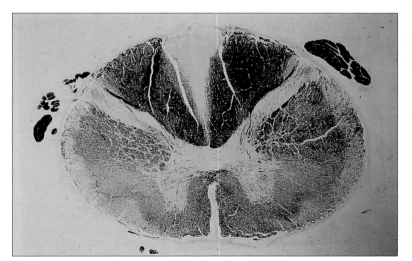

Fig. 16.16 Section through the upper cervical cord in tabes dorsalis. The cuneate fasciculi appear atrophic and depleted of myelinated fibers, reflecting disease in the lumbar region, whilst the gracile fasciculi are well preserved. (Loyez stain)

TABES DORSALIS

- The typical presentation is with 'lightning pains' or paresthesiae or both, in the distribution of the involved nerve roots.
- With progression, loss of pain and proprioceptive sensation may lead to recurrent joint trauma and degeneration (Charcot's joints) and ulceration of the feet.
- Patients develop a characteristic shuffling broad-based gait due to the proprioceptive deficit.

MACROSCOPIC AND MICROSCOPIC APPEARANCES

By the time that patients come to necropsy, the degree of inflammation is often quite mild, with scattered lymphocytes and plasma cells in the fibrotic spinal leptomeninges and dorsal root ganglia (**Fig. 16.14**). There is a moderate to marked loss of neurons from the dorsal root ganglia with an associated proliferation of satellite cells (forming nodules of Nageotte), depletion of dorsal root fibers (which may appear histologically unimpressive), and posterior column degeneration (**Figs 16.15, 16.16**). The changes are usually most marked in the lumbar region of the cord.

GUMMATOUS NEUROSYPHILIS

Gummas are a late manifestation of tertiary syphilis and only rarely involve the CNS as solitary space-occupying lesions (**Fig. 16.17**). As noted above, they resemble tuberculomas, but the central necrosis differs histologically because the reticulin is usually preserved.

CONGENITAL NEUROSYPHILIS

Invasion of the fetal CNS produces many of the changes of meningovascular and paretic neurosyphilis in adults, but developing over the course of the first decade of life. Untreated, the meningitis can lead to the development of obstructive hydrocephalus, and the chronic encephalitis to widespread loss of neurons, reactive gliosis, and a striking proliferation of microglia.

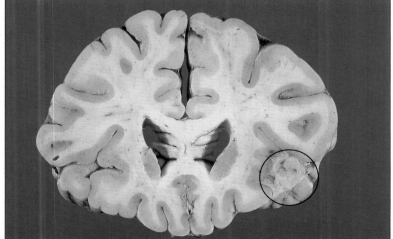

Fig. 16.17 Superficial gumma (encircled) in late tertiary syphilis.

LYME DISEASE

LYME DISEASE

- Lyme disease is named after the Connecticut town where it was first identified and is caused by *Borrelia burgdorferi*, a loosely coiled spirochete, 9–30 μm in length, that is transmitted by ticks.
- The same disease had long been recognized in Europe as Bannwarth's syndrome, which consists of lymphocytic meningitis, cranial nerve palsies, and polyradiculitis, and occurs several months after a skin rash known as erythema chronicum migrans. The disease has since been reported in most parts of the world, but is commonest in northern temperate regions.
- The principal vectors are *Ixodes* ticks, which parasitize deer, cattle, sheep, rodents, and a wide range of other animals, including domestic pets. Mice are particularly important reservoirs of infection. Transmission to humans is usually mediated by ticks in the nymph stage during the summer.
- Lyme disease is a multisystem disorder involving the skin, cardiovascular system, joints, and peripheral and central nervous systems. The lesions are largely caused by the inflammatory response to the spirochetes rather than the spirochetes themselves. Although initiated by the spirochetal infection, there is evidence that some aspects of the disease are due to autoimmunity.

MACROSCOPIC AND MICROSCOPIC APPEARANCES

Because Lyme disease is not usually fatal, data from necropsy studies are very limited. The spirochetes are demonstrable on biopsy of the leading edge of the maculopapular skin rash, and also in the brain and other tissues by silver impregnation (using the Warthin–Starry or modified Dieterle method), immunohistochemistry, or the polymerase chain reaction (PCR). Perivascular inflammation and, in chronic disease, axonal degeneration, have been noted in peripheral nerve biopsies (**Fig. 16.18**).

Lymphoplasmacytic infiltrates and microglial nodules have been described in the brain. Magnetic resonance imaging (MRI) may show lesions in the white matter resembling foci of demyelination. The pathologic counterpart of these imaging abnormalities has not been established.

LYME DISEASE

Like syphilis, Lyme disease has been subdivided into several stages, although the pathophysiologic basis of this staging has been questioned.
- Stage 1 is caused by proliferation of spirochetes at the site of inoculation (usually the thigh, groin, trunk, or armpit) and their subsequent systemic dissemination. The main feature is the enlarging maculopapular rash at the site of inoculation (erythema chronicum migrans) occurring within days to weeks of the tick bite. Typically, central clearing gives the rash a 'bull's eye' appearance. Spread of infection may cause lymphadenopathy, flu-like fever, chills, arthralgias, myalgias, and meningism.
- Stage 2 occurs several months after the initial infection and is characterized by the development of lymphocytic meningitis, polyradiculitis, and cranial nerve palsies. Rarer manifestations include transverse myelitis and encephalitis. Some patients develop myocarditis.
- Stage 3 occurs months or years after the initial infection and is marked by tertiary neurologic manifestations including axonal neuropathies, a low-grade encephalopathy, chronic progressive encephalomyelitis, and strokes due to cerebral angiopathy. Symptoms and signs include ataxia, gait spasticity, dysarthria, optic atrophy, incontinence, and cognitive decline. The other principal features of tertiary disease are recurrent monoarthritis or polyarthritis, predominantly involving large joints, and acrodermatitis chronica atrophicans.

Lyme disease has a fairly broad differential diagnosis encompassing other chronic bacterial infections, viral meningoencephalitides, and collagen–vascular and autoimmune disorders. The disease is usually confirmed by serology, though this may be negative in the early stages, and responds well to antibiotic treatment.

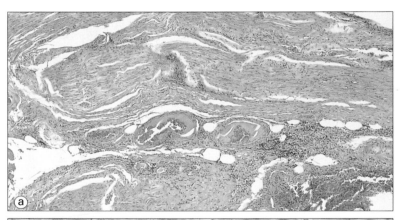
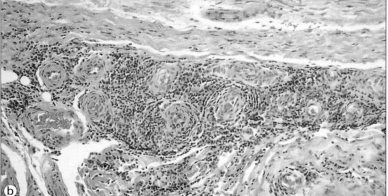

Fig. 16.18 Peripheral nerve involvement in Lyme disease. (a) and **(b)** This patient had acrodermatitis chronica atrophicans, a chronic cutaneous disorder associated with Lyme borreliosis; for details see Kristoferitch *et al*, 1988. Note the mononuclear cell infiltration of the epineurium which is accentuated in perivascular regions; both micrographs are from the same specimen. (Courtesy of Professor H. Budka, University of Vienna, Austria)

NEUROSARCOIDOSIS

Sarcoidosis is an inflammatory disorder of unknown etiology. The nervous system is involved in approximately 5% of patients: 50% of these patients present with neurologic disease and most later develop systemic manifestations, but in about 10% the disease remains confined to the nervous system.

MACROSCOPIC APPEARANCES
The distribution of lesions is variable. There is often yellowish-gray thickening of the leptomeninges over the base of the brain, particularly around the infundibular stalk and optic chiasm (Figs 16.19, 16.20a). The meninges covering the brain stem, cerebellum and, less commonly, the cerebral convexities, may also show macroscopic involvement, as

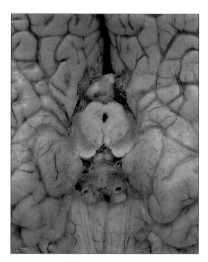

Fig. 16.19 Neurosarcoidosis. Thickening of the leptomeninges over the floor of the hypothalamus and around the optic chiasm.

may those around the spinal cord and nerve roots. In some cases, sectioning of the brain reveals gelatinous gray material in the walls of the ventricles and in the choroid plexus (Fig. 16.20b). This may be associated with obstructive hydrocephalus.

MICROSCOPIC APPEARANCES
Histology reveals granulomatous inflammation in the meninges, ventricles, and adjacent brain or cord parenchyma. Although the granulomas are classically noncaseating (Fig. 16.21), they may show central fibrosis and, rarely, necrosis. The floor of the hypothalamus and the infundibulum are often extensively involved. There may be large granulomatous masses in the choroid plexus (Fig. 16.22). The inflammatory infiltrate can involve the optic nerves (Fig. 16.23) and chiasm, the facial, auditory, vestibular, and other cranial nerves (16.24), and the spinal nerve roots (Fig. 16.25). Small veins and arteries may be incorporated within the granulomas. Rarely, this leads to fibrinoid necrosis (Fig. 16.26) and even thrombosis.

NEUROSARCOIDOSIS

- The most commonly clinical manifestation is facial nerve palsy.
- Patients may develop deafness, vertigo, aseptic meningitis, hydrocephalus, diabetes insipidus, or hypopituitarism.
- Optic atrophy, ataxia, hemiparesis, and epilepsy are rare manifestations.
- CNS disease is quite commonly associated with involvement of the peripheral nervous system and muscle.

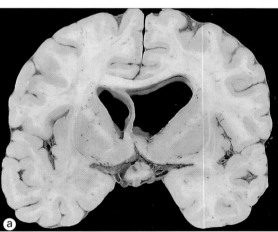
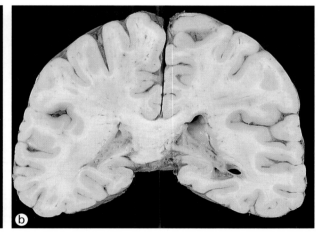

Fig. 16.20 Neurosarcoidosis. (a) The optic chiasm is encased in gelatinous gray tissue. The ventricles are asymmetrically dilated, and lined by gelatinous material. **(b)** Gelatinous gray material is present in the choroid plexus and in the walls of the ventricles.

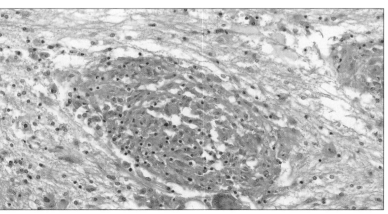

Fig. 16.21 Noncaseating sarcoid granuloma in the hypothalamus.

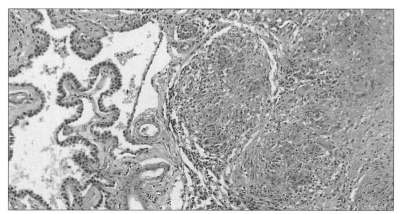

Fig. 16.22 Sarcoid granulomas in choroid plexus.

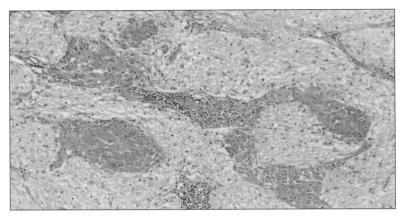

Fig. 16.23 Neurosarcoidosis. Granulomatous infiltrate within the optic nerve.

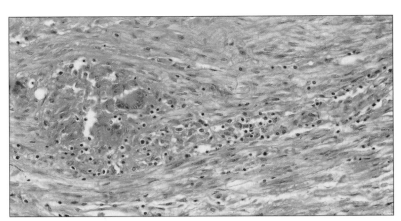

Fig. 16.24 Neurosarcoidosis. Oculomotor nerve containing sarcoid granuloma.

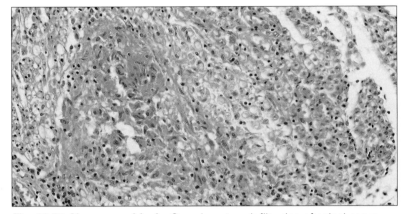

Fig. 16.25 Neurosarcoidosis. Granulomatous infiltration of spinal nerve roots.

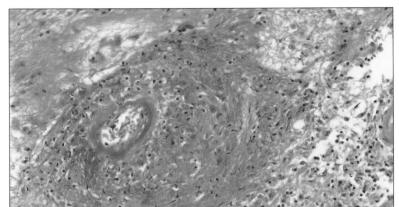

Fig. 16.26 Neurosarcoidosis. Fibrinoid necrosis of small artery within a sarcoid granuloma.

DIFFERENTIAL DIAGNOSIS OF SARCOIDOSIS

The diagnosis of sarcoidosis is to some extent one of exclusion since its appearance, particularly in a small biopsy, may simulate granulomatous inflammation due to tuberculosis (see p. 16.1) or fungal infection. For discussion of the differential diagnosis of infectious granulomatous meningitides, see under tuberculous meningitis on p. 16.2. The principal noninfectious differential diagnoses are Wegener's disease, idiopathic hypertrophic pachymeningitis, and isolated angiitis of the CNS.

- Wegener's disease can usually be distinguished on the basis of its systemic and serologic manifestations and the prominence of the necrotizing vasculitis.
- Idiopathic hypertrophic pachymeningitis, another diagnosis of exclusion, causes more extensive meningeal fibrosis (occasionally with focal necrosis) and less prominent granulomatous inflammation. There is no deep parenchymal or systemic involvement.
- In the absence of systemic sarcoidosis, differentiation from isolated angiitis of the CNS may be difficult, particularly on the basis of a biopsy, although isolated angiitis usually presents differently (see chapter 9) and the granulomatous inflammation is largely restricted to blood vessels. In addition, the vascular necrosis is more prominent than in neurosarcoidosis.

WHIPPLE'S DISEASE

WHIPPLE'S DISEASE

- This chronic multisystem illness is caused by the Gram-positive bacillus *Tropheryma whippelii*, large numbers of which accumulate within macrophages in the mucosa of the small intestine and in other affected tissues.
- Attempts to culture the bacilli have been unsuccessful, but a specific bacterial 16S ribosomal RNA (rRNA) sequence can be detected in infected tissues by PCR amplification.
- The pathogenesis of infection by this bacillus is not known.

WHIPPLE'S DISEASE

- This is typically a disease of middle-aged white males. It usually involves the intestine, producing malabsorption, weight loss, and diarrhea. Other manifestations include fever, arthritis, and lymphadenopathy.
- Varied symptoms and signs occur with CNS involvement, including ophthalmoplegia, oculomasticatory myorhythmia, facial or ocular myoclonus, sleep disturbances, confusion, dementia, and evidence of raised intracranial pressure. Contrast-enhancing space-occupying lesions may be demonstrable on computerized tomography (CT) or MRI.
- Intestinal or other systemic involvement is usually evident if there is disease of the CNS.
- Biopsy of the small intestinal mucosa, which is infiltrated by macrophages containing gram-positive bacilli and staining strongly with PAS is usually diagnostic.
- The 16S bacterial rRNA has been amplified from the CSF by the polymerase chain reaction (PCR).
- Whipple's disease usually responds well to prolonged antibiotic treatment. Antibiotics should be used that are able to cross the blood–brain barrier (most often a combination of sulfamethoxazole and trimethoprim) since the CNS is the commonest site of relapse.

MACROSCOPIC AND MICROSCOPIC APPEARANCES

Foci of granular yellow discoloration may be macroscopically discernible in the thalamus, hypothalamus, cerebellar dentate nuclei, and around the aqueduct. Microscopy reveals meningeal and parenchymal clusters of macrophages containing PAS-positive, diastase-resistant material (**Fig. 16.27**). The bacilli are gram positive, but this may be difficult to demonstrate because of degenerative changes. They can be demonstrated reasonably well by methenamine silver impregnation (**Fig. 16.28**). There is usually a scanty lymphocytic infiltrate. Thickening and fibrosis of the walls of arteries and arterioles in affected parts of the brain may lead to the development of small infarcts.

Electron microscopy reveals rod-shaped intracellular bacilli (**Fig. 16.29**), many of which may be degenerating, as well as accumulations of membranous material.

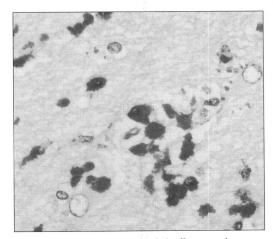

Fig. 16.27 Cerebral Whipple's disease. A cluster of macrophages containing PAS-positive, diastase-resistant cytoplasmic material.

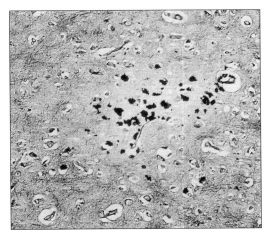

Fig. 16.28 Cerebral Whipple's disease. The bacilli are demonstrable by methenamine silver impregnation.

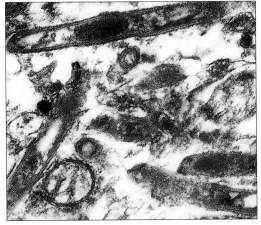

Fig. 16.29 Cerebral Whipple's disease. Electron microscopy reveals the intracellular bacilli.

REFERENCES

al Deeb SM, Yaqub BA, Sharif HS, Motaery KR (1992) Neurotuberculosis: a review. *Clin Neurol Neurosurg* 94(Suppl): S30–S33.

Alba D, Molina F, Vazquez JJ (1995) Manifestaciones neurologicas de la enfermedad de Whipple. *An Med Interna* 12: 508–512.

Cintron R, Pachner AR (1994) Spirochetal diseases of the nervous system. *Curr Opin Neurol* 7: 217–222.

Dastur DK, Manghani DK, Udani PM (1995) Pathology and pathogenetic mechanisms in neurotuberculosis. *Radiol Clin North Am* 33: 733–752.

Duray PH, Steere AC (1988) Clinical pathologic correlations of lyme disease by stage. *Ann NY Acad Sci* 539: 65–79.

Fantry GT, James SP (1995) Whipple's disease. *Dig Dis* 13: 108–118.

Garcia–Monco JC, Benach JL (1995) Lyme neuroborreliosis. Ann Neurol 37: 691–702.

Halperin JJ, Pachner AR, Nadelman RB (1995) Neuroborreliosis. *Am J Med* 98: 4A52S–4A59S.

Heck AW, Phillips LH (1989) Sarcoidosis and the nervous system. *Neurol Clin* 7: 641–654.

Johnson RA, White M (1992) Syphilis in the 1990s: cutaneous and neurologic manifestations. *Semin Neurol* 12: 287–298.

Kristoferitsch W, Sluga E, Graf M, Neumann R, Stanek G, Budka H. (1988). Neuropathy associated with titis chronica atrophicans. *Ann N Y Acad Sci* 539: 35–45.

Meier C, Grahmann F, Engelhardt A, Dumas M (1989) Peripheral nerve disorders in Lyme-borreliosis. Nerve biopsy studies from eight cases. *Acta Neuropathol* 79:271–278.

Oksanen V (1986) Neurosarcoidosis: clinical presentations and course in 50 patients. *Acta Neurol Scand* 73: 283–290.

Relman DA, Schmidt TM, MacDermott RP, Falkow S (1992) Identification of the uncultured bacillus of Whipple's disease. *N Engl J Med* 327: 293–301.

Scheck DN, Hook EW (1994) Neurosyphilis. *Infect Dis Clin North Am* 8: 769–795.

Stern BJ, Krumholz A, Johns C, Scott P, Nissim J (1985) Sarcoidosis and its neurological manifestations. *Arch Neurol* 42: 909–917.

Wolf B, Kalangu K (1993) Congenital neurosyphilis revisited. *Eur J Pediatr* 152: 493–495.

Wroe SJ, Pires M, Harding B, Youl BD, Shorvon S (1991) Whipple's disease confined to the CNS presenting with multiple intracerebral mass lesions. *J Neurol Neurosurg Psychiatry* 54: 989–992.

17 Fungal infections

Fungi are responsible for an increasing proportion of CNS infections. Contributory factors include:
- the widespread use of immunosuppressive drugs
- an increase in the relative number of elderly individuals in many Western populations, and an associated increase in the incidence of certain malignant diseases
- the spread of AIDS

Most fungi live in the soil or on vegetation and infect humans only occasionally, by inhalation or through puncture wounds. *Candida* species are part of the normal intestinal flora. Fungi are common in the environment, but most are not usually pathogenic. Only a few fungi, such as *Blastomyces dermatitidis* and *Coccidioides immitis*, are capable of causing disease in the absence of known predisposing factors.

Mycotic diseases of the CNS are almost invariably due to spread, usually hematogenous, from a primary focus of infection elsewhere in the body. A small proportion complicate direct extension of infections of the sinuses or bone.

The commonest presentations are:
- basal meningitis
- intraparenchymal abscesses

Candidiasis, cryptococcosis, aspergillosis, and mucormycosis have become the most common fungal infections of the CNS.

The manifestations of CNS infection partly reflect the form and size of the organism involved:
- Yeasts are not large enough to occlude capillaries and tend to produce leptomeningitis.
- Hyphal forms obstruct large and medium-sized arteries and cause extensive infarcts, such as occur in aspergillosis and phycomycosis.
- Pseudohyphae, such as those of *Candida*, occlude small parenchymal blood vessels (arterioles), producing immediately adjacent small infarcts that rapidly evolve into microabscesses.

As fungal infections progress, granulomatous inflammation develops in the adjacent leptomeninges, neural parenchyma, or both. The type and extent of reaction will depend on the underlying immunologic status of the patient.

Rare opportunistic CNS mycoses include allescheriosis, cephalosporiosis, chromoblastomycosis, rhinosporidiosis, and sporotrichosis.

Staining techniques such as the periodic acid–Schiff (PAS) method and methenamine silver impregnation are valuable for identifying fungi in tissue sections. More recently, immunohistochemical reagents that facilitate accurate diagnosis of some fungal infections have become available.

CONDITIONS PREDISPOSING TO OPPORTUNISTIC FUNGAL INFECTIONS

- corticosteroids or other immunosuppressive therapy
- HIV infection
- neoplasms (especially lymphomas and leukemias)
- diabetes mellitus
- chronic pulmonary disease
- organ transplantation
- neutropenia
- hepatic failure
- cardiovascular surgery
- alcoholism
- intravenous drug abuse
- malnutrition
- burns

FORMS OF FUNGI IN CNS INFECTION

Yeasts
- Up to 20 μm in diameter.
- Examples are *Blastomyces, Candida, Coccidioides, Cryptococcus, Histoplasma, Paracoccidioides, Sporotrichum,* and *Torulopsis.*

Branching hyphae
- May be regular in caliber and septate (e.g. *Aspergillus, Cladosporium*).
- May be irregular and non-septate (e.g. *Mucor* and related species).

Pseudohyphae
- Larger and more irregular in shape than yeasts.
- Smaller than true hyphae.
- Include *Candida* species.

FILAMENTOUS FUNGI (MOLDS)

ASPERGILLOSIS

This is one of the commoner mycotic infections of the nervous system. It occurs worldwide and its incidence is increasing in many countries as the number of immunocompromised patients has increased.

PATHOGENESIS OF CNS ASPERGILLOSIS

- Most cases are due to *Aspergillus fumigatus* or *Aspergillus flavus*, which have dichotomously branching, septate hyphae, 4–12 µm in width. The branches emerge at an acute angle and grow in the same direction as the main hyphae.
- Airborne spores derived from soil, water, or decaying vegetation usually gain entrance to the body through the lungs. Other portals of entry are the nose or paranasal sinuses, the external ear, the eye, and the skin and adnexa. *Aspergillus* may also be introduced during cardiovascular or other surgery or as a result of trauma.
- The fungus spreads intrabronchially and along blood vessels and lymphatics. Invasion of arteries and veins produces a necrotizing angiitis and leads to hematogenous spread to the heart, brain, kidneys, gastrointestinal tract, liver, and other organs.
- CNS aspergillosis can result from hematogenous dissemination from the lungs; direct extension from the paranasal sinuses, middle ears, or orbit; and cranial trauma.

MACROSCOPIC APPEARANCES

Hematogenous dissemination generally leads to multiple lesions, which vary from a few millimeters to several centimeters in diameter. These often occur in the anterior and middle cerebral artery distributions and involve the cerebral cortex (**Figs 17.1, 17.2**), white matter, and basal ganglia, but brain stem and cerebellar structures (**Fig. 17.3**) may also be affected.

Early lesions often resemble hemorrhagic infarcts (see Fig. 17.2). These may form abscesses, although a thick fibrous capsule only rarely develops. In other lesions, there are foci of non-suppurative white or yellow necrotic material admixed with a variable amount of hemorrhagic tissue (**Fig. 17.4**). Much less frequently the fungus produces intraparenchymal granulomas or even meningitis. *Aspergillus* granulomas are usually a feature of chronic infection, but may be solitary lesions.

CEREBRAL ASPERGILLOSIS

- The manifestations of cerebral aspergillosis depend on the mode of entry of fungus into the central nervous system, and the distribution and extent of the lesions.
- Common presentations include headache, hemiparesis and other focal neurological deficits, seizures, cranial nerve palsies, and signs of increased intracranial pressure.
- The cerebrospinal fluid shows mild to moderate pleocytosis but only rarely contains organisms.

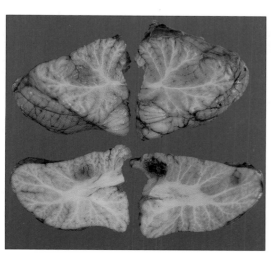

Fig. 17.1 CNS aspergillosis. Scattered foci of softening and hemorrhage on the external surface of the brain from a leukemic patient with *Aspergillus* infection.

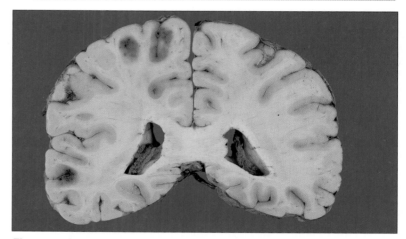

Fig. 17.2 *Aspergillus* lesions in the cerebral cortex. The necrotic lesions resemble foci of acute infarction.

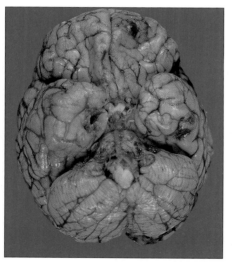

Fig. 17.3 Cerebral involvement in aspergillosis. Hemorrhagic *Aspergillus* lesions are present in the cerebellum.

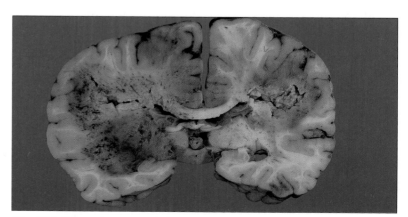

Fig. 17.4 Extensive necrosis in cerebral aspergillosis. Foci of yellow necrotic material surrounded by dusky brown hemorrhagic tissue.

Aspergillus that enters the cranial cavity as a result of direct rather than hematogenous spread usually causes chronic, relatively localized infection with a tendency to fibrosis and granuloma formation.

MICROSCOPIC APPEARANCES

Prominent microscopic features are:

- infiltration of blood vessels by fungal hyphae
- vascular thrombosis, hemorrhage, and infarction
- a variable inflammatory infiltrate

Hyphae are found in the lumen, the wall and adjacent tissue of blood vessels of varying caliber (**Fig. 17.5**). Although they are faintly visible in hematoxylin and eosin preparations (see Fig. 17.5d) and stain with the PAS technique (see Fig. 17.5c), the hyphae are most clearly demonstrated by methenamine silver impregnation. Because *Aspergillus* is morphologically similar to several other molds, a diagnosis of 'invasive septate hyphae consistent with aspergillosis' is the most accurate diagnosis that can be obtained by histopathology alone.

Neutrophils predominate in the early phase of disease and macrophages at later stages. In abscesses, frank pus can be seen in the center of the lesion and abundant neutrophil infiltration at the edges, in some cases accompanied by granulomas. Necrotizing non-suppurative lesions include zones of coagulative necrosis with scanty neutrophil reactions and hemorrhage. Both types of acute lesion are associated with vasculitis, vascular necrosis, and thrombosis (**Fig. 17.6**).

Granulomatous lesions consist of aggregates of lymphocytes, plasma cells, epithelioid macrophages, Langhans'-type multinucleated giant cells, and variable amounts of collagen and necrotic tissue (**Fig. 17.7**).

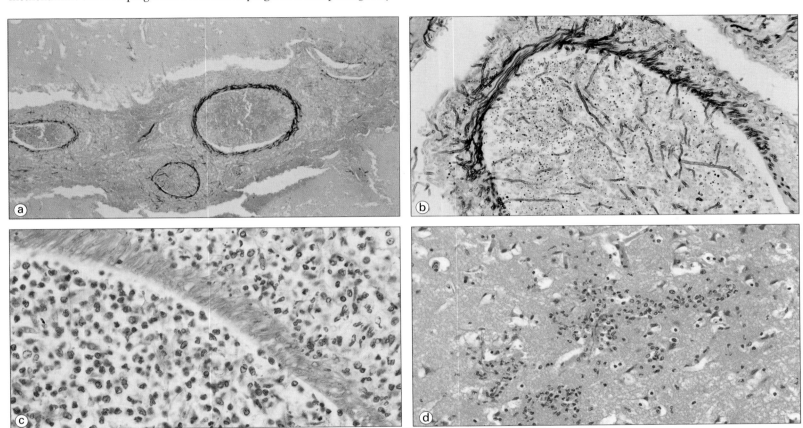

Fig. 17.5 *Aspergillus* invasion of blood vessels. (a) Extensive infiltration of the walls of leptomeningeal blood vessels by *Aspergillus* hyphae. (Methenamine silver) **(b)** Vascular invasion by *Aspergillus* admixed with thrombus in the lumen, infiltrating the vessel wall and extending into adjacent tissue. (Methenamine silver) **(c)** *Aspergillus* hyphae in the wall of an artery. Numerous hyphae are also visible within the adjacent inflammatory infiltrate that consists largely of macrophages. (PAS) **(d)** Spread of infection along small parenchymal blood vessels.

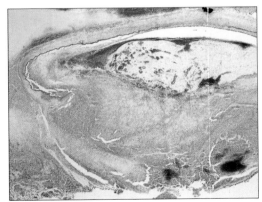

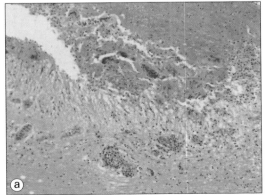

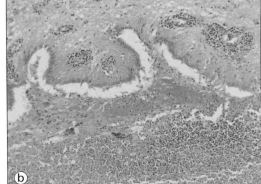

Fig. 17.6 Arterial thrombosis in aspergillosis. Inflammation and thombosis of a branch of the middle cerebral artery that had been infiltrated by *Aspergillus*. (Luxol fast blue/cresyl violet)

Fig. 17.7 Granulomatous inflammation due in aspergillosis. (a) and **(b)** show granulomatous periventricular and intraventricular inflammation due to *Aspergillus*. The inflammatory infiltrate includes multinucleated giant cells.

Chronic abscesses may develop a dense collagenous connective tissue capsule (**Fig. 17.8**) without a granulomatous tissue reaction. The amount of inflammation varies from patient to patient and may be scanty in treated cases.

MUCORMYCOSIS

Mucormycosis is caused by ubiquitous fungi of several genera in the family Mucoraceae, such as *Rhizopus* (accounting for 95% of cases), *Mucor*, and *Absidia*. The terms phycomycosis and zygomycosis are often used interchangeably with mucormycosis. The fungal hyphae are broad and non-septate and measure 6–20 μm in diameter and up to 200 μm in length. Branches emerge at right angles to the main hyphae.

MACROSCOPIC APPEARANCES

In rhinocerebral mucormycosis, foci of hemorrhagic necrosis are most prominent in the orbital part of the frontal lobes (**Fig. 17.9**). Necrotic, hemorrhagic tissue is present in the nasopharynx, orbit, and adjacent skull base. There may be thrombosis in the cavernous sinus or carotid artery. When CNS involvement results from hematogenous dissemination, lesions tend to be concentrated in the basal ganglia.

PATTERNS OF MUCORMYCOSIS ASSOCIATED WITH DIFFERENT PREDISPOSING CONDITIONS

Rhinocerebral mucormycosis

- This results from spread of infection from the skin of the face or the nasal or nasopharyngeal mucosa, through the cribriform plate, into the brain. The sphenoid sinus and the floor of the pituitary fossa may also be involved.
- This is the most common form of mucormycosis (unlike most other mycoses, in which cerebral involvement is secondary to a primary focus in the lung).
- Most patients have poorly controlled diabetes and associated ketoacidosis.
- The fungus tends to spread to the cavernous sinus, the arteries of the orbit, and the internal carotid arteries, with eventual thrombosis. It may also invade through the roof of the orbit into the frontal lobes.

Hematogenous dissemination of mucormycosis

- This may complicate infection at extracranial sites such as the lungs.
- Predisposing conditions include acidosis due to diarrhea and dehydration in children, organ transplantation, immunosuppressive therapy for hematologic malignancies, and intravenous drug abuse (mucormycosis has been reported in patients with AIDS, but some of these were also drug abusers).

Cerebral mucormycosis does very occasionally occur in previously healthy individuals. Rarely, it complicates cranial trauma or neurosurgery.

MUCORMYCOSIS

- Rhinocerebral mucormycosis usually starts with nasal or unilateral facial swelling and hyperemia.
- There may be focal ulceration and necrosis of the skin or mucosa.
- The infection extends rapidly into the orbit, producing unilateral ophthalmoplegia, proptosis, edema of the lids, corneal edema, and, blindness in some cases.
- Meningeal infiltration causes severe headaches and nuchal rigidity, which are usually prominent features.
- Spread of rhinocerebral or hematogenously-derived mucormycosis within cerebral blood vessels may result in seizures, aphasia, hemiplegia, lethargy, disorientation, and coma.
- The illness tends to run an acute fulminating course, leading to death within a few days. Survival is possible with aggressive surgical clearance and antifungal therapy.
- Antemortem diagnosis of rhinocerebral mucormycosis can be made by histologic examination of antral scrapes or biopsies.

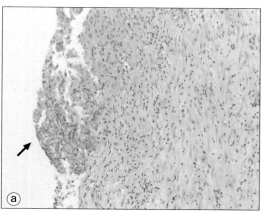
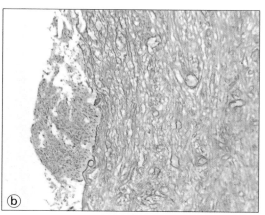
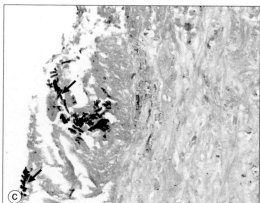

Fig. 17.8 Adjacent sections through a chronic *Aspergillus* abscess. (a) The abscess cavity contains necrotic debris (arrow). The wall consists of multiple layers of fibroblasts and collagen, and contains scattered lymphocytes and macrophages. **(b)** Abundant intercellular reticulin in the abscess wall. (Reticulin silver impregnation) **(c)** Fungal hyphae (arrows) can be demonstrated amongst the necrotic debris within the abscess cavity. (Methenamine silver)

MICROSCOPIC APPEARANCES

The diagnostic broad non-septate hyphae vary in caliber and branch at irregular intervals. They can be seen in and around the walls of blood vessels in the meninges and brain (**Fig. 17.10**). Admixed hyphae and thrombus occlude the lumina (see Fig. 17.10a) and are associated with extensive hemorrhagic infarction (**Fig. 17.11**). The hyphae, which may be relatively sparse, are best demonstrated by methenamine silver impregnation (**Fig. 17.12**). A mixed or predominantly neutrophil inflammatory response may occur around the infiltrated blood vessels and where hyphae extend into adjacent brain tissue. Multinucleated giant cells are occasionally seen, but granulomas are not a typical feature.

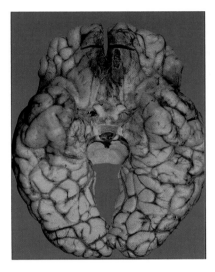

Fig. 17.9 Rhinocerebral mucormycosis.
Hemorrhagic necrosis of the medial orbital region of the frontal lobes.

PSEUDOALLESCHERIA BOYDII INFECTION

Cerebral allescheriosis (also called monosporiosis) is rare and usually occurs in immunocompromised individuals. The fungus, *Allescheria boydii*, belongs to the class Ascomycetes, and has a worldwide distribution. It forms septate hyphae, similar to those of *Aspergillus*. The CNS is usually involved as a result of hematogenous spread from a pulmonary infection. This, in turn, tends to be associated with other diseases of the respiratory system, including sarcoidosis, chronic bronchitis, and emphysema, or can occur as a complication of near-drowning.

MACROSCOPIC AND MICROSCOPIC APPEARANCES

The hyphae invade blood vessels and, admixed with thrombus, occlude vascular lumina, causing hemorrhagic infarcts. These tend to evolve into cerebral abscesses, which are usually associated with granulomatous inflammation in the surrounding brain parenchyma and leptomeninges.

CEREBRAL ALLESCHERIOSIS

- causes symptoms and signs of meningeal inflammation, focal neurologic deficits, and raised intracranial pressure.
- may be associated with the presence of hyphae in the cerebrospinal fluid (CSF).

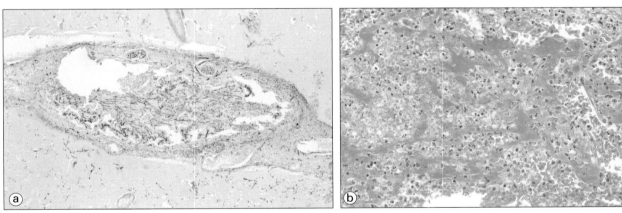

Fig. 17.10 Hyphae in rhinocerebral mucormycosis. (a) Thrombosed artery in which thrombus is admixed with fungal hyphae. Hyphae are also present in the adjacent necrotic brain tissue. (Methenamine silver) **(b)** Broad irregular hyphae admixed with fibrin and macrophages in rhinocerebral mucormycosis.

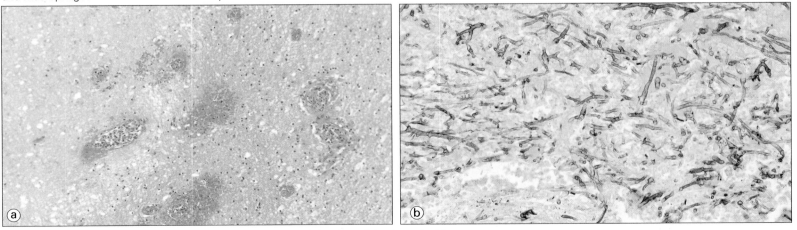

Fig. 17.11 Rhinocerebral mucormycosis. (a) Hemorrhagic infarction of the frontal white matter.
(b) Broad non-septate hyphae that vary in caliber. (Methenamine silver)

CHROMOBLASTOMYCOSIS

Chromoblastomycosis (chromomycosis) is a chronic, usually cutaneous, mycosis caused by pigmented fungi of the genera *Cladosporium*, *Hormodendrum*, and *Phialophora*. Of these, *Cladosporium trichoides* (*bantianum*) is the fungus most frequently isolated from the brain (in which case the disease is usually referred to as cladosporidiosis). These fungi are found as saprophytes in soil and decaying vegetation, and usually infect barefoot workers in the tropical regions of America and Africa. The fungus comprises slender branching hyphae, 2–3 μm in thickness, with indentations every 3–15 μm, and unicellular elliptical conidia.

PATHOGENESIS OF CNS CHROMOBLASTOMYCOSIS

- The usual form of chromoblastomycosis is a chronic, cutaneous, mycosis, affecting adult male field and forest workers, who develop, on their lower extremities, warty, black or brown pigmented lesions that may coalesce (to produce 'Madura foot').
- The fungi have also been isolated from conjunctiva, lymph nodes, oropharynx, upper respiratory, intestinal and urinary tracts.
- Cerebral chromoblastomycosis is usually caused by hematogenous spread of fungus to the brain but has, rarely, complicated cranial trauma.
- Rarely, the CNS is the only demonstrable site of infection.
- Although *C. trichoides* is considered to be a primary pathogen, cases of cladosporidiosis have been reported in patients receiving immunosuppressive treatment.

MACROSCOPIC APPEARANCES

The frontal lobe is most often involved, but lesions can occur anywhere in the brain. Foci of infarction and necrosis occur that cavitate and become encapsulated to form single or multiple abscesses (**Fig. 17.12a**). These may extend into the subarachnoid space or ventricles, producing leptomeningitis or ventriculitis. The characteristic brown color of the mycelia can be recognized macroscopically.

MICROSCOPIC APPEARANCES

Histology reveals septic infarcts and intraparenchymal abscesses. There may be a chronic meningitis and ventriculitis. The abscesses contain necrotic debris and branching fungal hyphae with prominent elliptical conidia (**Fig. 17.12b–d**). Both the conidia and the hyphae are pigmented, and can be stained with PAS and methenamine silver impregnation. Because the pigment may be obscured by staining, unstained sections should also be examined. The parenchymal inflammatory reaction is variable. In some cases the necrotic tissue and fungi are surrounded by neutrophils, lymphocytes, histiocytes and multinucleated giant cells, and there is prominent fibrosis and reactive gliosis. In other cases the reaction may be minimal.

CNS CHROMOBLASTOMYCOSIS

- The usual form of CNS involvement is abscess formation with or without meningitis.
- Patients develop headache and fever, often associated with localizing neurologic signs and evidence of raised intracranial pressure.
- The onset of symptoms and signs of CNS infection may be insidious, over weeks or months.

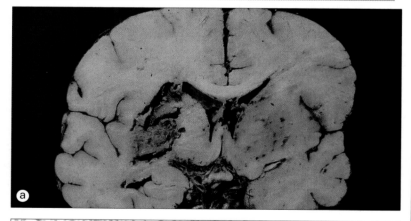

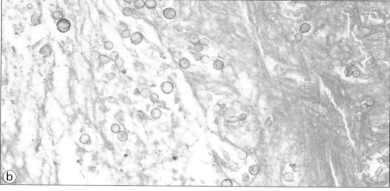

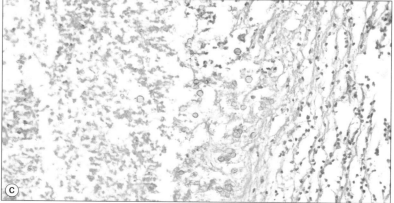

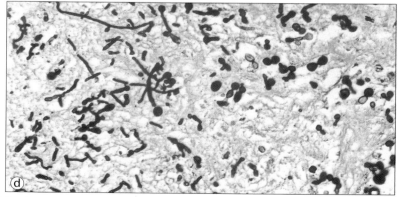

Fig. 17.12 CNS Chromoblastomycosis caused by *C. trichoides* (cladosporidiosis). (a) A coronal section through the cerebral hemispheres shows a large focus of necrosis and early encapsulation in the left basal ganglia. The brown discoloration of the material within the abscess is partly due to the pigmentation of the fungi. There is also infarction and dusky discoloration of the right basal ganglia and insula. **(b)** The brown pigmentation of the fungal hyphae and conidia is clearly visible in this tissue section. **(c)** Mononuclear inflammation and early encapsulation at the edge of the abscess. **(d)** The hyphae and elliptical conidia are strikingly demonstrated by methenamine silver impregnation. (Courtesy of Dr Luciano Queiroz)

YEASTS

CRYPTOCOCCOSIS

Cryptococcosis (in the past referred to as torulosis or European blasto-mycosis) is a deep visceral, systemic, or generalized mycosis caused by the fungus *Cryptococcus neoformans*. This is a spherical budding yeast that measures 5–20 m m in diameter. Pathogenic strains have a thick polysaccharide capsule and grow in culture media both at room temperature and at 37°C. *C. neoformans* has a worldwide distribution, occurring in both the soil and bird excreta.

MACROSCOPIC APPEARANCES

Macroscopic changes may be minimal. However, in most cases the meninges over the base of the brain and cerebellum are moderately thickened and opacified (**Fig. 17.13**). In cases of particularly florid infection, the large number of organisms gives the surface of the specimen a slimy consistency. Rarely, small granulomas 2–3 mm in diameter and similar to those of tuberculous meningitis are seen (see Fig. 17.13a). In some patients with AIDS, there is a yellow–gray exudate in the ventricles and perivascular spaces as well as in the leptomeninges.

Subacute or chronic cryptococcal meningitis produces leptomeningeal fibrosis (**Fig. 17.14**) and is often associated with hydrocephalus (see Fig. 17.15c).

FORMS OF CRYPTOCOCCAL INFECTION OF THE CNS

The two main forms of CNS infection are:
- meningitis, with or without parenchymal cysts
- cryptococcal abscesses (cryptococcomas)

In both forms of disease, the primary infection is usually pulmonary with subsequent hematogenous spread to the CNS. The pulmonary lesions have often resolved before the neurologic disease manifests.

- *C. neoformans* is the commonest cause of fungal meningitis.
- This may occur in previously healthy people, but is usually a complication of immunosuppression or debilitating illnesses.
- The disease is most frequent in the fourth to sixth decades of life, but the incidence in children seems to be increasing.
- Cryptococcal infections are more common in males than females.
- Cryptococcomas are much less common than cryptococcal meningitis and usually occur in patients who are not immunocompromised.
- In a small proportion of patients, cryptococcomas and cryptococcal meningitis occur together.

CRYPTOCOCCAL INFECTION OF THE CNS

Cryptoccal meningitis
- The presentation is very variable.
- Patients usually develop a low-grade fever, debility, and headache, which may be associated with other features of meningeal irritation or raised intracranial pressure.
- Irritability, insomnia, and mild cognitive impairment are common.
- The course is unpredictable. Symptoms may worsen over a period of weeks, months, or years, with the development of more pronounced mental disturbances, cranial nerve palsies, and seizures. Periods of remission and relapse are common, even in untreated cases.
- Cryptococci are often identifiable in preparations of CSF mixed with India ink. This provides a dark background against which the thick capsule around each organism can be clearly seen. In most cases the diagnosis can be confirmed by CSF culture or cryptococcal antigen assay.

Cryptococcomas
- Patients develop nonspecific features of chronic infection and raised intracranial pressure, which may be associated with focal neurologic deficits.
- Cryptococcomas are occasionally asymptomatic and found incidentally at necropsy.

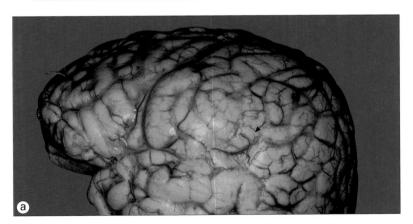
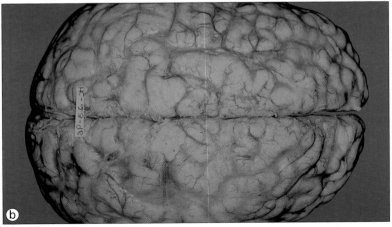

Fig. 17.13 Cryptococcal meningitis. (a) and **(b)** The meninges are slightly thickened opacified. A few small granulomas are visible in (a) (arrow).

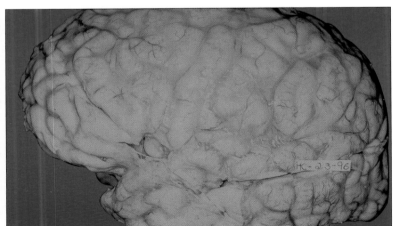

Fig. 17.14 Chronic cryptococcal meningitis. Markedly fibrotic leptomeninges in chronic cryptococcal meningitis. Hydrocephalus is usually also present.

Approximately 50% of cases show multiple intraparenchymal cysts that resemble soap bubbles (**Fig. 17.15**) in addition to meningeal involvement. These are related to the exuberant capsular material produced by proliferating cryptococci in perivascular spaces in the gray matter. Cryptococcal cysts are often prominent in the basal ganglia. The dura mater is occasionally involved, particularly in the spinal canal.

Cryptococcomas have a variable appearance. Some are solid gelatinous or granulomatous lesions, while others resemble bacterial abscesses. They can occur in the meninges, parenchyma, adjacent to ependymal surfaces, or in the choroid plexus (**Fig. 17.16**).

MICROSCOPIC APPEARANCES

The organisms appear as singly budding yeast forms. They have a round body, 4–7 μm in diameter, and are surrounded by a capsule 3–5 μm thick, which stains strongly with Alcian blue or mucicarmine (**Fig. 17.17**). The fungi can also be visualized by PAS staining or methenamine silver impregnation. Shrinkage of the capsule during paraffin embedding may leave a clear 'halo' around the stained organisms. The staining reactions are similar to those of corpora amylacea, with which cryptococci can be confused.

Leptomeningeal inflammation is usually scant. When present, it comprises collections of lymphocytes, plasma cells, eosinophils, fibroblasts, and multinucleated giant cells. The nuclei of the giant cells are generally located more centrally than in Langhans'-type giant cells (**Figs 17.18, 17.19**). Cryptococci, with or without capsules, are often visible in the cytoplasm of the giant cells (Fig. 17.19).

Granulomas are found only rarely. They consist of fibroblasts, giant cells, massive aggregates of organisms, and areas of necrosis. Many of the organisms are found within multinucleated giant cells and show scant encapsulation.

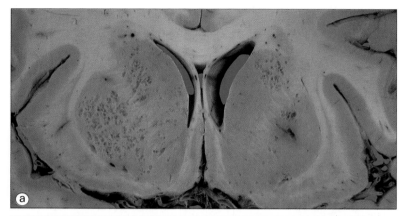

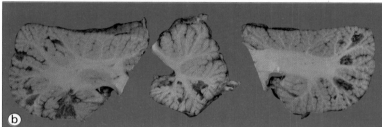

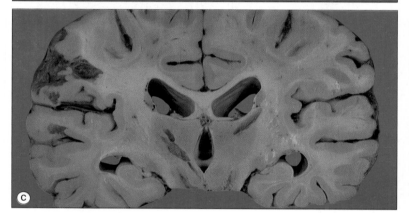

Fig. 17.15 Cryptococcosis with multiple small cysts. (a) In the basal ganglia. **(b)** In the cerebellum. **(c)** In the thalamus and cerebral cortex. Note the hydrocephalus.

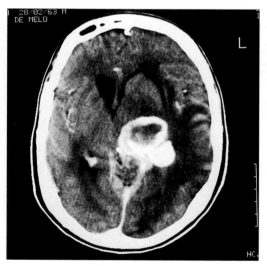

Fig. 17.16 Computerized tomographic scan of a large intracerebral cryptococcoma.

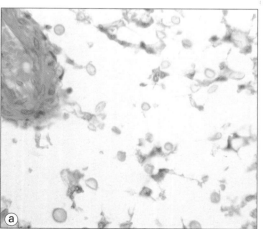
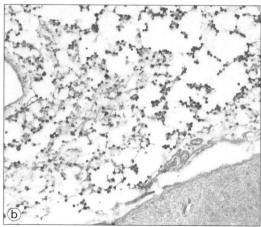
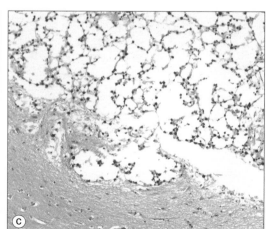

Fig. 17.17 Sections showing cryptococci, demonstrated with different stains. (a) In sections stained with hematoxylin and eosin, cryptococci appear as spherical basophilic bodies, that may resemble corpora amylacea. **(b)** The yeast capsule stains strongly with mucicarmine. **(c)** The yeasts are well visualized by PAS staining.

The gelatinous parenchymal lesions consist of colonies of cryptocci, which fill and expand the perivascular spaces. There is usually little or no surrounding inflammation and gliosis (**Fig. 17.20**).

Cryptococcomas: The histologic appearance of cryptococcomas varies from lesions containing numerous organisms and a relatively scanty infiltrate of mononuclear cells to those with a densely fibrosing granulomatous reaction and containing few organisms (**Fig. 17.21**).

CANDIDIASIS

Candida species are normal intestinal and skin commensals. The commonest form of candidiasis (also known as moniliasis) is thrush, which is an infection of the mucous membrane of the oral cavity or vagina. *Candida* can also infect the skin and viscera, and candidiasis has become the commonest mycotic infection of the CNS.

Candida species are budding round or oval yeasts, 2–3 μm in length. The yeasts may cohere after budding to form chains or pseudohyphae. These represent a succession of individual cells, which unlike true hyphae or filaments are separated by periodic constrictions marking the intercellular junctions. *Candida albicans* can also produce true hyphae.

MACROSCOPIC APPEARANCES

In some cases there are no macroscopic abnormalities. The meninges usually appear normal. Scattered hemorrhagic infarcts may involve any part of the CNS, but occur most often in the perfusion territories of the anterior and middle cerebral arteries. The infarcts evolve into small abscesses (**Fig. 17.22**) or granulomas.

PATHOGENESIS OF CNS CANDIDIASIS

- Systemic candidiasis may complicate intestinal overgrowth of *Candida* caused by antibiotics, immunosuppression, or debilitation. Alternatively, the fungus may invade the blood during intravenous catheterization or injection, or surgery.
- Cerebral lesions are a relatively late manifestation of systemic candidiasis and are usually associated with cardiac and renal lesions.
- CNS candidiasis rarely occurs in previously healthy persons.

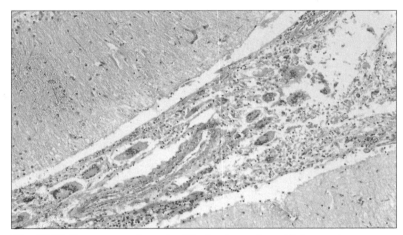

Fig. 17.18 Cryptococcal meningitis. Leptomeningeal inflammatory infiltrate including several multinucleated giant cells.

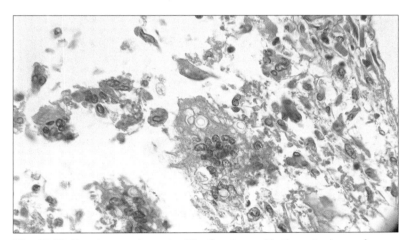

Fig. 17.19 Cryptococcal meningitis. Cryptococci in the cytoplasm of multinucleated giant cells. Note the clear halos due to shrinkage of the capsule around many of the cryptococci.

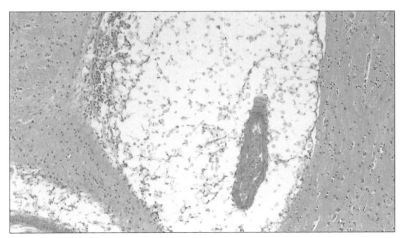

Fig. 17.20 Cryptococcal cyst. Enlarged perivascular space containing numerous cryptococci.

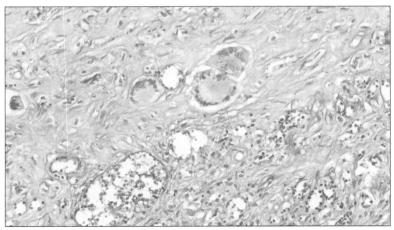

Fig. 17.21 Cryptococcoma. Section through part of a cryptococcoma showing dense fibrosis, multinucleated giant cells, and a moderate number of organisms. (PAS)

MICROSCOPIC APPEARANCES

The budding yeasts and pseudohyphae are faintly basophilic in sections stained with hematoxylin and eosin (**Fig. 17.23**), stain intensely with PAS (**Fig. 17.24**), and are also well visualized with methenamine silver impregnation (**Fig. 17.25**). They are demonstrable in and around blood vessels and in and adjacent to foci of necrosis. There may be thrombosed blood vessels with adjacent hemorrhage and infarction.

There is usually only scanty lymphocytic infiltration of the meninges.

The cellular response to the fungus in the brain parenchyma is variable. There may be:

- no reaction
- formation of microabscesses with an accumulation of mononuclear and polymorphonuclear leukocytes
- formation of small granulomas (**Figs 17.26, 17.27**) associated with lymphocytes, macrophages, plasma cells, and occasional multinucleated giant cells

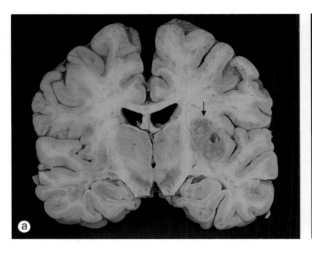
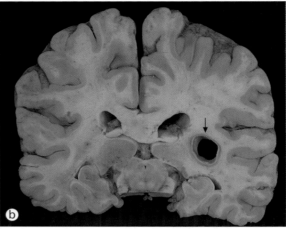

Fig. 17.22 (a, b) CNS candidiasis. *Candida* abscesses (arrows) in the brain of a patient with AIDS.

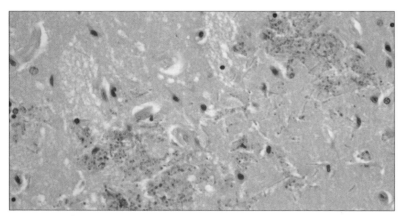

Fig. 17.23 CNS candidiasis. Basophilic *Candida* yeasts and pseudohyphae. The surrounding brain tissue shows changes of acute infarction.

CNS CANDIDIASIS

- *Candida* infection of the CNS is usually associated with oral thrush and acute or subacute lesions in the vagina, skin, nails and lungs.
- Patients may develop symptoms and signs of a low-grade meningitis or present non-specifically with drowsiness and confusion.
- Focal neurological signs usually indicate abscess formation.
- Diagnosis depends on clinical suspicion and the isolation of *Candida* from urine, sputum, bone marrow or other sites. Culture of cerebrospinal fluid only rarely yields *Candida*.

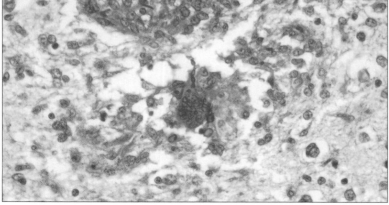

Fig. 17.24 Demonstration of *Candida* in tissue sections. The yeasts stain strongly with PAS. Here they are surrounded by an infiltrate of lymphocytes and macrophages.

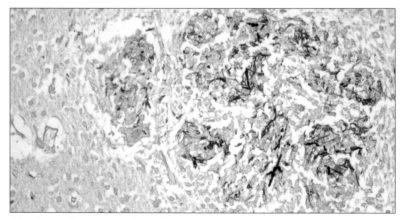

Fig. 17.25 Demonstration of *Candida* in tissue section. Silver methanin impregnation of *Candida* fungi within a focus of granulomatous inflammation.

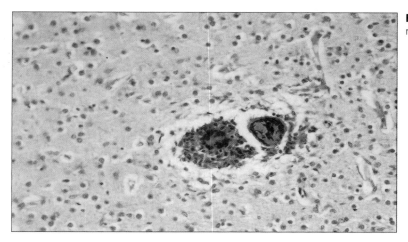

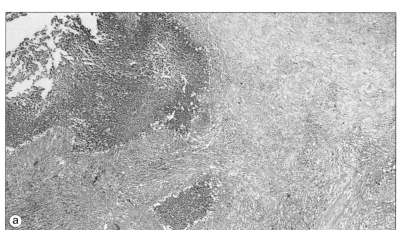

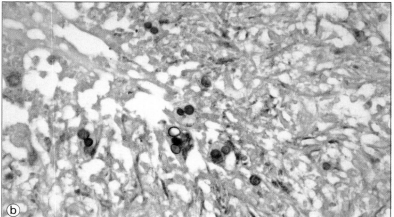

Fig. 17.26 *Candida* granuloma. Small *Candida* granuloma containing multinucleated giant cells.

Fig. 17.27 *Candida* granulomas. (a) Foci of necrosis surrounded by dense fibrosis with large numbers of inflammatory cells, including multinucleated giant cells. **(b)** Demonstration of *Candida* yeasts within the granulomas by silver methenamine impregnation.

DIMORPHIC FUNGI

These fungi are called dimorphic because they form mycelia at room temperature, but grow as yeasts at 37°C.

NORTH AMERICAN BLASTOMYCOSIS

The causative agent of North American blastomycosis is *Blastomyces dermatitidis* This is found in the soil and possibly in decaying wood. Blastomycosis is endemic in the southeastern United States, but occurs less frequently in most parts of the world. Men are predominantly affected. *B. dermatitidis* grows at 37°C as a spherical yeast with a diameter of 10–25 μm. It has a thick refractile wall and forms single buds with a broad neck. The CNS is involved in fewer than 5% of cases, by hematogenous spread from the lungs. The risk seems not to be increased by immunosuppression or debilitating disease.

MACROSCOPIC APPEARANCES

In most cases there is patchy thickening and opacity of the meninges due to a combination of purulent exudate and fibrosis, which may cause hydrocephalus. Small abscesses or granulomas are often present in the underlying brain parenchyma or in the subdural space. Solitary or multiple, larger abscesses or granulomas (blastomycomas) can occur in any part of the CNS.

MICROSCOPIC APPEARANCES

Although usually visible in hematoxylin and eosin-stained sections, the fungi are best demonstrated with PAS or methenamine silver impreg-

nation (**Fig. 17.28c**). *B. dermatitidis* elicits a mixed granulomatous and purulent reaction in varying combinations. Neutrophils, lymphocytes, plasma cells, and macrophages surround necrotic tissue containing variable numbers of yeasts. Older abscesses develop a thick collagenous capsule (**Fig. 17.28a,b**). The lesions may resemble tuberculous granulomas with central caseous necrosis and Langhans'-type multinucleated giant cells.

CNS BLASTOMYCOSIS

- Most patients also have symptoms of pulmonary disease.
- Involvement of the CNS is usually signalled by the development of headaches, a stiff neck, and other evidence of meningitis.
- Occasionally, patients develop intracranial blastomycomas (blastomycotic abscesses or granulomas), which produce focal neurologic signs and evidence of increased intracranial pressure.
- Antemortem diagnosis usually requires biopsy of a lesion, as the fungi can only rarely be isolated from the CSF.

COCCIDIOIDOMYCOSIS

The causative organism is *Coccidioides immitis*, which is endemic in southwestern parts of the United States (especially in the San Joaquin Valley and Arizona), Mexico, and South America (particularly Argentina and Paraguay). At body temperature *Coccidioides* forms large round spherules or sporangia, which are 20–35 mm in diameter and have a thick refractile capsule. Within the spherules are endospores, which are 2–5 mm in diameter. These are released into the tissue when the spherules rupture.

MACROSCOPIC APPEARANCES

An exudate is usually visible in the cerebral sulci or over the base of the brain. As the exudate organizes the leptomeninges thicken and opacify. Small granulomas may be discernible, particularly in the thickened basal meninges. Sectioning of the brain usually reveals scattered small granulomas or, less commonly, abscesses. There may be ischemic lesions, infarcts, or multifocal encephalomalacia due to the development of endarteritis.

MICROSCOPIC APPEARANCES

The spherules and enclosed endospores usually appear basophilic when stained with hematoxylin and eosin (**Fig. 17.29**), but are better demonstrated by methenamine silver impregnation. The spherules are surrounded by varying numbers of lymphocytes, plasma cells, epithelioid cells, multinucleated giant cells, and fibroblasts (**Figs 17.30, 17.31**). These may be aggregated to form small granulomas with central caseous necrosis. The inflammatory reaction resembles that of a tuberculous infection. On rupture of the spherules, however, the endospores tend to elicit a more acute inflammatory response with neutrophils and microabscess formation. Extension of the acute inflammation into the meninges may produce a florid but localized meningoencephalitis (see Fig. 17.31).

CNS COCCIDIOIDOMYCOSIS

- CNS infection manifests as acute, subacute, or chronic meningitis.
- Transient focal deficits such as aphasia or hemiparesis may occur.
- The meningitis is sometimes complicated by acute hydrocephalus.
- Extensive spinal meningitis or granulomas can produce spinal cord compression.
- The diagnosis can be made by microscopy and culture of CSF.

PATHOGENESIS OF CNS COCCIDIOMYCOSIS

- Pulmonary infection usually occurs in the absence of underlying disease, but is associated with occupations involving exposure to large amounts of dust. It is usually mild and self-limiting, although there may be residual fibrosis and calcification.
- Hematogenous spread is rare and usually occurs in the context of pregnancy, diabetes mellitus, or immunosuppression.
- Involvement of the CNS is a late, usually terminal, event.

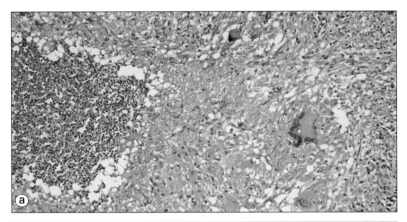
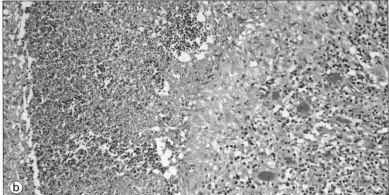
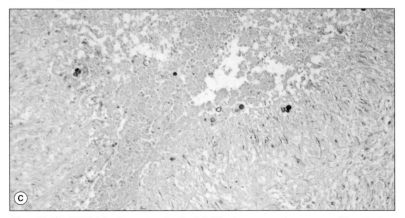

Fig. 17.28 CNS blastomycosis. (a, b) *Blastomyces* abscess cavities that contain necrotic debris and are surrounded by a granulomatous inflammatory infiltrate, with scattered multinucleated giant cells. **(c)** The *Blastomyces* yeasts are demonstrated by methenamine silver impregnation. (Courtesy of Dr Sydney Schochet, West Virginia University, USA).

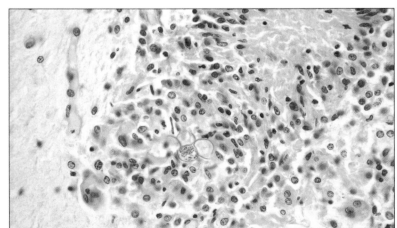

Fig. 17.29 CNS coccidioidomycosis. *Coccidioides* spherules with enclosed endospores are visible in a focus of granulomatous inflammation with central necrosis.

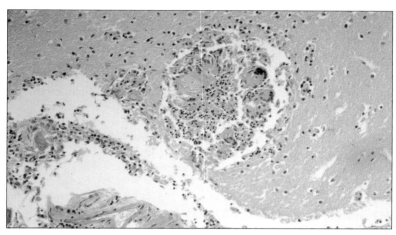

Fig. 17.30 CNS coccidiodomycosis. Small *Coccidioides* granuloma with multinucleated giant cells present in the cerebral cortex.

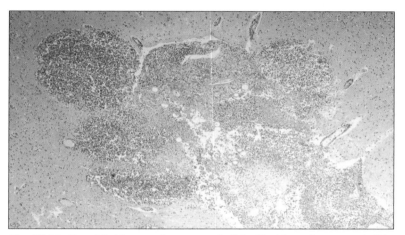

Fig. 17.31 *Coccidioides* meningoencephalitis. Florid meningoencephalitis in a patient with coccidioidomycosis.

HISTOPLASMOSIS

The causative organism is *Histoplasma capsulatum*, which grows at 37°C as budding yeasts with a diameter of 2–5 mm. It grows in soil contaminated by chicken, bird, or bat excreta.

MACROSCOPIC APPEARANCES

Lesions in the CNS consist of thickened leptomeninges, especially around the base of the brain, miliary granulomas, and small foci of necrosis. A yellowish gray exudate may accumulate within the cerebral sulci and basal meninges (**Fig. 17.32a,b**). The granulomas often involve the ependyma and choroid plexus.

MICROSCOPIC APPEARANCES

Diagnosis depends on identifying the organisms by staining or culture since the lesions closely resemble those of other granulomatous fungal infections and tuberculosis.

The 2–5 mm yeasts are best visualized with PAS or methenamine silver impregnation (**Figs. 17.32c, 17.33a**). The fungi appear much smaller on hematoxylin and eosin staining (**Fig. 17.33b**), which reveals only the basophilic yeast cytoplasm and not the surrounding cell wall. The cyto-

PATHOGENESIS OF CNS HISTOPLASMOSIS

- Histoplasmosis occurs worldwide, but the incidence is particularly high in the Ohio, Mississipi, and St Lawrence river valleys of North America, where an estimated 25% of the population has a positive histoplasmin skin test, and in parts of Central and South America.
- The portal of entry is usually the lung, where acute self-limited or chronic cavitary infection ensues.
- CNS histoplasmosis is relatively rare and usually occurs in the context of disseminated infection, either in infancy or childhood, or in adults with immunosuppression or debilitating illnesses.

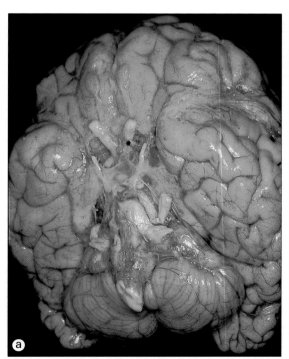

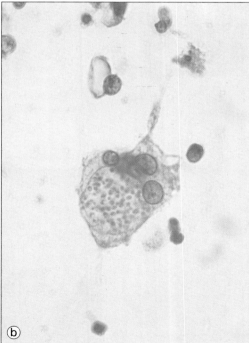

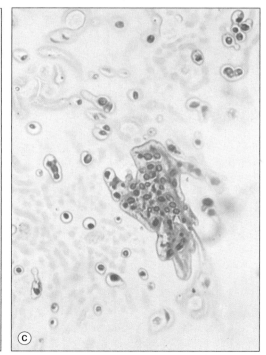

Fig. 17.32 CNS histoplasmosis. (a) Yellowish gray exudate over the base of the brain, particularly around the optic chiasm and over the left temporal pole. **(b)** A smear of the meningeal exudate contains multinucleated cells within which are many small, round, basophilic *Histoplasma* yeasts. **(c)** Intracellular and extracellular yeasts are well demonstrated by methenamine silver impregnation.

CNS HISTOPLASMOSIS

- Disseminated histoplasmosis manifests with fluctuating pyrexia, malaise, weight loss, and splenomegaly, which are usually associated with a persistent cough.
- CNS involvement produces confusion, seizures, and signs of raised intracranial pressure.
- Focal neurologic findings are rare.
- Rarely, histoplasmosis causes cord compression and paraplegia as a result of vertebral infection.
- CNS infection can usually be diagnosed by culturing the fungi from CSF.

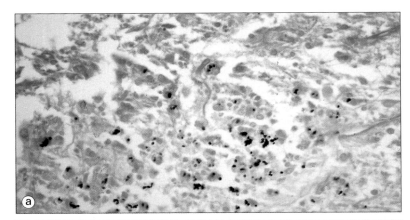

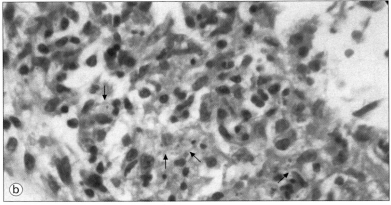

Fig. 17.33 CNS histoplasmosis (a) *Histoplasma* yeasts in macrophages and lying extracellularly in the brain of a patient with AIDS. (Methenamine silver) **(b)** *Histoplasma* yeasts appear as small spherical basophilic structures (arrows) just discernible within the cytoplasm of macrophages. Shrinkage of the yeast cytoplasm away from the surrounding wall gives the appearance of a capsule in sections stained with hematoxylin and eosin.

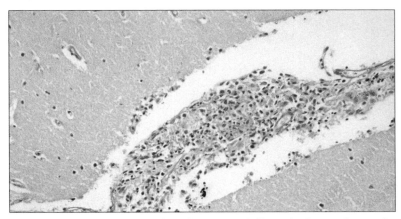

Fig. 17.34 CNS histoplamosis. Inflammatory infiltrate in the meninges of a patient with CNS histoplasmosis.

plasm tends to shrink away from the cell wall during tissue processing to produce a halo, which on cursory examination resembles a capsule.

Lesions range from small nodular aggregates of macrophages to classical caseating or non-caseating granulomas containing epithelioid cells and Langhans' giant cells. The yeasts are usually found aggregated within the cytoplasm of macrophages (see Fig. 17.33), but may be sparse.

The meningeal infiltrate (**Fig. 17.34**) resembles that of tuberculous meningitis, with lymphocytes, macrophages, and plasma cells, and occasional granulomas. The inflammation can extend into the walls of blood vessels, causing focal vascular necrosis.

PARACOCCIDIOIDOMYCOSIS

Paracoccidioidomycosis (also known as South American blastomycosis) is caused by *Paracoccidioides brasiliensis*. It is a disease of the New World, occurring in countries from Mexico to Argentina (with the exceptions of Chile, El Salvador, and Panama), and is the mycosis most frequently encountered in Brazil, Venezuela, and Colombia. The fungi probably live in soil or vegetation. At 37°C, they grow as thick-walled yeasts with round to oval bodies, which are 10–20 mm in diameter and give rise to single or multiple thin-necked buds.

Paracoccidioidomycosis is a chronic granulomatous disease that affects the lungs and the nasal and oropharyngeal mucosa and adjacent tissues, spreading to lymph nodes, the adrenal glands, and other viscera, including, in some patients, the CNS.

MACROSCOPIC APPEARANCES

The more frequent form of CNS paracoccidioidomycosis is the pseudotumorous form, which results from the formation of one or more paracoccidioidomycomas. These well-circumscribed necrotic nodules vary from a few millimeters to several centimeters in diameter (**Figs 17.35, 17.36**) and are usually situated in the cerebral cortex. Similar lesions can occur in the spinal cord. Paracoccidioidomycomas in the dura mater may simulate meningiomas both clinically and macroscopically. The leptomeningitis is granulomatous, predominantly basal, and may cause obstructive hydrocephalus.

CNS PARACOCCIDIOIDOMYCOSIS

- Manifests with symptoms and signs of space-occupying lesions in the brain or spinal cord (the pseudotumorous form of CNS paracoccidioidomycosis) or of meningitis (the meningitic form).
- Is often accompanied by evidence of raised intracranial pressure.

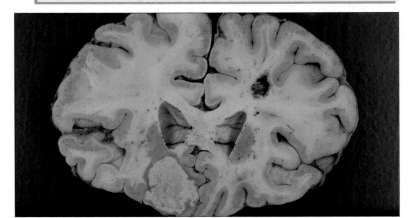

Fig. 17.35 CNS paracoccidioidomycosis. Paracoccidioidomycomas in the cerebral cortex and white matter.

MICROSCOPIC APPEARANCES

The granulomas are formed from lymphocytes, macrophages, epithelioid cells, and Langhans'- or foreign body-type giant cells (**Fig. 17.37**). The granulomas may have a necrotic center and resemble tubercles, but thick-walled budding yeasts are usually demonstrable in sections stained with hematoxylin and eosin, PAS (**Fig. 17.38a**), or methenamine silver impregnation (**Figs 17.38b,c**). There may be a chronic inflammatory infiltrate in the leptomeninges. The meningeal infiltrate tends to extend along the perivascular (Virchow–Robin) space into the underlying brain parenchyma, particularly in the hypothalamus and the lateral fissures.

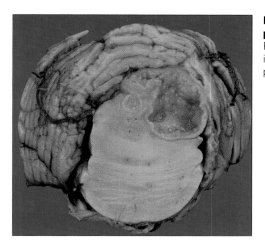

Fig. 17.36 CNS paracoccidioidomycosis. Paracoccidioidomycomas in the pons and adjacent part of the cerebellum.

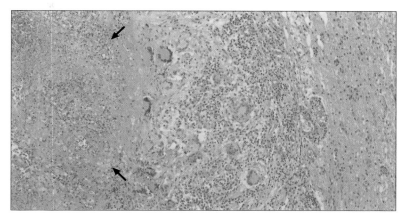

Fig. 17.37 CNS paracoccidioidomycosis. Paracoccidioidomycoma with central necrosis (arrows) and surrounding inflammation, including multinucleated giant cells.

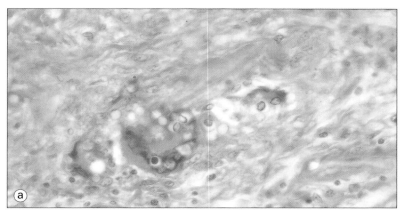

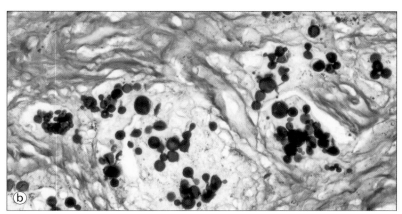

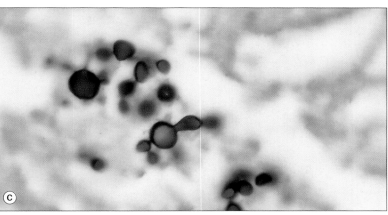

Fig. 17.38 *Paracoccidioides* yeasts. (a) PAS-stained yeasts in the cytoplasm of multinucleated cells. **(b)** The yeasts within a paracoccidioidomycoma are well demonstrated by methenamine silver impregnation. **(c)** High magnification view of budding *Paracoccidioides* yeasts. (Methenamine silver)

REFERENCES

Baker LH, Baker AB. (1994) Nonviral forms of encephalitis. In RJ Joynt (ed.) *Clinical Neurology. Volume 2*. pp.1–116. Philadelphia: Lippincott.

Dauserman SC, Schochet SS Jr. (1993) In JS Nelson, JE Parisi, SS Schochet Jr (eds) pp. 42–74. London: Mosby.

Kirkpatrick JB. (1997) Neurologic infections due to bacteria, fungi, and parasites. In RL Davis and DM Robertson (eds) *Textbook of Neuropathology. Third edition.* pp. 823–925. Baltimore: Williams & Wilkins.

Scaravilli F, Cook GC. (1997) Parasitic and fungal infections. In DI Graham, PL Lantos (eds) *Greenfield's Neuropathology. Sixth edition*, vol. II. pp. 65–111. London: Arnold.

Boes B, Bashir R, Boes C, Halm F, McConnell JR, McComb R. (1994) Central nervous system aspergillosis. Analaysis of 26 cases. *J Neuroimaging* **4**: 123–129.

Nussbaum ES, Hall WA. (1994) Rhinocerebral mucormycosis: changing patterns of disease. *Surg Neurol* **41**: 152–156.

Mitchell DH, Sorrell TC, Allworth AM, Heath CH, McGregor AR, Papanaoum K, Richards MJ, Gottlieb T. (1995) Cryptococcal disease of the CNS in immunocompetent hosts: influence of cryptococcal variety on clinical manifestations and outcome. *Clin Infect Dis* **20**: 611–616.

Hussain S, Salahuddin N, Ahmad I, Salahuddin I, Jooma R. (1995) Rhinocerebral invasive mycosis: occurrence in immunocompetent individuals. *Eur J Radiol* **20**: 151–155.

18 Parasitic infections

AMEBIC INFECTIONS

The main types of amebic infection of the central nervous system (CNS) in man are cerebral amebic abscess and the diseases caused by free-living amebae (i.e. primary amebic meningoencephalitis and granulomatous amebic encephalitis).

CEREBRAL AMEBIC ABSCESS
MACROSCOPIC APPEARANCES

The cerebral lesion is usually single and located in the cortical gray matter, basal ganglia, or at the junction between cortex and white matter. Early lesions appear as small foci of hemorrhagic softening. These become necrotic, with yellow–green centers, and later cavitate. The walls are irregular and there is no evidence of encapsulation. Occasionally there are multiple abscesses.

MICROSCOPIC APPEARANCES

Cerebral amebic abscesses contain inflamed necrotic tissue and it may be difficult to distinguish *E. histolytica* trophozoites within this tissue from macrophages. The trophozoites are spherical or oval, 15–25 μm in diameter, and have vacuolated cytoplasm and a single nucleus; occasionally pseudopodia can be seen. In routinely stained sections, the nuclei are round and have a small central karyosome and peripheral chromatin. The cytoplasm contains abundant glycogen (**Fig. 18.1**).

Trophozoites can usually be identified in the abscess wall, which has an inner zone of necrotic tissue and a broad outer zone with prominent congestion and vascular proliferation. A reactive gliosis and an infiltrate of lymphocytes, plasma cells, macrophages, and some neutrophils are seen in the surrounding brain.

PATHOGENESIS OF CEREBRAL AMEBIC ABSCESS

- The etiologic agent is *Entamoeba histolytica* and is a common intestinal parasite, particularly in tropical and subtropical climates.
- The organisms exist in two forms: trophozoites and cysts (spherical structures up to 25 μm in diameter which contain 4–8 nuclei).
- Trophozoites are found in the colon while cysts are excreted in the feces. Trophozoites invade the brain through hematogenous routes from a primary intestinal, pulmonary, or hepatic focus.
- Very occasionally, amebic abscesses of the brain develop without an obvious extraneural infection.

CEREBRAL AMEBIC ABSCESS

- This is a rare and late complication of intestinal, pulmonary, or hepatic amebiasis, and is usually fatal.
- Patients present with a combination of nonspecific features of encephalitis or meningoencephalitis, and manifestations of a mass lesion.
- Severe headaches tend to be a particularly prominent symptom.

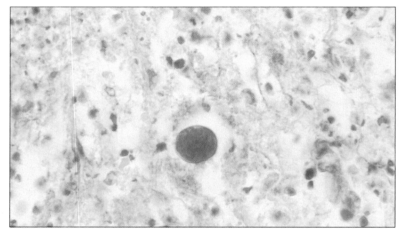

Fig. 18.1 *E. histolytica* **surrounded by necrotic debris in a cerebral abscess.** A PAS stain reveals abundant glycogen within the cytoplasm of the parasite.

PRIMARY AMEBIC MENINGOENCEPHALITIS
MACROSCOPIC APPEARANCES
The brain is swollen and there is a hemorrhagic exudate in the meninges over the cerebrum, brain stem, and cerebellum. The olfactory bulbs and tracts and the adjacent parts of the frontal and temporal lobes contain areas of hemorrhagic necrosis (**Figs 18.2, 18.3**).

MICROSCOPIC APPEARANCES
A scanty mononuclear inflammatory infiltrate (**Fig 18.4**) with focal hemorrhage is seen in the meninges, and there is usually extensive necrosis of brain parenchyma. *N. fowleri* amebae are present in the sub-arachnoid space and around vessels in the necrotic parenchyma (**Fig 18.5**). Their diameter, of 8–15 μm, is slightly less than that of *E. histolytica*. They resemble macrophages, but can be distinguished from them by their vesicular nucleus with its large central nucleolus.

PRIMARY AMEBIC MENINGOENCEPHALITIS

- This is usually acquired by swimming, diving, or water-skiing in fresh water, and is not associated with any predisposing medical condition.
- The presentation is of an acute, fulminant, rapidly fatal illness that usually affects previously healthy children and young adults.
- Patients develop a meningitis that rapidly progresses to coma and death within 48–72 hours. There may be seizures or focal neurologic signs.

*PATHOGENESIS OF
PRIMARY AMEBIC MENINGOENCEPHALITIS*

- This rare form of hemorrhagic meningoencephalitis has been recognized in most parts of the world.
- The etiologic agent, *Naegleria fowleri*, has been isolated from fresh water, soil, sewage, heating, ventilation and air conditioning units, dental units, gastrointestinal washings, and dust.
- The organisms infect the nasal cavity after inhalation of dust, contact with contaminated water, or inhalation of aerosols containing the trophozoites or cysts, which spread to the CNS through the cribriform plate.

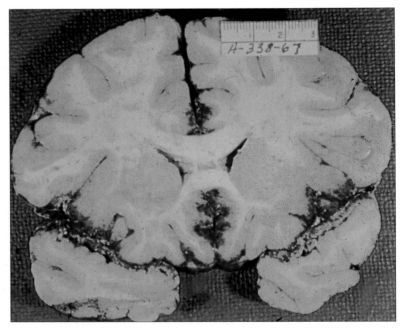

Fig. 18.2 Primary amebic meningoencephalitis.
A hemorrhagic exudate is present in the meninges. There is also hemorrhagic necrosis of the underlying temporal, inferior frontal, and cingulate cortex. (Courtesy of Dr A J Martinez, University of Pittsburgh, USA)

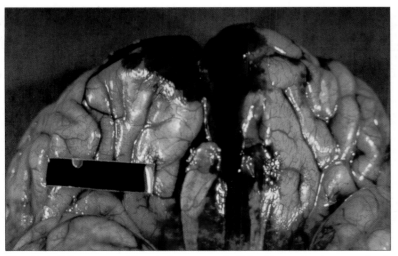

Fig. 18.3 Primary amebic meningoencephalitis. Hemorrhagic necrosis of the frontal poles, olfactory bulbs and tracts, and the underlying inferior frontal cortex. (Courtesy of Dr A J Martinez, University of Pittsburgh, USA)

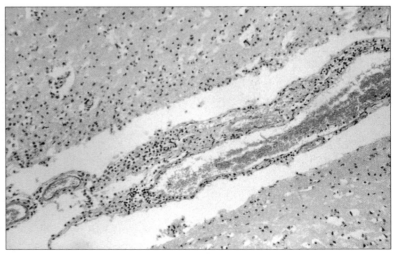

Fig. 18.4 Primary amebic meningoencephalitis. Scanty inflammatory infiltrates are present in the meninges.

GRANULOMATOUS AMEBIC ENCEPHALITIS
MACROSCOPIC APPEARANCES
The brain is usually swollen, covered by a diffuse leptomeningeal exudate, and shows foci of softening, hemorrhage, and necrosis, particularly in the anterior part of the cerebral hemispheres, the thalamus (**Fig. 18.6**), brain stem, and cerebellum (**Fig. 18.7**).

PATHOGENESIS OF GRANULOMATOUS AMEBIC ENCEPHALITIS

- Granulomatous amebic encephalitis is usually caused by various species of *Acanthamoeba*, which have a worldwide distribution and can be found in the same locations as *Naegleria*.
- The route of invasion and penetration into the brain is hematogenous, probably from a primary focus in the lower respiratory tract or the skin.
- The infection is predominantly encountered in chronically ill and debilitated or immunosuppressed individuals.
- In recent years, other free-living amebae have also been recognized as causes of granulomatous amebic encephalitis. They belong to the order Leptomyxida and have been classified as *Balamuthia mandrillaris*. Although the organisms and the lesions are morphologically identical to those of *Acanthamoeba*, the organisms can be distinguished immunohistochemically.

GRANULOMATOUS AMEBIC ENCEPHALITIS

- Patients present with headache, fever, stiff neck, focal neurologic abnormalities, and seizures.
- Granulomatous amebic encephalitis has a subacute or chronic course and is usually fatal, although there are rare reports of successful treatment with surgery and ketoconazole.

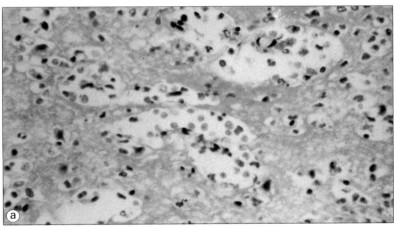
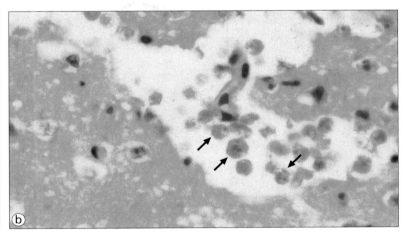

Fig. 18.5 Perivascular amebae in primary amebic meningoencephalitis.
(a) The perivascular amebae bear some resemblance to macrophages, but at higher magnification (arrows) (b) can be distinguished by their vesicular nucleus which has a large central nucleolus.

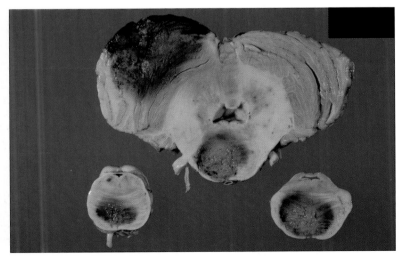

Fig. 18.6 Granulomatous amebic encephalitis. Medial temporal and adjacent thalamic necrosis in granulomatous amebic encephalitis caused by *B. mandrillaris*.

Fig. 18.7 Hemorrhagic necrosis in granulomatous amebic encephalitis. Foci of brain stem and cerebellar necrosis in *Acanthamoeba castellani* encephalitis. Courtesy of Dr A J Martinez, University of Pittsburgh, USA).

MICROSCOPIC APPEARANCES

The brain shows foci of chronic inflammation centered around arteries and veins. The inflammation is typically granulomatous and includes lymphocytes, macrophages, plasma cells, and multinucleated giant cells, but may be necrotizing. There is also a chronic inflammatory infiltrate in the meninges (**Fig. 18.8**). *Acanthamoeba* or *Balmuthia* trophozoites and cysts may be found in and around the walls of affected blood vessels (**Fig. 18.9**), and also in areas relatively free of inflammation (**Figs 18.10, 18.11**). The amebae are 15–40 μm in diameter and have a prominent vesicular nucleus with a dense central nucleolus. The cysts are surrounded by a double membrane.

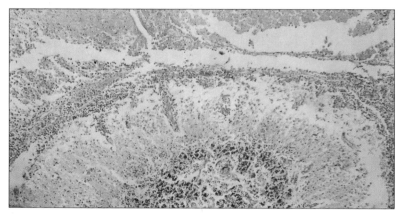

Fig. 18.8 Granulomatous amebic encephalitis. Meningeal and perivascular inflammation with necrosis of adjacent cerebellar tissue.

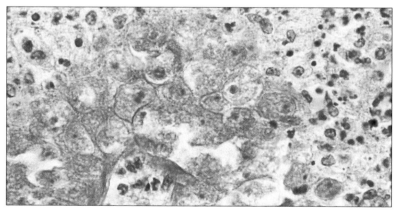

Fig. 18.9 Perivascular trophozoites and cysts in granulomatous amebic encephalitis. This section shows perivascular *Balamuthia* trophozoites and cysts with surrounding inflammation and necrosis. The amebae have a prominent vesicular nucleus with a dense central nucleolus.

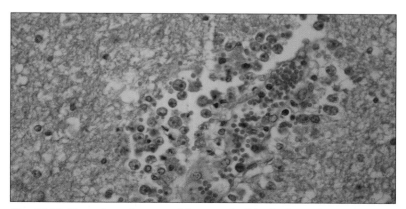

Fig. 18.10 Granulomatous amebic encephalitis. Perivascular *Acanthameba* trophozoites and scanty mononuclear inflammatory cells in the cerebral white matter.

CEREBRAL MALARIA

Malaria remains a major cause of morbidity and mortality. It is endemic in many tropical and subtropical regions and can also affect travelers from or through these regions.

PATHOGENESIS OF CEREBRAL MALARIA

- Malaria is caused by four species of *Plasmodium*: *P. falciparum*, *P. vivax*, *P. malariae*, and *P. ovale*, the first two being responsible for 95% of cases.
- Cerebral malaria occurs in 1–10% of patients infected with *P. falciparum* and is commonest in individuals who are not immune to the parasite (i.e. children between six months and four years of age and foreign visitors to endemic areas).
- Sickle cell trait or disease provides some protection.
- Malaria is acquired by the bite of an infected *Anopheles* mosquito, which inoculates the sporozoites into the blood stream. The sporozoites are then carried to the liver, where they penetrate hepatocytes and develop into merozoites, which rupture the hepatocytes, enter the blood stream, and invade red blood cells (**Fig. 18.12**). The merozoites develop into trophozoites, which subsequently produce schizonts. After maturation the schizont splits into merozoites. These are liberated when the red blood cells rupture and enter other red blood cells to repeat the schizogonic cycle.

A key event in the development of cerebral malaria is the occlusion of capillaries by red blood cells containing P. falciparum, *which is facilitated by several factors, including:*

- The formation of 40–80 nm knob-like protrusions by the schizont-infested red blood cells, and endothelial pseudopodia by cerebral blood vessels.
- Deposition of antigen–antibody complexes, with endothelial damage and platelet aggregation.
- A cell-mediated immune response, associated with the release of tumor necrosis factor (TNF) and other cytokines, an increase in vascular permeability, exudation of serum, and diapedesis of leukocytes and red blood cells.
- Increased expression of several cell adhesion molecules including intercellular adhesion molecule-1 (ICAM-1), endothelial leukocyte adhesion molecule-1 (ELAM-1), and vascular cell adhesion molecule-1 (VCAM-1).

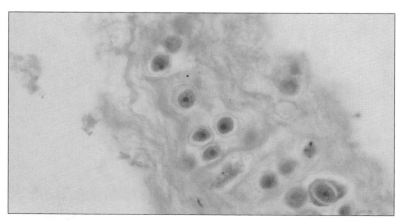

Fig. 18.11 Granulomatous amebic encephalitis. Encysted amebae in the wall of a leptomeningeal blood vessel.

CEREBRAL MALARIA

- The incubation period is 1–3 weeks.
- Patients present with fever, severe headache, somnolence, disorientation, backache, photophobia, and vomiting.
- Seizures are common, especially in children.
- The symptoms and signs vary according to which part of the CNS is involved: meningitic, encephalitic, cerebellar, myelitic, and hemiplegic forms are described, and almost any combination of focal neurologic deficits can occur.
- Rapid progression to coma occurs in the absence of prompt treatment.
- The outcome is fatal in 20–50% of patients but disease progression may be halted by the administration of corticosteroids and antimalarial drugs.

MACROSCOPIC APPEARANCES

The brain is usually swollen with congested leptomeninges. The cerebral cortex may have an abnormal dusky pink color due to marked congestion or a slate gray color due to the presence of abundant malarial pigment (**Fig. 18.13**). The white matter often contains petechial hemorrhages.

MICROSCOPIC APPEARANCES

The small vessels are engorged by red blood cells, which may have a ghost-like appearance with poor staining of hemoglobin (**Fig. 18.14**). Many of these cells, particularly in the gray matter, contain malaria parasites and/or granules of dark malarial pigment, which is related to hematin. Marginated aggregates of red blood cells may appear to be adherent to the vascular endothelium (**Fig. 18.15**).

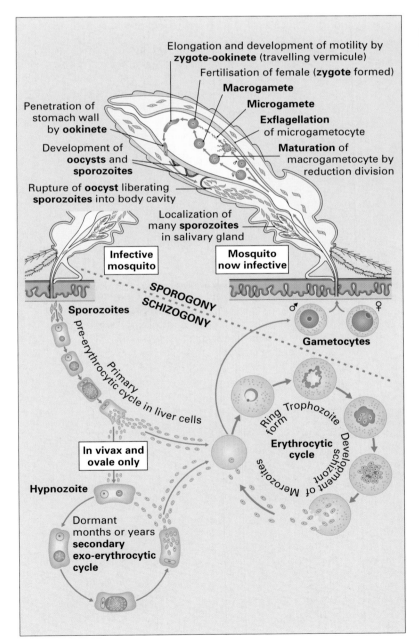

Fig. 18.12 Life cycle of malarial parasites.

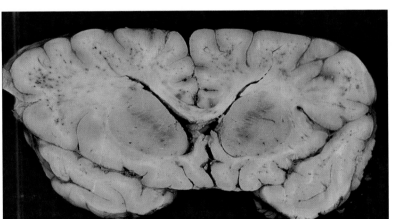

Fig. 18.13 Slate gray brain in cerebral malaria. Blood vessels in the white matter are congested and some are surrounded by small hemorrhages.

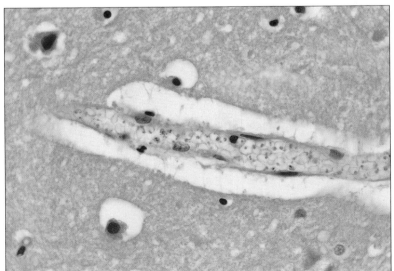

Fig. 18.14 Parasitized blood cells. Ghost-like red blood cells contain malaria parasites.

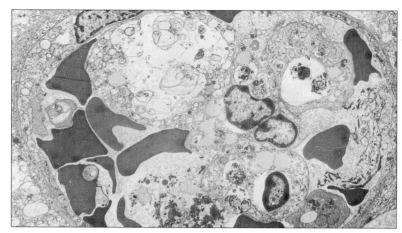

Fig. 18.15 Endothelial adherence of parasitized red blood cells.
Electron micrograph showing a capillary occluded by macrophages with osmiophilic granular pigment and red blood cells containing *P. falciparum* schizonts. Note that the parasitized red blood cells have knob-like protrusions that are attached to the endothelium. (Courtesy of Dr JEH Pittella, Department of Pathology, Santa Casa de Sao Paulo, Brazil)

Edema, capillary necrosis, and perivascular hemorrhages are usually evident, and there may be parenchymal and meningeal infiltration by lymphocytes and macrophages. Petechial or larger hemorrhages can occur in any part of the brain, but are most common in the white matter and may surround necrotic arterioles and veins (**Figs 18.16**). Patients with longer survival may harbor foci of softening and gliosis. Collections of microglia and astrocytes, the so-called Dürck granulomas, are probably related to resorption of ring hemorrhages (**Fig. 18.17**). The microglia contain iron pigment and lipid.

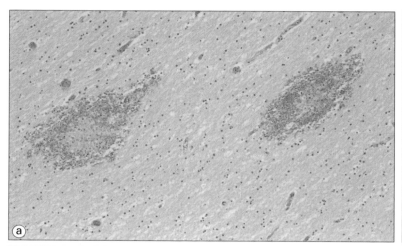

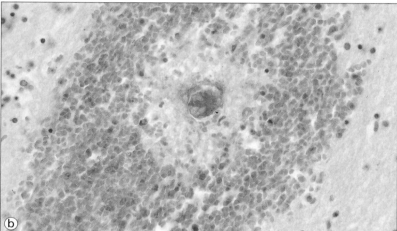

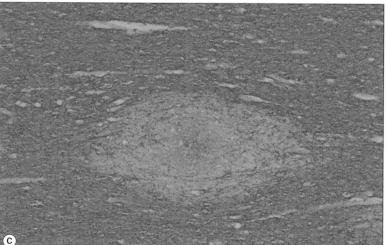

Fig. 18.16 Perivascular hemorrhages and necrosis in the cerebral white matter in cerebral malaria. (a) and **(b)** show white matter hemorrhages. In **(b)**, the hemorrhage is clearly centered on a necrotic blood vessel.
(c) Perivascular necrosis with fragmentation of myelinated nerve fibers in cerebral malaria. (Luxol fast blue/cresyl violet)

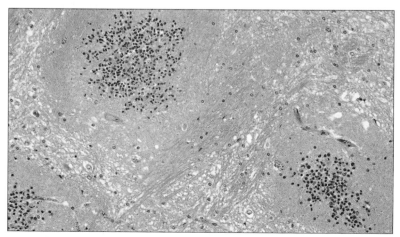

Fig. 18.17 Dürck granulomas. Accumulations of mononuclear cells, predominantly macrophages, related to the resorption of ring hemorrhages.

CEREBRAL TOXOPLASMOSIS

POSTNATALLY-ACQUIRED CEREBRAL TOXOPLASMOSIS
MACROSCOPIC APPEARANCES

The brain typically contains multifocal necrotic lesions of variable size (**Figs 18.18, 18.19**). There may be associated hemorrhage. Older abscesses contain collections of small cystic spaces produced by resorption of necrotic material (see Fig. 18.19). The basal ganglia are often involved, but any part of the brain may be affected. Occasionally brain involvement results in an encephalitic process without focal lesions on macroscopic examination.

MICROSCOPIC APPEARANCES

Necrotizing abscesses or foci of coagulative necrosis are surrounded by mononuclear and polymorphonuclear inflammatory cells, newly formed capillaries, reactive astrocytes, and microglia (**Figs 18.20, 18.21**).

PATHOGENESIS OF CEREBRAL TOXOPLASMOSIS

- Toxoplasmosis is caused by the coccidian *Toxoplasma gondii*.
- The definitive hosts for this parasite are domestic cats and other feline species.
- Human infection is usually acquired by consumption of undercooked meat or cat feces containing parasitic cysts.
- The prevalence of *T. gondii* seropositivity varies widely, ranging from 20–40% in the United States to approximately 70% in Haiti and Brazil.
- *T. gondii* is an obligate intracellular parasite with a propensity to infect the nervous system.
- Most primary infections in immunocompetent individuals are asymptomatic. Some people develop lymphadenopathy, but although the protozoa may encyst and remain dormant in the CNS, symptomatic neurologic disease is rare.
- Neurologic disease in adults is much more commonly associated with depression of cell-mediated immunity, particularly in AIDS, and is probably due to reactivation of dormant infection.
- Congenital toxoplasmosis results from transplacental spread of protozoa and is almost always due to primary maternal infection during pregnancy. The risk of congenital infection is greater during the latter part of pregnancy, but infection during the earlier months leads to more severe involvement of the CNS and eyes.

CEREBRAL TOXOPLASMOSIS

- The clinical presentation of symptomatic disease of the CNS is variable and may include headaches, drowsiness, disorientation, nonspecific features of raised intracranial pressure, and progressive focal neurologic deficits.
- Computerized tomography and magnetic resonance imaging usually reveal multiple ring-enhancing lesions.

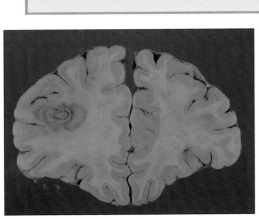

Fig. 18.18 *Toxoplasma* abscess. A solitary lesion is present in the frontal white matter.

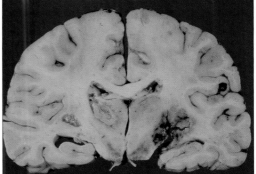
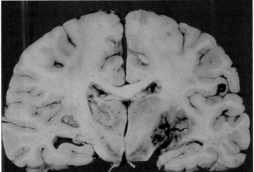

Fig. 18.19 *Toxoplasma* lesions of differing ages. Several lesions are visible in this brain slice. Some are hemorrhagic. Older lesions are partly cavitated.

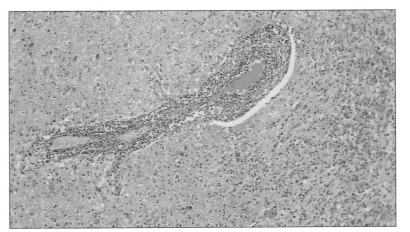

Fig. 18.20 Inflammation adjacent to a *Toxoplasma* abscess. A dense perivascular and intestitial infiltrate of inflammatory cells, predominantly lymphocytes and macrophages, is present in the adjacent brain tissue.

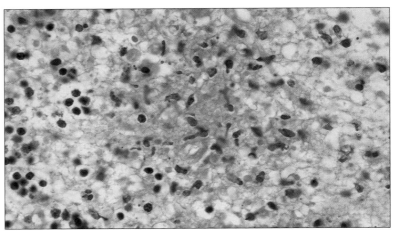

Fig. 18.21 Toxoplasmosis involving the cerebellar cortex. Note the proliferation of microglia and the presence of extracellular *Toxoplasma* tachyzoites.

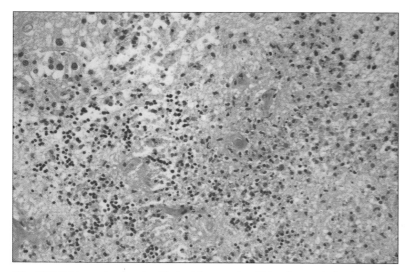

Fig. 18.22 Toxoplasmosis. Fibrinoid necrosis of blood vessels in the cerebellum in *Toxoplasma* infection.

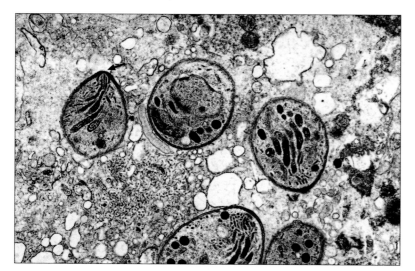

Fig. 18.23 Ultrastructual appearance of Toxoplasma tachyzoites. This Electron micrograph shows several *Toxoplasma* tachyzoites, each surrounded by a double-layered pellicle. The conoid is clearly visible (arrow) in one of the tachyzoites.

Infiltrates of lymphocytes and macrophages surround the blood vessels (see Fig. 18.20). Other findings include intimal proliferation and thrombosis, fibrinoid necrosis (**Fig. 18.22**), and perivascular hemorrhage.

Intracellular and extracellular *Toxoplasma* tachyzoites (also known as endozoites or trophozoites) are usually abundant. They are oval- or crescent-shaped and measure 2–4 × 4–8 μm (**Fig. 18.23**). Those within cells may be clustered together (in vacuoles or larger pseudocysts) or may appear to lie free in the cell cytoplasm. They can be seen reasonably well when stained with hematoxylin and eosin, but are more readily identified and distinguished from other protozoa immunohistochemically (**Fig. 18.24**). Cysts measuring 20–100 μm in diameter and containing large numbers of bradyzoites (also known as cystozoites) may occur within, or at the periphery of, the necrotic areas (**Figs 18.24, 18.25**).

Chronic lesions consist of cystic spaces containing macrophages and only very rare tachyzoites. Cerebral toxoplasmosis occasionally causes a diffuse non-necrotizing inflammatory process with scattered microglial nodules and astrocytic gliosis involving both gray and white matter.

CONGENITAL TOXOPLASMOSIS
MACROSCOPIC APPEARANCES
Macroscopic abnormalities occur in the more severe cases and include:
- multifocal or confluent areas of necrosis, particularly in the periventricular and subpial regions (**Fig. 18.26**)
- hydrocephalus or even hydranencephaly (**Fig. 18.27**)
- foci of calcification scattered throughout the brain (see Fig. 18.26) in contrast to the predominantly periventricular calcification of congenital cytomegalovirus encephalitis
- microcephaly

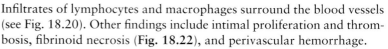

CONGENITAL TOXOPLASMOSIS

- The severity of congenital toxoplasmosis is highly variable.
- The classic triad of hydrocephalus, cerebral calcifications, and chorioretinitis is seen in a minority of cases.
- Seizures are often a prominent early feature.
- Infants who appear to be mildly affected at birth may develop significant neurologic deficits later in life.

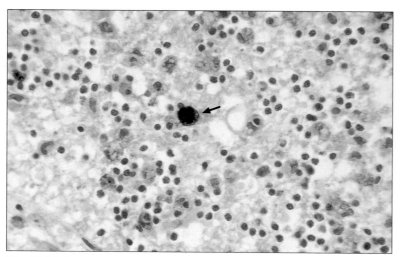

Fig. 18.24 Immunohistochemical demonstration of *Toxoplasma*. Immunostained Toxoplasma protozoa are visible within a cyst (arrow) and in the cytoplasm of macrophages.

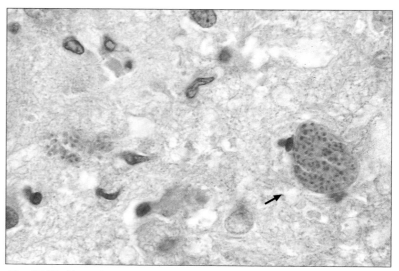

Fig. 18.25 *Toxoplasma* cyst. The cyst (arrow) in this section contains large numbers of *Toxoplasma* bradyzoites.

MICROSCOPIC APPEARANCES

Active lesions in congenital toxoplasmosis show extensive coagulative necrosis. They are usually associated with lipid-laden macrophages, lymphocytes, and a few neutrophils, which are also present in the lepto-meninges (**Fig. 18.28**). The adjacent brain tissue may contain microglial nodules. *Toxoplasma* tachyzoites and cysts can be seen in the meningeal exudate, around (rather than within) the necrotic lesions, and are particularly numerous near the ventricular cavities (**Fig. 18.29**).

The foci of necrosis eventually tend to undergo mineralization (**Fig. 18.30**, see also Fig. 18.26). Residual *Toxoplasma* cysts can usually be found (**Fig. 18.31**). Ependymal granulations and gliosis may lead to aqueduct stenosis and obstructive hydrocephalus.

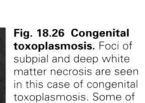
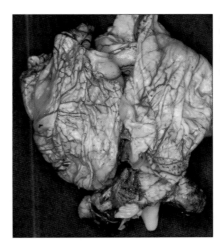

Fig. 18.26 Congenital toxoplasmosis. Foci of subpial and deep white matter necrosis are seen in this case of congenital toxoplasmosis. Some of the subpial foci are partly calcified.

Fig. 18.27 Congenital toxoplasmosis. Collapsed cerebral hemispheres of a severely hydrocephalic brain in congenital toxoplasmosis.

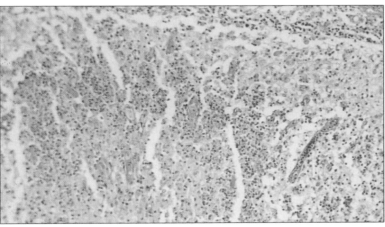

Fig. 18.28 Congenital toxoplasmosis. Focal cortical necrosis with inflammation of the adjacent brain tissue and overlying leptomeninges.

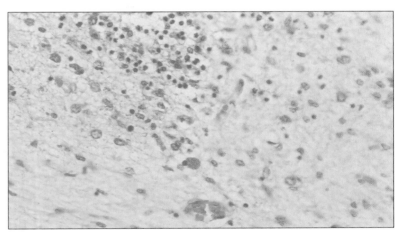

Fig. 18.29 Congenital toxoplasmosis. A cyst and scattered tachyzoites are present at the periphery of a necrotic lesion.

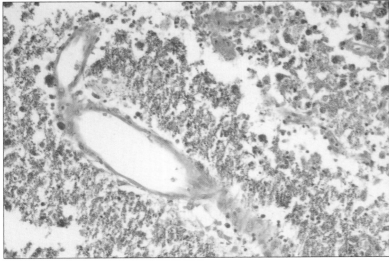

Fig. 18.30 Congenital toxoplasmosis. The foci of necrosis tend eventually to undergo mineralization, as illustrated here.

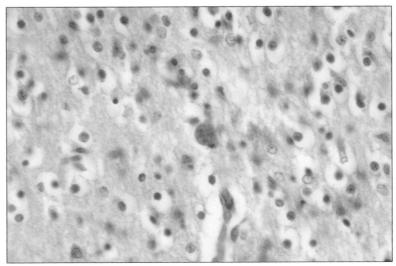

Fig. 18.31 Congenital toxoplasmosis. Residual *Toxoplasma* cyst.

TRYPANOSOMIASIS

Trypanosomes are hemoflagellates and are important causes of disease in large, but geographically restricted, parts of the world.

PATHOGENESIS OF AFRICAN TRYPANOSOMIASIS

- African trypanosomiasis is caused by subspecies of *Trypanosoma brucei* (i.e. *T. b. rhodesiense* and *T. b. gambiense*). Both forms are transmitted to humans and animals by the tsetse fly.
- Both *T. b. rhodesiense* and *T. b. gambiense* cause a meningoencephalitis, the so-called African sleeping sickness.
- Infection with *T. b. rhodesiense* found in east and southeast Africa tends to be relatively fulminant.
- *T. b. gambiense* occurs predominantly in western and sub-Saharan regions and causes subacute or chronic meningoencephalitis.

AFRICAN TRYPANOSOMIASIS

- Meningoencephalitis is characteristic of the late phase of the disease.
- Affected patients show slow gait, mask-like facies, somnolence (or sometimes insomnia), psychiatric disturbances ranging from subtle alterations in personality to florid psychoses, and terminally, extrapyramidal dysfunction, seizures, papilledema, stupor, and coma.

AFRICAN TRYPANOSOMIASIS (SLEEPING SICKNESS)
MACROSCOPIC APPEARANCES
The leptomeninges may be cloudy and the brain swollen and congested. Sometimes the brain is macroscopically normal. Patients who have been treated with melarsoprol may develop acute hemorrhagic leuko-encephalopathy (**Fig. 18.32**) (see chapter 20).

MICROSCOPIC APPEARANCES
Lymphocytes, macrophages, and plasma cells surround the cerebral blood vessels and infiltrate the subarachnoid space (**Fig. 18.33**). Some of the plasma cells contain multiple intracytoplasmic globules of immunoglobulin. These 'morular cells' (**Fig. 18.34**) are characteristic,

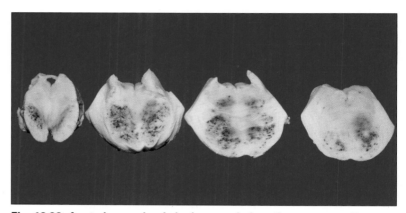

Fig. 18.32 Acute hemorrhagic leukoencephalopathy may complicate melarsoprol treatment. Petechial hemorrhages and surrounding gray discoloration in the brain stem of a patient with acute hemorrhagic leukoencephalopathy. This was due to melarsoprol treatment of trypanosomiasis. (Courtesy of Professor JH Adams, Southern General Hospital, Glasgow)

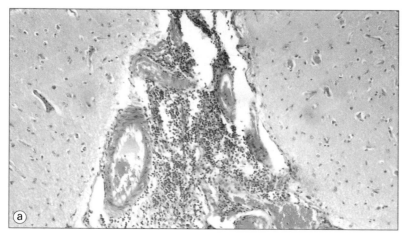

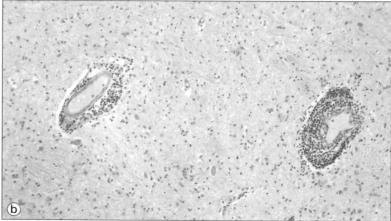

Fig. 18.33 African trypanosomiasis. (a) Meningeal and **(b)** perivascular parenchymal infiltrates of mononuclear inflammatory cells in trypanosomiasis. Note the diffuse reactive gliosis. (Courtesy of Professor JH Adams, Southern General Hospital, Glasgow)

but not specific. Other features include a reactive gliosis (see Fig. 18.33). Clusters of mononuclear inflammatory cells (**Fig. 18.35**) or typical microglial nodules may be abundant, especially in *T. b. rhodesiense* encephalitis, and are often associated with lymphophagocytosis. Trypanosomes are rarely demonstrable in the histologic sections.

AMERICAN TRYPANOSOMIASIS (CHAGAS' DISEASE)
MACROSCOPIC AND MICROSCOPIC APPEARANCES

Acute phase: The brain appears swollen and congested, with scattered petechial hemorrhages. Amastigote (*Leishmania*-like) forms of the parasites are present within glial cells (**Fig. 18.36**) or less frequently at the center of microglial nodules, which are scattered within the brain

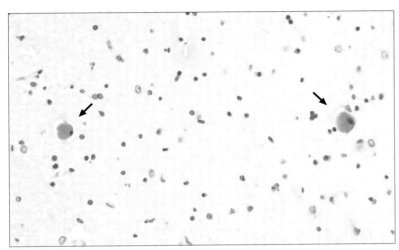

Fig. 18.34 African trypanosomiasis. Scattered morular cells (arrows) are characteristic. (Courtesy of Professor JH Adams, Southern General Hospital, Glasgow)

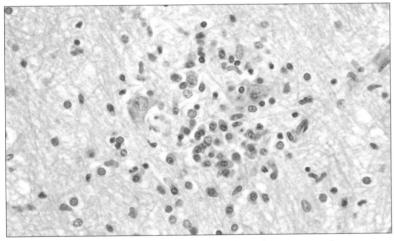

Fig. 18.35 African trypanosomiasis. Parenchymal aggregate of mononuclear inflammatory cells. (Courtesy of Professor J H Adams, Southern General Hospital, Glasgow)

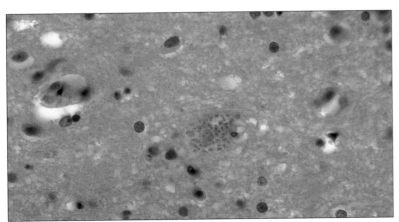

Fig. 18.36 *T. cruzi* encephalitis. Amastigote parasites within a glial cell.

PATHOGENESIS OF AFRICAN TRYPANOSOMIASIS

- This disease is found predominantly in South America (especially Brazil) and Central America.
- The infection is usually acquired during childhood and is caused by *Trypanosoma cruzi*, which is transmitted by reduviid bugs. These bugs carry the parasites in their feces. As they bite they defecate and parasites enter their victim through the skin wound.
- Transmission can also occur by blood transfusion, breast feeding, and across the placenta.

AMERICAN TRYPANOSOMIASIS

The clinical manifestation of T. cruzi *infection can be subdivided into those due to acute infection, those due to chronic infection, and those caused by reactivation of dormant infection.*

Acute infections:
- Most acute infections by *T. cruzi* involve infants or small children, and are asymptomatic.
- In under 1/3 of cases, the acute (parasitemic) phase of infection manifests with fever, swollen eyelids and face, and conjunctivitis. Hepatosplenomegaly may also occur.
- Symptomatic acute illness may be complicated by the development of encephalitis or myocarditis. Manifestations can include seizures and focal neurologic defects.

Chronic infections:
- The chronic phase of infection predominately affects adults. Circulating protozoa are rarely detected during this phase.
- The major clinical manifestations of the chronic phase of infection are due to the damage to the autonomic nervous system – megaesophagus, megacolon, cardiomyopathy.
- Secondary ischemic or embolic disease of the CNS may complicate the cardiomyopathy but encephalitis is seldom associated with this phase of the disease.

Reactivated infection:
- Rarely patients develop granulomatous or necrotizing lesions in the CNS that present with focal deficits or mass effect. This pattern of disease occurs almost exclusively in immuno-compromized patients and probably reflects reactivation of dormant infection.

parenchyma (**Fig. 18.37**). The identity of the parasite can be confirmed immunohistochemically (**Fig. 18.38**).

Chronic phase: The brain usually appears normal. A few glial nodules and aggregates of lymphoid cells may be found, but no parasites.

Reactivated disease takes the form of granulomatous or multifocal necrotizing encephalitis (**Figs 18.39, 18.40**) with abundant amastigote parasites (**Fig. 18.41**, see **Fig. 18.38**).

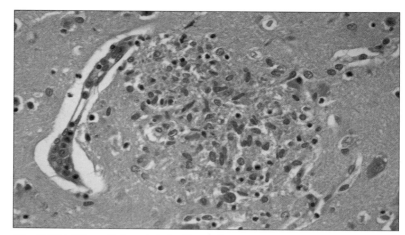

Fig. 18.37 Microglial nodule in *T. cruzi* encephalitis.

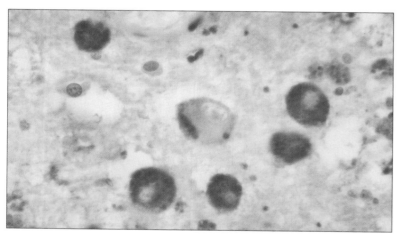

Fig. 18.38 Immunohistochemical confirmation of the identity of *T. cruzi* parasites. Abundant parasites are present in this patient with AIDS.

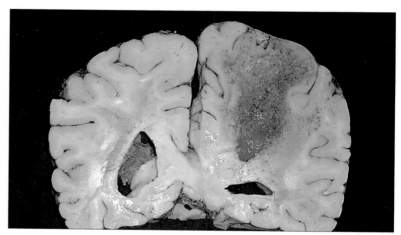

Fig. 18.39 Necrotizing *T. cruzi* infection. Large necrotic lesion in the brain of a patient with AIDS and *T. cruzi* encephalitis.

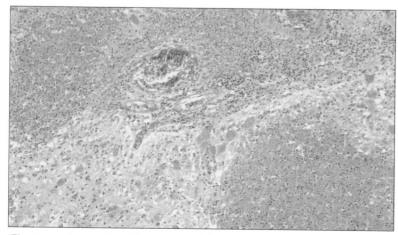

Fig. 18.40 *T. cruzi* mutifocal necrotizing encephalitis. This pattern of infection is restricted to immunocompromized patients.

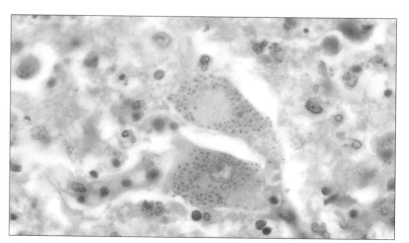

Fig. 18.41 *T. cruzi* infection in an AIDS patient. Abundant amastigote parasites, most of which appear to be in astrocytes and macrophages.

HELMINTHIC INFECTIONS

The cestodes (tapeworms) and the trematodes (flukes) are two major groups of Platyhelminthes (flatworms) and may cause serious neurologic disease. A wide variety of nematodes (roundworms) may also occasionally involve the nervous system and produce disease.

CESTODES
Cysticercosis
In global terms cysticercosis is the commonest parasitic infection of the CNS. Although relatively uncommon in most parts of the United States, it is an important infection in California and states bordering Mexico, as well as in other parts of the world, such as South America, India,

and certain European countries. In Brazil, the prevalence in unselected autopsies varies from 0.7–3.6%.

MACROSCOPIC APPEARANCES
The number of cysts within the CNS varies from one to several hundred (**Fig. 18.43**). They occur in the parenchyma (especially the gray matter), meninges, or ventricles (**Figs 18.44, 18.45**). The viable intraparenchymal cysticerci are usually 1–2 cm in diameter and contain a single invaginated scolex. After degeneration they become fibrotic and represented by a firm white nodule (**Fig. 18.46**) which eventually calcifies. The spinal cord is rarely involved.

PATHOGENESIS OF CYSTICERCOSIS

- The etiologic agent of cysticercosis is *Cysticercus cellusosae*, the larval form of the pork tapeworm, *Taenia solium.*
- Humans are the definitive hosts of *T. solium* and usually become infected by consuming inadequately cooked pork containing encysted larvae. The ingested cysticercus develops an invaginated scolex that attaches to the jejunal mucosa and develops into an adult worm. Periodically, proglottids containing ova are shed from the terminal segment of the adult tapeworm.
- Proglottids are ingested by a suitable intermediate host, usually a pig. The ova then develop into larvae that penetrate the intestinal wall, invade the lymphatics and veins, and disseminate to skeletal muscle and other tissues, including the CNS (**Fig. 18.42**).

Cysticercosis occurs when a human serves as the intermediate host.

Human acquisition of the larval forms that produce cysticercosis occurs:
  - By ingestion of food contaminated with *T. solium* ova from infected feces (fecal-oral contamination by carriers of the adult tapeworm may result in autoinfection).
  - Possibly by regurgitation/reverse peristalsis and swallowing of intestinal ova.
- As in the pig, the ova hatch in the small intestine, disseminate to other tissues and mature within 12 weeks to form cysticerci, which are oval, translucent cysts containing a single scolex bearing four suckers.
- Cysticerci occur most commonly in skeletal muscle. Other sites include the brain, eyes, liver, lung and subcutaneous tissue.

CNS CYSTICERCOSIS

- The clinical features are very varied depending upon the number and location of the cysts.
- Manifestations include focal and generalized seizures, papilledema, headache, vomiting and ataxia (which may be intermittent), vertigo produced by abrupt movements of the head, focal motor and sensory deficits, dementia, acute hydrocephalus due to obstruction of the ventricular system, and occasionally, sudden death.
- Often cerebral cysticerci cause no symptoms and are discovered only at autopsy.

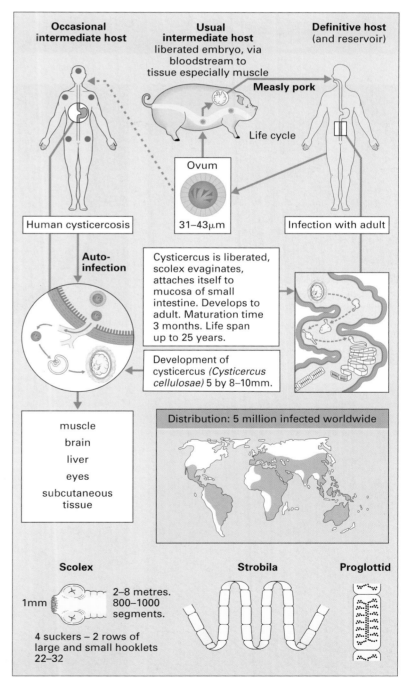

Fig. 18.42 Diagram summarizing the life cycle and geographical distribution of cysticercosis.

The meningeal cysts are small and colorless. They adhere to the pia or float freely in the subarachnoid space (**Fig. 18.47**), particularly in the Sylvian fissure (see **Fig. 18.44**). With time, basal cysts tend to shrink, and the meninges become thickened and fibrotic (**Fig. 18.48**).

Racemose cysticerci are large multiloculated grape-like clusters of cysts that lack an invaginated scolex. They are usually found in the basilar cisterns or within the ventricular system (**Fig. 18.49**), especially the fourth ventricle.

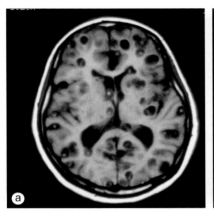
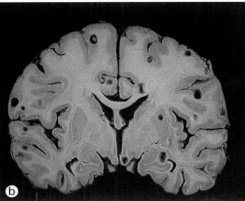

Fig. 18.43 Brains with large numbers of parenchymal cysticerci. (a) Axial magnetic resonance image of the brain of a patient with cysticercosis. There are multiple visible cysticerci (low signal intensity lesions) and degenerating parasites (producing cysts with higher signal intensity). The small foci of high signal intensity in several of the cysts are caused by the scolex. **(b)** This coronal brain slice contains multiple cysts in the cortex and white matter, some of them with a scolex. (Courtesy of Dr JEH Pittella, Department of Pathology, Santa Casa de Sao Paulo, Brazil)

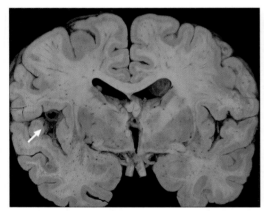

Fig. 18.44 Cysticercosis. Intraventricular and leptomeningeal (arrow) cysticerci.

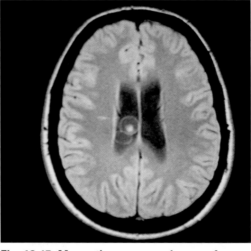

Fig. 18.45 Magnetic resonance image of intraventricular cysticerci. Two cysticerci are visible in one lateral ventricle. A scolex is visible in the larger cyst. The increased signal intensity of the cyst membranes indicates that they are degenerating. (Courtesy of Dr JEH Pittella, Department of Pathology, Santa Casa de Sao Paulo, Brazil)

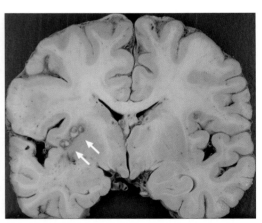

Fig. 18.46 Degenerate cysticerci in the brain parenchyma. After degeneration, the cysticerci become firm white or grey nodules (arrows) that are partly calcified.

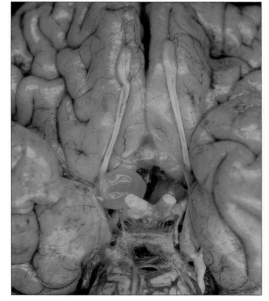

Fig. 18.47 Cysticerci in the leptomeninges. In this brain, meningeal cysticerci are visible anterior to the optic chiasm.

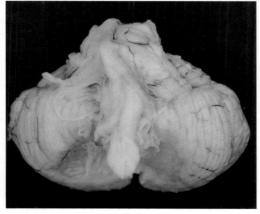

Fig. 18.48 Chronic basal cysticerci. Thickened basal meninges due to longstanding cysticercosis.

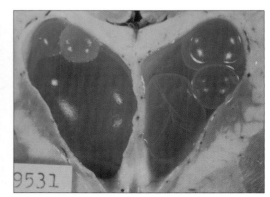

Fig. 18.49 Racemose cysticerci. The cysticerci are forming grape-like clusters in the lateral ventricles. (Courtesy of Dr JEH Pittella, Department of Pathology, Santa Casa de Sao Paulo, Brazil)

MICROSCOPIC APPEARANCES

Each scolex has a rostellum with four suckers and a double row of 22–32 hooklets (**Fig. 18.50**). The cyst wall is sparsely cellular and consists of three histologically distinct layers (**Fig. 18.51**):

- an outer or cuticular layer, which is about 3 mm thick, is eosinophilic, and has hair-like protrusions called microtricha.
- a middle cellular layer with a pseudoepithelial appearance.
- an inner reticular or fibrillary layer, which may contain fine mineral concretions.

While encysted larvae are viable, the surrounding parenchyma shows minimal reaction. Shortly after the cysticerci die, they are surrounded by neutrophils, lymphocytes, macrophages, foreign body giant cells, and eosinophils (**Figs 18.52, 18.53**), and then enclosed by a zone of granulation tissue, which eventually produces a dense collagenous capsule (**Fig. 18.54**). The lesion may include necrotic tissue and cholesterol clefts. Old nodules may be entirely fibrotic. Eventually some of the cysts become mineralized (see Fig. 18.54).

Ventricular cysticerci usually cause a granular ependymitis. Degeneration of racemose cysticerci in the ventricles or subarachnoid space may provoke a florid granulomatous inflammatory reaction (**Fig. 18.55**).

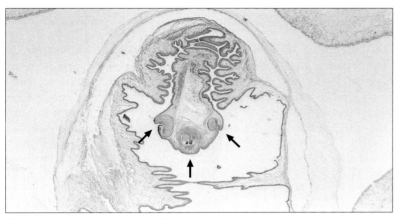

Fig. 18.50   *T. solium* scolex. The rostellum, with suckers (arrowheads) and hooklets (arrows), is clearly visible.

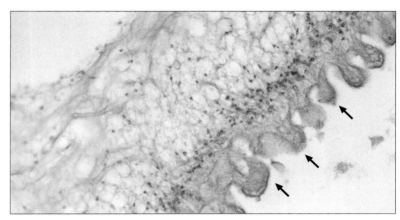

Fig. 18.51   Section through a cyst wall. This consists of a cuticular layer with hair-like protrusions (microtricha) (arrows), a middle cellular layer, and an inner reticular layer.

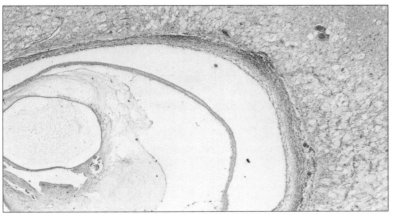

Fig. 18.52   Dead cysticercus. An intense inflammatory reaction is present around the dead parasite.

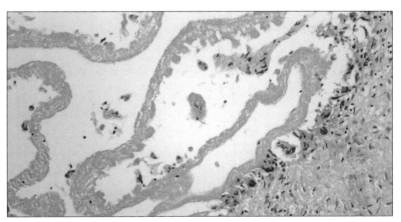

Fig. 18.53   Dead cysticercus. The necrotic cyst wall is abutted by a row of foreign body giant cells. There are scattered lymphocytes and microglia in the surrounding brain tissue.

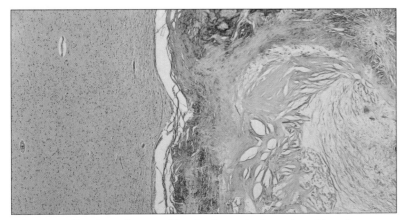

Fig. 18.54   Dead cysticercus. The dead parasite is enclosed in a dense, focally calcified, collagenous capsule.

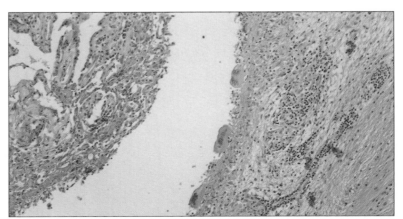

Fig. 18.55   Degeneration of ventricular cysticerci. This has provoked florid granulomatous inflammation in the choroid plexus and periventricular tissue.

Hydatid disease (echinococcosis)
MACROSCOPIC APPEARANCES

Hydatid cysts in the CNS are usually solitary, spherical, and unilocular. The commonest sites are in the perfusion territory of the middle cerebral artery. Skull and vertebral involvement have been reported. The cysts contain clear colorless fluid and a granular deposit of protoscoleces, the so-called hydatid sand.

MICROSCOPIC APPEARANCES

The wall of a cyst (**Fig. 18.56**) is 2–3 mm thick and consists of:
- an outer layer of fibrous tissue, derived from the host.
- an intermediate laminated, chitinous or cuticular layer.
- an inner germinal layer to which oval capsules are usually attached.

The interior of the cyst contains numerous small protoscoleces in brood capsules (**Fig. 18.57**). Apart from mild gliosis and lymphocytic cuffing of blood vessels in the immediate vicinity, there is little other reaction to the cysts.

PATHOGENESIS OF HYDATIDOSIS

- Hydatid disease is caused by larvae of *Echinococcus granulosus* and related species. These are small tapeworms found primarily in dogs. The usual intermediate hosts are sheep. The disease occurs in sheep-rearing countries and has been reported in Australia, New Zealand, Uruguay, and Argentina. In the UK most cases occur in Wales and the Shetland Islands.
- The life cycle of the parasite is similar to that of *T. solium*, but the dog is the definitive host of the adult worm. The ova are excreted with feces, infect herbage, and are eaten by sheep or, accidentally, by humans.
- Hatched embryos infiltrate the wall of the duodenum and reach the veins of the portal system, the liver, and lungs, and via the systemic circulation, other tissues. There they form enlarging cysts that contain budding protoscoleces in brood capsules. Cyst rupture leads to the formation of daughter cysts from the extruded protoscoleces.

HYDATIDOSIS

- usually occurs in children.
- results from accidental ingestion of the ova, usually due to close contact with dogs.
- is associated with the development of larval cysts, usually in the liver and lungs and only rarely in the CNS.
- produces CNS effects according to the location of the larval cysts. Such effects may be seizures, focal neurologic deficits, or spinal cord compression.

Coenurosis
MACROSCOPIC AND MICROSCOPIC APPEARANCES

The cysts are usually unilocular and measure up to 5 cm in diameter. They are found in the ventricles, usually the fourth, or in the subarachnoid space. Unlike hydatid cysts, the walls of a coenurus are thin and milky-white and are not laminated. There is no surrounding fibrous capsule. The cysts contain multiple scoleces, which project from the inner surface into the lumen. The head of each scolex carries a rostellum armed with a double row of hooklets. There is reactive gliosis and chronic inflammation with occasional giant cells in the adjacent brain tissue.

PATHOGENESIS OF COENUROSIS

- Coenurosis is a rare parasitic disease of humans caused by *Coenurus cerebralis*, the larvae of various dog tapeworms, especially *Multiceps multiceps (Taenia multiceps)*, a parasite with a life cycle similar to that of *E. granulosus*. The disease has been recognized in the Caribbean and in South Africa. Most cases occur in tropical Africa, but cerebral involvement has been reported only in temperate climates.
- The definitive hosts are dogs, and the usual intermediate hosts are sheep. Human infection results from accidental ingestion of ova from food contaminated with canine feces.
- After ingested ova have hatched in the intestinal walls, the larvae migrate to various tissues and metamorphose into coenurus. The cysts develop predominantly in the subcutaneous tissue, muscle, eye, and CNS.

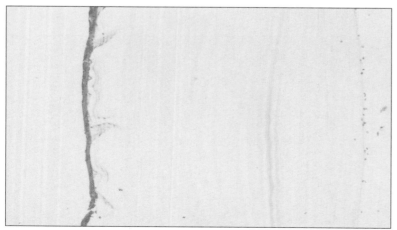

Fig. 18.56 Section through hydatid (echinoccocal) cyst wall. This comprises a thick laminated cuticular layer and a relatively thin germinal layer. The outer adventitial layer is not shown.

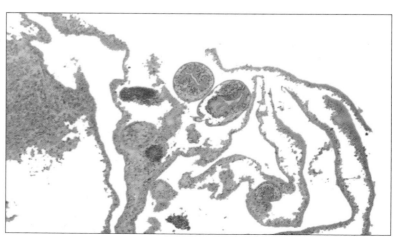

Fig. 18.57 Hydatid cyst. Protoscoleces surrounded by fragments of brood capsule.

NEMATODES
Angiostrongyliasis
MACROSCOPIC AND MICROSCOPIC APPEARANCES
Reported findings include:
- subarachnoid hemorrhage.
- meningitis with lymphocytes, plasma cells, and eosinophils.
- worm tracks.
- identifiable larvae surrounded by granulomatous inflammation with giant cells.
- vascular necrosis, thrombosis, and infarction.

ANGIOSTRONGYLIASIS

- Angiostrongyliasis is caused by *Angiostrongylus cantonensis*, a nematode that in its adult form lives in the pulmonary arteries of rats and other rodents. It occurs in southeast Asia and the Pacific islands. The larvae migrate through the respiratory passages into the pharynx, are swallowed, and eliminated with the feces.
- Humans generally acquire the infection from accidental or intentional ingestion of the intermediate hosts (terrestrial snails or slugs) or of leafy vegetables or strawberries that have been soiled by the slime tracks of these mollusks.
- The larvae penetrate the wall of the stomach and reach the general circulation through the portal vein and liver. They have an unexplained predilection for the CNS, which they reach either hematogenously or by way of a peripheral nerve after invading other tissues.
- The life cycle cannot be completed in the accidental human hosts.

Trichinosis
MACROSCOPIC AND MICROSCOPIC APPEARANCES
Reported lesions include:
- petechial or larger hemorrhages.
- perivascular and leptomeningeal inflammation.
- very rarely, granulomas around larvae.

TRICHINOSIS

- Trichinosis is caused by *Trichinella spiralis*, which has no free-living stage in its life cycle.
- Although trichinosis is usually an infection of animals, humans may act as both intermediate and final hosts, harboring the adult nematode temporarily and the larvae for longer periods.
- The infection is acquired by ingesting undercooked meat (usually pork) containing encysted *T. spiralis*.
- The adult nematodes are found in the duodenum and jejunum. Newly formed motile larvae migrate from the intestine to various tissues, but can mature only in skeletal muscle where they may encyst and remain dormant for years.
- They rarely invade the nervous system.

Strongyloidiasis
MACROSCOPIC AND MICROSCOPIC APPEARANCES
Pathologic findings may include:
- the presence of larvae in the leptomeninges (**Fig. 18.58**) or with microinfarcts that result from capillary obstruction by the parasites.
- conversion of microinfarcts to brain abscesses.
- bacterial meningitis.

STRONGYLOIDIASIS

- Strongyloidiasis is caused by *Strongyloides stercoralis*, a nematode with a wide geographic distribution, but commonest in the tropics.
- The worms have a free-living phase in damp warm soil, where they deposit eggs that give rise to rhabditiform larvae. Under adverse conditions they become filariform larvae, which can infect humans by penetrating the skin.
- The larvae pass through the lungs and mature in the duodenum and jejunum. During systemic migration, the larvae may end up in ectopic sites, including the CNS.
- The endogenous cycle is completed by the production of rhabditiform larvae by female nematodes. These larvae can reinfect their human host through the colon or anus.
- The major CNS complications are associated with immunosuppression, which causes massive intestinal overgrowth of the nematodes, colonic ulceration and septicemia.

NEMATODE INVOLVEMENT OF THE CNS

CNS angiostrongyliasis
- The presentation varies from a mild meningitis to severe radiculomyeloencephalitis.
- Patients may develop symptoms and signs of raised intracranial pressure.
- The cerebrospinal fluid contains many eosinophils.

CNS trichinosis
- CNS involvement is signaled by the development of meningism, features of raised intracranial pressure and focal neurological deficits deficits 2–4 weeks after the onset of the systemic illness.
- CNS lesions are evident as small hypodensities in the cortex and white matter on computerized tomography.
- In severe cases, confusion progresses to delirium, coma, and death after about six weeks.

CNS strongyloidiasis
- Patients may develop symptoms and signs of brain abscess formation or bacterial meningitis, because bacteria (usually *Escherichia coli* or other enteric bacteria) are carried into the brain or subarachnoid space with the larvae, or enter the circulation through colonic ulcerations.

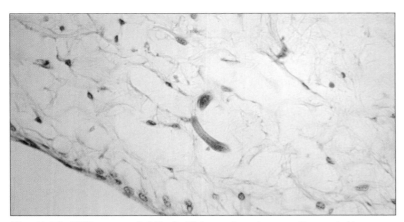

Fig. 18.58 CNS strongyloidiasis. This section shows a *Strongyloides stercoralis* larva in the leptomeninges.

Visceral larva migrans
MACROSCOPIC AND MICROSCOPIC APPEARANCES
In the brain the larvae produce small necrotic and inflammatory lesions containing macrophages, lymphocytes, neutrophils, and eosinophils. Dead larvae are usually surrounded and partly engulfed by giant cells (**Fig. 18.59**).

VISCERAL LARVA MIGRANS

- This disorder results from accidental human infection with various nematodes that usually infect non-human hosts. The disease is relatively common in the southern United States, where it is generally due to the dog ascarid, *Toxocara canis*. Less commonly, the cat ascarid, *Toxocara cati*, or the raccoon ascarid, *Bayliascaris procyonis*, is responsible. The adult nematode lives in the animal's intestines and eggs are excreted in the feces.
- Children acquire the infection by ingesting ova from contaminated soil.
- The parasites are unable to complete their life cycle in humans. The larvae are released and migrate through the intestinal mucosa to other organs, especially the liver and lungs. The resulting clinical syndrome is called visceral larva migrans. Rarely, the larvae migrate to the CNS.

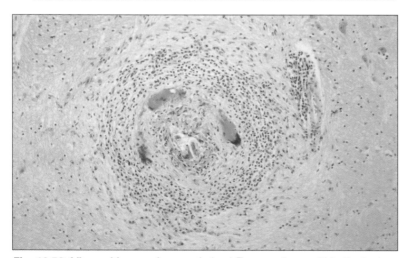

Fig. 18.59 Visceral larva migrans. A dead *Toxocara* larva within the brain is surrounded by a chronic inflammatory infiltrate with foreign body giant cells. (Courtesy of the estate of the late Dr C Scholz)

TREMATODES
Schistosomiasis
MACROSCOPIC APPEARANCES
Miliary granulomas may be seen scattered throughout the brain, but are most numerous in the cerebral and cerebellar cortex and the deep gray matter. Sometime the lesions are solitary and mimic a tumor. Spinal schistosomiasis can cause marked swelling of the affected cord segments (**Fig. 18.61**). Granulomas may be studded over the surface of the brain or cord, or agglomerated to form nodules up to 3 cm in diameter, which protrude from the surface and occasionally invade the dura.

MICROSCOPIC APPEARANCES
The histologic reaction to the ova varies from nothing to florid granulomatous inflammation with multinucleated giant cells, marked fibrosis, and adjacent gliosis (**Figs 18.62–18.64**). Eosinophils are usually present. Some patients develop focal arteritis.

SCHISTOSOMIASIS

- Several species, including *Schistosoma japonicum* (endemic in China, Philippines, Japan, Thailand, and Laos), *S. mansoni* (in South America, Puerto Rico, the West Indies, the Middle East, and Africa) and *S. haematobium* (in Africa and the Middle East) are important causes of the disease.
- Man is the definitive host and the adult schistosomes inhabit blood vessels: *S. japonicum* and *S. mansoni* live predominantly in the superior and inferior mesenteric veins whereas *S. haematobium* is usually found in the veins around the urinary bladder.
- Large numbers of ova are deposited in the blood and lodge in venules. Some rupture through the venule wall and into the urinary bladder or bowel, eventually being excreted in the urine or feces.
- Once in water, miracidia hatch from the eggs and penetrate a snail. Fork-tailed cercariae then develop in this intermediate host, emerge into the water, and swim in search of their definitive host, entering through the skin. The cercariae invade blood vessels and eventually lodge in the mesenteric or vesical veins to mature into adult male or female trematodes (**Fig. 18.60**).

- CNS involvement is uncommon, the risk probably depending on the level of immunity and the magnitude of the schistosomal invasion.
- The ova reach the CNS by retrograde passage through the pelvic veins and the valveless vertebral venous plexus of Batson. The distribution of the embolized ova is related to their size and shape.

SCHISTOSOMIASIS AND THE NERVOUS SYSTEM

- Cerebral schistosomiasis is commonest in infections by *S. japonicum*, which has the smallest eggs and an inconspicuous terminal spine.
- *S. haematobium* may cause cerebral disease, but more commonly affects the spinal cord.
- Embolization of *S. mansoni* ova is impeded by their size and their large lateral spine. As a result this species usually causes lumbosacral myelopathy.

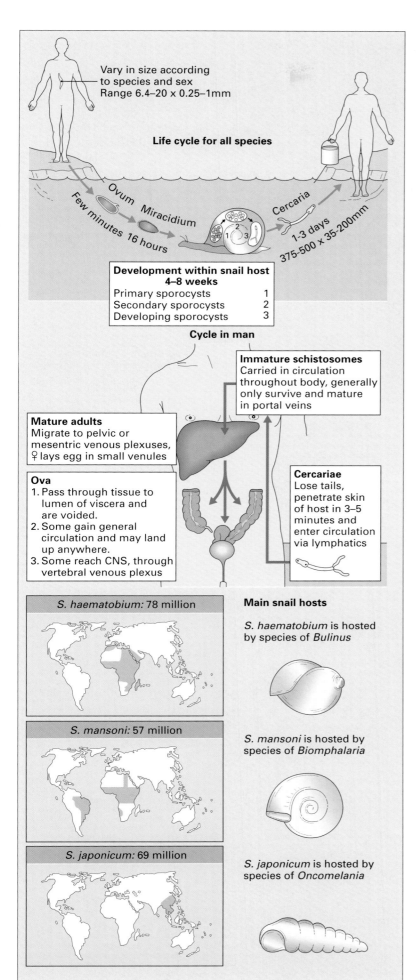

Vary in size according to species and sex
Range 6.4–20 x 0.25–1mm

Life cycle for all species

Ovum Miracidium
Few minutes 16 hours
Cercaria
1-3 days
375-500 x 35-200mm

**Development within snail host
4–8 weeks**
Primary sporocysts   1
Secondary sporocysts   2
Developing sporocysts   3

Cycle in man

Immature schistosomes
Carried in circulation throughout body, generally only survive and mature in portal veins

Mature adults
Migrate to pelvic or mesentric venous plexuses, ♀ lays egg in small venules

Ova
1. Pass through tissue to lumen of viscera and are voided.
2. Some gain general circulation and may land up anywhere.
3. Some reach CNS, through vertebral venous plexus

Cercariae
Lose tails, penetrate skin of host in 3–5 minutes and enter circulation via lymphatics

S. haematobium: 78 million

S. mansoni: 57 million

S. japonicum: 69 million

Main snail hosts

S. haematobium is hosted by species of *Bulinus*

S. mansoni is hosted by species of *Biomphalaria*

S. japonicum is hosted by species of *Oncomelania*

Fig. 18.60 Diagram summarizing the trematode life cycle and geographical distribution.

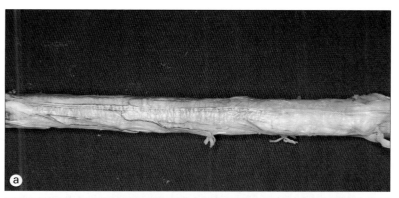

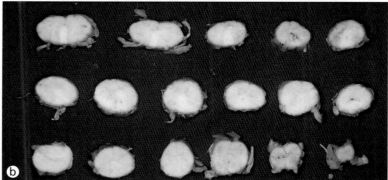

Fig. 18.61 Spinal schistosomiasis due to *S. mansoni*. (a) There is marked swelling of the thoracic cord, with thickening of the surrounding leptomeninges. **(b)** The swelling of the thoracic cord (second row) is clearly visible in these transverse sections.

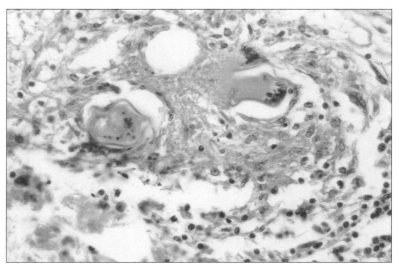

Fig. 18.62 Schistosomiasis. Moderate inflammatory reaction to *Schistosoma* ova.

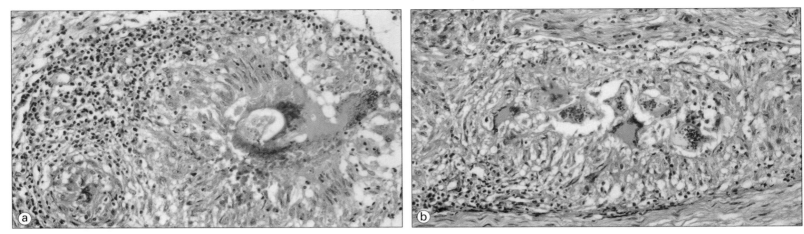

Fig. 18.63 Spinal schistosomiasis. *Schistosoma* ova with surrounding granulomatous inflammation in the spinal cord **(a)** and nerve roots **(b)**.

REFERENCES

Bauserman SC, Schochet SS Jr. (1993) In *Bacterial fungal and parasitic diseases of the central nervous system*. eds Nelson JS, Parisi, Schochet Jr SS. Mosby: London. pp 42–74

Cameron ML, Durack DT. (1991) Helminthic infections of the central nervous system. In *Infections of the central nervous system*. eds Scheld WM, Whitely RJ, Durack DT. Raven Press: New York. pp 825-858.

Cegielski JP, Durack DT. (1991) Protozoal infections of the central nervous system. In *Infections of the central nervous system*. eds Scheld WM, Whitely RJ, Durack DT. Raven Press: New York. pp 767–800

Chimelli L, Mahler-Araujo MB. (1997) Fungal Infections. *Brain Pathology* 7: 613–627.

Dukes CS, Luft BJ, Durack DT. (1991) Toxoplasmosis of the central nervous system. In *Infections of the central nervous system*. eds Scheld WM, Whitely RJ, Durack DT. Raven Press: New York. pp 801–824.

Kirkpatrick JB. (1997) Neurologic infections due to bacteria, fungi and parasites. In *Textbook of Neuropathology* (3rd edition) eds Davis RL and Robertson DC. Williams and Wilkins, Baltimore. pp 823–925.

Martinez AJ, Visvesvara GS. (1997) Free living, amphizoic and opportunistic amebas. *Brain Pathology* 7: 583–598.

Pentreath VW. (1995) Trypanosomiasis and the nervous system. Pathology and immunology. *Trans R Soc Trop Med Hyg* 89: 9–15.

Pittella JEH. (1997) Neuroschistosomiasis. *Brain Pathology* 7: 649–662.

Pittella JEH. (1997) Neurocysticercosis. *Brain Pathology* 7: 681–693.

Rocha A, Meneses ACO, Silva AM, Ferreira MS, Nishioka SA, Burgarelli MKN, Almeida E, Turkato Jr G, Metze K, Lopes ER. (1994) Pathology of patients with Chagas' disease and acquired immunodeficiendcy syndrome. *Am J Trop Med Hyg* 50: 261–268.

Scaravilli F, Cook GC. (1997) Parasitic and fugal infections. In *Greenfield's Neuropathology* volume II (6th edition). eds Graham DI, Lantos PL. Arnold: London. pp 65–111.

Scrimgeour EM, Gajdusek DC. (1985) Involvement of the central nervous system in *Schistosoma mansoni* and *S. hematobium*. A review. *Brain* 108: 1023– 1038.

Taratuto AL, Venturiello SM. (1997) Trichinosis. *Brain Pathology* 7: 663–672.

Taratuto AL, Venturiello SM. (1997) Echinococcosis. *Brain Pathology* 7: 673–679.

Turner G. (1997) Cerebral malaria. *Brain Pathology* 7: 569–582.

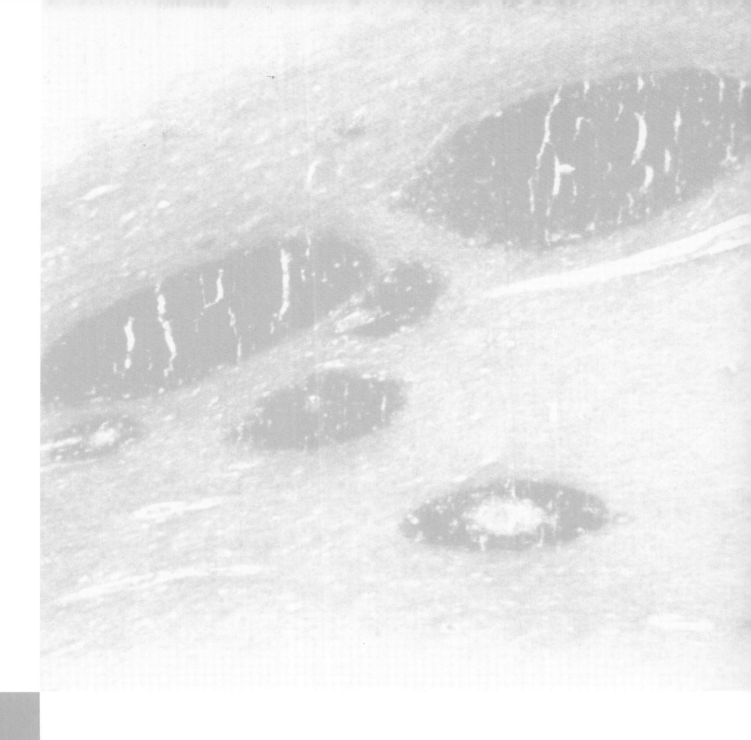

6 Demyelinating diseases

19 Multiple sclerosis

Demyelination is characterized by destruction of normal myelin with relative preservation of axons. By convention, the term demyelination excludes disorders in which there is a failure to form myelin normally (dysmyelination) or a loss of myelin as a result of axonal degeneration. The central nervous system (CNS), peripheral nervous system, or both, may be affected by demyelinating diseases. Disorders characterized by a loss of myelin due to an inherited defect of metabolism are considered in Chapter 22.

EPIDEMIOLOGIC ASPECTS OF MULTIPLE SCLEROSIS

- Commoner in men than women (male:female ratios range from 1.4:1 to 3.1:1 in different studies).
- Peak age of onset is 20–40 years; onset before puberty or after 60 years of age is rare.

Geographic and migration studies
- Incidence is greatest in North America, northern Europe, southeast Australia, and New Zealand.
- Clustering of cases in some places (e.g. in the Faroe Islands and Orkneys).
- Migration before 15 years of age from a high- to a low-incidence area reduces the likelihood of developing MS.
- Migration before 15 years of age from a low- to a high-incidence area probably increases the risk of developing MS.
- Migration after 19 years of age does not affect the risk of developing MS.

Family, twin, racial, and HLA studies
- The risk of developing MS is increased 15–20-fold in first-degree relatives of patients with this disorder.
- The concordance rate of MS is significantly higher in monozygotic twins than in dizygotic twins.
- The incidence is low in some racial groups, including African blacks, Japanese and Chinese (and probably other oriental populations), and Asians from (and probably those living in) India and Pakistan.
- There are significant associations with HLA-A3 and HLA-B7, HLA-DR15, HLA-DQ-6 and particularly with HLA-DR2.

MULTIPLE SCLEROSIS (MS)

This is the commonest demyelinating disease of the CNS. Demyelination is typically multifocal with lesions of different ages. The classic form of the disease usually follows a relapsing and remitting or a progressive course over many years. The cause is not known, but:
- Geographic and migration studies suggest an environmental etiologic agent.
- Family, twin, racial, and human leukocyte antigen (HLA) studies indicate that genetic factors play a role.
- Immunologic studies provide evidence of an autoimmune disorder, possibly precipitated by a viral infection.

Classification
There are four main types of MS: classic (Charcot type), acute (Marburg type), neuromyelitis optica (Devic's disease), and concentric sclerosis (Baló's disease).

CLASSIC (CHARCOT-TYPE) MS

MACROSCOPIC APPEARANCES
In fixed tissue the patches of demyelination appear as well-demarcated regions of gray discoloration (plaques), that:
- vary in size, shape, number, and distribution (**Fig. 19.1**)
- may extend to the surface of the brain stem and spinal cord, forming gray depressions on external examination (**Fig. 19.2**)

IMMUNOLOGIC ASPECTS OF MULTIPLE SCLEROSIS

- Patients have significantly greater antibody levels to measles virus than controls. Antibody titers to several other viruses are also elevated, but less consistently.
- When compared with their unaffected monozygotic twins, patients with MS show restricted expression of certain T-cell receptor genes.
- There are reports that patients with MS show abnormal T-cell responses to several white matter antigens, including myelin basic protein, myelin oligodendrocyte glycoprotein, and αB-crystallin.
- αB-crystallin is expressed by oligodendroglia and astrocytes in MS plaques, but not in normal white matter.

MULTIPLE SCLEROSIS (MS)

- commonly presents with weakness, paresthesia, and sensory loss involving one or more limbs, optic neuritis, diplopia, incoordination, and vertigo
- can also cause loss of vision, dysarthria, disturbances of micturition, constipation, painful muscle spasms, trigeminal neuralgia, cognitive impairment, seizures, and Lhermitte's sign
- is usually associated with demonstrable foci of demyelination on magnetic resonance imaging (MRI)
- is often associated with delayed visual evoked responses
- is usually associated with oligoclonal bands of immunoglobulins on electrophoresis of the cerebrospinal fluid
- can produce clinical features and CT scan and MRI appearances that mimic those of a brain neoplasm and lead to biopsy
- often pursues a relapsing and remitting course, but can be progressive from the outset or become progressive after initial remissions. The interval between relapses is variable, and the latent phase between the onset of disease and the first relapse can be many years.

- may be seen in the olfactory tracts and are frequently present in the optic nerves (**Figs 19.3, 19.4**)
- are often present adjacent to the lateral angles of the lateral ventricles on sectioning the cerebrum (**Figs 19.5, 19.6**)
- can occur anywhere in the white matter, at the junction between the cerebral gray and white matter (**Fig. 19.7**), and within the cortical gray matter and deep gray nuclei (**Fig. 19.8**), which include myelinated axons as well as neuronal somata and dendrites
- may occur in the cerebellar white matter and peduncles, in the floor of the fourth ventricle, elsewhere in the brain stem (**Fig. 19.9**, see also Fig. 19.2a), and in the spinal cord (**Fig. 19.10**, see also Fig. 19.3)

Brain stem and spinal plaques are usually more difficult to see by macroscopic inspection than those in the cerebral white matter.

Plaques containing many lipid-laden macrophages may appear slightly yellow or chalky white rather than gray (**Fig. 19.11**), while old plaques and, rarely, fulminant acute plaques may contain foci of cavitation (**Fig. 19.12**).

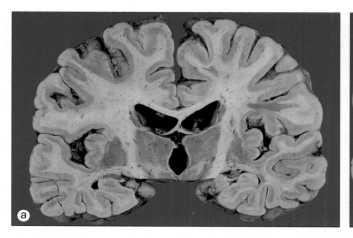

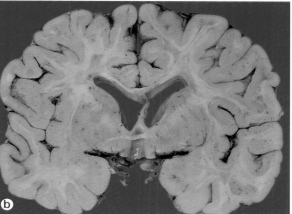

Fig. 19.1 Plaques in MS. (a, b) Scattered plaques of varying shapes, sizes, and locations in coronal brain slices from two patients with MS.

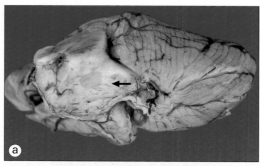

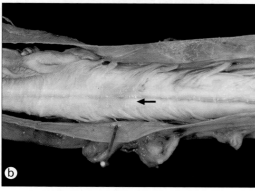

Fig. 19.2 Plaques in MS. (a) On the surface of the pons (arrows). **(b)** On the surface of the spinal cord (arrows).

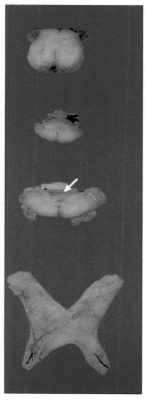

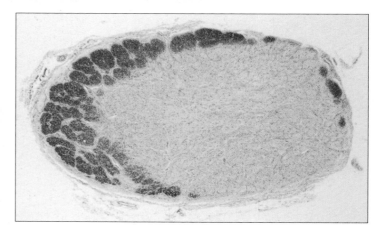

Fig. 19.4 Optic nerve in MS. Transverse section through optic nerve in which only a peripheral crescent of myelin can still be stained. (Solochrome cyanin)

Fig. 19.3 Optic chiasm in MS. Grayish brown discoloration and atrophy of demyelinated optic chiasm and spinal white matter, most marked in the posterior cervical columns (arrow).

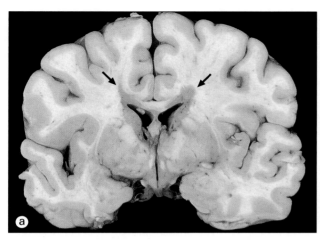
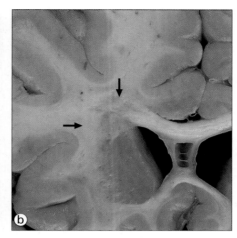
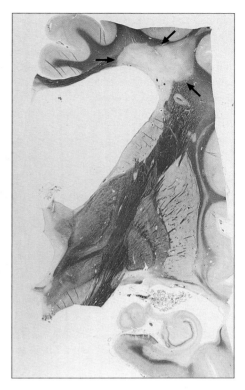

Fig. 19.5 Plaques adjacent to the lateral angles of the lateral ventricles. (a) and **(b)** In MS, plaques are often found around the lateral angles of the lateral ventricles (arrows).

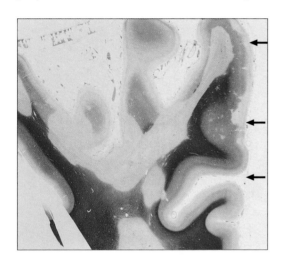

Fig. 19.7 Subpial and junctional plaques. Multiple plaques of demyelination. Here occurring in the subpial region (arrows) and at the junction between cerebral cortex and white matter. (Luxol fast blue/cresyl violet)

Fig. 19.6 Demyelination at the angle of the lateral ventricle. A well-circumscribed zone of pallor (arrows) in this section stained for myelin. (Luxol fast blue/cresyl violet)

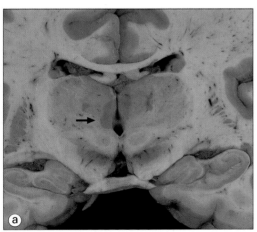

Fig. 19.8 Multiple plaques in the deep cerebral grey matter. (a) and **(b)** These appear as dark gray-brown patches within the the basal ganglia and thalamus (arrows to some)

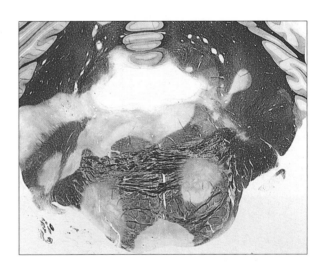

Fig. 19.9 Plaques of demyelination in the base and tegmentum of the pons. Histology often reveals involvement of the brain stem in MS although the plaques may be difficult to discern on gross examination of the fixed brain. (Luxol fast blue/cresyl violet)

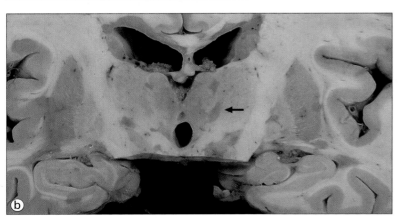

MICROSCOPIC APPEARANCES

The plaques vary in appearance according to their age, the disease activity, and the presence or absence of remyelination (**Fig. 19.13**). The evolution of the earliest demyelinating lesions is still debated. It is probable that perivascular inflammation consisting of lymphocytes and macrophages occurs at a very early stage, as does disruption of the blood–brain barrier, resulting in a high signal on MRI enhanced with gadolinium–DTPA and an inter-

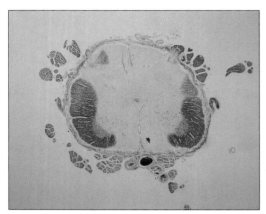

Fig. 19.10 Extensive demyelination in the lumbar spinal cord. Note the preservation of anterior horn cells. (Luxol fast blue/cresyl violet)

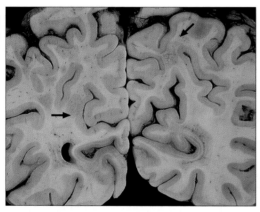

Fig. 19.11 Plaques of active demyelination in the parieto-occipital region. Plaques containing large numbers of lipid-laden macrophages tend to have a yellow hue and may have a slightly granular texture (arrows to some).

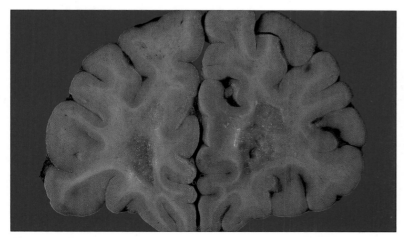

Fig. 19.12 Plaque cavitation. Cavitated plaques in the frontal white matter in longstanding MS.

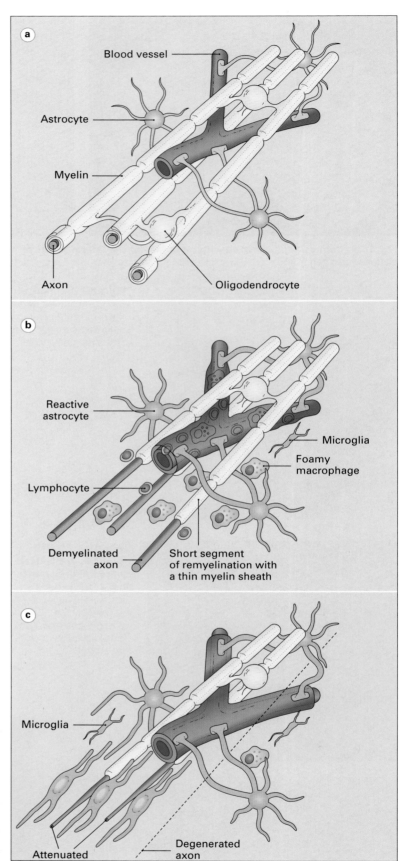

Fig. 19.13 Different stages of disease activity in multiple sclerosis plaques. (a) Normal white matter. **(b)** During active demyelination, there is perivascular and parenchymal infiltration by lymphocytes and macrophages. Many of the macrophages are distended by lipid material and appear 'foamy'. Remyelinating activity probably commences at an early stage. **(c)** Inactive plaques are hypocellular, most of the cells within them being astrocytes, there is some loss of axons and those that remain have a reduced caliber.

stitial accumulation of serum proteins that can be demonstrated immuno-histochemically (**Fig. 19.14**). It is widely believed that inflammation and disruption of the blood–brain barrier precede myelin destruction.

Established lesions can be subdivided into active, inactive, and shadow plaques. The features of the different plaque types may overlap in any single lesion.

Active plaques are hypercellular lesions containing a relatively dense perivascular and parenchymal infiltrate of lymphocytes and macrophages (**Figs 19.15–19.18**), and scattered reactive astrocytes, which may be quite pleomorphic (**Figs 19.19, 19.20**). The inflammation tends to be greatest towards the edge of the plaque and in the contiguous intact white matter. The lymphocytes in these regions are mostly T cells (see **Fig. 19.18**). CD4-positive (helper) cells predominate in earlier lesions and the actively

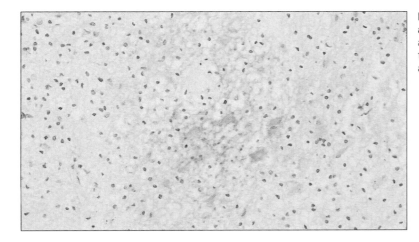

Fig. 19.14 Perivascular transthyretin (prealbumin) immunoreactivity in an active plaque. Enhancement of vascular permeability to serum proteins occurs at an early stage of demyelination, and immunoreactivity for albumin transthyretin, and other proteins can be demonstrated in the interstitium of active plaques.

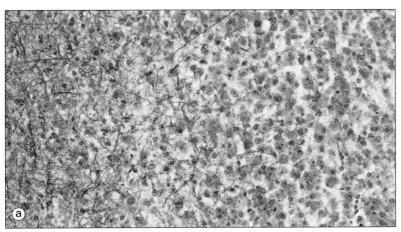

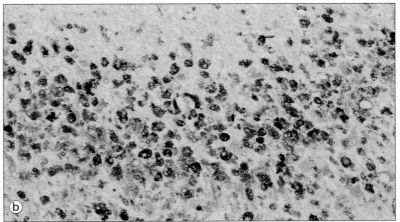

Fig. 19.15 Active MS plaque. (a) Sheets of foamy macrophages towards the margin of an active plaque. Some contain granules of dark blue (luxophilic) myelin debris. (Luxol fast blue/cresyl violet) **(b)** CD68 immunoreactivity of macrophages in an active plaque.

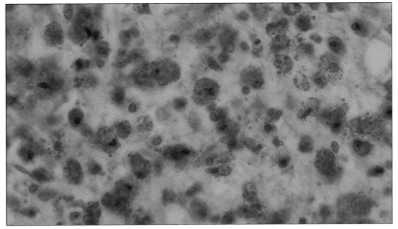

Fig. 19.16 Macrophages in an active MS plaque. The foamy macrophages contain numerous lipid droplets, stained here with oil red-O.

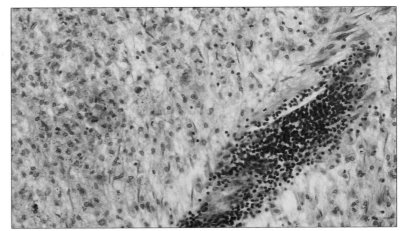

Fig. 19.17 Perivascular and scattered interstitial lymphocytes in an active plaque. The lymphocytic inflammation tends to be most prominent in regions of active demyelination.

demyelinating regions of older lesions, while CD8-positive (suppressor/cytotoxic) cells are more numerous in less active regions.

The cytoplasm of the macrophages appears foamy towards the edge of the plaque owing to their accumulation of material that reacts strongly with oil red O (see Figs 19.14, 19.16) and with stains for myelin (see Fig. 19.14). The macrophages express major histocompatibility complex (MHC) class II antigens, as do some astrocytes in zones of active demyelination. MHC class II antigen expression is not a feature of normal CNS tissue, but occurs in several inflammatory disorders including MS.

The disease activity can vary considerably in different parts of the same plaque (**Figs 19.21, 19.22**). Silver impregnation usually reveals preservation of most axons (**Fig. 19.23**), and this is confirmed by electron microscopy, which reveals that most myelin destruction appears

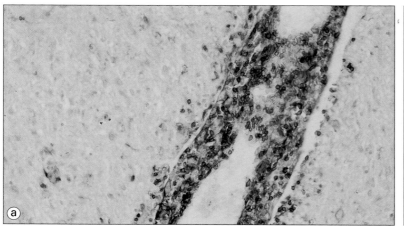
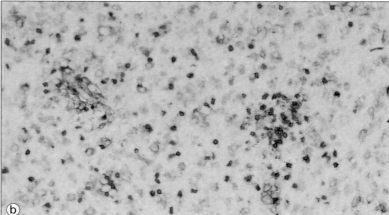

Fig. 19.18 Lymphocytic inflammation in MS. Most of the perivascular **(a)** and interstitial **(b)** lymphocytes are T cells, as shown by their CD45RO immunoreactivity.

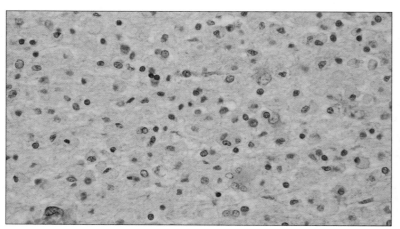

Fig. 19.19 Reactive astrocytes in MS plaque. Reactive astrocytes with abundant homogeneous eosinophilic cytoplasm are scattered among macrophages and lymphocytes. Note that one of the astrocytes is multinucleated.

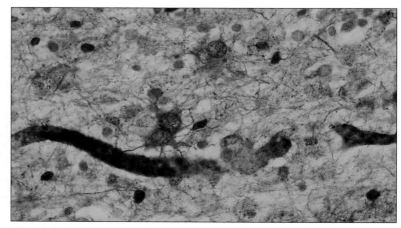

Fig. 19.20 Large reactive astrocytes. These are clearly demonstrated in a Holzer-stained section of this MS plaque.

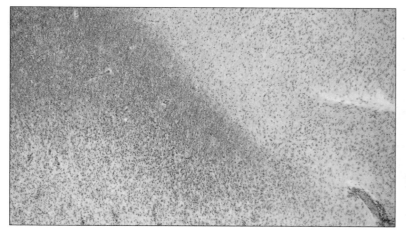

Fig. 19.21 Variation in disease activity in am MS plaque. Marked variation in the density of the cellular infiltrate in two contiguous regions of demyelination. (Luxol fast blue/cresyl violet)

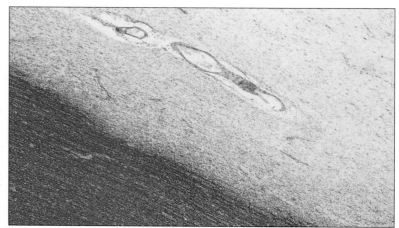

Fig. 19.22 Variation in disease activity in an MS plaque. Chronic plaque with a hypocellular center, but a densely cellular actively demyelinating periphery. (Luxol fast blue/cresyl violet)

to be mediated by macrophages (**Fig. 19.24**). The neurons are preserved within plaques involving gray matter. (**Fig. 19.25**).

In active MS there may be a patchy infiltrate of lymphocytes and macrophages in the leptomeninges, especially those overlying plaques (**Fig. 19.26**).

Inactive plaques are hypocellular, densely gliotic lesions showing a marked loss of oligodendrocytes (**Fig. 19.27**). Stains for myelin usually show that the plaque margins are sharply defined. There is a reduction in caliber and variable depletion of axons, the extent of which is less marked at the periphery of the plaque (**Fig. 19.28**). MRI and ultrastructural studies have shown that the loss of axons is associated with a concomitant increase in the amount of extracellular space. Severe axonal loss may be associated with cavitation (see Fig. 19.12).

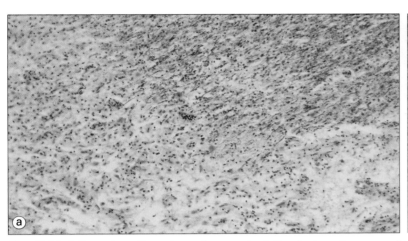
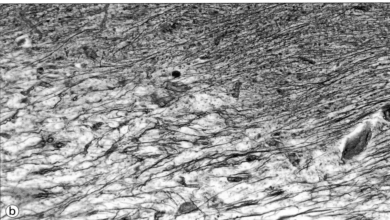

Fig. 19.23 Adjacent sections through a poorly defined edge of an area of active demyelination. **(a)** A luxol fast blue/cresyl violet stain shows loss of myelin. Silver impregnation of axons in an adjacent section **(b)** shows that they are relatively well preserved within the plaque.

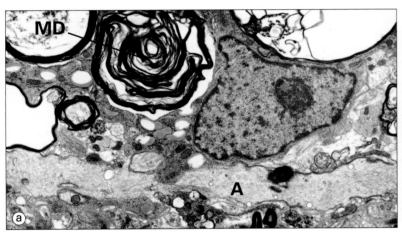
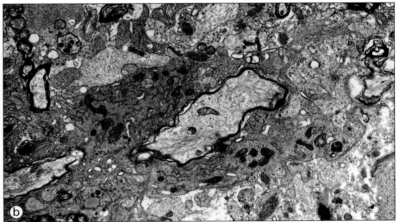

Fig. 19.24 Electron micrographs of an active plaque. (a) Demyelinated axon (A) in contact with a macrophage containing myelin debris (MD). **(b)** Myelinated fiber completely surrounded by a macrophage. (Courtesy of JW Prineas)

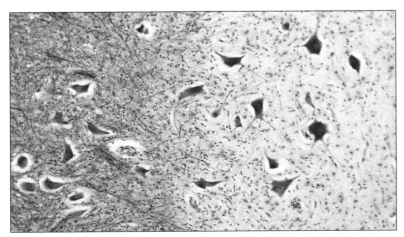
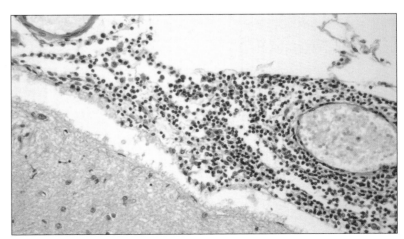

Fig. 19.25 Preservation of neurons in a pontine plaque. (Luxol fast blue/cresyl violet)

Fig. 19.26 Lymphocytic infiltrate in the leptomeninges of a patient with MS.

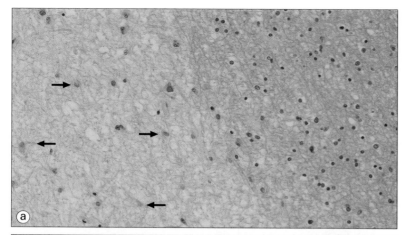

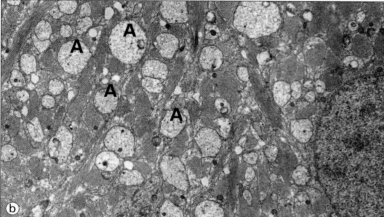

Fig. 19.27 Inactive plaques. (a) A markedly hypocellular inactive plaque with obvious loss of oligodendrocytes. Most of the cells within the plaque are astrocytes (arrows). **(b)** Electron micrograph showing chronic inactive plaque of demyelination. The axons (A) are separated by astrocyte processes containing large numbers of glial intermediate filaments. (Courtesy of JW Prineas)

DIFFERENTIAL DIAGNOSIS OF MS

- Many disorders can simulate MS clinically, including cerebrovascular diseases (Chapters 9 and 10), neoplasms (Chapters 34–47), Chiari malformation, cervical spondylosis, vestibular neuronitis, and Lyme disease, but their pathologic processes are easily distinguishable
- The lesions of subacute combined degeneration of the spinal cord may superficially resemble those of MS, but the symmetry of involvement, the spongy appearance of the white matter, the early loss of axons, and the clinical circumstances in which the lesions occur are different.
- Similarly, the vacuolar myelopathy of AIDS (see chapter 13) and the early lesions of HAM (see p. 13.3) bears some histologic resemblance to spinal demyelination in MS, but occurs in a different clinical context.
- The pattern of demyelination in adrenoleukodystrophy, adrenomyeloneuropathy, and other leukodystrophies is more diffuse and symmetric (Chapter 6).
- Marchiafava–Bignami disease is characterized by foci of demyelination in the corpus callosum and elsewhere, but occurs almost exclusively in the context of chronic severe alcoholism.
- The clinical circumstances and distribution of demyelination in central pontine and extrapontine myelinolysis are usually distinctive.
- Inflammatory demyelination is rarely a so-called 'early delayed' manifestation of radiation injury to the CNS.
- The clinical course and pathologic findings in acute disseminated encephalomyelitis are considered on in chapter 13
- Leber's hereditary optic neuropathy is caused by specific point mutations of mitochondrial DNA (see chapter 24) and can cause a neurologic syndrome that is clinically indistinguishable from MS. It is associated with multifocal white matter lesions demonstrable by MRI that have not been well characterized pathologically.
- Inflammatory demyelination has rarely been reported as a complication of treatment with 5-fluorouracil and its derivatives.

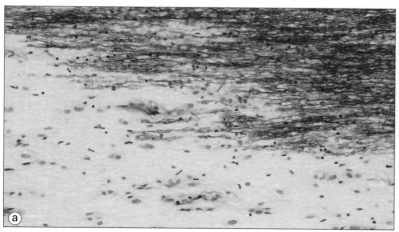

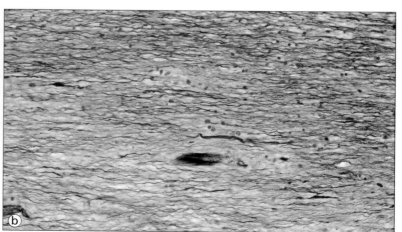

Fig. 19.28 Adjacent sections through an inactive plaque. (a) Loss of myelin. (Luxol fast blue/cresyl violet) **(b)** Silver impregnation shows that the axons within the plaque are attenuated in comparison with those in the adjacent white matter.

Shadow plaques are recognized by light microscopy as plaques with reduced but not absent myelin staining (**Fig. 19.29**). Examination of well-preserved resin-embedded material has shown that shadow plaques contain remyelinated axons, with relatively thin myelin sheaths and moderate to large numbers of oligodendrocytes (**Fig. 19.30**). The zone of remyelination that constitutes a shadow plaque often appears to be confined to part of a larger zone of demyelination (**Fig. 19.31**). Remyelination probably commences within weeks of demyelination. Demyelination and remyelination can occur repeatedly and even concurrently in the same plaque (**Fig. 19.32**). Foci of remyelination in the brain stem and spinal cord may occasionally be mediated by invading Schwann cells rather than oligodendrocytes (**Fig. 19.33**).

Peripheral nervous system involvement

MS is usually regarded as a disorder that exclusively affects the CNS. However, chronic inflammatory demyelinating polyneuropathy with onion-bulb formation has been reported in a small number of patients. An association between acute inflammatory demyelinating polyneuropathy and MS has also been described in a few rare cases.

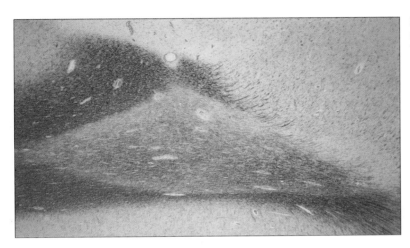

Fig. 19.29 Well-defined shadow plaque. The fibers stain for myelin albeit less intensly than in the adjacent subcortical white matter. (Luxol fast blue/cresyl violet)

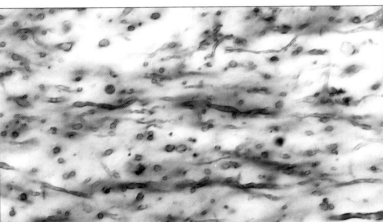

Fig. 19.30 Semithin resin-embedded section through the center of a shadow plaque containing many thinly remyelinated axons. (Courtesy of JW Prineas)

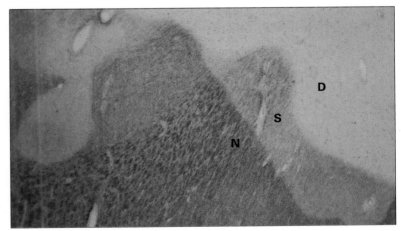

Fig. 19.31 Remyelination at the periphery of a large plaque. Adjacent zones of complete demyelination (D), shadow plaque (S), and normal myelin staining (N). (Luxol fast blue/cresyl violet)

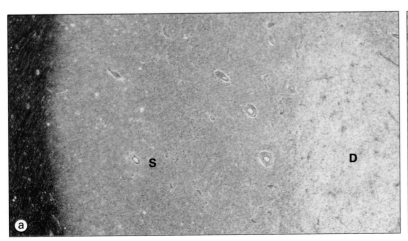

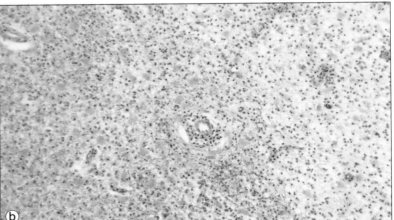

Fig. 19.32 Concurrent demyelination and remyelination. Sections through a shadow plaque (S) with central active demyelination **(D)**. **(a)** Low magnification. **(b)** Higher magnification. (Luxol fast blue/cresyl violet)

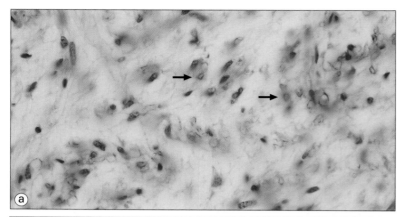

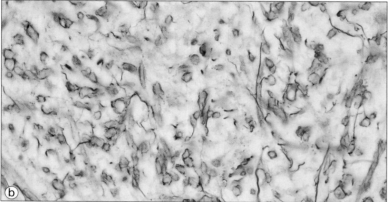

Fig. 19.33 Schwann cell-mediated remyelination. Part of a plaque in the medulla. **(a)** This contains thinly scattered remyelinated fibers (arrows). **(b)** Reticulin impregnation reveals the basal lamina of the Schwann cells responsible for the remyelination.

ACUTE (MARBURG-TYPE) MS

This designation is given to MS that follows a rapidly progressive monophasic course and is usually fatal within a few months and always within one year of onset. It is said to be most common in children and young adults, but this variant has also been described in older patients.

MACROSCOPIC AND MICROSCOPIC APPEARANCES

Sections contain multiple active plaques, all of which are hypercellular, with prominent perivascular lymphocytic cuffing, numerous foamy macrophages, and scattered pleomorphic reactive astrocytes (**Figs 19.34–19.37**). The edges of the plaques tend to be poorly defined and some plaques are difficult to see macroscopically (see Fig. 19.34). Occasionally, edema in the surrounding white matter produces a significant mass effect, simulating a neoplasm.

NEUROMYELITIS OPTICA (DEVIC'S DISEASE)

This is characterized by the development of optic neuritis and acute transverse myelitis within weeks of each other. Approximately two-thirds of patients present with visual loss and subsequently develop paraplegia and sensory loss, but in the remaining third the order may be reversed. Some patients die during or soon after the acute syndrome, but others, although severely incapacitated, survive for many years, during which time they may develop other symptoms of MS.

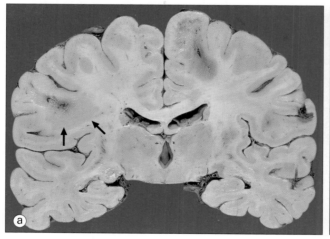

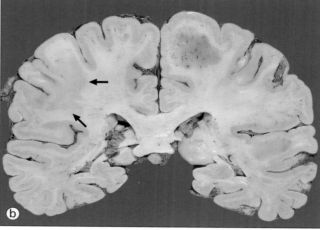

Fig. 19.34 Acute MS. **(a)** and **(b)** Adjacent coronal slices through the brain of a patient with acute MS. Note the multiple large plaques, some of which are quite poorly defined (arrows).

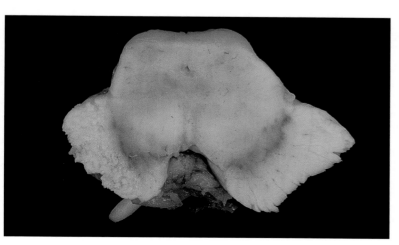

Fig. 19.35 Acute MS. Granular, yellow appearance or right cerebral peduncle in a patient with acute MS.

MACROSCOPIC APPEARANCES

The optic nerves and affected region of the spinal cord are swollen and congested in patients who die during or soon after the acute presentation. The cord may appear necrotic on sectioning (**Fig. 19.38**). In patients who survive longer, the optic nerves become thin and gray-brown in color, while the cord shows similar discoloration (**Fig. 19.39**) and may also appear attenuated.

MICROSCOPIC APPEARANCES

The optic nerves and spinal cord show extensive demyelination (**Fig. 19.40**).

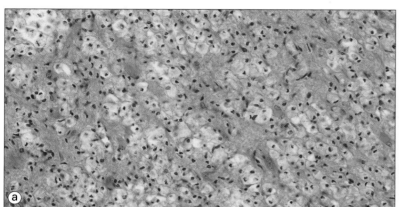

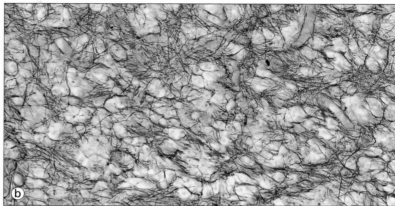

Fig. 19.36 Adjacent sections through a plaque in acute MS. (a) This shows the features of active demyelination (i.e. sheets of foamy macrophages and scattered reactive astrocytes). **(b)** Axons are relatively well preserved. (Bielschowsky silver impregnation)

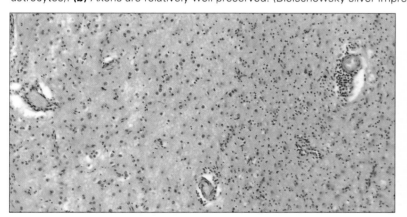

Fig. 19.37 Plaque in acute MS. Many of the macrophages at the plaque edge contain luxophilic (dark blue) granules of myelin debris. (Luxol fast blue/cresyl violet)

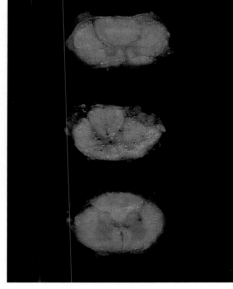

Fig. 19.38 Acute neuromyelitis optica. Extensive softening of the spinal white matter and necrosis of the gray matter can be seen. The thoracic region (center section) is most severely affected.

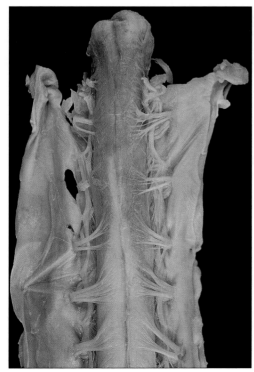

Fig. 19.39 Neuromyelitis optica. Brown discoloration of the upper part of the cervical cord in long-term survivor of neuromyelitis optica.

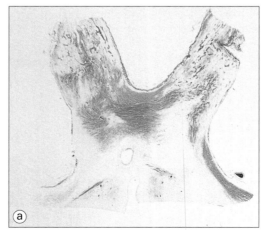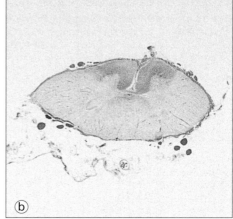

Fig. 19.40 Histology of neuromyelitis optica. Sections showing extensive demyelination in neuromyelitis optica. **(a)** Through the optic chiasm. **(b)** Through the spinal cord. (Luxol fast blue/cresyl violet)

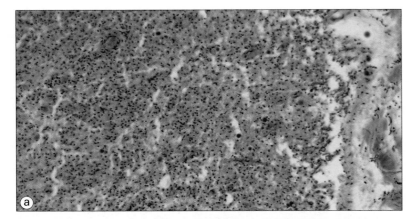

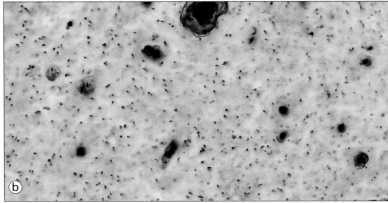

Fig. 19.41 The spinal white matter in acute neuromyelitis optica. (a) This shows spinal white matter largely replaced by sheets of foamy macrophages. (Luxol fast blue/cresyl violet) **(b)** A few surviving axons are demonstrable by silver impregnation.

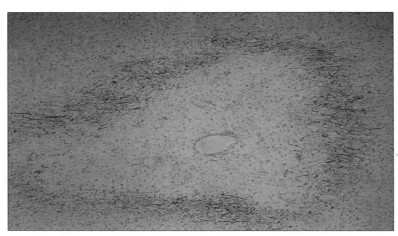

Fig. 19.43 Preserved perivascular ring of myelinated white matter in classic MS. This appearance is seen much more often than the multiple concentric zones of myelination and demyelination of full-blown concentric sclerosis. (Luxol fast blue/cresyl violet)

In the acute phase, involved segments of the spinal cord and optic nerve are inflamed, and the cord in particular may be partly necrotic (**Fig. 19.41**). These lesions become cavitated and gliotic in those patients who survive the acute stage, and there may be associated degeneration of ascending and descending tracts.

Typical MS plaques are usually present elsewhere in the CNS, but may be small and sparsely distributed.

CONCENTRIC SCLEROSIS (BALÓ'S DISEASE)
This is a rare variant of MS that is usually monophasic, rapidly progressive, and diagnosed at necropsy.

MACROSCOPIC AND MICROSCOPIC APPEARANCES
The white matter usually contains multiple large plaques, some with central necrosis. The characteristic histologic feature is the presence of plaques composed of alternating, more or less concentric rings of demyelinated and myelinated white matter (**Fig. 19.42**). The plaques are usually hypercellular, with perivascular lymphocytic cuffing, foamy macrophages, and reactive astrocytes. Cases with typical Baló-type plaques are rare, but plaques containing bands or islands of preserved myelin are occasionally seen in classic MS (**Fig. 19.43**).

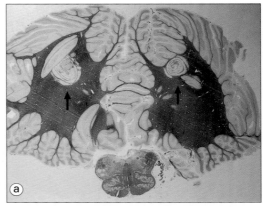

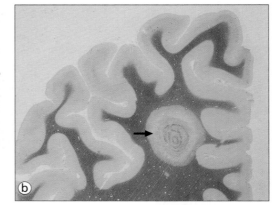

Fig. 19.42 Concentric sclerosis (Baló's disease). Concentric rings of demyelinated and myelinated white matter (arrows). **(a)** In the cerebellum. **(b)** In the cerebrum. (Loyez stain)

REFERENCES

Matthews WB (ed) (1991) *McAlpine's Multiple Sclerosis. Second edition.* Edinburgh, London, Melbourne and New York: Churchill Livingstone.

McDonald WI, Miller DH, Barnes D (1992) The pathological evolution of multiple sclerosis. *Neuropathol Appl Neurobiol* 18: 319–334.

McDonald WI (1994) Rachelle Fishman–Matthew Moore lecture: The pathological and clinical dynamics of multiple sclerosis. *J Neuropathol Exp Neurol* 53: 338–343.

Prineas JW, Barnard RO, Kwon EE, Sharer L, Cho E–S (1993) Multiple sclerosis: remyelination of nascent lesions. *Ann Neurol* 33: 137–151.

Prineas JW, Barnard RO, Kwon EE, Sharer L, Cho E–S (1993) Multiple sclerosis — pathology of recurrent lesions. *Brain* 116: 681–693.

Prineas JW, McDonald WI. (1997) Demyelinating diseases. In Graham DI, Lantos PL (eds) *Greenfield's Neuropathology.* Sixth edition. vol. 1 pp 813–896. London:Arnold.

Raine CS (1991) Demyelinating diseases. In RL Davis, DM Robertson (eds) *Textbook of Neuropathology.* Second edition. pp. 535–620. Baltimore: Williams & Wilkins.

Raine CS (1994) Presidential address. Multiple sclerosis: immune system molecule expression in the central nervous system. *J Neuropathol Exp Neurol* 53: 328–337.

20 *Other idiopathic demyelinating diseases*

Acute disseminated encephalomyelitis and acute hemorrhagic leuko-encephalopathy are covered in this chapter. Demyelinating diseases of known etiology or that occur only in specific clinical contexts are included in other chapters: progressive multifocal leukoencephalopathy in chapter 14, central pontine myelinolysis and multifocal necrotizing leukoencephalopathy in chapter 22, and Marchiafava–Bignami disease in chapter 25. The leukoencephalopathies associated with lysosomal and peroxisomal disorders are covered in chapter 23.

ACUTE DISSEMINATED ENCEPHALOMYELITIS (ADEM)

This is a multifocal inflammatory disorder of the CNS. It is usually preceded by a systemic viral infection or, more rarely, vaccination and is believed to be due to a T cell-mediated hypersensitivity reaction. It resembles experimental allergic encephalitis induced in animals by immunization with any of several myelin antigens. Although some vaccination-related cases are attributable to contamination of the

vaccines by neural tissue and amino acid homologies have been identified between certain viruses and myelin proteins, in most cases the cause of ADEM is not known.

MACROSCOPIC APPEARANCES

Apart from some congestion and swelling, the brain and spinal cord may look macroscopically normal. In some cases, scattered small foci of gray-brown discoloration, some obviously centered on a small blood vessel, are evident in the white matter. The gray matter may also be involved, although usually to a lesser degree.

ACUTE DISSEMINATED ENCEPHALOMYELITIS

- The latent period between the preceding infectious illness (or vaccination) and the development of neurologic symptoms is usually a few days, but may be up to 3 weeks.
- Typical manifestations include sudden headache, vomiting, and fever, with subsequent rapid development of weakness, sensory loss, ataxia, visual impairment, incontinence, and stupor. Seizures may occur. Symptoms of spinal cord involvement may predominate.
- The symptoms and signs usually resolve over several weeks, allowing a good recovery in most patients. The recovery may be accelerated by administration of corticosteroids or, possibly, by plasmapheresis. Some patients are left with permanent neurologic deficits and approximately 20% die during the acute illness.
- Relapses are very rare. A recurrent form of demyelinating perivenous encephalomyelitis has been reported in association with familial erythrophagocytic lymphohistiocytosis.
- Very rarely ADEM is associated with the development of concurrent Guillain–Barré syndrome (acute inflammatory demyelinating peripheral neuropathy).

ACUTE DISSEMINATED ENCEPHALOMYELITIS

Preceding infections
- The most commonly implicated preceding viral infections are measles, mumps, chickenpox (varicella), German measles (rubella), influenza, and infectious mononucleosis (caused by Epstein–Barr virus).
- Other implicated preceding infections include *Mycoplasma pneumoniae*, *Campylobacter jejuni*, and group A streptococci infections.
- Symptoms of previous infection are not reported in all cases or may be mild and nonspecific.

Preceding vaccinations
- The best documented implicated preceding vaccinations are smallpox vaccination and the use of a rabies vaccine contaminated by neural tissue, which are now largely of historic interest.
- ADEM has been reported as a rare complication of influenza vaccination.
- Although chronic neurologic disease has occurred after whooping cough (pertussis) vaccination, in most cases this is due not to ADEM but to cerebral hypoxic injury complicating seizures.

Iatrogenic
- There are very occasional reports of ADEM in patients receiving sicca-cell preparations, gold, levamisole in combination with 5-fluorouracil, and levamisole alone.

MICROSCOPIC APPEARANCES

Many small veins and venules within the brain parenchyma are surrounded by an infiltrate of lymphocytes, macrophages, and occasional plasma cells. The inflammatory infiltrate extends a variable distance into the surrounding tissue (**Fig. 20.1**) and is associated with a corresponding zone of demyelination (**Figs 20.2, 20.3**). There may be small perivascular hemorrhages. Although loss of myelin predominates, there may be some axonal destruction. Arteries are relatively free of inflammation (see Fig. 20.1), but there are often inflammatory cells in the leptomeninges. Subpial inflammation and demyelination may occur in the brain stem and spinal cord.

ACUTE HEMORRHAGIC LEUKOENCEPHALOPATHY (AHL)

ACUTE HEMORRHAGIC LEUKOENCEPHALOPATHY

- Patients present with headache, pyrexia, vomiting, drowsiness, and generalized weakness, proceeding rapidly to coma.
- Seizures may be a prominent feature.
- AHL is usually fatal within days.

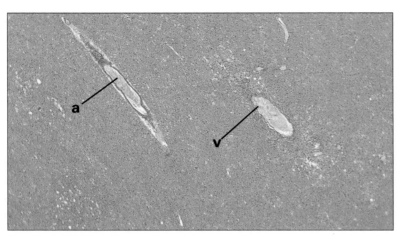

Fig. 20.1 ADEM. Infiltrate of lymphocytes and macrophages around a vein (v) in the cerebral white matter. Note the paucity of inflammation in relation to the adjacent artery (a).

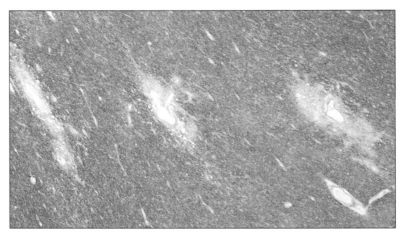

Fig. 20.2 ADEM. A zone of demyelination surrounds the affected blood vessels. (Solochrome cyanin)

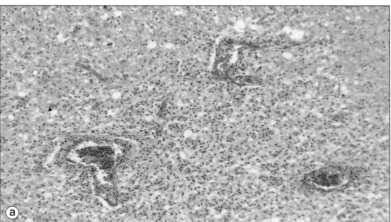

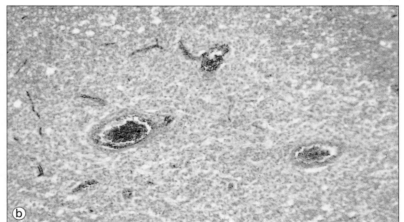

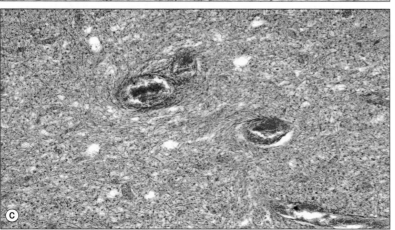

Fig. 20.3 Perivenous inflammation and demyelination in ADEM. (a) A solochrome cyanin preparation reveals confluent perivenous demyelination. **(b)** A corresponding zone of infiltration by lymphocytes and macrophages is seen in an adjacent section stained with hematoxylin and eosin. **(c)** Silver impregnation reveals relative preservation of axons in the demyelinated white matter.

ETIOLOGIC ASPECTS OF AHL

- Like ADEM, AHL may be preceded by a systemic viral or respiratory infection such as measles or primary atypical pneumonia (caused by *M. pneumoniae*).
- AHL has also been described in ulcerative colitis and Crohn's disease, in the context of septicemia associated with immune complex deposition, in methanol poisoning, and as a reaction to the treatment of trypanosomiasis with melarsoprol, which contains an organic arsenic compound.

This is a fulminant, usually fatal, disorder, regarded by some as a hyper-acute form of ADEM.

MACROSCOPIC APPEARANCES

The brain is soft and swollen. Sectioning reveals numerous small and occasional larger foci of hemorrhage, which are most prominent in the cerebral and cerebellar white matter and in the pons (**Figs 20.4, 20.5**).

MICROSCOPIC APPEARANCES

Many small blood vessels undergo fibrinoid necrosis and are surrounded by a narrow zone of necrotic tissue containing nuclear debris and a larger zone of hemorrhage (**Fig. 20.6**). The classic description is of ring- and ball-shaped perivascular hemorrhages. Other blood vessels are still recognizable as veins or venules, but are surrounded by fibrin and a mixed inflammatory infiltrate, including neutrophils and mononuclear cells (**Fig. 20.7**). Some fibers within the infiltrates are demyelinated, but many show axonal fragmentation (**Fig. 20.8**).

DIFFERENTIAL DIAGNOSIS OF AHL

Fibrinoid necrosis and widely scattered hemorrhages may also be seen in:
- fat embolism.
- thrombotic thrombocytopenic purpura.
- disseminated intravascular coagulation.

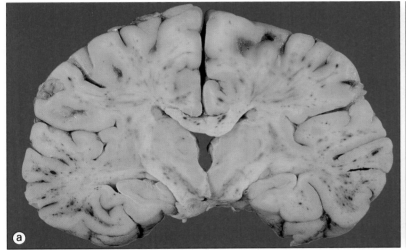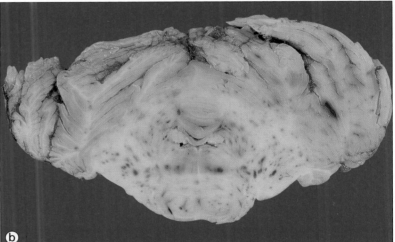

Fig. 20.4 AHL. Sections through the cerebrum (**a**) and the cerebellum and pons (**b**) of a patient with Crohn's disease who developed AHL. Perivascular hemorrhages and foci of gray-brown discoloration are scattered throughout the white matter in the cerebrum, and the brain stem and cerebellum. (Figures courtesy of Dr DA Hilton, Derriford Hospital, Plymouth, UK)

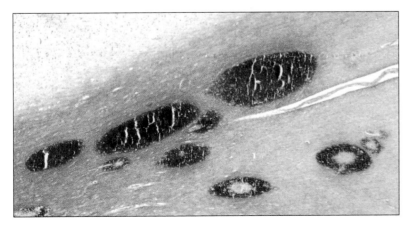

Fig. 20.5 AHL. Scattered ring- or ball-shaped perivascular hemorrhages in the white matter. (Luxol fast blue/cresyl violet)

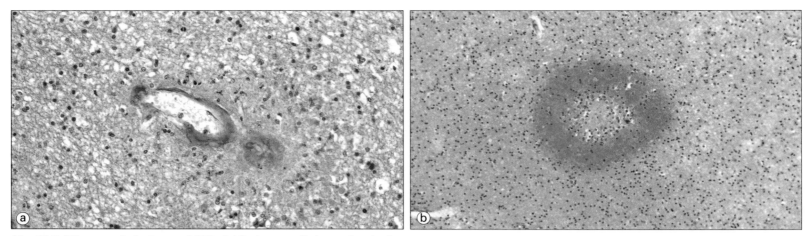

Fig. 20.6 Microscopic features of AHL. (a) Perivenous fibrin exudate (red), inflammatory cell infiltrate, and scanty hemorrhage in a case of AHL. (Martius–scarlet blue) **(b)** Ring-shaped hemorrhage around a zone of fibrinoid necrosis.

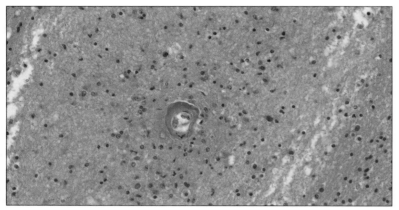

Fig. 20.7 AHL. Blood vessel showing fibrinoid necrosis and surrounded by a zone of hemorrhagic tissue with a predominantly mononuclear cell inflammatory infiltrate.

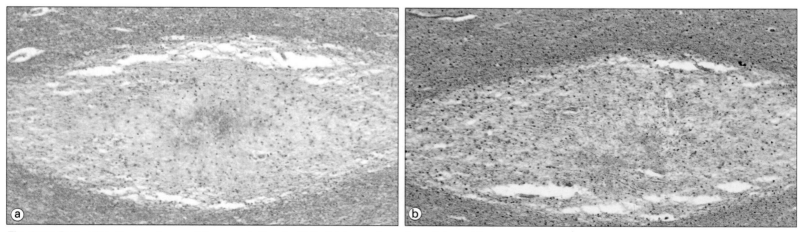

Fig. 20.8 Demyelination and axonal fragmentation in AHL. (a) Loss of myelin staining with a zone of perivascular hemorrhage in AHL. **(b)** Although a few axons appear to be preserved, most are fragmented. (Palmgren silver impregnation)

REFERENCES

Adams JH, Haller L, Boa FY, Doua F, Dago A, Konian K (1986) Human African trypanosomiasis (*T.b. gambiense*): A study of 16 fatal cases of sleeping sickness with some observations on acute reactive arsenical encephalopathy. *Neuropathol Appl Neurobiol* **12**: 81–94.

Graham DI, Behan PO, More IAR (1979) Brain damage complicating septic shock. Acute haemorrhagic leukoencephalitis as a complication of the generalised Schwartzman reaction. *J Neurol Neurosurg Psychiat* **42**: 19–28.

Prineas JW, McDonald WI (1977) Demyelinating diseases. In DI Graham, PL Lantos (eds) *Greenfield's Neuropathology. Sixth Edition.* pp. 813–896. London: Edward Arnold.

Raine CS (1991) Demyelinating diseases. In RL Davis, DM Robertson (eds) *Textbook of Neuropathology. Second edition.* pp. 535–620. Baltimore: Williams & Wilkins.

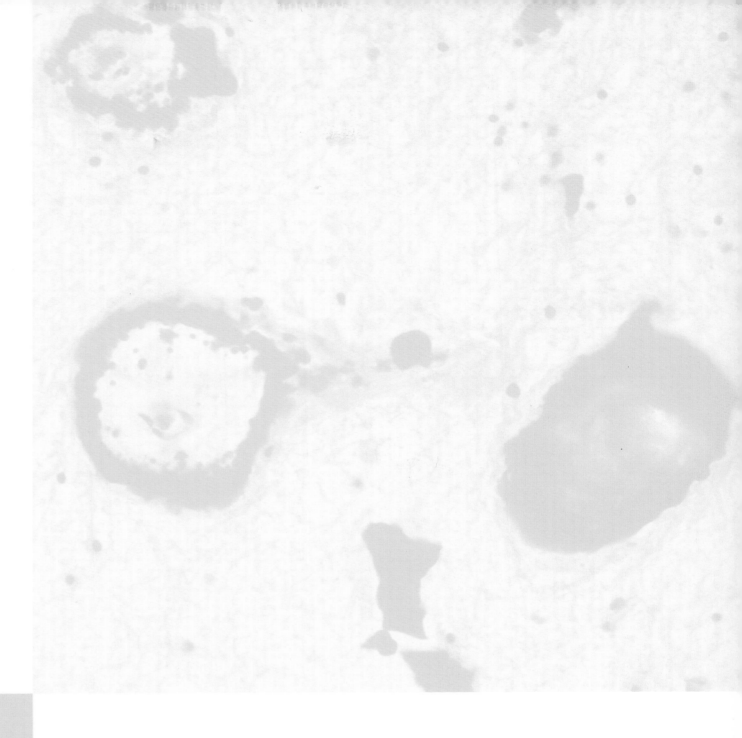

7 Nutritional and Metabolic Disorders

21 Vitamin deficiencies

Vitamin deficiencies are a significant cause of neurologic disease in developing countries and in certain high-risk groups in developed countries (i.e. chronic alcoholics, patients with gastrointestinal diseases, and patients receiving long-term parenteral nutrition with inadequate vitamin supplementation).

THIAMINE DEFICIENCY AND WERNICKE'S ENCEPHALOPATHY

MACROSCOPIC APPEARANCES

Lesions are usually discernible in the mamillary bodies (**Figs 21.1–21.5**), but may also involve other parts of the hypothalamus (see Figs 21.3,

21.4), the medial thalamic nuclei, the floor of the third ventricle, the periaqueductal region (**Fig. 21.6**), the colliculi (Fig. 21.6), the nuclei in the pontomedullary tegmentum (Fig. 21.6) (particularly the dorsal motor nuclei of the vagus), the inferior olives, and the cerebral cortex. Typically, the involved regions are slightly shrunken and show brown

WERNICKE'S ENCEPHALOPATHY

- Thiamine deficiency causes Wernicke's encephalopathy and beri-beri.
- Wernicke's encephalopathy usually complicates chronic alcoholism, but can be associated with gastrointestinal disorders.
- Thiamine pyrophosphate is a cofactor of the pyruvate dehydrogenase complex, α-ketoglutarate dehydrogenase, and transketolase.
- The encephalopathy is probably due to the energy deficit that results from impaired enzyme activity.

WERNICKE'S ENCEPHALOPATHY

- This usually manifests acutely with gaze palsies and ataxia, which rapidly respond to thiamine administration.
- Apathy and confusion may form part of the initial presentation, though these symptoms often develop later if the encephalopathy is left untreated for more than a few days.
- Wernicke's encephalopathy is sometimes associated with Korsakoff's psychosis, which is characterized by retrograde and anterograde amnesia (i.e. impaired recall of events before the onset of illness and of new information) and confabulation. This does not respond to thiamine and is usually irreversible. The combination of Korsakoff's psychosis with Wernicke's encephalopathy is known as Wernicke–Korsakoff syndrome.
- Post-translationally modified variants of transketolase with a reduced affinity for thiamine pyrophosphate have been described in some chronic alcoholics with Wernicke–Korsakoff syndrome.

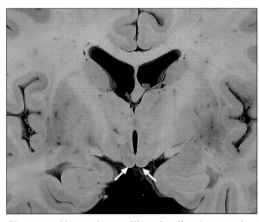

Fig. 21.1 Normal mamillary bodies (arrows).

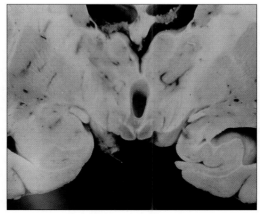

Fig. 21.2 Wernicke's encephalopathy. The mamillary bodies are slightly shrunken, and brown.

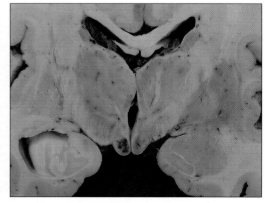

Fig. 21.3 Wernicke's encephalopathy. Petechial hemorrhages are present in the mamillary bodies. Further lesions are barely visible in the walls of the third ventricle.

discoloration due to hemosiderin deposition (see Fig. 21.2), and there may be petechial hemorrhages (see Figs 21.3, 21.6). The periventricular and periaqueductal lesions often spare a slender strip of subependymal tissue.

In some patients, particularly those with previously treated disease, the mamillary bodies may be only mildly discolored and other lesions may be inconspicuous (see Figs 21.4, 21.5).

MICROSCOPIC APPEARANCES

Acute lesions are edematous with relative preservation of neurons, variable necrosis of intervening tissue (**Fig. 21.7**), and loss of myelinated fibers. Capillaries may appear strikingly prominent due to endothelial hyperplasia and cuffing by macrophages (**Fig. 21.8**), but this is not a constant feature. There may be petechial hemorrhages and hemosiderin-laden macrophages (**Fig. 21.9**). Astrocytes show reactive changes.

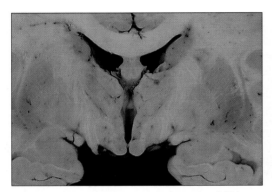

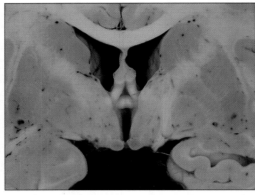

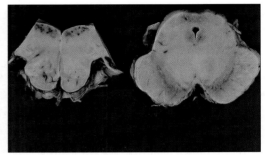

Fig. 21.6 Wernicke's encephalopathy. Brown discoloration and petechial hemorrhages in the periaqueductal region, colliculi, and floor of the fourth ventricle.

Fig. 21.4 Wernicke's encephalopathy. Mild macroscopic changes are visible in the mamillary bodies and scattered lesions elsewhere in the hypothalamus.

Fig. 21.5 Wernicke's encephalopathy. Only mild discoloration is seen in the mamillary bodies.

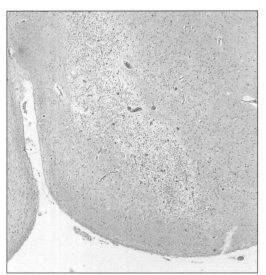

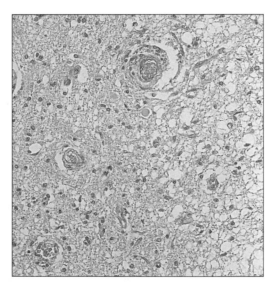

Fig. 21.7 Histology of Wernicke's encephalopathy. Necrosis in the mamillary body, with sparing of neurons and capillaries and accumulation of macrophages.

Fig. 21.8 Histology of Wernicke's encephalopathy. Capillary endothelial hyperplasia and cuffing by macrophages in the mamillary body of a patient with acute Wernicke's encephalopathy.

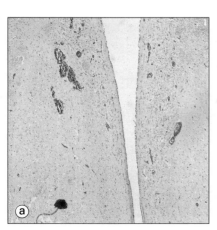

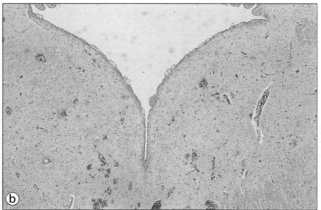

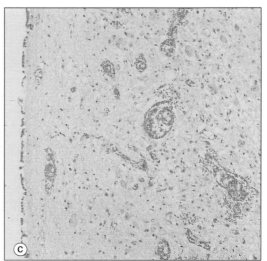

Fig. 21.9 Hypothalamic and periaqueductal lesions in acute Wernicke's encephalopathy.
(a) Petechial hemorrhages in the hypothalamus, and **(b)** periaqueductal gray matter. **(c)** Higher magnification view of petechial hemorrhages in the hypothalamus.

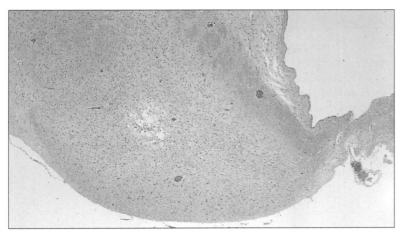

Chronic lesions usually appear gliotic and slightly spongiotic (**Figs 21.10, 21.11**), with a mild loss of neurons, depletion of myelinated fibers (**Fig. 21.11b**), and scattered hemosiderin-laden macrophages and astrocytes (**Fig. 21.12**).

The histologic changes in Wernicke's encephalopathy and Wernicke–Korsakoff syndrome are essentially identical. Studies suggest that Korsakoff's psychosis occurs in those patients who have lesions involving the medial dorsal (or possibly other medial thalamic) nuclei (**Fig. 21.13**).

Fig. 21.10 Chronic Wernicke's encephalopathy. Mild focal spongiosis of the mamillary body.

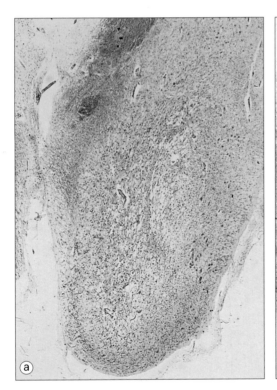

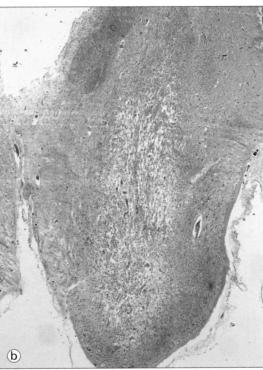

Fig. 21.11 Chronic Wernicke's encephalopathy. (a) Marked shrinkage and spongy gliosis of the mamillary body. **(b)** The mamillary body is depleted of myelinated fibers. (Luxol fast blue/cresyl violet)

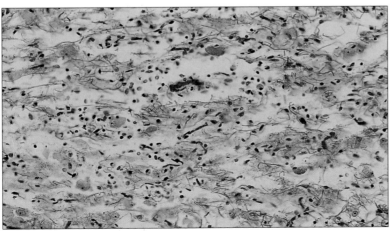

Fig. 21.12 Chronic Wernicke's encephalopathy. Gliotic mamillary body containing scattered hemosiderin-laden macrophages. Note the preserved neuronal somata. (Phosphotungstic acid/hematoxylin)

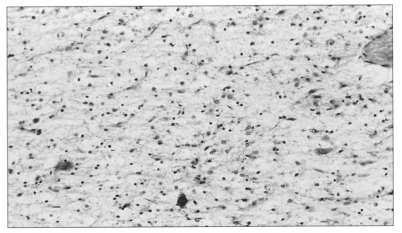

Fig. 21.13 Wernicke–Korsakoff syndrome. Rarefied gliotic dorsomedial thalamic nucleus from a patient with Wernicke–Korsakoff syndrome. (Luxol fast blue/cresyl violet)

NICOTINIC ACID DEFICIENCY AND PELLAGRA

MACROSCOPIC AND MICROSCOPIC APPEARANCES

The brain and spinal cord appear macroscopically normal. Histologic changes in the CNS occur predominantly in the later stages of pellagra. Betz cells (**Fig. 21.14**) and neurons in the pontine (**Fig. 21.15**) and cerebellar dentate nuclei show striking chromatolysis without associated microglial or astrocytic changes. Other neurons in the brain stem (**Fig.** 21.16) and the anterior horn cells of the spinal cord (**Fig. 21.17**) may also be affected. Symmetric degeneration of the dorsal columns, especially the gracile funiculi, and, to a lesser extent, of the corticospinal tracts, has been observed.

◼ NICOTINIC ACID DEFICIENCY AND PELLAGRA

Pellagra is caused by a deficiency of nicotinic acid or its amino acid precursor (i.e. tryptophan). Although fortification of bread and cereals with niacin has greatly reduced its prevalence, pellagra still occurs in developing countries where the primary source of calories is unfortified maize. Other causes include:
- Chronic alcoholism.
- Hartnup disease, which is an autosomal recessive disorder characterized by defective monoaminomonocarboxylic amino acid transport across the intestinal mucosa (and renal tubules).
- Certain antituberculous drugs (especially isoniazid, but also cycloserine, ethionamide and pyrazinamide), which interfere with conversion of tryptophan to niacin (see chapter 25).
- Chronic intestinal disorders.

◼ PELLAGRA

The classic clinical triad of dermatitis, diarrhea, and dementia is often present only in part. The range of manifestations includes:
- cutaneous-atrophy, hyperpigmentation, and eventually ulceration of sun-exposed skin
- gastrointestinal-glossitis, stomatitis, vomiting, and diarrhea
- neurologic-irritability, depression, apathy, impaired memory, delirium and seizures, myelopathy with spastic weakness, and peripheral neuropathy

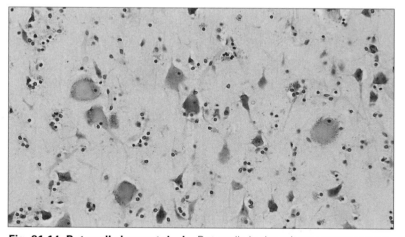

Fig. 21.14 Betz cell chromatolysis. Betz cells in the primary motor cortex are particularly susceptible to chromatolysis in pellagra. (Cresyl violet)

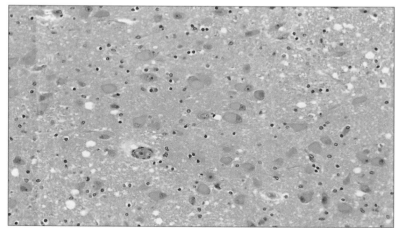

Fig. 21.15 Pellagra. Widespread chromatolysis of neurons in the pontine nuclei.

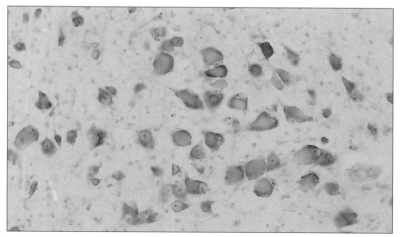

Fig. 21.16 Pellagra. Chromatolysis of neurons in the hypoglossal nucleus. (Cresyl violet)

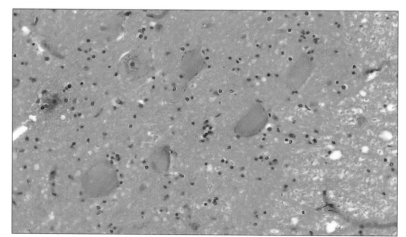

Fig. 21.17 Spinal cord in pellagra. Most of the anterior horn cells are chromatolytic.

PYRIDOXINE (VITAMIN B₆)

Pyridoxine is present in most foods, and nutritional deficiency is rare. A functional deficiency can occur in patients receiving isoniazid or other pyridoxine antagonists (see chapter 25).

PYRIDOXINE DEFICIENCY

- Pyridoxine deficiency can cause irritability and seizures in children.
- Symptoms of pellagra may occur because pyridoxine deficiency impairs the synthesis of niacin from tryptophan.
- A specific syndrome of pyridoxine-dependent seizures occurs in infancy. This is thought to be due to defective binding of pyridoxal phosphate to glutamate decarboxylase, which is the rate-limiting enzyme in the synthesis of the inhibitory neurotransmitter γ-aminobutyric acid. The resulting γ-aminobutyric acid deficiency causes severe epilepsy, which responds to large doses of pyridoxine.

MACROSCOPIC AND MICROSCOPIC APPEARANCES

Neuropathologic data are lacking, but hypodense white matter and increased T2 signal intensity have been reported in neuroimaging studies of infants with pyridoxine-dependent seizures.

VITAMIN B₁₂ (COBALAMIN) DEFICIENCY AND SUBACUTE COMBINED DEGENERATION (SACD)

MACROSCOPIC APPEARANCES

The spinal cord of patients with long-standing, severe disease, may be mildly shrunken with discolored posterior and lateral columns, especially in the lower cervical and thoracic regions.

VITAMIN B₁₂ DEFICIENCY

- Neurologic disease (which can occur in the absence of hematologic abnormalities) develops in approximately 40% of patients with untreated pernicious anemia.
- Early manifestations include paresthesiae in the lower limbs, progressing to loss of fine touch, vibration, and position sense.
- Further progression leads to spastic paraparesis, ataxia, and anesthesia of the lower limbs and trunk. The upper limbs are usually less severely affected.
- Less common neurologic disturbances include visual impairment, depression, irritability, confusional states, and dementia ('megaloblastic madness').

MICROSCOPIC APPEARANCES

Early lesions consist of spongy vacuolation and degeneration of myelin sheaths in the thoracic region, initially in the posterior columns and later in the corticospinal and spinocerebellar tracts in the lateral columns (**Figs 21.18–21.21**). The lesions are approximately symmetric. The disease is not a system degeneration in the sense of involving specific nuclei and their related pathways, and the extent of individual lesions in cross-sections through the cord does not necessarily correspond to that of specific fiber tracts. As the disease progresses myelin breakdown is followed by axonal degeneration, macrophage infiltration, and astrocytic gliosis (**Figs 21.20–21.22**). The severity of the lesions usually diminishes towards the cervical and lumbar regions, but these show changes of secondary ascending and descending tract degeneration. In severe cases the anterior columns are also involved (**Fig. 21.23**). Rarely, the lesions extend rostrally into the medulla.

The cerebral white matter and optic nerves may contain small, often perivascular, foci of demyelination or fiber degeneration with an accumulation of lipid-laden macrophages (**Fig. 21.24**). Rarely, the cerebral lesions are more extensive than those in the spinal cord.

VITAMIN B₁₂ DEFICIENCY

Vitamin B₁₂ deficiency can cause SACD of the spinal cord, and peripheral neuropathy, as well as megaloblastic anemia, glossitis, and gastrointestinal disturbances. Vitamin B₁₂ is present only in animal foods such as meat, dairy products, and yeasts, is released during gastric digestion, and must bind to intrinsic factor (a glycoprotein produced by gastric parietal cells) before it can be absorbed in the distal ileum.
SACD is believed to result from defective methylation of myelin basic protein and other CNS proteins. The synthesis of the methyl donor (i.e. S-adenosylmethionine) is wholly dependent on methionine synthase (at least in the CNS), which is itself dependent on vitamin B₁₂.
Vitamin B₁₂ deficiency is usually due to autoimmune atrophic gastritis resulting in inadequate production of intrinsic factor by the gastric parietal cells in patients with pernicious anemia.

Other causes of vitamin B₁₂ deficiency are:
- Strict vegetarianism (veganism).
- Partial or complete gastrectomy or gastric neoplasms that interfere with intrinsic factor production.
- Other causes of intestinal malabsorption.
- Competitive uptake of the vitamin by fish tapeworm infestation or bacterial overgrowth in small intestinal blind loops or diverticula.
- Abnormalities of vitamin B₁₂ metabolism in HIV infection.

Other causes of SACD are:
- Nitrous oxide abuse (see chapter 25).
- Folate deficiency (see p 21.7), which affects methionine synthase activity.
- Inherited defects of methylation (rare).
- Abnormal plasma vitamin B₁₂-binding protein (very rare).

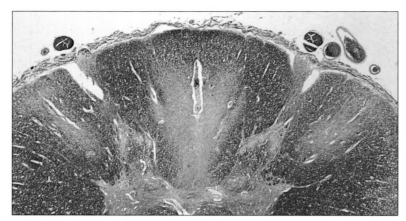

Fig. 21.18 Early SACD. There is symmetric loss of myelin staining in part of the posterior and lateral columns. (Luxol fast blue/cresyl violet)

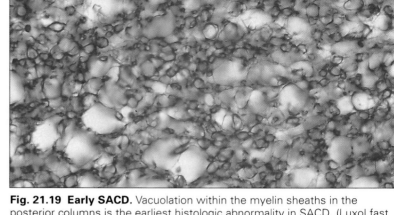

Fig. 21.19 Early SACD. Vacuolation within the myelin sheaths in the posterior columns is the earliest histologic abnormality in SACD. (Luxol fast blue/cresyl violet)

Fig. 21.20 SACD. These lesions show early infiltration by macrophages. (Luxol fast blue/cresyl violet)

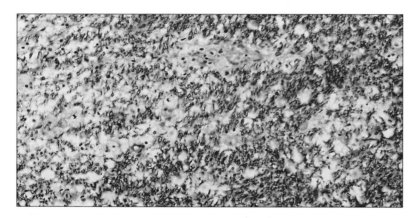

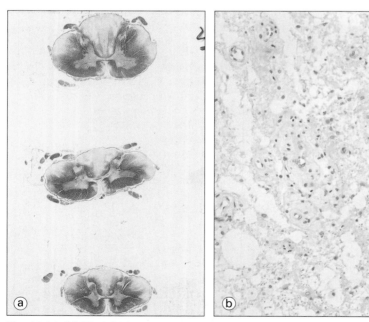

Fig. 21.21 SACD. (a) Myelin pallor in the posterior and lateral columns in the cervical and upper thoracic spinal cord in advanced SACD. There is also some anterior column involvement. (Luxol fast blue/cresyl violet) **(b)** Higher magnification view showing spongy vacuolation of white matter in the posterior column, loss of myelin staining, perivascular macrophages, and some reactive astrocytes. Note the punctate cross-sectional profiles of some axons that are still intact, particularly towards the bottom left of the illustration. (Luxol fast blue/cresyl violet)

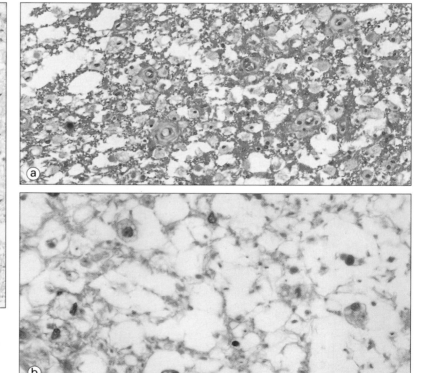

Fig. 21.22 Advanced SACD. (a) and **(b)** show coarse vacuolation of the affected spinal white matter, and infiltration by macrophages.

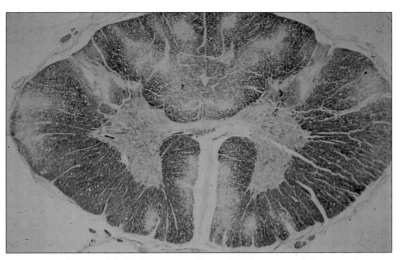

Fig. 21.23 Severe SACD. This case shows involvement of the anterior columns as well as the posterior and lateral columns. (Loyez myelin stain)

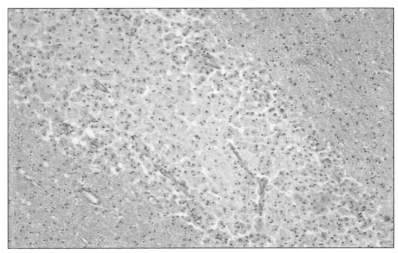

Fig. 21.24 Cerebral lesions in SACD. Perivascular lesion with accumulation of foamy macrophages in the cerebral white matter of a patient with SACD.

FOLIC ACID DEFICIENCY

MACROSCOPIC AND MICROSCOPIC APPEARANCES

The neuropathologic findings in acquired folate deficiency are presumed to resemble those of SACD due to vitamin B_{12} deficiency, but scanty human data are available. There are reports that inborn errors of folate metabolism cause typical SACD of the cord and leukoencephalopathy, with foci of perivascular demyelination or fiber degeneration.

FOLIC ACID DEFICIENCY

- Folic acid is present in many foods, but particularly leafy vegetables, legumes, yeasts, and liver. It is a cofactor of enzymes involved in nucleotide synthesis and methylation. N_5-methyltetrahydrofolate donates a methyl group to the vitamin B_{12}-dependent enzyme, methionine synthase, for the conversion of homocysteine to methionine.
- Folic acid deficiency is usually due to malnutrition or malabsorption.
- Several drugs, including phenytoin, primidone, phenobarbitone, estrogens, alcohol, methotrexate, trimethoprim, and triamterene, are folate antagonists and can produce signs of deficiency, particularly when associated with other predisposing factors.
- Rare inborn errors of folate metabolism (e.g. an inherited defect of folate transport across the intestine and the blood–brain barrier, methylenetetrahydrofolate reductase deficiency, methionine synthase deficiency, and glutamate formiminotransferase-cyclodeaminase deficiency) cause severe disease of the CNS from an early age.

FOLIC ACID DEFICIENCY

- Although most of the clinical effects of folic acid deficiency are related to the development of megaloblastic anemia, patients occasionally also develop neurologic disease.
- Peripheral nerve and myelopathic disturbances can occur that are similar to those associated with vitamin B_{12} deficiency (i.e. paresthesiae, sensory impairment, and weakness predominantly involving the lower limbs), but unresponsive to vitamin B_{12} administration.
- Confusion and cognitive impairment have been reported.
- The rare inborn errors of folate metabolism (see box on left) result in varying degrees of megaloblastic anemia, mental and physical retardation, extrapyramidal disorders, and seizures.
- Folate deficiency has been associated with abnormal fetal development, particularly neural tube defects. Administration of supplementary folate to pregnant women (even those with normal serum folate levels) who have already had a child with a neural tube defect probably reduces the risk that a similar defect will affect the fetus *in utero*.

VITAMIN A DEFICIENCY AND INTOXICATION

Vitamin A is the precursor of the light-sensitive retinal pigment rhodopsin. It is ingested in animal tissues or synthesized from carotenoids in fruits and vegetables.

Vitamin A deficiency usually results from intestinal malabsorption with steatorrhea, though inadequate dietary intake is another cause, particularly in developing countries. It causes night blindness, corneal keratinization, and dryness and hyperkeratosis of the skin. Increased intracranial pressure has been reported as a rare manifestation of deficiency in infancy.

Vitamin A toxicity usually results from taking excessive vitamin supplements. It causes liver disease and brain swelling, leading to the symptoms and signs of raised intracranial pressure.

VITAMIN E (α-TOCOPHEROL)

MACROSCOPIC AND MICROSCOPIC APPEARANCES

The brain and spinal cord appear macroscopically normal. Histology reveals swelling and degeneration of the distal part of longer axons in peripheral nerves and the posterior spinal, spinocerebellar, and corticospinal tracts (see chapter 25). Axonal swellings are particularly prominent in the gracile and, to a lesser extent, cuneate funiculi and nuclei (**Figs 21.26, 21.27**), but may also be seen in other brain stem nuclei and in the basal ganglia. The axons show dystrophic ultrastructural changes with an accumulation of filaments, membranes, tubules, degenerate mitochondria, and osmiophilic debris.

Neuronal loss may be evident in the dorsal root ganglia and occasionally in the brain stem sensory and oculomotor nuclei, the anterior spinal horn, and Clarke's column. There may be prominent neuronal lipofuscinosis.

VITAMIN E (α-TOCOPHEROL)

- Vitamin E is present in vegetable oils and leafy vegetables, and its absorption depends on normal biliary, pancreatic, and small intestinal function.
- Vitamin E is transported to the liver in chylomicrons, and in the systemic circulation in very-low-density and low-density lipoproteins. Its incorporation into lipoproteins in the liver depends on the presence of functional α-tocopherol transfer protein.
- Vitamin E is an important biologic antioxidant and as such prevents phospholipid peroxidation in biologic membranes. Deficiency causes neurologic disease and acanthocytosis (i.e. spiny deformity of red blood cells, resulting in a diminished lifespan, **Fig. 21.25**) and is most commonly due to malabsorption associated with liver or pancreatic disease.
- Cystic fibrosis is an important cause of vitamin E deficiency in children.
- Two inherited metabolic disorders that produce deficiency are:
  - Ataxia with isolated vitamin E deficiency, which is an autosomal recessive disease caused by mutations in α-tocopherol transfer protein.
  - Bassen–Kornzweig syndrome (abetalipoproteinemia), which is an autosomal recessive disorder in which there is a failure of apoprotein B incorporation into very-low-density and low-density lipoproteins, probably due to a deficiency of microsomal triglyceride transfer protein.

INTESTINAL ABSORPTION OF FAT-SOLUBLE VITAMINS, INCLUDING VITAMINS A AND E

- Absorption of fat-soluble vitamins depends on normal biliary, pancreatic, and small intestinal function.
- Absorption is impaired by diseases such as biliary obstruction, pancreatic insufficiency, tropical sprue, celiac disease, multiple intestinal resections, and radiation injury, in which there is steatorrhea with defective fat absorption. These conditions are the commonest causes of deficiencies of these vitamins.

VITAMIN E DEFICIENCY

- Hematologic manifestations are acanthocytosis and hemolytic anemia of varying severity.
- Neurologic manifestations are peripheral neuropathy and spinocerebellar dysfunction that may closely resemble Friedreich's ataxia (see chapter 29), with ataxia, impaired vibration and position sense, absent tendon reflexes, weakness, dysarthria, and nystagmus.
- Patients with abetalipoproteinemia also develop pigmentary retinopathy with macular degeneration.

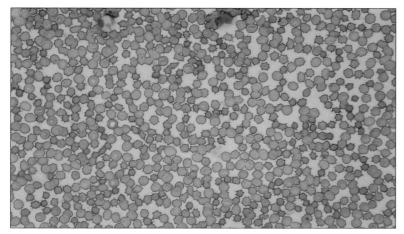

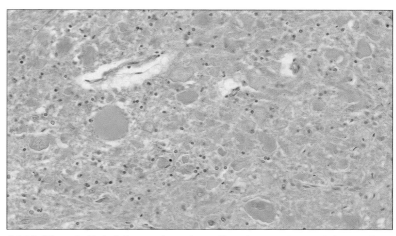

Fig. 21.25 Acanthocytosis due to vitamin E deficiency. Blood smear showing the surface of the red blood cells to have the characteristic spiny protuberances of acanthocytes. (Giemsa)

21.26 Vitamin E deficiency. Axonal swellings in rostral part of the gracile funiculus.

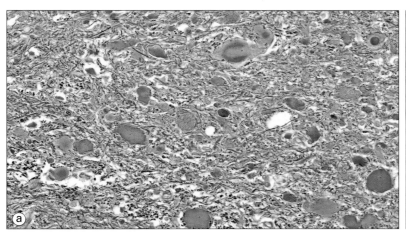

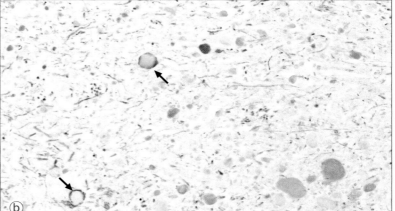

21.27 Vitamin E deficiency. The swollen axons in the gracile funiculus are moderately argyrophilic **(a)** and show variable neurofilament immunoreactivity **(b)**, in some cases confined to the subsarcolemmal region (arrows).

REFERENCES

Greenberg DA (1993) Ethanol and sedatives. In *Neurologic Complications of Drug and Alcohol Abuse. Neurologic Clinics* **11**(3): 523–533.

Harper C, Butterworth R (1996) Nutritional and metabolic disorders. In DI Graham, PL Lantos (eds) *Greenfield's Neuropathology.* (6th Edition). pp. 601–655. London: Edward Arnold.

Kierbutz K, Feigin A (1994) Neurologic manifestations of vitamin and mineral disorders. In Robert J Joynt (ed.) *Clinical Neurology. Volume 4.* pp.1–19. Philadelphia: Lippincott.

Schochet Jr SS (1993) Intoxications and metabolic diseases of the central nervous system. In JS Nelson, JE Parisi, SS Schochet Jr (eds) *Principles and Practice of Neuropathology.* pp. 302–343. London: Mosby.

Schochet Jr SS, Nelson J (1991) Exogenous toxic–metabolic diseases including vitamin deficiency. In RL Davis, DM Robertson (eds) *Textbook of Neuropathology.* (Second Edition). pp. 428–460. Baltimore: Williams & Wilkins.

Victor M (1994) Neurologic disorders due to alcoholism and malnutrition. In Robert J Joynt (ed.) *Clinical Neurology. Volume 4.* pp. 1–94. Philadelphia: Lippincott.

Victor M (1993) Persistent altered mentation due to ethanol. In *Neurologic Complications of Drug and Alcohol Abuse. Neurologic Clinics* **11**(3): 639–661.

22 Systemic metabolic disease

HYPOGLYCEMIA

ETIOLOGY OF HYPOGLYCEMIC BRAIN INJURY

- The principal source of energy in the CNS is glucose. Its uptake by nerve cells is independent of insulin. Neuronal stores of glucose and glycogen are relatively small and the requirement practically continuous. During periods of fasting, adults and, to a lesser extent, children are able to obtain some energy from metabolism of ketones, but a blood glucose level of less than 1.5 mmol/l (25–30 mg/100 ml) leads to brain damage within 1–2 hours.
- The commonest cause of hypoglycemia sufficiently severe to cause CNS damage is an excess of exogenous insulin or other hypoglycemic drugs. Other causes include:
  - primary hyperinsulinism (usually due to an islet cell adenoma)
  - severe liver disease
  - adrenal insufficiency
  - nesidioblastosis (in neonates).
- The effects of hypoglycemia are not solely due to the energy deficit. Experimental studies have demonstrated release of aspartate, and to a lesser extent glutamate, which probably cause selective neuronal excitotoxic damage.

HYPOGLYCEMIA

- Patients typically present with headache, confusion, irritability, incoordination, and lethargy, leading to stupor, and coma.
- Seizures are common, especially in children under 1 year of age.
- Prolonged or frequent episodes of hypoglycemia result in permanent CNS dysfunction.

MACROSCOPIC APPEARANCES

The brain is usually congested and mildly swollen. There may be little else of note or, in some cases, ill-defined dusky discoloration of the cerebral cortex, caudate nucleus, and putamen.

MICROSCOPIC APPEARANCES

The lesions are similar to those of acute hypoxia–ischemia (see chapter 8), but not identical. In general, the pattern of injury is that of isolated neuronal necrosis rather than frank infarction. Affected neurons are shrunken with hypereosinophilic cytoplasm. The nuclei are initially pyknotic, but later become more eosinophilic and appear to blend in with the cytoplasm (nuclear dropout) (**Fig. 22.1**). As in hypoxia, the subiculum and CA1 field of the hippocampus are particularly vulnerable, while CA3 and 4 are less and CA2 is least vulnerable. In the cerebral neocortex, the large neurons in laminae 3, 5, and 6 are most likely to be involved. The caudate nucleus and putamen, particularly the small neurons, are highly vulnerable to hypoglycemia. The dentate nucleus is usually affected (**Fig. 22.2**), but in contrast to hypoxic–ischemic brain injury, Purkinje cells are relatively spared.

Infants dying from hypoglycemia may show widespread neuronal degeneration throughout the brain.

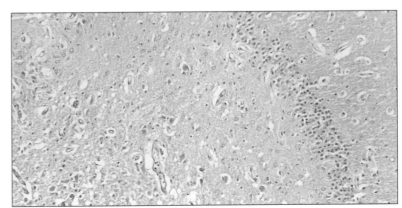

Fig. 22.1 Severe hypoglycemic hippocampal injury due to insulin overdose. Most of the nuclei in the dentate fascia are shrunken and pyknotic. Many of the large neurons in the end folium (CA3/4) show nuclear dropout.

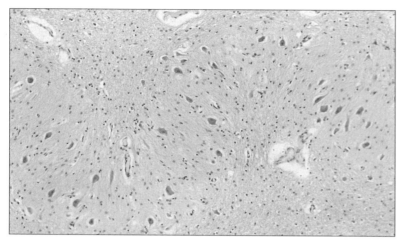

Fig. 22.2 Hypoglycemic injury. Hypereosinophilic neurons in the dentate nucleus of an infant with fatal hypoglycemia due to nesidioblastosis.

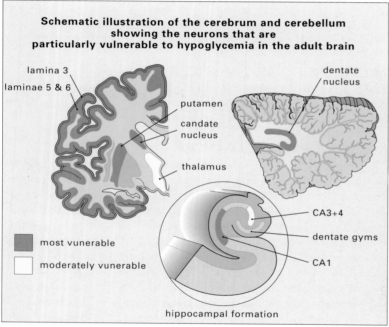

Fig. 22.3 Regions of the brain that are particularly vulnerable to hypoglycemia.

Schematic illustration of the cerebrum and cerebellum showing the neurons that are particularly vulnerable to hypoglycemia in the adult brain

lamina 3
laminae 5 & 6
putamen
candate nucleus
thalamus
dentate nucleus
CA3+4
dentate gyms
CA1
most vunerable
moderately vunerable
hippocampal formation

FINDINGS IN LONG-TERM SURVIVORS OF SEVERE HYPOGLYCEMIA

MACROSCOPIC APPEARANCES

The cerebral cortex may appear thinned and the hippocampi shrunken and discolored (**Fig. 22.4**). The white matter is reduced in bulk and the ventricles are dilated. There may be marked atrophy of the caudate nucleus and putamen (**Fig. 22.5**).

MICROSCOPIC APPEARANCES

The cerebral cortex shows laminar neuronal loss and gliosis associated with capillary proliferation (**Fig. 22.6**). There is often dense subpial gliosis. The hippocampal pyramidal cell layer and subiculum are replaced by a loose meshwork of glial tissue (**Fig. 22.7**). The white matter is usually rarefied and gliotic. The caudate nucleus and putamen are diffusely gliotic (**Fig. 22.8**). The globus pallidus is relatively spared. Moderate neuronal loss and gliosis may be evident in the thalamus. As in acute hypoglycemia, the cerebellar cortex, including the Purkinje cells, is relatively spared (**Fig. 22.9**).

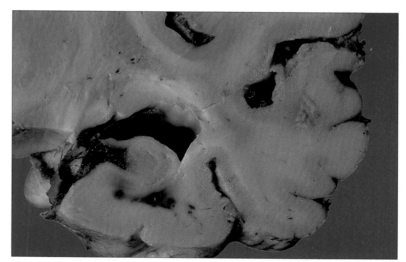

Fig. 22.4 Macroscopic findings in long-term survivor of severe hypoglycemia. Granular and atrophic neocortex in a survivor of an insulin overdose. The hippocampus and tail of the caudate nucleus are also severely shrunken.

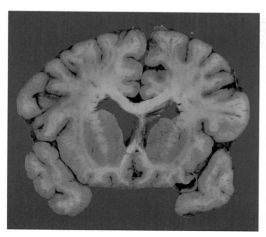

Fig. 22.5 Macroscopic features several weeks after an insulin overdose. The cerebral cortex is congested and focally thinned, particularly in the orbital frontal region and in the depths of sulci over the cerebral convexities. The corpus striatum is congested and there is irregular shrinkage of the caudate nucleus so that the medial surface is uneven.

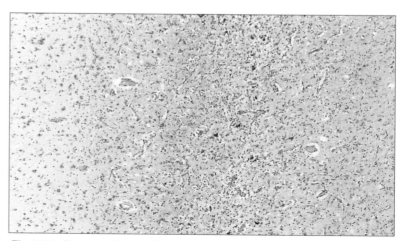

Fig. 22.6 Chronic effects of severe hypoglycemia. The cerebral cortex shows laminar neuronal loss, gliosis, and capillary proliferation. Several remaining neurons are mineralized.

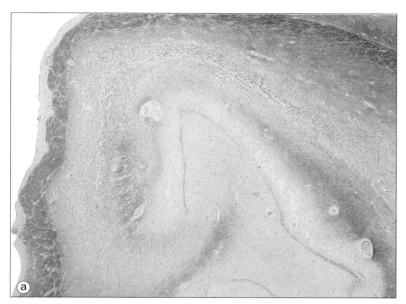
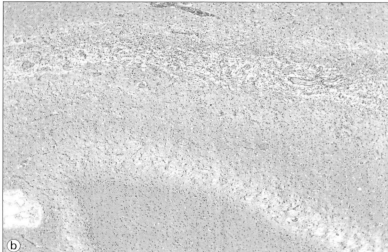

Fig. 22.7 Microscopic features 6 weeks after an insulin overdose.
(a) The hippocampal pyramidal cell layer and subiculum are replaced by a loose meshwork of glial tissue and capillaries. (Luxol fast blue/cresyl violet)
(b) Higher magnification view of the pyramidal cell layer and the dentate fascia (below), which is also severely gliotic.

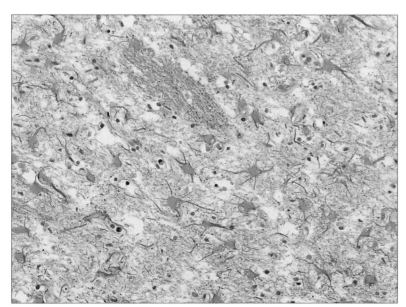

Fig. 22.8 Chronic hypoglycemic injury. Diffuse gliosis of the putamen after severe hypoglycemia. (Phosphotungstic acid/hematoxylin)

DISTURBANCES OF BODY TEMPERATURE

HYPOTHERMIA
This may cause apathy, confusion, obtundation, and coma. Choreoathetosis has been reported in a small proportion of patients after deliberate induction of deep hypothermia with cardiopulmonary bypass for cardiac surgery. No consistent neuropathologic abnormalities have been described.

HYPERTHERMIA
This is most commonly due to strenuous physical exertion under hot and humid conditions, but may also be a consequence of an infection or drug reaction. Predisposing conditions include diabetes mellitus, alcoholism, intoxication with certain drugs (3,4–methylenedioxymethamphetamine (Ecstasy), other amphetamines) and disorders in which there is impaired sweating (e.g. anhidrotic ectodermal dysplasia).

Malignant hyperthermia is an autosomal dominant disorder in which high fever, muscle rigidity, and rhabdomyolysis may be precipitated by inhalational anesthetics and depolarizing muscle relaxants.

MACROSCOPIC AND MICROSCOPIC APPEARANCES
The brain often appears normal or only mildly edematous. Some patients develop a bleeding diathesis, which may be associated with parenchymal or meningeal hemorrhages. Other described abnormalities are similar to those of hypoxic–ischemic damage (see chapter 8) and probably result from a combination of cardiovascular collapse and an increased metabolic rate (**Fig. 22.10**).

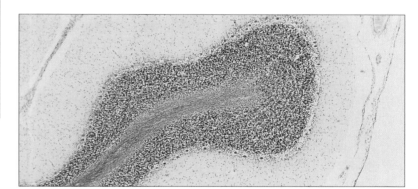

Fig. 22.9 Relative sparing of the cerebellar cortex, including the Purkinje cells, after hypoglycemia. This is from the same case as shown in Fig. 22.6. (Luxol fast blue/cresyl violet)

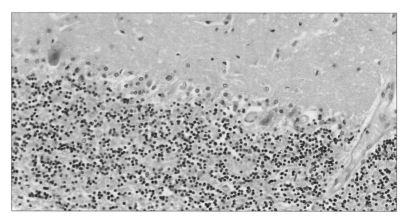

Fig. 22.10 Cerebellar cortex from a patient who collapsed and later died after spending several hours in a steam tent. The systemic necropsy findings were in keeping with heat stroke. Examination of the brain revealed changes indistinguishable from those of acute hypoxic neuronal injury, as illustrated by these shrunken Purkinje cells with hypereosinophilic cytoplasm.

DISORDERS OF SERUM ELECTROLYTES

HYPONATREMIA

Hyponatremia may be caused by:

- Excessive water ingestion in psychogenic polydipsia.
- Infusion of hypotonic fluids intravenously, especially when replacing electrolyte-rich fluids in gastrointestinal or renal disease.
- Use of hypotonic fluids for bladder or endometrial irrigation (e.g. during transcervical endometrial resection).
- Inappropriate antidiuretic hormone secretion.
- Drugs (e.g. oxcarbazepine).
- Adrenal insufficiency, cirrhosis, renal failure, or congestive cardiac failure.

Patients develop lethargy, headache, and nausea and vomiting, and if severe, seizures and coma leading to death.

MACROSCOPIC AND MICROSCOPIC APPEARANCES

Neuropathologic examination shows brain swelling due to intracellular accumulation of fluid (cytotoxic edema).

HYPERNATREMIA

Hypernatremia usually results from inadequate replacement or excessive loss of water in incapacitated patients (e.g. patients with burns). Other causes include:

- Diabetes insipidus (renal or hypothalamic).
- Osmotic diuresis (e.g. in uncontrolled diabetes mellitus).
- Rarely, excessive salt administration (as has occurred after accidental substitution of salt for sugar in infant feed).

The CNS adapts to chronic hypernatremia by increased synthesis of 'idiogenic' osmoles, which are amino acids, polyols, and trimethylamines that retain intracellular water. Symptoms are more likely in acute hypernatremia and include confusion, lethargy, stupor, seizures, and, rarely, coma.

MACROSCOPIC AND MICROSCOPIC APPEARANCES

Limited neuropathologic data are available. Findings in infants given hypernatremic feeds and adults with excessive water loss have included cerebral venous thromboses and hemorrhages. These probably result from a combination of blood hyperviscosity and shrinkage of brain tissue.

CENTRAL PONTINE AND EXTRAPONTINE MYELINOLYSIS

Central pontine myelinolysis (CPM) is a monophasic demyelinating disease that predominantly involves the basis pontis. It usually occurs as a complication of rapid correction of hyponatremia. The mechanism of the demyelination is poorly understood.

MACROSCOPIC APPEARANCES

Typically, the basis pontis includes a fusiform region of gray discoloration, which is abnormally soft and appears granular on sectioning (**Fig. 22.11**). The extent of the lesion is variable. Its cross-sectional area is usually greatest in the upper part of the pons, where only a narrow

CPM

- CPM usually manifests with rapid onset of confusion, limb weakness (often progressing to quadriparesis), conjugate gaze palsies, dysarthria (or mutism), dysphagia, and hypotension.
- Movement disorders (dystonia and choreoathetosis) occur in some patients and have been attributed to extrapontine myelinolysis.
- Until relatively recently a definite diagnosis of CPM could be made only at necropsy, but the diagnosis can now often be made during life by magnetic resonance imaging.
- In most cases CPM is fatal within a few weeks, but there are increasing numbers of well-documented cases of partial or complete neurologic recovery which occurs over a period of weeks or months.

ETIOLOGY OF CPM

- Most predisposing conditions are associated with hyponatremia (i.e. alcoholic liver damage, extensive skin burns, inappropriate secretion of antidiuretic hormone, psychogenic polydipsia, hyperemesis gravidarum).
- CPM occasionally develops in patients with a normal serum sodium concentration.
- The incidence of CPM is relatively high in liver transplant patients.
- Most studies have shown that the risk of developing CPM is related to the severity, duration, and speed of correction of the hyponatremia.
- CPM has occurred after infusion of hypertonic saline into normonatremic patients.

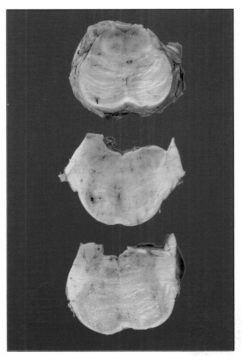

Fig. 22.11 CPM. Transverse sections through the brain stem in CPM showing gray discoloration and slight granularity of much of the basis pontis.

rim of subpial tissue may be spared (**Fig. 22.12**). It may involve the middle cerebral peduncles, but rarely extends rostrocaudally beyond the confines of the pons and lower midbrain. The lesion may be asymmetric, being largely or completely confined to one side of the pons.

The reported frequency of extrapontine lesions varies, but careful examination will reveal lesions in other parts of the CNS such as the cerebellum (Fig. 22.13), lateral geniculate body, capsula externa or extrema, subcortical cerebral white matter (Fig. 22.14), basal ganglia, thalamus, or internal capsule in 25–50% of cases. In up to 25% of patients the lesions may be exclusively extrapontine.

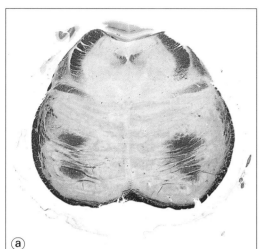
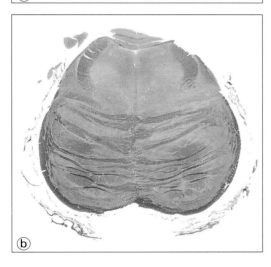

Fig. 22.12 Sections of the pons in CPM. (a) There is extensive loss of myelin. Note the sparing of myelin in a narrow rim of subpial tissue and in small 'islands' within the base of the pons. (Solochrome cyanin) **(b)** In an adjacent section, axons are seen to be well preserved. (Palmgren silver impregation)

DIFFERENTIAL DIAGNOSIS OF CPM

- The distribution of lesions, their identical age (if multiple), the paucity of lymphocytic inflammation, and clinical circumstances should allow this disorder to be distinguished from multiple sclerosis.
- Poor myelin staining of the deeper part of the pons due to inadequate fixation may on cursory examination lead to a misdiagnosis of CPM.

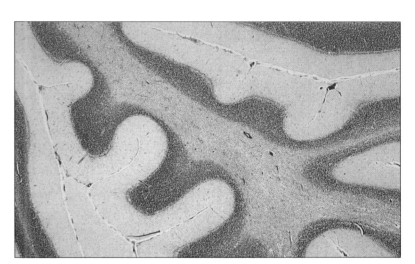

Fig. 22.13 Extrapontine demyelination. This section shows extrapontine demyelination in the white matter in the cerebellum. (Luxol fast blue/cresyl violet)

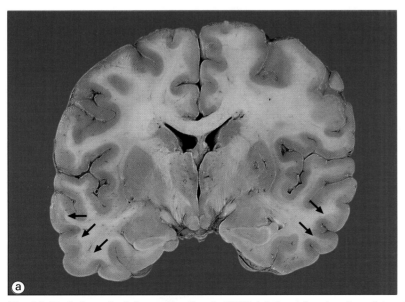
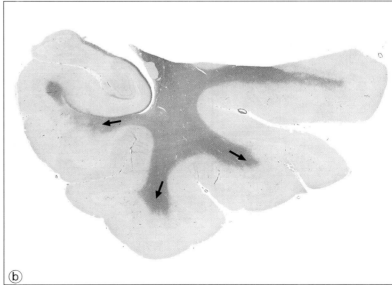

Fig. 22.14 Subcortical demyelination in CPM. (a) Gray discoloration of the demyelinated subcortical white matter (arrows) in a case of extrapontine myelinolysis associated with CPM. **(b)** Solochrome cyanin staining confirms the presence of subcortical demyelination involving white matter in the crests of gyri (arrows).

MICROSCOPIC APPEARANCES

The microscopic appearances of CPM are of active demyelination (**Fig. 22.15**). The lesions contain reactive astrocytes and large numbers of foamy lipid-laden macrophages (**Fig. 22.16**), but only very scanty lymphocytes. Silver impregnation may reveal some axonal fragmentation, but most neuronal somata and axons are intact (see Figs 22.12 and 22.15). Within the lesions, cranial nerves or central 'islands' of transverse pontine fibers or corticospinal tracts may be preserved (see Fig. 22.12).

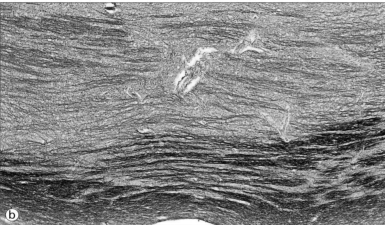

Fig. 22.15 Preservation of neuromal somata and axons in CPM. (a) Section of pons stained to show myelin. (Luxol fast blue/cresyl violet) **(b)** Section of pons adjacent to (a) stained for axons. There is good preservation of neuronal somata and axons within the zone of demyelination. (Palmgren silver impregation)

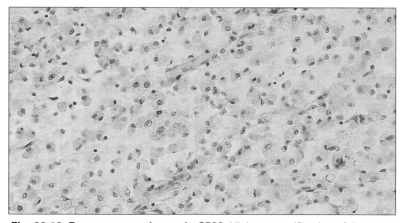

Fig. 22.16 Foamy macrophages in CPM. Higher magnification of the zone of demyelination in CPM reveals large numbers of foamy macrophages. (Luxol fast blue/cresyl violet)

CALCIUM DISTURBANCES AND FAHR'S DISEASE

Fahr's disease (non-arteriosclerotic cerebral calcification) is a heterogeneous group of disorders characterized by extensive calcification involving the basal ganglia, dentate nucleus, cerebral cortex, subthalamus, and red nucleus (in approximately decreasing order of frequency and severity).

FAHR'S DISEASE

- Fahr's disease may be inherited as an autosomal recessive or, rarely, autosomal dominant, disorder.
- Many patients have hypoparathyroidism, but a few have pseudohypoparathyroidism, pseudopseudohypoparathyroidism or hyperparathyroidism.
- In some cases the disorder has been attributed to intrauterine infection of undetermined etiology.

FAHR'S DISEASE

- The clinical manifestations depend on the specific etiology, age of onset, and associated disorders, but can include choreoathetosis, ataxia, spastic paraplegia, and dementia.
- Fahr's disease may also be associated with microcephaly, optic atrophy, and glaucoma.
- The intracranial calcification is readily demonstrable radiologically.

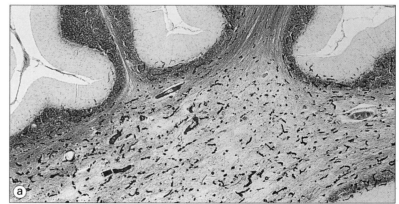

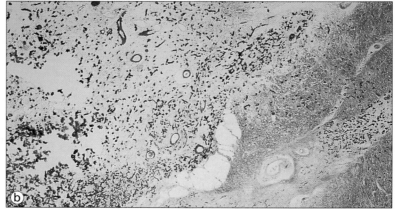

Fig. 22.17 Vascular and parenchymal mineralization in Fahr's disease. (a) In the cerebellar cortex and white matter. **(b)** In the caudate nucleus. (Luxol fast blue/cresyl violet)

MACROSCOPIC AND MICROSCOPIC APPEARANCES

Vascular calcification and scanty parenchymal mineral deposits are a common incidental finding in the pallidum and, to a lesser extent, in the hippocampus and dentate nucleus, particularly in old age. The mineralization in Fahr's disease is, however, much more extensive and can involve the cerebral sulci, basal ganglia, dentate nucleus, subthalamus, red nucleus, and other regions (**Fig. 22.17**). The concretions contain iron, magnesium, aluminum, and glycoproteins, in addition to calcium. The calcification of the media and adventitia of blood vessels may be associated with intimal fibrosis and narrowing, in some cases completely occluding the lumen (**Fig. 22.18**). The extent of associated neuronal degeneration and gliosis is variable and may be partly related to the degree of ischemia.

LIVER DISEASE

ACQUIRED HEPATIC ENCEPHALOPATHY
MICROSCOPIC APPEARANCES

The only consistent finding in acute hepatic encephalopathy is the presence of Alzheimer type II astrocytes. These have an enlarged vesicular nucleus with marginated chromatin, and scanty cytoplasm with little or no demonstrable glial fibrillary acid protein. Alzheimer type II astrocytes occur in the:
- Deep layers of the cerebral cortex.
- Caudate nucleus and putamen (**Fig. 22.19**).

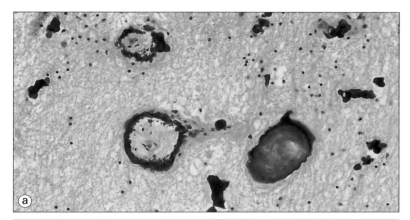

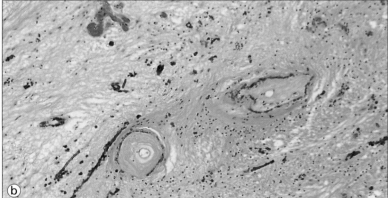

Fig. 22.18 Vasculopathy changes in Fahr's disease. (a, b) Vascular mineralization and the associated intimal fibrosis may stenose or occlude the lumen of affected blood vessels in Fahr's disease.

ACQUIRED HEPATIC ENCEPHALOPATHY

- This is a complication of severe liver disease or chronic portacaval shunting.
- The pathogenesis is not fully understood. The typical astroglial abnormalities are largely due to the hyperammonemia, which is probably also directly or indirectly responsible for many of the neurologic disturbances.
- Other factors that have been implicated include:
  - Elevated levels of benzodiazepine-like substances that bind to part of the γ-aminobutyric acid receptor.
  - Alterations in glutamatergic and serotoninergic transmission.

ACQUIRED HEPATIC ENCEPHALOPATHY

- Inattentiveness and impairment of short-term memory are typical early manifestations.
- Later features include confusion, which is often associated with asterixis (a flapping tremor of the outstretched hands), drowsiness, stupor, and coma.
- Patients often have a musty breath odor (*fetor hepaticus*), and a tendency to hyperventilation, resulting in respiratory alkalosis.
- Repeated episodes of hepatic encephalopathy may lead to neuropsychiatric disturbances, dysarthria, ataxia, and choreoathetosis.

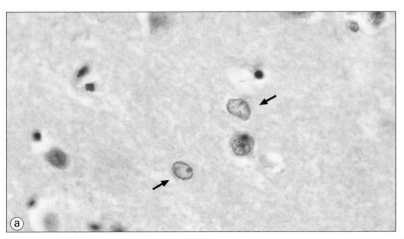

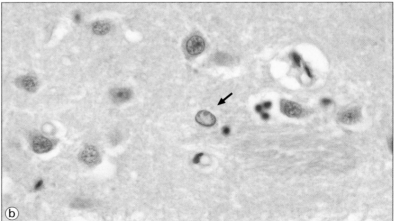

Fig. 22.19 Alzheimer type II astrocytes (arrows) in the putamen (a, b). They have an enlarged vesicular nucleus and scanty cytoplasm.

- Pallidum (where they are often particularly prominent) (**Fig. 22.20**).
- Thalamus, subthalamus, and hypothalamus.
- Dentate nucleus of the cerebellum.
- Brain stem.

Alzheimer type II astrocytes in the cerebral cortex, striatum, thalamus, and hypothalamus tend to have round nuclei, while those in the pallidum, subthalamus, dentate nucleus, and brain stem are often irregularly lobulated.

Chronic or recurrent hepatic encephalopathy may also cause:

- Patchy pseudolaminar necrosis and microcavitation in the depths of sulci at the junction of cerebral cortex and white matter (**Fig. 22.21**). The necrosis may extend into the cerebral white matter and can also involve the cerebellar white matter in severe cases.
- Neuronal loss, gliosis and, in severe cases, microcavitation, which are most prominent in the dorsal pole of the putamen (**Fig. 22.22**).

Although they are more usually associated with Wilson's disease (see below), Opalski cells may also be seen in non-Wilsonian chronic hepatic encephalopathy (**Fig. 22.23**).

HEPATOLENTICULAR DEGENERATION (WILSON'S DISEASE)

ETIOLOGY OF HEPATONLENTICULAR DEGENERATION (WILSON'S DISEASE)

- This autosomal recessive disorder is caused by mutations in a copper-transporting ATPase (ATP7B) gene encoded on chromosome 13 (13q14.3).
- ATP7B is expressed most strongly in liver and brain and may be necessary for the export of copper from the cell.
- ATP7B shares over 80% amino acid identity with ATP7A, the copper-transporting ATPase that is believed to be defective in Menkes' disease (see chapter 6) and is probably involved in the import of copper into the cell.

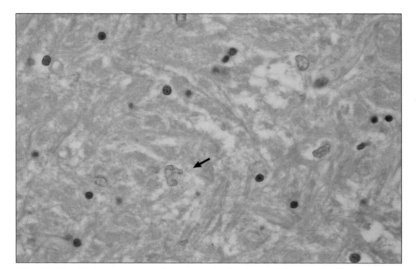

Fig. 22.20 Alzheimer type II astrocytes in the pallidum. These tend to have an irregularly lobulated nucleus (arrow).

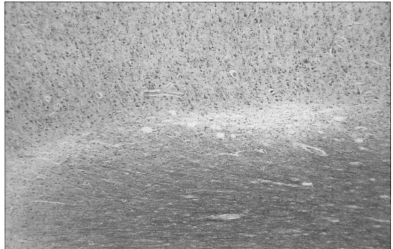

Fig. 22.21 Chronic hepatic encephalopathy. Microcavitation at the junction of cerebral cortex and white matter in chronic hepatic encephalopathy. (Luxol fast blue/cresyl violet)

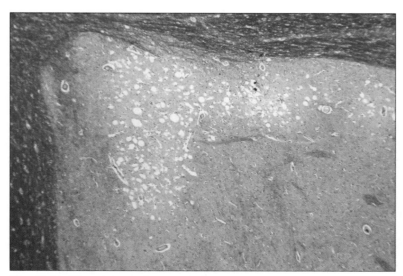

Fig. 22.22 Chronic hepatic encephalopathy. Neuronal loss and microcavitation in the dorsal pole of the putamen in chronic hepatic encephalopathy. (Phosphotungstic acid/hematoxylin)

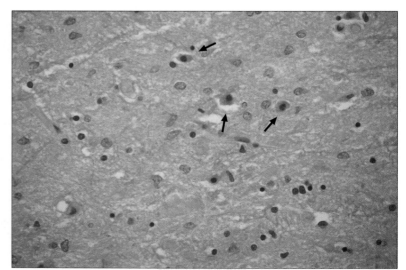

Fig. 22.23 Opalski cells in the subthalamus in hepatic encephalopathy due to portacaval shunting. These cells have a small hyperchromatic nucleus and abundant granular deeply eosinophilic cytoplasm (arrows). Note also the presence of numerous Alzheimer type II astrocytes with irregularly lobulated nuclei.

HEPATOLENTICULAR DEGENERATION

- This usually presents towards the end of the second decade, but patients with mutations that severely disrupt the ATP7B gene may develop cirrhosis and liver failure in early childhood.
- Neurologic disease develops only after adolescence in patients with less severe mutations, and can include dysarthria, dysphagia, dystonia and painful muscle spasms, coarse tremor, and dementia.
- Other findings are the presence of Kayser–Fleischer rings and azure lunulae, due to corneal and finger nail deposition of copper.
- Biochemical manifestations include low serum ceruloplasmin concentration and increased secretion of copper in the urine.
- The chelating agents D-penicillamine and triethylenetetramine dihydrochloride are used to reduce tissue deposition of copper. Zinc acetate is also administered, to induce hepatic metallothionein, which sequesters copper in a non-toxic form.

MACROSCOPIC AND MICROSCOPIC APPEARANCES

The putamen and caudate nucleus appear brown and shrunken, particularly the middle third of the putamen (**Fig. 22.24**). The putamen may be centrally cavitated. Histology of these nuclei reveals neuronal loss, scattered lipid- and pigment-laden macrophages, and many fibrillary astrocytes (**Fig. 22.25**). Alzheimer type II astrocytes (see

acquired hepatic encephalopathy above) are abundant. The globus pallidus, subthalamic nucleus, thalamus, and brain stem are often involved, but less severely.

A distinctive but not entirely specific feature (see acquired hepatic encephalopathy above) is the presence of Opalski cells, particularly in the globus pallidus. These are round cells with a small central nucleus and abundant, finely granular, deeply eosinophilic cytoplasm (**Fig. 22.26**). Expression of glial antigens has been noted in some studies. Other cells showing more varied degenerative nuclear and cytoplasmic changes are often found in the basal ganglia, thalamus, and zona reticulata of the substantia nigra (**Fig. 22.27**).

Other abnormalities that may be present include foci of spongy degeneration in the cerebral cortex and white matter.

HEREDITARY CERULOPLASMIN DEFICIENCY

This is included here because it shares some of the metabolic abnormalities of Wilson's disease. Unlike Wilson's disease, however, cirrhosis does not occur and the neuropathologic findings are not related to liver dysfunction.

Hereditary ceruloplasmin deficiency is an autosomal dominant disorder caused by mutation of the ceruloplasmin gene on chromosome 3q21-24. It usually presents in middle age with varying combinations of choreoathetosis, blepharospasm, ataxia, dementia, retinal degeneration, and diabetes mellitus. Kayser–Fleischer rings develop. Serum iron concentration is low and ferritin concentration is high.

Copper and iron accumulate in the liver, pancreas, and brain, particularly in the basal ganglia, red nucleus, and dentate nucleus, which show neuronal loss and gliosis.

Wilson's disease: distribution of abnormalities within the cerebrum

- lateral ventricle
- caudate nucleus
- pallidum
- thalamus
- third ventricle
- putamen (atrophy of the middle third of the putamen gives the nucleus a "Cupid's bow" appearance)

■ severely affected

☐ mildly affected

Fig. 22.24 Wilson's disease. Distribution of abnormalities within the cerebrum.

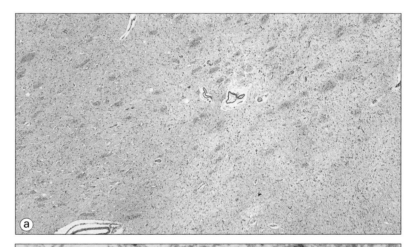
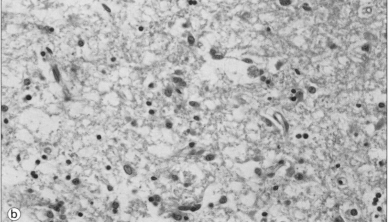

Fig. 22.25 Histology of the putamen in Wilson's disease. (a) and **(b)** show neuronal loss, pigment-laden macrophage, and gliosis of the putamen in a case of Wilson's disease.

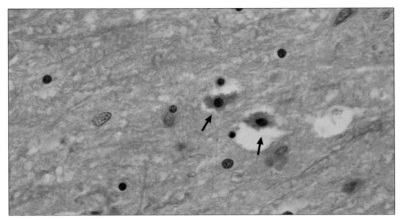

Fig. 22.26 Opalski cells. These cells have small darkly stained nuclei and granular eosinophilic cytoplasm (arrows).

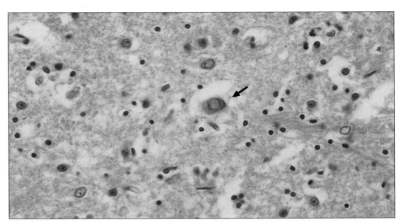

Fig. 22.27 Putamen in Wilson's disease. The arrow indicates a cell with the nuclear features of an Alzheimer type II astrocyte, but the granular eosinophilic cytoplasm of an Opalski cell.

REYE'S SYNDROME

Reye's syndrome is an acute non-inflammatory encephalopathy associated with fatty degeneration of the viscera, particularly the liver. It is predominantly a disease of children and is commonest in the USA and UK. Its incidence has declined in recent years.

MACROSCOPIC APPEARANCES

Macroscopic examination often shows only cerebral congestion and brain swelling. In some cases reduced cerebral perfusion may produce obvious watershed infarcts. More severe raised intracranial pressure can cause global brain ischemia, resulting in widespread cortical laminar necrosis and hemorrhagic infarcts in the cortex, basal ganglia, diencephalon, and brain stem.

MICROSCOPIC APPEARANCES

Histology reveals brain edema and ischemic changes of varying severity, but no inflammation. Electron microscopy has been reported to show features of cytotoxic edema with swollen astrocyte foot processes. In some reports mitochondrial abnormalities have been described, but these may be at least partly attributable to the effects of ischemia.

The liver shows diffuse microvesicular steatosis and, in fatal cases, usually includes large foci of coagulative necrosis. Like the brain, it is not inflamed.

REYE'S SYNDROME

- This is usually preceded by a flu-like or exanthematous viral illness.
- The encephalopathy and hepatocellular dysfunction manifest acutely with vomiting, anorexia, and lethargy, progressing to stupor, convulsions, and coma.
- There may be obvious hepatomegaly.
- Biochemical investigation reveals hyperammonemia, elevated serum transaminase concentrations, and varying degrees of hypoglycemia.
- Neurologic sequelae in survivors include spasticity, choreoathetosis, and mental retardation.

ETIOLOGY OF REYE'S SYNDROME

- Multiple precipitating factors have been implicated including viral infections (most often influenza, parainfluenza, or varicella), drugs, especially acetylsalicylic acid (aspirin), and aflatoxin (derived from peanuts and grain contaminated by the fungus *Aspergillus flavus*).
- The syndrome is thought to be due to injury to mitochondria, particularly in the liver, resulting in acute hyperammonemia as well as accumulation of other toxic metabolites. The severity of disease correlates well with the degree of hyperammonemia.
- The liver dysfunction and hyperammonemia probably contribute to the development of cerebral edema, but mitochondrial damage in endothelial cells and astrocytes may also play a role.

DIFFERENTIAL DIAGNOSIS OF REYE'S SYNDROME

Several inherited disorders of metabolism can simulate Reye's syndrome:

- Medium-chain acyl-CoA dehydrogenase (MCAD) deficiency, an autosomal recessive disorder, is probably most often misdiagnosed as Reye's syndrome. A codon 329 lysine-to-glutamic acid substitution in the MCAD gene has recently been identified as the cause of approximately 90% of mutant MCAD alleles in Caucasians.
- Other disorders that may cause Reye's syndrome-like attacks include deficiency of long-chain acyl-CoA dehydrogenase, primary carnitine deficiency, carnitine palmitoyl transferase I deficiency, 3-hydroxy-3-methylglutaryl-coenzyme A lyase deficiency, mitochondrial trifunctional protein α-subunit deficiency, and glutaric aciduria.

PORPHYRIA

Hepatic porphyrias		
All are autosomal dominant disorders		
Subtype	Enzyme defect	Locus
Acute intermittent	Phorphobilinogen deaminase	11q24
Coproporphyria	Coproporphyrinogen III oxidase	3q12
Variegate porphyria	Protoporphyrinogen oxidase	1q22
Δ-aminolevulinic acid dehydrate deficiency		9q34

Fig. 22.28 Enzyme defects and genetic loci in hepatic porphyrias.

The porphyrias are inherited defects of metabolism characterized by over-production and excretion of porphyrins or their precursors (**Fig. 22.28**):

- In the erythropoietic porphyrias, porphyrins accumulate in normo-blasts and red blood cells.
- In the hepatic porphyrias, porphyrins or their precursors are over-produced by the liver.

Only the hepatic porphyrias produce neurologic disease.

The symptoms and signs of hepatic porphyrias are summarized in **Fig. 22.29**. They rarely begin before puberty. Factors that may precipitate acute disease include:

- Certain drugs (e.g. barbiturates, sulphonamides, griseofulvin, meprobamate, phenytoin, succinimides, steroids).
- Infections.
- Starvation.
- Menstruation (some women experience attacks just before menstruation).

Fig. 22.29 Clinical features of hepatic porphyrias.

Clinical features of hepatic porphyrias				
Clinical features	Acute intermittent porphyria	Coproporphyria	Variegate porphyria	Δ-ALA dehydratase deficiency
CNS	Confusion Psychosis Delirium Focal deficits Seizures	*Rarely:* Psychosis Seizures	Confusion Psychosis Delirium Focal deficits Seizures	*Rarely:* Psychosis Seizures

PNS	Neuropathy -
	   motor>sensory
		Rarely:
		Neuropathy
			Neuropathy -
			   motor>sensory	

Autonomic	Abdominal pain Nausea and vomiting Ileus Urinary retention Tachycardia Hypertension Sweating	*Rarely:* Colic Constipation	Abdominal pain Nausea and vomiting Ileus Urinary retention Tachycardia Hypertension Sweating	*Rarely:* Colic Constipation
Skin	No photosensitivity	*Rarely:* Photosensitivity	Photosensitivity Hyperpigmentation	*Rarely:* Photosensitivity
Other	Normal fecal coproporphyrin excretion between attacks (unlike other hepatic porphyrias)	May present perinatally with hepatosplenomegaly, jaundice and hemolysis	Common form of porphyria in South Africa	May present perinatally with hepatosplenomegaly, jaundice and hemolysis

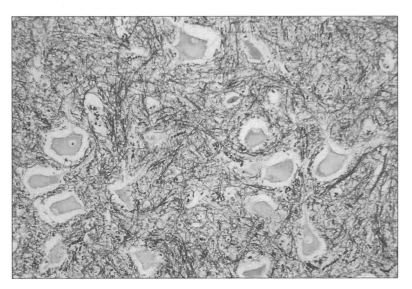

Fig. 22.30 Chromatolysis of lower motor neurons in porphyria.
Chromatolytic cervical anterior horn cells in the spinal cord from a patient with acute intermittent porphyria. (Luxol fast blue/cresyl violet)

MACROSCOPIC AND MICROSCOPIC APPEARANCES

The autonomic, somatomotor, and sensory disturbances are due to an axonal neuropathy. Motor neurons in the spinal cord and brain stem nuclei may appear chromatolytic (**Fig. 22.30**). Distal degeneration of posterior column fibers has been reported in some cases.

No structural lesions have been identified to account for the CNS disturbances. The hypertension of acute attacks may be complicated by the development of hemorrhages or infarcts.

PANCREATIC DISEASE

PANCREATIC ENCEPHALOPATHY
This is thought to be due to the release of vasoactive peptides, hormones, and enzymes in acute pancreatitis and is characterized by delirium, hallucinations, seizures, and multifocal neurologic deficits 2–5 days after the onset of acute pancreatitis.

MACROSCOPIC AND MICROSCOPIC APPEARANCES
The brain is swollen. Petechial hemorrhages may be present in the basal ganglia and periventricular regions.

Histology reveals pericapillary hemorrhages, edema, and reactive gliosis. There may also be foci of infarction.

CYSTIC FIBROSIS
The ataxia, impaired vibration and position sense, absence of tendon reflexes, weakness, and other neurologic disturbances that may occur in this condition are largely attributable to malabsorption of vitamin E and are discussed in chapter 21.

GASTROINTESTINAL DISORDERS

CELIAC DISEASE

ETIOLOGY OF CELIAC DISEASE

- Celiac disease is characterized by jejunal villous atrophy and circulating antibodies to gliadin and reticulin. It is thought to be due to interaction between HLA class II D gene products and gliadin proteins in gluten, possibly because of their homology with an intestinal virus.
- A specific HLA-DQ heterodimer is found in 95% of patients.
- The mucosal changes respond to treatment with a gluten-free diet.
- A small proportion (less than 10%) of patients with celiac disease develop neurologic complications. These respond to dietary manipulation only if is this is started soon after their onset.

CELIAC DISEASE

- Usually presents with malabsorption and diarrhea, but gastrointestinal symptoms may be mild or absent.
- Can cause a variety of CNS manifestations including progressive cerebellar ataxia, myoclonic epilepsy, complex partial seizures, which are occasionally associated with transient blindness, and dementia.
- Is accompanied by radiologically-demonstrable parieto-occipital calcifications in some cases.
- Rarely, results in myelopathy or peripheral neuropathy due to malabsorption and vitamin deficiency, particularly of vitamin E (see chapter 21).

MACROSCOPIC AND MICROSCOPIC APPEARANCES
The most consistent neuropathologic abnormality is cerebellar atrophy with loss of Purkinje cells, Bergmann cell gliosis, and a variable loss of granule cells (**Fig. 22.31**). There may be diffuse neuronal loss and gliosis in the dentate and inferior olivary nuclei (**Fig. 22.32**). Perivascular lymphocytic infiltrates have been described in the cerebellum in some cases, and probably represent an early phase of the cerebellar lesions in celiac disease. Focal neuronal loss and gliosis are occasionally seen in the basal ganglia, diencephalon, and brain stem nuclei. Little has been published on the neuropathologic findings associated with the cortical and subcortical parieto-occipital calcification that may occur in this disorder.

CROHN'S DISEASE AND ULCERATIVE COLITIS
Focal neurologic disturbances occasionally complicate these inflammatory bowel diseases. In some cases MRI has revealed white matter lesions thought to be due to vasculitis.

Neuropathologic data are lacking. Rarely, patients have developed cerebral infarcts or venous sinus thrombosis. As in other causes of malabsorption, neurologic disease may complicate nutritional deficiencies.

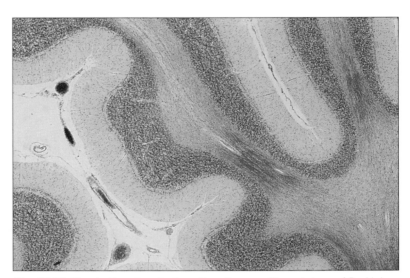

Fig. 22.31 Cerebellar atrophy in celiac disease. There is loss of Purkinje cells, Bergmann cell hyperplasia, and rarefaction of the white matter. (Luxol fast blue/cresyl violet)

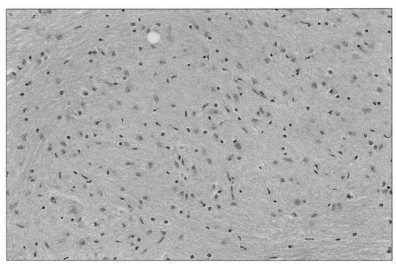

Fig. 22.32 Inferior olive in celiac disease. The olive is depleted of neurons and severely gliotic.

RENAL DISEASE

UREMIC ENCEPHALOPATHY

Patients with uremia may develop an encephalopathy in which apathy, fatigue, incoordination, and twitching are prominent features. The pathogenesis is poorly understood, but presumably involves the accumulation of neurotoxic products of metabolism that are normally excreted in the urine.

Nonspecific neuropathologic abnormalities have been described, including cerebral atrophy, gliosis, and foci of perivascular necrosis with accumulation of macrophages. Patients may also develop changes of hypertensive encephalopathy (see chapter 10).

DIALYSIS ENCEPHALOPATHY

Two distinct CNS disorders have been associated with dialysis for end-stage renal disease:
- Dialysis dysequilibrium syndrome.
- Dialysis dementia.

Dialysis dementia is thought to be due to aluminum toxicity (see chapter 25). Dialysis dysequilibrium syndrome is more commonly caused by hemodialysis than peritoneal dialysis. It consists of acute headache, nausea, muscle cramps, asterixis, myoclonus, and seizures, and is believed to be due to cerebral water intoxication caused by hypo-osmolality.

MULTIFOCAL NECROTIZING LEUKOENCEPHALOPATHY (MNL)

This is characterized by the development of multiple, usually microscopic, foci of necrosis with calcification, predominantly in the white matter. The basis pontis is often affected and the condition used to be known as focal pontine leukoencephalopathy. The pathogenesis of MNL is not known, but it occurs predominantly in immunosuppressed patients. The most commonly associated diseases are AIDS and leukemia. X-irradiation, amphotericin B, methotrexate, and various other cytotoxic drugs have been implicated in some cases (see chapter 25).

MNL has no consistent clinical correlate and is often diagnosed only at necropsy. Most patients have complex neurologic abnormalities and have been critically ill for extended periods of time.

MACROSCOPIC AND MICROSCOPIC APPEARANCES

The brain usually appears macroscopically normal. Ill-defined foci of chalky white discoloration may be visible in the pons or cerebral white matter (**Fig. 22.33**). Rarely, the pons is diffusely swollen, simulating a mass lesion.

In general, the likelihood of identifying MNL depends on how extensively the brain is examined histologically. Microscopically, the lesions consist of well-demarcated areas of spongy vacuolation (**Fig. 22.34**) and loss of myelin staining, containing swollen fragmented axons (**Fig. 22.35**),

which are often calcified, and scattered macrophages. The lesions are most consistently found in the basis pontis, especially in the transverse pontine fibers. There are also extrapontine foci in some patients.

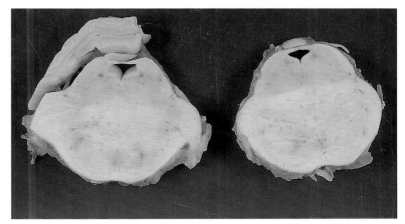

Fig. 22.33 Multifocal necrotizing leukoencephalopathy. The base of the pons is slightly swollen and includes an ill-defined central zone of chalky white discoloration.

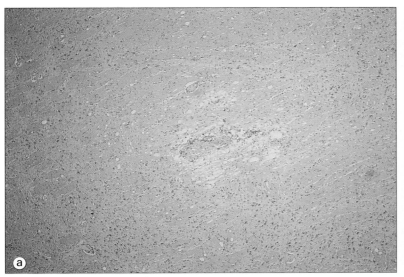
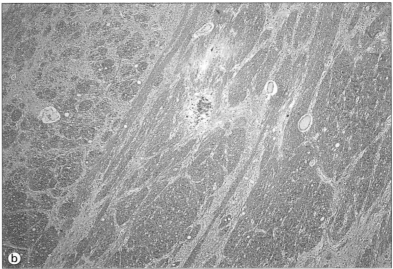

Fig. 22.34 MNL (a, b). Foci of spongy vacuolation with calcification in the base of the pons in MNL. (Luxol fast blue/cresyl violet)

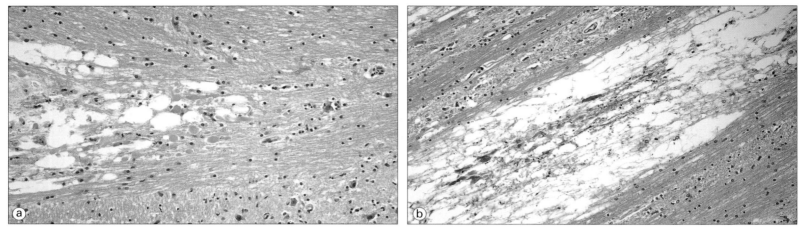

Fig. 22.35 MNL. Foci of necrotizing leukoencephalopathy with swollen axons. **(a)** This lession is infiltrated by macrophages. **(b)** The swollen axons tend to calcify, and become deeply hematoxyphilic.

REFERENCES

Anders KH *et al.* (1993) Multifocal necrotizing leukoencephalopathy with pontine predilection in immunosuppressed patients: A clinicopathologic review of 16 cases. *Hum Pathol* **24**: 897–904.

Harper C, Butterworth R (1997) Nutritional and metabolic disorders. In DI Graham, PL Lantos (eds) *Greenfield's Neuropathology. Sixth edition.* pp. 601–655. London: Arnold.

Kierbutz K, Feigin A (1994) Neurologic complications of vitamin and mineral disorders. In Robert J Joynt (ed.) *Clinical Neurology. Volume 4.* pp.1–19. Philadelphia: Lippincott.

Norenberg MD, Bruce–Gregorios J (1991) Nervous system manifestations of systemic disease. In RL Davis, DM Robertson (eds) *Textbook of Neuropathology. Second edition.* pp. 461–534. Baltimore: Williams & Wilkins.

Pincus JH, Cohan SL, Glaser GH. *Neurologic Complications of Internal Disease. Volume 4.* pp. 1–76.

Schochet SS, Nelson J (1991) Exogenous toxic-metabolic diseases including vitamin deficiency. In RL Davis, DM Robertson (eds) *Textbook of Neuropathology. Second edition.* pp. 428–560. Baltimore: Williams & Wilkins.

Tanzi RE *et al.* (1993) The Wilson disease gene is a copper transporting ATPase with homology to the Menkes disease gene. *Nature Genet* **5**: 344–350.

Verbalis JG, Martinez AJ, Drutarosky MD (1991) Neurological and neuropathological sequelae of correction of chronic hyponatremia. *Kidney Int* **39**: 1274–1282.

23 Lysosomal and peroxisomal disorders

This chapter deals first with the lysosomal disorders that principally affect gray matter and then with those involving white matter (leukodystrophies). Lastly the chapter covers the peroxisomal disorders, which include adrenoleukodystrophy. Other leukodystrophies are considered in chapter 5. Chapter 5 also covers comparative aspects of all of the leukodystrophies, and an approach to their differential diagnosis.

LYSOSOMAL DISORDERS

A huge, complex and still increasing array of inborn errors of metabolism is now known to be associated with defective lysosomal activity and abnormal lysosomal storage. Multiple genes affect the synthesis, stability, and activity of lysosomal enzymes and their essential cofactors. Defects of any of these may be responsible for vacuolation and storage of abnormal material in neurons and other cells.

G_{M2} GANGLIOSIDOSIS

In this group of disorders there is an excess of normal ganglioside in the brain, and occasionally in other organs. Many variants are known and all show autosomal recessive inheritance. They are diagnosed by enzyme assay using leukocytes, serum or fibroblasts, or by histochemistry on frozen sections of a suction rectal biopsy.

MACROSCOPIC APPEARANCES

In the infantile forms, the brain size varies from excessively small to overlarge, but gyral atrophy and loss of white matter are evident. Changes are much less dramatic in the juvenile and adult variants, and amount at most to mild atrophy.

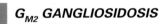

G_{M2} GANGLIOSIDOSIS

Infantile G_{M2} gangliosidosis (Tay–Sachs disease)
- Onset: psychomotor retardation evident by 4 months. Features during the first year include progressive retardation, hypotonia, spasticity, blindness, and cherry red spots in the macula.
- Course: cachexia and decerebration by 3 years of age and death at around 5 years of age.

Late-infantile G_{M2} gangliosidosis
- Onset: abnormal startle and regression from 18 months of age.
- Course: appearance of cherry red spots in the macula, epilepsy.

Juvenile G_{M2} gangliosidosis
- Onset: slowly progressive dementia commencing at 4–6 years of age.
- Course: spasticity, epilepsy, and death within 10 years.

Adult G_{M2} gangliosidosis
- Slowly progressive dementia, which may begin in childhood.
- Course: ataxia, dystonia, choreoathetosis, peripheral neuropathy, and psychosis.

ETIOLOGY OF OF G_{M2} GANGLIOSIDOSIS

Infantile Tay–Sachs disease, type B
- Enzyme deficiency: lack of hexosaminidase A.
- Cause: faulty synthesis of α-subunit.

Infantile Tay–Sachs disease, type O (Sandhoff disease)
- Enzyme deficiency: lack of both hexosaminidases A and B.
- Cause: faulty synthesis of β-subunit.

Infantile Tay–Sachs disease, type AB
- Enzymes present.
- Cause: lack of activator protein.

Late-infantile, juvenile, and adult forms of G_{M2} gangliosidosis, type B
- Enzyme deficiency: lack of hexosaminidase A.
- Cause: mutations in α-subunit.

Late-infantile, juvenile, and adult forms of G_{M2} gangliosidosis, type B1
- Enzyme deficiency: low hexosaminidase A.
- Cause: defective α-subunit.

MICROSCOPIC APPEARANCES

In the older patients neuronal storage of excessive lipofuscin is confined to the basal ganglia, brain stem, cerebellum, and spinal cord. In infantile G_{M2} gangliosidosis, ballooned neurons are found throughout the CNS and the peripheral nervous system. The foamy nerve cells stain strongly with luxol fast blue and Sudan black, and in frozen sections the soluble ganglioside is periodic acid–Schiff (PAS)-positive (**Fig. 23.1**). Microglia are also PAS-positive, retaining stored material even in paraffin sections. Ultrastructural studies show membranous cytoplasmic bodies (MCBs) within neuronal somata.

G_{M1} GANGLIOSIDOSIS

In this autosomal recessive disorder approximately four times the normal amount of G_{M1} ganglioside accumulates in the brain. As with other lysosomal diseases, there are several subtypes with different clinical presentations. They are diagnosed by enzyme assay using leukocytes or fibroblasts, or frozen sections of a suction rectal biopsy. In blood films there are lymphocytes with vacuoles in type 1 G_{M1} gangliosidosis only.

MACROSCOPIC AND MICROSCOPIC APPEARANCES

Mild gyral atrophy is present in all three subtypes (**Fig. 23.2a,b**). Ballooned neurons with staining characteristics virtually identical to those seen in G_{M2} gangliosidosis are widespread in the cerebrum (**Fig. 23.2c,d**), brain stem and spinal cord, and in autonomic ganglia (in subtypes 1 and 2).

ETIOLOGY OF G_{M1} GANGLIOSIDOSIS

- The accumulation of G_{M1} ganglioside is due to deficiency of β-galactosidase activity.
- Functional defects occur as a result of mutations of the β-galactosidase gene on chromosome 3, or of its protector protein gene on chromosome 20.

Ballooned neurons are confined to the striatum and pallidum in the adult form. Ultrastructural studies show membranous cytoplasmic bodies.

Visceral pathology

In type 1 G_{M1} gangliosidosis only, highly water-soluble oligosaccharide storage produces vacuolation of hepatocytes, liver, spleen and lymph node histiocytes, renal glomerular epithelium, and endothelial cells.

G_{M1} GANGLIOSIDOSIS

Type 1: Infantile G_{M1} gangliosidosis
- Onset: failure to thrive evident from birth, hepatosplenomegaly, bony changes and dysmorphism similar to those of mucopolysaccharidoses, cardiomyopathy, peripheral edema.
- Course: psychomotor retardation and epilepsy, cherry red macular spots, death before 2 years of age.

Type 2: Late-infantile and juvenile G_{M1} gangliosidosis
- Onset: at 1–5 years of age with progressive psychomotor retardation, epilepsy, spastic tetraplegia, cerebellar signs, no visceral changes, and bony changes confined to the vertebrae.
- Course: decerebrate rigidity and death at 3–10 years of age.

Type 3: Adult G_{M1} gangliosidosis
- Starting during the first decade, patients develop slowly progressive weakness, ataxia, extrapyramidal signs, myoclonus, dysarthria. There are no bony changes.

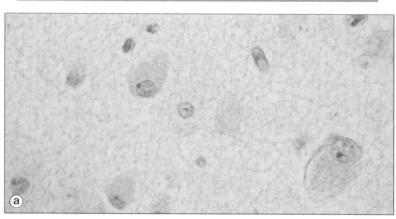

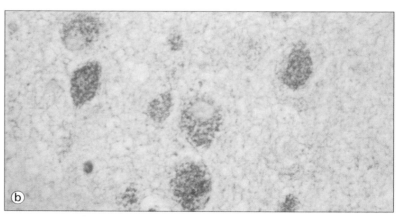

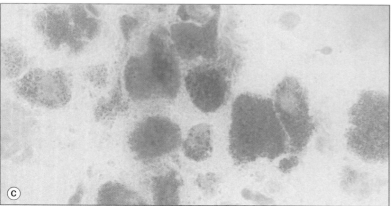

Fig. 23.1 G_{M2} gangliosidosis. (a) Ballooned cortical neurons with foamy cytoplasm and marginated nuclei are negative with PAS in routine paraffin sections. **(b)** These neurons are, however, strongly stained with luxol fast blue. **(c)** The stored ganglioside can be demonstrated in cryostat sections stained with PAS, in this example protected by celloidinization prior to staining.

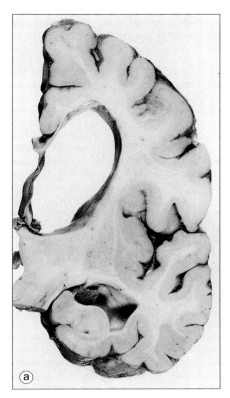

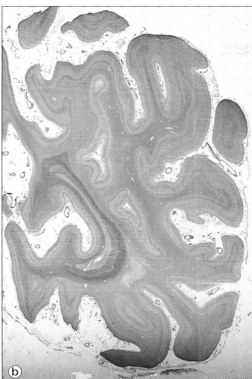

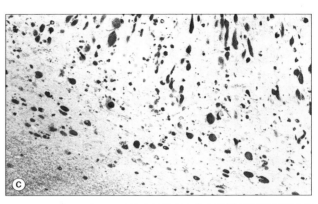

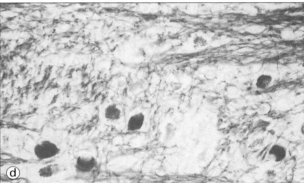

Fig. 23.2 GM₁ gangliosidosis. (a) Coronal section of cerebral hemisphere from a patient with the type 2 (late-infantile and juvenile) form of G_{M1} gangliosidosis, who died aged 10 years. There is mild cortical atrophy and ventricular dilatation. **(b)** Cortical atrophy and poverty of myelination are more evident in a stained section from the occipital lobe. (Luxol fast blue/cresyl violet) **(c)** In the cerebral cortex there is extensive neuronal and glial storage. The granular storage bodies fill the neuronal cytoplasm and distend the proximal dendrites. Note also the myelin pallor. (Luxol fast blue/cresyl violet) **(d)** Heavy neuronal storage is also present in the pontine nuclei.

BATTEN'S DISEASE OR NEURONAL CEROID LIPOFUSCINOSIS (NCL OR CLN)

This group of disorders has a confusing set of eponyms (**Fig. 23.3**), classification is further complicated by newer terminology related to the molecular genetics of the disorders. The classification used here combines clinical presentation, age of onset, pathology, and electrophysiology. The diagnosis is most readily obtainable for all forms except Kufs'

**Fig. 23.3
Classification scheme
for Batten's disease.**

Classification scheme for Batten's disease	
Type	Synonym
Infantile (CLN1)	Hagberg–Santavuori, Infantile NCL
Late–infantile (CLN2)	Bielschowsky–Jansky, Late–infantile NCL
Juvenile (CLN3)	Batten, Batten–Mayou, Spielmeyer–Vogt, Juvenile NCL
Adult (CLN4)	Kufs'
Variant forms of late–infantile (CLN5 and CLN6)	
Early juvenile	Lake–Cavanagh
Juvenile with granular osmiophilic deposits (GRODs)	
Congenital	Norman–Wood

ETIOLOGY OF BATTEN'S DISEASE

- All subtypes show recessive inheritance except for some families with an autosomal dominant form of Kufs' disease (CLN4).
- All subtypes are accompanied by increased tissue levels of dolichol and dolichyl pyrophosphoryl oligosaccharides and affected cells contain saposins A and D.

Infantile (CLN1)
- Gene locus: 1p32, encoding palmitoyl-protein thioesterase.
- Comment: storage of glycosphingolipids.

Classic late–infantile (CLN2)
- Gene locus: 11p15.
- Comment: high level of the proteolipid subunit C of mitochondrial ATP synthase.

Juvenile (CLN3)
- Gene locus: 16p12.1-11.2.
- Comment: high level of the proteolipid subunit C of mitochondrial ATP synthase.

Adult (CLN4)
- Gene locus: unknown.
- Comment: some patients withe this diagnosis may represent late onset forms of juvenile Batten's disease (CLN3).

Finnish variant late–infantile (CLN5)
- Gene locus: 13q21.1-32.

Indian variant late–infantile (CLN6)
- Gene locus: 15q21-23.

disease by cutting cryostat sections of a suction rectal biopsy to examine neurons and other cell types (i.e. smooth muscle, histiocytes, vascular endothelium).

MACROSCOPIC APPEARANCES

Cerebral atrophy is always present, but is at its most severe in the infantile form (**Fig. 23.4a–c**), manifesting as a walnut brain with shriveled cortex and rubbery white matter encased in a markedly thickened skull. Atrophy may also be considerable in infantile and juvenile Batten's disease, and increases with the length of survival. In adult cases (Kufs' disease), atrophy is more limited, and predominantly in frontal and cerebellar regions.

MICROSCOPIC APPEARANCES

The stored material, which is insoluble and therefore readily detectable in paraffin as well as frozen sections, is widespread in the nervous system and in many other tissues. Its tinctorial properties vary slightly

BATTEN'S DISEASE

Infantile (CLN1)
- Onset: at 8–18 months with rapidly progressive psychomotor retardation, irritability, visual failure, hypotonia, ataxia.
- Course: myoclonic jerks, hyperkinesia, microcephaly, flat electroencephalogram (EEG) by 3 years of age, and death at 3–10 years of age.

Late–infantile (CLN2)
- Onset: at 18 months–4 years of age with epilepsy.
- Course: regression, visual failure, spastic tetraplegia, bulbar paresis, characteristic EEG with large polyspike response to low rates of photic stimulation, attenuated electroretinogram (ERG) and enlarged visual evoked potential (VEP); death at 4–10 years of age.

Juvenile (CLN3)
- Onset: at 4–9 years of age with deteriorating vision and pigmentary retinopathy.
- Course: dementia, epilepsy, gait disorder, and dysarthria; hallucinations in older patients; attenuation of ERG and VEPs; death at 15–30 years of age.

Adult (CLN4)
- Onset: at about 30 years of age — either type A with progressive myoclonic epilepsy, dementia, and ataxia, or type B with behavioral disturbance, dementia, motor disorder, and facial hyperkinesia.
- Course: may survive for several decades.

Finnish variant late–infantile (CLN5)
- Onset: at 4–7 years of age with clumsiness, retardation, and visual failure.
- Course: ataxia, myoclonic epilepsy, and cerebellar signs. Electrophysiology similar to that of CLN2; death by early 20s.

Early juvenile
- Onset and course: similar to those of CLN5, but a wider age range of onset.

Juvenile with GROD
- Onset and course: similar to those of CLN3 despite differing pathology.

between the various subtypes of the disease (**see Fig. 23.5**). In infantile Batten's disease, storage is evident in CNS neurons, astrocytes, and macrophages, and in autonomic ganglia from an early stage, but neuronal loss is relatively subtle to begin with, becoming obvious after two years. By four years of age virtually all cortical neurons have disappeared, and there is dense astrocytic gliosis, and myelin loss. Some astrocytes contain storage material.

In late–infantile and juvenile Batten's disease (**Fig. 23.4d,e**) neuronal loss is less severe and myelin loss, if present, is slight. The rarity of adult cases and the accumulation of lipofuscin during normal ageing have impeded the formulation of a consensus view of the histology of Kufs' disease, although widespread storage is the principal element (**Fig. 23.4f,g**).

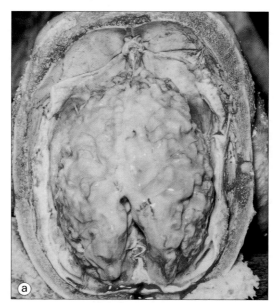

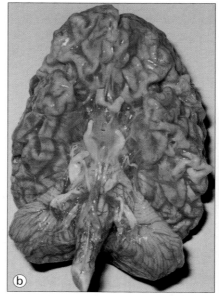
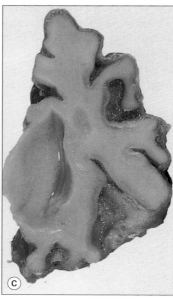

Fig. 23.4 Batten's disease. (a) Infantile Batten's disease in a boy aged 9 years. The extremely atrophied brain (300 g weight) is covered by gelatinous leptomeninges and markedly thickened dura and surrounded by greatly thickened calvaria. **(b)** Viewed from below, the cerebral convolutional atrophy is marked and widespread, but the cerebellum and brain stem are relatively spared. **(c)** A coronal slice of frontal lobe shows a very thin cortical ribbon and tough rubbery white matter. **(d)** Juvenile Batten's disease. Neuronal storage material reacts strongly with Sudan black in the cortex. **(e)** Juvenile Batten's disease. Neuronal storage material reacts strongly with PAS in hippocampal pyramidal cells. **(f)** Kufs' disease. In the rare adult form of NCL there is similar widespread neuronal storage material, which stains strongly with PAS. **(g)** Neuronal storage material in Kufs' disease also reacts strongly with PAS. **(h)** Blood film of a patient with juvenile Batten's disease showing a vacuolated

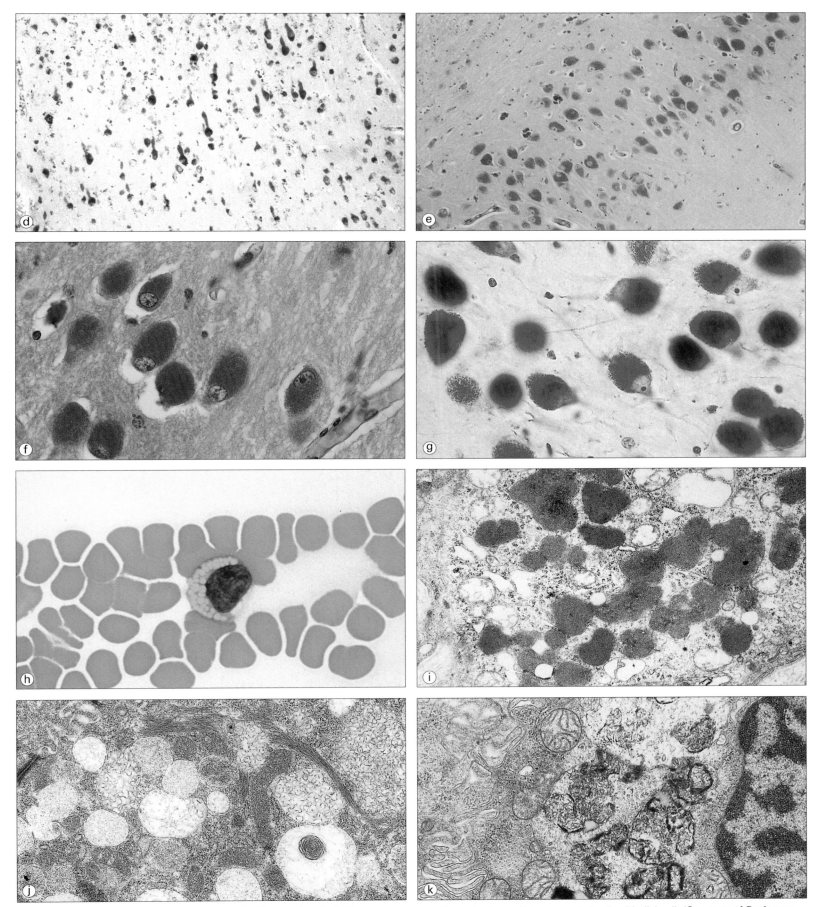

lymphocyte with characteristic large uniform 'bold' vacuoles. A similar appearance is seen in GM$_1$ gangliosidosis. (Courtesy of Professor B. Lake, Great Ormond Street Hospital, London). **(i)** Ultrastructural appearance in infantile Batten's disease showing granular osmiophilic deposits in a neuron. (Courtesy of Professor B. Lake, Great Ormond Street Hospital, London). **(j)** Ultrastructural appearance in late–infantile Batten's disease showing curvilinear bodies within a sweat gland epithelial cell. (Courtesy of Professor B. Lake, Great Ormond Street Hospital, London). **(k)** Ultrastructural appearance in juvenile Batten's disease (similar in early juvenile and Finnish variant late–infantile Batten's disease) showing a sweat gland epithelial cell containing mixed curvilinear and fingerprint bodies. (Courtesy of Professor B. Lake, Great Ormond Street Hospital, London)

Histochemical and ultrastructural abnormalities in Batten's disease			
Type	Staining of CNS neuronal storage material	Histology of other tissues	Ultrastructure
Infantile	Sudan black, PAS, silvery autofluorescence (UV)	Storage material is seen in autonomic neurons, macrophages in spleen/lymph nodes, smooth/cardiac/skeletal muscle, renal glomeruli and distal tubules, vascular endothelium, testis, thyroid, sweat gland epithelium, and Kupffer cells	Globular osmiophilic deposits with a granular matrix (Fig. 23.4j) either single, or aggregated and surrounded by a unit membrane, and known as 'granular osmiophilic deposits'(GRODs) or 'Finnish snowballs.'
Late–infantile	Luxol fast blue, Sudan black, PAS, bright yellow autofluorescence (UV)	Tissue involvement as above, but staining differs: PAS pale, Sudan black staining gray	Cytoplasmic curvilinear bodies (Fig. 23.4k)
Juvenile	Luxol fast blue, Sudan black, PAS, yellow autofluorescence (UV)	Tissue involvement and staining are similar to late–infantile. Lymphocytes with multiple clear cytoplasmic vacuoles are present in blood films	Gastrointestinal neurons contain only fingerprint bodies, while CNS neurons show a mixture of fingerprint and curvilinear inclusions as do other tissues and lymphocytes (Fig. 23.4). However, in skeletal muscle there are only rare rectilinear profiles
Adult	Luxol fast blue, Sudan black, PAS, yellow autofluorescence (UV)	Gastrointestinal neurons, Kupffer cells, hepatocytes, splenic macrophages, muscle, pancreas and kidney may show storage	Curvilinear bodies, fingerprint bodies, rectilinear profiles, and GRODs have all been reported

Fig. 23.5 Histochemical and ultrastructural abnormalities in Batten's disease.

NIEMANN–PICK DISEASE

This comprises autosomal recessive disorders that show common clinical features, but a diversity of underlying biochemical mechanisms. There are two main groups:
- sphingomyelinase deficient
- not sphingomyelinase deficient (**Fig. 23.6**)

This classification incorporates the earlier four alphabetically defined groups.

MACROSCOPIC AND MICROSCOPIC APPEARANCES

Niemann–Pick disease group I: While hepatosplenomegaly is striking in both types, CNS abnormalities are not found in type B. In type A, cerebral atrophy may be slight or absent. Microscopically (**Fig. 23.7**), there is generalized enlargement of neurons and glia, and storage extends to white matter, which is demyelinated and gliotic. Gastrointestinal tract neuronal plexuses are also affected. Sudananophilic foamy histiocytes containing cholesterol esters, but not

ballooned neurons, are numerous in the globus pallidus, substantia nigra, and dentate nucleus. Niemann–Pick cells (see Fig. 23.7b) are present throughout the mononuclear phagocyte system, and can fill the alveolar spaces of the lungs. The lymphocytes of patients with type A

ETIOLOGY OF NIEMANN–PICK DISEASE

- Group I patients have a profound deficiency of lysosomal sphingomyelinase activity. The gene for lysosomal sphingomyelinase is located at 11p15.1-15.4.
- A defect in cholesterol esterification has been demonstrated in cells cultured from group II patients; the cells accumulate excessive free cholesterol in response to a lipoprotein load.
- The defect in type C and D forms of disease has been linked to chromosome 18q11-12.

NIEMANN–PICK DISEASE

Group I
- The onset of type A is in the first year, with hepatosplenomegaly and failure to thrive, followed by mental retardation. Other common findings are cherry red macular spots and diffuse pulmonary infiltration. Survival is uncommon beyond four years of age, but in longer survivors neurologic symptoms of dementia, spasticity, and epilepsy may be delayed beyond 5 years of age.
- The chronic non-neuropathic visceral form (type B) presents with hepatosplenomegaly in later childhood or adulthood and often has a benign course.

Group II
- Type C has a variable presentation, and features include congenital ascites, neonatal failure to thrive, hepatosplenomegaly, and prolonged neonatal obstructive jaundice, insidious onset of dementia and ataxia in childhood, various forms of psychosis in adolescence and early adulthood and dystonia and loss of vertical eye movements in early adulthood or middle age.

Niemann–Pick disease contain cytoplasmic vacuoles, which are small and discrete. In contrast, in patients with type B there is minimal or no lymphocytic vacuolation. Bone marrow aspirates show collections of Niemann–Pick cells in patients with type A and in younger patients with type B. In older patients with type B disease there are fewer foamy Niemann–Pick cells, and more prominent 'sea-blue histiocytes,' in which the cytoplasm is filled with small granules that stain intensely blue with the Giemsa or Wright histochemical method.

Sphingomyelin and cholesterol are extracted during routine processing, but the lipid deposits can be detected in frozen or cryostat sections using the ferric–hematoxylin method, while Sudan black stains the cells and deposits, which in polarized light show red birefringence.

Ultrastructurally, the neuronal inclusions are membrane-bound vacuoles containing irregular, loosely packed osmiophilic lamellae.

Niemann–Pick disease group II: Despite the diverse chemical abnormalities, the morphologic features are fairly uniform. Cerebral atrophy and sclerotic firm white matter are evident. Microscopically, widespread neuronal ballooning is particularly noticeable in the basal ganglia, brain stem, and spinal cord. In addition to finely granular storage material, neuroaxonal dystrophy and Alzheimer-type neurofibrillary tangles are also observed (**Fig. 23.8**). Neurons, including those of the gastrointestinal tract, store a substance that is lost during routine processing. In frozen sections the substance is only weakly sudanophilic, but includes phospholipid and a PAS-positive sugar-containing compound.

The numerous foam cells present in the spleen have similar staining characteristics to those of the neurons.

Ultrastructurally, the neuronal storage material consists of membrane-bound polymorphous cytoplasmic bodies that contain loosely packed lamellae. These are concentric in some planes of section. Dense osmiophilic inclusions are also commonly found.

Classification of Niemann–Pick disease

Group I: sphingomyelinase deficient	Group II: not sphingomyelinase deficient
Type A: neurovisceral (infantile, juvenile, and adult)	Types C and D (Nova Scotia): neurovisceral
Type B: visceral only (infantile, juvenile, and adult)	Possible pure visceral form

Fig. 23.6. Classification of Niemann–Pick disease.

GAUCHER'S DISEASE
This is an autosomal recessive disorder and occurs in three main forms. Types 2 and 3 are neuronopathic.

MACROSCOPIC AND MICROSCOPIC APPEARANCES
The characteristic Gaucher cell (**Fig. 23.9**) is present in many tissues, is large (20–100 μm), and has one or more nuclei. Its cytoplasm is filled

ETIOLOGY OF GAUCHER'S DISEASE

- Deficient activity of glucocerebrosidase produces a marked increase in tissue glucocerebroside, especially in the spleen, where its concentration is 100-times normal.
- In some patients, deficiency of a cofactor, saposin C, is responsible for Gaucher's disease.
- The gene for glucocerebrosidase is located at 1q21.
- Prosaposin, the precursor of saposin C, is encoded on chromosome 10 at q21.

GAUCHER'S DISEASE

- Type 1: chronic non-neuronopathic Gaucher's disease can begin at any age from birth to adulthood. An early onset is associated with massive splenomegaly and some hepatomegaly.
  In older children and adolescents, bone pain and fractures of the femur are common, and vertebral collapse may lead to spinal cord compression.
- Type 2: acute neuronopathic Gaucher's disease begins in infancy with hepatosplenomegaly, opisthotonos, and failure to thrive. Delayed motor milestones, cranial nerve palsies, and extrapyramidal tract involvement follow. Death, usually from pulmonary infection, occurs before two years of age.
- Type 3: (Norrbottnian) subacute or juvenile neuronopathic Gaucher's disease presents with hypersplenism and intellectual deterioration at around five years of age. This is followed by myoclonic epilepsy, spasticity, and the development of bone necrosis and fractures.

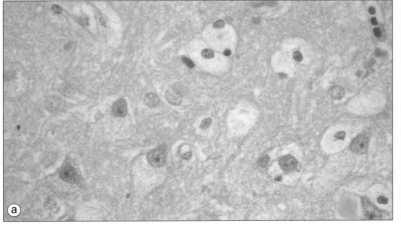
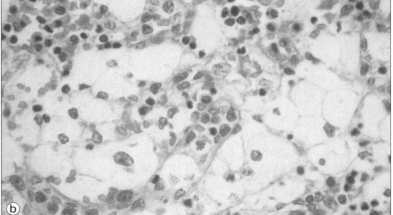

Fig. 23.7 Niemann–Pick disease type A. (a) Prominent neuronal and glial ballooning are seen in the cortex. **(b)** Large mulberry-like storage cells filling the red pulp of the spleen contain a single nucleus, uniform vacuoles, and occasional red cell debris.

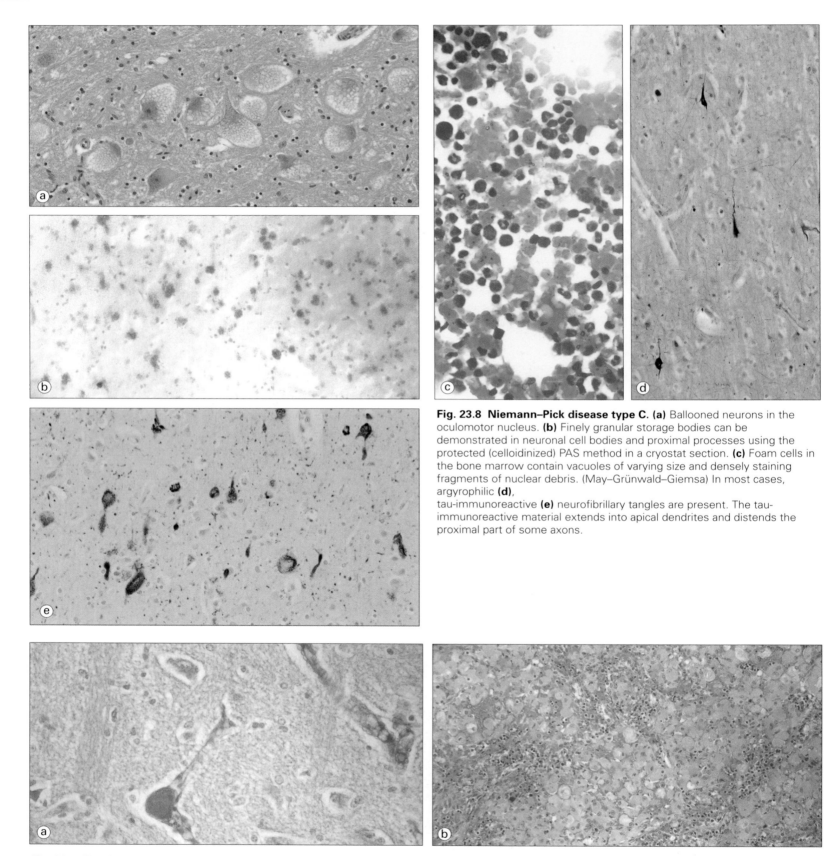

Fig. 23.8 Niemann–Pick disease type C. (a) Ballooned neurons in the oculomotor nucleus. **(b)** Finely granular storage bodies can be demonstrated in neuronal cell bodies and proximal processes using the protected (celloidinized) PAS method in a cryostat section. **(c)** Foam cells in the bone marrow contain vacuoles of varying size and densely staining fragments of nuclear debris. (May–Grünwald–Giemsa) In most cases, argyrophilic **(d)**,
tau-immunoreactive **(e)** neurofibrillary tangles are present. The tau-immunoreactive material extends into apical dendrites and distends the proximal part of some axons.

Fig. 23.9 Gaucher's disease. (a) A PAS-positive Gaucher cell close to a capillary in the striatum.
(b) Groups of Gaucher cells are present in the spleen. The cytoplasm of these cells may have a vacuolar or fibrillar appearance.

with finely or coarsely fibrillar material. The appearance of the cytoplasm in histologic sections has been likened to crumpled tissue paper. Gaucher cells are PAS-positive, negative with lipid stains, and sometimes contain iron pigment. Ultrastructurally, the fibrillar inclusions are membrane-bound elongated bodies containing a tubular arrangement of the glucocerebroside.

Gaucher cells are numerous in the spleen, lymph nodes, bone marrow and hepatic sinusoids (hepatocytes themselves being spared), pancreas, thyroid, and lung.

Findings in the neuronopathic forms of Gaucher's disease (types 2 and 3) are similar. Macroscopic changes are minimal. Perivascular clusters of Gaucher cells are present in the subcortical white matter and cerebellum, and are sometimes associated with myelin loss and gliosis. Gaucher cells are also prominent in the thalamus, hippocampus, and pons. Neuronal loss occurs in the cortex, cerebellum, and brain stem, and may be particularly severe in the cochlear nuclei, olives, and vestibular and cuneate nuclei. Neuronal storage is not detected by light microscopy.

In some cases of the non-neuronopathic form (type 1), perivascular Gaucher cells can be found in the brain, cord, and pituitary.

MUCOPOLYSACCHARIDOSES (MPSs)

The classification of the MPSs incorporates historic eponyms, specific enzyme defects, and the analysis of urinary excretion of glycosaminoglycans (GAGs) (**Fig. 23.10**). Inheritance is autosomal recessive, except for MPS II (Hunter's syndrome), which is transmitted as an X-linked recessive trait.

MACROSCOPIC AND MICROSCOPIC APPEARANCES

There is intralysosomal storage of mucopolysaccharides within most types of cell and there may also be storage of gangliosides within neurons. The mucopolysaccharides are not protein-bound and are extremely water-soluble, and therefore not demonstrable in fixed tissue.

Macroscopic appearances are usually nondescript, but there may be considerable widening of the skull, dural and meningeal thickening, and sometimes cerebral atrophy. Hydrocephalus may occur (see chapter 4). A characteristic finding in sectioned brain is the presence of small perivascular cavities in the white matter (**Fig. 23.11a–d**), which are shown microscopically to contain foamy macrophages.

Neuronal storage (**Fig. 23.11e–g**) is very variable, but usually parallels the severity of mental retardation. The stored material in neurons is ganglioside, and therefore PAS-positive, sudanophilic, and strongly positive with luxol fast blue. However, neuronal storage of mucopolysaccharide cannot be demonstrated.

In other tissues, cryostat sections of snap-frozen tissue are required to demonstrate stored mucopolysaccharide in vacuolated cells by a suitable metachromatic method, but this is hampered by the tendency of the material to diffuse into surrounding tissue. Storage is especially marked

MUCOPOLYSACCHARIDOSES

- There are many clinical similarities between the different types of MPS, including coarse features, mild to severe skeletal changes (occasionally causing cord compression), hepatosplenomegaly, and mild to severe mental retardation.
- Carpal tunnel syndrome, cardiomyopathy, and aortic and mitral valve incompetence are common.
- Corneal clouding is a feature of MPS I, IV, VI, and VII.
- Patients with MPS 1S, IV, VI have normal intelligence, while those with MPS III rarely show skeletal dysplasia but develop severe mental retardation and behavioral disturbances.

Fig. 23.10 Classification and etiology of the mucopolysaccharidoses.

Classification and etiology of the mucopolysaccharidoses

Type	Eponym	Subtype	Urinary GAGs	Enzyme defect	Gene location
MPS IH	Hurler		Dermatan sulfate	α-L-iduronidase	4p16.3
1S	Scheie			α-L-iduronidase	
1H/S	Hurler–Scheie			α-L-iduronidase	
MPS II	Hunter	A Severe	Dermatan sulfate	Iduronate sulfatase	Xq27-28
	Hunter	B Mild		Iduronate sulfatase	
MPS III	Sanfilippo	A	Heparan sulfate	Heparan N-sulfatase	
	Sanfilippo	B	Heparan sulfate	α-N-acetyl-glucosaminidase	
	Sanfilippo	C	Heparan sulfate	Acetyl CoA:α-glucosaminide acetyl transferase	
	Sanfilippo	D	Heparan sulfate	N-acetylglucosamine-6-sulfatase	12q14
MPS IV	Morquio	A Severe		galactose-6-sulfatase	16q24
	Morquio	B Mild		β-galactosidase	
MPS VI	Maroteaux–Lamy	A Severe	Dermatan sulfate	N-acetylgalactosamine-4-sulfatase	5q13-q14
	Maroteaux–Lamy	B Mild	Dermatan sulfate	N-acetylgalactosamine-4-sulfatase	
MPS VII	Sly		Dermatan and heparan sulfate	β-glucuronidase	7q21.1-q22

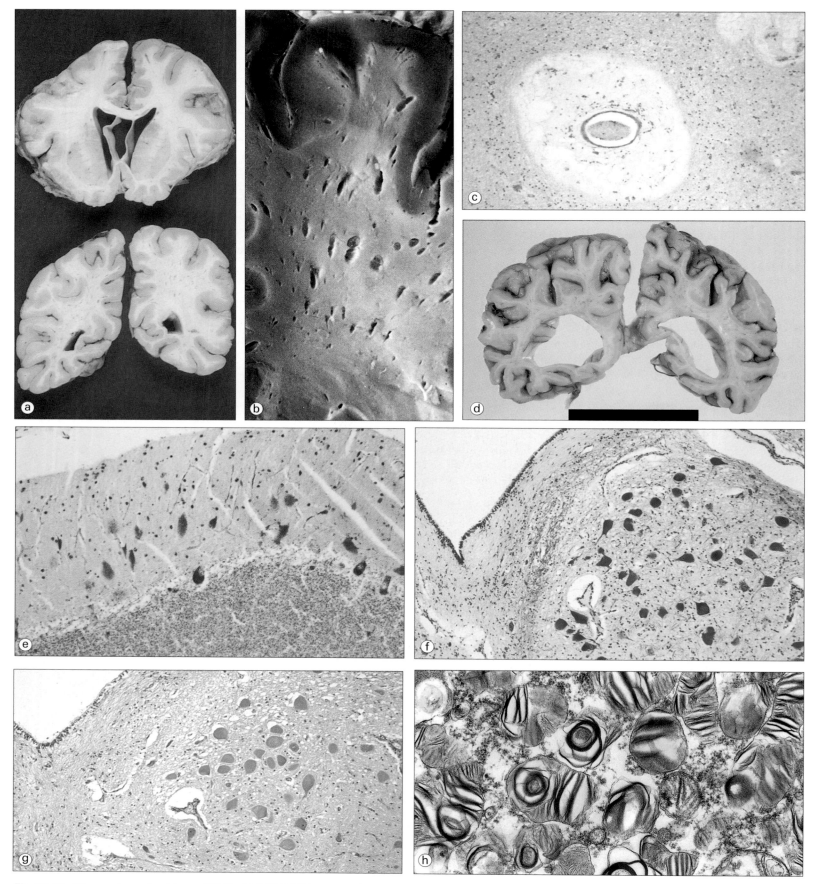

Fig. 23.11 Mucopolysaccharidoses (MPS). (a) MPS VI (Maroteaux–Lamy): the white matter is studded with fine pits. **(b)** On closer inspection the fine pits are perivascular. **(c)** These perivascular pits are filled with foamy macrophages containing water-soluble mucopolysaccharide, which accounts for their empty appearance in routinely processed sections. **(d)** MPS IIIa (Sanfillipo A) in an 11-year-old boy: a coronal section of the brain shows severe cerebral atrophy. Neuronal storage of ganglioside is present throughout the brain. **(e)** In the cerebellar cortex of the patient shown in (d), Purkinje cells and their dendrites are filled with granules. (Luxol fast blue/cresyl violet) **(f)** MPS IH: storage of ganglioside in neurons of the twelfth cranial nerve nucleus stained with luxol fast blue. **(g)** Same as (f), but stained with PAS. **(h)** Ultrastructurally, the stored material forms membrane stacks or 'zebra' bodies ..

in hepatocytes and Kupffer cells, cartilage, lymph nodes, tonsils, spleen, kidney, heart (notably the valves), fibroblasts in skin, conjunctiva, cornea, and vascular endothelial cells.

In blood, Alder granulation, which is a coarse reddish violet granulation in neutrophils stained with May–Grünwald–Giemsa or Wrightstain is found in MPS VI and MPS VII.

Ultrastructurally, large membrane-bound vacuoles in many tissues are usually empty, but some fine granular material and lamellae are occasionally noted. Various neuronal storage bodies are seen including MCBs, and loosely arranged parallel lamellae juxtaposed with spaces to form 'zebra' bodies (**Fig. 23.11h**).

MANNOSIDOSIS

α-mannosidosis and β-mannosidosis are two different lysosomal disorders with similar presentations. They show autosomal recessive transmission and are due to defects in lysosomal α-mannosidase and β-mannosidase respectively, resulting in an accumulation of mannose-rich oligosaccharides. The α-mannosidase gene has been sequenced and maps to chromosome 19cen-q12. The β-mannosidase gene is probably on chromosome 4.

MANNOSIDOSIS

- α-mannosidosis presents in two ways: a severe infantile form (type I) and a milder juvenile or adult form (type II).
- Features of both forms are psychomotor retardation, coarse facies, dysostosis multiplex, and gingival hyperplasia.
- Frequent bacterial infections, hepatosplenomegaly, deafness, and corneal opacities are common features.
- β-mannosidosis presents with mental retardation, deafness, and mild dysmorphic features.

MACROSCOPIC AND MICROSCOPIC APPEARANCES

In α-mannosidosis, vacuolated neurons are plentiful in the cerebral cortex, brain stem, and spinal cord, and in the peripheral nervous system. Astrocytes, endothelial cells, and pericytes are also vacuolated. Gliosis, myelin depletion, and cerebellar degeneration may also occur.

The stored mannose-rich oligosaccharides are so water-soluble that they can be demonstrated only in cryostat sections of snap-frozen tissue stained by the alcoholic PAS reaction or after previous protection with celloidin.

Lymphocytes have large or small discrete vacuoles, both in peripheral blood and in bone marrow aspirates, which also contain large foamy storage cells.

Morphologic descriptions of β-mannosidosis are sparse, but vacuolated lymphocytes are not found.

FUCOSIDOSIS
MICROSCOPIC APPEARANCES

Granulovacuolar storage is present in many tissues, including kidney, spleen, lymph nodes, lungs, heart, endocrine glands, hepatocytes, Kupffer cells, vascular endothelial cells, fibroblasts, and sweat glands. There are foam cells in the bone marrow. The stored material is extremely soluble, and impossible to characterize histochemically.

Neurons in many areas of the CNS are vacuolated and enlarged. The olives and thalamus are particularly affected. Purkinje cells may be depleted. In some cases, the white matter is extensively demyelinated and gliotic, and the presence of many Rosenthal fibers (**Fig. 23.12**) produces an appearance reminiscent of Alexander's disease.

Ultrastructurally, there are membrane-bound vacuoles, which are either empty or contain parallel or concentric lamellae at their periphery.

FUCOSIDOSIS

- Two forms have been described, but they may not be truly distinctive and can both occur within one family.
- In type I, presentation is in the first year with respiratory infections and psychomotor regression. Hepatomegaly may be evident, and dysostosis multiplex resembling that of MPS type I is found. Death occurs in the first decade.
- Type II has a more slowly progressive course: mental retardation beginning in the second year, bony and facial changes like those of MPS type I, and angiokeratomas are the principal features.

FABRY'S DISEASE
MICROSCOPIC APPEARANCES

ETIOLOGY OF FABRY'S DISEASE

- α-galactosidase A deficiency is present, leading to the accumulation of ceramide-trihexoside and ceramide dihexoside with terminal α-galactosyl residues.
- The gene is located at Xq22.1 and variable manifestations are found in female heterozygotes.

FABRY'S DISEASE

- Presenting features, usually in childhood, are clusters of punctate red–black telangiectases in the bathing trunk area and on mucous membranes (angiokeratoma corporis diffusum), and proteinuria.
- Renal failure eventually follows.
- Other features include retinal, conjunctival, and corneal abnormalities, paresthesiae, and autonomic dysfunction.
- Isolated hypertrophic cardiomyopathy is a rare but important presentation.

In frozen sections vascular endothelium and smooth muscle contain PAS- and Sudan black-positive birefringent deposits. Although deposits in all sites are generally removed during processing, frozen or cryostat sections retain considerable material, and sometimes there is residual staining in paraffin sections.

Similar storage is present in renal glomerular and tubular epithelia, which are vacuolated. Urinary deposit derived from desquamated distal tubules contains intensely PAS-positive, mulberry-like cells, which can be analysed biochemically. Glomerular sclerosis supervenes in the later stages of the disease.

Cardiac muscle, cells of the mononuclear/phagocyte system, and peripheral nervous system ganglion cells also exhibit storage.

Neuronal storage is notable in the amygdala, hypothalamus, brain stem, and cord, but neuropathology is largely the consequence of vasculopathy, which manifests as small infarcts.

Ultrastructurally, cytoplasmic inclusions are composed of tightly packed concentric or parallel lipid lamellae arranged in stacks or as interwoven curved segments.

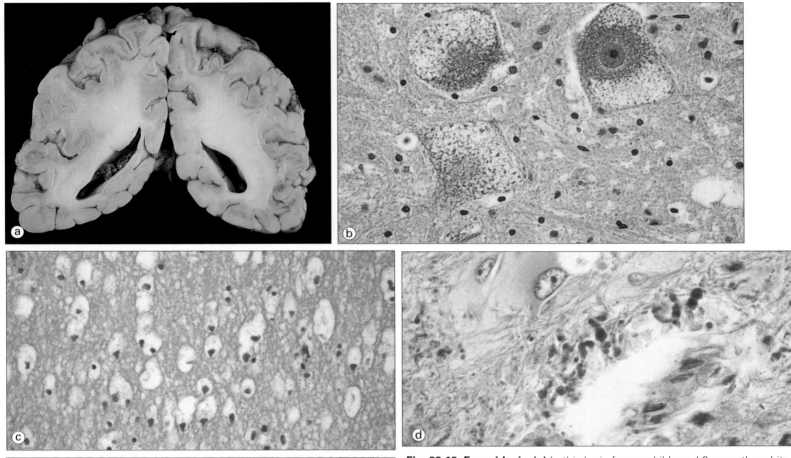

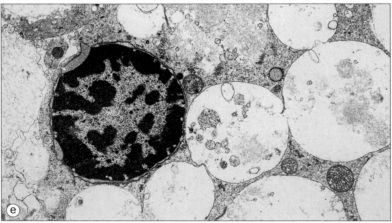

Fig. 23.12 Fucosidosis. (a) In this brain from a child aged 6 years the white matter is strikingly firm and white. **(b)** Ballooned anterior horn cells. **(c)** Cortical neurons are distended, but empty of the highly soluble stored fucose compounds. **(d)** In some patients the white matter is extremely rich in Rosenthal fibers, which as in Alexander's disease cluster around blood vessels. **(e)** The stored material is so soluble that only empty vacuoles can be demonstrated ultrastructurally. (Courtesy of Professor B. Lake).

TYPE II GLYCOGENOSIS (POMPE'S DISEASE)

Type II glycogenosis is an autosomal recessive deficiency of acid α-1,4-glucosidase (acid maltase). Deficiency of acid α-1,4-glucosidase can be caused by several mutations of chromosome 17q23.

TYPE II GLYCOGENOSIS

- There is neonatal onset of hypotonia, cardiomegaly, hepatomegaly, and, occasionally, macroglossia.
- Death is usually before 2 years of age from cardiac dysfunction or respiratory failure secondary to muscle weakness.
- A juvenile form presents with weakness of limb girdle and trunk muscles, and respiratory problems.
- An adult form presents in the second or third decade with weakness of skeletal muscles, particularly the muscles of respiration.

MICROSCOPIC APPEARANCES

The hallmark of the disease is a vacuolar degeneration of skeletal myofibers: extreme in infants, moderate in juveniles, and modest or mild in adults. The vacuoles contain excessive soluble β-particle glycogen and strong acid phosphatase activity. Excess glycogen is also present in capillary endothelium and smooth muscle, and in the infantile form in cardiac muscle fibers in association with cardiomegaly. Neuronal glycogen storage is a feature of the infantile and juvenile forms, but not the adult-onset form. It is found in anterior horn cells (**Fig. 23.13**) and motor cranial nerve nuclei, basal ganglia, and gastrointestinal tract plexuses. Glycogen is also abundant in astrocytes in the cerebral cortex.

In blood films, lymphocytes have small discrete cytoplasmic glycogen-containing vacuoles.

FARBER'S DISEASE

Deficiency of lysosomal ceramidase leads to a marked increase in ceramide concentration with hydroxylated forms in the liver, brain, and kidney, but non-hydroxylated forms exclusively in subcutaneous nodules.

FARBER'S DISEASE

- Onset in infancy with painful swollen joints associated with subcutaneous nodules, a hoarse cry, respiratory and feeding difficulties, and psychomotor retardation.
- Survival is rarely longer than 2 years.

MICROSCOPIC APPEARANCES

Neuronal loss and gliosis are associated with marked neuronal storage in the basal ganglia, brain stem, and anterior horns, and to a lesser degree in the cerebral cortex and gastrointestinal tract plexuses. The stored material is strongly PAS-positive, weakly sudanophilic, and bire-fringent in polarized light.

Foamy cells are numerous in the spleen, lungs, and lymph nodes. The subcutaneous nodules are aggregates of foam cells or granulomas with macrophages, lymphocytes, and multinucleate giant cells. Granulomas may also be present in the lungs.

Neurons and endothelial cells contain zebra bodies. Hepatocytes contain membrane-bound collections of lipid lamellae. Subcutaneous foam cells contain small curvilinear tubular structures (Farber bodies or banana bodies).

KRABBE'S LEUKODYSTROPHY
MACROSCOPIC APPEARANCES

The changes are similar in both the typical infantile form and in the rarer examples with late or adult onset. Externally there is moderate to severe atrophy, widened sulci and marked weight reduction, while on palpation the firm white matter surrounded by normal cortex gives the impression of an 'iron fist in a velvet glove'. On cut section the white matter is extensively discolored and grayish, though subcortical white fibers are spared, and the ventricles are dilated (**Fig. 23.14a**). Cerebellar white matter is similarly affected.

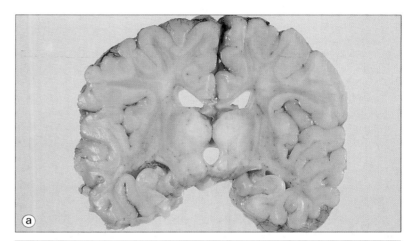

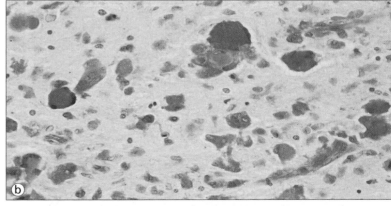

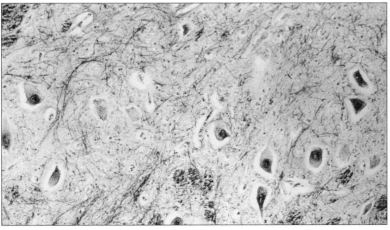

Fig. 23.13 Type II glycogenosis (Pompe's disease). Distended neurons in the twelfth cranial nerve nucleus

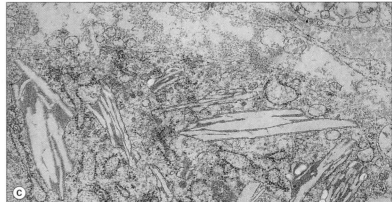

Fig. 23.14 Krabbe's globoid cell leukodystrophy. (a) Coronal section through cerebrum. The subcortical U-fibers are generally spared, but the centrum semi-ovale is gray and firm, so the intact brain has the texture of an 'iron fist in a velvet glove'. **(b)** The demyelinated matter contains both mononuclear and multinucleated macrophages (globoid cells) which are strongly PAS-positive. (Midbrain section stained with PAS)
(c) Ultrastructure of a globoid cell/macrophage. There are numerous curved or straight tubular inclusions with a crystalloid appearance.

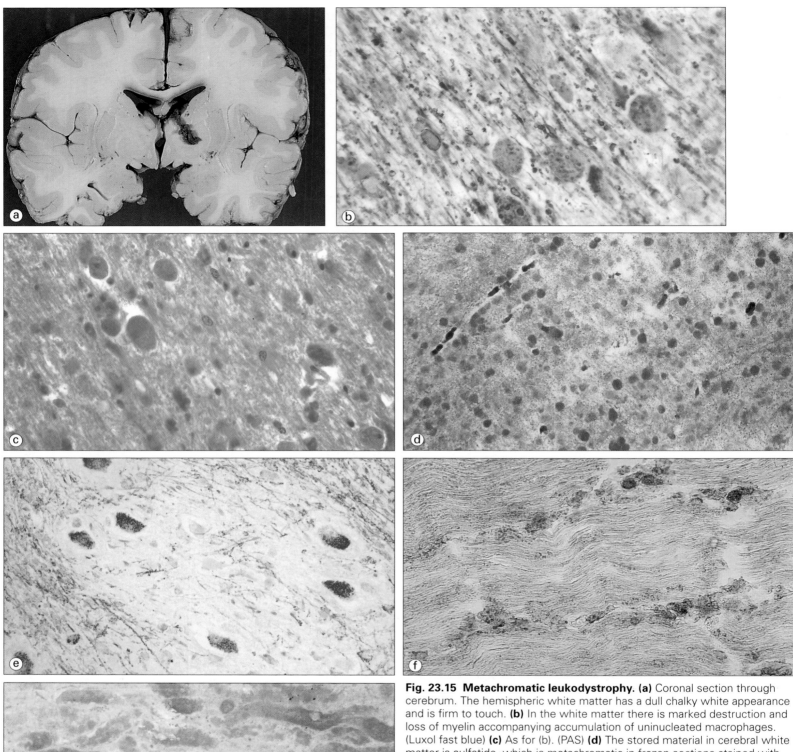

Fig. 23.15 Metachromatic leukodystrophy. (a) Coronal section through cerebrum. The hemispheric white matter has a dull chalky white appearance and is firm to touch. **(b)** In the white matter there is marked destruction and loss of myelin accompanying accumulation of uninucleated macrophages. (Luxol fast blue) **(c)** As for (b). (PAS) **(d)** The stored material in cerebral white matter is sulfatide, which is metachromatic in frozen sections stained with thionin or acidified cresyl violet. **(e)** Neuronal storage of sulfatide in the cerebellar dentate nucleus. (Luxol fast blue/cresyl violet) **(f)** Sulfatide in peripheral nerve. **(g)** Sulfatide in renal tubular epithelium.

MICROSCOPIC APPEARANCES

Principal changes are extensive myelin and oligodendrocyte loss, astrocytic gliosis, and the pathognomonic presence of globoid macrophages which early in the course of the disease are mononuclear but later form perivascular clusters of multinucleated cells with as many as 20 peripheral nuclei. Eventually myelin, axons, and even globoid cells may disappear leaving only an intense gliosis. Globoid cells are PAS-positive, faintly sudanophilic, but not metachromatic (**Fig. 23.14b**). They show strong acid phosphatase activity, and ultrastructurally contain straight or curved tubular profiles which are irregularly crystaloid on cross-section (**Fig 23.14c**). Demyelination affects most of the cerebral white matter, usually the optic tracts, and the brain stem and cord variably with preservation of cranial and spinal roots. There is no neuronal storage but there may be severe neuronal loss from the dentate and olivary nuclei, and more moderate involvement of other brain stem nuclei and Purkinje cells. Peripheral nerves also show demyelination, fibrosis, and the presence of macrophages containing tubular inclusions.

KRABBE'S DISEASE AND METACHROMATIC LEUKODYSTROPHY (MLD)

Krabbe's disease

- Presentation in infancy — irritability, developmental failure, deteriorating motor function, tonic spasms, myoclonic jerks, hyperpyrexia, blindness, bulbar paralysis
- Presentation in childhood — gait disorder, progressive spasticity, peripheral neuropathy, visual disturbance

Metachromatic leukodystrophy

- Presentation in infancy — progressive motor disability
- Presentation in childhood — behavioral and educational, problems, gait disorder
- Presentation in adults — psychosis, behavioral problems

METACHROMATIC LEUCODYSTROPHY (MLD)

MACROSCOPIC APPEARANCES

In the late infantile form the brain may appear externally normal, slightly enlarged or atrophic (changes are slight in juvenile and adult cases). On section the white matter is a dull chalky white, firm to touch, and sharply demarcated from the cortex (**Fig. 23.15a**). Cerebellar atrophy may also occur.

MICROSCOPIC APPEARANCES

Demyelination and considerable axon loss are extensive in cerebral and cerebellar white matter and corticospinal tracts. There is oligodendrocyte loss, intense astrogliosis, and accumulation of PAS and luxol fast blue positive macrophages which, in frozen sections, demonstrate brown metachromasia with acidified cresyl violet toluidine blue or thionine (**Fig. 23.15c,d**). This sulfatide deposition also occurs in neurons in the basal ganglia, dentate nucleus, some brain stem nuclei and dorsal root ganglia, as well as within macrophages and Schwann cell, in peripheral nerves, within renal tubular epithelium, macrophages in lymph nodes and spleen, liver, Kuppfer cells, biliary duct epithelium, adrenal medulla, islets of Langerhans, and many other organs. Ultrastructurally, there are three types of inclusion: prismatic, tuffstone and laminated.

LYSOSOMAL ENZYME DEFECTS CAUSING LEUKODYSTROPHY

Krabbe's disease

- Galactocerebroside–β–galactosidase deficiency
- Gene locus 14q31
- Transmission AR

Metachromatic leukodystrophy

- Most cases due to aryl sulfatase A deficiency; rarely caused by deficiency of sphingolipid activator protein-1 (SAP-1; saposin B)
- Aryl sulfatase A gene locus 22q13; SAP-1 gene locus 10q22.1
- Transmission AR; rarely AD

PEROXISOMAL DISORDERS

Peroxisomes are tiny organelles, 0.05–0.2 μm in diameter in the cytoplasm of all nucleated cells (in the liver and kidney they are ~10× larger). They are identified by their structure, positive histochemical reaction for catalase (**Fig. 23.18a**), or immunohistochemistry. New peroxisomes form by budding from existing peroxisomes. Peroxisomal proteins, both enzymes and membrane proteins, are encoded by nuclear genes and imported via special receptors into the organelle. The many functions of peroxisomes are listed in **Fig. 23.16**.

A classification of peroxisomal disorders is given in **Fig. 23.17**. Although this is a long list and probably still far from complete, morphologic data remain scanty for many of these conditions. Disorders with significant neurologic disturbance and well-documented neuropathology are fewer: in particular, the adrenoleukodystrophies and Zellweger syndrome and its variants.

Functions of peroxisomes

Processes integral to normal metabolism of the nervous system, adrenals, and liver

- Plasmalogen biosynthesis (important components in cell membranes and myelin)
- Cholesterol biosynthesis
- Bile acid biosynthesis
- β-oxidation of fatty acids (including very long chain fatty acids)

Other functions

- Dolichol synthesis (through action of mevalonate kinase)
- Glyoxalate transamination
- Peroxide-based respiration/peroxidatic oxidation
- Pipecolic acid oxidation
- Glutaric acid oxidation
- Phytanic acid α-oxidation
- Alcohol dehydrogenase (medium chain)

Fig. 23.16 Functions of peroxisomes.

Classification of peroxisomal disorders

1. Peroxisomes absent or severely reduced (defective peroxisomal membrane synthesis or import of matrix proteins results in defective peroxisomal assembly and generalized enzyme defects)

- Zellweger cerebrohepatorenal syndrome
- Neonatal adrenoleukodystrophy
- Infantile Refsum's disease
- Zellweger-like syndrome
- Rhizomelic chondroplasia punctata (classic form)
- Pseudo-infantile Refsum's disease

2. Peroxisomes present, but may be structurally abnormal (single peroxisomal enzyme defect)

- X-linked adrenoleukodystrophy
- Pseudo-neonatal adrenoleukodystrophy
- Rhizomelic chondroplasia punctata
- Bifunctional enzyme deficiency
- Pseudo-Zellweger syndrome
- Trihydroxycholestanoic acidemia
- Pipecolic acidemia (isolated)
- Refsum's disease
- Atypical Refsum's disease
- Glutaric aciduria type III
- Primary hyperoxaluria type I
- Acatalasemia
- Mevalonic aciduria
- Sjögren–Larsson syndrome

Fig. 23.17 Classification of peroxisomal disorders.

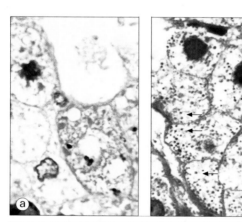
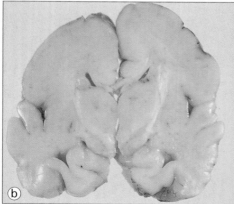
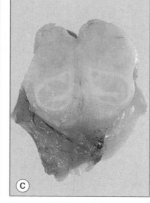

Fig. 23.18 Zellweger cerebrohepatorenal syndrome. (a) Peroxisomes are readily demonstrated in liver by catalase histochemistry. They appear as darkly stained bodies (arrows) in a normal control (right panel), but are absent in Zellweger syndrome (left panel). Courtesy of Professor B. Lake. **(b)** Macrogyric convolutions and thickened cortical ribbon in a neonate with Zellweger syndrome. **(c)** Horizontal slice through the medulla showing the dysplastic inferior olivary nuclei, which are coarse, thickened dorsally, and can be partially fragmented.

ZELLWEGER CEREBROHEPATORENAL SYNDROME

ZELLWEGER SYNDROME

- Onset at birth with severe hypotonia and characteristic dysmorphic features (i.e. high forehead, large fontanelles, epicanthic folds, shallow supraorbital ridges, micrognathia, abnormal ears, and high arched palate). There is often stippled calcification of the patella.
- The further course includes epilepsy, failure to thrive, psychomotor retardation, pigmentary retinopathy, and abnormal liver function.
- Death occurs at about 5 months of age.
- Biochemical abnormalities include abnormal plasma bile acids, increased very long chain fatty acids, and defective plasmalogen synthesis indicated by deficient activity of dihydroxyacetone-phosphate acyl transferase, and accumulation of pipecolic acid and phytanic acid in body fluids.

MACROSCOPIC AND MICROSCOPIC APPEARANCES

The weight of the brain is often increased and there are widespread gyral abnormalities with both widened pachygyric convolutions and polymicrogyria (**Fig. 23.18b**).

Extensively deranged cortical migration manifests as pachygyria, polymicrogyria, and neuronal heterotopias (see chapter 3). Focal gray heterotopias are present in cerebellar white matter, the dentate nucleus is dysplastic, and the inferior olivary nuclei show a characteristic malformation (**Fig. 23.18c**) (see chapter 3). The white matter shows decreased myelin and evidence of myelin breakdown with lipid deposition (cholesterol esterified to very long chain fatty acids) in astrocytes and macrophages in some cases. A neuronal lipidosis and neuroaxonal dystrophy in the spinal nucleus of Clarke and in the lateral cuneate nucleus have also been reported.

Ultrastructural examination shows that macrophages in white matter contain lipid clefts, lamellae, and lamellar lipid profiles.

The adrenal gland may show striated cortical cells, which ultrastructurally contain trilaminar and lamellar lipid profiles. In the kidney, there may be renal cysts, which are mostly dilatations of Bowman's space of the glomerulus, lined by flat or cuboidal epithelium. Hepatic pathology varies, but usually there is progressive fibrosis leading to micronodular cirrhosis, and sometimes cholestasis, giant cell change, or paucity of bile ducts. Peroxisomes are absent. Ultrastructurally, some angular lysosomes include trilaminar bodies.

Zellweger variants

Infantile Refsum's disease presents with a mild Zellweger phenotype and survival into adolescence. The liver shows absent peroxisomes and micronodular cirrhosis. Cerebellar cortical atrophy has been reported in one case.

Pseudo-Zellweger syndrome: Despite the clinical and pathologic features of classic Zellweger syndrome, there are abundant hepatic peroxisomes. The typical histology of Zellweger syndrome is found in the brain, adrenals, and kidneys.

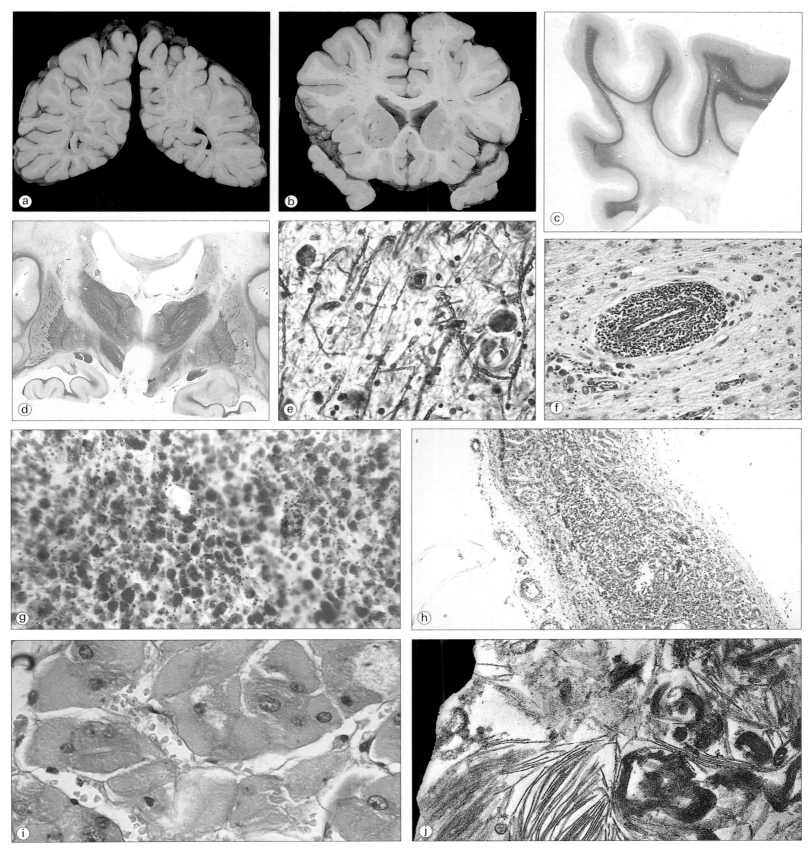

Fig. 23.19 Adrenoleukodystrophy. Macroscopically, the affected white matter is firm and gray, and is usually more severely affected posteriorly **(a)** than anteriorly **(b)**. **(c)** Section through the frontal lobe showing extensive myelin loss from the centrum semiovale and corpus callosum, but with sparing of the U-fibers. (Luxol fast blue/cresyl violet) **(d)** Section through the basal ganglia at the level of the amygdala showing extensive myelin loss from the centra semiovalia, corpus callosum, and internal capsules, but with sparing of the U-fibers. (Luxol fast blue/cresyl violet) **(e)** Myelin fragmentation and a sparse infiltrate of macrophages are found at the advancing edge of the demyelinating process. (Luxol fast blue/cresyl violet) **(f)** In the center of the demyelinated areas there are prominent perivascular collections of lymphocytes and groups of PAS-positive macrophages. **(g)** These macrophages may form large aggregates. **(h)** The adrenal gland is usually severely atrophic and may be difficult to find at necropsy. **(i)** The remaining adrenocortical cells are enlarged, eosinophilic, and show prominent striations. **(j)** The lipid deposits contain very long chain fatty acids and appear ultrastructurally as needle-like trilaminar bodies up to 7 nm long and 10 nm wide.

ETIOLOGY OF ZELLWEGER SYNDROME (ZWS) AND PSEUDO-ZWS

This syndrome can be caused by defects of several proteins involved in the assembly of peroxisomes.
- ZWS1 has been localized to 7q11.23.
- ZWS2 is due to defective peroxisomal membrane protein-1 (PXMP1). Gene locus 1p21-22.
- ZWS3 is due to defective peroxisomal assembly factor-1 (PAF1; also known as peroxisomal membrane protein-3). Gene locus 8q21.1.
- ZWS can also be caused by defective peroxisomal assembly factor-2 (PAF2; also known as peroxisome-type ATPase). Gene locus 6p11-22.
- At least one form of pseudo-ZWS is due to peroxisomal 3-oxoacyl-CoA thiolase deficiency. Gene locus 3p22-23.

ADRENOLEUKODYSTROPHY
MACROSCOPIC APPEARANCES

Externally relatively normal, the sliced brain shows an extensive symmetric white matter abnormaly which in the fixed state is firm and gray. There is a caudal to rostral gradient of severity with the frontal areas often less severely involved (**Fig. 23.19a,b**).

MICROSCOPIC APPEARANCES

Demyelination is severe in the central cerebral white matter, optic nerves, internal capsule, and commissures, while U-fibers and stria of Gennari are relatively spared (**Fig. 23.19c,d**). There may be some involvement of the descending brain stem tracts (much more evident in the adrenomyeloneuropathy variant). Histologically, three zones of abnormality may be discerned. In the most recent there is demyelination with preservation of axons, and scattered sudanophilic PAS–positive macrophages (**Fig. 23.19e**). Older lesions also demonstrate a pronounced perivascular mononuclear infiltrate and numerous macrophages (**Fig. 23.19f,g**). The most ancient lesions are without macrophage or inflammatory activity, depleted of axons and oligodendroglia, and heavily gliotic.

Adrenal atrophy may cause severe difficulty in identifying the adrenals at autopsy: histologically, ballooned cells wth striated cytoplasm replace the cortex (**Fig. 23.19h,i**). With electron microscopy, adrenal, testis, peripheral nerves, and brain show cytoplasmic inclusions comprising needle-like trilaminar bodies of very long chain fatty acid esters (**Fig. 23.19j**).

ADRENOLEUKODYSTROPHY (ALD)

- Presentation in infancy – hypertonia, seizures, failure to thrive, deafness, retinal degeneration
- Presentation in childhood – loss of skills, educational problems, dementia, problems with hearing and vision, progressive pyramidal, extrapyramidal, or cerebellar disorder
- Presentation in adulthood – clumsiness and spasticity, schizophrenia-like syndrome, dementia

PEROXISOMAL DEFECTS CAUSING ADRENOLEUKODYSTROPHY (ALD)/ADRENOMYELONEUROPATHY

Adrenoleukodystrophy/adrenomyeloneuropathy
- Single peroxisomal enzyme defect of an ATP-binding cassette transporter reduces the capacity to form the coenzyme A derivative of very long chain fatty acids
- Gene locus Xq28
- Transmission X-linked; female carriers may manifest

Neonatal adrenoleukodystrophy
- Defective peroxisomal assembly results in absent or severely reduced numbers of peroxisomes and loss of multiple peroxisomal functions
- Transmission AR

REFERENCES:

Fournier B *et al.* (1994) Peroxisomal disorders. A review. *J Inher Metab Dis* **17**: 470–486.
Goebel HH. (1995) The neuronal ceroid-lipofuscinoses. *J Child Neurol* **10**: 424–437.
Lake B. (1997) Lysosomal and peroxisomal disorders. In Graham D, Lantos P (eds) *Greenfield's Neuropathology. Sixth edition.* pp. London: Arnold.
Love S, Bridges LR, Case CP. (1995) Neurofibrillary tangles in Niemann–Pick disease type C. *Brain* **118**: 119–129.
Online Mendelian Inheritance in Man OMIN (TM). Center for Medical Genetics, John J Hopkins University (Baltimore, MD) and National Center for Biotechnology Information, National Library of Medicine (Bethesda, MD), 1966. World Wide Web URL: http://www3.ncbi.nlm.nih.gov/omim/.

Powers JM. (1985) Adreno-leukodystrophy (Adreno-testiculo-leuko-myelo-neuropathic complex). *Clin Neuropathol.* **4**:181–199, .
Scriver CR, Beaudet AL, Valle D, Sly WS (1995) *The Metabolic and Molecular Basis of Inherited Disease. Seventh edition.* New York: McGraw-Hill Inc.
Sharp JD *et al.* (1977) Loci for classical and variant late infantile neuronal ceroid lipofuscinosis map to chromosomes 11p15 and 15q21-23. *Hum Molec Genet* **6**: 591–595.

24 *Mitochondrial encephalopathies*

The mitochondrial genome is a circular molecule of DNA (mitochondrial DNA; mtDNA) comprising 16,569 base pairs. Each mitochondrion contains 2–10 copies of the genome, which encodes 22 transfer RNAs (tRNAs), two ribosomal RNAs (rRNAs), and 13 subunits of the respiratory chain (**Fig. 24.1**). Since spermatozoa do not contribute mitochondria during fertilization, mitochondria and their genomes are all maternally inherited.

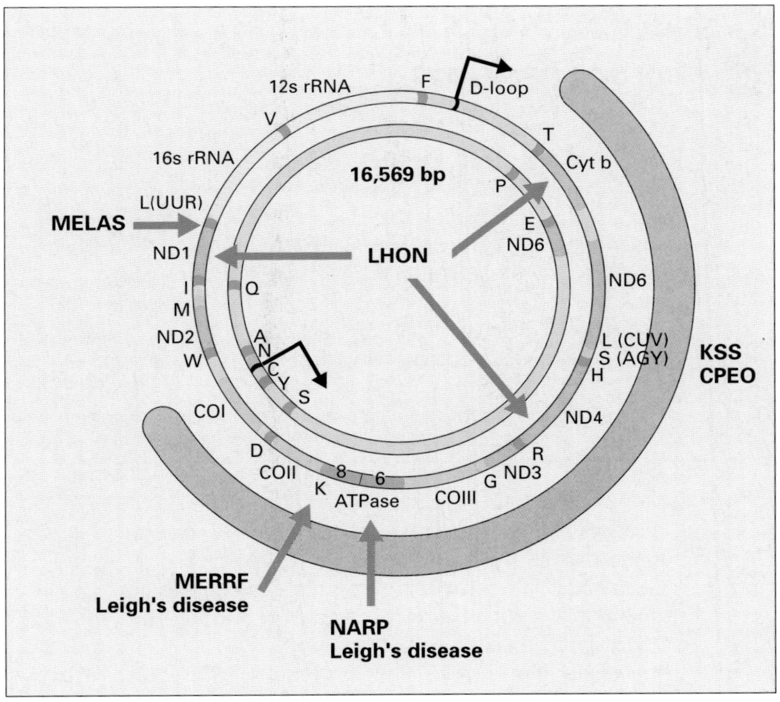

A wide range of disorders affecting the central nervous system (CNS) is attributable to defective mitochondrial function. This chapter covers only those encephalopathies and encephalomyopathies that are due to abnormalities of mtDNA. These mtDNA abnormalities may be the primary genetic defect or secondary to mutations of nuclear DNA (**Fig. 24.2**). Mitochondrial disorders that do not involve the CNS are not considered in this book. Disorders of mitochondrial metabolism in which the primary defect involves proteins encoded by nuclear DNA and in which there is no secondary abnormality of the mitochondrial genome (e.g. Alpers' syndrome, Menkes' syndrome, some forms of Leigh's disease, and several defects of fatty acid, amino acid, and pyruvate metabolism) are described separately in chapters 6 and 7.

Most mtDNA defects are heteroplasmic (i.e. cells contain a mixture of mutant and wild-type mitochondria within their cytoplasm). As mitochondria are randomly segregated during mitosis, the proportion of mitochondria containing mutant genomes varies from cell to cell.

Fig. 24.1 Diagram of human mtDNA. The outer and inner circles represent the heavy and light strands respectively. The genes encoding the mitochondrial rRNAs are shown as 12s and 16s rRNA, those encoding the reduced form of nicotinamide adenine dinucleotide dehydrogenase (NADH) subunits as ND1–6, the cytochrome oxidase subunits as COI–III, and cytochrome b as Cyt b. Also shown are the genes encoding subunits 6 and 8 of adenosine triphosphatase (ATPase). Conventional single letter amino acid abbreviations are used to indicate the tRNA genes. The broad gray arc shows the region involved to a greater or lesser extent in most deletions of mtDNA. The blue arrows indicate the main sites of point mutations or deletions in mitochondrial disorders that affect the CNS.

Classification of mitochondrial encephalopathies

Cause	Examples
Mutation in mtDNA	
• point mutations	• MELAS, MERRF, LHON, NARP, some cases of Leigh's disease
• deletions	• KSS, CPEO
Mutation in nuclear DNA	
• producing deletions of mtDNA	• mtDNA breakage syndrome, some cases of MNGIE
• producing depletion of mtDNA	• mtDNA depletion syndrome

Fig. 24.2 Classification of mitochondrial encephalopathies. Encephalopathies in which there are primary or secondary defects of mtDNA. (MELAS=mitochondrial myopathy, encephalopathy, lactic acidosis, and stroke-like episodes; MERRF=mitochondrial epilepsy with 'ragged-red' fibers; LHON=Leber's hereditary optic neuopathy; NARP=neuropathy, ataxia, and retinitis pigmentosa; KSS=Kearns–Sayre syndrome; CPEO=chronic progressive external ophthalmoplegia; MNGIE=myoneurogastrointestinal encephalopathy.)

MITOCHONDRIAL MYOPATHY, ENCEPHALOPATHY, LACTIC ACIDOSIS, AND STROKE-LIKE EPISODES (MELAS)

MELAS

- MELAS is usually a disorder of children and young adults.
- The syndrome has a variable presentation, which may include sudden onset of headache, vomiting, seizures, hemiplegia, hemianopia, and occasionally, loss of consciousness. Milder attacks may simulate migraine.
- There is often some neurologic recovery between attacks, but the natural history is of recurrent stroke-like episodes leading to increasing impairment.
- The degree of lactic acidosis is variable, and the myopathy may be mild.
- MELAS due to the nucleotide 3243 mutation, may be associated with sensorineural hearing loss, pigmentary retinal degeneration, migraine, hypothalamic hypogonadism, hypertrophic cardiomyopathy, and noninsulin-dependent diabetes mellitus.

MACROSCOPIC APPEARANCES

Scattered foci of necrosis and cavitation are usually evident in the cerebral cortex (**Fig. 24.3**). These infarct-like lesions may be of varying ages. Although they can occur in any part of the cerebral cortex, the occipital lobe is often most severely affected. The basal ganglia, thalamus, and cerebellum are much less commonly involved.

MICROSCOPIC APPEARANCES

The necrotic foci are histologically indistinguishable from infarcts of various ages (**Fig. 24.4**), although their distribution does not correspond to that of any particular arterial perfusion territory (**Fig. 24.5**; and also **Fig. 24.3**) and the crests of gyri are often more extensively affected than the depths of sulci. As with infarcts, there is capillary proliferation around and within the lesions. In many cases there is also mineralization in and around the walls of blood vessels in the globus pallidus, and occasionally in the cerebral white matter, thalamus, and dentate nucleus. This may be associated with fibrous thickening of the affected blood vessels and severe narrowing of the lumen. There may be spongy vacuolation of cerebral and cerebellar white matter, but this is unusual. Histology, histochemistry, and electron microscopy of skeletal muscle reveal 'ragged-red' fibers containing accumulations of morphologically abnormal mitochondria, some with paracrystalline inclusions. There are also accumulations of mitochondria in the endothelium and smooth muscle of intramuscular blood vessels (**Fig. 24.6**).

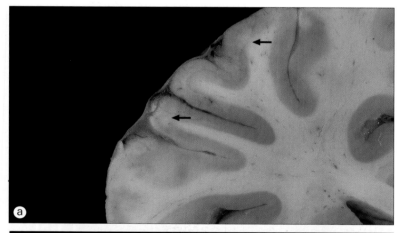

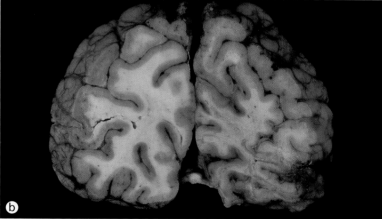

Fig. 24.3 **MELAS.** Infarct-like lesions of varying ages. **(a)** Recent lesions (arrows) in the frontal cortex. The distribution is not typical of hypoxic/ischaemic damage in that the crests of gyri are more extensively affected than the depths of sulci. The occipital lobes **(b)** are often severely affected in this case by lesions of differing ages. The older lesions have produced shrinkage and brown discoloration of the cortical ribbon.

ETIOLOGY OF MELAS

- In over 80% of cases, MELAS is caused by an A-to-G transition at nucleotide 3243 in the mitochondrial tRNA$^{Leu(UUR)}$ gene. This transition is within the region of termination of transcription of the mitochondrial rRNAs, but whether this is relevant to the genesis of MELAS lesions is uncertain.
- Less commonly, MELAS is due to a T-to-C transition at nucleotide 3271 in the tRNA$^{Leu(UUR)}$ gene.
- Occasionally, MELAS has been attributed to an A-to-G transition at nucleotide 11,084 in the ND4 gene, but other evidence suggests that this may be a normal polymorphism.

- The lesions of MELAS probably result from defective mitochondrial metabolism, although some researchers have suggested that the stroke-like lesions are due to impaired cerebral blood flow resulting from an accumulation of mitochondria within the cerebrovascular endothelium and smooth muscle cells.
- The likelihood of developing symptomatic MELAS is related to the proportion of mtDNA that contains the mutation. However, there is wide variation in the degree of heteroplasmy in different tissues and in most cases the precise correlation between the distribution of lesions and that of the mutant mtDNA is relatively poor.
- *In vitro* studies have shown that the mutant mtDNA replicates more efficiently than wild-type mtDNA and therefore tends to increase as a proportion of total mtDNA with time.

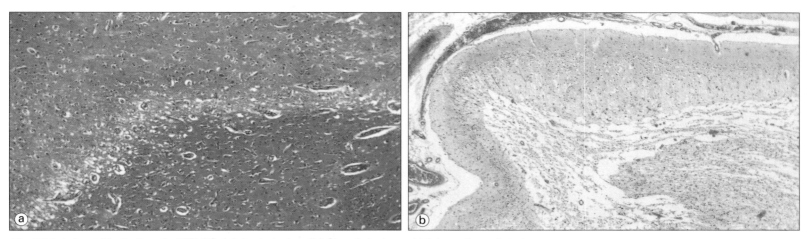

Fig. 24.4 Infarct-like lesions in MELAS. (a) Acute lesion. **(b)** Chronic lesion, which is partly cavitated.

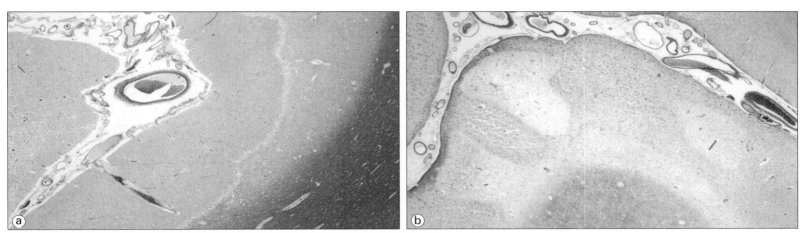

Fig. 24.5 Histology of lesions in MELAS. (a) A serpiginous boundry is visible between the acutely affected superficial cortex and the intact deeper cortex. **(b)** 'Punched-out' chronic lesions within cortex that is gliotic and depleted of nervous tissue. (Phosphotungstic acid/hematoxylin)

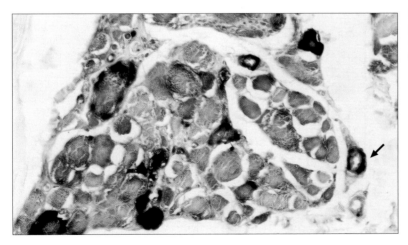

Fig. 24.6 Skeletal muscle in MELAS. Demonstration of abnormal accumulations of mitochondria in paraffin sections of muscle from a patient with MELAS by in situ-hybridization with probes to mitochondrial rRNA. An abnormally strong signal is also present in some of the blood vessels (arrow).

MITOCHONDRIAL EPILEPSY WITH RAGGED-RED FIBERS (MERRF)

▮ *MERFF*

Patients present in childhood or early adulthood with:
- myoclonic epilepsy of increasing severity.
- proximal myopathy.
- mental deterioration.
- Patients with MERRF/MELAS overlap syndromes may also develop lactic acidosis and stroke-like episodes.
- Other less common features include short stature, hearing loss, and ataxia. The A-to-G transition of nucleotide 8344 can also cause Leigh's disease (see below).

▮ *ETIOLOGY OF MERFF*

- An A-to-G transition at nucleotide 8344 in the mitochondrial tRNA^{Lys} gene is demonstrable in 80–90% of cases.
- Less common mutations producing MERRF include a C-to-T transition at nucleotide 3256 in the tRNA$^{Leu(UUR)}$ gene, and MERRF/MELAS overlap syndromes have been associated with T-to-C transitions at nucleotide 8356 in the tRNA^{Lys} gene or at nucleotide 7512 in the tRNA^{Ser} gene.
- In most studies, the correlation between the proportion of mtDNAs carrying the mutation in different tissues and the clinical manifestations has been relatively poor.

MACROSCOPIC AND MICROSCOPIC APPEARANCES

The brain usually appears unremarkable macroscopically, but there may be obvious brown discoloration and shrinkage of the dentate nuclei (**Fig. 24.7**) and inferior olives. Microscopy reveals neuronal loss and gliosis, which is most severe in the dentate nuclei (**Figs 24.8**), inferior olivary nuclei, substantia nigra, red nuclei, and basal ganglia (**Figs 24.9, 24.10**). The gracile and cuneate nuclei and Clarke's column in the spinal cord may also be affected. Blood vessels in the basal ganglia and cerebral white matter may show mineralization (**Fig. 24.11**). Skeletal muscle reveals histologic and histochemical changes of mitochondrial myopathy, with 'ragged-red' fibers containing accumulations of morphologically abnormal mitochondria, some with paracrystalline inclusions.

The findings in Leigh's disease, which is occasionally caused by an A-to-G transition at nucleotide 8344 in the mitochondrial tRNA^{Lys} gene, are considered in chapter 7.

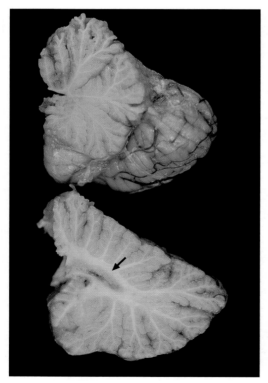

Fig. 24.7   MERRF. Shrinkage and brown discoloration of the dentate nucleus (arrow).

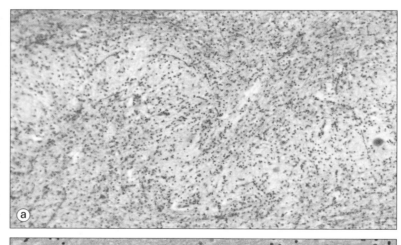

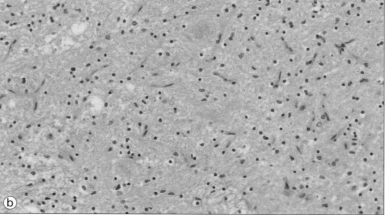

Fig. 24.8 Dentate nucleus in MERRF.
(a) Loss of neurons from the ribbon of the nucleus and of myelinated fibers from the hilum. (Luxol fast blue/cresyl violet)
(b) Higher magnification of the ribbon of the dentate nucleus shown in (a) revealing neuron depletion.

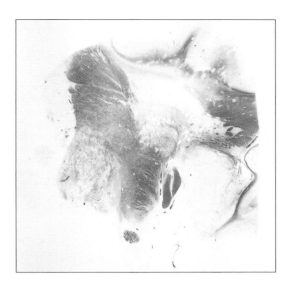

Fig. 24.9 Histology of MERFF. Marked pallor of myelin staining in the putamen in a case of MERRF. (Luxol fast blue/cresyl violet) (Courtesy of Professor F Scaravilli, Institute of Neurology,London, U.K.)

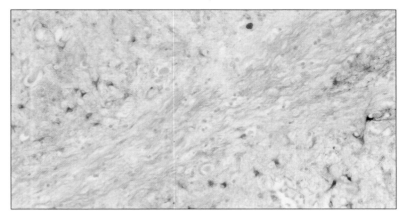

Fig. 24.10 Histology of MERFF. Gliosis of the putamen in a case of MERRF. The gliosis has been demonstrated by immunostaining for Glial fibrillary acidic protein immunoreactivity. (Courtesy of Professor F Scaravilli, Institute of Neurology, London, U.K.)

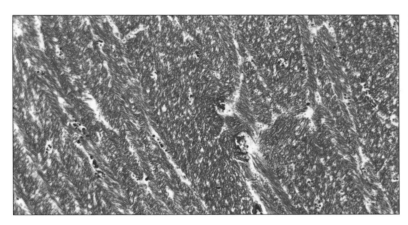

Fig. 24.11 Histology of MERFF. Mineralized blood vessels in the internal capsule in MERRF. (Luxol fast blue/cresyl violet) (Courtesy of Professor F Scaravilli, Institute of Neurology, London, U.K.)

LEBER'S HEREDITARY OPTIC NEUROPATHY (LHON), INFANTILE BILATERAL STRIATAL NECROSIS AND MARSDEN SYNDROME

ETIOLOGY OF LEBER'S HEREDITARY OPTIC NEUROPATHY

- Over 90% of families with LHON have mis-sense G-to-A mutations at nucleotides 11,778, 3460, or 14,484, although to date there are reports of a further 5 mutations that may cause LHON and a further 10 that influence the severity of the disease caused by the primary LHON mutations.
- Some of the mutations are heteroplasmic, affecting only a proportion of the mitochondrial genomes; others are homoplasmic.
- An A-to-G mutation at nucleotide 14,459 is responsible for a severe form of LHON and has been reported in some cases of infantile bilateral striatal necrosis.
- All the mutations affect mitochondrial genes encoding subunits in complexes I, III, IV, or V of the respiratory chain, and defective functioning of this chain is thought to cause the manifestations of this disease. However, several aspects of the pathophysiology remain unclear, including:
  - the factors determining the timing and close concordance of onset between the two eyes.
  - the considerably greater risk of visual loss in males than in females, which may lead to its being mistakenly attributed to X-linked recessive disorder.

LHON

- LHON usually presents in the third or fourth decade with acute or subacute loss of central vision.
- Both eyes are affected simultaneously, or sequentially over a period of up to 2 years.
- Variable recovery of vision occurs depending on the site of the mutation, with the mutation at nucleotide 11,778 having the worst prognosis.
- LHON is associated with non-ophthalmologic manifestations, including cardiac conduction defects and lesions involving the brain and spinal cord.
- If due to the 11,778 mutation or, rarely, the 3460 mutation, LHON may be associated with a multiple sclerosis-like disease (see chapter 19). The MRI characteristics of this condition are strongly suggestive of foci of demyelination in the cerebral white matter.
- If due to the 11,778 mutation LHON may be associated with neuropathy, ataxia, dystonia, and the development of lesions in the basal ganglia.

LEBER'S HEREDITARY OPTIC NEUROPATHY
MACROSCOPIC AND MICROSCOPIC APPEARANCES

Abnormalities of the white matter, including myelin sheath vacuolation and demyelination, are well recognized in KSS (see below) and, to a lesser extent, in other mitochondrial encephalopathies. However, the changes in the brain and spinal cord in LHON with multiple sclerosis-like lesions on magnetic resonance imaging are poorly documented.

INFANTILE BILATERAL STRIATAL NECROSIS (IBSN) AND MARSDEN SYNDROME

IBSN is a rare disorder that is often preceded by a febrile illness, and manifests with choreoathetosis, abnormal eye movements, seizures and mental retardation. At least some cases are due to the A-to-G nucleotide 14,459 mutation that can also cause severe LHON. CT scans reveal bilateral striatal lucencies. There is clinical and radiological overlap between infantile bilateral striatal necrosis and a rare familial disorder in which bilateral striatal lucencies are associated with dystonia, optic atrophy and visual failure (Marsden Syndrome); this is due to the same nucleotide 14,459 mutation in at least some families.

MACROSCOPIC AND MICROSCOPIC APPEARANCES

The putamen and, less consistently, the caudate nucleus and intervening white matter, are symmetrically cavitated (**Fig. 24.12**). Histology reveals accumulation of lipid laden macrophages, and surrounding gliosis (**Fig. 24.13**).

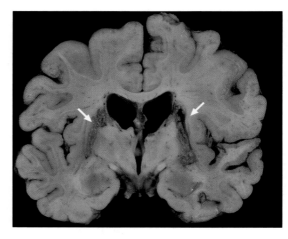

Fig. 24.12 Infantile bilateral striatal necrosis. (arrows)

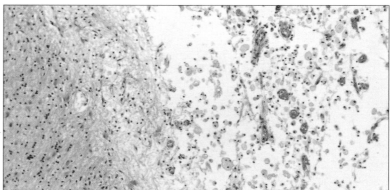

Fig. 24.13 Infantile bilateral striatal necrosis. Accumulation of lipid-laden macrophages in the putamen.

NEUROPATHY, ATAXIA, AND RETINITIS PIGMENTOSA (NARP) AND LEIGH'S DISEASE DUE TO NT8993 MUTATIONS

Leigh's disease is most commonly due to defects in nuclear DNA (resulting in pyruvate carboxylase or cytochrome *c* oxidase deficiency or reduced thiamine triphosphate synthesis), but may also be caused by either a T-to-C transition or a T-to-G transversion at nucleotide 8993 in the mitochondrial ATPase 6 gene. In some patients the latter mutation produces a syndrome of sensory neuropathy, cerebellar ataxia, retinitis pigmentosa (NARP), and mental retardation. Scant information is available concerning the histologic changes in the CNS. Biopsies of skeletal muscle from patients with NARP have been reported not to show 'ragged red' fibers but to contain accumulations of lipid and glycogen within vacuoles. The clinical and neuropathologic findings in Leigh's disease are considered in chapter 6.

KEARNS–SAYRE SYNDROME (KSS) AND ITS RELATIONSHIP TO OTHER CHRONIC PROGRESSIVE EXTERNAL OPHTHALMOPLEGIA (CPEO) SYNDROMES

MACROSCOPIC AND MICROSCOPIC APPEARANCES

The commonest neuropathologic abnormality in KSS is vacuolation of the white matter in the brain stem, cerebellum, and cerebrum (in decreasing order of frequency). Myelinated fibers in the deep gray nuclei and spinal cord may also be involved. This change is usually not discernible on macroscopic examination. On microscopy the affected white matter has a spongy appearance (**Fig. 24.14**) due to separation of myelin lamellae by clear vacuoles (**Fig. 24.15**), which are elongated in the long axis of the nerve fibers. Occasionally, severe spongiform vacuolation in the brain stem or cerebellum leads to oligodendrocyte degeneration and rather poorly demarcated foci of demyelination.

Mineral deposits are found in the walls of blood vessels in the globus pallidus, thalamus, dentate nucleus, mid brain, and medulla in approximately one-third of cases. There may be associated fibrous thickening of the vessel walls and severe narrowing of the lumina.

Histologic, histochemical, and electron microscopic examination of

KEARNS–SAYRE SYNDROME

- KSS presents in childhood or adolescence.
- KSS is characterized by:
  - progressive external ophthalmoplegia
  - pigmentary degeneration of the retina
  - cardiomyopathy with conduction defects
  - various combinations of short stature, proximal myopathy, high levels of protein in the cerebrospinal fluid (CSF), deafness, and electroencephalographic abnormalities.

skeletal muscle usually reveals 'ragged-red' fibers (**Figs 24.16, 24.17**) containing accumulations of morphologically abnormal mitochondria, some with paracrystalline inclusions (**Fig. 24.18**).

ETIOLOGY OF KSS AND CPEO

- CPEO is a component of KSS but often occurs without other features of that syndrome.
- KSS is usually associated with mtDNA deletions, which vary in size in different patients.
- In most cases the deletions are bracketed by direct repeats of 13–18 nucleotides, suggesting that the deletions occur as a result of a recombinational event during replication of mtDNA.
- An identical 4977 base pair deletion is present in approximately one-third of patients with KSS and most patients with 'pure' CPEO due to mitochondrial disease. This same deletion also occurs in patients with Pearson pancreas–marrow syndrome, some of whom eventually develop KSS.
- Differential tissue distribution of the deleted and wild-type mtDNAs in these disorders may partly account for the differences in phenotype.
- Recent research indicates that tandem duplication of the abnormal mtDNA occurs in KSS but not 'pure' CPEO. The functional significance of this is uncertain.
- Other rare causes of CPEO include mitochondrial DNA breakage syndrome (see below), MNGIE (see below), and point mutations of mtDNA.
- A syndrome of CPEO, proximal myopathy, psychiatric disturbances, and sudden death has been reported in association with an A-to-G transition at nucleotide 3251 of the mitochondrial tRNA^{Leu} gene.
- CPEO may also be a manifestation of several neuromuscular disorders that are not due to a defect in mitochondrial DNA.

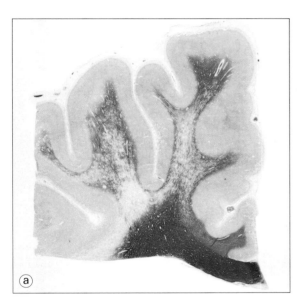

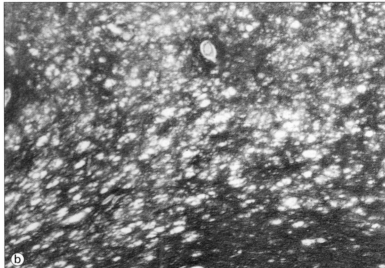

Fig. 24.14 KSS. (a) and **(b)** show the typical spongy vacuolation of the white matter. (Luxol fast blue/cresyl violet)

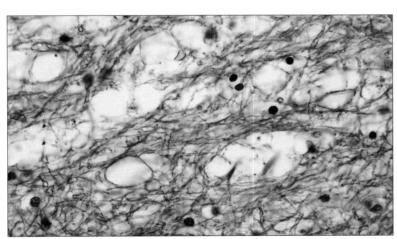

Fig. 24.15 KSS. At higher magnification of Fig. 24.14 some of the vacuoles can be seen to be within the myelin sheaths. (Phosphotungstic acid/hematoxylin)

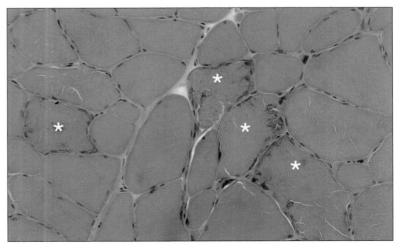

Fig. 24.16 'Ragged red' muscle fibers (asterisks) in KSS. (Modified Gomori trichrome preparation)

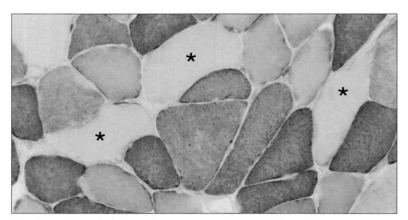

Fig. 24.17 Muscle biopsy in a patient with KSS. Many of the muscle fibres are deficient in cytochrome oxidase activity (asterisks).

MITOCHONDRIAL DNA DEPLETION SYNDROME

This syndrome is a rare, autosomally inherited disease associated with a depletion of mtDNA from some tissues of up to 98%. It presents in infancy or childhood with severe myopathy, liver failure, or nephropathy. Patients may show CNS lesions due to liver failure. In a personal case this syndrome was also associated with neuropathologic abnormalities resembling those in Leigh's disease (**Fig. 24.20**). The syndrome may be due to a deficiency of mitochondrial transcription factor A in some families.

Two other disorders associated with a depletion of mtDNA are:
• azidothymidine myopathy, in which there is a reduction of up to 70–80% in the amount of mtDNA
• inherited myopathy due to focal depletion of mitochondria.
In neither of these has CNS involvement been reported.

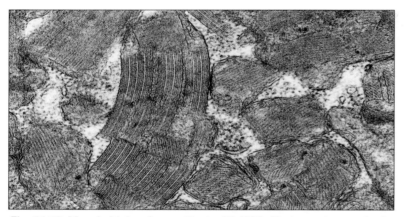

Fig. 24.18 Muscle biobsy in a patient with KSS. Electron micrograph of part of a muscle fibre with enlarged mitochondria containing paracrystalline inclusions.

MITOCHONDRIAL DNA BREAKAGE SYNDROME

This is a rare disorder with autosomal dominant transmission and characterized by accumulation of multiple deletions of mtDNA. Its pathogenesis is unknown. Clinical features include CPEO, proximal myopathy, dysphagia, cataracts, lactic acidosis, and early death.

MYONEUROGASTROINTESTINAL ENCEPHALOPATHY (MNGIE) SYNDROME

MNGIE is also known as polyneuropathy, ophthalmoplegia, leukoencephalopathy and intestinal pseudo-obstruction (POLIP). It is an uncommon syndrome and its main clinical features are encapsulated in the two acronyms by which it is usually known. Some cases are due to point mutations affecting mitochondrial tRNA genes, and a combination of MELAS and MNGIE has been described in association with an A-to-G transition at nucleotide 3243 in the mitochondrial tRNA$^{Leu(UUR)}$ gene. Other cases are associated with a progressive depletion of mtDNA and may be autosomal recessive disorders. Patients with the latter condition have diffusely abnormal white matter on MRI, but the histologic substrate of the abnormality is poorly documented.

The diagnosis of mitochondrial disorders

Important investigations

In many cases coming to autopsy the precise genetic abnormality will not have been determined. If a mitochondrial disorder is suspected it is advisable to:

• sample skeletal muscles for histology and, if possible, enzyme histochemistry and electron microscopy
• examine the heart, eyes, and peripheral nerves

Findings suggestive of mitochondrial disorder

The morphologic findings on examination of the CNS may suggest or indicate a mitochondrial disorder although without genetic analysis precise classification is often difficult. There is extensive overlap between the neuropathologic findings in different mitochondrial disorders. Features suggestive of a mitochondrial disorder include:

• intramyelinic edema or spongy vacuolation of white matter (but see also differential diagnosis on p. 25.5)
• extensive calcification in the basal ganglia or cerebral white matter, thalamus, dentate nucleus, and brain stem (but see chapter 1 and Fahr's disease on p. 22.6)
• neuronal loss and gliosis involving the dentate nucleus, inferior olives, striatum, and gracile and cuneate nuclei. Differential diagnoses include Friedreich's ataxia and other system degenerations (see chapters 27, 29, and 30)
• rarefaction and coarse vacuolation of gray matter with preservation of neurons, particularly in the striatum, brain stem, and dentate nucleus (see also Wernicke's encephalopathy on p. 21.1 and Leigh's disease on p. 6.12)

Fig. 24.19 The diagnosis of mitochondrial disorders.

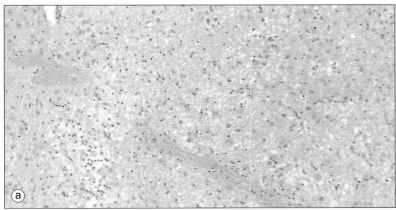

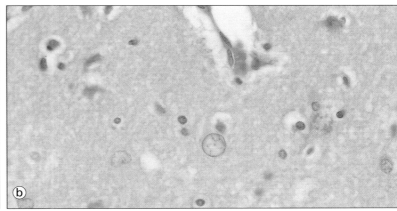

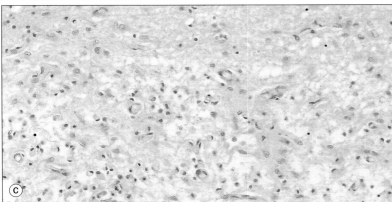

Fig. 24.20 CNS abnormalities in mtDNA depletion syndrome. (a) Coarse vacuolation and focal cavitation of the putamen. **(b)** Vascular proliferation within the vacuolated neuropil. **(c)** Scattered Alzheimer type II astrocytes, due to liver failure.

REFERENCES

De Vivo DC, DiMauro S. (1990) Mitochondrial encephalomyopathies. *International Pediatrics*; 5: 112–20.

DiMauro S, Moraes CT. (1993) Mitochondrial encephalomyopathies. *Archives of Neurology*; 50: 1197–208.

Harding AE, Sweeney MG, Miller DH, Mumford CJ, Kellarwood H, Menard D, McDonald WI, Compston DAS. (1992) Occurrence of a multiple sclerosis-like illness in women who have a Leber's hereditary optic neuropathy mitochondrial-DNA mutation. *Brain*; 115: 979–89.

Jun AS, Brown MD, Wallace DC. (1994) A mitochondrial DNA mutation at nucleotide pair 14459 of the NADH dehydrogenase subunit 6 gene associated with maternally inherited Leber hereditary optic neuropathy and dystonia. *Proc. Natl. Acad. Sci.* 91: 6206–6210.

Love S, Hilton DA (1996) Assessment of the distribution of mitochondrial ribosomal RNA in MELAS and in thrombotic cerebral infarcts by in situ hybridisation. *J. Pathol.* 178: 182–189.

Marsden CD, Lang AE, Quinn NP, McDonald WI, Abdallat A, Nimri S. Familial dystonia and visual failure with striatal CT lucencies. *J. Neurol. Neurosurg. Psychiat.* 49: 500–509.

Mito T, Tanaka T, Becker L E, Takashima S, Tanaka J. (1986) Infantile bilateral strialtal necrosis: clinicopathological classification. *Arch. Neurol.* 43: 677–680.

Sparaco M, Bonilla E, DiMauro S, Powers J. (1993) Neuropathology of mitochondrial encephalomyopathies due to mitochondrial DNA defects. *Journal of Neuropathology and Experimental Neurology* 52: 1–10.

Zeviani M, Antozzi C. (1992) Defects of mitochondrial DNA. *Brain Pathology*; 2: 121–32.

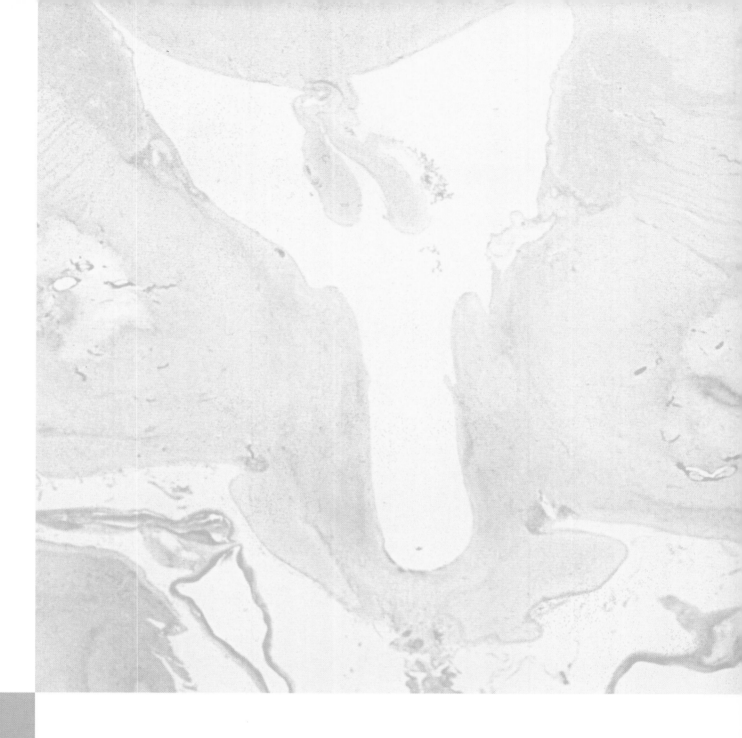

8 Toxic Injury

25 Toxic injury of the CNS

Toxin-induced injuries of the central nervous system (CNS) are an increasing clinical problem. Contributing factors include:
- The ubiquity of industrial waste and the cost and difficulties in disposing of it.
- The continued development of novel chemical compounds and their growing use for therapeutic and recreational purposes.

This chapter covers toxins that are known to produce lesions of the CNS. Some of them also cause peripheral neuropathy, but this will be mentioned only briefly.

METAL TOXICITY IN THE CNS

ALUMINUM TOXICITY

Aluminum toxicity is most common in patients undergoing chronic hemodialysis and is due to high concentrations of aluminum in water used for the dialysis. It manifests clinically as dialysis encephalopathy syndrome, which is characterized by a combined dysarthria and apraxia of speech, myoclonus, gait disturbance, focal seizures, and dementia.

MACROSCOPIC AND MICROSCOPIC APPEARANCES

In most cases, the brain appears macroscopically normal and scant abnormalities (mild cortical gliosis, slight prominence of microglia) are demonstrable by conventional staining. Use of appropriate silver impregnation techniques reveals argyrophilic material containing aluminum in the choroid epithelium and to a lesser extent in the glia and neurons, particularly in the brain stem nuclei.

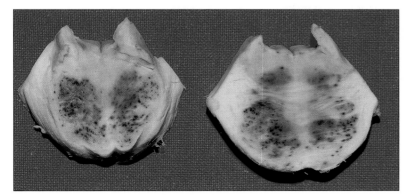

Fig. 25.1 Acute hemorrhagic encephalopathy complicating melarsoprol treatment. Petechial hemorrhages and surrounding gray discoloration in the pons. This patient developed acute hemorrhagic leukoencephalopathy as a reaction to melarsoprol treatment. (Courtesy of Professor Hume Adams)

ARSENIC TOXICITY

ARSENIC EXPOSURE

- Arsenicals are rapidly absorbed from mucous membranes or through the skin, but do not cross the blood–brain barrier into the CNS to any significant extent.
- Trivalent arsenicals have often been associated with deliberate poisoning. The arsenic interferes with pyruvate decarboxylation by binding to the sulfhydryl groups of the cofactor, lipoic acid, resulting in gastrointestinal, cardiac, and cutaneous disturbances. Chronic intoxication causes a distal peripheral axonal neuropathy, probably reflecting the permeability of blood vessels in the dorsal root ganglia. It does not cause a specific encephalopathy.
- Organic pentavalent arsenicals are present in some drugs used to treat trypanosomiasis, and are used in insecticides and weed killers. Ingestion may produce an acute hemorrhagic leukoencephalopathy, which is thought to be an immune reaction to the organic compound rather than a direct toxic effect of the arsenic. Approximately 2–5% of patients with trypanosomiasis who are treated with melarsoprol develops acute hemorrhagic leukoencephalopathy (see chapter 20).

MACROSCOPIC AND MICROSCOPIC APPEARANCES

The peripheral neuropathy associated with chronic trivalent arsenical intoxication may be associated with chromatolysis and loss of anterior horn cells. In patients with acute hemorrhagic leukoencepalopathy complicating organic pentavalent arsenical administration, the brain is swollen and contains numerous small and occasional larger foci of hemorrhage (**Fig. 25.1**). Histology reveals fibrinoid necrosis of many parenchymal blood vessels and hemorrhage into the surrounding tissue (**Fig. 25.2**). Some of the blood vessels are surrounded by a fibrin exudate containing a mixed inflammatory infiltrate. The findings are described in more detail in chapter 20.

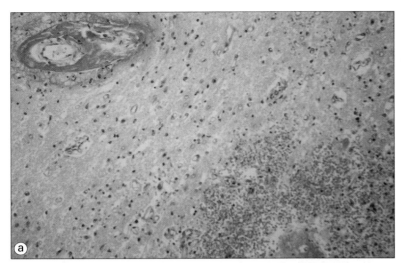

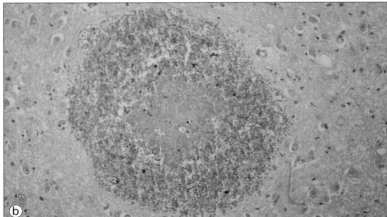

Fig. 25.2 Acute hemorrhagic encephalopathy complicating melarsoprol treatment. (a) and **(b)** Histology reveals fibrinoid necrosis of blood vessels and hemorrhage into the surrounding white matter.

BISMUTH TOXICITY

BISMUTH EXPOSURE

- Bismuth encephalopathy is usually caused by excessive intake of inorganic salts. These are used for some chronic gastrointestinal disorders, including the treatment of *Helicobacter pylori* infection.
- Toxicity has also occurred following bismuth absorption from BIPP (bismuth iodoform paraffin paste), which is used for surgical dressings.

BISMUTH TOXICITY

- Patients develop anxiety, depression, and insomnia, progressing in some cases to confusion, myoclonic jerks, dysarthria, and gait disturbance.
- The symptoms resolve after withdrawing the bismuth, but continued exposure can cause coma and death.
- The manifestations may simulate Creutzfeldt–Jakob disease.

MACROSCOPIC AND MICROSCOPIC APPEARANCES

Descriptions of the neuropathologic findings of bismuth toxicity are sparse. Most of the described abnormalities such as a loss of Purkinje cells and degeneration of pyramidal cells in the hippocampus are probably due to hypoxia.

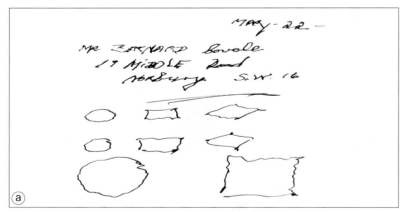

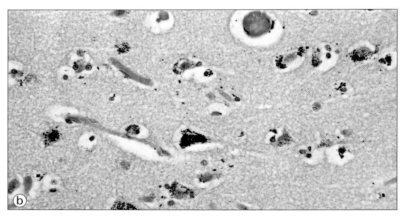

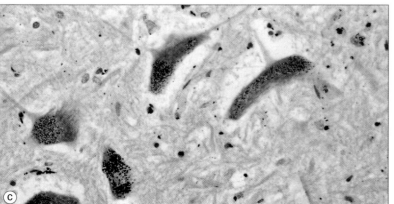

Fig. 25.3 Mercury poisoning. (a) Examples of the handwriting and drawing of a patient who 16 years previously had worked for about 18 months filling mercury thermometers and had developed metallic mercury poisoning. **(b)** Demonstration of intralysosomal mercury in the cerebral cortex. **(c)** Demonstration of intralysosomal mercury in spinal motor neurons. (b) and (c) Silver precipitation method of Danscher and Schroeder, see *Histochemistry* (1979) **60**: 1–7.

LEAD TOXICITY

LEAD EXPOSURE

Inorganic lead intoxication
- Common sources of inorganic lead include lead paint, pottery with lead glazes, herbal and traditional medicines or cosmetics, discarded car batteries, soft water collected in leaded conduits or containers, and alcohol and illicit drugs distilled using lead pipes.
- The lead is absorbed through the gastrointestinal and respiratory tracts.
- Motor vehicle emissions may contribute to chronic low-level toxicity in some communities.

Organic lead intoxication
- The main source of organic lead is the tetraethyl lead used as an anti-knock agent in gasoline (petrol).
- Exposure may be occupational or a consequence of deliberate sniffing of petrol fumes to induce euphoria.

LEAD INTOXICATION

Inorganic lead intoxication
- This can cause encephalopathy, peripheral neuropathy, or both, with encephalopathy being a common manifestation in children.
- Acute encephalopathy produces symptoms of increased intracranial pressure and may simulate a posterior fossa mass lesion or acute hydrocephalus. The encephalopathy responds to removal of the source of lead, and the administration of chelating agents, but there may be long-term intellectual and motor impairment.
- Intoxication can manifest more insidiously in adults and produce lethargy, abdominal cramps, weight loss, a predominantly motor mononeuropathy, seizures, and psychiatric disturbances.
- Adverse effects on cognitive and motor skills have been noted after chronic low-level exposure.
- Other abnormalities include basophilic stippling of red blood cells and 'lead lines' in radiographs (due to skeletal lead deposition).

Organic lead intoxication
- This produces headache, insomnia, confusion, delirium, hallucinations, and a variety of extrapyramidal movement disorders.
- The intoxication usually responds to sedation and chelation therapy, but can lead to permanent damage.

MACROSCOPIC AND MICROSCOPIC APPEARANCES

The macroscopic appearances are brain swelling and congestion, and in some cases petechial hemorrhages or hydrocephalus.

Microscopically, the endothelial cells appear swollen, and capillary necrosis or thrombosis has been reported. There is a proteinaceous exudate in the perivascular spaces extending into the adjacent brain tissue. Periodic acid–Schiff (PAS) positive globules may be seen within the exudate and in astrocytes. Other findings include widespread gliosis, and, in some cases, foci of necrosis or spongiosis.

MANGANESE TOXICITY

MANGANESE EXPOSURE

- This may result from inhaling dust in manganese mines, or vapor released during ferromanganese smelting or the production of chlorine gas, storage batteries, paints, varnish, and enamel.
- Manganese toxicity has also been reported in agricultural workers exposed to the fungicide maneb (manganese-ethylene-bisdithiocarbamate) and in patients who have taken certain Chinese herbal medicines.

Clinical manifestations include extrapyramidal movement disorders that may resemble Parkinson's disease, transient psychiatric disturbances, and intellectual impairment.

MACROSCOPIC AND MICROSCOPIC APPEARANCES

In contrast to idiopathic Parkinson's disease (see p. 28.1), the substantia nigra is preserved, but there is gliosis and a loss of neurons from the pallidum and subthalamic nucleus and, to a lesser extent, from the caudate and putamen.

MERCURY TOXICITY

MERCURY EXPOSURE

Both inorganic and organic mercury are potentially toxic.
- Inorganic mercury is a waste product of paper manufacture and chloralkali production. Metallic mercury is volatile at room temperature and symptoms of neurotoxicity may develop after inhaling the vapor.
- Organic mercury intoxication is usually caused by ingestion of contaminated food such as bread made from grain treated with an organic mercury fungicide, and fish. Fish contaminated by factory effluent caused a disastrous outbreak of poisoning in Japan in 1900. Some microorganisms in the water can convert inorganic mercury salts into methylmercury, which then accumulates in fish.
- Upon ingestion of the contaminated bread or fish, methylmercury is absorbed and readily enters the CNS, where it is mostly transformed into inorganic mercury.
- Mercury probably produces its toxic effects by combining with sulfhydryl groups and interfering with protein synthesis. The consequences are most devastating during embryogenesis.

MERCURY TOXICITY

- Acute toxicity, can produce a range of symptoms including hypersalivation, abdominal cramps, diarrhea, and halitosis which is often described as 'metallic'. Headache, tiredness, and emotional and psychiatric disturbances may be early manifestations. Other symptoms include tremor (**Fig. 25.3a**), ataxia, vertigo, nystagmus, choreoathetosis, weakness, blurred vision with constricted visual fields, and a sensory neuropathy.
- Chronic exposure can cause mental retardation, cortical blindness, and quadriplegia.
- Exposure *in utero* causes profound psychomotor retardation.

MACROSCOPIC APPEARANCES

There are no reports of macroscopic abnormalities in the brain following exposure to inorganic mercury. Survivors of methylmercury intoxication develop moderate to marked brain atrophy, particularly of the calcarine cortex and cerebellum.

MICROSCOPIC APPEARANCES

There is a preferential loss of small neurons, particularly of the granule cell layer of the cerebellum and the primary visual, auditory, and somatosensory regions of the cerebral cortex, in which small neurons predominate. In severe cases, particularly in children, neuronal loss is more extensive and there is spongiform cortical degeneration. Other features include an associated gliosis and, in acute lesions, infiltration by macrophages. Degeneration of dorsal root ganglion cells results in some loss of nerve fibers from the posterior columns of the spinal cord. Sprouting of Purkinje cell dendrites is a prominent feature in long-term survivors, in whom granular deposits of mercury are demonstrable in astrocytes, microglia, and neurons (**Fig. 25.3b,c**).

Fetal intoxication can cause neuronal heterotopia and cortical dysplasia in addition to degenerative lesions.

THALLIUM TOXICITY

Most cases of thallium intoxication result from accidental or deliberate ingestion of thallium-containing pesticides or rodenticides. The clinical picture resembles that of trivalent arsenical poisoning. The only consistent abnormalities in the CNS are those related to the sensorimotor distal axonopathy, which are:
- chromatolysis of motor neurons (**Fig. 25.4a**)
- degeneration of posterior column fibers (**Fig. 25.4b**)

TIN TOXICITY

ORGANIC TIN EXPOSURE

Inorganic tin is not neurotoxic, but two organotin compounds, triethyltin and trimethyltin, are:
- Triethyltin poisoning occurred in France in patients who used Stalinon to treat furunculosis.
- Trimethyltin is generated during the production of dimethyltin dichloride, which is used in the manufacture of plastic and for strengthening glass. Trimethyltin intoxication has occurred as a result of occupational exposure.

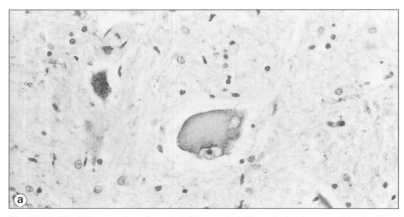

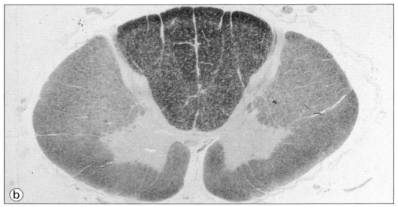

Fig. 25.4 Thallium poisoning. (a) Chromatolytic anterior horn cell in thallium poisoning. (Cresyl violet) **(b)** Degenerating posterior column fibers in a case of thallium poisoning. (Marchi preparation) (Both illustrations courtesy of Professor John Cavanagh)

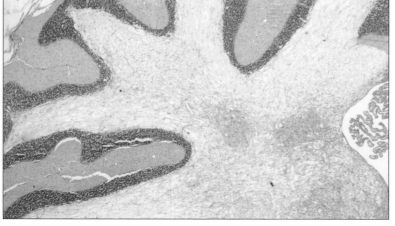

Fig. 25.5 Triethyltin intoxication. Widespread vacuolation of the cerebellar white matter in experimental triethyltin intoxication. (Courtesy of Professor John Cavanagh)

ORGANOTIN TOXICITY

- Triethyltin poisoning causes signs and symptoms of raised intracranial pressure and flaccid paraparesis.
- Trimethyltin poisoning causes confusion, confabulation, and amnesia.

MACROSCOPIC AND MICROSCOPIC APPEARANCES

Triethyltin causes striking white matter edema (**Fig. 25.5**) due to the accumulation of fluid in vacuoles within the myelin sheaths (**Fig. 25.6**). The vacuoles are formed by separation of myelin along intraperiod lines (**Fig. 25.7**). Trimethyltin does not cause intramyelinic edema, but is toxic to neurons in the hippocampus, entorhinal cortex, and amygdala.

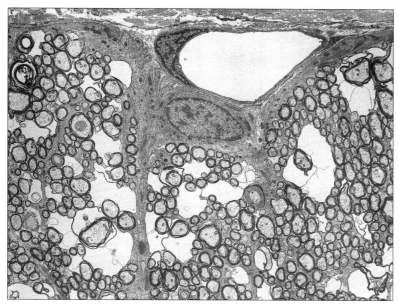

Fig. 25.6 Experimental triethyltin intoxication. Electron microscopy reveals accumulations of fluid within the myelin sheaths. (Courtesy of Professor John Cavanagh)

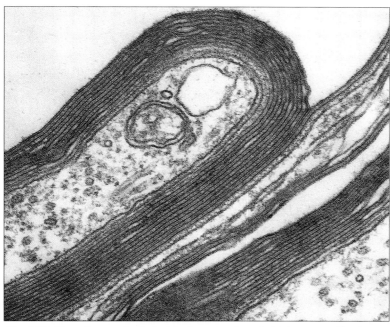

Fig. 25.7 Experimental triethyltin intoxication. At higher magnification, the myelin is seen to have separated along intraperiod lines. (Courtesy of Professor John Cavanagh)

CAUSES OF INTRAMYELINIC EDEMA

Toxic causes

- hexachlorophane/hexachlorophene
- triethyltin
- 5-fluorouracil, tegofur, and carmofur
- lithium

Nutritional deficiencies

- subacute combined degeneration (vitamin B_{12} deficiency)

Metabolic causes

- mitochondrial encephalopathies
- Canavan's disease (aspartoacylase deficiency)
- several other disorders of amino acid metabolism

Infective causes

- vacuolar myelopathy in HIV infection
- HTLV-1-associated myelopathy (HAM)

CNS TOXICITY DUE TO OTHER INDUSTRIAL AND ENVIRONMENTAL CHEMICALS

ACRYLAMIDE TOXICITY

Acrylamide polymers are widely used in industry as flexible sealants and grouting agents. Although the polymers are non-toxic, the acrylamide monomer from which they are formed is a potent neurotoxin. Prolonged low-level exposure causes peripheral neuropathy. Heavier exposure can cause tremor, ataxia, dysarthria, and mental disturbances.

CAUSES OF DISTAL DEGENERATION OF LONG AXONS IN THE CNS

Toxic causes

- acrylamide (the distal axonal swellings contain accumulations of neurofilaments)
- carbon disulfide
- cisplatinum (involves posterior columns only)
- clioquinol
- hexacarbon solvents (*n*-hexane and methyl *n*-butyl ketone)
- organophosphorus (in the early stages distal axonal swellings contain accumulations of smooth endoplasmic reticulum)
- thallium
- neurolathyrism (involves corticospinal tracts only)

System degenerations

- motor neuron disease
- familial spastic paraplegia
- Friedreich's ataxia

Nutritional deficiencies

- vitamin E deficiency
- pellagra (which is also associated with chromatolysis of Betz cells, neurons in the brain stem, and anterior horn cells in the spinal cord)
- subacute combined degeneration due to vitamin B_{12} deficiency (in which the axonal degeneration is secondary to the myelinopathy)

MACROSCOPIC AND MICROSCOPIC APPEARANCES

The brain and spinal cord appear macroscopically normal. Histology reveals swelling and degeneration of the distal part of longer axons in peripheral nerves and the posterior spinal, spinocerebellar, and corticospinal tracts. The swellings contain accumulations of neurofilaments.

CARBON DISULFIDE

CARBON DISULFIDE EXPOSURE

- Carbon disulfide is used in the manufacture of viscose, rayon, cellophane, and adhesives, and can be absorbed by inhalation or skin contact.
- Experimental studies have shown that, like the hexacarbon solvents (see below), carbon disulfide causes cross-linking of proteins, including neurofilaments.

CARBON DISULFIDE TOXICITY

- Chronic exposure results in fatigue, headache, intellectual impairment, peripheral and cranial neuropathy, and altered lipid metabolism (leading to increased atheroma and predisposing to cardiovascular disease).
- Acute intoxification can cause agitation, psychosis, and delirium.

CARBON TETRACHLORIDE TOXICITY

CARBON TETRACHLORIDE EXPOSURE

- Carbon tetrachloride (tetrachlormethane) is used in the manufacture of refrigerants and aerosols, as a dry-cleaning fluid, and as a component in fire extinguishers, insecticides, and shampoos.
- Acute intoxication has resulted from inhaling carbon tetrachloride, and from swallowing it in shampoo.

CARBON TETRACHLORIDE (TETRACHLORMETHANE) TOXICITY

- Headaches, drowsiness, abdominal pain, nausea, vomiting, and diarrhea are presenting symptoms.
- Vertigo, gait ataxia, confusion, lethargy, seizures, and coma follow severe intoxication.
- Optic neuritis is an occasional complication.
- Patients may recover from the acute neurologic manifestations, only to develop hepatic and renal toxicity.
- Mental confusion, polyneuritis, and parkinsonism have been reported in patients with chronic exposure to carbon tetrachloride.

MACROSCOPIC AND MICROSCOPIC APPEARANCES

The brain and spinal cord appear macroscopically normal, and histologic changes are sparsely documented. In the peripheral nervous system, carbon disulfide intoxication results in axonal swellings (**Fig. 25.8**), which contain abnormal accumulations of neurofilaments, and distal nerve fiber degeneration. Described CNS abnormalities include distal axonal spinocerebellar degeneration and increased cerebral atherosclerosis. Spinal long tracts contain neurofilamentous axonal swellings (**Fig. 25.9**). The distal axonopathy is probably secondary to progressive cross-linking and accumulation of neurofilaments during their anterograde transport in long axons.

MACROSCOPIC AND MICROSCOPIC APPEARANCES

Published descriptions of the pathologic features of carbon tetrachloride toxicity are scarce. Brain edema, hemorrhages, focal vascular necrosis, venous thromboses, and hemorrhagic infarcts have been reported.

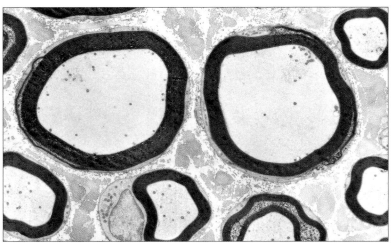

Fig. 25.8 Experimental carbon disulfide intoxication. Ultrathin section of peripheral nerve showing distension of axons by neurofilaments in experimental carbon disulfide intoxication. (Courtesy of Professor John Cavanagh)

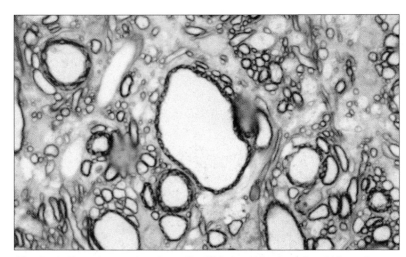

Fig. 25.9 Experimental carbon disulfide intoxication. Semithin resin-embedded section showing swollen CNS axons in experimental carbon disulfide intoxication. (Courtesy of Professor John Cavanagh)

ETHYLENE GLYCOL TOXICITY

ETHYLENE GLYCOL EXPOSURE

- Ethylene glycol is extensively used as a solvent, and an antifreeze in automobile and aeroplane coolants.
- Intoxication is usually caused by its ingestion as an inebriant.
- Hepatic and renal oxidation produces several toxic metabolites, including glycoaldehyde, glycolic acid, glyoxylic acid, and oxalic acid.

ETHYLENE GLYCOL TOXICITY

- Patients show agitation, ataxia, and drowsiness, progressing to stupor and coma.
- Metabolic acidosis is usually severe.
- Later complications are cardiorespiratory and renal failure.
- Oxalic acid crystals can be detected in the urine.

MACROSCOPIC AND MICROSCOPIC APPEARANCES

Acute intoxication produces meningeal congestion and cerebral edema, and, occasionally, petechial hemorrhages. Microscopically, birefringent calcium oxalate deposits can usually be demonstrated by polarized light microscopy (**Figs 25.10, 25.11**) in and around vessels in the meninges, brain parenchyma, and choroid plexus. Neurons may show hypoxic change and there is often white matter edema. Scanty perivascular acute inflammatory infiltrates may be seen (see Fig. 25.12), but these are not consistently related to the calcium oxalate deposits and may be a reaction to hypoxic brain injury.

ETHYLENE OXIDE TOXICITY

This gas is used in the production of various industrial chemicals and to sterilize heat-sensitive medical supplies. Chronic exposure can cause peripheral sensorimotor neuropathy, cognitive impairment, dysarthria, and parkinsonism, but neuropathologic data on intoxication are lacking.

HEXACARBON SOLVENT (*n*-HEXANE AND METHYL *n*-BUTYL KETONE) TOXICITY

n-HEXANE AND METHYL *n*-BUTYL KETONE EXPOSURE

- These hexacarbons are used as paint, varnish, and glue solvents.
- Exposure can occur in a wide range of industries. Intoxication was until recently a particular occupational hazard of shoe-making, which used glues containing hexacarbon solvents.
- Both *n*-hexane and methyl *n*-butyl ketone are converted to 2,5-hexanediol, which causes cross-linking of neurofilaments and other proteins, at lysine moieties.

HEXACARBON SOLVENT TOXICITY

- Chronic exposure produces a sensorimotor peripheral neuropathy and, in severe cases, symptoms of CNS disease (i.e. dysarthria, ataxia of gait, blurred vision).
- Lower limb spasticity may become evident after recovery from the peripheral neuropathy.

MACROSCOPIC AND MICROSCOPIC APPEARANCES

The brain and spinal cord appear macroscopically normal. Histologic changes in the human CNS are sparsely documented, but there are many experimental studies demonstrating the formation of neurofilamentous axonal swellings (**Fig. 25.12**) and distal degeneration of nerve fibers in long ascending (spinocerebellar and posterior column) and descending (corticospinal) spinal tracts, as occur in the peripheral nerves. As in carbon disulfide intoxication, the changes are probably due to progressive cross-linking and accumulation of neurofilaments during their anterograde transport.

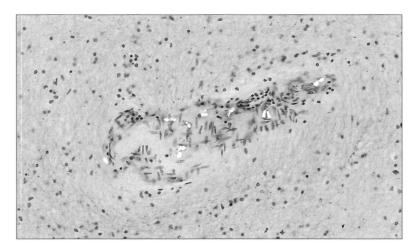

Fig. 25.10 Ethylene glycol poisoning. Birefringent calcium oxalate deposits (arrows) associated with ethylene glycol poisoning. Viewed under polarized light.

Fig. 25.11 Ethylene glycol poisoning. Scanty perivascular inflammation and birefringent calcium oxalate deposits in ethylene glycol poisoning. Viewed under polarized light. The surrounding white matter is edematous. (Luxol fast blue/cresyl violet)

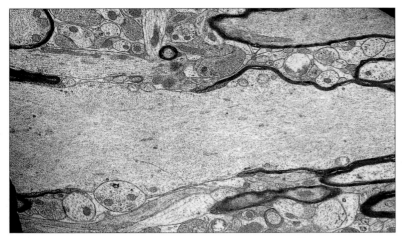

Fig. 25.12 Experimental 2,5-hexanediol intoxication. Electron micrograph showing marked neurofilamentous distension of an axon at a node of Ranvier. (Courtesy of Professor John Cavanagh)

METHANOL TOXICITY

METHANOL EXPOSURE

- Methanol (methyl alcohol) is widely used as a solvent.
- Poisoning is usually a consequence of its ingestion as a cheap inebriant or an adulterant of liquor.
- Methanol toxicity is believed to be due to the formaldehyde and formic acid that are produced when it is oxidized in the liver.

METHANOL TOXICITY

- The manifestations of acute toxicity are delayed for several hours, until after the methanol has been metabolized to form formaldehyde and formic acid.
- Patients develop headache, abdominal pain, nausea, vomiting, and generalized weakness.
- Loss of vision is a common, usually permanent, complication.
- Severe intoxication may cause delirium, convulsions, coma, cardiorespiratory failure, and death.

MACROSCOPIC AND MICROSCOPIC APPEARANCES

In acute methanol intoxication the brain is usually edematous and shows features of global hypoxic injury (see chapter 8). There may be scattered petechial hemorrhages and larger, symmetric foci of hemorrhagic infarction in the putamen and claustrum (**Fig. 25.13**). Residual foci of cavitation and yellow discoloration are present in longer-term survivors (**Figs 25.14, 25.15**). Some patients develop extensive white matter necrosis. Degeneration of retinal ganglion cells results in optic nerve atrophy and gliosis.

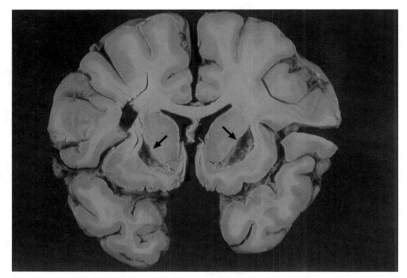

Fig. 25.13 Methanol toxicity. Bilateral cavitation (arrows) of medial part of putamen and anterior fibers of internal capsule in methanol poisoning. (The cavitation of the left centrum semiovale is artefactual.)

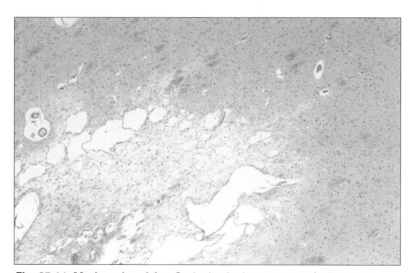

Fig. 25.14 Methanol toxicity. Cavitation in the putamen of a long-term survivor of methanol poisoning.

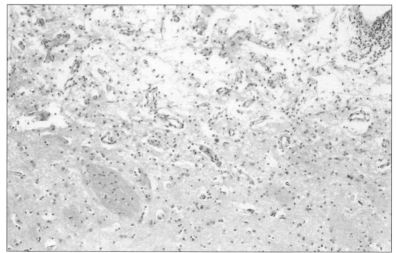

Fig. 25.15 Methanol poisoning. Higher magnification view of the cavitated putamen, which contains scattered macrophages and shows some neovascularization.

ORGANOPHOSPHATE TOXICITY

ORGANOPHOSPHATE EXPOSURE

- These chemicals are powerful inhibitors of acetylcholinesterase.
- Alkyl organophosphates in insecticides are responsible for most cases of poisoning, and exposure may occur during manufacture, mixing, or spraying.
- There are several reports of deliberate suicidal ingestion of concentrated insecticide.
- Poisoning has also followed adulteration of cooking oil or alcohol with aryl organophosphates, most notoriously in 1930, when thousands of Americans were poisoned by an illicit extract of Jamaica ginger ('jake'), which was used to circumvent the prohibition laws and contained triorthocresyl phosphate.

ORGANOPHOSPHATE TOXICITY

- Acute anticholinesterase effects consist of headache, abdominal pain, vomiting, sweating, miosis, and muscular twitching.
- 1–3 days after recovery from the acute effects, a small proportion of patients develops an intermediate syndrome of proximal limb, neck flexor, respiratory weakness and paralysis, and cranial motor nerve palsies.
- After 1–3 weeks, some patients develop a predominantly motor axonal neuropathy. As the nerve fibers regenerate and the peripheral neuropathy slowly resolves, a chronic myelopathy with spasticity and brisk tendon reflexes may develop.

MACROSCOPIC AND MICROSCOPIC APPEARANCES

The brain and spinal cord appear macroscopically normal. Histology reveals swelling and degeneration of the distal part of longer axons, particularly in peripheral nerves, but also in the posterior spinal, corticospinal, and spinocerebellar tracts.

N-3-PYRIDYLMETHYL-*N'*-P-NITROPHENYL UREA (PNU) TOXICITY

PNU is the active component of the rodenticide, Vacor. It is chemically and toxicologically similar to alloxan and streptozotocin, which are both toxic to β cells in the pancreatic islets. Acute features of intoxication are hypoglycemia, vomiting, lethargy, and seizures. Survivors may develop a sensory and autonomic neuropathy and an encephalopathy. There is a lack of neuropathologic data on PNU intoxication.

TOLUENE TOXICITY

TOLUENE EXPOSURE

- Toluene is widely used as a solvent in paints, varnishes, thinners, dyes, and glues, and as a constituent of motor and aviation fuels.
- Toluene is also used in histology laboratories.
- Toluene is volatile and readily absorbed through the respiratory tract.

TOLUENE TOXICITY

- Excessive exposure causes dizziness, exhilaration, confusion, ataxia, and dizziness.
- Severe intoxication, which is usually intentional and caused by glue sniffing with the head in a plastic bag, can cause psychotic behavior, unconsciousness, and death.
- Patients exposed repeatedly to toluene may develop tremulousness, unsteadiness, emotional lability, and insomnia.
- Persistent cerebellar ataxia, visual, cognitive and motor abnormalities, and peripheral neuropathy have also been reported.

MACROSCOPIC AND MICROSCOPIC APPEARANCES

Cerebellar atrophy has been demonstrated by computerized tomography and an increase in the water content of white matter is suggested by some findings on magnetic resonance imaging. No information is available about the pathologic substrate of these abnormalities.

TOXIC OIL SYNDROME AND EOSINOPHILIA–MYALGIA SYNDROME

ETIOLOGY OF TOXIC OIL SYNDROME AND EOSINOPHILIA–MYALGIA SYNDROME

- These two syndromes have virtually identical clinical and pathologic features and are probably etiologically related.
- The toxic oil syndrome affected more than 20,000 people and was caused by the ingestion of aniline-denatured rape seed cooking oil in Spain in 1981.
- Eosinophilia–myalgia syndrome affected over 1500 people and resulted from the ingestion of impure preparations of L-tryptophan, in the United States in late 1989 and early 1990. (L-tryptophan is used to treat a variety of disorders including mild depressive illness and premenstrual syndrome.)
- Recent studies suggest that contaminating aniline derivatives were responsible for both syndromes.

TOXIC OIL SYNDROME AND EOSINOPHILIA–MYALGIA SYNDROME

The clinical presentation is biphasic.
- The acute manifestations are fever, headache, pruritic or tender rashes, and dyspnea, associated with systemic hypereosinophilia. Death has occurred in a few cases, due to respiratory failure or thromboembolic disease.
- The second phase commences 3–6 weeks later and is characterized by paresthesiae and dysesthesiae, sensory loss, myalgias, weakness, scleroderma-like rashes, and severe weight loss. Occasionally, patients have developed an encephalopathy with impaired memory and cognition, focal deficits, or signs of increased intracranial pressure.

MACROSCOPIC AND MICROSCOPIC APPEARANCES

No macroscopic changes have been reported. Striking inflammatory and vasculitic abnormalities affect peripheral nerves and skeletal muscle, but tend to spare the CNS. Large neurons in the spinal cord and brain stem may be chromatolytic or, in some cases, vacuolated and distended by argyrophilic masses composed of neurofilaments.

TRICHLORETHYLENE (TCE) TOXICITY

TCE is an organic solvent used for dry cleaning, degreasing metal parts, extracting oils and fats from vegetable products, and in leather adhesives. It has also been used as a general anesthetic. Toxicity may result from chronic occupational exposure or deliberate inhalation of TCE for its euphoric effects. The earliest manifestation of toxicity is trigeminal neuropathy, and facial nerve palsy and other cranial and peripheral neuropathies may occur.

Neuropathologic features are axonal degeneration in the affected cranial nerves associated with a loss of neurons from the corresponding brain stem nuclei.

TOXIC GASES

CARBON MONOXIDE

CARBON MONOXIDE EXPOSURE

- Carbon monoxide is a colorless and odorless gas produced by incomplete combustion of carbon fuels. It is a relatively common cause of fatal poisoning, either accidental (e.g. due to inadequate venting of fumes from domestic gas heaters) or suicidal (e.g. due to inhalation of automobile exhaust fumes).
- Carbon monoxide prevents the binding of oxygen to hemoglobin by competing for the same binding site with 200-fold greater affinity to form carboxyhemoglobin. It also interferes with the release of oxygen from oxyhemoglobin. Both actions impair tissue oxygenation. Further toxicity may result from the interaction of carbon monoxide with other heme-containing proteins such as myoglobin, cytochromes, catalases, and peroxidases.

CARBON MONOXIDE TOXICITY

- The clinical manifestations depend on the concentration of carboxyhemoglobin in the blood. This is influenced by the duration of exposure and the concentration of carbon monoxide in the environment.
- Symptoms range from headache and dizziness, through nausea, confusion, and visual disturbances, to convulsions, coma, and death.
- Survivors may experience a persistent tremor, psychiatric disturbances, and intellectual impairment, in some cases after an initial clinical recovery.

MACROSCOPIC APPEARANCES

During the first few hours, the brain is swollen, congested, and cherry-red in color, though this is less striking after prolonged formalin fixation. After 24–48 hours of survival, scattered petechial hemorrhages may be seen in the white matter and larger hemorrhages in the pallidum (**Fig. 25.16**). These usually involve the dorsal part of the inner segment of the pallidum, but may extend laterally into the outer segment or dorsomedially into the internal capsule. The pallidal lesions are often asymmetric (**Fig. 25.17**) and may be unilateral or absent. In some cases there are hemorrhages in the hippocampus and cerebral cortex. Following survival of several days or weeks, the lesions in the pallidum appear necrotic or cavitated (**Fig. 25.17**). Discrete or confluent foci of necrosis may also be evident in the white matter (**Figs 25.18, 25.19**, see also Fig 25.17). These tend to spare the arcuate fibers (see Fig. 25.19).

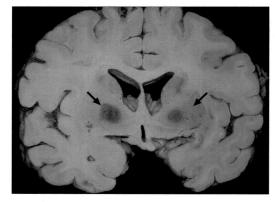

Fig. 25.16 Acute carbon monoxide poisoning. Hemorrhagic discoloration (arrows) of the pallidum in carbon monoxide poisoning. The dorsal part of the nucleus is most severely affected.

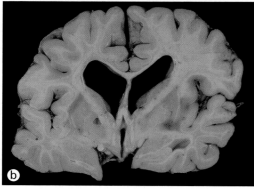
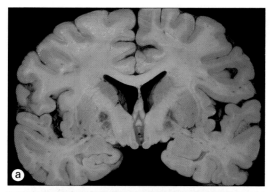

Fig. 25.17 Sequelae of carbon monoxide poisoning. Cavitation of the dorsomedial part of the pallidum in survivors of acute carbon monoxide poisoning. **(a)** Symmetric cavitation. **(b)** Asymmetric cavitation. Note the gray discoloration of the cerebral white matter and thinning of the corpus callosum.

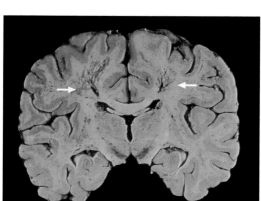

Fig. 25.18 White matter necrosis due to carbon monoxide poisoning. Cavitated necrosis (arrows) in the cerebral white matter in a survivor of acute carbon monoxide poisoning.

Although pallidal necrosis is typical of delayed death from carbon monoxide poisoning, it is not unique to this condition and can occur in other hypoxic states, methanol toxicity (see page 25.8), or cyanide toxicity (see below).

MICROSCOPIC APPEARANCES

In the acute stage there may be foci of necrosis and/or perivascular hemorrhage in the affected parts of the gray and white matter. Within days, these foci accumulate numerous lipid- or hemosiderin-laden macrophages. Lesions in longer-term survivors are cavitated (**Fig. 25.20**) or rarefied and gliotic. Typical changes of global brain hypoxia-ischemia of varying severity (see chapter 8) are usually seen. The white matter lesions may be small and discrete, extensive, or even confluent. In some cases there is a loss of myelin, but relative preservation of axons in the deep white matter. This pattern tends to be associated with a delayed clinical deterioration. Arcuate fibers are usually spared (**Fig. 25.21**).

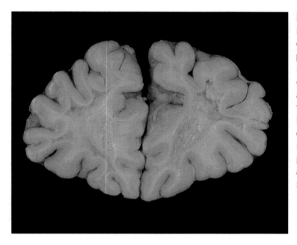

Fig. 25.19 White matter lesions in carbon monoxide poisoning. White matter with a gelatinous gray appearance and focal cavitation in a long-term survivor of carbon monoxide poisoning. The arcuate fibers are spared.

CAUSES OF BILATERAL BASAL GANGLIA NECROSIS

Toxic or hypoxic injury

- carbon monoxide
- cyanide
- methanol
- Marchiafava–Bignami disease (usually associated with chronic alcoholism)
- heroin and other causes of global cerebral hypoxia

Metabolic disorders

- Leigh's disease (see chapters 6 and 24)
- infantile bilateral striatal necrosis (see chapter 24)
- mitochondrial myopathy, encephalopathy, lactic acidosis, and stroke-like episodes (MELAS) and other mitochondrial disorders (see chapter 24)
- Wilson's disease (see chapter 22)

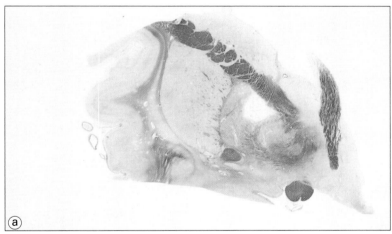

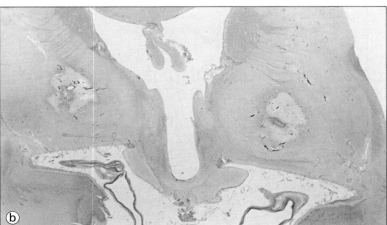

Fig. 25.20 Histology of the globus pallidus in survivors of acute carbon monoxide poisoning. (a) Cavitation confined to the dorsomedial part of the globus pallidus. (Luxol fast blue/cresyl violet) **(b)** More extensive bilateral pallidal cavitation.

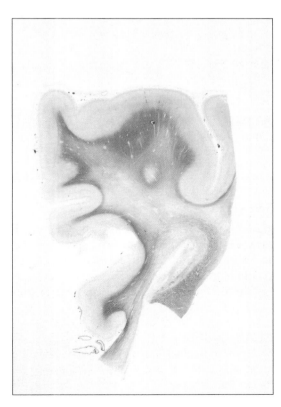

Fig. 25.21 Extensive loss of myelinated fibers caused by carbon monoxide poisoning. Note the sparing of the subcortical arcuate fibers. (Luxol fast blue/cresyl violet)

CYANIDE TOXICITY

CYANIDE EXPOSURE

- Cyanide binds strongly to the trivalent iron in cytochrome oxidase, thereby preventing oxidative phosphorylation. Because the cells are therefore unable to use oxygen, this type of toxicity has been termed cytotoxic hypoxia.
- Potassium cyanide, sodium cyanide, and hydrocyanic acid have all been used as suicidal or homicidal agents.
- Industrial exposure can occur during electroplating and gold or silver ore extraction.
- Domestic poisoning has been caused by ingesting acetonitrile-containing false-nail removers, also metal-cleaning solutions.
- Hydrogen cyanide is released from many building materials and furnishings during fires.
- Cyanide intoxication has also resulted from prolonged administration of sodium nitroprusside to control hypertension and from the ingestion of cyanogenic glycosides including amygdalin (Laetrile) and cassava derivatives (cassava is the tuberous root of the shrub-like plant *Manioc palmata*).
- Cassava-induced cyanide toxicity and malnutrition may both contribute to the development of ataxic polyneuropathy in Nigeria and some other parts of Africa.

CYANIDE TOXICITY

- Acute intoxication due to inhalation of cyanide causes death within minutes.
- Oral intake of cyanide causes hyperventilation and agitation, followed by headache, nausea, and vertigo. These symptoms are usually followed by profound dyspnea, convulsions, coma, and death within hours.
- Survivors may develop parkinsonism and/or dystonia. In these patients, neuroimaging reveals destructive lesions in the external segment of the pallidum and medial part of the putamen.
- Chronic low-level exposure can cause optic atrophy, nerve deafness, myelopathy with posterior and lateral column dysfunction, cerebellar ataxia, mental changes, and polyneuropathy.

MACROSCOPIC APPEARANCES

After acute intoxication, the brain usually appears normal, but if death is delayed by a few hours, there may be edema and small subarachnoid and petechial parenchymal hemorrhages. Necrotic foci have been noted in the white matter and pallida in the rare cases that survive days or weeks. These lesions are similar to those associated with carbon monoxide poisoning (see above).

MICROSCOPIC APPEARANCES

Relevant data are sparse. Reported findings in patients surviving days or weeks include white matter and pallidal necrosis, gliosis of the cerebral cortex, and loss of cerebellar Purkinje cells.

SAFETY PRECAUTIONS WHEN PERFORMING A NECROPSY IN A CASE OF ACUTE CYANIDE INGESTION

The prosector is at risk of intoxication by cyanide fumes. The risk is usually greatest when the stomach is opened. The stomach should therefore be tied off at its proximal and distal ends and opened under a safely vented laminar flow hood.

NITROUS OXIDE TOXICITY

NITROUS OXIDE EXPOSURE

- Nitrous oxide is used as an anesthetic agent, particularly in obstetric and dental practice.
- Chronic exposure inactivates cobalamin (probably by oxidizing cobalt) and inhibits methionine synthase, as also occurs in vitamin B_{12} deficiency (see chapter 21).
- Neurotoxicity has usually resulted from chronic abuse of nitrous oxide, mostly by dentists or dental nurses, but has occasionally complicated repeated inadvertent exposure in poorly ventilated surgeries.

NITROUS OXIDE TOXICITY

- Patients present with a clinical picture resembling that of subacute combined degeneration and neuropathy associated with vitamin B_{12} deficiency. Manifestations include ataxia, leg weakness, impotence, sphincter disturbances, and sensorimotor peripheral neuropathy.
- In patients with subclinical vitamin B_{12} deficiency, nitrous oxide anesthesia may precipitate subacute combined degeneration.

MACROSCOPIC AND MICROSCOPIC APPEARANCES

Human data are lacking, but administration of nitrous oxide to animals has produced neuropathologic changes resembling those of subacute combined degeneration (see chapter 21).

CNS TOXICITY PRODUCED BY ANTIVIRAL, ANTIBACTERIAL, ANTIFUNGAL, AND ANTIPROTOZOAL DRUGS

AMPHOTERICIN B TOXICITY

The neurotoxic effects of the antifungal drug amphotericin B are associated with intrathecal or high-dose systemic administration. Rarely, radiculopathy, myelopathy, and encephalopathy with parkinsonian features have been reported. Neuroimaging has shown cerebellar, cerebral, and basal ganglia atrophy and white matter abnormalities.

MACROSCOPIC AND MICROSCOPIC APPEARANCES

Data on human intoxication are sparse. In experimental animals, amphotericin B produces a leukoencephalopathy with a loss of oligodendrocytes, axon swelling or fragmentation, gliosis, and an accumulation of lipid-laden macrophages. A multifocal necrotizing leukoencephalopathy has also been reported in humans.

CLIOQUINOL TOXICITY

CLIOQUINOL EXPOSURE

- Clioquinol, a halogenated hydroxyquinoline, has been used for amebic and other intestinal infections, particularly in Japan. It has also been prescribed for children with acrodermatitis enteropathica.
- A disorder known as subacute myelo-optic neuropathy (SMON) can complicate ingestion of large amounts of clioquinol, and numerous cases (estimates range from 10,000 to 100,000) occurred in Japan between 1955 and 1970, though there is some doubt as to whether these were all due to clioquinol.

SUBACUTE MYELO-OPTIC NEUROPATHY (SMON)

- The full-blown syndrome of SMON is relatively uncommon and comprises impaired vision with optic atrophy, subacute myelopathy with prominent spasticity and dysesthesiae affecting the lower limbs and trunk, and peripheral neuropathy.
- Many patients develop isolated optic atrophy or a combination of optic atrophy and myelopathy.
- High doses of clioquinol can produce an acute encephalopathy with transient global amnesia.

MACROSCOPIC AND MICROSCOPIC APPEARANCES

The brain and spinal cord appear macroscopically normal. Histology reveals degeneration of the distal part of longer axons in:
- the optic pathways (i.e. in the optic tract near the lateral geniculate body)
- the posterior spinal and corticospinal tracts in the cervical and lumbosacral regions, respectively

Other abnormalities that may be seen include:
- chromatolysis of lumbosacral anterior horn cells
- degeneration of dorsal root ganglion cells with proliferation of satellite cells and the formation of nodules of Nageotte
- neuronal loss and gliosis affecting the inferior olivary nuclei
- cerebral edema and white matter gliosis.

HEXACHLOROPHENE (USA)/HEXACHLOROPHANE (UK) TOXICITY

Hexachlorophene is a phenolic antiseptic widely used to sterilize the skin pre-operatively and to prevent neonatal sepsis, and is present in some cosmetics. It can, however, be absorbed in toxic quantities through the mucous membranes and skin, particularly of premature infants and burns patients. Excessive absorption may cause irritability, nausea and vomiting, visual disturbances, drowsiness and convulsions, and, in severe poisoning, coma and death.

MACROSCOPIC AND MICROSCOPIC APPEARANCES

Poisoning causes spongy degeneration of the white matter due to intramyelinic edema (see p. 25.7), which is most marked in the brain stem. Necrosis of the optic nerves, chiasm, and tracts has also been reported.

MELARSOPROL TOXICITY

Melarsoprol is an organic pentavalent arsenical-containing drug used for the treatment of trypanosomiasis and its neurotoxicity is described in the section on arsenic (see p. 25.1).

VIDARABINE (ADENINE ARABINOSIDE, ARA-A) TOXICITY

Vidarabine is a purine analog used to treat herpes simplex encephalitis and disseminated varicella–zoster infection. Neurotoxicity causes tremor, encephalopathy, and myoclonus. Reported neuropathologic findings include chromatolysis and degeneration of neurons, particularly in the brain stem.

TOXICITY OF OTHER ANTIBIOTICS

Encephalopathy is a rare complication of therapy with several antibiotics and is usually reversible. Very rarely, neuropathologic changes have been reported. Various antibiotics can case adverse neurologic effects:
- Chloramphenicol may cause optic atrophy and peripheral neuropathy after prolonged high-dose administration.
- Cycloserine, ethionamide, and pyrazinamide may cause a pellagra-like syndrome similar to that associated with isoniazid toxicity (see below).
- Gentamicin is a rare cause of encephalopathy. Foci of white matter necrosis and calcification have been observed in the midbrain and pons after intrathecal administration. The aminoglycosides, including gentamicin, are all ototoxic.
- Overdosage is a particular risk in slow acetylators of the antituberculous drug isoniazid (isonicotinic acid hydrazide, INH), and especially in patients with impaired renal function. INH chelates pyridoxal phosphate and the resulting inhibition of pyridoxal phosphokinase and impaired conversion of tryptophan to niacin produces an acute pellagra-like syndrome, which responds to pyridoxine (vitamin B_6) administration. The occurrence of seizures is thought to be due to inhibition of the synthesis of the inhibitory neurotransmitter γ-aminobutyric acid. Visual disturbances and optic atrophy have been reported.
- Ethambutol can cause visual disturbances and optic atrophy.
- Metronidazole can cause a reversible encephalopathy in high doses.
- Penicillins can cause seizures, partly because the β-lactam ring binds to γ-aminobutyric acid receptors. Hydrophobic penicillins such as cloxacillin and dicloxacillin are most likely to be neurotoxic.
- Sulfonamides (USA)/sulphonamides (UK) very rarely cause acute psychosis, meningism, and myelitic symptoms. Neuropathologic examination of fatal cases has shown vascular endothelial swelling and necrosis, and scattered foci of necrosis with or without hemorrhage in the gray and white matter.

ANTINEOPLASTIC AGENT TOXICITY IN THE CNS

ALKYLATING AGENT TOXICITY

Alkylating agents, including cyclophosphamide, ifosfamide, mechlorethamine (nitrogen mustard), procarbazine, and spiromustine, are used as antineoplastic and, in the case of cyclophosphamide, immunosuppressive agents. Neurotoxicity has most often been associated with ifosfamide, although all these alkylating agents can cause encephalopathy, which is usually but not always reversible and is occasionally fatal. White matter edema and necrosis have been described after intra-arterial mechlorethamine. Pediatric administration of ifosfamide has caused progressive brain atrophy.

L-ASPARAGINASE TOXICITY

L-asparaginase, a bacterial enzyme used primarily in the treatment of leukemias, can produce an encephalopathy when used in high doses. However, human neuropathologic data are lacking.

1,3-BIS(2-CHLOROETHYL)-1-NITROSOUREA (BCNU) TOXICITY

Intra-arterial or high-dose intravenous administration of BCNU (carmustine), in most cases to treat malignant gliomas, can cause a multifocal necrotizing leukoencephalomyelopathy with vascular injury and calcification, resembling that associated with methotrexate (see below).

METHOTREXATE TOXICITY

Methotrexate is a folic acid antagonist used to treat leukemias and lymphomas as well as some solid tumors. Neurotoxicity is associated with high dosage or intrathecal administration, particularly in conjunction with craniospinal X-irradiation.

METHOTREXATE TOXICITY

- Acute symptoms include headache, confusion, seizures, and, rarely, transient hemiplegia.
- Some days or weeks after administration, patients may develop:
  - a subacute encephalopathy characterized by a gradual onset of drowsiness, irritability, mental deterioration, cerebellar dysfunction, parkinsonian features, and seizures.
  - myelopathy with paraplegia or quadriplegia.
    These subacute complications are usually irreversible and may be fatal.
- Computerized tomography reveals low-density white matter lesions, calcification, and atrophy.
- Other subacute or chronic manifestations of neurotoxicity include optic atrophy and growth retardation.

MACROSCOPIC APPEARANCES

Multiple discrete or confluent foci of necrosis may be evident in the cerebral and/or spinal white matter. The lesions may be periventricular in patients given intraventricular methotrexate. In longer-term survivors the white matter is gliotic and atrophic.

MICROSCOPIC APPEARANCES

There is a loss of myelin and swelling and fragmentation of axons within foci of coagulative necrosis in the white matter (**Figs 25.22, 25.23**).

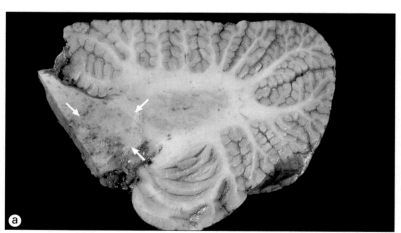

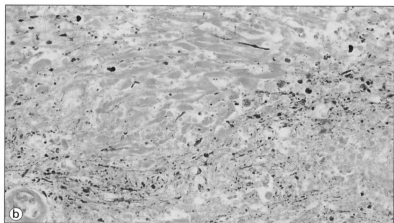

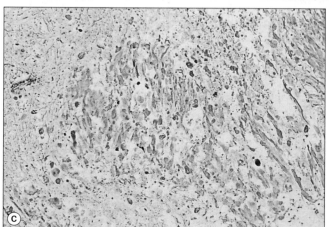

Fig. 25.22 Methotrexate toxicity. (a) Large focus of necrosis (arrows) in the middle cerebellar peduncle of a 6-year-old girl who had received repeated intrathecal methotrexate for leukemia with CNS relapses. **(b)** Histology shows that the lesion contains swollen axons, many of which are mineralized. **(c)** Bodian silver impregnation of the swollen axons. (Courtesy of Professor E Tessa Hedley-Whyte, Massachusetts General Hospital)

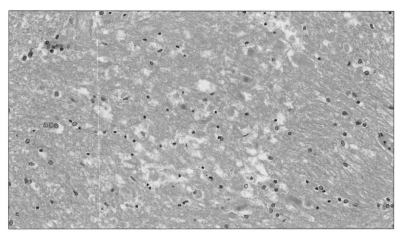

Fig. 25.23 Methotrexate toxicity. Swollen and fragmented axons in the cerebral white matter of a child, who died shortly after completing a course of chemotherapy that included high-dose systemic methotrexate for the treatment of lymphoma.

The axonal swellings and other cellular debris tend to calcify. Lipid-laden macrophages are plentiful in the early stages. In longer-term survivors the white matter may be reduced to an attenuated layer of gliotic, focally calcified tissue. Vascular abnormalities are present in some cases and include perivascular fibrin exudates, fibrinoid vascular necrosis, and a non-inflammatory mineralizing angiopathy, which is most severe in the lenticular nuclei. Intra-arterial methotrexate administration has caused multiple hemorrhagic infarcts due to fibrinoid necrosis and thrombosis of small blood vessels.

CISPLATIN TOXICITY

Like carboplatin, which is much less neurotoxic, cisplatin is a platinum (II) complex with two ammonia groups in the *cis* position. It is used for treating ovarian carcinomas, head and neck cancers, malignant gliomas, and small-cell carcinomas of the lung. Cisplatin therapy is frequently complicated by a distal sensory neuropathy affecting both peripheral and central (posterior column) projections of the dorsal root ganglia. Intra-arterial administration in the treatment of head and neck cancers can produce a neuropathy involving the cranial nerves. Cisplatin can also cause an acute reversible encephalopathy and, very rarely, necrotizing leukoencephalopathy.

CAUSES OF MULTIFOCAL NECROTIZING LEUKOENCEPHALOPATHY (MNL) (SEE ALSO p. 22.13)

- amphotericin B
- BCNU
- cisplatin
- cytosine arabinoside
- methotrexate
- X-irradiation
- AIDS

The white matter abnormalities in patients with previous carbon monoxide, cyanide, or methanol poisoning, global cerebral hypoxia, and mitochondrial disorders can be confused with MNL but are usually less circumscribed, and tend not to contain prominent axonal swellings or to calcify.

PYRIMIDINE ANALOG TOXICITY

Cytosine arabinoside (ara-C) is used to treat leukemia. Neurotoxicity is rare. The risk increases with age and is greater after intrathecal than after systemic administration.

5-fluorouracil and its derivatives tegafur and carmofur are used in the treatment of various gastrointestinal, breast, and ovarian carcinomas.

CYTOSINE ARABINOSIDE TOXICITY

- The most common neurotoxic manifestation is cerebellar dysfunction with ataxia, nystagmus, and dysarthria, and, in some cases, ophthalmoplegia.
- Other complications include optic atrophy, anosmia, parkinsonism, hemiparesis, and paraplegia.

TOXICITY OF 5-FLUOROURACIL (AND ITS DERIVATIVES)

- Neurotoxic manifestations include acute encephalopathy, memory loss, focal stroke-like deficits, and cerebellar ataxia.
- Computerized tomography has shown white matter hypodensities that may enhance with contrast.
- The neurotoxicity is thought be due to a common degradation product, possibly α-fluoro-β-alanine.

MACROSCOPIC AND MICROSCOPIC APPEARANCES

Reported findings in cases of cytosine arabinoside toxicity include cerebellar cortical degeneration and karyorrhexis of brain stem tegmental and spinal motor neurons associated with perikaryal accumulation of masses of neurofilaments. White matter vacuolation and loss of nerve fibers have been noted in the spinal cord.

Experimentally, 5-fluorouracil and its derivatives cause intramyelinic edema and foci of gray matter softening and necrosis in the cerebellum and brain stem. Findings in human intoxication have included neuronal degeneration involving Purkinje cells and the dentate and inferior olivary nuclei, and an inflammatory cerebral demyelinating disease.

VINCRISTINE TOXICITY

The vinca alkaloids, vincristine and vinblastine, bind to and prevent polymerization of microtubule proteins. This interferes with mitotic spindle formation and with axonal transport. Vincristine causes a dose-related peripheral, predominantly sensory and autonomic, neuropathy, and, rarely, encephalopathy has complicated its systemic administration. Accidental intrathecal administration has produced ascending myelopathy, respiratory failure, and death.

MACROSCOPIC AND MICROSCOPIC APPEARANCES

Neuropathologic findings in the CNS have included distension of neurons in the spinal cord and brain stem by abnormal aggregates of neurofilaments and, in one case, eosinophilic intracytoplasmic crystals, which may have been composed of microtubule proteins.

MISCELLANEOUS THERAPEUTIC OR DIAGNOSTIC DRUGS CAUSING CNS TOXICITY

LITHIUM TOXICITY

Lithium carbonate is used to treat and prevent mania, manic-depressive illness, and episodic depression. Patients vary widely in their sensitivity to lithium and in their threshold for neurotoxicity. Intoxication can cause encephalopathy, and sometimes coma. Recovery is usual, but some patients have permanent neurologic sequelae, of which cerebellar dysfunction is often prominent.

MACROSCOPIC AND MICROSCOPIC APPEARANCES

Neuropathologic examination has shown neuronal loss and gliosis in the cerebellar cortex and dentate nuclei, and spongy vacuolation of the cerebellar white matter.

METRIZAMIDE TOXICITY

Metrizamide is used as a contrast medium for myelography. However, a small proportion of patients has developed an encephalopathy, and in some cases this is associated with radiologic evidence of metrizamide entry into brain tissue.

MACROSCOPIC AND MICROSCOPIC APPEARANCES

Mononuclear inflammatory infiltrates around blood vessels in the periventricular region were noted in a patient who died after intraventricular instillation of metrizamide.

PHENYTOIN TOXICITY

PHENYTOIN EXPOSURE

- The principal use of phenytoin (diphenylhydantoin) is as an anticonvulsant, but it has also been used to treat trigeminal neuralgia and ventricular arrhythmias.
- Administration, usually over several years, can cause cerebellar degeneration. Although some authors have suggested that this results from hypoxia during repeated seizures, it should be noted that the cerebellar degeneration:
  - has occurred in patients who have never had seizures, to whom phenytoin was given for cardiac arrhythmias or prophylactically after uncomplicated subarachnoid hemorrhage
  - is not related to the frequency or total number of seizures
  - can occur in patients treated for partial seizures and not just in those subject to generalized tonic–clonic convulsions

PHENYTOIN TOXICITY

- Acute phenytoin toxicity causes nystagmus, diplopia, dysarthria, and ataxia, which are usually reversible.
- Chronic intoxication can cause permanent cerebellar dysfunction, mental deterioration, and a mild, predominantly sensory, peripheral neuropathy.

MACROSCOPIC AND MICROSCOPIC APPEARANCES

There may be obvious atrophy of the cerebellar vermis and hemispheres (**Fig. 25.24**). Microscopic findings are relatively nonspecific, with severe loss of Purkinje, and usually, granule cells (**Fig. 25.25**). There is marked proliferation of Bergmann astrocytes, with associated isomorphic gliosis (**Fig. 25.26**). The cerebellar cortical degeneration is usually diffuse, but may be patchy.

ANTIEPILEPTIC DRUGS AND FETAL DEVELOPMENT

- Most of the commonly used antiepileptic drugs are teratogenic, especially in high doses, if used in combination, and if administered during the first trimester. Overall, the risk of major fetal malformations is increased by about 3–5%.
- Phenobarbitone (phenobarbital), phenytoin, and, to a lesser extent, carbamazepine, are particularly associated with craniofacial malformations, including microcephaly.
- Valproate administration carries an approximately 2% risk of spina bifida.

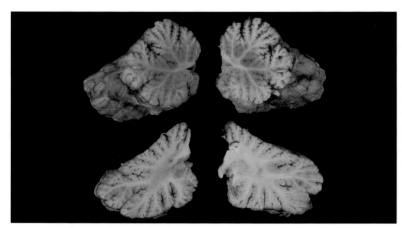

Fig. 25.24 Phenytoin toxicity. Atrophy of the cerebellar vermis and hemispheres in a well-controlled epileptic patient who had been taking phenytoin for many years.

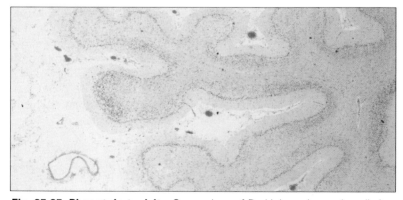

Fig. 25.25 Phenytoin toxicity. Severe loss of Purkinje and granule cells in phenytoin toxicity. The superficial parts of the folia are most severely affected.

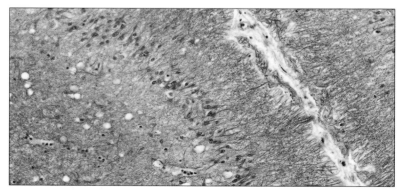

Fig. 25.26 Phenytoin toxicity. Proliferation of Bergmann astrocytes with associated isomorphic gliosis. (Phosphotungstic acid/hematoxylin)

CNS TOXICITY OF STREET DRUGS

AMPHETAMINE TOXICITY

This group includes amphetamine itself and related non-catecholamine sympathomimetic drugs with central stimulant activity (including methamphetamine, and 3,4-methylenedioxymethamphetamine or 'ecstasy'). Routes of administration may be oral, intravenous, or nasal, and clinical manifestations of overdosage range from headaches, panic, paranoia, and psychosis, to delirium, seizures, coma, and death. In some cases of 'ecstasy' intoxication, death has been due to hyperthermia.

MACROSCOPIC AND MICROSCOPIC APPEARANCES

Neuropathologic complications include arterial or venous infarcts and subarachnoid or parenchymal hemorrhages. In a few cases histology has shown a necrotizing vasculitis, predominantly of small blood vessels, but larger arteries and veins may also be involved.

COCAINE TOXICITY

Neurologic complications may result from intravenous or intramuscular injection, smoking, or snorting of cocaine. Alkaloidal forms (i.e. 'crack') are increasingly responsible. Neurologic manifestations of toxicity range from mydriasis with blurred vision, headache, vomiting, and vertigo, to stereotyped repetitive movements, dystonia, hypereflexia, myoclonus, seizures, coma, and death. The presentation may resemble neuroleptic malignant syndrome. Migraine-like headaches with transient hemiparesis or focal or generalized seizures can occur without other signs of toxicity.

MACROSCOPIC AND MICROSCOPIC APPEARANCES

Neuropathologic complications include arterial infarcts, and subarachnoid or parenchymal hemorrhages (**Fig. 25.27**):
* Some are embolic secondary to cardiomyopathy.
* Some have been attributed to small vessel angiitis characterized by a mixed inflammatory infiltrate but not usually fibrinoid necrosis.
* Some have been attributed to cerebral vasospasm.
The spinal cord may be affected.

Rupture of saccular (berry) aneurysms (see chapter 10) is a well-documented complication of cocaine abuse in young adults and is thought to be due to the transient, but occasionally marked, hypertension.

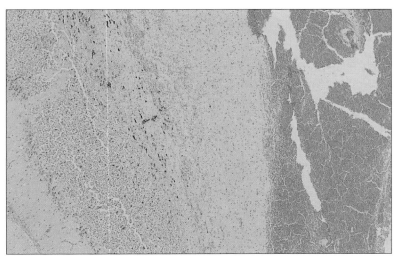

Fig. 25.27 Cerebellar hemorrhage in a young woman with a history of cocaine and amphetamine abuse. The blue reaction product reveals abundant hemosiderin pigment relating to previous hemorrhage. There was no underlying vascular malformation or other explanation for the recurrent hemorrhage apart from the history of drug abuse. (Perl's stain)

The vasoconstrictive action of chronic intranasal cocaine can cause local soft tissue and bony erosion. Rarely this results in CSF rhinorrhea and secondary bacterial or fungal infection.

CEREBROVASCULAR COMPLICATIONS OF 'RECREATIONAL' DRUGS

The commonest CNS complications of 'recreational' drugs are cerebrovascular infarcts and hemorrhages, either parenchymal or subarachnoid.

These may be caused by:
* emboli associated with cardiac arrhythmias, myocardial infarction, or endocarditis.
* vasospasm either due to the pharmacologic action of drugs such as amphetamines, cocaine, phencyclidine, lysergic acid diethylamide (LSD), and mescaline, or secondary to subarachnoid hemorrhage.
* vasculitis, which is a reported complication of many drugs, including amphetamines, phenylpropanolamine, heroin, methylphenidate, ephedrine, pseudoephedrine, pentazocine and tripelennamine, and cocaine. The diagnosis has often been based on angiographic demonstration of segmental narrowing and dilatation of distal intracerebral arteries. Supporting histologic data are relatively scanty.

ABUSE OF VASOACTIVE DRUGS DURING PREGNANCY

* A range of CNS abnormalities has been associated with abuse of cocaine and other vasoactive drugs such as amphetamine and phenylpropanolamine during pregnancy.
* The CNS abnormalities include periventricular leukomalacia, cerebral infarction, intraventricular hemorrhage, parenchymal hemorrhage, agenesis of the corpus callosum, septo-optic dysplasia, schizencephaly, hydranencephaly, congenital hydrocephalus, porencephaly, holoprosencephaly, microcephaly, and spinal abnormalities.

HEROIN (DIAMORPHINE) TOXICITY

Heroin is usually injected intravenously or snorted. Neurologic manifestations of toxicity range from anorexia, nausea, and vomiting, to cardiorespiratory depression, coma, and death. Ischemic CNS complications include cerebral infarcts, ischemic myelopathy, and global hypoxic-ischemic brain injury (**Figs 25.28, 25.29**).

MACROSCOPIC AND MICROSCOPIC APPEARANCES

Angiographic findings have been suggestive of a small vessel angiitis in some patients. However, the predominant findings have been watershed infarcts, laminar sclerosis, and bilateral infarcts of the globus pallidus, all presumably due to a combination of reduced cerebral perfusion and global hypoxia. The spinal cord may be affected. Refractile embolic particles of foreign material have been observed in the skin, and rarely in the spinal cord of heroin users, but not in the brain.

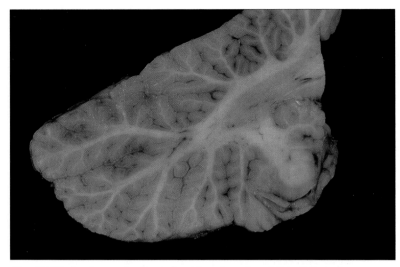

Fig. 25.28 Acute cerebellar infarct in a heroin addict. Folia in the superior part of the cerebellar hemisphere show dusky discoloration, and loss of definition of the white matter.

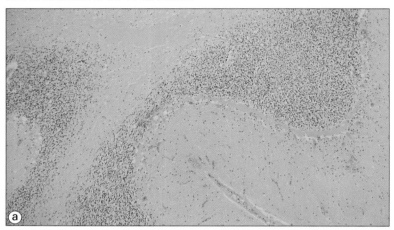

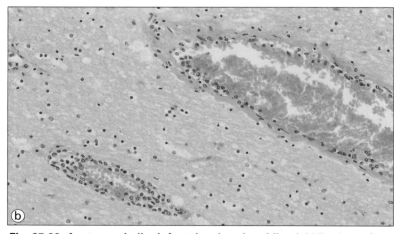

Fig. 25.29 Acute cerebellar infarct in a heroin addict. (a) Histology of the cerebellum shown in Fig. 25.28, confirming acute infarction with congestion and edema. **(b)** Blood vessels in the adjacent white matter show margination and scanty perivascular cuffing by mononuclear inflammatory cells, but no vasculitis.

MPTP (1-METHYL-4-PHENYL-1,2,3,6-TETRAHYDROPYRIDINE) TOXICITY

MPTP

- MPTP is a thermal breakdown product and contaminant of the pethidine (meperidine) analog, 1-methyl-propionoxy-pyridine and causes L-dopa-responsive parkinsonism.
- It is converted by monoamine oxidases (MAO A and B) to 1-methyl-4-phenyl-2,3-dihydropyridinium ($MPDP^+$), which undergoes further oxidation to 1-methyl-4-phenylpyridinium (MPP^+).
- The mechanism of neurotoxicity is still unclear. MAO A and B are irreversibly inactivated by MPTP and $MPDP^+$, resulting in an extracellular accumulation of dopamine and other biologic amines. MPP^+ is taken up by catecholaminergic nerve terminals. Experimental studies have shown that MPTP administration results in the generation of hydroxyl and other free radicals and inhibits mitochondrial oxidation in the striatum.

CAUSES OF IRREVERSIBLE, DRUG-INDUCED PARKINSONISM

As a major manifestation of neurotoxicity

- manganese (the substantia nigra is preserved, but there is gliosis and loss of neurons from the pallidum and subthalamic nucleus, and, to a lesser extent, from the caudate and putamen)
- MPTP (the pattern of neuronal loss closely resembles that of idiopathic Parkinson's disease)

As a rare manifestation of neurotoxicity

- amphotericin B
- cytosine arabinoside
- carbon tetrachloride
- cyclophosphamide
- ethylene oxide
- haloperidol
- methotrexate

MACROSCOPIC AND MICROSCOPIC APPEARANCES

Neuropathologic examination reveals nigrostriatal neuronal degeneration in a pattern closely resembling that of idiopathic Parkinson's disease (see Chapter 29). Typical Lewy bodies are, however, not seen. In experimental studies:

- inclusion bodies have been noted within distorted mitochondria in the substantia nigra and locus ceruleus after acute intoxication.
- eosinophilic cytoplasmic inclusions composed of randomly oriented, thick filamentous or tubular structures have been seen after chronic administration.

ALCOHOL-ASSOCIATED CNS TOXICITY

Ethanol affects the nervous system through a variety of direct and indirect mechanisms, the latter including metabolic disturbances produced by ethanol-induced organ (especially liver) damage and various nutritional deficiencies that tend to complicate chronic alcohol abuse. In addition, alcoholism predisposes to infections, is associated with an increased likelihood of sustaining traumatic injuries, and increases the risk of hemorrhagic strokes. Alcoholism and the associated nutritional deficiencies are important causes of peripheral neuropathy. Some of the direct and indirect toxic effects of ethanol on the CNS are discussed below, while Wernicke–Korsakoff syndrome and pellagra are discussed in the context of nutritional deficiencies (see chapter 21). Central pontine myelinolysis is considered with other metabolic disorders in chapter 22.

CNS EFFECTS OF ACUTE ETHANOL INTOXICATION
Acute intoxication produces varying degrees of exhilaration and excitement, loss of restraint, loquacity, slurred speech, impaired coordination, aggressiveness, irritability, drowsiness, stupor, coma, and, in severe intoxication, death from cardiorespiratory depression.

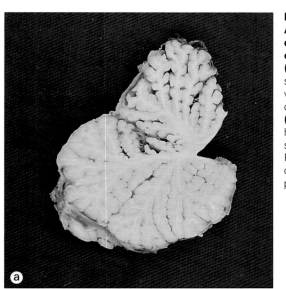

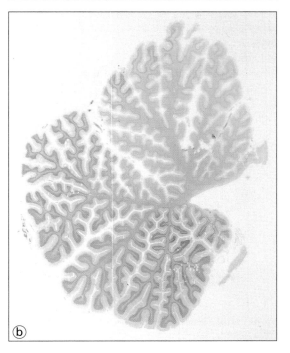

Fig. 25.30 Alcoholic cerebellar degeneration.
(a) Atrophy of the superior part of the vermis complicating chronic alcoholism.
(b) Corresponding histologic section, showing loss of Purkinje and granule cells in the superior part of the vermis.

MACROSCOPIC AND MICROSCOPIC APPEARANCES
Fatal acute intoxication may produce cerebral congestion, edema, and diffuse petechial hemorrhages. Occasionally, a massive hemorrhage or infarct is encountered, usually in the context of pre-existing arteriosclerosis or hypertension.

CNS EFFECTS OF CHRONIC ALCOHOLISM
CNS effects include cerebral atrophy, cerebellar degeneration, Marchiafava–Bignami disease, Morel's laminar sclerosis, and fetal alcohol syndrome. Chronic alcoholism also predisposes to a range of other disorders including Wernicke's encephalopathy, Wernicke–Korsakoff syndrome, and pellagra (see Chapter 21), and central pontine myelinolysis (see Chapter 22).

CEREBRAL ATROPHY
Enlargement of the lateral ventricles and widening of the cerebral sulci have been documented in neuroimaging studies of chronic alcoholics.

MACROSCOPIC AND MICROSCOPIC APPEARANCES
Postmortem morphometric analysis has shown that the loss of volume predominantly involves the white matter. The neuropathologic findings, however, are nonspecific and correlate poorly with the cognitive decline that tends to be associated with chronic alcoholism.

CEREBELLAR DEGENERATION
The clinical manifestations of cerebellar degeneration in alcoholics evolve over months or years and include truncal instability, a broad-based stance, and gait ataxia. Men are more often affected than women.

MACROSCOPIC AND MICROSCOPIC APPEARANCES
Neuropathologic examination reveals atrophy of the superior part of the vermis and adjacent regions of the cerebellar hemispheres, with atrophy of the folia and widening of the sulci (**Figs 25.30, 25.31**). In contrast to the pattern of degeneration resulting from hypoxia, the crests of the folia tend to be more severely affected than the depths of the sulci. There

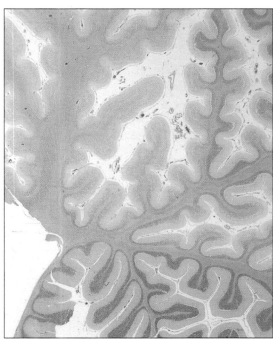

Fig. 25.31 Alcoholic cerebellar degeneration. The crests of the folia are usually more severely affected than the depths of the sulci in chronic alcoholism, but the distribution of degeneration may be rather patchy.

is a loss of Purkinje cells, a patchy loss of granular cells with resulting atrophy of the molecular layer, and proliferation of Bergmann glia (**Fig. 25.32**). Neuronal loss and gliosis are usually evident in the dorsal layer of the inferior olivary nuclei (**Fig. 25.33**). The vestibular, fastigial, globose, and emboliform nuclei may show mild degenerative changes.

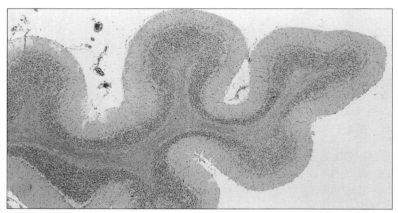

Fig. 25.32 Alcoholic cerebellar degeneration. Loss of Purkinje cells with thinning of the molecular layer and proliferation of Bergmann glia, in chronic alcoholism.

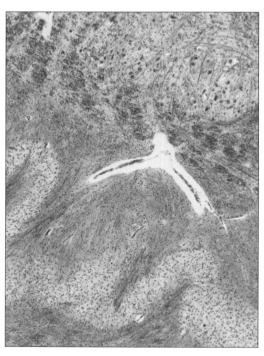

Fig. 25.33 Neuronal loss and gliosis in the dorsal layer of the inferior olivary nucleus in chronic alcoholism. In contrast, the dorsal accessory olivary nucleus (towards the top of the figure) is well preserved. (Luxol fast blue/cresyl violet)

MARCHIAFAVA–BIGNAMI DISEASE

Although originally reported to affect poorly nourished Italian males who had consumed large amounts of crude red wine over many years, this rare disorder has since been described in chronic alcoholics in other populations and even in malnourished non-alcoholics. The pathogenesis is unknown.

Marchiafava–Bignami disease is commonly associated with other manifestations of chronic alcohol abuse such as Wernicke's encephalopathy, central pontine myelinolysis, and Morel's laminar sclerosis.

MARCHIAFAVA–BIGNAMI DISEASE

- Although left-sided apraxia, hemidyslexia, and other callosal disconnection syndromes have been reported, the clinical features are variable and often nonspecific. They include tremor, unsteadiness of gait, and confusion, and, in acute cases, convulsions progressing to coma.
- The disease is often fatal, though spontaneous recovery may occur.
- The lesions are readily demonstrable by contrast-enhanced computerized tomography or magnetic resonance imaging.

MACROSCOPIC APPEARANCES

Macroscopically, the central part of the corpus callosum appears shrunken, and dusky gray or yellow, depending on the age of the lesion (**Fig. 25.34**), and there may be cavitation. Similar lesions are occasionally seen in the optic chiasm, anterior and posterior commissures, and middle cerebellar peduncles. Striatal necrosis is an inconstant finding.

MICROSCOPIC APPEARANCES

Histologically, the disorder is characterized by variable combinations of necrosis and demyelination. These most consistently involve the genu and body of the corpus callosum and spare a thin layer of myelinated fibers along the dorsal and ventral surfaces (**Figs 25.35, 25.36**). Other white matter structures may be involved, as noted above. Macrophages are abundant in the early stages, but lymphocytic inflammation is not a feature. Oligodendrocytes are markedly reduced in number, and astrocytes generally show only modest reactive changes. A striking feature is the proliferation and hyaline thickening of small blood vessels.

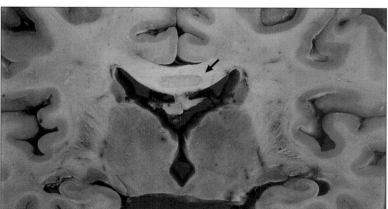

Fig. 25.34 Marchiafava–Bignami disease. Gray central discoloration of the corpus callosum (arrow) due to demyelination.

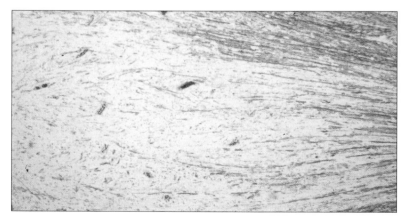

Fig. 25.35 Marchiafava–Bignami disease. Focal demyelination in the corpus callosum in Marchiafava–Bignami disease. (Luxol fast blue/cresyl violet)

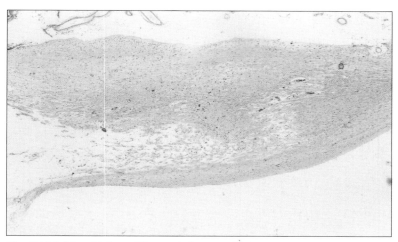

Fig. 25.36 Marchiafava–Bignami disease. Cavitated corpus callosum in chronic Marchiafava–Bignami disease.

MOREL'S LAMINAR SCLEROSIS

This is characterized by a band of spongiosis and gliosis involving the third (and, in some cases, the fourth) layer of the frontal and temporal cortex. It is usually associated with, and may be secondary to, the callosal lesions of Marchiafava–Bignami disease, but has rarely been reported as an isolated finding in chronic alcoholics.

FETAL ALCOHOL SYNDROME

This term refers to the poor intrauterine growth and postnatal development, craniofacial abnormalities, and, less consistently, limb, cardiac, and other malformations, that occur in varying combinations in infants born to mothers who maintain a high alcohol intake during pregnancy. CNS abnormalities can include microcephaly, cerebellar dysplasias, and hypoplasia. Neuroglial heterotopias are particularly common in the periventricular region and in the leptomeninges, where the heterotopic tissue may be extensive. A wide range of rarer brain stem, cerebellar and cerebral malformations has also been reported.

BIOLOGIC TOXINS AFFECTING THE NERVOUS SYSTEM

CLOSTRIDIUM BOTULINUM EXOTOXIN

This is the most potent bacterial neurotoxin. Neurotoxicity results from inhibition of acetylcholine release at the neuromuscular junction. There are no specific CNS abnormalities.

LYSOGENIC STRAINS OF *CORYNEBACTERIUM DIPHTHERIAE* EXOTOXIN

This produces a non-inflammatory demyelination of peripheral nerves and cardiac conduction disturbances. Rarely, patients develop a 'toxic' encephalopathy; however, there are no specific pathologic abnormalities in the CNS.

CLOSTRIDIUM TETANI EXOTOXIN

Clostridium tetani is an anaerobic soil saprophyte that produces exotoxin in soil-contaminated wounds. The toxin gains access to the nervous system by retrograde axonal transport and once in the nervous system inhibits the inhibitory neurotransmitters γ-aminobutyric acid and glycine. The incubation period is usually 5–25 days, but may be shorter. Rare sources of infection are unclean needles used by drug addicts and dung applied to the stump of the umbilical cord. The clinical manifestations are muscle spasms and rigidity, often including trismus at an early stage (lock-jaw), low-grade pyrexia, sweating, and autonomic disturbances.

MICROSCOPIC APPEARANCES

Histologic changes in the CNS are sparse if death occurs before the fifth day of the illness. Thereafter neurons in the cerebral cortex and brain stem in particular become swollen and chromatolytic. Brain edema, focal vascular necrosis, and perivascular hemorrhages have been reported.

CYCAD TOXIN

It has been suggested that environmental factors (possibly the local use of seeds of the indigenous cycad, *Cycas circinalis*, in food and medicine) are involved in the development of the distinct variants of amyotrophic lateral sclerosis (ALS) and parkinsonism–dementia syndrome that are particularly prevalent in Guam and other Western Pacific islands (see chapter 28). The cycad's seeds contain the amino acid L-β-methylaminoalanine, which has been reported to produce a disorder resembling motor neuron disease in rhesus monkeys.

LATHYRUS TOXIN

Neurolathyrism occurs in India, parts of North Africa, and Europe, and is caused by the consumption of certain varieties of the hardy chick pea, *Lathyrus*, usually in times of drought or famine. The excitotoxic amino acid β-N-oxalylamino-L-alanine is thought to be responsible. Patients develop a spastic paraplegia without sensory loss. In severe cases, the upper limbs may also be involved.

MICROSCOPIC APPEARANCES

Histology reveals symmetric degeneration of the corticospinal tracts in the lumbosacral and, to a lesser extent, thoracic regions of the cord. Posterior column degeneration and filamentous and paracrystalline inclusions in anterior horn cells have been noted in a patient who developed neurolathyrism 30 years earlier.

SNAKE AND SCORPION VENOMS

Many snake and scorpion venoms have peripheral neurotoxic or myotoxic effects that are not considered here. Parenchymal or subarachnoid hemorrhage may complicate the coagulopathy caused by envenomation by several snakes, such as the brown snakes (of the genus *Pseudonaja*), the tiger snake (*Notechis scutatus*), and many species of viper. Cerebral infarction related to coagulopathy, hypotension, or vasculopathy has been reported after scorpion stings.

REFERENCES

Abou-Donia MB, Lapadula DM. (1990) Mechanisms of organophosphorus ester-induced delayed neurotoxicity: type I and type II. *Annu Rev Pharmacol Toxicol* **30**: 405–440.

Baumgartner G *et al.* (1979) Neurotoxicity of halogenated hydroxyquinolines: clinical analysis of cases reported outside Japan. *J Neurol Neurosurg Psychiatry* **42**: 1073–1083.

Cavanagh JB (1990) Toxic and deficiency disorders. In RO Weller (ed.) *Systemic Pathology. Third Edition, Volume 4. Nervous System, Muscle and Eyes.* pp. 244–308. Edinburgh: Churchill Livingstone.

Chang LW. (1990) The neurotoxicology and pathology of organomercury, organolead, and organotin. *J Toxicol Sci*; **15** Suppl 4: 125–151.

Choi BH, Lapham LW, Amin-Zaki L, Saleem T. (1979) Abnormal neuronal migration, deranged cerebral cortical organization, and diffuse white matter astrocytosis of human fetal brain: a major effect of methylmercury poisoning in utero. *J Neuropathol Exp Neurol* **37**: 719–733.

Eto K, Takeuchi T. (1978) A pathological study of prolonged cases of Minamata disease. With particular reference to 83 autopsy cases. *Acta Pathol Jpn.* **28**: 565–84.

Forno LS, DeLanney LE, Irwin I, Langston JW. (1993) Similarities and differences between MPTP-induced parkinsonism and Parkinson's disease. Neuropathologic considerations. *Adv Neurol.* **60**: 600–608.

Forrest AR, Galloway JH, Slater DN. (1992) The cyanide poisoning necropsy: an appraisal of risk factors. *J Clin Pathol.* **45**: 544–545.

Liu HM, Maurer HS, Vongsvivut S, Conway JJ. (1978) Methotrexate encephalopathy. A neuropathologic study. *Hum Pathol.* **9**: 635–648.

Louis-Ferdinand RT. (1994) Myelotoxic, neurotoxic and reproductive adverse effects of nitrous oxide. *Adverse Drug React Toxicol Rev* **13**: 193–206.

Mayeno AN, Benson LM, Naylor S, Colberg–Beers M, Puchalski JT, Gleich GJ. (1995) Biotransformation of 3-(phenylamino)-1,2-propanediol to 3-(phenylamino)alanine: a chemical link between toxic oil syndrome and eosinophilia-myalgia syndrome. *Chem Res Toxicol* **8**: 911–916.

McLain LW Jr, Martin JT, Allen JH. Cerebellar degeneration due to chronic phenytoin therapy. *Ann Neurol* 7: 18–23.

Morgan JP, Penovich P. (1978) Jamaica ginger paralysis. Forty-seven-year follow-up. *Arch Neurol* 35: 530–532.

Mott SH *et al.* (1995) Encephalopathy with parkinsonian features in children following bone marrow transplantations and high-dose amphotericin B. *Ann Neurol* **37**: 810–814.

Ney GC, Lantos G, Barr WB, Schaul N. (1994) Cerebellar atrophy in patients with long-term phenytoin exposure and epilepsy. *Arch Neurol* **51**: 767–771.

Ochs JJ. (1989) Neurotoxicity due to central nervous system therapy for childhood leukemia. *Am J Pediatr Hematol Oncol* **11**: 93–105.

Reusche E, Seydel U. (1993) Dialysis-associated encephalopathy: light and electron microscopic morphology and topography with evidence of aluminum by laser microprobe mass analysis. *Acta Neuropathol* **86**: 249–258.

Ricoy JR, Cabello A, Rodriguez J, Tellez I. (1983) Neuropathological studies on the toxic syndrome related to adulterated rapeseed oil in Spain. *Brain* **106**: 817–835.

Schneider JA, Mirra SS. (1994) Neuropathologic correlates of persistent neurologic deficit in lithium intoxication. *Ann Neurol* **36**: 928–931.

Schochet SS Jr, Nelson J. (1987) Exogenous toxic-metabolic diseases including vitamin deficiency. In Davis RL and Robertson DM (eds) *Textbook of Neuropathology.* pp.511–546. Baltimore: Williams & Wilkins.

Singer TP, Salach JI, Castagnoli N Jr, Trevor A. (1984) Interactions of the neurotoxic amine 1-methyl-4-phenyl-1,2,3,6-tetrahydropyridine with monoamine oxidases. *Biochem J* **235**: 785–789.

Spencer PS, Schaumburg HH. (1975) Nervous system degeneration produced by acrylamide monomer. *Environ Health Perspect* **11**: 129–133.

Uitti RJ, Rajput AH, Ashenhurst EM, Rozdilsky B. (1985) Cyanide-induced parkinsonism: a clinicopathologic report. *Neurology* **35**: 921–925.

Verity MA. (1997) Toxic disorders. In *Greenfield's Neuropathology*, Sixth Edition. Graham DI and Lantos PL (eds) pp.755–811. London: Arnold .

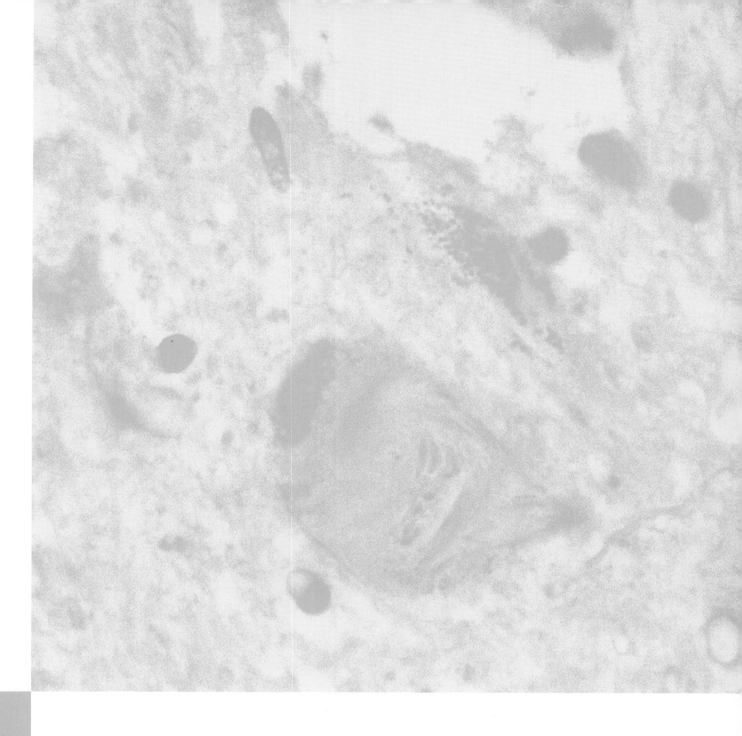

9 Neurodegenerative Diseases

26 Classification and pathogenesis of neurodegenerative diseases

The neurodegenerative diseases are characterized by the progressive dysfunction and death of neurons. The degeneration often affects specific systems, implying some form of selective neuronal vulnerability. Diseases with a known vascular, toxic, metabolic, infective, or autoimmune cause are by convention excluded from this group.

CLASSIFICATION

The main neurodegenerative diseases manifest with movement disorder, cognitive disturbance (dementia), or a mixture of features (**Fig. 26.1**).

Clinicopathologic studies have shown that apparently distinct clinical phenotypes are associated with several different types of pathologic abnormality. For example:

- The syndrome of progressive supranuclear palsy can be associated with neurofibrillary tangles in neurons, Lewy body pathology, or cerebrovascular disease.
- The clinical features of Parkinson's disease are most commonly due to Lewy body pathology, but can also be caused by multiple system atrophy or by several disorders characterized by neurofibrillary tangle formation.
- The syndrome of frontal dementia can be associated with several distinct neuropathologic patterns of neurodegenerative disease.

With the recognition of distinctive histologic changes and specific genetic defects in several neurodegenerative diseases it has become clear that the same process of neurodegeneration can have several clinical phenotypes. The region affected by disease determines the clinical manifestations. For example:

- The entity of multiple system atrophy as defined by the presence of large numbers of glial inclusions can present with parkinsonism, laryngeal palsy, autonomic failure, cerebellar ataxia, or a combination of features.
- Lewy body pathology can cause Parkinson's disease, cortical dementia, autonomic failure, focal dystonia, or isolated dysphagia.
- The pathologic changes of corticobasal degeneration can produce an akinetic rigid syndrome, a cortical dementia, primary aphasia, or a mixture of manifestations.

Different types of neurodegenerative disease.

Movement disorders

Type	Features	Cause
Akinetic and rigid	Predominantly extrapyramidal deficits	Degeneration involving the substantia nigra and basal ganglia
Hyperkinetic	Dysregulation of movement	Degeneration involving the basal ganglia
Ataxic	Cerebellar ataxia	Degeneration involving the cerebellum and its connecting tracts
Motor neuron disorders	Motor weakness	Degeneration of motor systems

Cognitive disturbance (dementia)

Type	Features	Cause
Temporal and parietal degenerations	Memory disturbance with parietal lobe dysfunction	Degeneration of hippocampal and cortical neurons
Frontotemporal degenerations	Apathy, disinhibition, depression, memory disturbance	Degeneration of frontal and temporal cortical neurons
Multifocal degenerations	Variable cortical and subcortical deficits	Degeneration of cortical and subcortical neurons

Fig. 26.1 Different types of neurodegenerative disease.

PATHOGENESIS

Most neurodegenerative diseases are of unknown cause, but recent work has provided some insights into the mechanisms of neurodegeneration. Many environmental factors, such as toxins and viruses, have been considered as possible causes of neurodegenerative diseases (**Fig. 26.2**), but the search for such factors has been largely disappointing and none has been established as causative.

PROTEIN ACCUMULATIONS

These are a key feature of several neurodegenerative diseases. The accumulations of abnormal proteins occur either intracellularly as inclusion bodies or extracellularly. Cellular inclusion bodies have long been recognized as characteristic of certain degenerative processes, and in many cases are core features for the histologic diagnosis of specific diseases. The most important examples of inclusions are:
- the neurofibrillary tangles of Alzheimer's disease
- Lewy bodies of Parkinson's disease

Most inclusions were originally defined by special tinctorial staining techniques. Cellular and molecular biologic studies have characterized the constituent proteins of most inclusions and defined many of the steps involved in their biogenesis. Most of the intracellular inclusions of degenerative diseases are derived from cytoskeletal or cytoskeleton-related proteins, in many instances modified by abnormal patterns of phosphorylation. A practical consequence of these insights is the increasing use of specific immunohistochemical techniques to detect inclusions rather than empirical stains such as various types of silver impregnation.

The accumulation of abnormal extracellular proteins in the form of amyloid is a characteristic feature of Alzheimer's disease as well as prion diseases. The pathogenesis of the accumulation of amyloid is beginning to be uncovered. Amyloids are extracellular fibrillar proteins defined by their physicochemical characteristics, including:
- an affinity for Congo red (and related stains)
- a yellow–green birefringence when the stained material is viewed under polarized light

These properties are due to the arrangement of the constituent peptides in an antiparallel β-pleated sheet into which the Congo red intercalates in a precise orientation.

The formation of amyloid is facilitated by:
- the overproduction of precursor peptide
- the presence of accessory proteins, which promote nucleation of the β-pleated sheet
- possible inbalances in the systems that regulate extracellular proteolysis (**Fig. 26.3**)

Environmental factors in neurodegenerative disease		
Environmental factor	Agent	Links
Physical	Trauma	Epidemiologically linked to Alzheimer's disease and motor neuron disease
Toxin	Metals	Several implicated in Alzheimer's disease and motor neuron disease but none shown to be causative
	Dietary excitotoxic amino acids	Implicated in endemic forms of motor neuron disease but none shown to be causative
Infection	Bacterial	Direct or immune-mediated responses to unusual infections but none implicated in disease after investigation
	Viral	Several linked to Alzheimer's disease and motor neuron disease but none shown to be causative

Fig. 26.2 Environmental factors in neurodegenerative diseases.

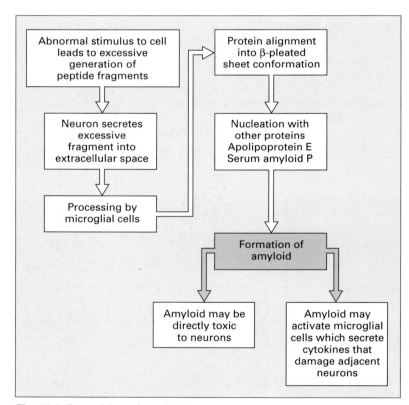

Fig. 26.3 Deposition of amyloid.

EXCITOTOXICITY

Neuronal death may be induced by excessive glutamatergic stimulation of neurons, a process termed excitotoxicity, which has been implicated in the pathogenesis of several degenerative diseases. There are several forms of glutamate receptor and these are characterized by their responses to different pharmacologic agonists (**Fig. 26.4**). In neurodegenerative disease, the vulnerability of certain neuronal systems to damage has been linked to the expression of certain types of glutamate receptor that render neurons vulnerable to excitotoxic damage (**Fig. 26.5**).

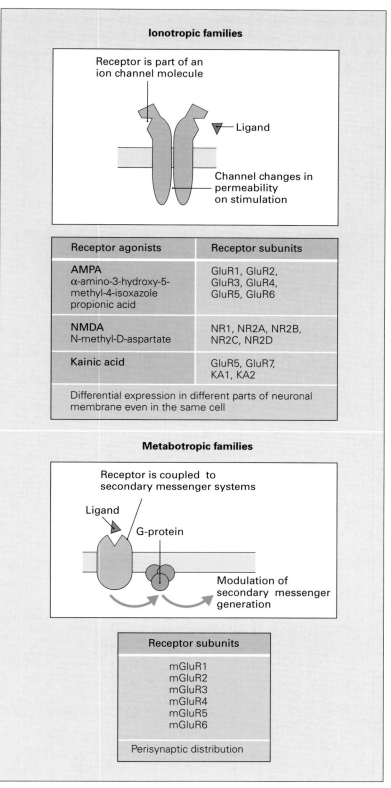

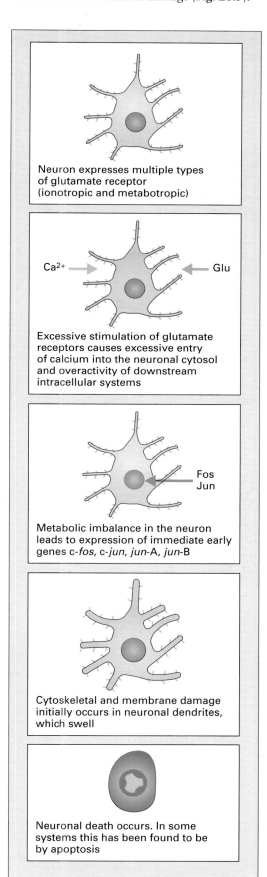

Fig. 26.5 Excitotoxicity.

Fig. 26.4 Glutamate receptors. There are two main families of glutamate receptor. They have been characterized by differential responses to pharmacologic agonists. One explanation for the selective vulnerability of certain neurons in degenerative disease is expression of certain combinations of glutamate receptors by the cells susceptible to excitotoxic damage.

INDUCTION OF PROGRAMMED CELL DEATH

The death of neurons in at least some neurodegenerative diseases has been linked to the form of programmed cell death termed apoptosis (Fig. 26.6). The stimuli that triggers this in the different diseases are at present uncertain. Initiating factors under consideration include excitotoxicity, deprivation of neurotrophic growth factors, toxicity of local cytokines, and toxic effects of accumulated proteins.

ROLE OF CYTOKINES

The reactions of glial cells in some neurodegenerative diseases may include the production of cytokines and participation in an inflammatory response involving the activation of microglial cells and further stimulation of astrocyte proliferation. Increased local production of cytokines may contribute to neuronal dysfunction and death.

GENETIC FACTORS

Many genes responsible for neurodegenerative diseases have been characterized and the identification of such genes has led to major advances in the understanding of disease pathogenesis. Many neurodegenerative diseases are caused by single gene mutations. A genetic abnormality that underlies several neurodegenerative diseases is expansion of the number of tandem triplet repeats that occur in specific regions of certain genes (Fig. 26.7). Some neurodegenerative diseases result from interactions between multiple susceptibility factors (e.g. at

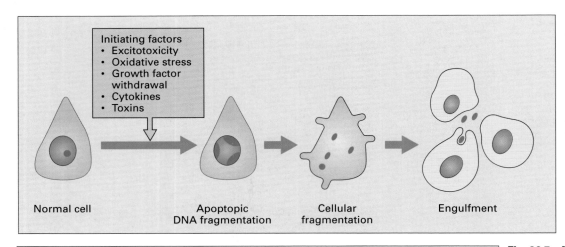

Fig. 26.6 Apoptosis. This is believed to be a common mode of cell death in many degenerative diseases. A variety of initiating stimuli can induce programmed cell death. In experimental systems, initiation is followed by reduced neuronal metabolism and expression of immediate early genes. Endonucleases are synthesized and cause nucleosomal fragmentation. The neuron undergoes fragmentation, and these fragments are removed by engulfment by adjacent cells.

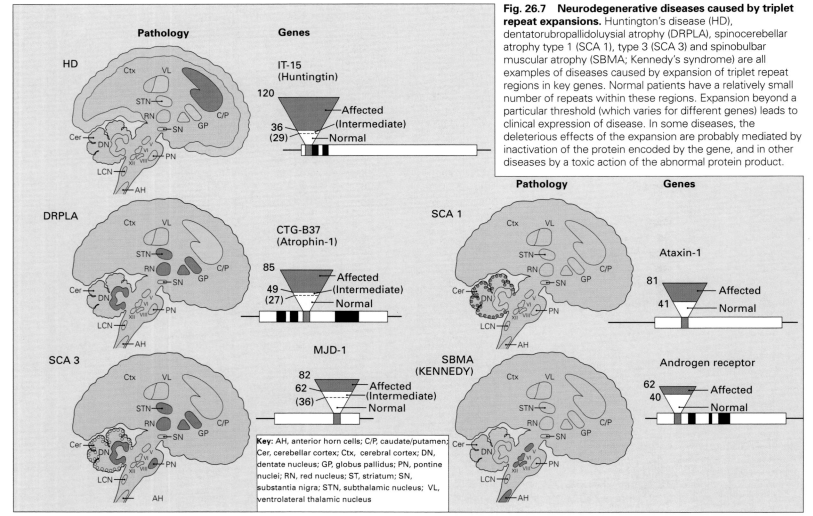

Fig. 26.7   Neurodegenerative diseases caused by triplet repeat expansions. Huntington's disease (HD), dentatorubropallidoluysial atrophy (DRPLA), spinocerebellar atrophy type 1 (SCA 1), type 3 (SCA 3) and spinobulbar muscular atrophy (SBMA; Kennedy's syndrome) are all examples of diseases caused by expansion of triplet repeat regions in key genes. Normal patients have a relatively small number of repeats within these regions. Expansion beyond a particular threshold (which varies for different genes) leads to clinical expression of disease. In some diseases, the deleterious effects of the expansion are probably mediated by inactivation of the protein encoded by the gene, and in other diseases by a toxic action of the abnormal protein product.

Key: AH, anterior horn cells; C/P, caudate/putamen; Cer, cerebellar cortex; Ctx, cerebral cortex; DN, dentate nucleus; GP, globus pallidus; PN, pontine nuclei; RN, red nucleus; ST, striatum; SN, substantia nigra; STN, subthalamic nucleus; VL, ventrolateral thalamic nucleus

least five genes in addition to environmental factors such as head injury are involved in the development of Alzheimer's disease) (**Fig. 26.8**).

AGING AND NEURODEGENERATION

The incidence of neurodegenerative diseases tends to increase with aging. This has been related to an age-related decline in the efficiency of certain metabolic pathways and cumulative damage resulting from lifetime exposure to potentially deleterious environmental factors. Possible consequences include:

- reduction in RNA synthesis
- inefficiency of protein degradative pathways with resulting accumulation of abnormal proteins
- insufficiency of trophic factors for survival of neurons in specific systems
- oxidative damage to mitochondrial enzymes and cytoplasmic neuronal proteins
- inappropriate triggering of programmed cell death.

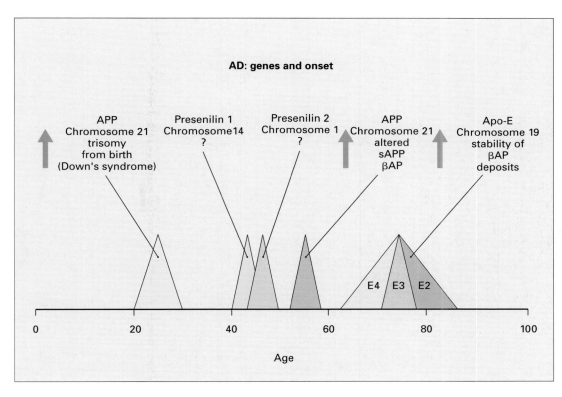

Fig. 26.8 Genes involved in Alzheimer's disease. Genetic factors are important in modulating degenerative diseases, as exemplified by recent understanding of the contribution of genetic factors to the etiology of familial and sporadic Alzheimer's disease. Trisomy 21 is believed to cause an accumulation of abnormal amyloid from about 20 years of age, predisposing to early-onset Alzheimer's disease in Down's syndrome. Mutations in three key genes, presenilin-1, presenilin-2, and APP predispose to early-onset Alzheimer's disease. The possession of an apolipoprotein ε4 allele is a risk factor for late-onset Alzheimer's disease.

REFERENCES

Ashley Jr CT, Waren ST. (1995) Trinucleotide repeat expansion and human expansion and human disease. *Ann Rev Gen* **29**: 703–728.

Burek MJ, Oppenheim RW. (1996) Programmed cell death in the developing nervous system. *Brain Pathol* **6**: 427–446.

Calne D. (1994) *Neurodegenerative diseases*. New York: Saunders.

Driscoll M. (1996) Cell death in C. *Elegans*: molecular insight into mechanisms conserved between nematodes and mammals. *Brain Pathol.* **6**: 411–425.

Lantos P and Graham D (eds) (1997) *Greenfield's Neuropathology* (6th Edition). Arnold: London.

Davis RL and Roberston DM. (eds) (1997) *Textbook of Neuropathology* (3rd edition) Baltimore: William & Wilkins.

27 Motor neuron disorders

CLASSIFICATION

Diseases that affect motor neurons can be classified as either primary, secondary, or multisystem (**Fig. 27.1**). The terms 'motor neuron diseases' and 'motor neuron disorders' are used to refer to any disease affecting motor neurons. The specific term 'motor neuron disease' is used in Europe as a synonym for amyotrophic lateral sclerosis (ALS) and related disorders.

AMYOTROPHIC LATERAL SCLEROSIS (ALS)

NOMENCLATURE

ALS, progressive bulbar palsy (PBP), and progressive muscular atrophy (PMA) are generally considered to be variants of a single clinicopathologic syndrome. Primary lateral sclerosis (PLS) is regarded by many workers as a distinct entity because there is no involvement of lower motor neurons. These conditions (**Fig. 27.2**) are characterized as follows:

- ALS is a neurodegenerative disorder affecting upper and lower motor neurons, and can be associated with variable pathology of non-motor systems.
- PBP is a syndrome of progressive dysarthria and dysphagia. Approximately 25% of patients who later develop other features of ALS initially present with PBP.
- PLS is a condition in which upper motor neuron signs occur in the absence of lower motor neuron signs, and pathologic changes are restricted to the motor cortex and corticospinal tracts.

Classification of disorders affecting motor neurons

Primary motor neuron disorders

Idiopathic	• Amyotrophic lateral sclerosis and variants • Monomelic motor neuron disease

Inherited	• Autosomal recessive
	    Spinal muscular atrophy
	    Neuroaxonal dystrophy
	    Fazio–Londe disease
	    Juvenile onset amyotrophic lateral sclerosis
	    Brown–Vialetto–van Laere syndrome
	• X-linked
	    Kennedy's syndrome
	• Autosomal dominant
	    Familial amyotrophic lateral sclerosis

Secondary motor neuron disorders

Infective	• Acute poliomyelitis • HIV infection • Human T cell leukemia/lymphoma virus (HTLV)-1 infection • Syphilis • Prion disease
Metabolic	• Hyperparathyroidism • Hyperthyroidism • Hypothyroidism • Hexosaminidase A deficiency
Immune	• Paraproteinemia • Dysimmune motor system degeneration (e.g. associated with anti-GM1 ganglioside antibodies)
Environmental	• Lead, arsenic, cadmium, thallium intoxication • Neurolathyrism
Vascular	
Paraneoplastic	• Hodgkin's disease • Non-Hodgkin's lymphoma

Multisystem neurodegenerative disease affecting motor neurons

- Western Pacific amyotrophic lateral sclerosis/parkinsonism-dementia complex
- Frontal dementia with motor neuron disease
- Spinocerebellar degeneration
- Neurocanthocytosis
- Machado–Joseph disease
- Huntington's disease
- Prion disease

Fig. 27.1 Classification of disorders affecting motor neurons.

Nomenclature of 'motor neuron disease'

Syndrome*	Site involved			
	Lower motor neuron	Upper motor neuron	Non-motor cortex	Other
ALS/PBP	+	+	+/ −	Substantia nigra Spinocerebellar tracts Dorsal columns Autonomic system
PMA	+	−	−	−
PLS	−	+	+/ −	−

*ALS: amyotrophic lateral sclerosis
PBP: progressive bulbar paresis
PMA: progressive muscular atrophy
PLS: primary lateral sclerosis

Fig. 27.2 Nomenclature of 'motor neuron disease'.

- PMA is a condition in which lower motor neuron signs correlating with a loss of anterior horn cells occur in the absence of upper motor neuron signs, and in which the upper motor neurons are preserved.

Clinical criteria for diagnosis divide cases into definite, probable, possible, and suspected ALS (**Fig. 27.3**). Variants of ALS have additional special features (**Fig. 27.4**). Since several diseases can be associated with motor neuron loss, secondary causes of motor neuron disease must be excluded. Typically, ALS progresses to death from respiratory failure or aspiration bronchopneumonia within 5 years of onset. Approximately 10–20% of patients develop disturbed frontal lobe cognition.

MACROSCOPIC APPEARANCES

The anterior nerve roots often appear shrunken and gray when compared with the posterior sensory roots (**Fig. 27.5**). The spinal cord may be atrophic. In most instances the brain is macroscopically normal, but in a small proportion of cases the precentral gyrus appears atrophic (**Fig. 27.6**). In patients with dementia the frontal and temporal lobes may be atrophied.

El Escorial diagnostic criteria for ALS	
Features that may be present	• Lower motor neuron signs, including electromyographic (EMG) features in clinically normal muscles • Upper motor neuron signs • Progression of the disorder
Features that may be absent	• Sensory signs • Sphincter disturbances • Visual and oculomotor disturbances • Autonomic dysfunction • Parkinson's disease • Alzheimer-type dementia • Exclusion of conditions that mimic ALS
Features supporting the diagnosis	• Fasciculation in one or more regions • Neurogenic changes in EMG studies • Normal motor and sensory nerve conduction (distal motor latencies may be increased) • Absence of conduction block
Diagnostic category	**Features**
Definite ALS	• Upper motor neuron plus lower motor neuron signs in three regions
Probable ALS	• Upper motor neuron plus lower motor neuron signs in two regions with upper motor signs rostral to lower motor neuron signs
Possible ALS	• Upper motor neuron plus lower motor neuron signs in one region, or upper motor neuron signs in two or three regions (e.g. monomelic ALS, PBP, PLS)
Suspected ALS	• Lower motor neuron signs in two or three regions (e.g. PMA and other motor syndromes)

Fig. 27.3 El Escorial diagnostic criteria for ALS.

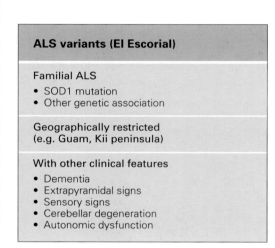

Fig. 27.4 ALS variants.

ALS variants (El Escorial)
Familial ALS • SOD1 mutation • Other genetic association
Geographically restricted (e.g. Guam, Kii peninsula)
With other clinical features • Dementia • Extrapyramidal signs • Sensory signs • Cerebellar degeneration • Autonomic dysfunction

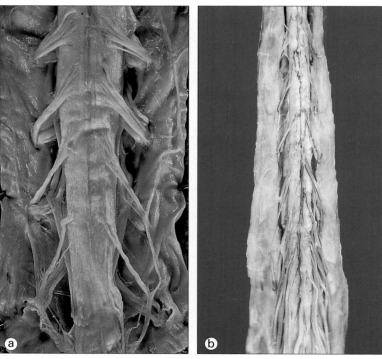

Fig. 27.5 Spinal cord from patients with ALS. **(a)** Cervical spinal cord. The upper motor (anterior) roots appear normal while the lower cervical anterior roots are severely atrophic. **(b)** Thoracolumbar spinal cord showing extensive atrophy of the anterior nerve roots.

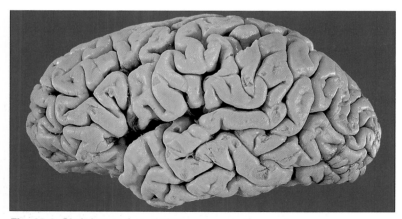

Fig. 27.6 Shrinkage of part of the precentral gyrus in severe amyotrophic lateral sclerosis. The leptomeninges have been stripped.

EPIDEMIOLOGY OF ALS

- Incidence is ~ 2/100,000
- Prevalence is ~ 5/100,000
- Mean age of onset of sporadic ALS is ~ 60 years
- Male:female ratio is 1.5:1

ETIOLOGY OF ALS

- The cause of ALS is unknown, but recent research has provided insights into the role of genetic factors and excitotoxic damage.
- Other possible etiologic factors include deficiencies of neurotrophic factors and autoantibodies to L-type calcium channels.

Genetic factors

- 5–10% of patients with ALS have an autosomal dominant inherited form of disease, and familial ALS typically starts 10 years earlier than sporadic disease.
- Mutations in Cu/Zn superoxide dismutase (SOD1, Cu/ZnSOD) gene on chromosome 21q account for about 25% of all familial cases. SOD1 has a role in removing superoxide radicals, but studies on mice transgenic for mutant human SOD1 suggest that the motor neuron degeneration results from the gain of a toxic property rather than impaired free radical scavenging.
- Mutations of the neurofilament heavy chain gene have been found in a few patients with apparently sporadic ALS. Transgenic mice with abnormal neurofilament protein expression have developed selective motor neuron degeneration.
- Tunisian ALS is an uncommon autosomal recessive disease linked to chromosome 2q33-q35.

Excitotoxic damage

- The excitotoxic neurotransmitter glutamate has been implicated in ALS, and riluzole, a glutamate release inhibitor and sodium channel blocker, has been shown to prolong patient survival.

NECROPSY IN CASES OF 'MOTOR NEURON DISEASE'

- The brain and spinal cord should be fixed intact.
- Skeletal muscles and peripheral nerves should be sampled for histology, and, if possible, enzyme histochemistry and electron microscopy as occasionally peripheral neuropathy or primary muscle disease is misdiagnosed as ALS.
- Postmortem blood samples should be taken for autoantibodies in appropriate cases.
- Material may be archived for DNA analysis, especially in familial cases.

DIFFERENTIAL DIAGNOSIS OF ALS (see also Fig. 27.1)

- It may be difficult clinically to distinguish the progressive lower motor neuron degeneration syndromes of late onset spinal muscular atrophy (SMA type III), X-linked bulbospinal neuronopathy (spinobulbar muscular atrophy; Kennedy's disease), and motor neuropathies associated with high titers of anti-ganglioside antibodies from variants of ALS.
- Guam-type motor neuron disease is associated with neurofibrillary tangles in the cerebral cortex and spinal cord.

MICROSCOPIC APPEARANCES

The most characteristic finding is loss of motor neurons and astrocytosis in the spinal cord, brain stem, and motor cortex (**Fig. 27.7**). The remaining motor neurons in the spinal cord and brain stem may show cytoskeletal abnormalities.

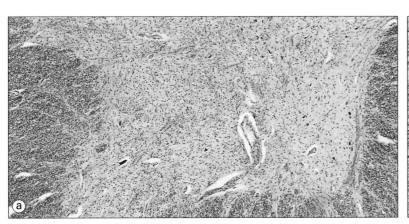 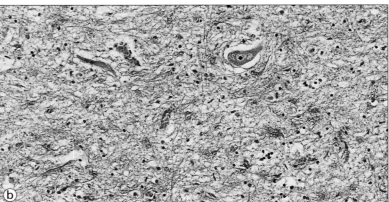

Fig. 27.7 Loss of neurons in ALS. (a) Marked depletion of neurons from the anterior horn of the spinal cord. (Luxol fast blue/cresyl violet) **(b)** Loss of neurons and gliosis of the hypoglossal nucleus. (Phosphotungstic acid/hematoxylin)

Inclusion bodies (**Figs 27.8–27.10**) may be seen in sections stained with hematoxylin and eosin (see Fig. 27.8), but the distinctive inclusions are more readily visualized by immunostaining for ubiquitin (Fig. 27.9). Inclusions are seen in both sporadic and familial ALS.

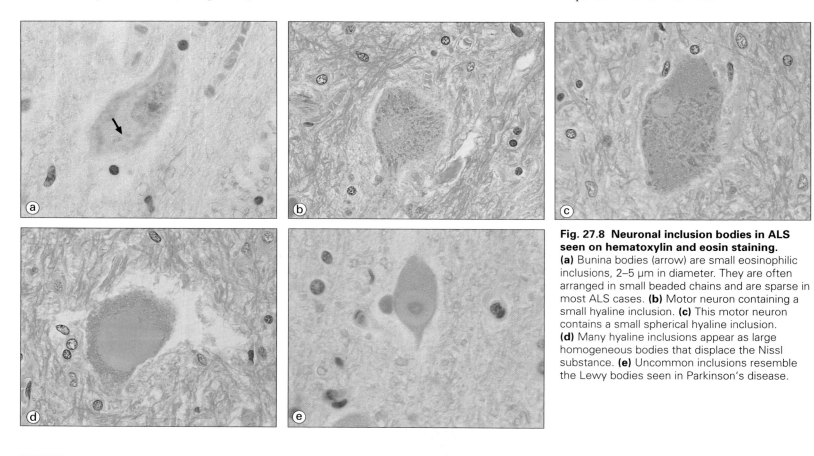

Fig. 27.8 Neuronal inclusion bodies in ALS seen on hematoxylin and eosin staining.
(a) Bunina bodies (arrow) are small eosinophilic inclusions, 2–5 μm in diameter. They are often arranged in small beaded chains and are sparse in most ALS cases. **(b)** Motor neuron containing a small hyaline inclusion. **(c)** This motor neuron contains a small spherical hyaline inclusion. **(d)** Many hyaline inclusions appear as large homogeneous bodies that displace the Nissl substance. **(e)** Uncommon inclusions resemble the Lewy bodies seen in Parkinson's disease.

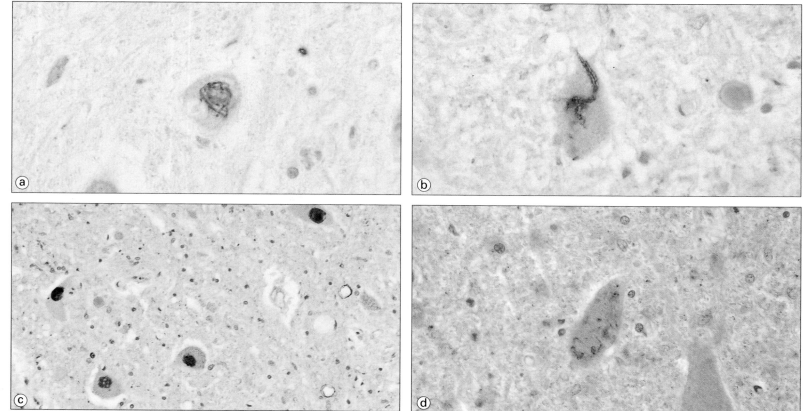

Fig. 27.9 Ubiquitin-immunoreactive neuronal inclusions in ALS.
(a) These skeins of thread-like structures are the commonest ubiquitin-immunoreactive neuronal inclusions in ALS. **(b)** In some neurons the skein inclusions extend into the nerve cell process. **(c)** Ubiquitinated spherical inclusions with a ragged filamentous margin correspond to the hyaline or Lewy body-like inclusions. **(d)** These scattered small granules or single threads are least common and may be the only inclusions left in cases with severe neuronal loss.

Spinal motor neurons may be ballooned due to an accumulation of phosphorylated neurofilaments, but this is a nonspecific finding (**Fig. 27.11**).

Axonal spheroids in the anterior horns (**Fig. 27.12**) are common, but are not specific to ALS.

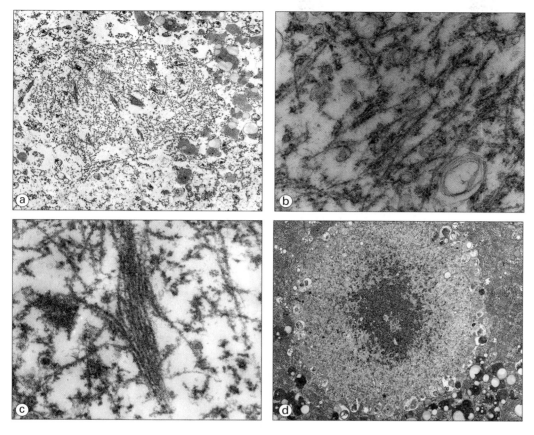

Fig. 27.10 Ultrastructure of ALS inclusions.
Ultrastructural examination of ALS inclusions shows that they consist of haphazard arrays of 10–15 nm filaments associated with granules. **(a)** Low magnification. **(b)** Higher magnification. **(c)** The filaments may form parallel bundles with intervening granular material. **(d)** Large spherical inclusions have a relatively electron-dense core and a peripheral zone of radially arranged filaments and granular material.

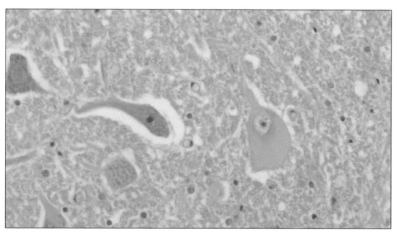

Fig. 27.11 Swollen achromasic neuron in ALS. This is a relatively nonspecific finding.

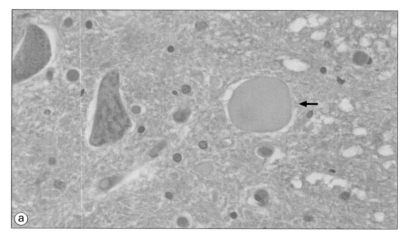

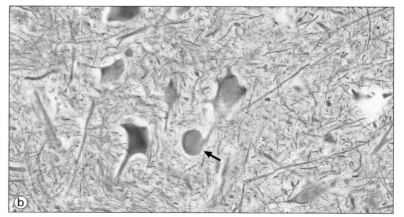

Fig. 27.12 Axonal spheroids (arrows) in the anterior horn in ALS.
(a) Hematoxylin and eosin. **(b)** Palmgren silver impregnation.

Motor neurons in the pons and medulla are often involved in the disease process and show histologic changes identical to those in the spinal anterior horn cells. The number of neurons in nuclei of the third, fourth, and sixth cranial nerves and Onufrowicz's nuclei in the sacral cord is usually normal, but the cells may contain ubiquitin-immunoreactive inclusions.

Loss of Betz cells may be evident in the motor cortex and be associated with astrocytic gliosis and microvacuolation (**Fig. 27.13**). Ubiquitin-reactive inclusions are rarely found.

Degeneration of myelinated fibers in the corticospinal tracts (**Figs 27.14, 27.15**) is usually more marked distally in the spinal cord than proximally in the internal capsule and cerebral peduncles. There may also be a loss of myelinated fibers from the spinocerebellar tracts and posterior columns and some workers suggest that this is characteristic of familial cases. The degeneration of anterior horn cells results in a loss of nerve fibers from the anterior roots with associated endoneurial fibrosis (**Fig. 27.16**).

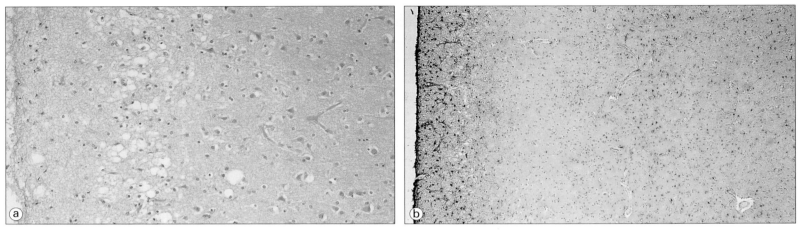

Fig. 27.13 Histology in ALS (a) Motor cortex showing microvacuolation and neuronal loss, mainly in the outer layers. **(b)** Astrocytic gliosis is predominantly in layers II/III and V/VI, as shown in this section immunostained for glial fibrillary acidic protein.

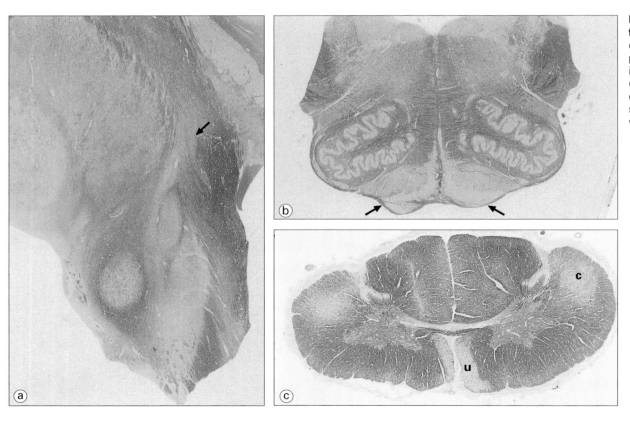

Fig. 27.14 Loss of corticospinal fibers in ALS. (a) The internal capsule (arrow) and cerebral peduncle. **(b)** Pyramids (arrows) in the medulla. **(c)** The crossed (c) and uncrossed (u) corticospinal tracts in the cervical spinal cord. (Luxol fast blue/cresyl violet)

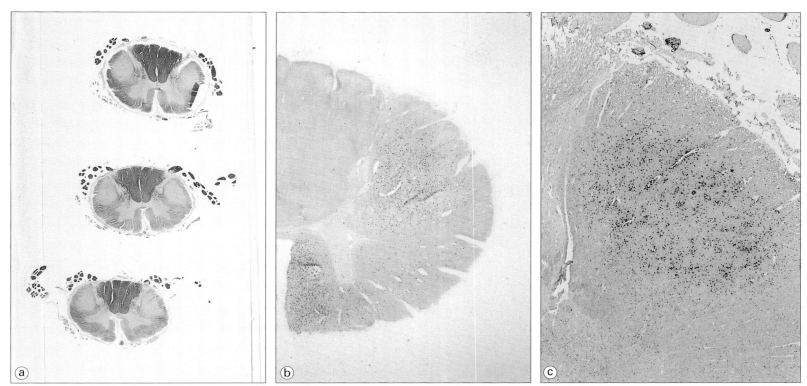

Fig. 27.15 Fiber degeneration in ALS. (a) Sections through the cervical cord showing predominantly lateral (crossed) corticospinal tract and anterior spinal nerve root degeneration. (Luxol fast blue/cresyl violet) **(b)** Marchi preparation demonstrating the products of fiber degeneration in the lateral and anterior corticospinal tracts. **(c)** Infiltration of the degenerating lateral corticospinal tract by CD68-immunoreactive macrophages.

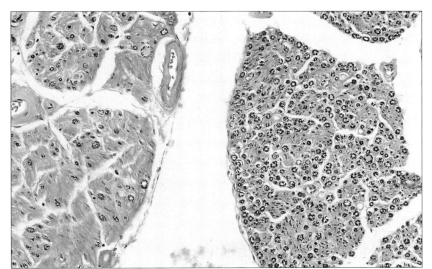

Fig. 27.16 Axon loss from nerve roots in ALS. The nerve fascicle on the right contains many myelinated axons and is part of a sensory nerve root. The nerve fascicle on the left is part of a motor root and shows severe loss of myelinated axons (PTAH).

EXTRA-MOTOR INVOLVEMENT IN ALS

- It is becoming increasingly apparent that ALS can be a multisystem disease with extra-motor involvement (**Figs 27.17, 27.18**). Affected nuclei may show variable neuronal loss and gliosis, and contain neurons with ubiquitinated inclusions.

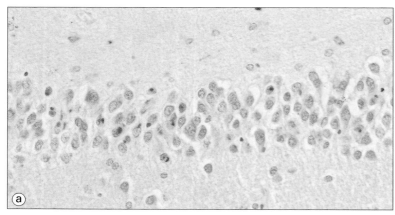

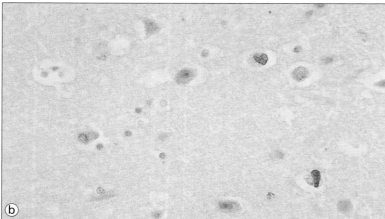

Fig. 27.18 Extra-motor inclusions in ALS. Inclusions are seen with anti-ubiquitin immunochemistry. **(a)** Dot-like inclusions in granule cells of the hippocarpal dentate fascia. **(b)** Small inclusions in neurons of layer II in the frontal cortex.

Extra-motor involvement in ALS
Spinal nuclei • Clarke's column • Dorsal root gangia • Onufrowicz's nucleus • Intermediolateral nucleus in the thoracic cord
Brain stem nuclei • Reticular formation • Locus ceruleus • Nuclei of pontine tegmentum • Substantia nigra • Red nucleus
Hemispheric nuclei • Basal ganglia • Thalamus • Subthalamic nucleus
Cerebellar nuclei • Dentate nucleus
Non-motor cerebral cortex • Temporal • Frontal • Insular • Hippocampal dentate granule cells

Fig. 27.17 Extra-motor involvement in ALS.

- Frontotemporal dementia with ALS inclusions in the non-motor cortex is now recognized as a common form of non-Alzheimer primary degenerative dementia (see chapter 32). In one family, motor neuron loss with frontotemporal dementia has been linked to chromosome 17.

X-LINKED BULBOSPINAL NEURONOPATHY (SPINOBULBAR MUSCULAR ATROPHY, KENNEDY'S DISEASE)

The disease is due to expansion of a tandem CAG repeat region in the first exon of the androgen receptor gene on the proximal part of the long arm of the X chromosome. Variable phenotypic expression between and within families is not clearly related to the size of the expansion.

X-LINKED BULBOSPINAL NEURONOPATHY (KENNEDY'S DISEASE)

- is an X-linked recessive disorder affecting males, usually around the third decade (a milder form of disease is reported in elderly males).
- causes slowly progressive lower motor neuron weakness of facial, bulbar, and proximal limb muscles, associated with gynecomastia
- is commonly associated with infertility and primary sensory neuronopathy

MACROSCOPIC AND MICROSCOPIC APPEARANCES

There is degeneration of facial, hypoglossal, and spinal cord motor neurons with neurogenic wasting of the corresponding skeletal muscles (particularly in the tongue). The third, fourth, and sixth cranial nerve nuclei are spared.

SPINAL MUSCULAR ATROPHY (SMA)

SMA is a disorder characterized by progressive lower motor neuron degeneration and four main features are used to subdivide SMA into different groups (**Figs 27.19, 27.20**).

Features used to classify SMA
Age of onset • Infantile • Juvenile • Adult
Distribution of weakness • Scapuloperoneal (proximal) • Distal • Complex
Severity and clinical progression • Acute (rapidly progressive to death) • Chronic (slowly progressive)
Pattern of inheritance • Autosomal recessive • Autosomal dominant • X-linked recessive

Fig. 27.19 Features used to classify SMAs.

AUTOSOMAL RECESSIVE SMA

Three main clinical patterns of autosomal recessive SMA have been defined. All are caused by abnormalities in the same gene. They are:

- SMA type 1 (SMA1)/acute infantile SMA (Werdnig–Hoffmann disease).
- SMA type 2 (SMA2)/chronic infantile SMA.
- SMA type 3 (SMA3)/chronic proximal SMA (Kugelberg–Welander disease).

MACROSCOPIC AND MICROSCOPIC APPEARANCES

Most descriptions are of SMA1, very few are of SMA2 or 3. The skeletal muscles and anterior nerve roots appear macroscopically atrophic. Histology reveals a loss of motor neurons from the spinal cord, most obviously in the cervical and lumbar regions, and from the hypoglossal and other motor nuclei in the medulla and pons. Some of the remaining motor neurons may appear swollen (**Fig. 27.21**) and contain accumulations of abnormally phosphorylated neurofilaments. There is peripheral granular immunoreactivity for ubiquitin, but no distinct inclusions.

Connective tissue stains show that the anterior spinal nerve roots are relatively fibrotic. In some cases there is obvious loss of anterior root axons. Loss of large myelinated axons may also be evident in peripheral nerves.

Skeletal muscle contains sheets of rounded atrophic fibers and scattered normal-sized or hypertrophic fibers (**Fig. 27.22**), often of histochemical type 1.

ADULT-ONSET SMA

This starts after the third decade with survival to 45–60 years of age. The inheritance is usually autosomal dominant, although autosomal recessive cases have been described. Kennedy's disease is likely if the inheritance is X-linked.

SPINAL MUSCULAR ATROPHY

SMA1
- may or may not be associated with congenital arthrogryposis
- causes neonatal hypotonia ('floppy baby')
- is characterized by severe progressive muscle weakness affecting the limbs and respiratory muscles
- usually results in death at 4–6 weeks from respiratory failure

SMA2
- onset between 3 and 15 months of age
- is typically associated with a survival of over 4 years
- frequently causes contractures and scoliosis

SMA3
- onset between 2 and 17 years of age
- causes atrophy and weakness of proximal limb muscles, and later involves distal and respiratory muscles
- is usually associated with survival beyond late adolescence.
- commonly causes contractures and scoliosis

GENETICS OF AUTOSOMAL RECESSIVE SMA

- SMA1, 2, and 3 have been linked to chromosome 5q.
- Mutations in two adjacent genes at 5q13 have been implicated:
  - survival motor neuron (SMN) — deletions occur in 93% of SMAs
  - neuronal apoptosis inhibitory protein (NAIP) — deletions occur in 37% of SMAs.

DIFFERENTIAL DIAGNOSIS OF SMA

- Lower motor neuron degeneration may be a component of metabolic diseases including hexosaminidase A deficiency, hydroxyisovaleric aciduria, and ceroid lipofuscinosis.
- Limb girdle weakness in SMA3 should be distinguished from dystrophin myopathy, metabolic myopathy, and limb girdle dystrophy.

Fig. 27.20 Classification of SMA.

Classification of SMA	
Type	**Inheritance**
Proximal SMAs	
1a Infantile, acute	AR
1b Infantile, chronic	AR
2 Onset 1–6 years, chronic	AR/AD
3 Onset 2–18 years, chronic	AR (AD rare)
4 Adult, chronic	AR
5 Adult, chronic	AD
Distal SMAs	
Juvenile	AD
Mild juvenile	AR
Adult	AD
Complex distribution SMAs	
Scapuloperoneal	AD/AR
Bulbospinal (Kennedy's syndrome)	XR
Fascioscapulohumeral	AD
Oculopharyngeal	AD
Bulbar	AR

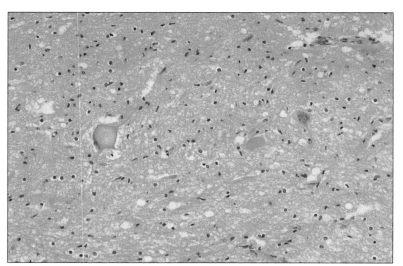

Fig. 27.21 A remaining spinal motor neuron in SMA1. It is swollen and there is peripheral displacement of Nissl substance by accumulations of phosphorylated neurofilaments.

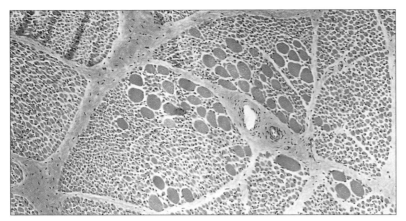

Fig. 27.22 Cryostat section of muscle in SMA. The muscle contains small numbers of normal-sized and hypertrophic fibers among sheets of rounded atrophic fibers. This appearance is typical of infantile SMA.

HEREDITARY PROGRESSIVE BULBAR PALSY

Loss of neurons from the lower cranial nerve nuclei leading to progressive bulbar paresis occurs in two very uncommon inherited disorders: Fazio–Londe disease and Brown–Vialetto–van Laere syndrome.

FAZIO–LONDE DISEASE

This condition is characterized by the onset of bulbar palsy at 2–5 years of age, and there are three subtypes (see also p 6.10):
- autosomal recessive with early respiratory symptoms and rapid progression
- autosomal recessive with an onset in mid-childhood and a long clinical course
- autosomal dominant

MACROSCOPIC AND MICROSCOPIC APPEARANCES

Neuropathologic examination shows severe loss of neurons from the hypoglossal, motor vagal, and facial nuclei, and moderate loss from the spinal anterior horns, and motor trigeminal and oculomotor nuclei.

BROWN–VIALETTO–VAN LAERE SYNDROME

This condition usually starts in the second decade and the inheritance is autosomal recessive. Patients develop sensorineural deafness followed by seventh, ninth, and twelfth cranial nerve palsies.

MACROSCOPIC AND MICROSCOPIC APPEARANCES

Neuropathologic examination shows a loss of cochlear nerve fibers and dense astrocytosis in the ventral cochlear nuclei. There is also neuronal loss from the motor nuclei of the lower cranial nerves and variable degeneration of the spinocerebellar tracts, Purkinje cells, posterior columns, Clarke's column, and anterior horn cells.

HEREDITARY SPASTIC PARAPARESIS

HEREDITARY SPASTIC PARAPARESIS

- Hereditary spastic paraparesis is a heterogeneous condition with autosomal dominant, autosomal recessive, and X-linked recessive types.
- These disorders can be classified into two main clinically defined groups: pure spastic paraparesis and complicated spastic paraparesis in combination with other neurologic features.

Pure spastic paraparesis:
- is slowly progressive
- is characterized by spasticity predominating over weakness
- is commonly associated with pes cavus
- is associated with a variety of late features including reduced vibration sense and disturbed micturition
- is usually inherited as an autosomal condition

Complicated spastic paraparesis in combination with other neurologic features:
- is associated with optic atrophy, amyotrophy, extrapyramidal disturbances, sensory neuropathy, and retinal degeneration
- is usually inherited as a sex-linked recessive condition

MACROSCOPIC AND MICROSCOPIC APPEARANCES

Neuropathologic examination shows predominantly distal degeneration of corticospinal and posterior column tracts (see chapter 25 for the differential diagnosis of distal degeneration of long axons in the CNS). In some cases this is associated with a loss of Purkinje cells and degeneration of cerebellar dentate nuclei.

GENETICS OF HEREDITARY SPASTIC PARAPARESIS

Autosomal dominant
- The commonest form of pure spastic paraparesis.
- Different subtypes are linked to markers on chromosome 14q and chromosome 2.

Autosomal recessive
- There is linkage to chromosome 8 in some families.

X-linked recessive
- Different subtypes are caused by mutation of the proteolipid protein (PLP) gene (other mutations of this gene cause Pelizaeus–Merzbacher disease, see Chapter 5), and the gene for L1 cell adhesion molecule (L1-CAM).

REFERENCES

Amato AA, Prior TW, Barohn RJ, Snyder P, Papp A, Mendell JR. (1993) Kennedy's disease: a clinicopathologic correlation with mutations in the androgen receptor gene. *Neurology* **43**: 791–794.

Deng H-X, Hentati A, Tainer J. (1993) Amyotrophic lateral sclerosis and structural defects in Cu,Zn superoxide dismutase. *Science* **261**: 1047–1051.

Figlewicz D *et al*. (1994) Variants of the heavy neurofilament subunit are associated with the development of amyotrophic lateral sclerosis. *Hum Mol Genetics* **3**: 1759–1761.

Hudson AJ, Kiernan JA, Munoz DG, Pringle CE, Brown WF, Ebers GC. (1993) Clinicopathological features of primary lateral sclerosis are different from amyotrophic lateral sclerosis. *Brain Res Bull* **30**: 359–364.

Lee M, Marszalek J, Cleveland D. (1994) A mutant neurofilament subunit causes massive, selective neuron death: implications for the pathogenesis of human motor neuron disease. *Neuron* **13**: 975–988.

Lefebvre S *et al.* (1995) Identification and characterization of a spinal muscular atrophy-determining gene. *Cell* **80**: 155–165.

Leigh P, Malessa S. (1995) Neurochemistry of motor neuron disease. In Leigh P, Swash M (eds) *Motor Neuron Disease: Biology and Management*. pp. 163–188. London: Springer–Verlag.

Lowe J. (1994) New pathological findings in amyotrophic lateral sclerosis. *J Neurol Sci* **124**(Suppl.): 38–51.

Rosen DR *et al*. (1993) Mutations in Cu/Zn superoxide dismutase gene are associated with familial amyotrophic lateral sclerosis. *Nature* **362**: 59–62.

Rowland L. (1994) Amyotrophic lateral sclerosis: theories and therapies. *Ann Neurol* **35**: 129–130.

Roy N *et al*. (1995) The gene for neuronal apoptosis inhibitory protein is partially deleted in individuals with spinal muscular atrophy. *Cell* **80**: 167–178.

Russman BS *et al*. (1992) Spinal muscular atrophy: new thoughts on the pathogenesis and classification schema. *J Child Neurol* **7**: 347–353.

Wong P *et al*. (1995) An adverse property of a familial ALS-linked SOD1 mutation causes motor neuron disease characterized by vacuolar degeneration of mitochondria. *Neuron* **14**:1105–1116.

World Federation of Neurology Research Group on Neuromuscular Diseases. (1994) Classification of neuromuscular disorders. *J Neurol Sci* **124**(Suppl.): 109–130.

Zeman S, Lloyd C, Meldrum B, Leigh P. (1994) Excitatory amino acids, free radicals and the pathogenesis of motor neuron disease. *Neuropath Appl Neurobiol* **20**: 219–231.

28 Parkinsonism and akinetic–rigid disorders

Akinetic–rigid disorders are characterized clinically by rigidity, bradykinesia, and resting tremor. The combination of these features is often termed parkinsonism, of which the commonest cause is Parkinson's disease (PD).

CAUSES OF PARKINSONISM

Common
- Parkinson's disease (PD)
  In necropsy studies, 20–30% of patients diagnosed clinically as having Parkinson's disease have been found to have an alternative cause for their parkinsonism.

Less common
- drug-induced parkinsonism
- multiple system atrophy (MSA)
- progressive supranuclear palsy (PSP)(Steele–Richardson–Olszewski syndrome)
- vascular causes

Rare
- corticobasal degeneration (CBD)
- Alzheimer's disease
- multisystem degenerations
- space-occupying lesions
- hydrocephalus
- frontotemporal neurodegenerative disorders
- Huntington's disease
- dementia pugilistica
- toxin-induced parkinsonism
- Wilson's disease

PARKINSON'S DISEASE (PD)

PARKINSON'S DISEASE

- For clinical diagnosis of PD, the patient should demonstrate at least two of the three cardinal features of bradykinesia, resting tremor, and rigidity.
- Commonly associated features include autonomic dysfunction, cognitive disturbance, or dysphagia.
- PD is the commonest of the Lewy body disorders.

The mean age of onset is 61 years and the mean duration of the disease is approximately 13 years. The incidence increases with age, and in North America and Europe is 7–19/100,000 population per annum. The prevalence is 30–190/100,000. Onset of PD under 40 years of age is uncommon, and during the first two decades very rare.

PARKINSON'S DISEASE

The manifestations of PD are largely attributable to reduced dopaminergic input into the striatum, due to degeneration of neurons in the pars compacta of the substantia nigra.
Several etiologic factors have been implicated or suggested, including:
- **Genetic factors.** PD is inherited as an autosomal dominant trait in some families. In addition, the frequency of a genetic marker of the debrisoquine hydroxylase 'poor metabolizer' phenotype is significantly increased in PD, as is a monoamine oxidase B polymorphism.
- **Free radical damage and defective oxidative phosphorylation.** Complex I defects in mitochondrial oxidative phosphorylation are more common in patients with PD than in controls and are believed to increase the production of free radicals, causing damage to mitochondrial DNA and other macromolecules.
- **Environmental agents.** There is a similarity between PD and the disorder produced by 1-methyl-4-phenyl-1,2,3,6-tetrahydropyridine (MPTP) intoxication (see chapter 25).

LEWY BODIES

The pathological hallmark of Parkinson's disease is the presence of intracellular inclusions in neurons called Lewy bodies. There are two main types, termed classical and cortical (**Fig. 28.1**), which are found in different locations. The presence of Lewy bodies defines several conditions, termed Lewy body disorders (**Fig. 28.2**).

Types of Lewy body		
	Classical (brain stem) Lewy bodies	Cortical Lewy bodies
Features	Neuronal inclusions that are usually roughly spherical with an eosinophilic core surrounded by a paler 'halo' (**Figs 28.3, 28.4**). One or more may be present in the cytoplasm of a single neuron.	Found in neurons in the deeper part of the cerebral cortex, particularly layers V and VI. Are less clearly defined than classical Lewy bodies in hematoxylin and eosin-stained sections, and consist of a homogeneous zone of hypereosinophilia that usually lacks a surrounding 'halo' (**Fig. 28.5**). Present in all cases of PD in small numbers, mainly in the limbic cortex but are usually more extensively distributed in Lewy body dementia (see chapter 32).
Main sites	Substantia nigra, locus ceruleus, substantia innominata, dorsal motor nucleus of the vagus, serotonergic raphe nuclei, thalamus and hypothalamus, intermediolateral column of the spinal cord, pedunculopontine nucleus, and Edinger–Westphal nucleus	In approximately decreasing order of frequency: entorhinal cortex, periamygdaloid cortex, cingulate gyrus, temporal cortex, insular cortex, frontal cortex, and parietal cortex
Less common sites	Peripheral sympathetic and parasympathetic neurons including the enteric ganglia (where their presence may be related to the gut dysmotility of many patients with PD)	
All Lewy bodies	Electron microscopy reveals an amorphous electron-dense core surrounded by a halo of radiating filaments amongst which are scattered granules of lipofuscin and neuromelanin, mitochondria, dense-core vesicles, and other organelles.	

Fig. 28.1 Types of Lewy body.

Distribution of Lewy bodies in different disorders		
Disorder	Main site of Lewy body pathology	Clinical correlate
Parkinson's disease	Substantia nigra	Akinetic–rigid syndrome
Dementia with cortical Lewy bodies	Cerebral cortex, substantia nigra	Dementia with akinetic–rigid syndrome
Autonomic failure	Sympathetic neurons in spinal cord	Autonomic failure
Lewy body dysphagia	Dorsal vagal nuclei	Dysphagia

Fig. 28.2 Distribution of Lewy bodies in different disorders.

LEWY BODIES

The formation of Lewy bodies may be cytoprotective: a means of removing damaged cytoskeletal proteins. Constituent proteins can be divided into two groups:
Functional proteins that make up the structure of the Lewy body:
- neurofilament proteins – these form the cytoskeleton of the inclusion
- ubiquitin, enzymes of the ubiquitin cycle, and proteosome subunits – involved in cytosolic proteolysis
- αB crystallin – a neurofilament chaperone protein
- kinases – that catalyse phosphorylation of neurofilament proteins

Incorporated proteins, probably in the process of being degraded:
- tubulin and microtubule-associated proteins
- β-amyloid precursor protein
- synaptic proteins

Immunohistochemical staining for ubiquitin is a sensitive way of detecting cortical Lewy bodies (Fig. 28.6). Pale bodies occur in neurons of the substantia nigra and locus ceruleus (Fig. 28.7) and have a similar immunohistochemical profile to Lewy bodies. Although not always associated with Lewy bodies, the latter should be carefully sought if pale bodies are present.

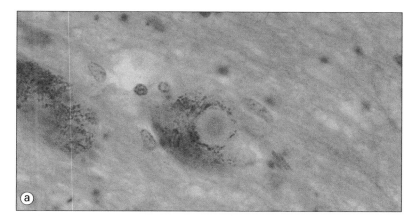
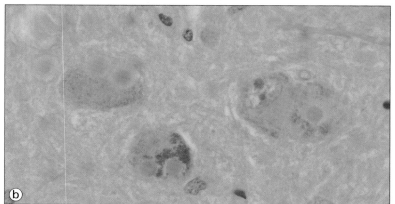

Fig. 28.3 Classical Lewy bodies. These are 8–30 µm in diameter, with a hyaline eosinophilic core and a pale halo. The core may comprise concentric lamellae of differing staining intensity. A single neuron may contain several Lewy bodies. **(a)** Shows a single Lewy body in a nigral neuron, with pronounced lamellation. **(b)** Lewy bodies may be found in large numbers and, as shown here, a neuron may contain more than one inclusion.

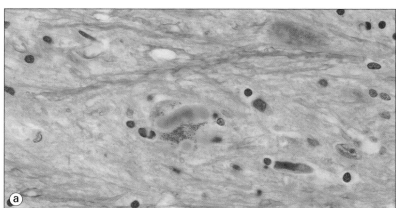
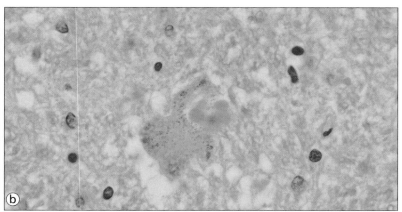
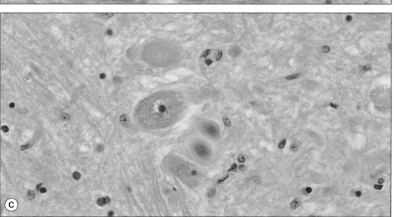

Fig. 28.4 Variant forms of classical Lewy bodies. (a) Here a Lewy body has an elongated form rather than the usual more or less spherical shape. **(b)** Agglomerated and serpiginous Lewy bodies are especially found in the nucleus basalis of Meynert. **(c)** Lewy bodies that are outside the neuronal perikaryon (though they may be within neurites) appear as circular hyaline eosinophilic profiles in the neuropil.

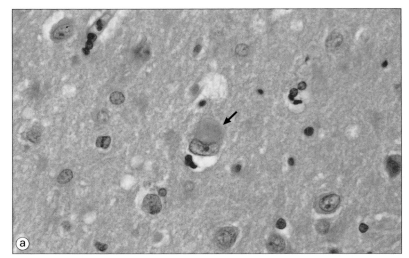

(a)

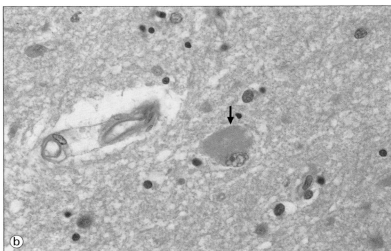

(b)

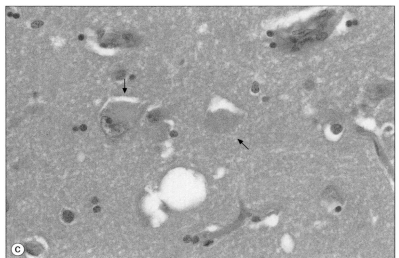

(c)

Fig. 28.5 Cortical Lewy bodies. These are homogeneous eosinophilic structures that have an ill-defined edge and usually lack an obvious halo (arrows). **(a)** Typically, a cortical Lewy body appears as an eosinphilic rounded inclusion which pushes the nucleus to one side of the cell. The nuclei of affected neurons usually appear somewhat vesicular with a prominent nucleolus. **(b)** Some cortical Lewy bodies appear in small swollen neurons, again displacing the nucleus to one side of the cell. **(c)** When the plane of section does not include the nucleus, cortical Lewy bodies (arrows) appear as rounded eosinophilic structures.

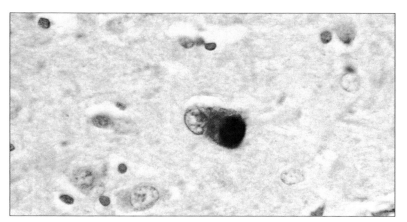

Fig. 28.6 Cortical Lewy body showing ubiquitin immunoreactivity.

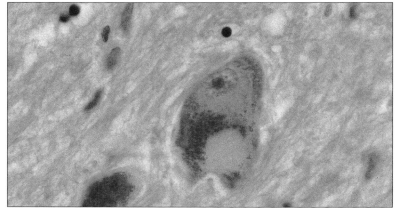

Fig. 28.7 A pale body. A rounded zone of granular palely eosinophilic material displaces the neuromelanin. In contrast to Lewy bodies, pale bodies have no halo.

MACROSCOPIC APPEARANCES

Sections through the midbrain and pons reveal loss of pigment from the substantia nigra and locus ceruleus (**Fig. 28.8**) (note that pallor of the substantia nigra is normal in childhood and adolescence, the slate-gray colour being acquired during early adulthood). The globus pallidus, putamen, and caudate nucleus appear normal.

MICROSCOPIC APPEARANCES

The substantia nigra and other pigmented brain stem nuclei show:

- cell loss (**Fig. 28.9**).
- accumulation of neuromelanin in macrophages (**Figs 28.10, 28.11**).
- astrocytic gliosis.
- Lewy bodies and pale bodies (see **Figs 28.5, 28.7**) in some remaining neurons.
- rarely, neuronophagia.

Lewy bodies must be found to make a diagnosis of PD. A reasonable approach is to examine two 7μm sections through the mid-level of the substantia nigra. If no Lewy bodies are found, two further sections should be examined. If Lewy bodies are still not seen a diagnosis of PD can usually be excluded and other causes of parkinsonism should be sought.

A distinctive form of neuritic degeneration demonstrable by immunostaining for ubiquitin but not by silver impregnation occurs in Lewy body diseases, including PD (**Fig. 28.12**). The ubiquitinated neurites may be detected in the substantia nigra, CA2/3 region of the hippocampus, dorsal motor nucleus of the vagus, nucleus basalis of Meynert, and amygdala.

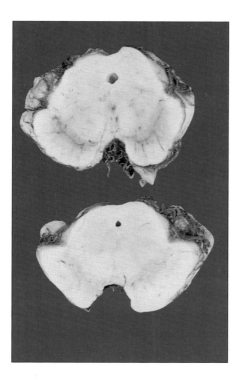

Fig. 28.8 Substantia nigra in Parkinson's disease. Sections through midbrain of normal control (top) and patient with PD (bottom), showing the abnormal pallor of the substantia nigra in PD.

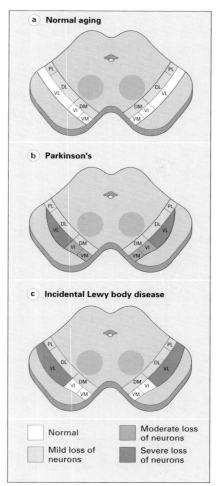

Fig. 28.9 Cell loss from the substantia nigra is not random, but occurs in a region-specific manner. The pars compacta of the substantia nigra can be divided into ventral and dorsal tiers, which project to different brain areas, and each tier can be further subdivided into regions (medial to lateral). **(a)** In normal aging, there is an estimated rate of cell loss from the dorsal tier in PD of the substantia nigra of 7% per decade, leading to 40–50% cell loss by 65 years of age. **(b)** In PD, cell loss is greatest in the ventrolateral tier (VL). Typically, 70–90% have been lost by the time a patient dies. The ventromedial tier (VM) is next most affected. Cell loss from the dorsal tier is not significantly different from that in normal aging. **(c)** It has been suggested that symptoms of PD occur only after 50% of ventral tier neurons have been lost. This is preceded by a subclinical phase that can be regarded as incidental Lewy body disease in which there is less pronounced cell loss, largely confined to the ventrolateral tier (VL). The age-specific prevalence of Lewy bodies rises from 3.8% to 12.8% between the sixth and ninth decades.

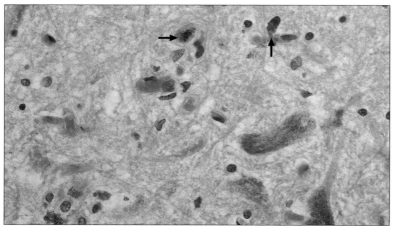

Fig. 28.10 Phagocytosis of neuromelanin. Neuromelanin from neurons that have degenerated is taken up into macrophages (arrows).

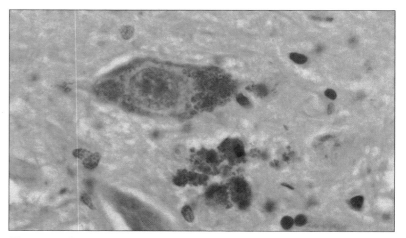

Fig. 28.11 A cluster of pigment-laden macrophages marks the site of degeneration of a nigral neuron.

JUVENILE PARKINSONISM

Rarely, PD develops in the first two decades of life, often as an autosomal dominant disorder associated with dystonia. There is clinical and pathologic overlap with dopa-responsive dystonia. Neuropathologic studies have shown numerous Lewy bodies in the brain stem and cerebral cortex in several cases. The condition may complicate other rare disorders, including neuroaxonal dystrophy and nuclear hyaline inclusion disease.

DRUG AND TOXIN-RELATED PARKINSONISM

Extrapyramidal movement disorders affect 10–15% of patients treated with neuroleptic drugs that block D2 dopamine receptors, and may persist after drug withdrawal.

Other causes of drug- and toxin-related parkinsonism are described in chapter 25.

PROGRESSIVE SUPRANUCLEAR PALSY (PSP) (STEELE–RICHARDSON–OLSZEWSKI SYNDROME)

The cause of PSP is not known. Approximately 1–8% of patients diagnosed clinically as having PD have PSP.

PROGRESSIVE SUPRANUCLEAR PALSY

- Patients present in later life (median age 64 years, range 50–77 years) with symmetrical akinesia and rigidity, which are most marked axially.
- Supranuclear gaze palsy is a characteristic feature.
- Other, variable features include dysarthria, dysphagia, and cognitive changes, that may progress to dementia.
- Death usually occurs after about 6–7 years from aspiration pneumonia.

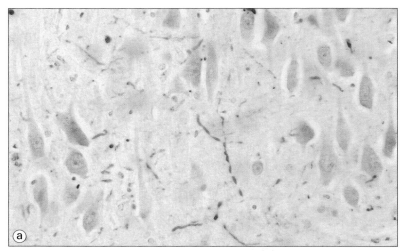
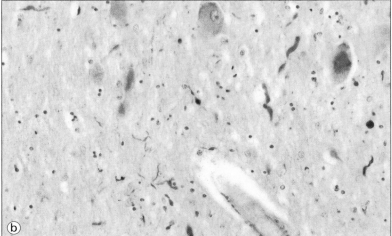
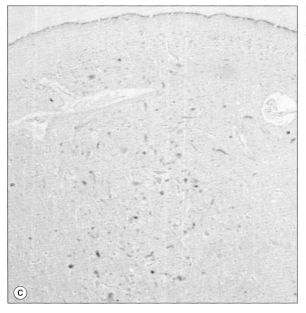

Fig. 28.12 Ubiquinated neurites with a distinctive swollen, beaded, or corkscrew appearance. (a) In the CA2/3 region of the hippocampus. **(b)** In the amygdala. **(c)** In the dorsal vagal nucleus. Restricted involvement of the dorsal vagal nucleus by Lewy bodies and neurites has been associated with isolated dysphagia in elderly patients. (Immunohistochemistry for ubiquitin)

MACROSCOPIC APPEARANCES

There is loss of pigment from the substantia nigra and locus ceruleus (**Fig. 28.13**), and, occasionally, atrophy of the midbrain, pontine tegmentum, and globus pallidus.

MICROSCOPIC APPEARANCES

Certain abnormalities are common to several regions of the central nervous system (CNS) (**Fig. 28.14**):

- Neuronal accumulation of abnormal tau protein (**Fig. 28.15**), either diffusely distributed and detectable only immunohistochemically, or aggregated into neurofibrillary tangles, many of which are also demonstrable by silver impregnation. The tangles stain poorly for ubiquitin.
- Glial cell filamentous inclusions showing tau immunoreactivity (**Fig. 28.16**).
- Neuronal loss and astrocytic gliosis.

The findings vary in different regions of the CNS:

- In the cerebral cortex there are commonly neuronal tangles, tau-reactive glia, and neuropil threads, particularly in the precentral gyrus, entorhinal cortex, and hippocampus. An occasional neuron in the cerebral cortex and basal ganglia may appear swollen and achromasic. An abundance of swollen neurons suggests corticobasal degeneration (CBD).
- In the substantia nigra neuronal loss may be severe, especially ventromedially. Other findings include basophilic globose neuronal tangles, astrocytic gliosis, conspicuous neuropil threads, and tau-reactive glia.
- The pontine nuclei, cerebellar dentate nucleus, striatum, globus pallidus, red nucleus, subthalamic nucleus, and brain stem nuclei contain neuronal tangles, conspicuous neuropil threads, astrocytosis, and tau-reactive glia.
- The cerebellar dentate nucleus may show grumose degeneration (i.e. accumulation of granular eosinophilic material, composed of swollen degenerating Purkinje cell axon terminals, around the neurons).
- The inferior olives often contain small numbers of neuronal tangles. Neuronal hypertrophy and vacuolation may occur in the olives owing to degeneration of neurons in the cerebellar dentate nuclei or central tegmental tracts.
- The spinal cord may conatain tau-immunoractive neuronal tangles, neuropil threads and glia, particularly in the dorsal horns.

Criteria for pathologic diagnosis of PSP have been proposed (see Fig. 28.18)

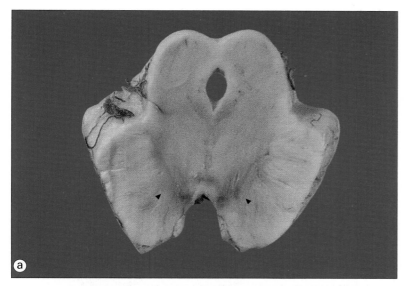

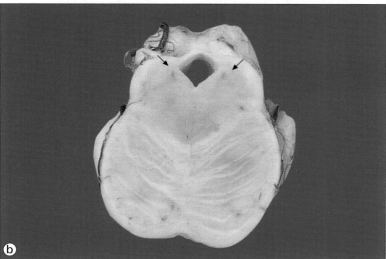

Fig. 28.13 PSP. (a) Atrophy of the midbrain and pallor of the substantia nigra (arrows). **(b)** Pallor of the locus ceruleus (arrows).

DIFFERENTIAL DIAGNOSIS OF PROGRESSIVE SUPRANUCLEAR PALSY

- Supranuclear palsy may be associated with several other neurologic diseases, including vascular disease, Lewy bodies, CBD, and Creutzfeldt–Jakob disease.
- Conversely, pathologic changes of PSP may be found in patients who have not had supranuclear palsy or other typical clinical features of PSP.
- Disorders with neurofibrillary tangles and similar neuronal inclusions and clinical features that can be confused with PSP include:
  - **Postencephalitic parkinsonism.** The distribution of tangles is similar to that in PSP. The clinical picture and history of encephalitis are important distinguishing features. Rarely, parkinsonian patients who have no history of encephalitis are found to have tangles restricted to the substantia nigra and locus ceruleus (tangle-only parkinsonism).
  - **CBD.** The inclusions are confined to the superficial part of the cerebral cortex and the locus ceruleus and substantia nigra, the medial part of which is relatively spared. Finding many swollen neurons in the cerebral cortex also favours a diagnosis of CBD.
  - **Alzheimer's disease.** Tangles may occur in the basal nuclei and brain stem, but are also present in a characteristic distribution in the cerebral cortex where they are accompanied by neuritic plaques (see chapter 32).

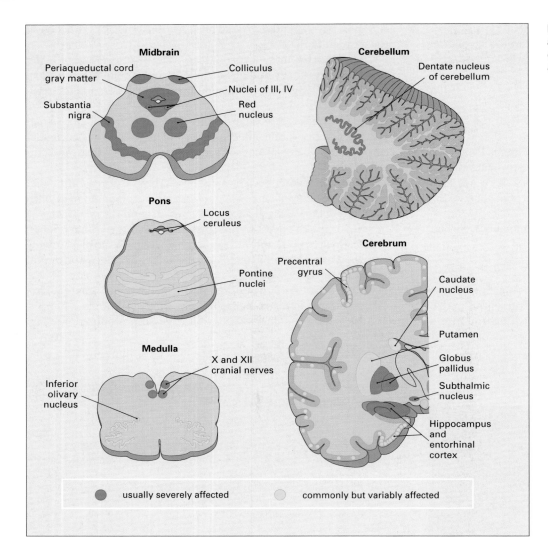

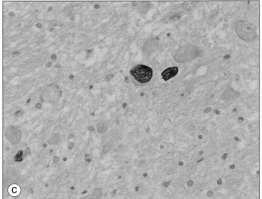

Fig. 28.14 Pathologic changes in PSP. The areas affected in PSP can be divided into those that are consistently and severely affected, and those that are less consistently affected.

Midbrain

Periaqueductal cord gray matter
Substantia nigra
Colliculus
Nuclei of III, IV
Red nucleus

Pons

Locus ceruleus
Pontine nuclei

Medulla

Inferior olivary nucleus
X and XII cranial nerves

Cerebellum

Dentate nucleus of cerebellum

Cerebrum

Precentral gyrus
Caudate nucleus
Putamen
Globus pallidus
Subthalmic nucleus
Hippocampus and entorhinal cortex

● usually severely affected   ○ commonly but variably affected

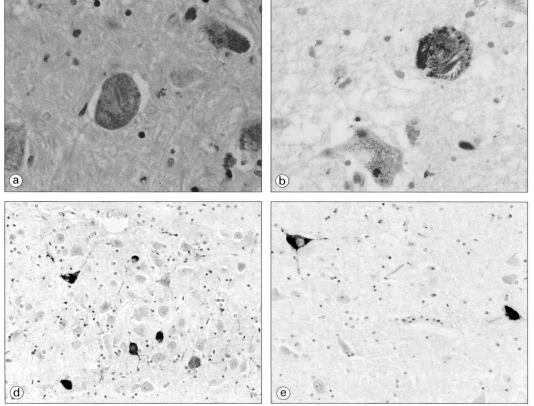

Fig. 28.15 Tangles in PSP. (a) Typical basophilic, rounded or globose tangle in the substantia nigra. **(b)** Gallyas silver impregnation is a sensitive method of detecting the tangles, as in this section of substantia nigra. **(c)** Tangles in the pontine nuclei. (Gallyas silver impregnation) **(d)** tau immunoreactivity is seen in many neurons, as shown here in the pontine nuclei. **(e)** Immunostaining for tau reveals abnormal neurons that do not contain argyrophilic material, especially in the cerebral cortex.

POSTENCEPHALITIC PARKINSONISM

This followed a pandemic of encephalitis lethargica (von Economo's disease) between 1915 and 1927. About 50% of those who survived the acute encephalitis developed an akinetic–rigid syndrome after a period of around 9 years. The nature of the infection remains uncertain.

MACROSCOPIC AND MICROSCOPIC APPEARANCES

Pigmentation of the substantia nigra and the locus ceruleus is reduced. There may be mild generalized cortical atrophy.

Histologically, the substantia nigra is gliotic and severely depleted

of neurons, the locus ceruleus moderately so. Neurofibrillary tangles composed of abnormal tau protein and biochemically and ultrastructurally identical to those in Alzheimer's disease (see chapter 31), are present in the remaining neurons in the substantia nigra (**Fig. 28.17**), and also in the locus ceruleus, hippocampus, and the entorhinal, temporal, frontal, parietal, and insular cortex. There are tau-immunoreactive glial cells in the affected regions.

POSTENCEPALITIC PARKINSONISM

- characterized by rigidity, bradykinesia, tremor with dystonia, pyramidal features, and delirium, which gradually worsen over several decades.
- not usually associated with dementia.

DIFFERENTIAL DIAGNOSIS OF POSTENCEPHALITIC PARKINSONISM

- There is considerable pathologic overlap between postencephalitic parkinsonism, PSP, and Guamanian parkinsonism and they may be indistinguishable on histologic grounds alone. Rarely, tangles confined to the substantia nigra and locus ceruleus occur in parkinsonian patients with no history of encephalitis (tangle-only parkinsonism).
- Nigral degeneration and parkinsonism are unusual complications of severe involvement of the substantia nigra by neurofibrillary tangles in Alzheimer's disease. Very rarely, severe Alzheimer-type nigral changes have been reported to cause parkinsonism without significant cognitive decline despite the presence of plaques and tangles in the cerebral cortex and striatum.

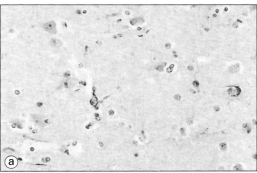

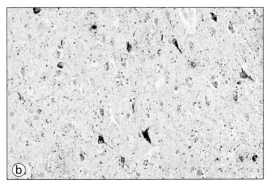

Fig. 28.16 Glial filamentous inclusions in PSP. These are often more obvious than the neuronal tangles. The inclusions extend into glial processes and contribute to the neuropil threads demonstrable by silver impregnation or, as illustrated in these sections of entorhinal cortex, by tau immunohisto-chemistry. **(a)** Shows many glial inclusions in the pontine nuclei. **(b)** Shows glial tau inclusions as well as neuronal inclusions in the cerebellar dentate nucleus.

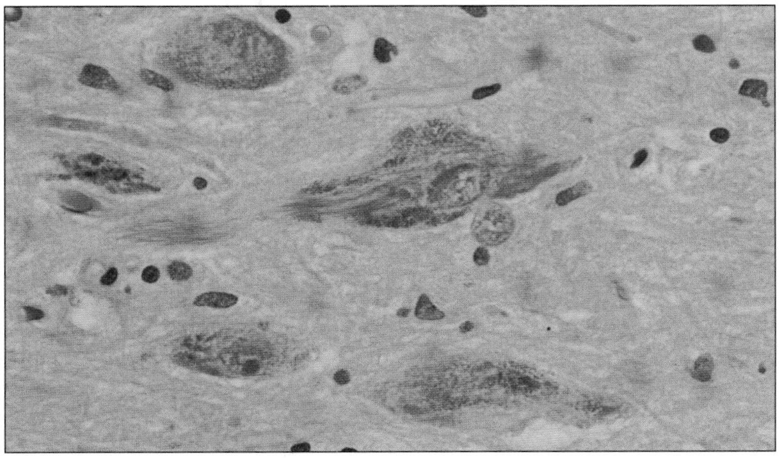

Validated National Institute of Neurologic Disorders and Stroke criteria for the pathologic diagnosis of PSP	
Typical PSP	• Two or more neurons containing a tangle in one microscopic field (x25 objective), and a high density of neutropil threads in at least three of the following regions: globus pallidus, subthalamic nucleus, substantia nigra, pons and • One or more neurons containing a tangle or a low-density of neutropil threads in at least three of the following regions: striatum, oculomotor complex, medulla, dentate nucleus and • Clinical history compatible with PSP (The presence of tau-reactive astrocytes in the affected brain regions supports the diagnosis)
Combined PSP	• Pathologic features of typical PSP as above and • Findings that are diagnostic of another condition affecting the brain stem, or basal ganglia, or both (e.g. infarcts, Lewy body pathology)

Fig. 28.18 Validated National Institute of Neurologic Disorders and Stroke criteria for the pathologic diagnosis of PSP. The criteria are based on histologic assessment of the globus pallidus, putamen, caudate nucleus, subthalamic nucleus, midbrain, pons, medulla, dentate nucleus, hippocampus, parahippocampal gyrus, and cerebral cortex from motor frontal and parietal regions in sections stained by silver impregnation or tau immunohistochemistry and examined at x250 magnification.

Fig. 28.17 Postencephalitic parkinsonism. Basophilic neurofibrillary tangles in the remaining neurons of the substantia nigra are a characteristic feature of postencephalitic parkinsonism.

MULTIPLE SYSTEM ATROPHY (MSA)

This term includes three disorders previously regarded as separate conditions, but unified by considerable clinical and pathologic overlap and the presence of very large numbers of distinctive inclusion bodies in glial cells. These disorders are:

- olivopontocerebellar atrophy (OPCA)
- Shy–Drager syndrome
- striatonigral degeneration

Of patients diagnosed clinically as having PD, 7–20% have MSA. The cause of MSA is not known.

MULTIPLE SYSTEM ATROPHY

- Patients usually presents between the fourth and sixth decades.
- The signs and symptoms relate to the systems involved (i.e. the specific ganglia and corresponding fiber tracts) and include parkinsonism, cerebellar ataxia, autonomic failure, laryngeal paresis, motor weakness, and cognitive decline.
- Death often results from the development of bulbar dysfunction and dysphagia, predisposing to aspiration pneumonia.
- In some patients sudden death may result from apnea due to involvement of the laryngeal muscles.

MACROSCOPIC APPEARANCES

Depending on the systems involved, there may be:

- atrophy of the cerebellum, middle cerebellar peduncles, and pons (**Fig. 28.19**).
- pallor of the substantia nigra and locus ceruleus (**Fig. 28.20**).
- atrophy and gray-brown discoloration of the putamen (**Fig. 28.21**).

Atrophy of the cerebral cortex, if present, is mild. The spinal cord is macroscopically normal, even in patients with autonomic failure.

MICROSCOPIC APPEARANCES

Several ganglia or regions of the CNS may show neuronal loss and astrocytic gliosis. The affected ganglia or regions are often in synaptic contact (e.g. the striatum and the substantia nigra, or the inferior olives and the Purkinje cells). However, the distribution is very variable and may include dorsolateral putamen, substantia nigra, locus ceruleus, the Purkinje cell layer of cerebellum, basis pontis, inferior olivary nucleus, dorsal motor nucleus of vagus, and intermediolateral column of the spinal cord.

The neuronal loss results in a corresponding loss of myelinated fibers from the external capsule, striatum and globus pallidus (striatopallidal fibers), cerebellar white matter, middle cerebellar peduncle, and basis pontis (transverse pontine fibers).

There are, in addition, four types of cytologic abnormality: glial cytoplasmic inclusions, neuronal cytoplasmic inclusions, nuclear inclusions, and neuropil threads.

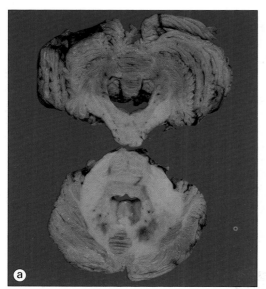

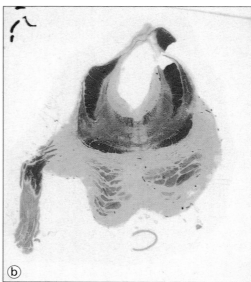

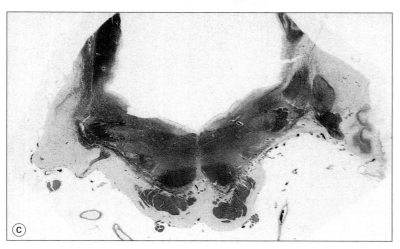

Fig. 28.19 MSA-OPCA pattern. (a) Horizontal sections through the pons and medulla of a patient with OPCA pattern of MSA (top) and a normal control (bottom). In OPCA there may be marked atrophy of the cerebellum, middle cerebellar peduncles, and base of the pons, the last two features giving the pons a 'beaked' appearance. **(b)** Marked atrophy of the base of the pons with loss of transverse pontine fibers. The superior cerebellar peduncles are preserved. (Loyez myelin stain) **(c)** Loss of pontocerebellar fibers, but preservation of the pontine tegmentum and superior cerebellar penduncles. (Loyez myelin stain)

Glial cytoplasmic inclusions:
- these inclusions are present in high density in MSA
- affect oligodendroglia in gray and white matter
- demonstrable by silver impregnation (Gallyas is particularly sensitive) (**Fig. 28.22a**)
- usually flame- or sickle-shaped
- immunoreactive for tau-protein, ubiquitin, tubulin, and αB-crystallin (**Fig. 28.22b,c**)
- electron microscopy shows randomly arranged 20–40 nm tubules or filaments associated with granular material on ultrastructural examination

Neuronal cytoplasmic inclusions:
- rounded filamentous structures, predominantly seen in the pontine nuclei, putamen, subthalamic nucleus, amygdala, hippocampus, dentate fascia, substantia nigra, inferior olivary nucleus, and the brain stem reticular formation
- demonstrable by silver impregnation (Gallyas is particularly sensitive)
- immunoreactive for ubiquitin
- ultrastructural examination reveals a meshwork of 18–28 nm filaments associated with granular material
- present in large numbers in the basis pontis and putamen only

Nuclear inclusions:
- sparse in most cases, these inclusions are seen predominantly in the basis pontis and putamen
- demonstrable in neuronal and glial nuclei by Gallyas silver impregnation
- evident as a web of fine fibrils beneath the nuclear membrane in neurons (**Fig. 28.23**) and evident as small rods in glia

Neuropil threads:
- numerous only in the basis pontis and putamen
- immunoreactive for ubiquitin, but not tau-protein

DIFFERENTIAL DIAGNOSIS OF MSA

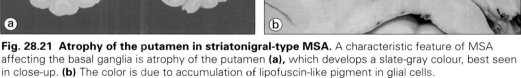

- MSA enters the differential diagnosis of parkinsonism, cerebellar ataxia, and autonomic failure.
- Relatively sparse glial cytoplasmic inclusions can occur in other degenerative diseases, especially CBD.
- An OPCA pattern of atrophy is often found in inherited or sporadic spinocerebellar ataxias.
- Shy–Drager syndrome can be caused by Lewy body pathology.
- Multiple system degeneration may occur in association with the inclusions of motor neuron disease.

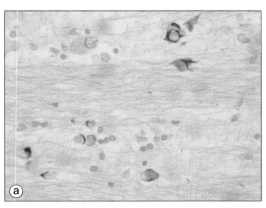
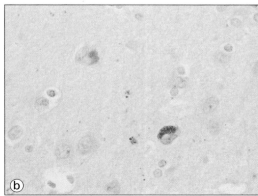
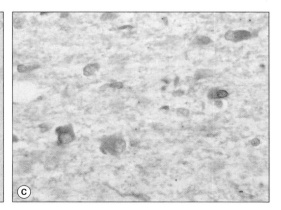

Fig. 28.20 Striatonigral-type MSA. Pallor of the substantia nigra in MSA, reflecting the loss of pigmented neurons. The loss of nigral neurons contributes in part to the extrapyramidal features of MSA.

Fig. 28.21 Atrophy of the putamen in striatonigral-type MSA. A characteristic feature of MSA affecting the basal ganglia is atrophy of the putamen **(a),** which develops a slate-gray colour, best seen in close-up. **(b)** The color is due to accumulation of lipofuscin-like pigment in glial cells.

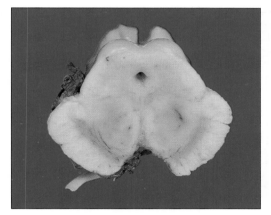
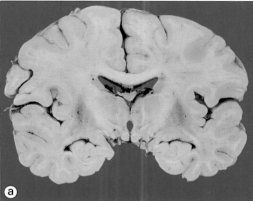
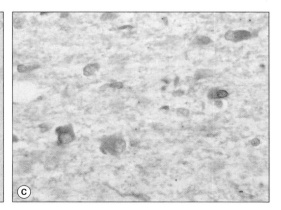

Fig. 28.22 Glial cytoplasmic inclusions in MSA. (a) Flame- or sickle-shaped glial cytoplasmic inclusions. (Gallyas silver impregnation) **(b)** Many of the glial cytoplasmic inclusions are immunoreactive for tau protein. **(c)** Glial cytoplasmic inclusions immunoreactive for ubiquitin.

CORTICOBASAL DEGENERATION (CBD)

This is a disorder of unknown etiology and is very rarely familial. Other terms for the same disorder include corticodentatonigral degeneration with neuronal achromasia, cortical–basal ganglionic degeneration, and corticonigral degeneration.

CORTICOBASAL DEGENERATION

- Average age of onset is approximately 60 years.
- Three phases of illness can usually be distinguished:
  - **Early phase** (years 1–3) asymmetric clumsiness, stiffness, or jerking of an arm or leg.
  - **Middle phase** (years 3–5) dystonic rigidity and akinesia of the limbs, 'alien limb' phenomenon, lower limb apraxia, pyramidal deficits, and cortical sensory disturbances.
  - **Late phase** (years 5–8) cognitive dysfunction and frontotemporal neurobehavioral disorder.
- Death is usually due to bronchopneumonia, in some cases related to bulbar dysfunction and aspiration.
- Can have atypical manifestations, which include primary aphasia, other circumscribed cortical dysfunction, and frontotemporal dementia.

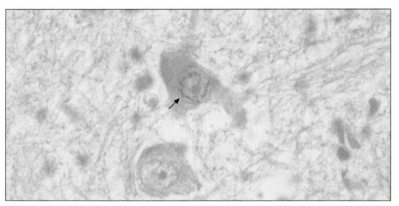

Fig. 28.23 Neuronal nuclear inclusion of MSA. This appears as a delicate web of argyrophilic intranuclear filaments (arrows). (Gallyas silver impregnation)

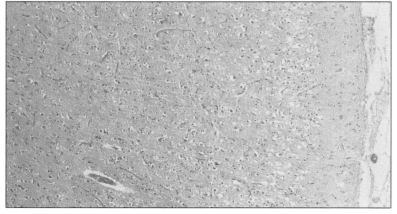

Fig. 28.24 CBD showing cortical microvacuolation. The microvacuolation is initially restricted to the superficial cortical layers. Later it affects all layers and is associated with marked gliosis.

MACROSCOPIC APPEARANCES

The posterior frontal, parietal, or the peri-Rolandic cortex shows atrophy, which is often asymmetric, relating to the distribution of limb and other involvement during life. The substantia nigra and locus ceruleus appear abnormally pale.

MICROSCOPIC APPEARANCES

The affected regions of cerebral cortex are usually well delimited and show neuronal loss and microvacuolation (**Fig. 28.24**), swollen neurons (**Fig. 28.25**), and astrocytic gliosis. Some neurons contain inclusion bodies (**Fig. 28.26**).

The substantia nigra is depleted of neurons and gliotic, especially laterally, with relative sparing of the medial nigra, and inclusions are present in some of the remaining neurons (**Fig. 28.27**).

Neuronal loss and astrocytosis with small numbers of swollen neurons may be seen in the globus pallidus, corpus striatum, subthalamic nucleus, thalamus, and red nucleus.

Deep to the affected parts of the cerebral cortex there is a loss of myelinated fibers from the hemispheric white matter and, in some cases, the corticospinal tracts. This may be associated with marked astrocytic gliosis.

All affected areas contain tau-immunoreactive glial cells (**Fig. 28.28**).

CLINICOPATHOLOGIC CORRELATIONS IN MSA

- Nigrostriatal degeneration causes parkinsonism that may be responsive to levodopa in the early stages.
- Degeneration of pontine nuclei and Purkinje cells results in progressive cerebellar ataxia.
- Degeneration of intermediolateral column neurons gives rise to autonomic disturbances related to loss of sympathetic function.
- Atrophy of the posterior cricoarytenoid (abductor) muscles causes laryngeal stridor.
- Loss of neurons from Onufrowicz's nucleus leads to sphincter disturbances.
- Frontal lobe dysfunction and dementia are related to involvement of the cerebral cortex.

DIFFERENTIAL DIAGNOSIS OF CBD

Prominent swollen cortical neurons are a feature of several neurodegenerative diseases.
- Large numbers of prominent swollen cortical neurons may be seen in Pick's disease with Pick bodies, CBD, and occasional cases of Creutzfeldt–Jakob disease.
- Small numbers of prominent swollen cortical neurons may be seen in Lewy body dementia, Alzheimer's disease, and motor neuron disease–inclusion dementia.
- Very occasional swollen cortical neurons are seen in PSP and Nasu–Hakola disease (membranous lipodystrophy).

There is considerable overlap in the distribution of basal and cortical tau-related pathology between CBD and PSP. The presence of large numbers of swollen cortical neurons, sparing of the cerebellar dentate nucleus, and a paucity of tangles in the pons and medulla favor a diagnosis of CBD rather than PSP.

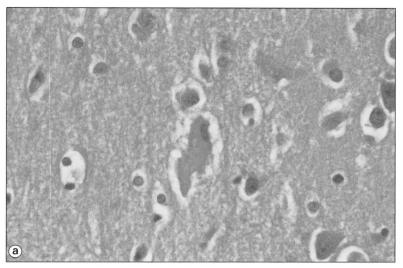

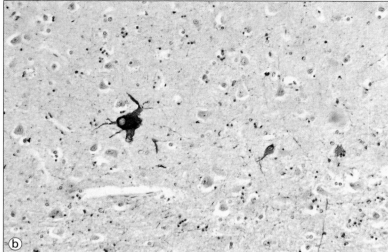

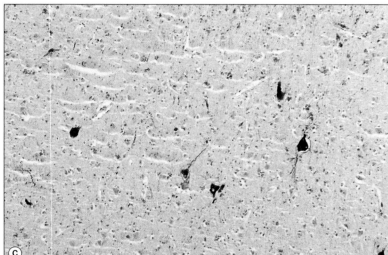

Fig. 28.25 Swollen cortical neurons (also termed achromasic or ballooned neurons) are a distinctive finding in CBD. (a) They are easily detected in hematoxylin and eosin-stained sections and are most frequent in layers III, IV, and VI, in the peri-Rolandic, posterior frontal, and parietal cortices. In advanced cases such swollen neurons may be seen in the insular and frontal cortex and the tip of the temporal lobe. **(b)** and **(c)** Cortex stained to show αB-crystallin. The swollen cells strongly express phosphorylated neurofilament proteins and αB-crystallin. Here immunostaining of αB-crystallin emphasizes the distortion of the axons and dendrites of the swollen neurons.

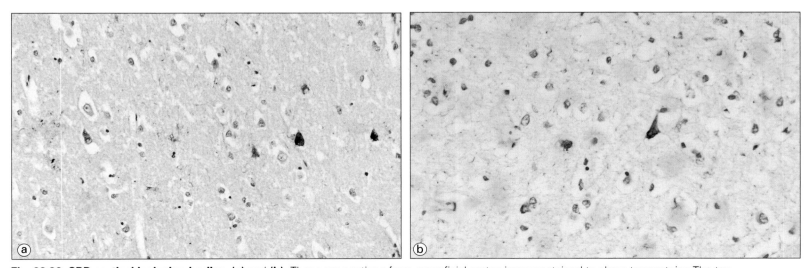

Fig. 28.26 CBD cortical inclusion bodies. (a) and **(b).** These are sections from superficial cortex immunostained to show tau-proteins. The tau-immunoreactive globular or angular inclusions (which are not ubiquitinated) are present in small numbers of neurons in the superficial cortex. The inclusions occur in residual neurons in areas of superficial microvacuolation, but may not be detectable in severely gliotic cortex.

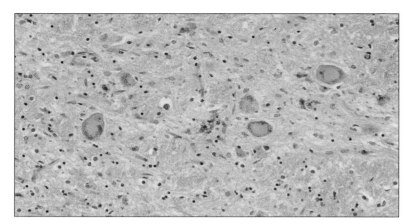

Fig. 28.27 Nigral neuronal loss and astrocytic gliosis in CBD. Argyrophilic filamentous inclusions termed 'corticobasal inclusions' are present in residual nigral neurons. In hematoxylin and eosin-stained sections the inclusions are moderately to weakly basophilic and displace the neuromelanin. Similar inclusions may be seen in the locus ceruleus. The inclusions are immunoreactive for tau-protein. Ultrastructurally, some consist of paired helical filaments, while others are composed of straight tubules and resemble the tangles of PSP.

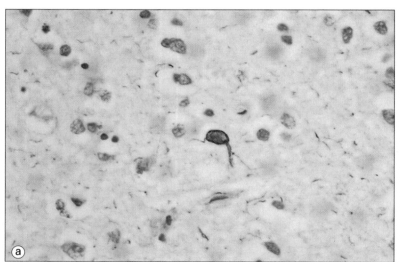

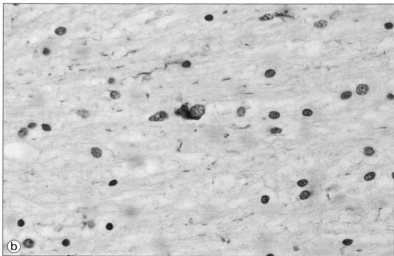

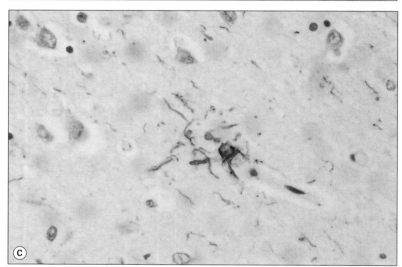

Fig. 28.28 Tau-immunoreactive glial inclusions in CBD. (a) Glial inclusions which are immunoreactive for tau protein are present in large numbers in CBD. Most appear as coils and grains as shown here. These can also be detected by Gallyas silver impregnation. **(b)** Some glial tau-reactive inclusions resemble those seen in MSA but are present in low density. **(c)** A feature of CBD is the formation of star-like tufts of glial processes detected either by IHC for tau protein (as here) or by Gallyas impregnation. These are seen in affected cortical regions.

ARTERIOSCLEROTIC PSEUDOPARKINSONISM

MACROSCOPIC AND MICROSCOPIC APPEARANCES

Pathologically, there are usually lacunar infarcts in the basal ganglia (**Fig. 28.29**) or ischemic lesions in the white matter of the frontal lobes (**Fig. 28.30**). Infarction of the substantia nigra is a very rare cause of parkinsonism.

ARTERIOSCLEROTIC PSEUDOPARKINSONISM

- This mainly affects the lower limbs, sparing the upper limbs and face.
- Bradykinesia and rigidity predominate. Tremor is unusual.
- Patients usually have risk factors for arteriosclerosis (e.g. hypertension, diabetes mellitus).

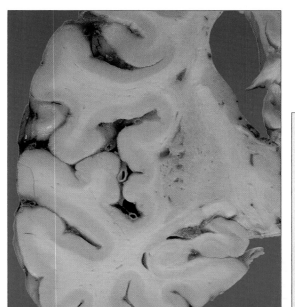

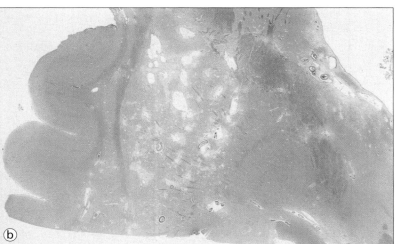

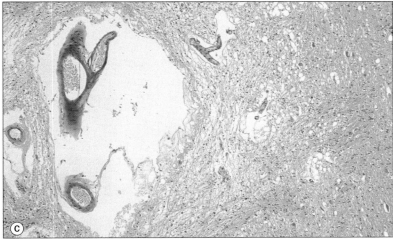

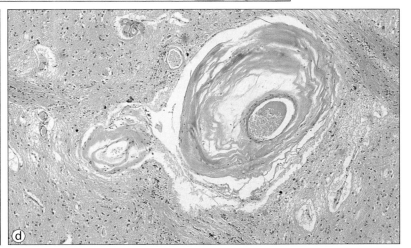

Fig. 28.29 Arteriosclerotic pseudoparkinsonism. (a) Multiple lacunar infarcts in the putamen. **(b)** Histology of basal ganglia shows dilated perivascular spaces with rarefaction of parenchyma. **(c)** Astrocytic gliosis is present around the dilated perivascular spaces. **(d)** Vessels in the basal ganglia are markedly arteriosclerotic.

Fig. 28.30 Patchy ischemic degeneration of frontal white matter. (Solochrome cyanin)

GUAM PARKINSONISM-DEMENTIA

This neurodegenerative disease occurs almost exclusively in the Western Pacific Marianas islands of Guam and Rota, and the Kii peninsula. The cause is not known. The incidence has been declining.

GUAM PARKINSONISM-DEMENTIA

- The manifestations are amyotrophic lateral sclerosis (ALS) and parkinsonism, in varying combination and usually with dementia.
- ALS may precede the development of parkinsonism–dementia by several years. Conversely, some patients develop ALS late in the course of the illness.
- The onset is usually in middle age.

MACROSCOPIC AND MICROSCOPIC APPEARANCES

The brain usually shows generalized atrophy, with pallor of the substantia nigra and locus ceruleus.

Histologically, neuronal loss and astrocytic gliosis are associated with neurofibrillary tangles in:
- hypocampus and amygdala
- the cerebral cortex (particularly in neurons in the superficial cortical laminae (**28.31a**), where the distribution of tangles may be patchy (**28.31b**) – the medial temporal cortex is usually severely affected
- basal ganglia
- thalamus
- hypothalamus
- substantia nigra (**28.31c**) (especially in patients with parkinsonian features)
- brain stem tegmental nuclei (**28.31d**)
- in small numbers, in anterior horn cells of the spinal cord (mainly in patients with features of MND)

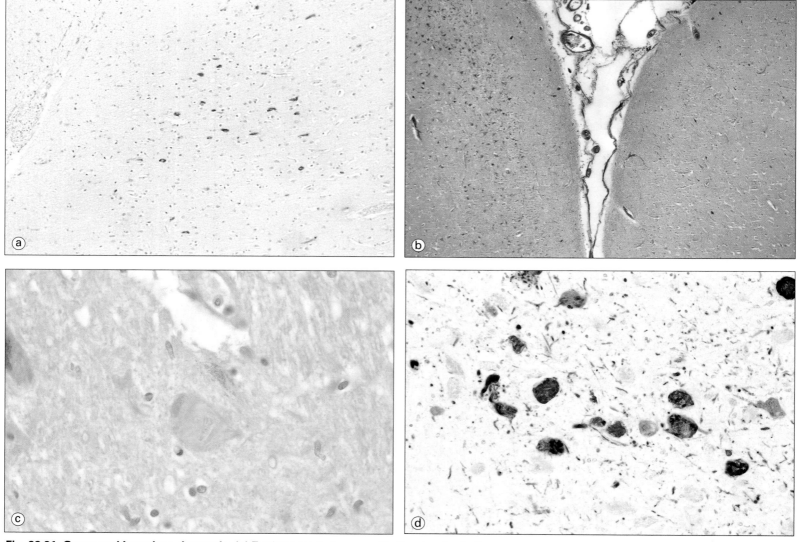

Fig. 28.31 Guam parkinsonism–dementia. (a) Tau-immunoractive neurofibrillary tangles in the superficial laminae of the neocortex. **(b)** Silver impregnation of two adjacent gyri reveals numerous tangles in one and relatively few in the other. **(c)** Tangle in a remaining neuron in the substantia nigra. **(d)** Numerous tau-immunoreactive tangles and neurites in the oculomotor nucleus.

DISEASES CHARACTERIZED BY ABNORMAL STIFFNESS

The rigidity of parkinsonian disorders should be distinguished from diseases in which stiffness is caused by continuous muscle activity.

Stiff man syndrome

- An autoimmune disease that presents in the fourth and fifth decades and results from reduced GABA-ergic inhibition in the spinal cord with a resulting increase in the activity of spinal flexor reflex pathways.
- Autoantibodies to glutamic acid decarboxylase are present in most patients.
- Antibodies to the synaptic vesicle-associated protein amphiphysin have been found in stiff man syndrome associated with breast cancer.
- Histology shows a loss of neurons and astrocytic gliosis in the medial motor nuclei of the spinal anterior horn and perivascular lymphocytic infiltration.

Progressive encephalomyelitis with rigidity (spinal interneuronitis)

- An idiopathic disorder of progressive muscle stiffness with multiple cranial nerve palsies.
- Histology shows neuronal loss and lymphocytic infiltration in the brain stem and spinal cord.

NECROPSY IN CASES OF AKINETIC–RIGID SYNDROME

- The brain should be fixed intact for neuropathologic examination.
- If sympathetic or motor neuron dysfunction has been a feature, the spinal cord should also be kept for examination of the intermediolateral columns and anterior horns.
- Regions of the CNS sampled for histology should include substantia nigra, pons (with locus ceruleus), medulla at the level of dorsal vagal nucleus, globus pallidus and putamen at the level of the lateral geniculate bodies, hippocampus and parahippocampal gyrus at the level of the lateral geniculate bodies, and any macroscopic focal abnormality.
- Assessment of the hippocampal and parahippocampal block, at least, should include stains and immunostains suitable for detecting neurofibrillary tangles.
- If examination of the substantia nigra and locus ceruleus reveals Lewy bodies and cell loss, and there are no other pathologic abnormalities, it is usually safe to make a diagnosis of idiopathic PD.
- Tangles in the substantia nigra suggest PSP, CBD, or postencephalitic parkinsonism, and additional blocks and stains will be needed for diagnosis.
- Neuronal loss and gliosis involving the substantia nigra, striatum, or pons suggest MSA. Additional blocks should be taken of regions likely to be affected and appropriate stains performed to detect glial cytoplasmic inclusions.
- Evidence of lacunar infarction and small vessel disease in the basal ganglia supports the possibility of vascular pseudoparkinsonism.
- In akinetic–rigid disease with cognitive decline, the brain should be examined as for dementia (see chapter 32), with particular emphasis on dementia with cortical Lewy bodies, Alzheimer's disease, and CBD.

REFERENCES

Arima K *et al.* (1994) Corticonigral degeneration with neuronal achromasia presenting with primary progressive aphasia: ultrastructural and immunocytochemical studies. *J Neurol Sci* **127**: 186–197.

Bancher C, Jellinger K (1994) Neurofibrillary tangle predominant form of senile dementia of Alzheimer type: a rare subtype in very old subjects. *Acta Neuropathol* **88**: 565–570.

Chang CM, Yu YL *et al.* (1992) Vascular pseudoparkinsonism. *Acta Neurol Scand* **86**: 588–592.

Forno LS (1996) Neuropathology of Parkinson's disease. *J Neuropathol Exp Neurol* **55**: 259–272.

Gearing M, Olson DA *et al.* (1994) Progressive supranuclear palsy: neuropathologic and clinical heterogeneity. *Neurology* **44**: 1015–1024.

Geddes JF, Hughes AJ *et al.* (1993) Pathological overlap in cases of parkinsonism associated with neurofibrillary tangles. A study of recent cases of postencephalitic parkinsonism and comparison with progressive supranuclear palsy and Guamanian parkinsonism–dementia complex. *Brain* **116**: 281–302.

Hughes AJ, Daniel SE *et al.* (1993) A clinicopathologic study of 100 cases of Parkinson's disease. *Arch Neurol* **50**(2): 140–148.

Lilienfeld D, Perl D *et al.* (1994) Guam neurodegeneration. In D Calne (ed.) *Neurodegenerative Diseases*. pp. 895–908. Philadelphia: WB Saunders.

Litvan I, Hauw JJ *et al.* (1996) Validity and reliability of the preliminary NINDS neuropathologic criteria for progressive supranuclear palsy and related disorders. *J Neuropath Exp Neurol* **55**: 97–105.

Lowe J (1994) Lewy bodies. In D Calne (ed.) *Neurodegenerative Diseases*. pp. 51–69. Philadelphia WB Saunders.

Meinck HM, Ricker K *et al.* (1994) Stiff man syndrome: clinical and laboratory findings in eight patients. *J Neurol* **241**: 157–166.

Mori H, Nishimura M *et al.* (1994) Corticobasal degeneration: a disease with widespread appearance of abnormal tau and neurofibrillary tangles and its relation to progressive supranuclear palsy. *Acta Neuropathol* **88**: 113–121.

Murrow RW, Schweiger GD *et al.* (1990) Parkinsonism due to a basal ganglia lacunar state: Clinicopathologic correlation. *Neurology* **40**: 897–900.

Papp MI, Lantos PL (1992) Accumulation of tubular structures in oligodendroglial and neuronal cells as the basic alteration in multiple system atrophy. *J Neurol Sci* **107**: 172–182.

Pollanen MS, Dickson DW *et al.* (1993) Pathology and biology of the Lewy body. *J Neuropathol Exp Neurol* **5**: 183–191.

Quinn N (1989) Multiple system atrophy—the nature of the beast. *J Neurol Neurosurg Psychiatry* **52** (Suppl.): 78–89.

Rinne JO, Lee MS *et al.* (1994) Corticobasal degeneration. A clinical study of 36 cases. *Brain* **117**(5): 1183–1196.

Stone R (1993) Guam: deadly disease dying out. *Science* **261**: 424–426.

Takahashi H, Ohama E *et al.* (1994) Familial juvenile parkinsonism: clinical and pathologic study in a family. *Neurology* **44**: 437–441.

Yoshimura N, Yoshimura I *et al.* (1988) Juvenile Parkinson's disease with widespread Lewy bodies in the brain. *Acta Neuropathol* **77**: 213–218.

29 *Ataxic disorders*

The spinocerebellar ataxias (SCAs) are a heterogeneous group of disorders characterized by progressive cerebellar ataxia, which is variably associated with other neurologic and systemic abnormalities. The pathologic substrate is degeneration of the cerebellum or its afferent and efferent tracts.

Cerebellar and spinocerebellar degenerations can be divided into two broad groups: primary and secondary (**Figs 29.1–29.3**). In addition to degenerative cerebellar ataxias, the cerebellum is affected in several malformations and developmental disorders (see chapter 3).

Secondary causes of cerebellar disease (i.e. toxic, nutritional, metabolic, inflammatory, infective, ischemic, and paraneoplastic) are dealt with in the relevant chapters elsewhere in this book.

Classification of spinocerebellar ataxias

Primary

- Inherited
  autosomal recessive
  autosomal dominant
  sex-linked
- Sporadic
  multiple system atrophy
  idiopathic cerebellar degeneration

Secondary

- Paraneoplastic
- Toxic/nutritional
- Vascular
- Infective/inflammatory
- Prion disease
- Metabolic diseases
- Mitochondrial diseases

Fig. 29.1 Classification of SCAs.

Classification of primary spinocerebellar ataxias

The eponymous conditions of early classification schemes were based on a mixture of pathologic and clinical criteria. Because of poor correlation between the clinical and pathologic features, and the inability to discriminate pathologically between different genetic disorders, these schemes have been largely abandoned in favor of a classification that places greater emphasis on clinical and genetic features.

The primary spinocerebellar ataxias fall into three broad groups:

- Familial spinocerebellar ataxias — subdivided according to a genetic classification that has been supported by the identification of many of the genes responsible for causing disease.
- Multiple system atrophy (chapter 2) can produce a pathologic picture of *cerebellar cortical atrophy* or *olivopontocerebellar atrophy*, with variable involvement of other regions of the CNS. These disorders can be distinguished from other types of cerebellar degeneration by recognition of the distinctive inclusion bodies.
- Other forms of sporadic idiopathic cerebellar degeneration
  – the commonest of which is of late onset and takes the form of isolated cerebellar cortical degeneration.

Fig. 29.2 Classification of primary SCAs. The eponymous conditions of early classification schemes were based on a mixture of pathologic and clinical criteria. These schemes have been largely abandoned in favor of a classification that places greater emphasis on clinical and genetic features.

Classification of inherited spinocerebellar and cerebellar ataxias

Autosomal recessive cerebellar ataxia
- Friedreich's ataxia
- SCA with retained reflexes
- SCA with isolated vitamin E deficiency
- Ataxia telangiectasia
- Rare recessive ataxias

X-linked cerebellar ataxia

Autosomal dominant cerebellar ataxia
- ADCA I
  SCA 1
  SCA 2
  SCA 3
  SCA 4
  SCA 5
  SCA 6
  SCA 7
- ADCA II
- ADCA III
- ADCA IV
- Dentatorubropallidoluysial atrophy (DRPLA)
- Episodic ataxias

Fig. 29.3 Classification of inherited spinocerebellar and cerebellar ataxias.

CEREBELLAR CORTICAL DEGENERATION

MACROSCOPIC AND MICROSCOPIC APPEARANCES

Cerebellar cortical degeneration is characterized macroscopically by atrophy of the cerebellar folia with widening of the intervening sulci and reduction in the amount of white matter (**Fig. 29.4a,b**).

The histologic changes are nonspecific and can be seen in diverse diseases that are clinically, metabolically, or genetically distinct. The Purkinje cells are reduced in number and may be absent from large lengths of cortex (**Fig. 29.4c,d**). There may also be a loss of granule cells, which is sometimes marked (see Fig. 29.4d). Surviving Purkinje cells frequently show axonal swellings ('torpedoes'). These are visible in the cerebellar granular layer as eosinophilic spheroids (see **Fig. 29.4d**),

but are better demonstrated by silver impregnation (**Fig. 29.4e,f**) or immunohistochemistry for neurofilament proteins. At the sites of loss of Purkinje cells the persisting basket cell fibers form 'empty baskets' that can be demonstrated by silver impregnation (**Fig. 29.4g**, see also **Fig. 29.4f**). With loss of Purkinje cells there is proliferation of Bergmann astrocytes at the junction of the granular and molecular layers (**Fig. 29.4h**). Bergmann astrocytes extend processes towards the pial surface in a regular radial pattern termed 'isomorphic gliosis' (**Fig. 29.4i**). Degeneration of Purkinje cells causes some loss of myelinated fibers from the cerebellar folia.

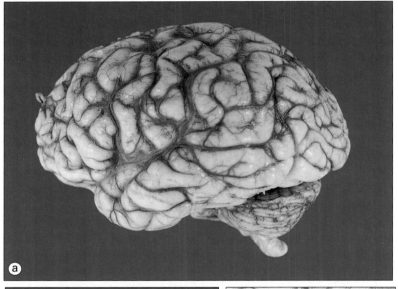

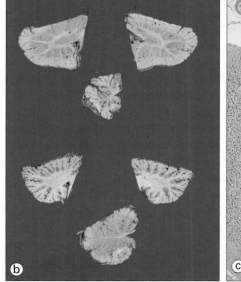

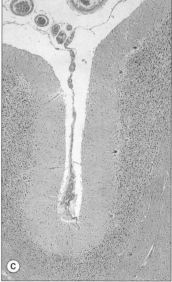

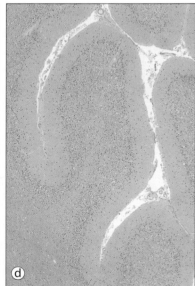

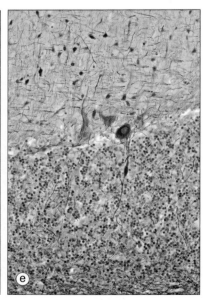

Fig. 29.4 Cerebellar cortical degeneration. (a) Lateral view of the brain from a patient with cerebellar cortical degeneration showing the marked atrophy of the cerebellum in relation to the size of the cerebrum. **(b)** Slices through the cerebellar hemispheres and vermis of a control brain (left) and a patient with cerebellar cortical degeneration (right). Note the reduction in the volume of cortical gray matter and the widening of the cerebellar sulci. **(c)** Patchy loss of Purkinje cells. **(d)** Severe diffuse loss of Purkinje cells. Note the eosinophilic Purkinje cell axonal swellings ('torpedoes') in the granule cell layer towards the top of the figure. There is also marked depletion of granule cells and proliferation of Bergmann astrocytes.

(e) The Purkinje cell axonal swellings are readily demonstrable by silver impregnation. **(f)** Note the 'empty basket' to the right of the axonal swelling. (Palmgren silver impregnation) **(g)** Several adjacent 'empty baskets' in cerebellar cortical degeneration. (Palmgren silver impregnation) **(h)** The degeneration of Purkinje cells is associated with proliferation of Bergmann astrocytes, at the junction of the granular and molecular layers. Note also the moderate loss of myelinated fibers from the white matter. (Luxol fast blue/cresyl violet) **(i)** Bergmann astrocytosis accompanied by isomorphic gliosis of the molecular layer. (Phosphotungstic acid/hematoxylin)

AUTOSOMAL RECESSIVE CEREBELLAR ATAXIA

This pattern of inheritance accounts for the majority of patients with early onset disease.

FRIEDREICH'S ATAXIA (FA)
MACROSCOPIC AND MICROSCOPIC APPEARANCES

The brain is generally macroscopically unremarkable, although cardiomyopathy may have caused ischemic damage. The spinal cord and dorsal roots are typically atrophic. Histologic abnormalities involve several regions of the CNS:

- The spinal cord shows degeneration and astrocytosis of the posterior columns, affecting the gracile more than the cuneate fasciculus, with distal degeneration of the pyramidal and spinocerebellar tracts (**Fig.** 29.5a,b). There is typically severe loss of neurons from Clarke's column.
- In the medulla, tract degeneration is accompanied by neuronal loss from the accessory cuneate and gracile nuclei, reflecting transneuronal degeneration. Cell loss and astrocytosis are seen in the vestibular and cochlear nuclei and in the superior olives. The inferior olives are generally normal.
- In the cerebellum the white matter may show astrocytic gliosis while the cerebellar cortex is usually normal. Hypoxic–ischemic damage caused by cardiomyopathy may produce secondary cerebellar cortical damage. Severe cell loss is seen in the dentate nuclei with marked atrophy of the superior cerebellar peduncle.
- In the cerebral cortex there are generally no specific pathologic

FRIEDREICH'S ATAXIA (FA)

- The prevalence is 1–2 per 100,000.
- Onset is usually before the age of 15 years and is rare after 25 years, although late onset cases have been identified by genetic studies.
- Patients typically present with ataxia of gait, and later, limb ataxia, dysarthria, loss of joint position and vibration sense in the lower limbs, generalized areflexia, pyramidal lower limb weakness, and extensor plantar responses. Ataxia is due to a combination of sensory neuropathy and the degeneration of cerebellar afferent and efferent fibers. Scoliosis and pes cavus are common.
- Over 60% of patients develop cardiomyopathy, and approximately 10% diabetes mellitus.
- Patients usually die by the end of their fourth decade.

GENETICS OF FA

- FA is caused by expansion of a GAA triplet repeat region in the gene that encodes a novel protein called frataxin. The gene has been mapped to a small centromeric region of chromosome 9q. The normal gene contains 10–21 repeats. In most patients with FA the number of repeats ranges from 200–900.
- This is the first recognized neurodegenerative disease that is caused by a triplet repeat expansion and also shows autosomal recessive inheritance.
- Expression studies have shown severe reduction in frataxin mRNA in the spinal cord and cerebellum of patients with FA, suggesting that the mutation causes abnormal transcription or processing of the mRNA.

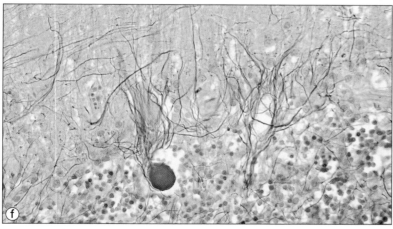

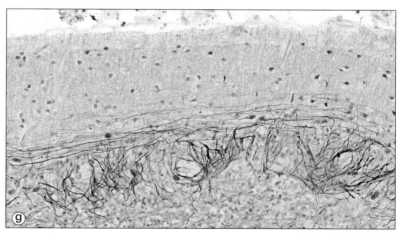

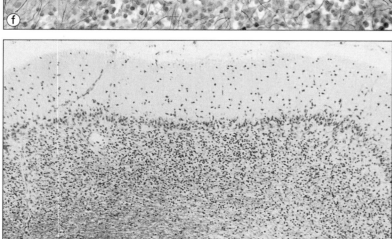

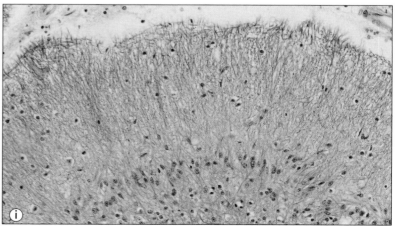

changes, but functional imaging studies have demonstrated cortical atrophy and reduced metabolism. Hypoxic–ischemic damage due to cardiomyopathy may produce secondary cortical damage.

- There may be neuronal loss from the globus pallidus and the subthalamic nuclei.
- Optic nerves and tracts usually show a slight loss of fibers.
- Peripheral nerves show a loss of dorsal root ganglion cells (**Fig. 29.5c**) associated with severe depletion of large myelinated axons from the posterior roots (**Fig. 29.5d**) and sensory nerves.

EARLY ONSET CEREBELLAR ATAXIA WITH RETAINED TENDON REFLEXES

This is probably genetically heterogeneous, some cases being phenotypic variants of FA and others not linked to chromosome 9. It is distinguished from FA by the retained tendon reflexes and the absence of significant peripheral neuropathy, optic atrophy, severe skeletal deformity, cardiomyopathy, or diabetes mellitus. The prognosis is substantially better than that of FA, with patients surviving into the fifth decade.

Neuroimaging shows more pronounced atrophy of the cerebellum and less of the spinal cord than in FA. There have been no definitive neuropathologic studies.

CEREBELLAR ATAXIA WITH ISOLATED VITAMIN E DEFICIENCY

This is caused by mutations of the gene encoding α-tocopherol transfer protein, which is needed for the absorption of dietary vitamin E. The manifestations are indistinguishable from those of FA (i.e. ataxia, areflexia, sensory loss, and pyramidal weakness, sometimes accompanied by cardiomyopathy), but progression can be prevented by vitamin E supplements. In North Africa AVED (ataxia with vitamin E deficiency) is as common as FA.

MACROSCOPIC AND MICROSCOPIC APPEARANCES

Scant information is available on the neuropathologic findings in this disorder, but they are presumably the same as in vitamin E deficiency due to malabsorption resulting from pancreatic, liver, or intestinal disease (see chapter 21).

ATAXIA–TELANGIECTASIA (AT)

This is the commonest cause of progressive ataxia in infancy, with an incidence of at least 1/80,000 live births.

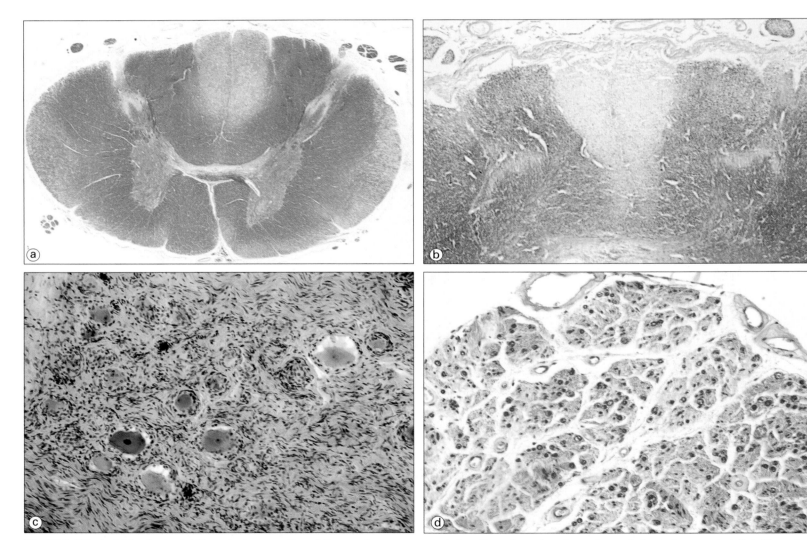

Fig. 29.5 Friedreich's ataxia. (a) There is degeneration of the gracile funiculi and spinocerebellar tracts in the upper cervical cord. As is often the case, at this level the pyramidal tracts are relatively spared. (Luxol fast blue/cresyl violet) **(b)** Degeneration of the gracile funiculi. (Palmgren silver impregnation) **(c)** Dense clusters of satellite cells (nodules of Nageotte) mark the sites where dorsal ganglion cells have degenerated. Satellite cells have proliferated to a varying extent around several of the remaining ganglion cells. (Hematoxylin/van Gieson) **(d)** Marked loss of nerve fibers from a posterior lumbar nerve root. (Phosphotungstic acid/hematoxylin)

MACROSCOPIC AND MICROSCOPIC APPEARANCES
The diverse multisystem abnormalities are summarized in **Fig. 29.7**.

CLINICAL FEATURES OF ATAXIA TELANGIECTASIA (AT)

Children typically manifest with early ataxia as soon as they begin to walk, and later dysarthria, chorea, and abnormal eye movements.

The characteristic telangiectasia, which affects the sclera and skin, becomes prominent by the end of the first decade. There may be progeric changes of hair and skin.

Other features include:
- *neurologic* — areflexia, distal wasting, weakness, sensory loss and cognitive slowing.
- *immunologic* — impairment of cell mediated and humoral immunity is common and predisposes to recurrent infections, although some patients have relatively normal immune function and survive well into adult life.
- *neoplasia* — patients are predisposed to develop malignancies, especially T cell leukemia and lymphomas, but also several types of carcinoma.

GENETICS AND PATHOGENESIS OF AT

- AT is caused by mutations in a single large gene (*AT-mutant*; *ATM*) of about 170 kb. The 350kDa protein product includes a carboxyl-terminal domain with homology to the signal transduction mediator, phosphatidylinositol 3′-kinase.
- The ATM gene is involved in multiple aspects of cell cycle control and DNA damage surveillance (**Fig. 29.6**).
- Cells from patients with AT are hypersensitive to radiation and exhibit chromosomal breakage, telomere shortening, and increased intrachromosomal recombination.
- 80–90% of patients with AT have mutations that are predicted to inactivate the ATM protein.
- 10–20% of AT families have a less severe clinical and cellular phenotype associated with mutations that do not completely inactivate the protein.

RARE RECESSIVE ATAXIAS
These include:
- Ataxia with learning disability, cataracts, short stature, and myopathy (Marinesco–Sjögren syndrome).
- Ataxia with hypogonadotrophic hypogonadism (Matthews–Rundle syndrome).
- Ataxia with learning disability, optic atrophy, and spasticity (Behr's syndrome).

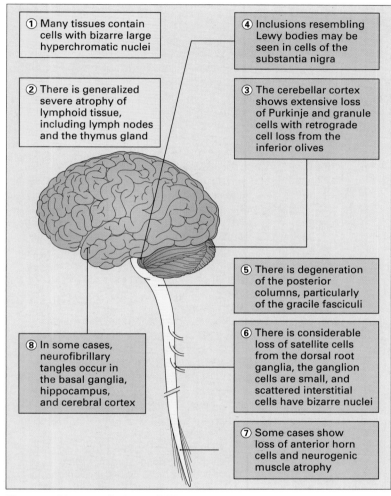

① Many tissues contain cells with bizarre large hyperchromatic nuclei

② There is generalized severe atrophy of lymphoid tissue, including lymph nodes and the thymus gland

④ Inclusions resembling Lewy bodies may be seen in cells of the substantia nigra

③ The cerebellar cortex shows extensive loss of Purkinje and granule cells with retrograde cell loss from the inferior olives

⑤ There is degeneration of the posterior columns, particularly of the gracile fasciculi

⑥ There is considerable loss of satellite cells from the dorsal root ganglia, the ganglion cells are small, and scattered interstitial cells have bizarre nuclei

⑧ In some cases, neurofibrillary tangles occur in the basal ganglia, hippocampus, and cerebral cortex

⑦ Some cases show loss of anterior horn cells and neurogenic muscle atrophy

Fig. 29.7 Neuropathology of AT.

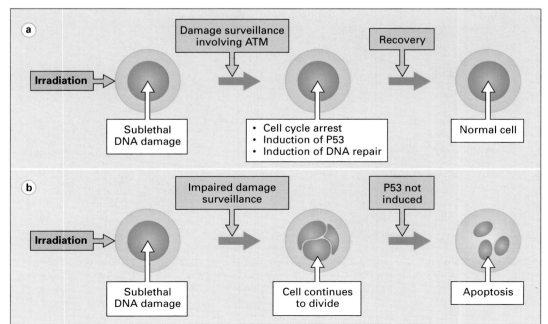

a

Irradiation → Sublethal DNA damage → Damage surveillance involving ATM → • Cell cycle arrest • Induction of P53 • Induction of DNA repair → Recovery → Normal cell

b

Irradiation → Sublethal DNA damage → Impaired damage surveillance → Cell continues to divide → P53 not induced → Apoptosis

Fig. 29.6 Pathogenetic mechanism of AT.
(a) In normal cells, cell cycle checkpoints at the G1, S, and G2 phases stop cell cycle progression after sublethal DNA damage, with induction of DNA-repair systems. ATM gene product is involved in surveillance of DNA damage. With cycle arrest there is induction of p53 protein and DNA repair can take place leading to recovery. **(b)** In AT cells, this process is defective and cells with damaged DNA can continue to divide. Induction of p53 protein associated with cell cycle arrest at the G1 checkpoint following DNA damage is impaired, leading to a disproportionate increase in apoptosis after low-level radiation damage. Initiation of inappropriate apoptosis in cells with non-lethal DNA damage is the probable reason for cell loss in the brain and lymphoid tissues.

AUTOSOMAL DOMINANT CEREBELLAR ATAXIA (ADCA)

Division of this group into clinical subtypes I to IV was proposed by Harding (1982), and has been supported by recent advances in molecular genetics. The subtypes are as follows:

- ADCA I is characterized by cerebellar ataxia with variable ophthalmoplegia, optic atrophy, cognitive impairment, parkinsonism, pyramidal signs, chorea, dystonia, and peripheral neuropathy, and includes at least seven genetic subtypes of spinocerebellar ataxia, SCA 1–6 and SCA8.
- ADCA II is characterized by ataxia, variable opthalmoplegia, and pigmentary macular degeneration leading to blindness.
- ADCA III is characterized by relatively pure cerebellar ataxia with some pyramidal signs and an onset after 50 years of age.
- ADCA IV is characterized by ataxia with additional features such as myoclonus, deafness, dementia, optic atrophy, myopathy, or neuropathy.

GENETICS OF ADCA

- ADCA I includes at least seven genetic subtypes:
  - SCA 1 caused by an unstable CAG triplet expansion in a gene coding for the protein ataxin-1 on chromosome 6p. Normal alleles have 6–39 repeats, SCA 1 alleles have 40–83. The CAG repeat codes for a polyglutamine tract. This disorder is also known as olivopontocerebellar atrophy type I (OPCAI).
  - SCA 2 caused by an unstable CAG triplet repeat expansion in a gene on chromosome 12. Normal alleles have 15–24 repeats, SCA 2 alleles have 35–59. The SCA 2 cDNA is predicted to code for 1313 residue protein, which is still of unknown function. This disorder is also known as olivopontocerebellar atrophy type II (OPCAII).
  - SCA 3 caused by an unstable CAG triplet expansion in a gene on chromosome 14. The same triplet expansion occurs in MJD. Normal alleles have 13–41 repeats, SCA 3 alleles have 62–80. Although there is considerable clinical overlap between the two diseases each has certain features that are distinctive. The reason for the phenotypic differences is not yet known.
  - SCA 4 linked to chromosome 16.
  - SCA 5 linked to chromosome 11.
  - SCA 6 is caused by an unstable CAG triplet expansion in a gene or chromosome 19p13 coding for the alpha (1A)-voltage-dependent Ca²⁺ channel.
  - SCA 8 (Infantile onset spinocerebellar ataxia) linked to chromosome 10q24.
- ADCA II linked to chromosome 3.
- SCA 7 is a form of ADCA II (and is also known as olivopontocerebellar atrophy type III; OPCA III), and has been linked to gene locus 3p21.1–p12
- ADCA III with genetic linkage not yet established.
- ADCA IV associated with mitochondrial abnormalities.

MACROSCOPIC AND MICROSCOPIC APPEARANCES

ADCA I, SCA 1, SCA 2, SCA 3 and Machado–Joseph disease (MJD): In the few genetically confirmed cases with necropsy data (**Fig. 29.8**) there are typically:

- Patchy cerebellar cortical atrophy with retrograde degeneration of the inferior olives.
- Degenerative changes in the pontine nuclei and their efferent tracts in the middle cerebellar peduncles.
- Variable, typically mild to moderate, neuronal loss and gliosis in the striatum, substantia nigra, Clarke's columns, the anterior spinal horns, brain stem motor nuclei, and sensory ganglia.
- Spinocerebellar and corticospinal tract degeneration.

In SCA 1 there is little or no pathology in the pars compacta of the substantia nigra or the locus ceruleus.

By comparison with SCA 2 and SCA 3 (see Fig. 29.8), SCA 1 is characterized by relatively severe degeneration of the olivocerebellar and dentatorubral fibers, more severe neuronal loss from the third and twelfth cranial nerve nuclei, and more extensive loss of spinal motor neurons.

In MJD there is relative sparing of the cerebello-olivary systems.

ADCA III: Cerebellar cortical atrophy and degeneration of the dentate nucleus have been reported in a single case.

ADCA IV: Findings include severe neuronal loss and gliosis in the dentate nucleus and inferior olives with milder degenerative changes in the cerebellar cortex. Other changes may be similar to those in Leigh's disease (see chapters 6 and 24). Muscle biopsy may or may not show ragged red fibers with pleomorphic mitochondria containing paracrystalline inclusions (see chapter 24).

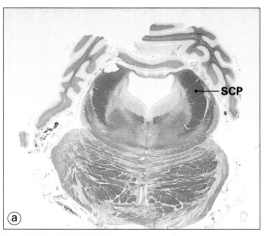 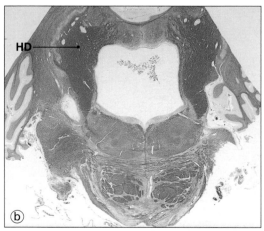 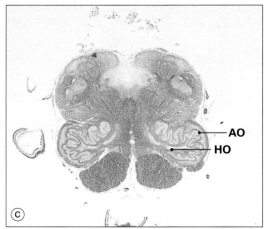

Fig. 29.8 ADCA I. The genetic subtype was not determined. **(a), (b)** This case shows degeneration of the pontine nuclei and transverse pontine fibers. **(c)** There is moderate depletion of neurons from the inferior olives, and loss of the corresponding afferent and efferent fibers from the amiculum (AO) and hilus (HO), which appear abnormally pale. The hilus of the dentate nucleus (HD) and the superior cerebellar peduncle (SCP) are relatively well preserved. (Luxol fast blue/cresyl violet)

DENTATORUBROPALLIDOLUYSIAL ATROPHY (DRPLA)

DRPLA is an autosomal dominant condition caused by an unstable CAG triplet repeat expansion in a gene on chromosome 12p. The normal gene includes 7–23 repeats. DRPLA alleles contain 49–75 repeats. The presentation is variable and may include ataxia, chorea, myoclonic epilepsy, and dementia. Since the identification of a genetic marker, the disease has been recognized as a cause of chorea and dementia that can simulate Huntington's disease.

MACROSCOPIC AND MICROSCOPIC APPEARANCES

Neuronal loss and astrocytic gliosis are most severe in the:

- dentate nucleus (**Fig. 29.9a,b**)
- external segment of the globus pallidus (**Fig. 29.9c**)
- subthalamus

There is mild to moderate cell loss from the red nucleus, with associated gliosis (**Fig. 29.9d**). Mild neuronal loss and gliosis are evident in the caudate nucleus, putamen, thalamus, substantia nigra (**Fig. 29.9e**), and inferior olives. The superior cerebellar peduncles containing the efferent tracts from the dentate nuclei are atrophic and depleted of myelinated fibers. There may be degeneration of the spinocerebellar tracts and posterior spinal columns (**Fig. 29.9f**).

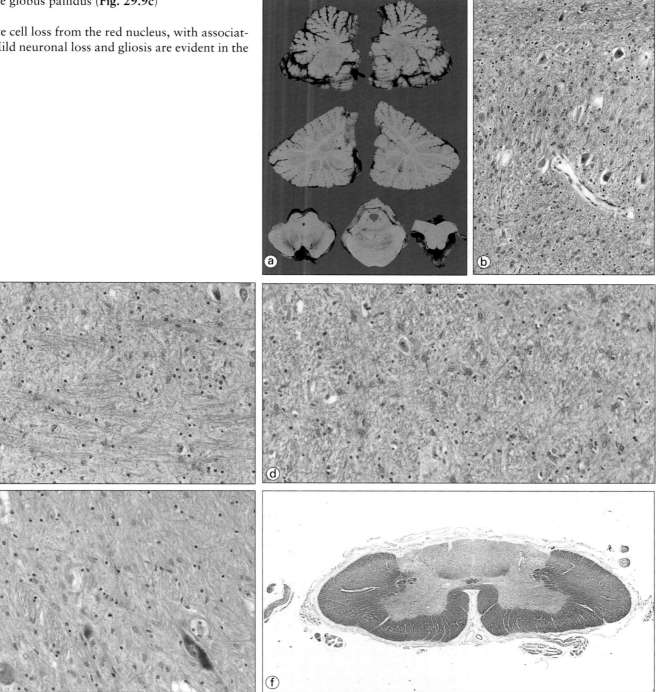

Fig. 29.9 DRPLA. (a) Atrophy and brown discoloration of the dentate nuclei in DRPLA. There is only mild cerebellar cortical atrophy. **(b)** There are a few remaining neurons in the dentate nucleus, which is severely gliotic. **(c)** Neuronal loss and gliosis involving the globus pallidus. **(d)** Neuronal loss and gliosis involving the red nucleus. (b–d all phosphotungstic acid/hematoxylin) **(e)** Neuronal loss and gliosis involving the substantia nigra. **(f)** Degeneration of the posterior funiculi of the spinal cord. (Luxol fast blue/cresyl violet)

SPORADIC IDIOPATHIC CEREBELLAR DEGENERATION

MULTIPLE SYSTEM ATROPHY OF OLIVOPONTOCEREBELLAR DISTRIBUTION

About 60% of cases of degenerative cerebellar ataxia presenting in people over 20 years of age are sporadic. The majority are due to multiple system atrophy of olivopontocerebellar distribution (see chapter 28, p. 28.10) and associated with the characteristic glial inclusions in high density.

IDIOPATHIC LATE ONSET CEREBELLAR ATAXIA

This is the second most frequent type of sporadic idiopathic cerebellar degeneration. It is characterized by an onset after 50 years of age and often manifests with a relatively pure midline cerebellar syndrome.

MACROSCOPIC AND MICROSCOPIC APPEARANCES

The neuropathologic findings are:
- cerebellar atrophy predominantly affecting the superior part of the cerebellum and often most severe in the vermis (**Fig. 29.10**)
- secondary atrophy of the inferior olives, predominantly involving the dorsal laminae
- variable spinocerebellar tract degeneration

SPORADIC CEREBELLAR ATAXIA

This is the least common type of sporadic idiopathic cerebellar degeneration. It is associated with severe resting, postural, and intention tremor, and occurs in people over 50 years of age. The associated neuropathologic findings are not well defined.

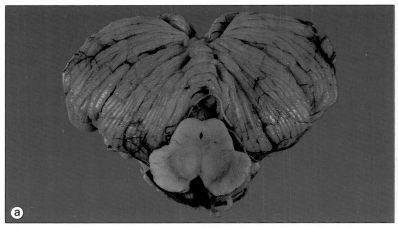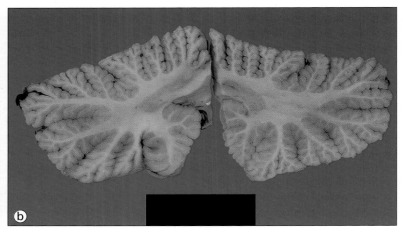

Fig. 29.10 Idiopathic late onset cerebellar ataxia. (a) Atrophy of the cerebellar folia and widening of the intervening sulci, particularly in the vermis. **(b)** The folia in the superior part of the cerebellar hemispheres are more atrophic than those in the inferior part.

REFERENCES

Banfi S, Zoghbi HY. (1994) Molecular genetics of hereditary ataxias. *Clin Neurol* **3**: 281–295.

Flanigan K, *et al*. (1996) Autosomal dominant spinocerebellar ataxia with sensory axonal neuropathy (SCA4): clinical description and genetic localization to chromosome 16q22.1 *Am J Hum Genet* **59**: 392–399.

Hammonds S. (1996) The inherited ataxias and the new genetics. *Journal of Neurol, Neurosurg and Psychiat* **61**: 327–332.

Harding A. (1982) The clinical features and classification of the late onset autosomal dominant cerebellar ataxias: a study of eleven families including descendants of the 'Drew family of Walworth'. *Brain* **105**: 1–28.

Hoffman P, Stuart W, Earle KM, Brody JA. (1971). Hereditary late-onset cerebellar degeneration. *Neurology* **21**: 771–777.

Nikali K, *et al*. (1997) Toward cloning of a novel ataxia gene: refined assignment and physical map of the IOSCA locus (SCA8) on 10q24. *Genomics* **39**: 185–191.

Rosenberg R (1995) Autosomal dominant cerebellar phenotypes: the genotype has settled the issue. *Neurology* **45**: 1–5.

Warner TT, Lennox GG, Janota I, Harding AE. (1994) Autosomal-dominant dentatorubropallidoluysian atrophy in the United Kingdom. *Movement Disorders* **9**: 289–296.

Zhuchenko O *et al*. (1997) Autosomal dominant cerebellar ataxia (SCA6) associated with small polyglutamine expansions in the alpha(1A)-voltage-dependent calcium channel. *Nature Genet* **15**: 62–69.

30 Hyperkinetic movement disorders

Several clinical conditions are characterized by the presence of excessive uncontrolled movements and are grouped as hyperkinetic movement disorders. These are chorea and ballismus, myoclonus, and dystonia. Tics can also be classed as hyperkinetic disorders, though pathologi studies of the commonest type (Gilles de la Tourette's syndrome) have not yet revealed significant abnormalities.

CHOREA

Chorea is characterized by the presence of non-rhythmic rapid involuntary movements and can be divided into sporadic and hereditary groups.

ETIOLOGY OF HUNTINGTON'S DISEASE (HD)

- The gene for Huntington's disease is located at the tip of the short arm of chromosome 4 and codes for the protein huntingtin, which is widely expressed in fetal and adult tissues. Its function is presently unknown.
- The huntingtin gene includes a CAG repeat sequence. The normal gene contains 9 to 37 CAG repeats (each encoding glutamine); in HD the number of repeats ranges from 37 to 100 or more. In general, the number of CAG repeats is inversely related to the age of onset and duration of the disease (the neurologic decline being most rapid in patients with early-onset HD). However, the correlation is insufficiently precise to allow reliable prediction of the course of disease in an individual patient.
- The disease shows *anticipation*: later generations are affected at an earlier age and more severely than earlier generations in the same family. This phenomenon is associated with a progressive increase in the length of CAG repeat sequences as the disease is passed on through successive generations. Very rare sporadic cases of HD are usually due to expansion of a 34 to 37 CAG repeat (intermediate allele) in an unaffected male patient.
- The polyglutamine resulting form transcription of the CAG repeat has been shown to bind to glyceraldehyde-3-phosphate dehydrogenase but whether this binding is involved in the pathogenesis of the disease is not yet known.

HUNTINGTON'S DISEASE (HD)

HD causes chorea, rigidity, and cognitive decline leading to dementia. The incidence of this disease is 4–7/100,00 in most populations. It is an autosomal dominant condition with a variable age of onset:

- Juvenile onset (4–19 years of age) accounts for 10% of cases and is particularly linked to paternal transmission.
- Early onset (20–34 years of age).
- Mid-life onset (35–49 years of age).
- Late onset (over 49 years of age) accounts for 25% of cases and is particularly linked to maternal transmission.

MACROSCOPIC APPEARANCES

Cerebral atrophy is usually present (**Fig. 30.1**) with a reduction in brain weight of approximately 30%. This is associated with a 21–29% loss of volume of the cerebral cortex and a 29–34% loss of white matter. The most characteristic macroscopic abnormality is atrophy of the caudate nucleus, putamen, and globus pallidus (**Fig. 30.1**).

CLINICAL VARIANTS OF HUNTINGTON'S DISEASE (HD)

Hyperkinetic HD

- This is the commoner variant of HD, and is the form of disease in almost all patients with mid-life or late-onset HD.
- Choreiform movements are prominent.
- Some patients, particularly those with late-onset disease, develop neuropsychiatric disease long before the onset of the movement disorder.
- The mean duration of disease is 17 years, with death usually occurring from cachexia and bronchopneumonia.

Akinetic-rigid HD

- This is an uncommon form of HD, seen in some patients with juvenile or early-onset disease.
- Rigidity and akinesia are prominent.
- Progression of disease is relatively rapid.

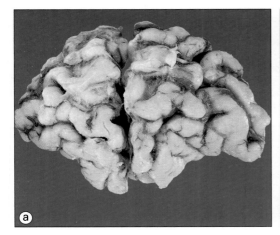

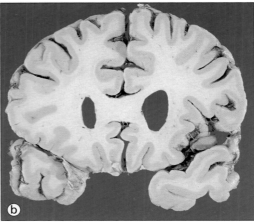

Fig. 30.1 Cerebral atrophy in HD.
(a) Surface of frontal lobe showing mild gyral atrophy. **(b)** Coronal section showing mild gyral atrophy.

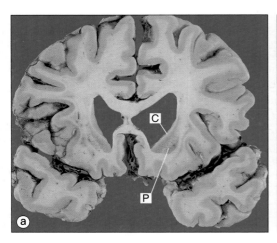

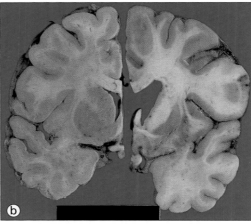

Fig. 30.2 Striatal atrophy in HD.
(a) Characteristic atrophy of the caudate nucleus (C) and putamen (P) in HD. There is also generalized widening of the cerebral sulci. **(b)** Comparison of a normal cerebral hemisphere (left) with that from a patient with HD (right) illustrating the severe atrophy of the basal ganglia.

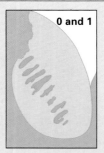

0 and 1

Grade 0 Macroscopically normal brain. Neuronal counts show 30–40% loss of neurons in striatum without gliosis.

Grade 1 Macroscopically normal brain. Moderate astrocytic gliosis in medial caudate and dorsal putamen. Neuronal counts show 50% loss of neurons in striatum.

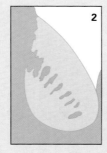

2

Grade 2 Macroscopically visible atrophy of head of caudate (which retains its convex medial contour) and putamen, with normal globus pallidus. Neuronal loss evident without quantitation in head, body, and tail of caudate and dorsal putamen. Associated astrocytic gliosis.

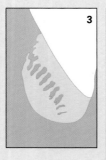

3

Grade 3 Macroscopically severe atrophy of head of caudate (which now has a flat medial contour) and putamen, with mild atrophy of globus pallidus. Neuronal loss evident without quantitation, in head, body, and tail of caudate and dorsal putamen, and associated astrocytic gliosis. Mild astrocytic gliosis in globus pallidus.

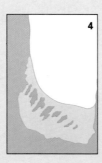

4

Grade 4 Macroscopically very severe atrophy of head of caudate (which now has a concave medial contour) and putamen, and severe atrophy of globus pallidus. Neuronal loss (>90%) evident without quantitation in head, body, and tail of caudate, and dorsal putamen. Severe associated astrocytic gliosis. Nucleus accumbens shows astrocytic gliosis.

Fig. 30.3 Grading of striatal atrophy in HD. The system of grading proposed by Vonsattel defines four degrees of severity of involvement in HD.

MICROSCOPIC APPEARANCES

The most marked histologic changes are seen in the basal ganglia where loss of neurons is associated with astrocytic gliosis in affected areas of the striatum (**Fig. 30.4**). In general, morphometric studies are required to show loss of large pyramidal neurons in the neocortex and hip-pocampus, which occurs in the absence of astrocytosis. Abnormal neurites have been shown to be widely distributed throughout the cortex in HD by immunostaining for ubiquitin (**Fig. 30.5**). Neuronal loss may also be found in the hypothalamus, substantia nigra, and cerebellar cortex, particularly in severe early-onset cases.

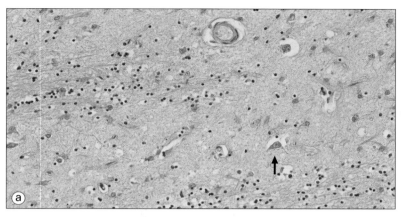

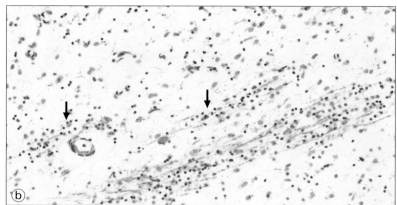

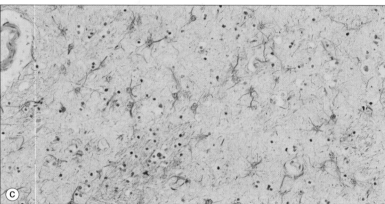

Fig. 30.4 (a) Rarefaction and gliosis of the putamen in HD of moderate severity. The smaller neurons are largely depleted, but some of the large neurons (arrow) are spared, as is usual until quite late in the disease. The smaller neurons normally outnumber the large neurons by 150–250-fold. **(b)** Loss of myelinated fibers (arrows). (Luxol fast blue/cresyl violet) **(c)** Astrocytic gliosis is quite marked. (Phosphotungstic acid/hematoxylin)

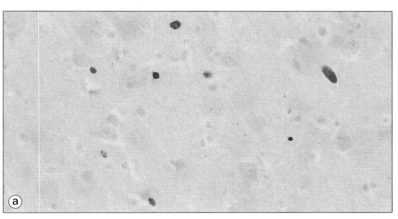

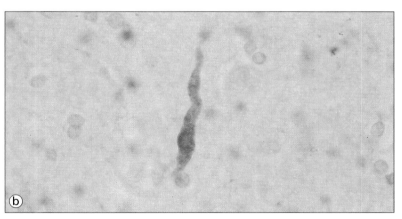

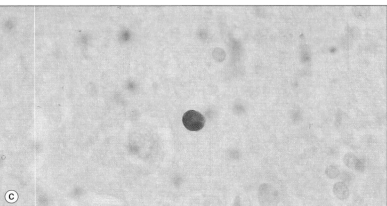

Fig. 30.5 Abnormal cortical neurites in HD revealed by ubiquitin immunohistochemistry. Their appearance depends upon the plane in which they have been sectioned. They are found in deeper cortical layers. **(a)** Oval and rounded structures. **(b)** Corkscrew-like and beaded neurite in longitudinal section. **(c)** Rounded profile with intense staining of periphery in cross-sectioned neurite.

The neuronal loss from the striatum preferentially affects certain neuronal subtypes. The normal striatum has two neuronal compartments:
- the patch (striosome) compartment composed mainly of neurons with spiny dendrites on Golgi staining (spiny neurons) containing gamma aminobutyric acid (GABA), enkephalin, dynorphin, and substance P
- the matrix compartment composed mainly of neurons with smooth dendrites on Golgi staining, that contain acetylcholinesterase (large aspiny neurons), or the reduced form of nicotinamide–adenine dinucleotide phosphate (NADPH), diaphorase (nitric oxide synthase), somatostatin, neuropeptide Y, and cholecystokinin (small aspiny neurons).

Spiny neurons are severely depleted in HD. Loss of aspiny neurons is much less marked and occurs in the late stages of the disease.

Pathologic grading of severity

The Vonsattel grading scheme for the severity of the atrophy of the basal ganglia correlates with the clinical severity of disease (**Fig. 30.5**).

NEUROACANTHOCYTOSIS

This term is applied to multisystem degenerative neurologic disorders, genetically heterogeneous, associated with acanthocytes in the blood. Inheritance is usually autosomal dominant but can be autosomal recessive.

Other causes of combined neurologic disease and acanthocytosis are:
- abetalipoproteinemia (see also vitamin E deficiency in chapter 21)
- Mcleod syndrome (an X-linked disorder in which striatal degeneration and myopathy are associated with absence of the Kx protein, and reduced Kell blood group antigenexpression).

MACROSCOPIC AND MICROSCOPIC APPEARANCES

The main findings are atrophy, neuronal loss, and astrocytic gliosis in various brain regions (**Fig. 30.6**). Examination of a fresh blood film

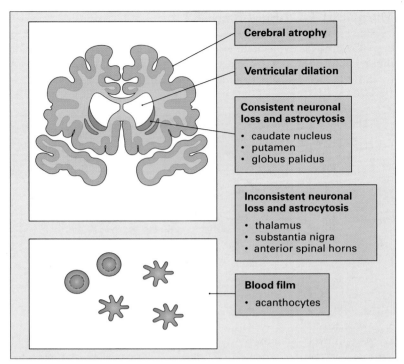

Fig. 30.6 Neuroacanthocytosis. Summary of main pathologic findings.

reveals acanthocytes. In some cases acanthocytes are not be easy to find and repeat examination or scanning electron microscopy of blood may be necessary for diagnosis.

NEUROACANTHOCYTOSIS

MYOCLONUS

Myoclonus is a nonspecific manifestation of many diseases of the central nervous system (CNS) and is characterized by rapid, shock-like, involuntary contractions of a single muscle or muscle group. It may be associated with other clinical features, the presence of which assist in the diagnosis (**Fig. 30.7**). The main types of myoclonus are focal myoclonus and arrhythmic myoclonus. For a discussion of the progressive myolonic epilepsies see chapter 7.

BALLISMUS AND HEMIBALLISMUS

Ballismus and hemiballismus are severe forms of chorea characterized by involuntary violent flinging movements of the limbs. Almost invariably this is caused by damage to the subthalamic nucleus (**Fig. 30.8**). The main causes are infarcts, small hemorrhages, infection, metastatic tumor, and demyelination. The neurochemical pathology is illustrated in **Fig. 30.9**.

DYSTONIA

This is characterized by sustained muscle contractions that cause abnormal postures or twisting, repetitive movements. Dystonia may be:

PRIMARY (IDIOPATHIC)
- inherited
  - primary torsion dystonia (autosomal dominant)
    DOPA-responsive dystonia (autosomal dominant)
    X-linked primary torsion dystonia
- sporadic (in some cases probably due to an autosomal dominant gene/genes, with incomplete penetrance)

SECONDARY (SYMPTOMATIC)
- due to a range of neurologic/neurometabolic diseases, including Wilson's disease, Hallevorden–Spatz disease, Lewy body disease, neuroacanthocytosis, perinatal brain injury, phenothiazine and other drug toxicity
- due to focal basal ganglia lesions (e.g. infarcts, tumors or trauma) — the dystonia is usually unilateral (hemidystonia)
- psychogenic

Dystonia is most often focal/multifocal, as in torticollis, blepharospasm, oromandibular dystonia, spastic dysphonia, and 'writer's cramp'. Several adjacent muscle groups may be involved, as in segmental craniofacial dystonia (Meige's syndrome). Generalized dystonia is rare and usually associated with familial disease.

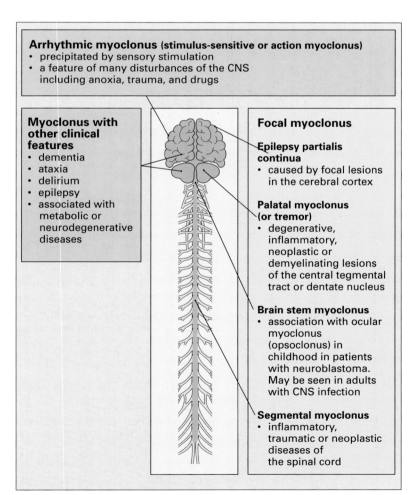

Arrhythmic myoclonus (stimulus-sensitive or action myoclonus)
- precipitated by sensory stimulation
- a feature of many disturbances of the CNS including anoxia, trauma, and drugs

Myoclonus with other clinical features
- dementia
- ataxia
- delirium
- epilepsy
- associated with metabolic or neurodegenerative diseases

Focal myoclonus

Epilepsy partialis continua
- caused by focal lesions in the cerebral cortex

Palatal myoclonus (or tremor)
- degenerative, inflammatory, neoplastic or demyelinating lesions of the central tegmental tract or dentate nucleus

Brain stem myoclonus
- association with ocular myoclonus (opsoclonus) in childhood in patients with neuroblastoma. May be seen in adults with CNS infection

Segmental myoclonus
- inflammatory, traumatic or neoplastic diseases of the spinal cord

Fig. 30.7 Myoclonus. Pathological associations with different types of myoclonus.

INHERITED FORMS OF PRIMARY DYSTONIA

Primary torsion dystonia
- This is an autosomal dominant disease with a relatively high incidence in Ashkenazi Jews. One responsible locus has been mapped to chromosome 9q34.
- The dystonia starts in childhood or adolescence and is initially restricted to the neck or trunk but becomes generalized over about 3 years.
- Reported neuropathologic findings are of neurofibrillary tangles in the brain stem, or cell loss and astrocytosis in the caudate and putamen.

Dopa-responsive dystonia (Segawa syndrome)
- This is an autosomal dominant disorder caused by a mutation in the gene for GTP cyclohydrolase I, the enzyme responsible for the rate-limiting step in the synthesis of tetrahydrobiopterin, a cofactor of tyrosine hydrolase. Reduced tetrahydrobiopterin levels cause diminished synthesis of dopamine.
- Symptoms develop gradually during the first decade, gait being affected at an early stage. Characteristically, the severeity of the dystonia fluctuates during the day. Patients also develop parkinsonism and, later, severe generalized dytonia. The disorder shows a striking and prolonged response to levadopa therapy.
- Reported neuropathologic findings include severe nigral degeneration and, in one case, Lewy bodies.

X-linked primary torsion dystonia
- This disorder occurring in the Filipino population (where it is called 'lubag') has been linked to a locus within Xq12-q13.1.
- Patients present at ~35 years with spasmodic eye blinking and parkinsonism.
- Reported neuropathologic findings are of striatal neuronal loss and astrocytosis.

There is a paucity of data on the pathogenesis and neuropathology of primary dystonia. In the event of an autopsy, the brain and spinal cord should be preserved for morphologic, neurochemical and genetic analysis

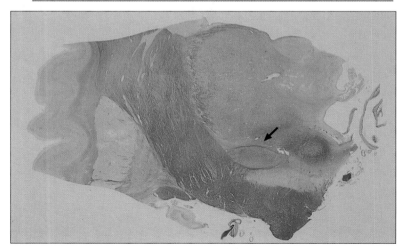

Fig. 30.8 Subthalamic nucleus. The subthalamic nucleus can be identified in a coronal slice through or just posterior to the plane of the mamillary bodies. The nucleus is biconvex (arrow) and lies above the substantia nigra and medial to the transition between the internal capsule and the cerebral peduncle.

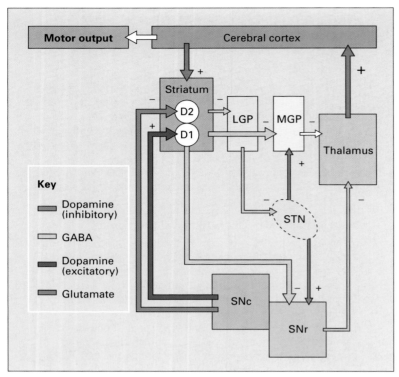

Fig. 30.9 Pathophysiology of ballismus. In the absence of the normal tonic excitation from the subthalamic nucleus, there is reduced output of the inhibitory neurotransmitter GABA from the medial segment of the globus pallidus and the substantia nigra to the thalamic nuclei. As a consequence, the thalamic nuclei release increased amounts of the excitatory neurotransmitter glutamate within the cerebral cortex. The increased cortical excitation causes a hyperkinetic movement disorder. LGP, lateral segment of globus pallidus; MGP, medial segment of globus pallidus; STN, subthalamic nucleus; SNc, pars compacta of the substantia nigra; SNr, pars reticulata of the substantia nigra; D1 and D2, dopamine receptors.

REFERENCES

Andrew SE et al. (1994) Huntington disease without CAG expansion: phenocopies or errors in assignment? Am J Hum Genet **54**(5): 852–863.

Calne D, Lang A. (1988) Secondary dystonias. In S Fahn, C Marsden, D Calne (eds), Advances in Neurology: Dystonia 2. pp. 9–33. New York: Raven Press.

de la Monte S, Vonsattel JP, Richardson EJ (1988) Morphometric demonstration of atrophic changes in the cerebral cortex, white matter, and neostriatum in Huntington's disease. J Neuropathol Exp Neurol **47**(5): 516–525.

Gibb WR, Kilford L, Marsden CD (1992) Severe generalised dystonia associated with a mosaic pattern of striatal gliosis. Mov Disord **7**(3): 217–223.

Gibb WR, Lees AJ, Marsden CD (1988) Pathological report of four patients presenting with cranial dystonias. Mov Disord **3**(3): 211–221.

Hardie RJ (1989) Acanthocytosis and neurological impairment. A review. Q J Med **71**(264): 291–306.

Hardie RJ et al. (1991) Neuroacanthocytosis. A clinical, haematological and pathological study of 19 cases. Brain **114**(1): 13–49.

Jackson M et al. (1995) The cortical neuritic pathology of Huntington's disease. Neuropathol Applied Neurobiol **21**: 18–26.

Kramer PL et al. (1990) Dystonia gene in Ashkenazi Jewish population is located on chromosome 9q32-34. Ann Neurol **27**: 114–120.

Kremer B et al. (1994) A worldwide study of the Huntington's disease mutation: the sensitivity and specificity of measuring CAG repeats. N Engl J Med **330**: 1401–1406.

Kupke K, Lee L, Viterbo G, Arancillo J, Donlon T, Muller U. (1990) X-linked recessive torsion dystonia in the Philippines. Am J Med Genet **36**: 237–242.

Mann DM, Oliver R, Snowden JS (1993) The topographic distribution of brain atrophy in Huntington's disease and progressive supranuclear palsy. Acta Neuropathol (Berl) **85**(5): 553–559.

Mark MH et al. (1994) Meige syndrome in the spectrum of Lewy body disease. Neurology **44**(8): 1432–1436.

Marsden CD, Rothwell JC (1987) The physiology of idiopathic dystonia. Can J Neurol Sci **14**(3S): 521–527.

Muller U, Haberhausen G, Wagner T, Fairweather N, Chelly J, Monaco A. (1994) DXS106 and DXS559 flank the X-linked dystonia-parkinsonism syndrome locus (DYT3). Genomics **23**: 114–117.

Ohye T et al. (1994) Hereditary progressive dystonia with marked diurnal fluctuation caused by mutations in the GTP cyclohydrolase I gene. Nature Genet **8**: 236–242.

Olsson JE, Brunk U, Linval B, Eeg O. (1992) Dopa-responsive dystonia with depigmentation of the substantia nigra and formation of Lewy bodies. J Neurol Sci **112**(1–2): 90–95.

Ozelius LJ et al. (1992) Strong allelic association between the torsion dystonia gene (DYT1) and loci on chromosome 9q34 in Ashkenazi Jews. Am J Hum Genet **50**: 619–628.

Padberg G, Bruyn G (1986) Chorea: differential diagnosis. In Extrapyramidal Disorders 5: 549–564 Amsterdam: Elsevier.

Segawa M, Hosaka A, Miyagawa F, Nomura Y, Imai H. (1976) Hereditary progressive dystonia with marked diurnal fluctuation. Adv Neurol **14**: 215–233.

Shefner J (1992) Ballism. In A Joseph, R Young (eds) Movement Disorders in Neurology and Neuropsychiatry. pp. 503–510 Oxford: Blackwell Scientific Publications.

Tolosa E, Marti MJ (1988) Blepharospasm–oromandibular dystonia syndrome (Meige's syndrome): clinical aspects. Adv Neurol **49**(1): 73–84.

Vonsattel JP, Myers RH, Stevens TJ, Ferrante RJ, Bird ED, Richardson EJ. (1985) Neuropathological classification of Huntington's disease. J Neuropathol Exp Neurol **44**(6): 559–577.

Waddy HM, Fletcher NA, Harding AE, Marsden CD (1991) A genetic study of idiopathic focal dystonias. Ann Neurol **29**(3): 320–324.

Waters CH, Takahashi H, Wilhelmsen KC, Shubin R, et al. (1993) Phenotypic expression of X-linked dystonia-parkinsonism (lubag) in two women. Neurology **43**(8): 1555–1558.

Zweig R, Hedreen C, Jankel W, Casanova M, Whitehouse P, Price D. (1988) Pathology in brainstem regions of individuals with primary dystonia. Neurology **38**: 702–706.

31 Dementias

Diseases causing dementia are among the commonest neurologic conditions encountered in clinical practice (**Fig. 31.1**). Our understanding of these disorders has been greatly extended in the past 10 years by immunohistochemical and molecular genetic advances. However, there is still uncertainty as to the precise incidence and prevalence of different types of dementia because:

- Most epidemiologic studies of dementia have been based on clinical diagnosis without pathologic validation.
- The clinical diagnosis of the type of dementia may be unreliable, particularly outside specialist units.
- Hospital-based series are biased to reflect patients with severe dementia requiring institutional care and probably do not reflect patterns of disease in the community.

- Different pathologic criteria for the diagnosis of degenerative diseases have been used in different studies.

Prevalence of dementia at different ages	
Age (years)	Prevalence (%)
<75	4%
80	12%
85	27%
90	40%

Fig. 31.1 Prevalence of dementia at different ages.

DEMENTIA

Definition

- Dementia can be defined as an impairment of previously attained occupational or social functioning due to an acquired and persistent impairment of memory associated with an impairment of intellectual function in one or more of the following domains — language, visuospatial skills, emotion, personality or cognition — in the presence of normal consciousness.
- The concept that a person has previously attained a high degree of occupational and social functioning separates dementia from mental retardation.
- Impairment in consciousness, such as develops in delirium or a confusional state, precludes a clinical diagnosis of dementia.
- Involvement of multiple domains of cognitive function separates dementia from focal neurobehavioral disorders (e.g. isolated amnesia due to bilateral hippocampal damage or isolated dysphasia due to a localized infarct).
- Dementia is predominantly caused by degenerative processes that evolve over many years (**Fig. 31.2**). Different diseases preferentially affect different brain regions and so distinctive clinical patterns of dementia can be recognized (**Fig. 31.3**). With progression of the disease, more cortical areas are often affected and a global deterioration in intellectual function ensues.

Certain clinical patterns of dementia are suggestive of particular disorders

- Frontotemporal dementias: behavioral disturbances of frontal lobe dysfunction, with later development of memory disturbances due to temporal lobe dysfunction; parietal lobe function is typically retained.
- Temporoparietal dementias: temporal lobe dysfunction with impairment of memory, and later parietal lobe dysfunction characterized by dysphasias and dyspraxias.
- Subcortical dementia: a syndrome of cognitive dysfunction characterized by slowing of thought processes; it is a feature of dementia related to diseases of the basal ganglia, such as that associated with parkinsonism.

Diagnosis

- The degenerative processes that cause cortical pathology may also affect subcortical structures and lead to other neurologic dysfunction, the most common of which is the development of parkinsonism. Identification of associated neurologic abnormalities may therefore help in establishing an accurate diagnosis.
- Several clinical bedside tests of cognitive function have been developed to assist in the diagnosing of dementia, but these mainly detect dysfunction of the temporal and parietal lobes, and are less sensitive to frontal lobe dysfunction.

The causes of dementia

Neurodegenerative diseases

Common
- Alzheimer's disease
- dementia with Lewy bodies

Less common
- dementia with MND inclusions
- dementia of frontal type (no inclusions)
- tangle-only dementia
- Huntington's disease
- progressive supranuclear palsy
- corticobasal degeneration

Uncommon
- Pick's disease
- multiple system atrophy

Rare
- multi-system degenerations
- chromosome 17-linked dementia

Cerebrovascular disease

Multi-infarct dementia, ischemic white matter degeneration or hippocampal sclerosis due to:
- atherosclerosis
- arteriolosclerosis
- vasculitis (several causes)
- amyloid angiopathy
- CADASIL

Hydrocephalus

- CSF resorption abnormality
- obstruction in CSF pathways

Toxic, metabolic and nutritional disorders

- drug-induced
- chronic alcoholism
- chronic hepatic encephalopathy
- vitamin deficiency (thiamine, B12, niacin)
- hypothyroidism
- neurometabolic storage diseases
- hypocalcemia
- hypoglycemia

Mitochondrial encephalopathy

- due to various mutations of mtDNA

Demyelinating and dysmyelinating diseases

- multiple sclerosis
- leukodystrophies

Head injury

- diffuse or focal brain damage
- subdural hematoma
- dementia pugilistica

Prion disease

- Creutzfeldt–Jakob disease (including vCTD)
- Kuru
- Gerstmann–Sträussler–Scheinker disease
- fatal familial insomnia

Infective disorders

- Whipple's disease
- neurosyphilis
- HIV infection
- HSV encephalitis
- SSPE
- PML

Neoplasia

- paraneoplastic encephalitis
- primary and secondary neoplasms

Fig. 31.2 Causes of dementia.

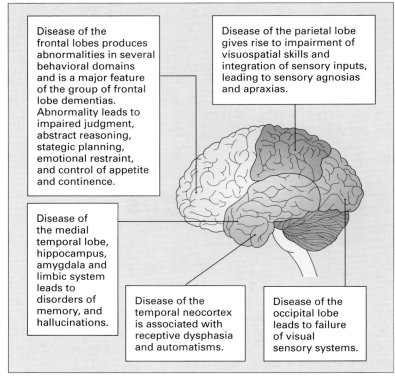

Fig. 31.3 Clinical features related to brain regions affected in dementia.

Disease of the frontal lobes produces abnormalities in several behavioral domains and is a major feature of the group of frontal lobe dementias. Abnormality leads to impaired judgment, abstract reasoning, stategic planning, emotional restraint, and control of appetite and continence.

Disease of the parietal lobe gives rise to impairment of visuospatial skills and integration of sensory inputs, leading to sensory agnosias and apraxias.

Disease of the medial temporal lobe, hippocampus, amygdala and limbic system leads to disorders of memory, and hallucinations.

Disease of the temporal neocortex is associated with receptive dysphasia and automatisms.

Disease of the occipital lobe leads to failure of visual sensory systems.

TEMPOROPARIETAL AND FRONTOTEMPOROPARIETAL DEMENTIAS

ALZHEIMER'S DISEASE (AD)

AD is the commonest cause of dementia and increases in incidence with age. It accounts for 50–75% of all cases of dementia, the precise figure depending on the criteria used to establish the diagnosis.

There are five main groups, with different molecular genetic associations (see p. 31.12).
- Sporadic late onset AD (commonest)
- Familial late onset AD (uncommon)
- Familial early onset AD (rare)
- Associated with Downs' syndrome
- Associated with other degenerative disease

About 10% of all cases have a strong family history of AD

MACROSCOPIC APPEARANCES

The brain weight is usually in the range of 900–1200 g. There is shrinkage of the cerebral gyri and widening of the sulci, most prominently in the medial temporal regions (particularly the hippocampus) but also affecting frontal and parietal regions. The occipital lobe and the motor

CLINICAL FEATURES OF ALZHEIMER'S DISEASE (SEE ALSO BOX ON DEMENTIA ON PAGE 31.1)

- AD typically presents with early memory dysfunction, later progressing to disorders of parietal lobe function with dysphasia and dyspraxia.
- In the late stages of disease the extensive involvement of cortical and subcortical regions renders patients immobile and mute.

cortex are generally spared. This pattern of atrophy may be present in diverse dementing diseases and is not specific for AD (**Fig. 31.4**).

In slices of fixed brain, the cortical mantle may appear to be thinned (**Fig. 31.5**). The white matter is of normal color and texture, but reduced in volume (see Fig. 31.5). There may be significant dilatation of the ventricular system, especially of the temporal horn of the lateral ventricles.

In the midbrain, the substantia nigra is normally pigmented. This is an important distinction from Lewy body dementia, discussed later. The locus ceruleus is often paler than normal.

Cerebral infarcts or hemorrhages in the brains of patients with AD may be related to cerebrovascular amyloid deposition.

MICROSCOPIC APPEARANCES

AD is characterized by the presence of several morphologic abnormalities, none of which is specific to this disease. Major pathologic changes are:

- Deposition of a specific amyloid in the brain as plaques. The amyloid is composed of Aβ peptide, derived by proteolytic breakdown from a normal neuronal membrane protein called amyloid precursor protein (APP).
- Intraneuronal filamentous inclusions termed neurofibrillary tangles (NFTs). These are composed of material which is generically termed paired helical filament protein (PHF). The main constituent of these filaments is the microtubule binding protein, tau.

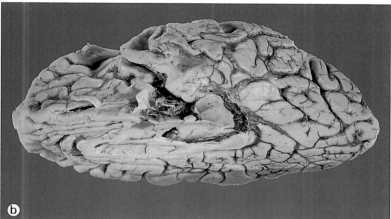

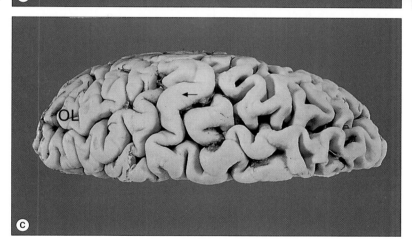

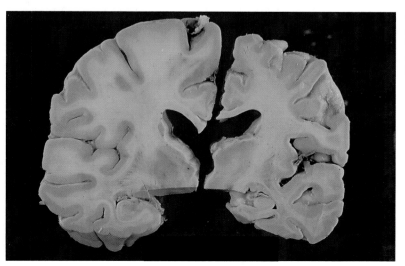

Fig. 31.4 Macroscopic appearance of brain in AD. The pattern of atrophy typically seen in AD is characteristic, but not specific for the disease. In this case the leptomeninges have been stripped from one half of a brain to show the regional atrophy clearly. **(a)** Lateral view showing severe atrophy of the temporal lobe with less severe atrophy of the parietal and frontal lobes. The occipital lobe is spared. **(b)** The severity of atrophy of the mesial temporal lobe structures is better appreciated in this view of the inferior surface. **(c)** Relative sparing of the primary motor cortex (arrow) and occipital lobe (OL) can be appreciated in this view of the superior surface.

Fig. 31.5 Macroscopic appearance of brain in AD. In this picture the slice on the left is from a normal patient aged 70, while the one on the right is from a patient with AD. Note that there is a reduction in the volume of white matter with cortical atrophy, mild sulcal widening and gyral thinning, the hippocampus is atrophic.

- Distortion of neuronal processes to form structures termed dystrophic neurites and neuropil threads (NTs). These structures also contain tau protein.
- Loss of synapses and, later, of neurons from the cerebral cortex.

Associated pathologic changes are:

- Amyloid (derived from Aβ peptide) deposition in arteries and arterioles in the cerebral and cerebellar cortex and leptomeninges (congophilic angiopathy) in most cases, although the extent of this is very variable (**Fig. 31.6**).
- Granulovacuolar degeneration (**Fig. 31.7**) affects greater numbers of hippocampal pyramidal neurons in AD than in age-matched controls and may also be seen in subcortical nuclei.
- Hirano bodies tend to be more numerous in AD in neurons in the hippocampal CA1 field and subiculum (see Fig. 31.7).
- There is increased accumulation of lipofuscin in neurons (see Chapter 1).
- Corpora amylacea may be seen in large numbers (see Chapter 1).

The structural changes seen in AD can be found in the brains of cognitively normal elderly individuals in low density or restricted distribution. The diagnosis of AD is based on the presence of lesions in high density and extended distribution in a patient with clinical evidence of dementia (see 'Pathologic diagnostic criteria for AD,' p. 31.16).

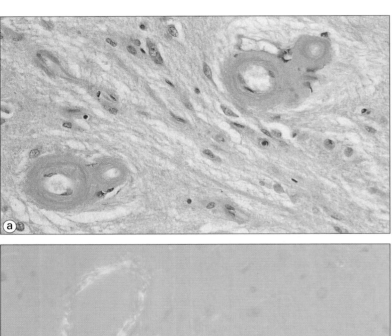

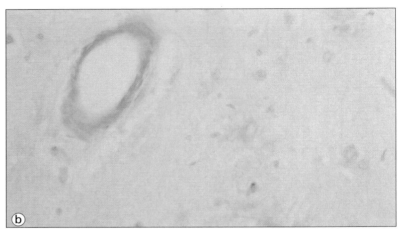

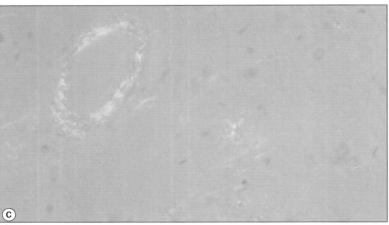

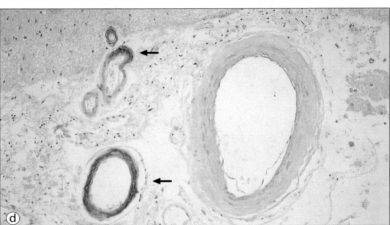

Fig. 31.6 AD congophilic angiopathy. (a) In hematoxylin and eosin-stained sections, as here, the vessels affected by amyloid are thick-walled and have a homogeneous pink appearance. **(b)** In this preparation stained with Congo red, amyloid in the wall of a vessel in the cerebral cortex stains orange.

(c) The amyloid nature can be confirmed by polarizing light microscopy, which will reveal apple-green birefringence and dichroism. (Congo red, polarized light) **(d)** The amyloid in the cerebral vessels shows Aβ peptide immunoreactivity (arrows).

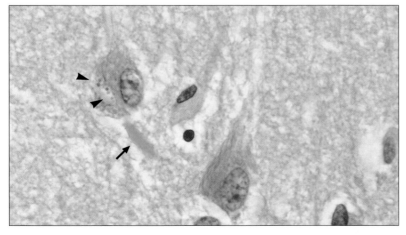

Fig. 31.7 Hirano body and granulovacuolar degeneration. This section of hippocampus includes a Hirano body (arrow) and a neuron showing granulovacuolar degeneration (arrowheads). The neuron towards the bottom of the figure contains a neurofibrillary tangle.

Amyloid plaques are extracellular proteinaceous deposits composed largely of Aβ peptide, either as amyloid filaments or in non-filamentous form, with variable associated abnormalities involving neuronal processes that traverse the abnormal region. The abnormal neuronal processes are termed dystrophic neurites. Plaques associated with abnormal neurites are termed neuritic plaques.

Plaques are widely distributed in the brain of patients with AD. The neocortex and hippocampus are always involved. Plaques may also be present in the basal ganglia, hypothalamus, the tegmentum of the midbrain and pons, and the subcortical white matter.

There are four main types of plaque:
- diffuse
- primitive
- classic (mature)
- burnt-out (end-stage) (**Fig. 31.11e**)

It is believed that there is progression from diffuse, through primitive to classic and finally burnt-out plaques, but there is no direct evidence for this.

Most neuritic plaques include tau-immunoreactive dystrophic neurites (see neuritic abnormalities in AD, p. 31.9) (**Fig. 31.11g**). In some neuritic plaques there are dystrophic neurites that contain chromogranin A and ubiquitin, but no neurites containing tau protein; of the sparse neuritic plaques that may be present in the brains of cognitively normal elderly subjects, this form predominates.

Fig. 31.8 Stains used in the histologic assessment of AD. Several different methods can be used for the assessment of histologic changes in Alzheimer's disease.

Stains used in the histologic assessment of Alzheimer's disease

Much of the pathology associated with Alzheimer's disease cannot be easily seen without special stains.

Silver stains are especially useful and can be divided into:
- Methods that are very sensitive for amyloid (e.g. modified methenamine silver techniques). These detect all plaques and a minority of tangles (Fig 31.9).
- Methods that are very sensitive for the detection of tangles and the abnormal nerve processes around plaques but do not tend to stain amyloid (eg, the Gallyas technique, several modifications of Palmgren's silver impregnation (Fig 31.10), and some modifications of Bodian and Bielschowsky methods).
- Methods that are optimized to detect both plaques and tangles. These tend to under-estimate the density of either plaques or tangles. This is true of most modified Bodian and Bielschowsky techniques, which underestimate the total amount of amyloid in sections.

Stains sensitive for amyloid can be used to detect plaques and tangles.
- Congo red stains amyloid cores and the periphery of many types of plaque. It will also detect a small proportion of neurofibrillary tangles.
- Thioflavin-S is a fluorescent dye which stains amyloid. Modified thioflavin-S staining techniques have been described that allow quite sensitive detection of different plaque types in addition to neurofibrillary tangles and abnormal neurites.

In many laboratories, specific staining of plaques and tangles is now performed by immunohistochemistry with commercially available antisera.
- Plaques are detected with antisera to Aβ peptide after formic-acid pretreatment of sections.
- Tangles are detected by immunostaining for phosphorylated tau protein, the main constituent of tangles.

An estimate of synaptic loss can be obtained by quantitative assessment of synaptophysin immunoreactivity in the cerebral cortex. Synaptophysin is a synaptic vesicle-associated glycoprotein.

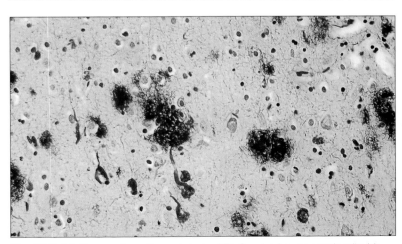

Fig. 31.9 Methenamine silver stain in AD. Cerebral cortex stained with methenamine silver to reveal plaques and NFTs. This technique provides a sensitive means of staining plaques. It is less effective for staining NFTs, and is relatively poor for demonstrating plaque-related neurites.

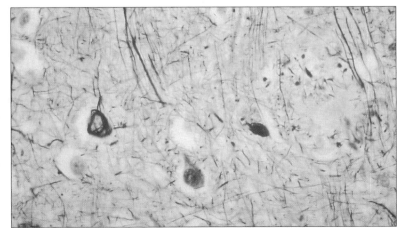

Fig. 31.10 Palmgren's stain in AD. Cerebral cortex impregnated by Palmgren's silver method to reveal a plaque and NFTs. This type of stain is not sensitive to amyloid, seen in the center of the plaque as a yellow background, but is good for detecting NFTs and plaque-related neurites.

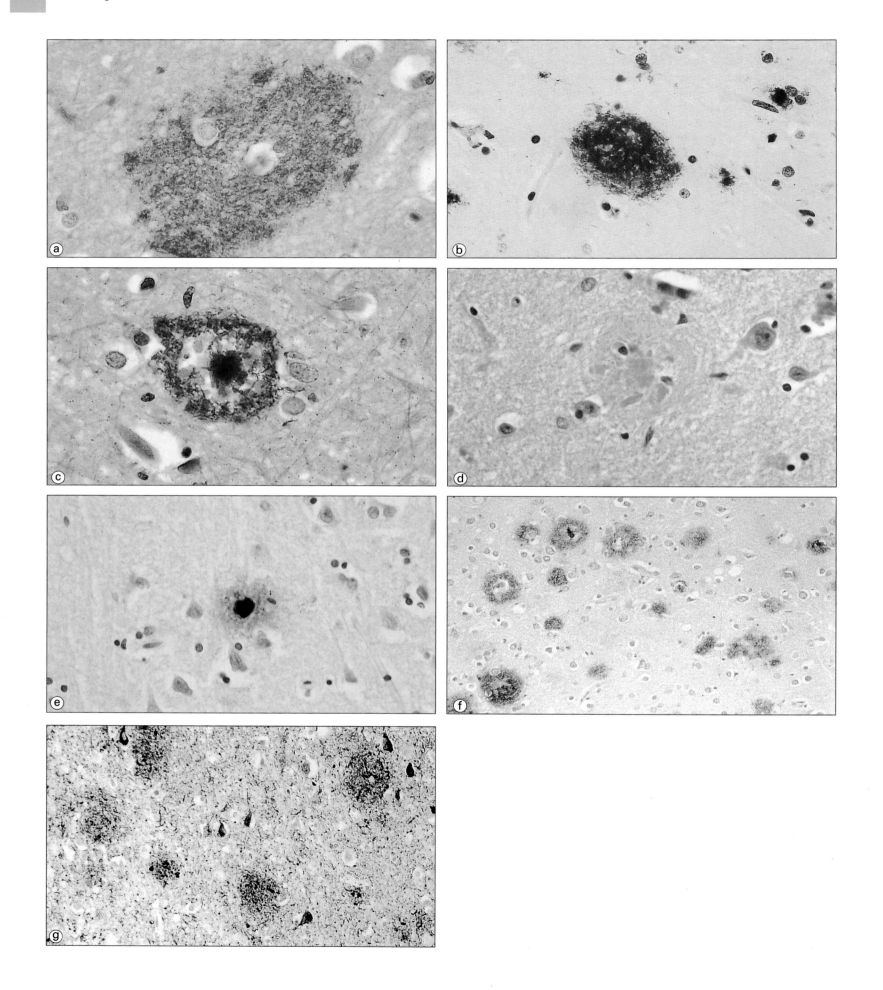

Fig. 31.11 Plaques in AD. (a) Diffuse plaques. These are extracellular ill-defined focal aggregates of amyloid and pre-amyloid material about 60–300 μm in diameter. Neuronal cell processes traversing the plaque appear normal and do not contain tau protein. Diffuse plaques may be detected using silver stains sensitive for amyloid, but are best demonstrated by immunohistochemistry for Aβ peptide after formic acid pretreatment of sections. **(b)** Primitive plaques. These are extracellular roughly spherical focal aggregates of amyloid and pre-amyloid material 60–120 μm in diameter. Neuronal cell processes traversing the plaque may be prominent on silver staining, but are not very dilated and do not contain tau protein on immunostaining. The plaque may be associated with reactive astrocytes as well as activated microglial cells. Primitive plaques may be detected using silver stains sensitive for amyloid, but are best demonstrated by immunohistochemistry for Aβ peptide after formic acid pretreatment of sections. **(c)** Classic (mature) or neuritic plaques. These are extracellular, roughly spherical, focal aggregates of amyloid material, 60–120 μm in diameter, that are often separated into dense core and peripheral halo regions. Neuronal cell processes traversing the plaque are prominent on silver staining and appear enlarged and distorted. Immunostaining (see (g)) shows processes containing tau protein, some of which are unequivocally neuronal, but others may be astroglial. There may be associated reactive astrocytes as well as activated microglial cells. **(d)** Mature plaque. In sections stained with hemotoxylin and eosin neuritic plaques are seen as an ill-defined area of condensation in the neuropil with an eosinophilic plaque core region. Nuclei of microglial or astrocytic cells may be seen radiating around the plaque periphery. **(e)** Burnt-out (end-stage) plaques. These are extracellular compact cores of aggregated amyloid material in the absence of abnormal neurites. They may be detected using silver stains, Congo red, thioflavin-S or immunohistochemistry for Aβ peptide. **(f)** Immunostaining for plaque amyloid. This can be achieved with antisera to Aβ peptide. Staining is enhanced by pretreatment of sections with formic acid and reveals the full range of morphologic plaque types. **(g)** Immunostaining for tau protein. This shows an accumulation of tau protein in abnormal nerve cell processes of neuritic plaques.

MOLECULAR PATHOLOGY OF PLAQUE AMYLOID

- APP is a normal transmembrane glycoprotein. The gene is located on chromosome 21, and several different mRNAs are generated through alternative splicing. The predicted structure of APP consists of three domains (**Fig. 31.12**): a small cytosolic domain; a transmembrane domain; and a large extracellular domain.
- The function of APP is uncertain, but there have been suggestions for a role in cell–cell and cell–matrix interactions.
- Aβ peptide in plaques (known previously as A4 protein, or β protein) is a 42 or 43 residue peptide (Aβ-42/43) derived from APP. 15 C-terminal residues are within the transmembrane domain of APP, the other 28 residues being derived from the extracellular domain (see Fig. 31.12).
- In many normal cells APP is cleaved around the middle of the Aβ region by an enzyme, not yet characterized, designated as α-secretase. This cleavage site precludes generation of Aβ (**Fig. 31.13**). APP is also cleaved by another uncharacterized enzyme, designated β-secretase, to generate the C-terminus of Aβ peptide. The N-terminus of Aβ peptide is generated when another enzyme, designated γ-secretase, cleaves APP within its transmembrane domain. Because this step involves an integral membrane domain, γ-secretase activity is likely to be within the endosome–lysosome compartment (see Fig. 31.14).
- A slightly shorter, 39/40 residue, Aβ peptide (Aβ-39/40) can be found in the CSF of normal patients, indicating that α- and γ-secretase cleavages of APP are normal events. Vascular amyloid in AD has been shown to be composed mainly of Aβ-39/40 while plaque amyloid consists mainly of Aβ-42/43 .
- Except in AD patients with Downs' syndrome, the expression of APP, unlike that of Aβ, is similar in AD and cognitively normal patients. The generation of plaque amyloid is thought to be due to abnormal processing of APP so that Aβ-42/43 is generated rather than the more soluble Aβ-39/40.

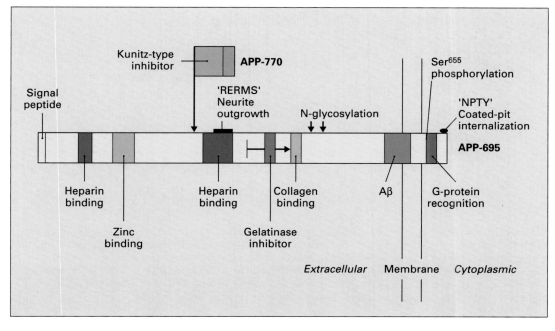

Fig. 31.12 Schematic illustration of amyloid precursor protein (APP). RERMS, neurotropic region; NPTY, coated pit internalisation sequence.

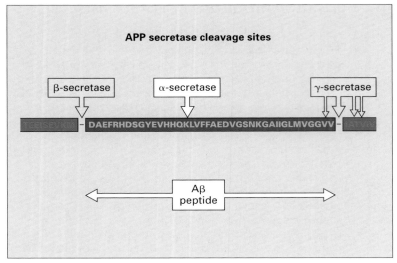

Fig. 31.13 Cleavage sites of APP. The action of α-secretase prevents the formation of Aβ peptide.

A variety of other plaque amyloid-related proteins can be demonstrated immunohistochemically, including apolipoprotein E (apoE), α1-antichymotrypsin, serum amyloid-P protein, growth factors, heparin sulfate, and complement factors.

NFTs are neuronal inclusions composed largely of filamentous aggregates of hyperphosphorylated tau proteins that are variably ubiquitinated and glycated. In sections stained with hematoxylin and eosin, intracellular NFTs are faintly basophilic and extracellular NFTs eosinophilic (**Fig. 31.15**). In silver or thioflavin-S preparations several morphologic forms of NFT can be identified, the shape of the NFT probably being determined by that of the neuron containing it. A multistage model of NFT formation has been proposed (**Fig. 31.16**).

Ultrastructural investigation reveals that NFTs are composed of PHFs with a maximum diameter of 20 nm and a periodic narrowing to 10 nm every 80 nm (**Fig. 31.17**). A small proportion of filaments is straight, with a diameter of 15 nm. Detailed examination of PHF preparations shows that the filaments have a dense core region with a surrounding fuzzy coat.

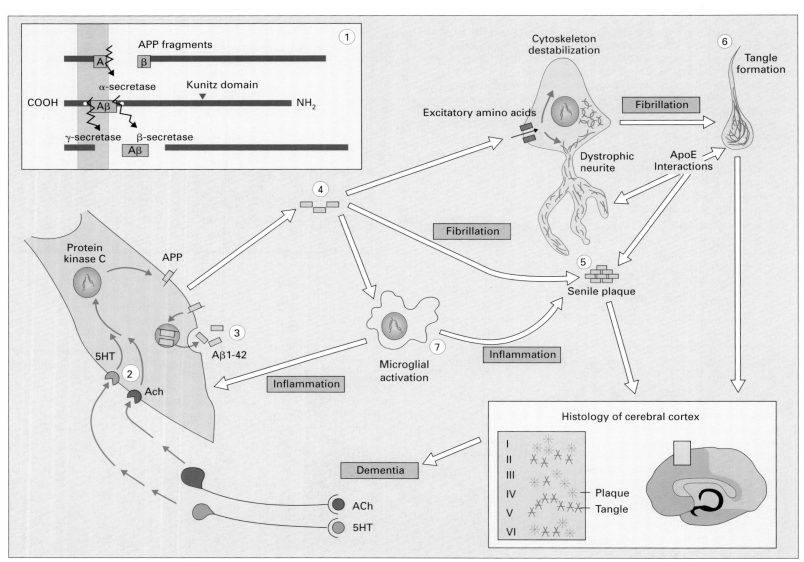

Fig. 31.14 Amyloid cascade model of AD. The general pattern of APP processing in neurons is shown (**1**). Non-amyloidogenic (α secretase) processing of APP can be modulated by stimulation of cholinergic (ACh) or serotinergic (5HT) receptors (**2**). Within the neuron PS1 associates with APP and traffics with it to an endosomal vesicle where Aβ1-42 can be generated (**3**). The Aβ1-42 is secreted and forms multimeric aggregates (**4**) which can activate microglia and can participate in excitotoxic reactions with neurons.

Fibrillar Aβ1-42 initiates senile plaque formation which involves dystrophic neurites, recruitment of activated microglia, interactions with ApoE and the deposition of β amyloid as plaque (**5**). Involvement in plaque formation results in the degeneration of susceptible neurons and tangle formation (**6**). Activated microglia act in a positive feedback loop to enhance Aβ1-42 generation from neurons, and plaque formation (**7**).

NFTs are readily detected by antisera directed against phosphorylated tau protein (**Fig. 31.18**). Early reports that NFTs were immunoreactive with antisera to neurofilament protein were the result of cross-reactivity. A few NFTs are immunoreactive for ubiquitin (**Fig. 31.19**).

Neuritic abnormalities in AD: There are two main forms:
- Plaque-related dystrophic neurites, which are abnormally dilated nerve cell processes running through Aβ plaque deposits. Some of the neurites contain increased amounts of lysosome-related dense

bodies, but no PHFs, and immunostain for chromogranin A and ubiquitin, but not tau. Other neurites contain PHFs and are immunoreactive both for tau protein and variably for ubiquitin.
- NTs, which are fine, distorted, and twisted nerve cell processes that can be detected by modified thioflavin-S or silver staining for NFTs and are immunoreactive for tau protein (**Fig. 31.21**) and variably for ubiquitin. Ultrastructural examination shows nerve cell processes that contain a mixture of PHF and straight filaments.

Golgi studies have shown a reduction in the dendritic arbor of cortical neurons, with a loss of dendritic spines.

THE AMYLOID CASCADE HYPOTHESIS OF AD

- Several lines of evidence point to a primary role for Aβ amyloid in the pathogenesis of AD:
  - Some mutations in the APP gene have been linked with rare familial forms of AD. The neuropathologic findings in these are indistinguishable from those of sporadic AD and include the presence of many NFTs.
  - Patients with Downs' syndrome (trisomy 21) are strongly predisposed to the development of AD by about 40 years. These patients have three APP genes with a commensurate increase in APP mRNA. Diffuse plaques are detectable in the brain of patients with Down's syndrome before the development of neuritic plaques and NFTs.
- The amyloid cascade model (**Fig. 31.14**) proposes a central role for Aβ amyloid in the pathogenesis of AD. The link between Aβ generation and the formation of NFTs is not known. Of possible relevance is the increased neuronal expression of a protein termed RAGE (Receptor for Advanced Glycation End-products and also a receptor for Aβ peptide) in AD, especially near deposits of amyloid.
- Arguments against the amyloid cascade model of AD are that cognitively normal individuals can have very large numbers of neocortical plaques, although predominantly of diffuse type, and only sparse NFTs, and also that the correlation between plaque density and the severity of dementia is relatively weak. Plaque formation in AD may be secondary to another, more fundamental, cellular pathologic process.

MOLECULAR PATHOLOGY OF TAU PROTEIN IN NFTs

- Normal tau proteins are microtubule binding proteins, predominantly axonal, that stabilize the microtubular neuronal cytoskeleton.
- There are several molecular forms of tau protein, all of which have tandem repeat regions that act as microtubule binding sites.
- In normal brain a proportion of potential phosphorylation sites on tau protein away from the microtubule binding sites is phosphorylated. This proportion is increased in tau protein derived from PHF in AD.
- The electron-dense core of PHF is probably composed of the self-aggregating microtubule binding domains of tau while the surrounding fuzzy coat is composed of the N- and C-terminal parts of the protein, heavily phosphorylated at serine–proline and threonine–proline sites (**Fig. 31.20**).
- In normal brain tau protein is also phosphorylated, but the phosphate groups are rapidly removed by phosphatases postmortem. In contrast, tau protein in PHF is relatively resistant to postmortem dephosphorylation, suggesting that defective dephosphorylation of tau may be a key event in its accumulation.

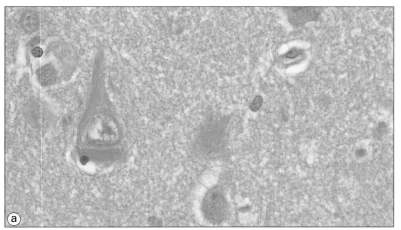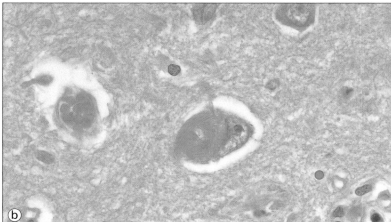

Fiig. 31.15 Neurofibrillary tangles. NFTs are typically faintly basophilic structures within the neuronal cytoplasm. **(a)** Some have a flame-shaped pattern, as here. **(b)** Others appear as globular filamentous structures.

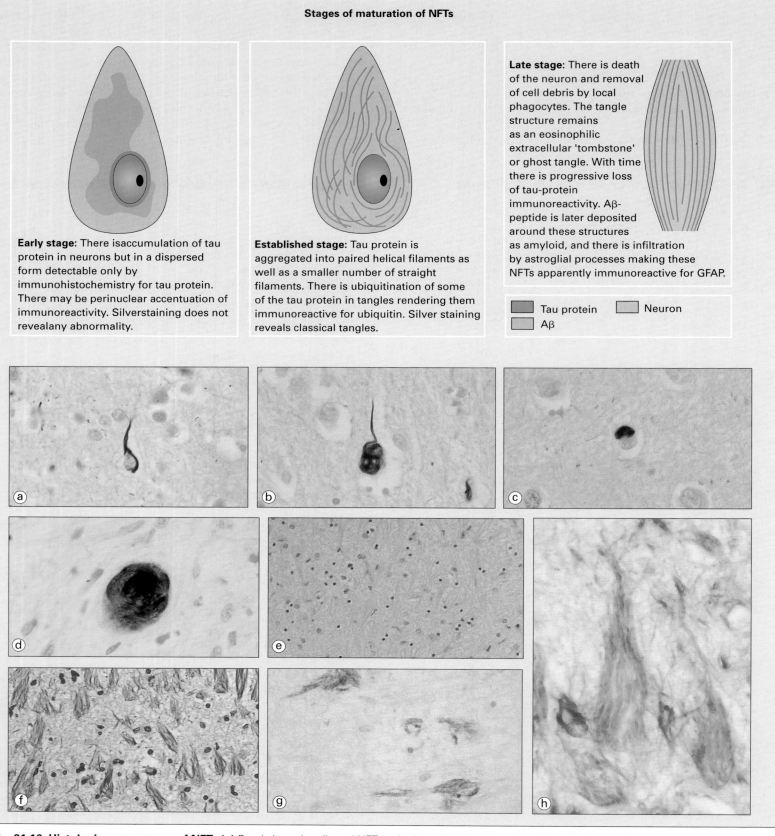

Stages of maturation of NFTs

Early stage: There isaccumulation of tau protein in neurons but in a dispersed form detectable only by immunohistochemistry for tau protein. There may be perinuclear accentuation of immunoreactivity. Silverstaining does not revealany abnormality.

Established stage: Tau protein is aggregated into paired helical filaments as well as a smaller number of straight filaments. There is ubiquitination of some of the tau protein in tangles rendering them immunoreactive for ubiquitin. Silver staining reveals classical tangles.

Late stage: There is death of the neuron and removal of cell debris by local phagocytes. The tangle structure remains as an eosinophilic extracellular 'tombstone' or ghost tangle. With time there is progressive loss of tau-protein immunoreactivity. Aβ-peptide is later deposited around these structures as amyloid, and there is infiltration by astroglial processes making these NFTs apparently immunoreactive for GFAP.

Tau protein   Neuron

Aβ

Fig. 31.16 Histologic appearances of NFTs (a) Band-shaped perikaryal NFT: a single well-defined band runs from the base of the neuron into the apical dendrite. This type of NFT is seen in both large and small pyramidal cells, and is perhaps an early stage of NFT formation. **(b)** Flame-shaped perikaryal NFT: a triangular mass of filaments, usually surrounding the nucleus and extending into the apical dendrite, and seen mainly in large pyramidal cells. **(c)** Small globose perikaryal NFT: a rounded mass of filaments displacing the nucleus to one side of the neuron. This type of NFT is seen in small cortical neurons, especially in layers 5 and 6 and in the periamygdaloid cortex. **(d)** Large globose NFTs: seen in the nucleus basalis of Meynert, periaqueductal gray matter, substantia nigra, locus ceruleus and raphe nuclei. **(e)** Ghost NFTs: faintly eosinophilic extracellular structures representing a stage after the death of the neuron. **(f)** Ghost NFTs: the extracellular ghost NFTs are moderately well seen on silver staining. **(g)** Ghost NFTs may become immunoreactive for Aβ peptide as a result of its deposition around them. **(h)** Ghost NFTs may seem to be immunoreactive for glial fibrillary acidic protein (GFAP) due to ingrowth of glial cell processes.

Neuronal and synaptic loss in AD: Of the order of a 30–40% loss of neocortical neurons can be demonstrated in AD, particularly in young onset patients. The neuronal loss is associated with astrocytic gliosis and, in some cases, microvacuolation — the latter often termed status spongiosus (**Fig. 31.22**). The vacuolation is coarser than that of prion disease (see Chapter 32) and is largely confined to the outer cortical layers.

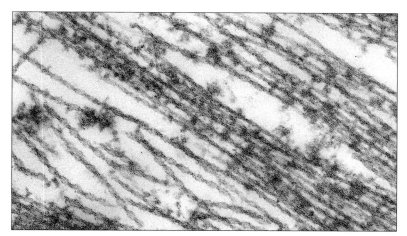

Fig. 31.17 Ultrastructure of NFT. NFTs are composed of paired helical filaments with a periodicity of 80 nm.

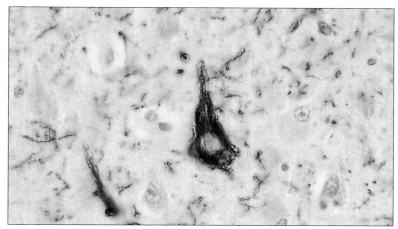

Fig. 31.18 NFT tau immunostaining. Immunostaining with antisera to phosphorylated tau protein is increasingly used as a routine method for detecting NFTs. Staining will detect established NFTs as well as dispersed tau protein prior to NFT formation. Many extracellular ('ghost') NFTs are, however, not immunoreactive for tau.

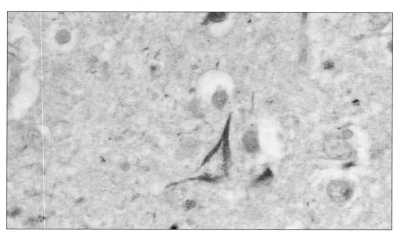

Fig. 31.19 NFT ubiquitin immunostaining. Only relatively few NFTs are immunoreactive for ubiquitin. It is of note that small globose NFTs are generally ubiquitinated and can therefore be almost indistinguishable from cortical Lewy bodies on ubiquitin immunohistochemistry.

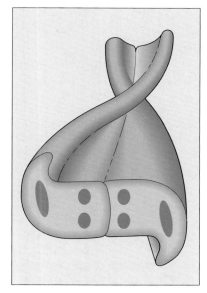

Fig. 31.20 PHF structure. Three-dimensional model of PHF based on denstiy coutour maps produced from isolated PHF. Three density peaks are present in each of the filaments, which twist round each other to produce a characteristic periodicity along their length. (Adapted from Crowther RA. Straight and paired helical filaments in Alzheimer's disease have a common structural unit (1991) *Proc Nat Acad Sci USA* **88:** 2288-2292.

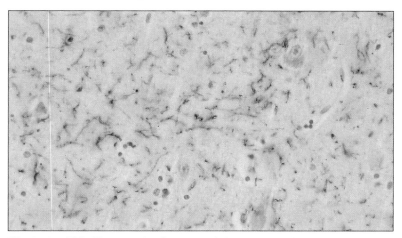

Fig. 31.21 NTs. The strands of tau protein immunoreactivity correspond to neuropil threads.

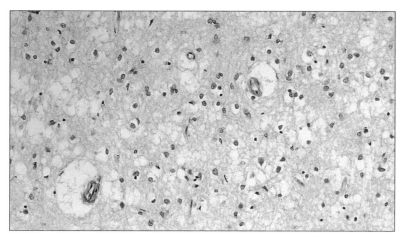

Fig. 31.22 Status spongiosus in AD. Severe neuronal loss from the cortex in AD, with associated astrocytic gliosis, results in irregular coarse vacuolation termed status spongiosus.

MOLECULAR GENETICS OF AD

Several genes play a central role in AD

The four genetic subtypes of AD

- AD1, due to APP gene mutations on chromosome 21.
- AD2, associated with the ApoE ε4 allele on chromosome 19.
- AD3, due to mutations in the presenilin-1 gene on chromosome 14.
- AD4, due to mutations in the presenilin-2 gene on chromosome 1.

AD1

Mutations in the APP gene on chromosome 21 account for about 10% of cases of familial early-onset AD (**Fig. 31.23**).

AD2

Apolipoprotein E (apoE) is a 4 kD protein the gene for which is on chromosome 19. There are three apoE isoforms, E2, E3, and E4, encoded by the alleles ε2, ε3, and ε4. The approximate relative frequency of the different apoE genotypes in Caucasians is:

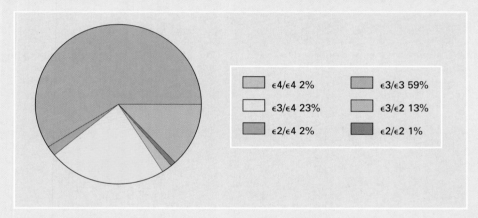

ε4/ε4 2%		ε3/ε3 59%
ε3/ε4 23%		ε3/ε2 13%
ε2/ε4 2%		ε2/ε2 1%

The risk of developing late-onset AD is increased by possession of an ε4 allele and reduced by possession of an ε2 allele. In Caucasian populations the relative risk of developing AD is approximately:

- 19-fold increased in ε4/ε4 homozygotes compared with ε3/ε3 homozygotes
- 4.5-fold increased in ε3/ε4 heterozygotes compared with ε3/ε3 homozygotes.
- 2-fold reduced in ε2/ε3 heterozygotes compared with ε3/ε3 homozygotes.
- very slightly reduced in ε2/ε4 heterozygotes compared with ε4/ε4 homozygotes.

It is important to note that some elderly ε4/ε4 homozygotes have been documented who do not have AD, indicating that this is a risk factor and not an inevitable cause of AD. The ε4 allele also confers an increased risk of cardiovascular disease compared to other apoE genotypes. Of possible relevance to the association of apoE ε4 and AD are observations that apoE:

- has been immunolocalized to plaque and vascular amyloid in AD.
- is involved in distributing membrane cholesterol and phospholipids in neurons.
- binds Aβ peptide, and the E4 isoform does so most strongly.
- promotes Aβ peptide polymerization to form amyloid fibrils

AD3

The gene for presenilin-1 (PS-1) is on chromosome 14 and encodes a 467-residue protein that has 6–9 possible transmembrane domains (probably seven) and is of unknown function.
Mutations in PS-1 account for about 50% of cases of early-onset familial AD (**Fig. 31.24**). The mutations alter the proteolytic processing of APP, enhancing production of the amyloidogenic Aβ 42/43 .

AD4

The gene for presenilin-2 (PS-2) is on chromosome 1 and encodes a 448-residue protein of unknown function that is homologous to PS-1 and also predicted to have between six and nine transmembrane domains. Mutations in PS-2 have been associated with late onset familial AD, originally described in a Volga German kindred. The mutations alter APP processing, enhancing Aβ 42/43 production. Some studies have linked PS-2 to apoptosis and PS-2 mutations to enhanced apoptosis.

α1-antichymotrypsin

α1ACT is a member of the serine protease inhibitor family and has been immunolocalized to plaque amyloid. Possession of a microsatellite marker (A10) linked to the α1ACT gene on chromosome 19 has been reported to increase the risk of AD independent of, and synergistic with, E4 status. The genetic basis for this remains to be determined as the A10 marker is not very close to the α1ACT gene. Earlier studies suggesting linkage with a polymorphism in the signal sequence for the α1ACT gene have not been confirmed.

In AD a synaptic loss of 30–50% can be demonstrated by quantitation of synapse-related proteins in affected cortical regions. The most widely used marker is synaptophysin, a glycoprotein associated with synaptic vesicles. The degree of synaptic loss correlates well with clinical scores of the severity of dementia.

NEUROCHEMICAL PATHOLOGY OF AD

- Neurochemical analysis of brains has shown widespread transmitter defects in the brains of patients with AD.
- There is a marked loss of acetylcholine from the cerebral cortex in AD. This is related to loss of neurons from the nucleus basalis of Meynert (in the basal forebrain), which is the major cholinergic input nucleus to the cerebral cortex. Several treatments augmenting cholinergic transmission are being used or tested in AD.
- There is loss of neurotransmitters associated with intrinsic neurons in the cerebral cortex, in keeping with neuronal and synaptic loss from these regions.
- 5-hydroxytryptamine (5-HT; seritonin) input to the cerebral cortex is reduced. This is related to a loss of neurons from the serotoninergic dorsal raphe nuclei and may correlate with depression in AD.
- Noradrenergic input to the cortex is reduced and related to a variable loss of neurons from the locus ceruleus.

Glial pathology in AD: Reactive astrocytes occur in and around neuritic plaques, and in areas of neuronal loss and cortical microvacuolation. Microglial activation occurs in relation to plaque amyloid. This close association has led to speculation that microglia are responsible for amyloidogenic processing of Aβ peptide. Aβ-induced activation of microglia may also lead to secretion of cytokines such as interleukin (IL)-1β and tumor necrosis factor (TNF)-α, and extracellular proteases, which are potentially neurotoxic.

White matter pathology in AD: Pallor of myelin staining of central hemispheric white matter is quite common in AD. In most cases this is probably related to microvascular changes of arteriolosclerosis. In a minority of cases pallor of myelin occurs in the absence of vascular abnormalities. This phenomenon in AD may have contributed to the overdiagnosis of vascular dementia on the basis of neuroimaging findings.

Subcortical involvement in AD: Many subcortical regions are involved by plaques, NFTs or NTs in AD (**Fig. 31.25**). Some regions, such as the dorsal raphe nucleus are affected at an early stage of disease. Involvement of the nucleus basalis of Meynert is especially important as this is the cholinergic projection nucleus to the cerebral cortex. Cell loss from this nucleus results in a severe cholinergic deficit in the cerebral cortex in AD.

Mutations in APP

	Mutation	Structural change	Phenotype	Functional effect in model system
London mutation	Point mutations at codon 717	Isoleucine, phenylalanine, glycine for valine substitution just beyond the γ-secretase cleavage site at the C-terminus of Aβ (1-42).	Early-onset AD	Associated with a 1.5- to 1.9-fold increase in the ratio of Aβ 42/43, to Aβ40 secretion
Swedish mutation	Double mutation at codons 670 and 671	Asparagine-leucine substitution for lysine-methionine just proximal to the N-terminal region of Aβ (1-42) near the β-secretase cleavage site of APP	Early-onset AD	Increased cellular secretion of Aβ peptide
Flemish mutation	Point mutation at codon 692	Alanine to glycine substitution	Familial early-onset dementia with neuritic plaques and cerebral amyloid angiopathy	
Dutch mutation	Codon 693	Glutamic acid to glutamine substitution near α-secretase cleavage site	Cerebral amyloid angiopathy with recurrent haemorrhagic strokes	
Late-onset Alzheimer mutation	Codon 665	Aspartate for glutamine substitution	Late-onset AD suggested in only one kindred	

Fig. 31.23 Mutations in APP. Several mutations have been characterised in APP and related to different AD phenotypes. In some, the functional effect of the mutation has been characterised.

Pathologic staging of AD

The evolution of pathologic changes in AD is fairly predictable and has been subdivided into several stages by Braak and Braak (1991).

Plaque stages correlate poorly with the severity of dementia (**Fig. 31.26**) and are:
- Stage A: low density of neuritic plaques in the neocortex, especially in the frontal, temporal, and occipital lobes.

- Stage B: neuritic plaques present in neocortical association areas and moderate hippocampal involvement.
- Stage C: neuritic plaques present in primary sensory and motor areas.

NFT stages correlate well with the severity of dementia (**Fig. 31.27**).

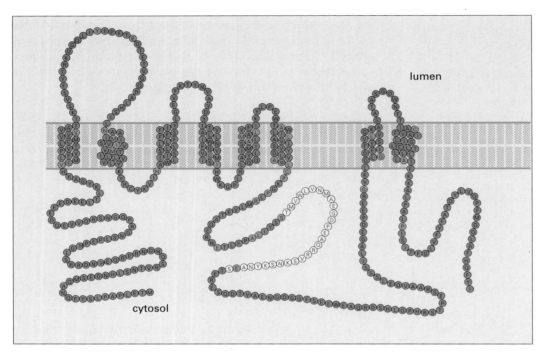

lumen

cytosol

Fig. 31.24 Mutations in presenilin-1 (PS-1). Schematic diagram of the presenilin 1 protein showing its probable topological orientation within the membrane of the endoplasmic reticulum. sites of amino acid mutations that cause early onset of familial Alzheimer's disease are shown in green. The region of PS1 deleted by the splice acceptor site mutation is shown in yellow (coded by exon 9).

Fig. 31.25 Non-cortical involvement in AD. Several subcortical regions may show involvment by plaques and/or NFTs.

Non-cortical involvement in AD		
Region	**Amyloid**	**Tangles**
Olfactory bulb	Small number of plaques in anterior olfactory nucleus	Many cells develop tangles with neuropil threads
Hypothalamus	Diffuse plaques in late stages	Few tangles in lateral, tuberal, and posterior nuclei Many tangles in tubero-mamillary nucleus
Thalamus	Diffuse plaques, small primitive plaques	Anterodorsal nucleus in early stages Less severe involvement of other nuclei , especially anteroventral nucleus, in late stages
Striatum	Many diffuse plaques	Very rare tangles in large neurons
Pallidum		Rare large globose tangles
Nucleus basalis of Meynert	Small numbers of plaques	Many large globose tangles, cell loss
Red nucleus	Small amyloid deposits	Large globose tangles and cell loss
Substantia nigra	Sparse amyloid deposits	Many globose tangles especially in advanced disease
Tectum of midbrain	Small amyloid deposits	
Dorsal raphe nucleus		Tangles early in disease, and cell loss
Locus Ceruleus		Globose tangles and cell loss
Cerebellum	Diffuse plaques in molecular layer	

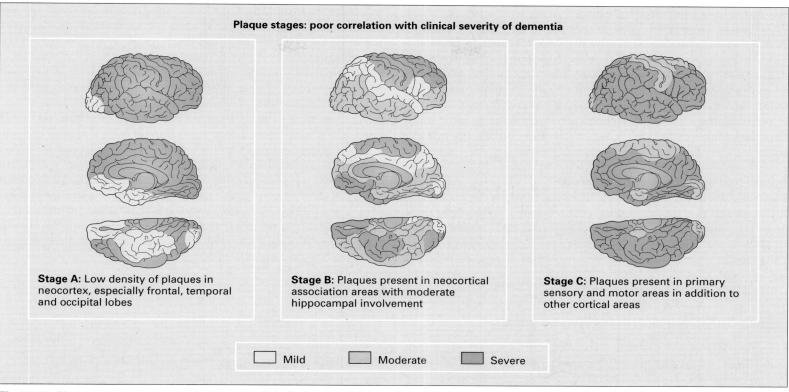

Plaque stages: poor correlation with clinical severity of dementia

Stage A: Low density of plaques in neocortex, especially frontal, temporal and occipital lobes

Stage B: Plaques present in neocortical association areas with moderate hippocampal involvement

Stage C: Plaques present in primary sensory and motor areas in addition to other cortical areas

☐ Mild   ◻ Moderate   ▨ Severe

Fig. 31.26 Plaque stages: poor correlation with clinical severity of dementia.

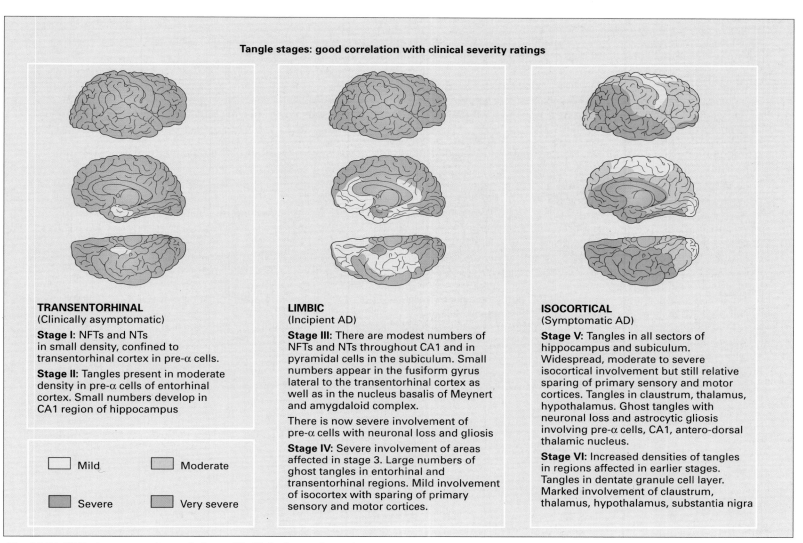

Tangle stages: good correlation with clinical severity ratings

TRANSENTORHINAL
(Clinically asymptomatic)

Stage I: NFTs and NTs in small density, confined to transentorhinal cortex in pre-α cells.

Stage II: Tangles present in moderate density in pre-α cells of entorhinal cortex. Small numbers develop in CA1 region of hippocampus

☐ Mild   ◻ Moderate

▨ Severe   ▨ Very severe

LIMBIC
(Incipient AD)

Stage III: There are modest numbers of NFTs and NTs throughout CA1 and in pyramidal cells in the subiculum. Small numbers appear in the fusiform gyrus lateral to the transentorhinal cortex as well as in the nucleus basalis of Meynert and amygdaloid complex.

There is now severe involvement of pre-α cells with neuronal loss and gliosis

Stage IV: Severe involvement of areas affected in stage 3. Large numbers of ghost tangles in entorhinal and transentorhinal regions. Mild involvement of isocortex with sparing of primary sensory and motor cortices.

ISOCORTICAL
(Symptomatic AD)

Stage V: Tangles in all sectors of hippocampus and subiculum. Widespread, moderate to severe isocortical involvement but still relative sparing of primary sensory and motor cortices. Tangles in claustrum, thalamus, hypothalamus. Ghost tangles with neuronal loss and astrocytic gliosis involving pre-α cells, CA1, antero-dorsal thalamic nucleus.

Stage VI: Increased densities of tangles in regions affected in earlier stages. Tangles in dentate granule cell layer. Marked involvement of claustrum, thalamus, hypothalamus, substantia nigra

Fig. 31.27 NFT stages: good correlation with clinical severity ratings.

AD pathology in normal aging

The histologic changes that affect AD patients may be found in a restricted distribution or low density in cognitively normal elderly individuals.

Plaques occur in the cortex with increased frequency in aging. In normal aging the plaques are mainly diffuse. There may be small numbers of neuritic plaques, most associated with ubiquitin- and chromogranin-immunoreactive neurites that do not contain tau protein.

NFTs may be seen in small numbers in the hippocampus and entorhinal cortex in the cognitively normal elderly. This corresponds to Braak stages I–III (see Fig 31.27).

Pathologic diagnostic criteria for AD

Difficulties in making a pathologic diagnosis of AD occur because the histologic changes are not entirely pathognomonic and overlap those in the cognitively normal elderly. The diagnosis of AD should be restricted to cases with both plaques and NFTs in the hippocampus and neocortex, and a history of dementia. Patients who have plaques and NFTs in a restricted distribution or who are not clinically demented are best classified as having 'Alzheimer changes' as this does not pre-judge the nature of their disease. Several different criteria have been proposed for the pathologic diagnosis for AD:

- The National Institutes of Ageing (Khachaturian) criteria are based on assessing the density of both diffuse and neuritic plaques in the cerebral cortex and allocating a score according to patient age. Application of these criteria probably leads to overdiagnosis of AD as diffuse plaques are a common feature of normal aging.
- The Consortium to Establish a Registry for Alzheimer's Disease (CERAD) Guidelines for the diagnosis of AD are widely used and are based on semi-quantitative assessment of neuritic plaque density by comparison with standard reference illustrations (**Figs. 31.28–31.32**). This has been shown to have good reproducibility between different laboratories. The patient's age and the clinical history of dementia are taken into account in determining the diagnostic category for each case.

DIFFICULTIES IN THE DIAGNOSIS OF AD

Some patients have clinical dementia and neuropathologic examination reveals the presence of NFTs in cortical and subcortical areas in the absence of significant numbers of plaques.
- PSP (see chapter 28) and CBD (see chapter 28 and p. 31.26) may both present as a dementia syndrome or a syndrome of parkinsonism and dementia. A search should be made of subcortical structures known to be affected in these disorders and cortical regions should be assessed for swollen neurons characteristic of CBD.
- Tangle-only dementia (see p. 31.28) is a rare but increasingly recognized disorder.

Some patients have an abundance of plaques but very few NFTs
- A careful search for cortical Lewy bodies should be made in cortical and subcortical regions, with a view to making a diagnosis of DLB, which accounts for many cases previously regarded as 'plaque-only AD'.
- If no cortical Lewy bodies are seen and the plaques are all diffuse, they may be incidental and other types of dementia (such as a frontotemporal dementia) should be considered and the relevant abnormalities sought (e.g. microvacuolation in layer II of the anterior temporal or frontal neocortex).

Some patients have Alzheimer changes in a restricted distribution or associated with other pathologic features. Consider the following:
- Limbic AD, which is characterized by clinical dementia and large numbers of NFTs restricted to the amygdala and hippocampus but with large numbers of neocortical plaques.
- Asymmetric AD. The changes of AD may rarely be asymmetric so that one hemisphere is preferentially affected.
- Posterior AD. Severe disease preferentially affecting the occipital and visual-association areas with pathologic features of AD has been reported.
- Frontal AD. AD pathology may be associated with the clinical features of frontotemporal dementia (see p. 31.22).
- Swollen neurons in AD. In a few cases swollen cortical neurons are a feature of disease that would otherwise be pathologically typical of AD. Care should be taken to ensure that the case does not meet criteria for CBD (see chapter 28 and p. 31.26).
- AD with other degenerative diseases. AD pathology occasionally occurs in association with other degenerative diseases such as Huntington's disease, Pick's disease, and Parkinson's disease.
- AD with vascular disease. There may be ischemic or hemorrhagic disease due to the cerebral and cerebellar amyloid angiopathy in AD (see chapter 10), and AD is often associated with atherosclerotic vascular disease of the brain; a diagnosis of mixed AD and vascular dementia is appropriate in some cases.

CERAD protocol for diagnosis of AD

Macroscopic appearance

The following features are noted:
- brain weight
- regional neocortical atrophy and ventricular enlargement (rated semiquantitatively as none, mild, moderate, severe)
- atrophy of the hippocampus and entorhinal cortex (present or absent)
- pallor of the substantia nigra and locus ceruleus (present or absent)
- atherosclerosis, significant obstruction or aneurysms of cerebral blood vessels (present or absent)
- lacunar infarcts, regional infarcts, hemorrhages (number, size, frequency, distribution, and laterality recorded).

Histologic sampling and staining

A minimum of six anatomic regions is designated for histologic examination (Fig. 31.29):
- middle frontal gyrus
- superior and middle temporal gyri
- anterior cingulate gyrus
- inferior parietal lobule
- hippocampus and entorhinal cortex
- midbrain including the substantia nigra.

Paraffin-embedded sections are cut at a thickness of 6–8μm and stained with:
- hematoxylin and eosin
- a silver stain, such as the modifed Bielschowsky impregnation, for the detection of neuritic plaques and neurofibrillary tangles

Thioflavin-S stained sections viewed under ultraviolet light can be used to assess plaques, tangles, and vascular amyloid.
A Congo red stain can be used for evaluating vascular amyloid.

Diagnostic classification

The CERAD classification is perfomed in three steps:
- A semiquantitative assessment is made of the density of neuritic plaques (i.e. that include thickened, silver-impregnated neurites) in the sections of neocortex. The density is scored by comparison with reference photomicrographs and diagrams, as *none*, *sparse*, *moderate*, or *frequent* (Fig. 31.30). The density of tangles is also estimated but this does not contribute to the diagnostic classification in the CERAD protocol.
- An age-related plaque score is obtained by relating the maximum plaque density in sections of frontal, temporal, or parietal neocortex, to the age of the patient at death (in the ranges <50, 50–75, or >75 years) (Fig. 31.31).
- The age-related plaque score is then integrated with the clinical presence or absence of dementia to allow cases to be categorised as *normal with respect to AD*, *possible AD*, *probable AD*, or *definite AD* (Fig. 31.32).

Fig. 31.28 CERAD protocol for diagnosis of AD.

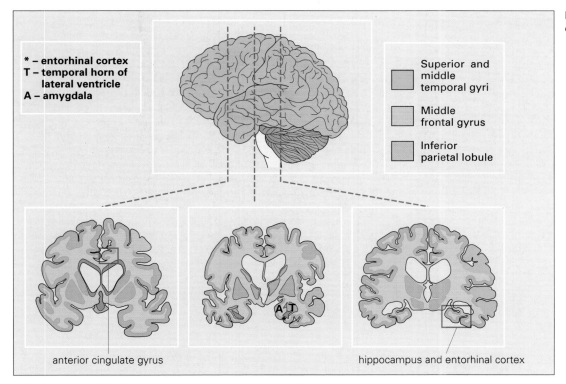

* – entorhinal cortex
T – temporal horn of lateral ventricle
A – amygdala

Superior and middle temporal gyri

Middle frontal gyrus

Inferior parietal lobule

anterior cingulate gyrus

hippocampus and entorhinal cortex

Fig. 31.29 Cortical sampling for CERAD diagnosis of AD.

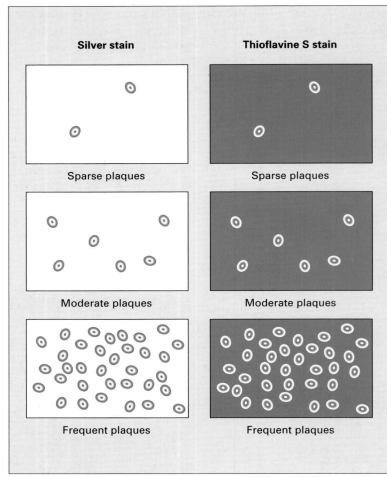

Silver stain | **Thioflavine S stain**

Sparse plaques | Sparse plaques

Moderate plaques | Moderate plaques

Frequent plaques | Frequent plaques

Fig. 31.30 CERAD plaque densities.

Age-related plaque score table

Age of patient at death (yrs)	Frequency of plaques			
	None	Sparse	Moderate	Frequent
<50	0	C	C	C
50–75	0	B	C	C
>75	0	A	B	C

The age-related plaque score corresponds to the following assessment:
O = No histologic evidence of Alzheimer's disease.
A = Histologic findings are UNCERTAIN evidence of Alzheimer's disease.
B = Histologic findings SUGGEST the diagnosis of Alzheimer's disease.
C = Histologic findings INDICATE the diagnosis of Alzheimer's disease.

Fig. 31.31 Age-related plaque scores table.

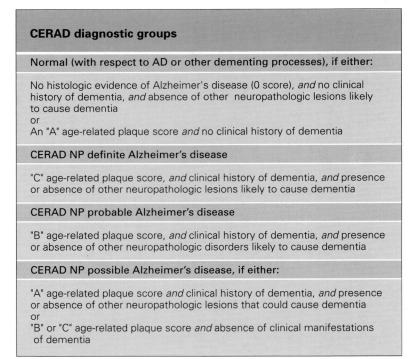

CERAD diagnostic groups

Normal (with respect to AD or other dementing processes), if either:

No histologic evidence of Alzheimer's disease (0 score), *and* no clinical history of dementia, *and* absence of other neuropathologic lesions likely to cause dementia
or
An "A" age-related plaque score *and* no clinical history of dementia

CERAD NP definite Alzheimer's disease

"C" age-related plaque score, *and* clinical history of dementia, *and* presence or absence of other neuropathologic lesions likely to cause dementia

CERAD NP probable Alzheimer's disease

"B" age-related plaque score, *and* clinical history of dementia, *and* presence or absence of other neuropathologic disorders likely to cause dementia

CERAD NP possible Alzheimer's disease, if either:

"A" age-related plaque score *and* clinical history of dementia, *and* presence or absence of other neuropathologic lesions that could cause dementia
or
"B" or "C" age-related plaque score *and* absence of clinical manifestations of dementia

Fig. 31.32 CERAD diagnostic groups.

DEMENTIA WITH LEWY BODIES (DLB)

DLB is now recognized as a common form of dementia. In several hospital-based series this form of dementia accounts for 10–25% of all cases making it second only to AD as a cause of dementia. The incidence of DLB in the community is unclear. The high frequency in hospital series may reflect a referral bias (e.g. due to frequent falls resulting in early hospitalization).

CLINICAL DIAGNOSIS OF DLB

- The central requirement is progressive cognitive decline of sufficient magnitude to interfere with normal social or occupational function. Prominent or persistent memory impairment may not necessarily occur in the early stages, but is usually evident with progression. Deficits on tests of attention and frontal subcortical skills and visuospatial ability may be prominent.
- In addition, two of the following are required for a probable and one for a possible diagnosis of DLB: fluctuating cognition with pronounced variations in attention and alertness; recurrent visual hallucinations (typically, these are well-formed and detailed); spontaneous motor features of parkinsonism.
- Features supportive of the diagnosis are repeated falls, syncope or transient loss of consciousness, neuroleptic sensitivity, systematized delusions, and non-visual hallucinations.
- A diagnosis of DLB is less likely in the presence of stroke disease, evident as focal neurologic signs or on brain imaging, or if there is evidence of any physical illness or other brain disorder sufficient to account for the clinical picture.

The hallmark of the disease is the presence of cortical Lewy bodies (see p. 31.20). In most affected patients there are also pathologic features of AD. Several terms have been used for DLB, the main ones being:

- diffuse Lewy body disease
- cortical Lewy body disease
- senile dementia of Lewy body type
- Lewy body variant of AD

The recommendation of an international workshop was that the preferred term should now be dementia with Lewy bodies (DLB).

MACROSCOPIC APPEARANCES

The macroscopic appearance is similar to that in AD, but atrophy of the frontal, temporal and parietal cortex is typically only mild to moderate (**Fig. 31.33a**) and the occipital lobe is spared. Atrophy of limbic structures is usually moderate to severe (**Fig. 31.33b**). There is pallor of the substantia nigra and locus ceruleus (**Fig. 31.33c**).

MICROSCOPIC APPEARANCES

The defining feature of DLB is the presence of Lewy bodies in several brain regions (**Fig. 31.34**). As in idiopathic Parkinson's disease, there is almost invariably a significant loss of neurons from the substantia nigra and locus ceruleus, but many of the residual neurons contain classic Lewy bodies (**Fig. 31.35**). There are also Lewy bodies in the cerebral cortex. Cortical Lewy bodies can be seen in sections stained with hematoxylin and eosin (**Fig. 31.36a–c**) but are better demonstrated by immunochemistry for ubiquitin (**Fig. 31.36d**). The inclusions are mainly concentrated in small neurons of the deep cortical layers. The limbic, insular, temporal, parietal, and frontal cortices may be involved, in decreasing order of frequency. The amygdaloid nuclei are usually affected. There is generally neuronal loss with Lewy bodies in the nucleus basalis of Meynert. This involvement causes a severe cholinergic deficit in the cerebral cortex in DLB.

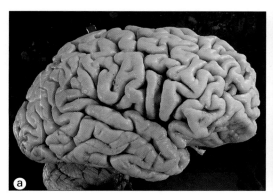 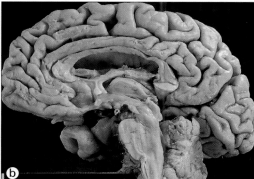 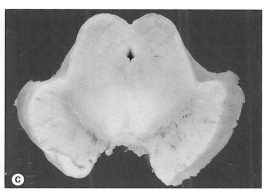

Fig. 31.33 Macroscopic appearances of DLB. (a) Cortical atrophy over the cerebral convexities is typically less severe than in a patient with AD of similar clinical severity. **(b)** There is typically significant atrophy involving the limbic system as seen here on the medial surface of the cerebral hemisphere. **(c)** The substantia nigra is abnormally pale in patients with DLB, due to loss of pigmented neurons.

Fig. 31.34 Pathologic features of DLB.

Pathologic features of DLB
Essential for diagnosis of DLB • Lewy bodies **Associated but not essential** • Lewy-related neurites • Plaques (all morphological types) • Neurofibrillary tangles • Regional neuronal loss - especially brain stem (substantia nigra and locus ceruleus) and nucleus basalis of Meynert • Microvacuolation (spongiform change) and synapse loss • Neurochemical abnormalities and neurotransmitter deficits

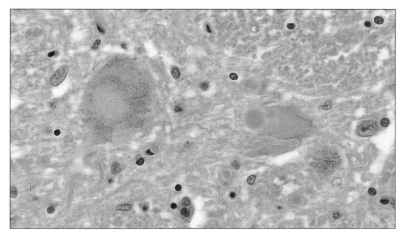

Fig. 31.35 Lewy bodies in substantia nigra in DLB. Lewy bodies and pale bodies are seen in residual neurons of the substantia nigra. The appearances are identical to those in Parkinson's disease.

Lewy-related neurites demonstrable by anti-ubiquitin but not anti-tau immunostaining may be present in the CA2–3 region of the hippocampus (**Fig. 31.37**) and in the subcortical nuclei affected by cell loss.

Transcortical microvacuolation resembling that in prion disease is seen in the mesial temporal lobe cortex in a small proportion of patients (**Fig. 31.38**).

Overlap with the pathology of AD is as follows:
- Approximately 80% of affected patients with DLB have numerous diffuse plaques and smaller numbers of neuritic plaques (**Fig. 31.39**). In many cases these patients fulfil pathologic diagnostic criteria for AD.
- Approximately 60% of patients have NFTs in the entorhinal cortex in moderate to severe density, and rare neocortical NFTs.

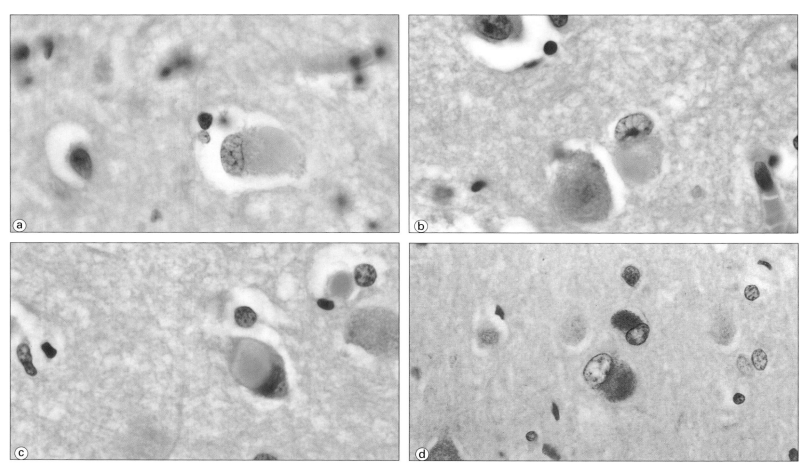

Fig. 31.36 Cortical Lewy bodies. Cortical Lewy bodies (arrows) have a variety of morphological appearances (**a–c**). Because the inclusions stain quite homogeneously and often have a poorly defined margin, cortical neurons that contain Lewy bodies may, on cursory examination, be confused with reactive astrocytes. Ubiquitin immuhistochemistry is the most sensitive way of detecting cortical Lewy bodies (**d**).

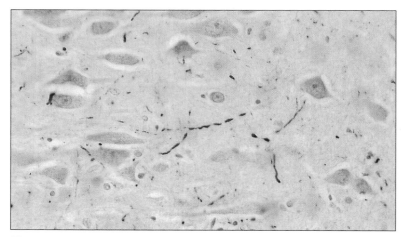

Fig. 31.37 Lewy-related neurites in the hippocampus. Lewy-related neurites are not visible on hematoxylin and eosin staining but are immunoreactive for ubiquitin, as shown here. They are also immunoreactive for NFP and PGP9.5.

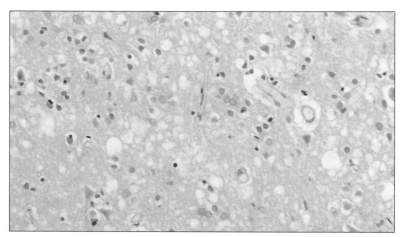

Fig. 31.38 Cortical microvacuolation in DLB. Fine transcortical vacuolation closely resembling that in prion disease may be present, but the distribution is largely restricted to the medial temporal neocortex and amygdala.

- Approximately 30% of patients with DLB, have florid AD-type changes, with many hippocampal and neocortical NFTs and a high density of neuritic plaques.
- A small proportion of DLB patients have cortical and brain stem Lewy body pathology in the complete absence of AD changes. This pattern is sometimes referred to as the pure form of DLB, while the more frequent combination of cortical and brain stem Lewy bodies in the presence of AD changes is referred to as the common form of DLB. Assessment of DLB is summarized in **Fig. 31.42**

NEUROCHEMICAL PATHOLOGY OF DLB

- There is a dopaminergic deficit in cortical and subcortical areas related to a loss of neurons from the substantia nigra.
- A severe cortical cholinergic deficit has been noted in DLB, more profound than in most cases of AD. Anecdotal reports have suggested that anticholinergic therapy may be particularly effective in delaying the progression of dementia in DLB patients.

GENETICS OF DLB

- The apoE ε4 allele is over-represented in patients with DLB at a level intermediate between that of populations with pure AD and non-demented populations. The ε4 allele frequency is probably normal in the pure form of DLB (as it is in Parkinson's disease).
- The frequency of the CYP2D6B allele of debrisoquine hydroxylase associated with a 'poor metabolizer' phenotype is increased in DLB (as it is in Parkinson's disease).
- Brain stem and cortical Lewy bodies have been found in some patients with familial AD due to a missense mutation at codon 717 of the APP gene.

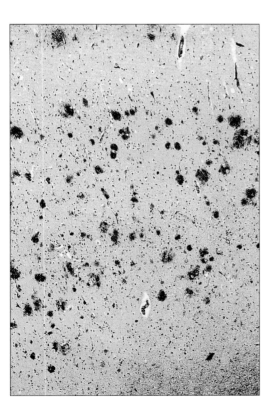

Fig. 31.39 Cortical plaques in DLB. Most patients with DLB have plaques in the neocortex, as shown here by silver impregnation. These tend to be predominantly of diffuse type.

Newcastle criteria for pathologic assessment of DLB

Pathologic criteria for the evaluation of dementia with Lewy bodies have been proposed. Cases are divided into three main subtypes according to a distribution of Lewy bodies in brain stem, limbic, and neocortical regions.

Histologic sampling and staining

The following areas should be sampled:

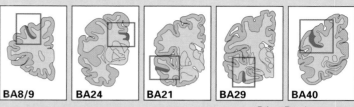

BA8/9   BA24   BA21   BA29   BA40

Sampling for diagnosis of DLB

BA = Brodmann area

Neocortical Regions
(i) Frontal BA8/9
     The middle frontal gyrus in the superior frontal sulcus at the plane just anterior to the temporal tip
(ii) Temporal BA21
     The superior sulcal margin (superior temporal sulcus) of the middle temporal gyrus at the plane of the mammillary body.
(iii) Parietal BA40
     The superior sulcal margin (intraparietal sulcus) of the parietal lobule at the plane 1cm posterior to the posterior pole of the splenium.

Limbic or Paralimbic Regions
(i) Anterior cingulate BA24
     In the plane of the anterior commissure approximately 2cm. posterior to the anterior pole of the genu.
(ii) Transentorhinal BA29
     The sulcal margin (collateral sulcus) of the parahippocampal gyrus in the plane of the red nucleus.

Brain Stem Regions
Substantia nigra, locus ceruleus and dorsal nucleus of vagus.

Paraffin-embedded sections are cut at a thickness of 6–8μm and stained with:
- hematoxylin and eosin
- anti-ubiquitin antibodies

Histologic assessment

In each of the designated areas, the total number of Lewy bodies should be counted within the full thickness of the cerebral cortex. The areas are delimited as follows:
- **Neocortical regions** — from base to crest along the indicated sulcus of the selected gyrus
- **Cingulate** — along the full length of the gyrus in the indicated coronal plane of section
- **Transentorhinal region** — along the collateral sulcus from base to crest of the parahippocampal gyrus

Semiquantitative scores are derived for each area:

Scoring of density of cortical Lewy bodies	
Score	Count (LB/area)
0	0
1	Up to 5
2	>5

The Lewy body scores for individual areas are summated and the final score is used to subclassify DLB into brain stem, limbic, or neocortical types:

Lewy Body Score						
Category	Transen-torhinal	Cingulate	Temporal	Frontal	Parietal	Total
Brain stem predominant	0–1	0–1	0	0	0	0–2
Limbic (transitional)	1–2	1–2	0–1	0–1	0	3–6
Neocortical	2	2	1–2	1–2	1–2	7–10

Fig. 31.40 Diagnosis of DLB. A scheme for the pathologic categorization of DLB into the brain stem predominant, limbic, and neocortical subtypes.

FRONTOTEMPORAL DEMENTIAS AND LOBAR ATROPHIES

Degenerative dementing diseases characterized by selective frontal and temporal lobe atrophy account for 12–20% of cases of dementia. The main diseases in this group are:

- Pick's disease
- dementia with motor neuron disease inclusions (MND–inclusion dementia)
- dementia with changes of corticobasal degeneration (CBD)
- dementia of frontal type (DFT) (also known as lobar degeneration without neuronal inclusions, or dementia lacking distinctive histologic features)
- chromosome 17-linked dementia.
- frontal AD.

In addition to these disorders, dementia with features of frontal lobe degeneration are seen late in the course of classic motor neuron disease/amyotrophic lateral sclerosis (ALS) (see Chapter 27), multiple system atrophy (see Chapter 28), and progressive supranuclear palsy (PSP) (see Chapter 28).

PICK'S DISEASE
MACROSCOPIC APPEARANCES

In Pick's disease atrophy of the frontal and temporal lobes is typically very severe, in some cases producing 'blade-like' or 'knife-edge' gyri (**Fig. 31.42**). The posterior part of the superior temporal gyrus is typically spared. In some cases of Pick's disease atrophy is only moderate. Whether atrophy of basal ganglia occurs is questionable as most descriptions of this relate to cases in which Pick bodies were not demonstrated.

MICROSCOPIC APPEARANCES

The cardinal histologic abnormality is the presence of Pick bodies. These are spherical inclusions in neuronal cell bodies. In contrast to Lewy bodies, Pick bodies are slightly basophilic and have a crisp margin (**Fig. 31.43a**). They are strongly argyrophilic (**Fig. 31.43b,c**) and may be seen in pyramidal neurons and dentate granule cells in the hippocampus and in affected regions of neocortex. Unlike Lewy bodies, Pick bodies are often numerous in cortical laminae II and III, as well as being present in the deeper laminae. They may be present in low density in subcortical nuclei (**Fig. 31.43d**).

Electron microscopy of Pick bodies shows that they contain intermediate filaments, 15 nm straight filaments, and some PHFs. Entrapped vesicular structures are also present. Immunohistochemistry shows

CLINICAL FEATURES OF FRONTOTEMPORAL DEMENTIA

- Clinical history is the mainstay of diagnosis. Physical examination and investigations are mainly of use to exclude non-neurodegenerative causes of frontotemporal dysfunction such as vascular dementia, hydrocephalus, and frontal neoplasms.
- The earliest manifestations are frontal deficits characterized by deterioration in personality and social function associated with neglect of personal hygiene, 'uncaring' incontinence, impaired judgement, disinhibition, and stereotyped behavior. Patients lack insight into their cognitive decline.
- Memory is preserved initially, but impaired as the disease progresses to affect temporal regions. Patients may become restless, or apathetic. Hyperorality and excessive eating are features of medial temporal involvement.
- Affective disorders, especially agitated depression are common. Late in the disease affect becomes shallow with emotional blunting.
- Excessive alcohol intake, caused by disinhibited behavior or hyperorality, may lead to a misdiagnosis of alcoholism as the cause of cognitive decline.
- With disease progression there is a decline in speech output, stereotypy of speech and eventual mutism.
- Frontal release signs such as forced grasping and palmomental, sucking, and rooting reflexes may be present.
- A significant proportion of patients has parkinsonian features. These can be difficult to evaluate and distinguish from the phenomenon of gegenhalten.
- Neuroimaging shows variable cerebral atrophy, which is most prominent in the frontal and temporal lobes and may be markedly asymmetric (**Fig. 31.41**)

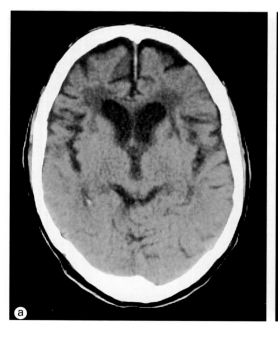

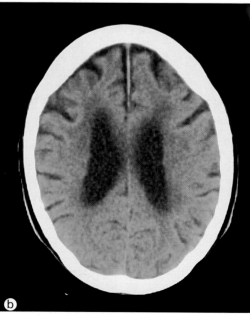

Fig. 31.41 Imaging in severe frontotemporal dementia. (a) and **(b)** CT scans from a patient with advanced frontotemporal dementia showing marked atrophy of the frontal lobes with ventricular dilatation and a low signal attenuation in the frontal white matter. **(a)** Horizontal scan at mid-thalamic level. **(b)** Horizontal scan at higher level, through body of lateral ventricles.

reactivity for phosphorylated neurofilament protein, tau protein (**Fig. 31.44**), ubiquitin, tubulin, and chromogranin-A. Cell biologic studies have shown that the tau protein in Pick bodies is similar to that which accumulates in PSP, and differs slightly from that in AD.

Neuronal loss relates to the degree of cortical atrophy present. In severe cases there is virtually complete neuronal loss with status spongiosus (**Fig. 31.45**). In cases with moderate cortical atrophy there is microvacuolation in layer II of the cortex and restricted neuronal loss. Astrocytic gliosis is present in areas of cortical neuronal loss as well as in white matter.

Swollen neurons are a typical feature of Pick's disease, but vary in number depending upon the severity of the neuronal loss. Swollen neu-

rons are argyrophilic and can be stained with antisera to phosphorylated neurofilament protein or αB crystallin (**Fig. 31.46**). Tau immunoreactivity may be present in some swollen neurons.

Pick's disease in relation to other diseases causing frontotemporal dementia

The several pathologic processes that underlie the clinical syndrome of frontotemporal dementia were formerly all included in the diagnostic category of Pick's disease, those cases lacking Pick bodies being designated as 'atypical' Pick's disease. Most workers now restrict the term Pick's disease to frontotemporal dementia with classic Pick bodies.

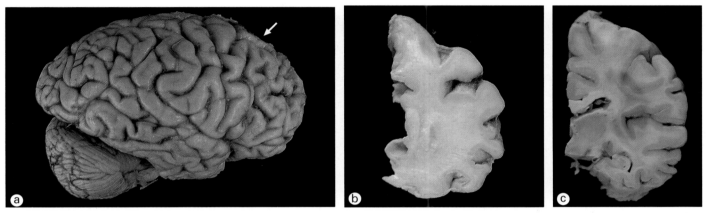

Fig. 31.42 Pick's disease macroscopic features. (a) Lateral view of brain. There is sharp demarcation (arrow) between the the atrophic frontal lobe and the posterior part of the cerebrum. Temporal atrophy is moderate in this case. **(b)** A coronal slice through the frontal lobe from the same brain reveals marked cortical atrophy, especially inferiorly and superomedially. The white matter has a gelatinous gray appearance. **(c)** There is good preservation of the cerebrum in the posterior frontal/anterior parietal region. The inferomedial temporal neocortex and subjacent white matter are atropic. No macroscopic abnormalities are discernible in the hippocampus.

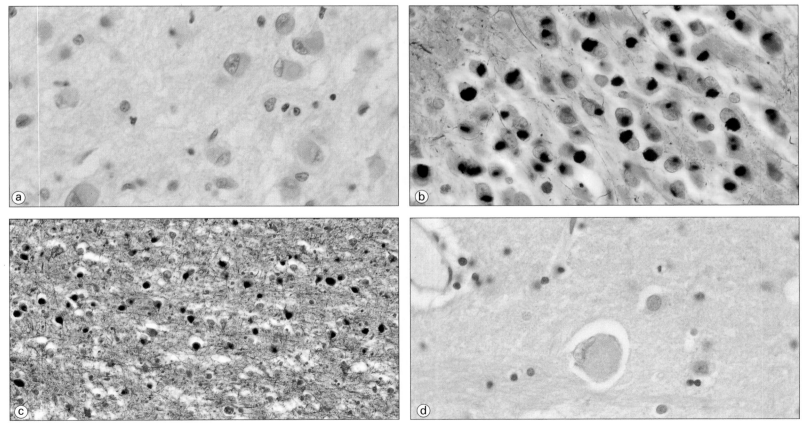

Fig. 31.43 Pick bodies. (a) In sections stained with hematoxylin and eosin, Pick bodies appear as well demarcated round, slightly basophilic inclusions in the neuronal cytoplasm. They are shown here in the amydala. **(b)** Bielschowsky impregnation of Pick bodies in neurons of the hippocampal dentate gyrus. **(c)** Silver impregnation of Pick bodies in the superficial frontal cortex. **(d)** Pick body in a large neuron in the putamen.

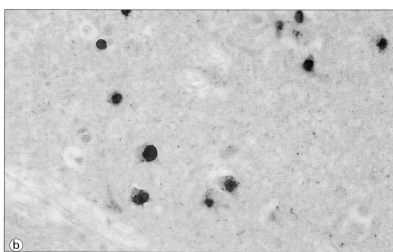

Fig. 31.44 Tau immunostaining of Pick bodies. (a) At low magnification one can see that Pick bodies are numerous in laminae II and III but are also present in the deeper parts of the cortex. (b) High magnification view of the immunostained spherical neuronal inclusions. Fine tau-immunoreactive neurites may also be present.

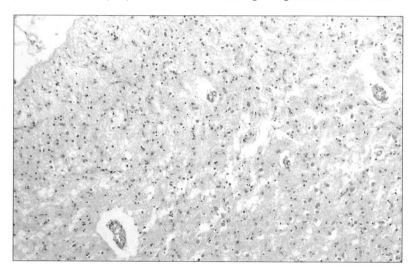

Fig. 31.45 Status spongiosus in Pick's disease. Severely affected frontal cortex showing transcortical neuronal loss with astrocytic gliosis and status spongiosus.

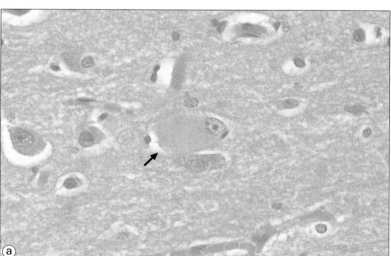

Fig. 31.46 Swollen neurons in Pick's disease. (a) Swollen neuron (arrow) with eosinophilic cytoplasm and eccentrically displaced nucleus. **(b)** αB-crystallin staining.

MND–INCLUSION DEMENTIA

Patients have clinical features of frontotemporal dementia but do not have clinical features of MND. This contrasts with the well-recognized syndrome of frontal dementia developing in patients with established MND (ALS).

MACROSCOPIC APPEARANCES

Frontal and temporal atrophy varies from moderate to very severe (**Fig. 31.47**). The basal ganglia may show mild to moderate atrophy, and the substantia nigra moderate pallor.

MICROSCOPIC APPEARANCES

In early disease neuronal loss and astrocytic gliosis are restricted to the superficial neocortical laminae, which show microvacuolation (**Fig. 31.48**). Variable numbers of swollen neurons are present. Severe disease is characterized by virtually complete transcortical loss of neurons from affected regions, with status spongiosus (**Fig. 31.49**). White matter myelin pallor and gliosis are usual.

Ubiquitin immunohistochemistry is the defining investigation and reveals characteristic cytoplasmic inclusions in dentate granule cells of the hippocampus, in the amydala, and in surviving superficial cortical neurons (**Fig. 31.50**). These inclusions are identical to those in patients with

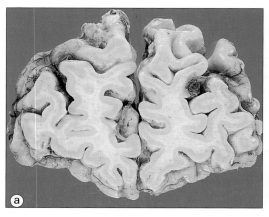
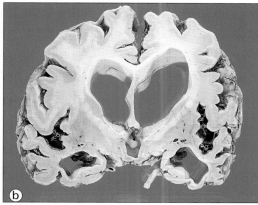

Fig. 31.47 Macroscopic features of MND–inclusion dementia. These slices are from a patient with clinical features of frontal lobe dementia, pathologically characterized as MND–inclusion dementia. **(a)** There is marked frontal lobe atrophy. **(b)** Further back there is marked ventricular enlargement, with atrophy of the temporal lobe and moderate atrophy of the basal ganglia.

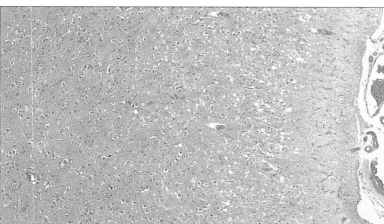

Fig. 31.48 Cortical microvaculation in MND–inclusion dementia. Superficial microvaculation with neuronal loss is seen in the affected frontal and temporal cortex.

Fig. 31.49 Status spongiosus in MND–inclusion dementia. In severe disease there is severe neuronal loss from the affected cortex, which becomes macroscopically shrunked and histologically replaced by astroglial cells, resulting in the appearances of status spongiosus.

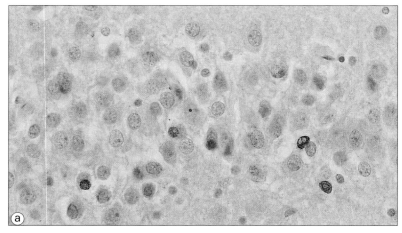
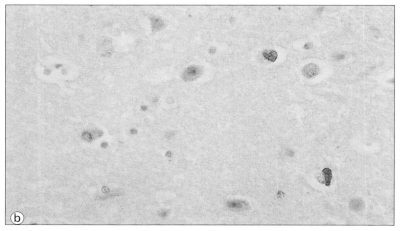

Fig. 31.50 Extramotor inclusions in MND–inclusion dementia. (a) Ubiquitinated cytoplasmic inclusions in hippocampal dentate granule cells. **(b)** Scattered layer II neurons of the frontal cortex contain ubiquitinated cytoplasmic inclusions.

classic ALS who later develop dementia. Ubiquitin-immunoreactive dystrophic neurites are seen in regions of neuronal loss, especially in regions of cortical microvacuolation (**Fig. 31.51**).

Neuronal loss and astrocytic gliosis may involve the basal ganglia and substantia nigra. There may also be loss of neurons from the hypoglossal nucleus.

DEMENTIA WITH CHANGES OF CBD
Most patients with CBD who develop DFT do so years after the development of the clinical movement disorder (see Chapter 28). However, some patients with CBD develop frontotemporal dementia in the absence of a movement disorder.

MACROSCOPIC APPEARANCES
There is typically mild or moderate atrophy of the frontal and temporal lobes. The basal ganglia may appear atrophic and the substantia nigra pale.

MICROSCOPIC APPEARANCES
Neuronal loss is usually mild or moderate and restricted to the superficial cortical layers, which show microvacuolation. Swollen neurons are present (**Fig. 31.52**). The subcortical white matter is gliotic, as may be the basal ganglia.

The substantia nigra shows variable cell loss. Some remaining neurons contain basophilic NFT-like inclusions (**Fig. 31.53**).

A key diagnostic feature is the presence of tau-immunoreactive neu-

ronal inclusions in cortical layer II (**Fig. 31.54**). Characteristic tau-reactive glial abnormalities may be seen in the abnormal cerebral cortex and substantia nigra as described in classic CBD (see chapter 28).

DFT (LOBAR DEGENERATION WITHOUT NEURONAL INCLUSIONS, DEMENTIA LACKING DISTINCTIVE HISTOLOGIC FEATURES
Patients usually present with frontal dementia, but clinical features of temporal degeneration may predominate (see Fig. 31.3).

MACROSCOPIC APPEARANCES
Frontal and temporal atrophy varies from moderate to severe (**Fig. 31.55**). The basal ganglia may appear atrophic and the substantia nigra pale.

MICROSCOPIC APPEARANCES
Neuronal loss and astrocytic gliosis are restricted to the superficial frontal and/or temporal neocortex, which is microvacuolated in early disease (**Fig. 31.56**). Variable numbers of swollen neurons are present. Severe disease is characterized by virtually complete transcortical loss of neurons from affected areas, with status spongiosus. The subcortical white matter shows myelin pallor and astrocytic gliosis. Neuronal loss and astrocytic gliosis may involve the basal ganglia and substantia nigra.

No inclusions are demonstrable with ubiquitin or tau protein antisera. Some workers have identified ubiquitin-immunoreactive dystrophic neurites in the regions of microvacuolation and neuronal loss.

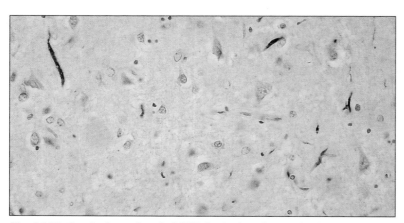

Fig. 31.51 Cortical neurites in MND–inclusion dementia. Fine dystrophic neurites are demonstrable by anti-ubiquitin staining in regions of cortical microvacuolation.

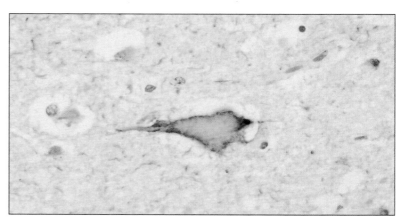

Fig. 31.52 Cortical swollen neuron in CBD. Swollen neurons are a prominent feature in the neocortex. They can be detected by immunostaining for neuroflament protein, αB-crystallin, or tau protein, as illustrated here.

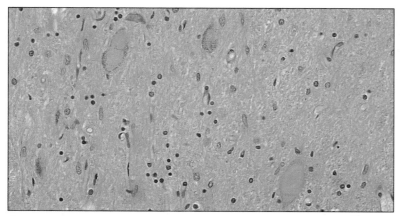

Fig. 31.53 Neuronal inclusions in the substantia nigra in CBD. Basophilic globose tangles are seen in residual neurons of the substantia nigra in CBD.

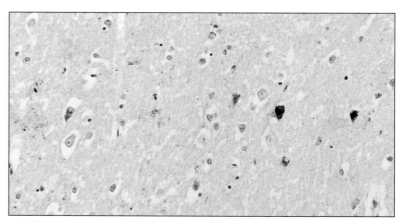

Fig. 31.54 Tau-reactive inclusions in the cortex in CBD. Small inclusions can be detected in residual neurons in superficial cortex with tau immunostaining. They are not immunoreactive for ubiquitin.

DFT AND PROGRESSIVE SUBCORTICAL GLIOSIS

Progressive subcortical gliosis is a term used to describe a pattern of neurodegeneration originally described by Neumann and Conn, and characterized by gliosis of frontal and temporal white matter, variable neuronal loss and microvacuolation of the superficial cerebral cortex, and variable gliosis and neuronal loss in subcortical nuclei. These findings are the same as those in DFT and the choice of terminology is largely a matter of personal preference.

Accumulations of prion protein in the form of diffuse plaques have been found in brains from two large kindreds with DFT/progressive subcortical gliosis. The disease was linked to chromosome 17 and not to chromosome 20 where the prion protein gene resides.

CHROMOSOME 17-LINKED DEMENTIA

Patients develop frontotemporal dementia with prominent parkinsonism, and amyotrophy. The disorder is linked to chromosome 17. At present the gene is not known.

MACROSCOPIC APPEARANCES

Atrophy affects the anterior and inferior parts of the temporal lobes, the frontal lobes, and the anterior part of the cingulate gyrus. There is relative sparing of hippocampal structures. The basal ganglia appear brown and atrophic, and the substantia nigra pale.

MICROSCOPIC APPEARANCES

Histology reveals marked gliosis, variable neuronal loss, and some swollen neurons in the atrophic cerebral cortex, which shows superficial microvacuolation. The basal ganglia and substantia nigra show neuronal loss and gliosis.

Argyrophilic inclusions, appearing as haphazardly oriented spicules, are present in the oculomotor nucleus, dorsal raphe nuclei, periaqueductal gray matter, substantia nigra, red nucleus, subthalamic nucleus, and globus pallidus. The inclusions are immunoreactive for phosphorylated neurofilament protein (NFP) and ubiquitin, but not tau protein.

The swollen neurons show variable tau immunoreactivity that corresponds ultrastructurally to lattices of 10–14 nm filaments. Many ubiquitin- and tau-immunoreactive oligodendroglia are demonstrable in the white matter.

There is no prion protein immunoreactivity.

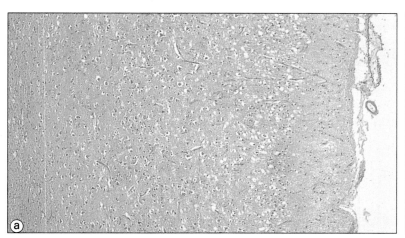
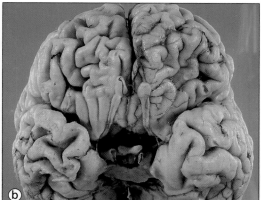
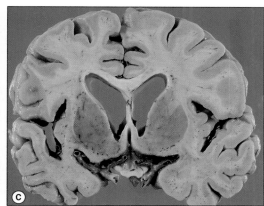

Fig. 31.55 Macroscopic appearances of brain in DFT. Superior **(a)** and inferior **(b)** views of the brain after stripping of the leptomeninges reveal moderate frontal and temporal atrophy. A coronal slice **(c)** shows, in addition, mild atrophy of the head of the caudate nucleus and anterior putamen.

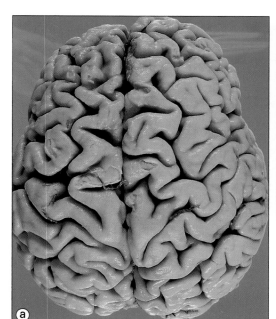
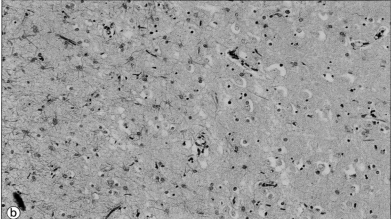

Fig. 31.56 Superficial microvacuolation and gliosis of DFT. (a) In DFT, the cortex shows superficial microvacuolation in the absence of ubiquitin- or tau-immunoreactive inclusions. **(b)** Higher magnification view of gliotic, vacuolated superficial cortex in DFT (phosphotungstic acid/hematoxylin).

FRONTAL ALZHEIMER'S DISEASE

GENETICS OF FRONTOTEMPORAL DEMENTIA

In different studies of so-called Pick's disease, now recognized to include several different pathologic entities, a high incidence of autosomal dominant transmission has been recorded. Families are described in which some members have classic ALS, some have ALS–dementia, and some have pure frontotemporal dementia. Precise genetic linkages are at present unclear.

DIFFERENTIAL DIAGNOSIS OF FRONTOTEMPORAL DEMENTIA

- In addition to the neurodegenerative disorders described above, the clinical syndrome of frontotemporal dementia may be caused by hydrocephalus, vascular dementia, and space-occupying lesions affecting the frontal lobes.
- There is pathologic overlap between CBD and PSP. The demonstration of large numbers of swollen neurons favors a diagnosis of CBD.
- Patients with classic MND may develop frontotemporal dementia with characteristic ubiquitin-immunoreactive intraneuronal inclusions in the hippocampal dentate granule cells and layer II of the frontal and temporal cortex.

NEUROPATHOLOGIC APPROACH TO FRONTOTEMPORAL DEMENTIA

The different degenerative conditions causing frontotemporal dementia can be distinguished by histologic examination of the anterior frontal cortex, hippocampus at the level of the lateral geniculate body, tip of the temporal lobe, and substantia nigra.

- Alzheimer-type changes should be sought in all cases, with appropriate stains (see earlier).
- If transcortical neuronal loss or superficial cortical microvacuolation and neuronal loss are noted in the frontal and/or temporal cortex, immunohistochemical studies (for tau protein, ubiquitin, aB crystallin, and NFP) are indicated.
- If no inclusions are seen, in the presence of cortical microvacuolation, a diagnosis of dementia of frontal type is appropriate.
- If argyrophilic inclusions staining for NFP and ubiquitin but not tau are seen, the possibility of a chromosome-17-linked dementia should be considered.
- If small ubiquitin-immunoreactive inclusions, not reactive for tau protein or NFP, are present in the hippocampal dentate granule cells and in small superficial neurons in the entorhinal cortex and layer II of the temporalneocortex, a diagnosis of MND-inclusion dementia is appropriate.
- The presence of argyrophilic, spherical, tau- and ubiquitin-immunoreactive inclusions with the morphology of Pick bodies, in the hippocampal dentate granule cells and/or neurons of the frontal and/or temporal cortex, indicate a diagnosis of Pick's disease.
- The presence of inclusions that are reactive with anti-tau in small neurons of the frontal and temporal cortex, and substantia nigra, suggests a diagnosis of corticobasal degeneration which is reinforced by the detection of swollen cortical neurons.

Some patients with frontotemporal dementia have histologic changes that satisfy criteria for AD. Swollen cortical neurons are often present in these cases.

PRIMARY PROGRESSIVE APHASIA (PPA)

This condition is characterized clinically by an isolated progressive aphasia. Imaging shows restricted cortical atrophy in the dominant cerebral hemisphere around the sylvian fissure.

Neuropathologic investigations in cases of PPA has shown a variety of changes:

- transcortical microvacuolation with severe neuronal loss
- transcortical microvacuolation with variable neuronal loss and swollen cortical neurons
- Alzheimer changes
- changes of CBD

The emerging perception is that PPA results from restricted expression of the same neurodegenerative diseases that can cause frontotemporal dementia. In some patients frontotemporal dementia is preceded by PPA.

INTERMITTENTLY RAISED PRESSURE HYDROCEPHALUS

Dementia associated with hydrocephalus accounts for about 2% of cases of dementia. Onset is generally after 70 years of age. Often no predisposing factor for the hydrocephalus is identified. Isolated measurements of CSF pressure at the time of lumbar puncture are typically within normal limits, so the term 'normal pressure hydrocephalus' has been applied to these patients. However, monitoring of CSF pressure over longer periods reveals that it is intermittently raised.

The dementia associated with hydrocephalus is characterized clinically by the triad of memory disturbance, early disturbance of gait, and early urinary incontinence. CT scans reveal ventricular dilatation and low-attenuation signal in periventricular white matter, without sulcal widening or other features of cortical atrophy.

MACROSCOPIC AND MICROSCOPIC APPEARANCES

Pathology confirms these imaging features (**Fig. 31.58**). There is symmetric dilatation of the lateral and third ventricles and good preservation of the cerebral cortex. The cerebral white matter appears macroscopically normal, but histology may reveal mild to moderate periventricular rarefaction and gliosis. Vascular dementia and primary neurodegenerative disease should be excluded by histologic examination.

If hydrocephalus is diagnosed in life a ventricular shunt is usually inserted. A frequent complication of this procedure in the elderly is the development of large subdural hematomas.

UNCOMMON DEGENERATIVE DEMENTIAS

TANGLE-ONLY DEMENTIA

Dementia may rarely be associated with NFTs in the hippocampal region, brain stem, and substantia nigra, in the absence of senile plaques — a condition termed tangle-only dementia (also known as AD with NFTs only, NFT-predominant AD, or mesolimbocortical dementia).

Most patients are female. The average age at onset is 80 years and at death, 85 years. In most reported cases the antemortem diagnosis has been AD. About 10% of patients have had parkinsonism.

MACROSCOPIC AND MICROSCOPIC APPEARANCES

Numerous tau-immunoreactive NFTs and NTs are present in the hippocampus, entorhinal cortex and amygdala, corresponding to Braak stage III (**Fig. 31.59**). In about 60% of reported cases plaques have been absent.

In others there have been only a few diffuse Aβ deposits, consistent with aging. The substantia nigra typically shows neuronal loss and NFT formation.

The distribution of NFTs has not been thought to conform to the diagnostic criteria for PSP.

The relationship between tangle-only dementia, AD, and PSP remains to be determined.

ARGYROPHILIC GRAIN DEMENTIA

This condition was described in a pathologic survey of patients diagnosed clinically as having AD.

MACROSCOPIC AND MICROSCOPIC APPEARANCES

Small spindle-shaped argyrophilic grains and coiled bodies or filaments are found in the hippocampus, entorhinal cortex and surrounding regions, and in some subcortical nuclei (**Fig. 31.60**). They are composed of tau-immunoreactive straight filaments with a diameter of about 9 nm.

Many patients in the original descriptions also had neocortical NFTs, NTs, and senile plaques. Recent observations of tau-immunoreactive glial inclusions in other neurodegenerative diseases have revealed pathologic overlap with PSP, CBD, and tangle-only dementia.

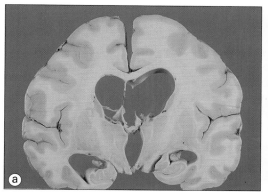
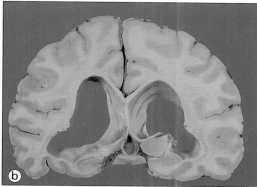

Fig. 31.58 Intermittently raised pressure hydrocephalus. Coronal slices **(a)** and **(b)** through the brain show dilation of the ventricular system. In contrast to the ventricular dilation that occurs with neurodegenerative diseases (hydrocephalus *ex vacuo*) there is no sulcal widening or cortical atrophy.

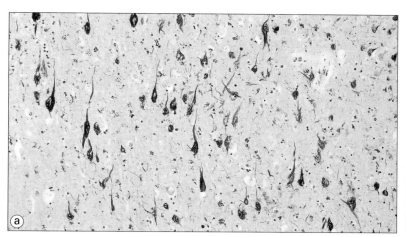
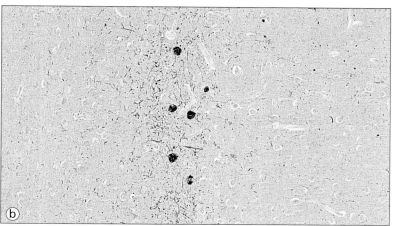

Fig. 31.59 Tangle-only dementia. (a) In tangle-only dementia the temporal cortex contains abundant NFT, demonstrated here by silver imoregnation, in the absence of plaques. (b) Tau-immunostaining sometimes shows a band of involved neurons in the entorhinal cortex, with abundant surrounding neuropil threads.

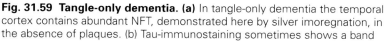

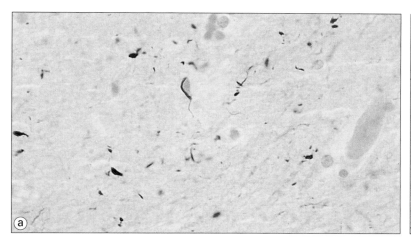
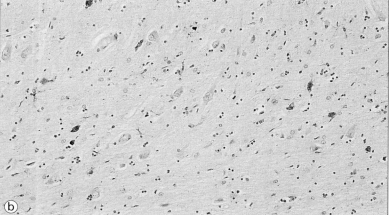

Fig. 31.60 Grain dementia. (a) Gallyas silver impregnation of coils and grains. **(b)** Tau immunostaining also highlights the coils and grains.

THALAMIC DEMENTIAS

Severe disturbance of memory and other cognitive functions amounting to a dementia syndrome may result from thalamic pathology. Neuronal loss and astrocytic gliosis affect the thalamus in a range of neurodegenerative disorders, including rare conditions regarded as primary thalamic degenerations.

VASCULAR DEMENTIA

Vascular dementia can be defined as an acquired intellectual impairment resulting from damage to the brain by cerebrovascular disease. Several difficulties arise in applying this broad definition:

CLINICAL FEATURES OF VASCULAR DEMENTIA

- Clinical diagnosis of vascular dementia is based on focal neurologic signs consistent with strokes, stepwise neurologic deterioration, and declining cognitive performance that may, however, fluctuate considerably on a day-to-day basis.
- Gait difficulties, urinary incontinence, parkinsonian features and pseudobulbar signs are common manifestations.
- The Hachinski score (**Fig. 31.61**) has been widely used to assess whether a patient has multi-infarct dementia, but leads to an inaccurate diagnosis in about 20% of cases. The clinical features in patients with both AD and strokes ('mixed' dementia) or with LBD, often simulate those of vascular dementia.
- Combined clinical, neuroimaging, and pathologic criteria have been proposed that allow diagnosis of vascular dementia with differing degrees of certainty for research studies (**Fig. 31.62**).

Hachinski score	
Clinical feature	**Score**
Abrupt onset	2
Stepwise deterioration	1
Fluctuating course	2
Nocturnal confusion	1
Relative preservation of personality	1
Depression	1
Somatic complaints	1
Emotional incontinence	1
History of hypertension	1
History of stroke	2
Clinical evidence of atherosclerosis	1
Focal neurologic symptoms	2
Focal neurologic signs	2

- A total score of 4 or less is suggestive of a degenerative cause of dementia such as Alzheimer's disease
- A score of 7 or more is suggestive of vascular dementia

Fig. 31.61 Hachinski score. (From Hachinski et al., 1975.)

- Cortical or subcortical damage due to cerebrovascular disease often results in circumscribed dysfunction in a cognitive domain related to the site of damage. Such restricted forms of cognitive dysfunction are best termed focal neurobehavioral disorders. Although it is possible to distinguish multiple forms of cognitive dysfunction in certain patients with severe cerebrovascular disease affecting several brain regions, the threshold at which the combined clinical effect is termed dementia is arbitrary.
- Some workers restrict the definition of vascular dementia to global cognitive decline caused by the cumulative effects of multiple episodes of cerebral ischemia. This definition excludes cases of diffuse cerebral damage caused by a single episode of severe hypoxia or global cerebral hypoperfusion, which are included by other workers.
- Neuroimaging and pathologic criteria of ischemic brain damage may diverge. The signal changes in deep hemispheric white matter that are often called 'leukoaraiosis' have been interpreted as ischemic, although the histologic correlates of these 'lesions' are inconsistent, and similar imaging abnormalities are frequently seen in cognitively normal elderly persons and in patients with neurodegenerative causes of dementia, such as AD.

NINDS–AIREN operational criteria for vascular dementia

Probable vascular dementia

1. Dementia must be present - defined as memory failure and other cognitive dysfunction in two or more domains (orientation, attention, language, visuospatial control, motor control, praxis, or executive function) leading to interference with activities of daily living.
2. Cerebrovascular disease is present as shown by compatible clinical features of focal neurologic deficits and by imaging.
3. Relationship between dementia and cerebrovascular pathology can be inferred or demonstrated:
   - onset of cognitive decline within 3 months of a stroke.
   - abrupt or stepwise deterioration in mental function consistent with causation by discrete events.
   - imaging evidence of damage to areas invoked in higher mental functioning

Supporting clinical features
- gait disturbance, falls, and urinary incontinence early in disease progression.
- pseudobulbar features.
- frontal lobe dysfunction.

Features making diagnosis unlikely
- Early and progressive onset of memory deficit with development of aphasia, apraxia or agnosia in the absence of corresponding focal lesions on imaging.
- Lack of focal neurologic signs other than memory disturbance.
- Lack of lesions of vascular disease on imaging.

Possible vascular dementia

1. Dementia involving memory failure and other cognitive dysfunction in two or more domains (orientation, attention, language, visuospatial control, motor control, praxis, or executrive function) and leading to interference with activities of daily living.
2. Cerebrovascular disease as shown by compatible clinical features of focal neurologic deficits, in the absence of confirmatory imaging or with lack of a temporal relationship between the onset of a stroke and the onset of dementia.

Definite vascular dementia

1. Clinical criteria of probable vascular dementia.
2. Histopathological evidence of cerebrovascular disease.
3. Absence of other clinical or pathological changes which may have resulted in dementia.

Fig. 31.62 NINDS–AIREN operational criteria for vascular dementia. (Adapted from Roman et al., 1992.)

For these reasons there are no widely accepted clinical or pathologic criteria for the diagnosis of vascular dementia. In recent studies vascular dementia has been cited as accounting for about 10% of all cases of dementia in developed countries whereas studies in the 1970s attributed a much higher proportion of cases to cerebrovascular disease. It is unclear to what extent this change is genuine (e.g. related to better medical treatment of hypertension and diabetes mellitus) or an artefact of changing clinical and pathologic definitions.

MACROSCOPIC AND MICROSCOPIC APPEARANCES
The pathology of vascular dementia (**Fig 31.63**) is quite varied and can be divided into lesions resulting from:
• small vessel disease
• large vessel disease
• global cerebral hypoperfusion
The abnormalities are also sometimes divided into those causing:
• cortical vascular dementia (i.e. due to infarcts mainly affecting the cerebral cortex)
• subcortical vascular dementia (i.e. due to ischemic white matter degeneration).
• lacunar dementia (i.e. due to multifocal infarction)

Small vessel disease: The most consistent finding in vascular dementia is hyaline arteriosclerosis and arteriolosclerosis affecting small vessels. This is strongly associated with hypertension and diabetes mellitus. Related neuropathologic abnormalities consist, in varying combination, of:
• Ischemic white matter degeneration. Macroscopically, the brain is usually of normal or slightly reduced weight with little external evidence of atrophy. The major cerebral arteries are usually atherosclerotic. The lateral and third ventricles are moderately dilated. The cerebral white matter often feels soft on sectioning. The cut surface appears slightly granular and may be pitted with small depressions (**Fig. 31.64**). Typically, these changes are most pronounced in the

MECHANISMS OF DEMENTIA IN CEREBROVASCULAR DISEASE

• The development of dementia has, in various studies, been correlated with the loss of a critical volume of brain substance or with the number of discrete lesions.
• It is likely that the most important factor is the extent of damage to the regions of brain involved in cognitive function (i.e. limbic regions, association areas, and the white matter that links the association areas).

deep frontal and temporal white matter. Coexistent lacunar infarcts are usually present in the basal ganglia, thalamus, pons, and, less often, the hemispheric white matter (**Fig. 31.65**). Histology reveals arteriosclerosis and arteriolosclerosis – hyalinization of small arteries and arterioles with loss of smooth muscle and replacement by collagen (**Fig. 31.66**). The white matter shows patchy pallor on myelin staining, axonal loss, reduction in the number of oligodendrocytes, and mild astrocytic gliosis (**Fig. 31.67**). Dementia with these changes has been termed lacunar dementia, Binswanger's disease, and subcortical arteriosclerotic encephalopathy.
Note that if histologic sampling is restricted to small blocks that include only 1–2 cm of subcortical white matter, significant deep white matter disease may well be missed.
• Cribriform atrophy of white matter. This appears as myriad fine pin-size holes in the white matter that are due to dilatation of perivascular spaces and most numerous in the anterior temporal and frontal regions. Histologically, hyalinized vessels are surrounded by a dilated perivascular space with surrounding myelin pallor and astrocytic gliosis that extend a small distance from the vessel (**Fig. 31.68**).
• Granular cortical atrophy. This is a relatively uncommon finding that may be associated with cognitive decline. Macroscopically, affected regions of cerebral cortex appear pitted by depressions 1–2 mm in diameter (**Fig. 31.69**). Histology shows these to correspond to numerous cortical microinfarcts, usually associated with hyaline arteriosclerosis of small vessels. Other diseases that involve small vessels can cause this pattern of lesions, the most notable example being the

Pathology of vascular dementia

Small vessel disease
• ischemic white matter degeneration
• cribriform atrophy of white matter
• lacunar infarction in subcortical nuclei and white matter
• granular atrophy of cortex

Large vessel disease
• very extensive or multifocal infarction (multi-infarct dementia)
• critically sited infarcts

Hypoperfusion lesions
• hippocampal sclerosis
• laminar cortical necrosis

Rare local vascular disorders
• CADASIL
• cerebral amyloidosis
• cerebral vasculitis
• antiphospholipid antibody syndrome

Fig. 31.63 Pathology of vascular dementia.

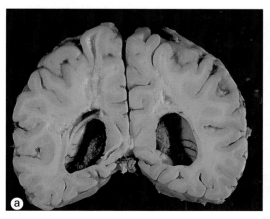 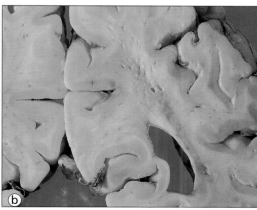

Fig. 31.64 Ischemic white matter degeneration. **(a)** Coronal slices show the parieto-occipital white matter to contain foci of granular gray discoloration that have sunken away from the cut surface. The sunken appearance and discoloration is seen at higher magnification in **(b)** which also demonstrates the 'pin-hole' effect caused by the dilatation of perivascular spaces.

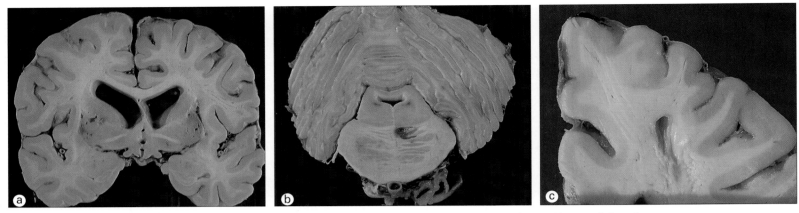

Fig. 31.65 Lacunar infarction. This is seen in association with small vessel disease of the brain. **(a)** Bilateral lacunar infacts in basal gaglia. **(b)** lacuna in pons. **(c)** Large lacuna in white matter.

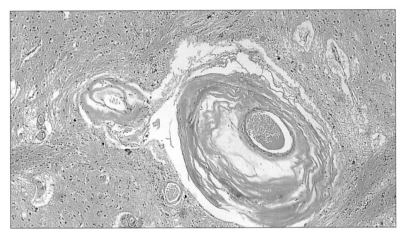

Fig. 31.66 Arteriosclerosis and arteriolosclerosis. The tunica media of small penetrating arteries and arterioles has been replaced by many layers of hyaline collagenous connective tissue.

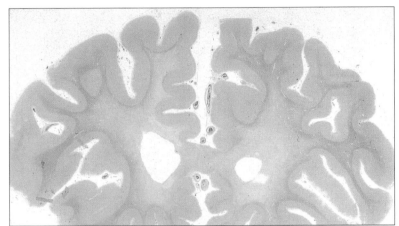

Fig. 31.67 Ischemic white matter degeneration. Whole mount of frontal lobes showing severe rarefaction of deep white matter with subcortical preservation.

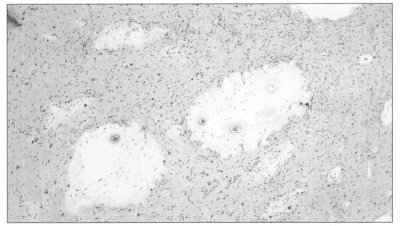

Fig. 31.68 Dilated perivascular spaces with surrounding gliosis in vascular dementia. A feature of vascular dementia is the prominent hyaline arteriosclerosis and dilation of perivascular spaces in the cerebral white matter. There is astrocytic gliosis of the surrounding white matter.

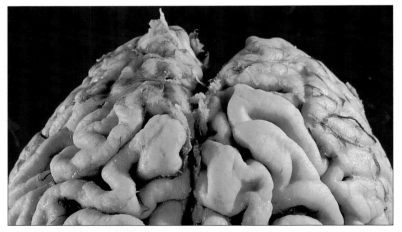

Fig. 31.69 Macroscopic appearances of granular cortical atrophy. Granular cortical atrophy is best seen after stripping the leptomeninges as numerous small depressions 1–2 mm across.

microvascular thrombosis associated with the antiphospholipid antibody syndrome.

Large vessel disease: Large regional cerebral infarcts rarely contribute significantly to global cognitive decline in the setting of a clinical dementia. Rarely, severe cognitive dysfunction is caused by bilateral small infarcts in critical sites such as the medial thalamus or hippocampal region (**Fig. 31.72**). Other reasons for the association of large vessel disease or regional cerebral infarcts with dementia are:

• the frequent coexistence of large vessel atherosclerosis with small vessel disease.
• the increased risk of AD in patients with the apoE ε4 allele, who are also predisposed to atherosclerosis.
• the increased risk of lobar hemorrhage and cerebral infarcts in patients with AD as a complication of amyloid angiopathy.

The causes and consequences of various forms of large vessel disease, including atherosclerotic and embolic disease, vasculitis, and CADASIL are considered in Chapter 9.

Global cerebral hypoperfusion: Conditions leading to cerebral hypoperfusion can cause ischemic injury to the hippocampus and watershed/boundary zone regions (see Chapters 8 and 9). Hippocampal sclerosis with clinical dementia is seen in some elderly patients (**Fig. 31.73**) and in most cases probably results from episodes of hypotension complicating cardiovascular disease. Boundary zone infarcts in the frontal and parietal cortex can also lead to dementia.

Infarcts causing dementia

Affected region	Clinical syndrome
Middle cerebral artery, lower division territory affecting angular gyrus	Fluent aphasia, alexia, agraphia. Memory disturbance, disturbed spatial awareness
Posterior cerebral artery territory, involving hippocampus	Amnesia, anomia, confusion, visual field impairment
Posterior cerebral artery territory, involving medial thalamic nuclei	Severe memory disturbance, inattention, clinical dementia
Anterior cerebral artery territory, involving medial frontal lobe	Frontal behavioral disturbance, memory disturbance, hemiparesis
Bilateral superior frontal and parietal convexity associated with boundary zone infarction	Amnesia, aphasia, apraxia, agnosia, visual disturbances, and hemineglect
Periventricular white matter or lesions in the capsular genu	Dementia caused by functional disconnection of cortical association or cortico-thalamic fibers

Fig. 31.70 Infarcts causing dementia.

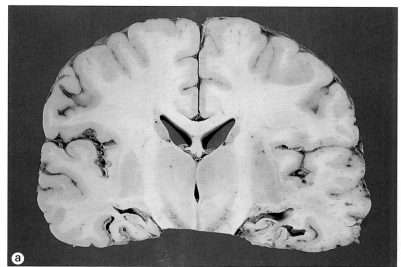

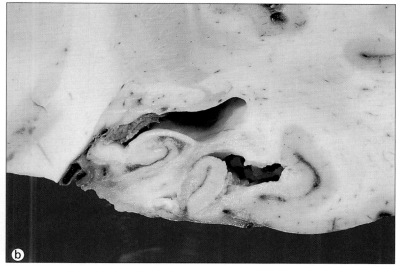

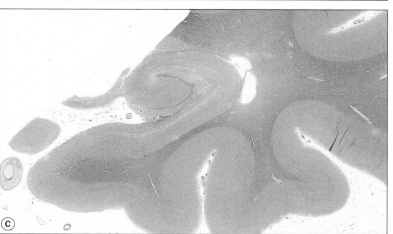

Fig. 31.71 Hippocampal sclerosis. (a) Macroscopic view showing bilateral hippocampal sclerosis. **(b)** The marked shrinkage of the hippocampus can be appreciated in this close-up view. **(c)** Histology shows extensive neuronal loss from the hippocampus with associated astrocytic gliosis.

SUBCORTICAL DEMENTIA

- This term has been applied to dementia characterized by the following four main features: some form of memory defect; general slowing of intellectual activity with a shortened attention span (bradyphrenia); alterations of personality, such as apathy; and impaired ability to manipulate acquired knowledge.
- This type of dementia involves a slowing in the rate at which the patient processes new information rather than a complete loss of competence to perform tasks. Language functions tend to be spared.
- There has been much debate over the pathologic and functional correlates of subcortical dementia. It is felt that disorders that affect the basal ganglia or non-cortical parts of the limbic system involved in thought processing lead to this clinical syndrome. These disorders include Wernicke's encephalopathy, hydrocephalus, vascular dementia due to ischemic white matter degeneration, PSP, Huntington's disease, and Parkinson's disease.
- Many of these disorders, which were previously regarded as primarily subcortical, show distinctive cortical abnormalities, and the relative contributions of subcortical and cortical pathology to the cognitive dysfunction remain unclear.

DEMENTIA ASSOCIATED WITH OTHER DEGENERATIVE DISEASES

Several diseases typically present as early onset degenerative diseases of the nervous system and but can present with a dementia syndrome in adult life. These have been comprehensively reviewed by Coker (**Fig. 31.74**).

Causes of dementia caused by degenerative diseases usually presenting in childhood

- mitochondrial cytopathy
- neuronal intranuclear inclusion disease
- Lafora body disease
- neuronal ceroid lipofuscinosis
- Wilson's disease
- Fabry's disease
- Krabbes disease
- metachromatic leukodystrophy
- Alexander's disease
- cerebrotendinous xanthomatosis
- Nasu Hakola Disease
- adrenoleukodystrophy
- GM_1 Gangliosidosis type III
- GM_2 Gangliosidosis
- Gaucher's disease
- Niemann Pick disease type C
- mucopolysaccharidosis type IIIB

Fig. 31.72 Degenerative diseases that cause dementia and usually present in childhood.

REFERENCES

Bancher C, Jellinger KA. (1994) Neurofibrillary tangle predominant form of senile dementia of Alzheimer type: A rare subtype in very old subjects. *Acta Neuropathol* 88: 565–570.

Braak B. (1991) Neuropathologic staging of Alzheimer related changes. *Acta Neuropathol* 82: 239–259.

Brun A. (1994) Pathology and pathophysiology of cerebrovascular dementia: pure subgroups of obstructive and hypoperfusive etiology. *Dementia* 5: 145–147.

Coker SB. (1991) The diagnosis of childhood neurodegenerative disorders presenting as dementia in adults. *Neurology* 41: 794–798.

Cooper PN, Jackson M, Lennox G, Lowe J, Mann DMA. (1995) Tau, ubiquitin, and αB-crystallin immunohistochemistry define the principal causes of degenerative frontotemporal dementia. *Arch Neurol* 52: 1011–1015.

Cruts M, Hendriks L, Van Broeckhoven C. (1996) The presenilin genes: A new gene family involved in Alzheimer disease pathology. *Hum Molecul Genet* 5: 1449–1455.

Cummings J, Benson D. (1984) Subcortical dementia. *Arch Neurol* 41: 874–879.

Dickson DW, et al. (1994) Hippocampal sclerosis: A common pathological feature of dementia in very old (>=80 years of age) humans. *Acta Neuropathol* 88: 212–221.

Gearing M, et al. (1995) The Consortium to Establish a Registry for Alzheimer's Disease (CERAD). Part X. Neuropathology confirmation of the clinical diagnosis of Alzheimer's disease. *Neurology* 45: 461–466.

Giannakopoulos P, Hof PR, Bouras C. (1994) Alzheimer's disease with asymmetric atrophy of the cerebral hemispheres: Morphometric analysis of four cases. *Acta Neuropathol* 88: 440–447.

Goedert M (1996) Tau protein and the neurofibrillary pathology of Alzheimer's disease. *Ann NY Acad Sci* 777: 121–131.

Hachinski VC et al. (1975) Cerebral blood flow in dementia *Arch Neurol* 32: 632–637

Ikeda K, et al. (1996) Corticobasal degeneration with primary progressive aphasia and accentuated cortical lesion in superior temporal gyrus: Case report and review. *Acta Neuropathol* 92: 534–539.

Katz DI, Alexander MP, Mandell AM (1987) Dementia following strokes in the mesencephalon and diencephalon. *Arch Neurol* 44(11): 1127–1133.

Kertesz A, Munoz D (1996) Clinical and pathological characteristics of primary progressive aphasia and frontal dementia. *J Neur Trans* 47(Suppl.): 133–141.

Kertesz A (1996) Pick complex and Pick's disease: The nosology of frontal lobe dementia, primary progressive aphasia, and corticobasal ganglionic degeneration. *Eur J Neurol* 3: 280–282.

Knopman D (1993). Overview of dementia lacking distinctive histology: Pathological designation of a progressive dementia. *Dementia* 4: 132–136.

McKeith IG, et al. (1996) Consensus guidelines for the clinical and pathologic diagnosis of dementia with Lewy bodies (DLB): Report of the consortium on DLB international workshop. *Neurology* 47: 1113–1124.

Mirra SS, et al. (1991) The Consortium to Establish a Registry for Alzheimer's Disease (CERAD). Part II. Standardization of the neuropathologic assessment of Alzheimer's disease. *Neurology* 41: 479–486.

Munoz DG (1991). The pathological basis of multi-infarct dementia. *Alzheimer Disease and Associated Disorders* 5: 77–90.

Perry R, McKeith I, Perry E (eds) (1996) *Dementia with Lewy bodies.* Clinical, Pathological and Treatment Issues. Cambridge : Cambridge University Press.

Rogaev EI, et al. (1995) Familial Alzheimer's disease in kindreds with missense mutations in a gene on chromosome 1 related to the Alzheimer's disease type 3 gene. *Nature* 376: 775–778.

Roman GC et al. (1993) Vascular dementia: diagnostic criteria for research studies. NINDS-AIREN Workshop. *Neurology* 43: 250–260.

Sima AAF et al. (1996) The neuropathology of chromosome 17-linked dementia. *Ann Neurol* 39: 734–743.

Terry RD, Katzman R, Bick KL (eds) (1994) *Alzheimer's disease.* New York: Raven Press.

Ulrich J, Spillantini M, Goedert M, Dukas L, Stähelin H (1992) Abundant neurofibrillary tangles without senile plaques in a subset of patients with senile dementia. *Neurodegeneration* 1: 257–264.

Van Duijn CM (1996) Epidemiology of the dementias: Recent developments and new approaches. *J Neurol Neurosurg Psychiatr* 60: 478–488.

Victoroff J, Ross GW, Benson DF, Verity MA, Vinters HV (1994) Posterior cortical atrophy: Neuropathologic correlations. *Arch Neurol* 51: 269–274.

Wolozin B, et al. (1996) Participation of presenilin 2 in apoptosis: enhanced basal activity conferred by an Alzheimer mutation. *Science* 274: 1710–1712.

Yamaoka LH, et al. (1996). Linkage of frontotemporal dementia to chromosome 17: Clinical and neuropathological characterization of phenotype. *Am J Hum Genet* 59: 1306–1312.

32 Prion diseases

The designation of prion diseases as a distinct nosologic category is based on the elucidation of a novel molecular pathology that is common to several disorders previously known as spongiform encephalopathies, unconventional viral infections, or transmissible dementias. These include the following human diseases:
- Creutzfeldt–Jakob disease (CJD).
- Gerstmann–Sträussler–Scheinker disease (GSS).
- Fatal familial insomnia (FFI).
- Kuru.

Common to all of these diseases are:
- An accumulation of an abnormal form of a cellular protein (prion protein).

- Neuronal death, synaptic loss, and microvacuolation (spongiform change) in the brain.
- Transmissibility to humans and other mammalian species.

Prion diseases occur in several mammalian species in addition to man, the most notable being scrapie in sheep and bovine spongiform encephalopathy (BSE) in cattle.

In approximately 85% of cases, human prion diseases are sporadic. Rarely, prion disease is transmitted by accidental inoculation during a therapeutic procedure (iatrogenic CJD), or by endocannibalism (kuru). In about 15% of cases, prion diseases are inherited in an autosomal dominant fashion.

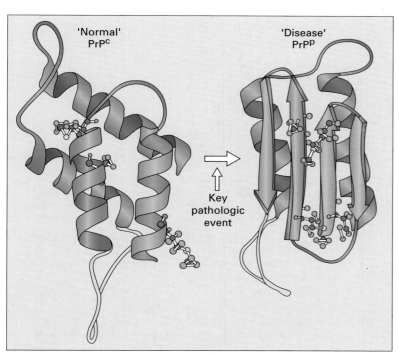

Fig. 32.1 Conformation of prion protein. Normal prion protein has an α-helical internal structure (coils). The protein can adopt a different stable conformation in which the α-helical structures are replaced by β-pleated sheets (arrows); this abnormal configuration is pathogenic.

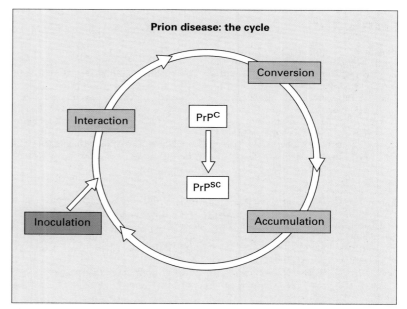

Fig. 32.2 Conversion of normal PrP to abnormal PrP. Endogenous or exogenous abnormal PrP can interact with normal PrP and induce it to adopt an abnormal pathogenic conformation. The abnormal form accumulates within cells, interacting with and converting more of the normal cell protein. In this way normal PrP^c is converted to PrP^p.

CELL BIOLOGY OF PRION PROTEIN AND PATHOGENESIS OF PRION DISEASE

*The prion diseases have a common molecular pathology that involves the conversion of a normal cellular protein called prion protein (PrP) into an abnormal isoform (**Fig. 32.1**). Most evidence implicates the abnormal protein as the transmissible factor; evidence is lacking for the involvement of DNA or RNA in the infective process.*

PrP

- is encoded by a normal cellular gene located on human chromosome 20.
- is a membrane-associated protein of uncertain function — a specific glycolipid is added to the carboxyl terminal of PrP to permit its attachment to the cell membrane.
- is normally expressed by cells, including neurons and glia, throughout life.

In prion disease

- PrP accumulates within cells, and also outside cells in the form of amyloid.
- The accumulated PrP is abnormal in that it is relatively resistant to degradation *in vitro* by proteinase K – this property is the basis of detection of abnormal PrP by immunochemical techniques. The normal isoform of PrP is often designated PrP^c and the abnormal and infectious isoform of PrP^c has been variably designated PrP*, PrP^p (for pathologic), PrP^{sc} (for scrapie, the spongiform encephalopathy of sheep), or PrP^{res} (for protease-resistant). The designation PrP^p is used in this chapter.

The two mechanisms believed to give rise to PrP^p

- Post-translational modification leading to an alteration in the conformation of the normal protein (**Fig. 32.2**). The most widely accepted hypothesis is that PrP^p serves as a template for the catalytic conversion of PrP^c into more PrP^p. Peripheral tissues (spleen, lungs, and gut) are probably the initial sites of conformational change of PrP^c into PrP^p in many cases.
- Mutations in the prion gene resulting in the translation of a protein with sequence abnormalities that predispose to the spontaneous adoption of an abnormal conformation (**Fig. 32.3**).

Prion strains

Distinct prion strains can be identified with characteristic patterns of pathology within the CNS, and distinct incubation times. Such strains can be stably propagated in experimental animals that are homozygous for their PrP genes.

Strain-specific differences in the pattern of PrP^p glycosylation

Research has revealed strain-specific differences in the pattern of PrP^p glycosylation in CJD and some related spongiform encephalopathies in animals. Western blot analysis of PrP from affected brain tissue shows three bands corresponding to protein with either two, one, or no attached polysaccharide chains. Four types of PrP^p that can be distinguished by western blot analysis are consistently associated with different patterns of disease:

- Types 1 and 2, with sporadic CJD.
- Type 3, with iatrogenic CJD.
- Type 4, with new variant CJD (vCJD, see p. 32.11).

PRP GENE AND PATHOGENESIS OF PRION DISEASE

*Several point mutations and insertions have been identified in the PrP gene that increase the susceptibility of PrP to assume a pathologic conformation (**Fig. 32.4**).*

Nomenclature of PrP gene mutations

This takes the form of disease phenotype (original amino acid, codon position, substituted amino acid), for example GSS (PRO102LEU) or GSS (P102L).

Polymorphism at codon 129 acting as a susceptibility factor

In addition to these pathogenic mutations, a polymorphism at codon 129 (which codes for either valine or methionine) acts as a susceptibility factor, modulating the facility with which PrP^C assumes an abnormal conformation when interacting with exogenous abnormal PrP^p (see below). The frequency of this polymorphism in Caucasian populations is:

- V V   12%
- MM   37%
- VM   51%

In the Japanese population the frequency is:

- V V   0%
- MM   92%
- VM   8%

In studies of the PrP genotype in sporadic CJD, over 90% of cases are homozygous for either M or V at 129, suggesting that this homozygosity confers relative susceptibility to disease. Having the same amino acid at this position may facilitate conversion of PrP^C to PrP^p when they interact.

EPIDEMIOLOGY OF CJD

- CJD occurs throughout the world and has an annual incidence of 1–2 cases/million population.
- Higher rates have been recorded in some regions or populations (e.g. Libyan Jews and in areas of central Slovakia, Hungary, and eastern England). Families with mutations in the prion gene account for these high local rates.
- Approximately equal numbers of men and women are affected.
- About 10% of cases are familial.
- The age of onset is usually 55–75 years with a peak incidence in the seventh decade.
- Rare cases with an onset as young as 16 or as old as 85 years have been reported.
- Epidemiologic data are largely based on clinical diagnostic criteria. The phenotype is, however, quite variable and these data may not be entirely accurate for all age groups; misdiagnosis is particularly likely in the elderly.

The commonest phenotype of prion disease is CJD. Patients typically present with subtle motor signs, which herald severe cerebellar ataxia, and progress to global dementia in under one year. Criteria for the clinical diagnosis of CJD have been proposed and widely adopted (**Fig. 32.5**).

Several phenotypes of prion disease other than CJD have been identified (**Fig. 32.6**). In all of these, the mainstay of diagnosis is clinical examination supplemented by additional radiologic, electrophysiologic and neuropathologic investigations (**Fig. 32.7**).

Many patients in the late stage of neurodegenerative disease develop myoclonus, but the length of the history usually contrasts with the rapid progression of classic CJD. Some patients who have dementia with cortical Lewy bodies deteriorate rapidly and develop myoclonus, in which case CJD enters the clinical differential diagnosis. The possibility that many cases of dementia of uncertain etiology or dementia with atypical features may be due to undiagnosed prion disease is not supported by comprehensive necropsy studies.

PATHOLOGY

The severity of abnormalities varies. In most cases, the pathologic changes described below are moderate to marked. Rarely, no abnormalities are demonstrable by standard histologic techniques. The neuropathologic manifestations depend upon whether the disease is sporadic, familial, or iatrogenic, and are modified by the nature of the PrP gene defect (if familial) and the codon 129 PrP genotype, and by the duration of the illness.

MACROSCOPIC APPEARANCES

The brain may appear macroscopically normal, even in cases with long clinical histories. Most cases, however, show some atrophy (**Fig. 32.8**) and this may be severe, with a reduction in brain weight to as low as 850 g. In such cases, ventricular enlargement is marked and the atrophy often includes the caudate nucleus and thalamus. The hippocampus may be relatively spared, even in cases with severe atrophy elsewhere.

Atrophy of the cerebellar folia is common and the brain stem may appear atrophic in some cases. In general, loss of brain substance appears to be confined to the gray matter, and white matter is relatively spared, although this is not always the case (see panencephalopathic CJD, p.32.12). Meninges and blood vessels appear normal.

MICROSCOPIC APPEARANCES

The histologic features of prion diseases are:
- spongiform change
- neuronal loss
- astrocytosis
- paucity of inflammation
- synaptic loss
- accumulation of PrP

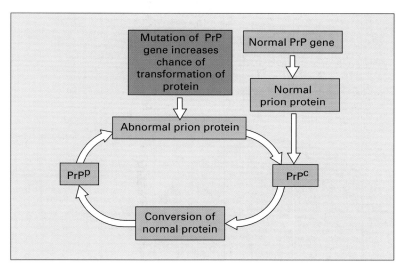

Fig. 32.3 Mutations in the prion gene predispose to the adoption of a pathogenic configuration by the protein.

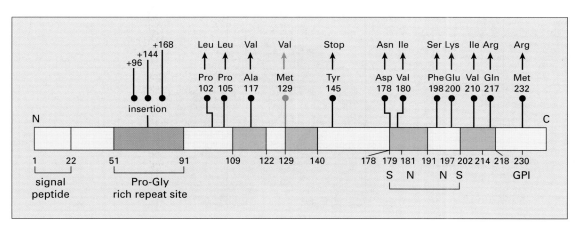

Fig. 32.4 Mutations in the prion gene. This diagram illustrates mutations that have been identified in familial forms of prion disease. Also shown (in blue) is the codon 129 polymorphism.

Clinical criteria for diagnosis of CJD

Diagnosis	Clinical criteria

Probable sporadic CJD	• Progressive dementia
	• Typical EEG
	• At least two of the following:
	   myoclonus
	   visual or cerebellar dysfunction
	   pyramidal or extrapyramidal dysfunction
	   akinetic mutism

Possible sporadic CJD	• Progressive dementia
	• Absence of typical EEG
	• At least two of the following:
	   myoclonus
	   visual or cerebellar dysfunction
	   pyramidal or extrapyramidal dysfunction
	   akinetic mutism
	• Duration of less than 2 years

Transmitted CJD	• Progressive cerebellar syndrome in a pituitary hormone recipient
	• Sporadic CJD associated with a known risk factor:
	   human dura mater transplant
	   neurosurgic instrumentation with known exposure

Familial CJD	• Definite or probable CJD in two or more first degree relatives • Neuropsychiatric disorder associated with a disease-related mutation in the PrP gene
New variant vCJD	• Psychiatric disease (anxiety, depression, or withdrawal) • Progressive cerebellar ataxia within weeks or months of presentation • Variable dysesthesia in limbs and face, chorea, extrapyramidal or pyramidal signs • Memory impairment with dementia in late stages • Myoclonus in late stages • EEG does not show changes typical of CJD • Necropsy confirmation mandatory for definite diagnosis

Fig. 32.5 Clinical criteria for the diagnosis of CJD.

Radiologic, electrophysiologic, and neuropathologic investigation of prion disease

Investigation	Findings
Imaging	• CT and MR show variable cerebral and or cerebellar atrophy
EEG	• Early disease: diffuse or focal slowing • Later disease: repetitive bilaterally synchronous sharp waves or slow spike and wave discharges • Finally: synchronous triphasic sharp wave complexes (1–2/s) superimposed on progressive suppression of cortical background activity
Brain biopsy	• Characteristic neuropathologic abnormalities (see main text) • Deposition of PrP detectable by immunohistochemistry (see main text) • These investigations may be supplemented by PrP immunoblotting, and by sequencing of the human PrP gene, *PRNP*, in some cases.

Fig. 32.7 Radiologic, electrophysiologic and neuropathologic investigation of prion disease.

Phenotypes of prion disease other than classic CJD

Prion disease	Phenotype
Ataxic Gerstmann–Sträussler–Scheinker disease (GSS)	• Autosomal dominant cerebellar disorder • Dementia tends to be mild. • Mean age of death around 50 years • Duration of illness 4–5 years
Fatal familial insomnia (FFI)	• Autosomal dominant disorder • Early sleep disturbances • Neuropsychiatric disease • Late dementia
Progressive spastic paraparesis	• Autosomal dominant disorder • Progressive spastic paraparesis • Cerebellar ataxia • Late dementia
New variant vCJD	• Presents as a sporadic neuropsychiatric disorder • Typically affects patients less than 45 years of age • Cerebellar ataxia • Dementia • Disease duration longer than that of classic CJD
Atypical prion dementia	• Sporadic late-onset-dementia syndrome • Clinically indistinguishable from Alzheimer's disease or dementia with Lewy bodies
Kuru	• Cerebellar ataxia associated with tremor and dementia, restricted to the Fore tribe of New Guinea • Runs a fulminating course leading to incapacitation and death within 1 year • Has virtually disappeared since the ending of particular funeral rites involving the handling or eating of brain tissue

Fig. 32.6 Phenotypes of prion disease other than classic CJD

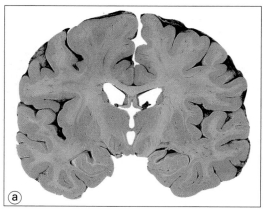
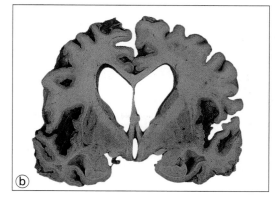

Fig. 32.8 CJD. (a) The brain may appear macroscopically normal, but there is usually some atrophy, as here. **(b)** Rarely, atrophy is marked.

Spongiform change

Microscopic examination of affected regions of the brain reveals vacuolation of the neuropil, an appearance termed spongiform change (**Fig. 32.9**). The vacuoles are typically round, relatively small (20–50 μm in diameter), and quite evenly distributed, but some can be large and irregular. The vacuoles are intracellular. Electron microscopy of early lesions shows that most of the vacuoles are within neuronal processes (**Fig.**

32.10). The vacuolation occurs mainly in gray matter. The distribution of pathology varies greatly between cases. The most consistently affected regions are the cerebral and cerebellar cortices, but the basal ganglia and thalamus are often involved. The distribution of lesions in the cerebral and cerebellar cortices is often patchy, affected regions alternating with seemingly unaffected areas, but may be confluent.

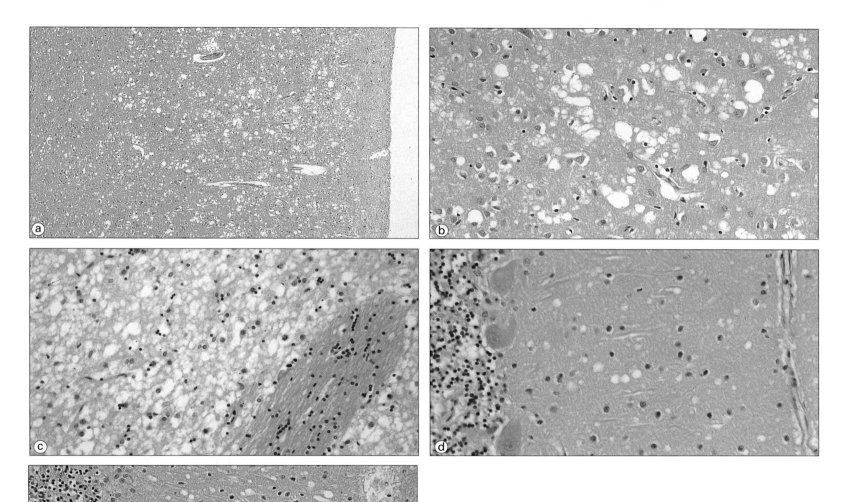

Fig. 32.9 Spongiform change. There is fine vacuolation of the neuropil, even well away from blood vessels and neuronal somata (where tissue shrinkage during processing may give an artefactual appearance of vacuolation). The fine round vacuoles in the affected cortex and deep gray matter are interspersed with coarser vacuoles, some of which appear to be formed by the coalescence of smaller ones. **(a)** Spongiform change affecting all layers of the cerebral cortex. **(b)** Some of the larger vacuoles appear to result from the coalescence of smaller ones **(c)** Spongiform change involving the putamen. **(d)** Spongiform change involving the cerebellum in which the small vacuoles are relatively sparse in the molecular layer. **(e)** Spongiform change involving the cerebellum in which there are numerous small vacuoles in the molecular layer. The cerebellar cortex is commonly, but not invariably, affected in prion disease.

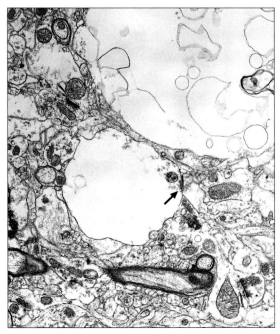

Fig. 32.10 Electron microscopic appearance of spongiform change. Dendrites and axons contain vacuoles, which appear empty apart from fragments of membrane and occasional wisps of amorphous material. Note the synaptic density (arrow). Small vacuoles may be enclosed by a membrane. Larger vacuoles are usually incompletely enclosed or lack any discernible surrounding membrane.

DIFFERENTIAL DIAGNOSIS OF SPONGIFORM CHANGE IN PRION DISEASES

- Microvacuolation may occur in other diseases and can be confused with the spongiform change of prion disease.
- Status spongiosus (**Fig. 32.11**) refers to the coarse microvacuolation that accompanies astrocytosis in association with severe neuronal loss. It is a nonspecific finding in several neurodegenerative diseases. It may be part of the pathology of prion disease in some cases, but is not a diagnostic feature.
- Superficial microvacuolation involving layers II and III of the frontal and temporal cortices is a feature of neurodegenerative diseases that present as frontotemporal dementias, especially dementia of frontal type, but also Pick's disease, dementia with motor neuron disease inclusions, and dementia associated with corticobasal degeneration (**Fig. 32.12**).
- Dementia with cortical Lewy bodies may be associated with transcortical microvacuolation very similar to that of prion disease (**Fig. 32.13**). This is localized to the medial temporal lobe structures and is not associated with an accumulation of PrP.
- Spongiform change in gray and white matter can occur in several metabolic encephalopathies, including aminoaciduria syndromes (**Fig. 32.14a**), Alpers' disease, and chronic hepatocerebral degeneration (**Fig. 32.14b**).
- Microvacuolation can occur in acute hypoxic–ischemic encephalopathy.
- Inadequate fixation or suboptimal processing of brain tissue during paraffin embedding can cause artefactual vacuolation of both gray and white matter.

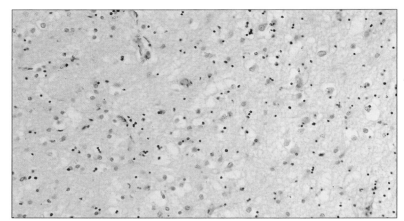

Fig. 32.11 Status spongiosus. Irregular vacuolation of gliotic cerebral cortex can be a feature of several degenerative disorders.

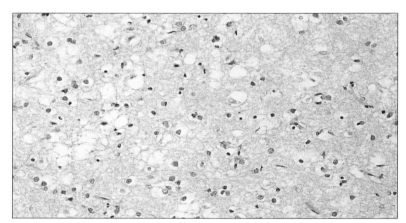

Fig. 32.12 Superficial microvacuolation in frontal dementia. Microvacuolation limited to the outer cortical laminae in the frontal and temporal lobes is a feature of several forms of neurodegenerative disorders (see Chapter 31) not related to prion disease. In contrast to prion disease, the vacuolation does not involve the full thickness of the cortex.

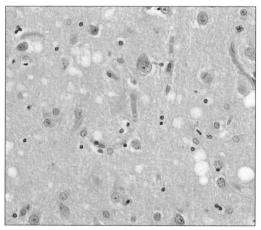

Fig. 32.13 Microvacuolation in Lewy body dementia. Spongiform change, which is transcortical, may be seen in Lewy body dementia, but the distribution is restricted to medial temporal lobe structures.

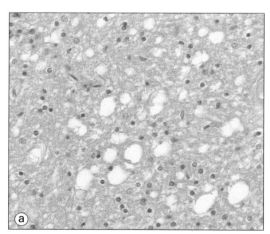
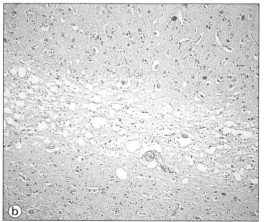

Fig. 32.14 Spongiform vacuolation in disorders other than prion disease. (a) Cortical vacuolation in aminoaciduria. **(b)** Coarse vacuolation at the junction of cerebral cortex and white matter in liver failure.

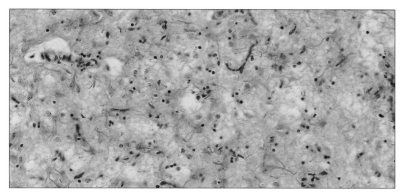

Fig. 32.15 Status spongiosus in CJD. Coarse vacuolation of the cortex in advanced CJD is a nonspecific finding. Similar changes occur in the later stages of other neurodegenerative diseases. (Phosphotungstic acid–hematoxylin)

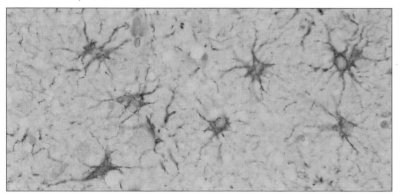

Fig. 32.16 Astrocytosis in CJD. Demonstration of astrocytic gliosis by glial fibrillary acidic protein (GFAP) immunohistochemistry in cerebral cortex affected by spongiform change.

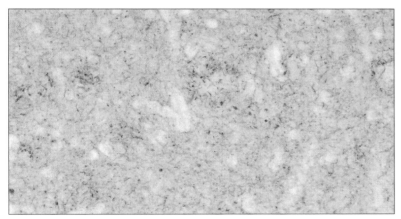

Fig. 32.17 Patchy reduction in synaptophysin immunoreactivity. This is an early feature in prion disease and indicates a loss of synapses.

Neuronal loss: In most cases there is a marked loss of neurons. This loss is greatest in cortical layers III–V and in focal regions of the caudate nucleus and thalamus. The pattern of loss is variable. There may be destruction of almost all neurons over large areas, causing a loss of lamination and coarse vacuolation (status spongiosus) (**Fig. 32.15**). Examination may reveal scattered shrunken remnants of neurons in the midst of apparently unaffected cells. In some cases residual neurons swell to form ballooned cells.

Astrocytosis: Loss of neurons is accompanied by massive activation and proliferation of astrocytes (**Fig. 32.16**). In severe cases, the neuronal component of cortical areas may have been replaced by reactive gliosis.

Paucity of inflammation: In contrast to most other infectious disorders, the neuronal destruction and gliosis of prion diseases are not accompanied by substantial inflammation. The spongiform degeneration and astrocytosis are associated with activation of microglia, but there is only a scanty infiltration of lymphocytes or accumulation of foamy macrophages.

Synaptic loss: Electron microscopy has shown that axons and dendrites are damaged early in the disease. Quantitative studies of synaptic density in cases with obvious spongiform change have estimated synaptic loss at about 30% in the cerebral cortex. A synaptic loss of approximately 20% has been shown in atypical cases lacking obvious pathology at the light microscopic level (**Fig. 32.17**).

Accumulation of PrP: PrP accumulates in the brain in prion diseases and can be detected by immunohistochemistry. There are several patterns of accumulation:
- a diffuse synaptic pattern (**Fig. 32.18**)
- perivacuolar deposits (**Fig. 32.19**)

Fig. 32.18 Synaptic PrP deposition. At low magnification deposition of PrP can be seen throughout the cerebral cortex. At higher magnification this diffuse staining pattern is seen to be due to fine punctate PrP immunoreactivity. Ultrastructural studies have shown this to be localized to synaptic structures.

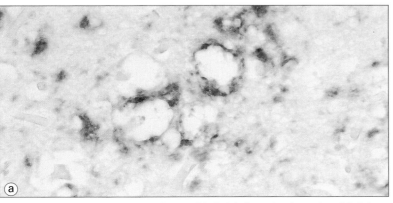

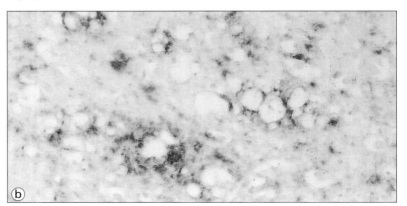

Fig. 32.19 Perivacuolar deposition of PrP. (a) Granular deposits of PrP immunoreactivity around areas of vacuolation. **(b)** Perivacuolar deposits and adjacent synaptic PrP immunostaining.

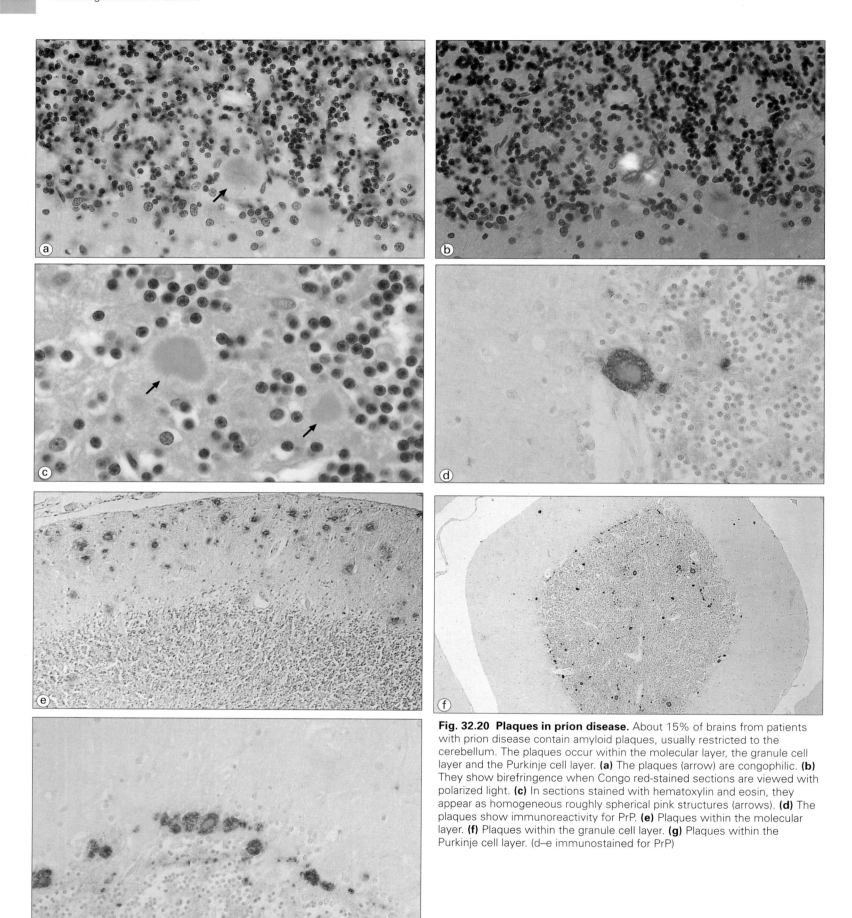

Fig. 32.20 Plaques in prion disease. About 15% of brains from patients with prion disease contain amyloid plaques, usually restricted to the cerebellum. The plaques occur within the molecular layer, the granule cell layer and the Purkinje cell layer. **(a)** The plaques (arrow) are congophilic. **(b)** They show birefringence when Congo red-stained sections are viewed with polarized light. **(c)** In sections stained with hematoxylin and eosin, they appear as homogeneous roughly spherical pink structures (arrows). **(d)** The plaques show immunoreactivity for PrP. **(e)** Plaques within the molecular layer. **(f)** Plaques within the granule cell layer. **(g)** Plaques within the Purkinje cell layer. (d–e immunostained for PrP)

- Larger deposits or plaques (**Fig. 32.20**) in which some of the PrP may be in the form of amyloid. There are five main types of plaque in prion disease:
  - Unicentric plaques, consisting of an amyloid core and radiating spicules of amyloid, which together form a spherical deposit. The amyloid is periodic acid–Schiff (PAS) positive. This type is often called a kuru plaque.
  - Multicentric plaques, consisting of several dense core regions of amyloid with radiating spicules, which form multilobed structures as if made by the fusion of many unicentric plaques. The amyloid is PAS positive. This form is characteristic of GSS.
  - Unicentric plaques, consisting of a dense amyloid core that lacks surrounding radiating spicules of amyloid material. The amyloid is PAS positive.
  - Florid plaques, appearing as unicentric amyloid deposits with radiating spicules of amyloid and a surrounding rim of spongiform change. The amyloid is PAS positive. This type is characteristic of vCJD.
  - Diffuse plaques consisting of large (100–200 μm diameter) ill-defined areas of PrP deposition visible on immunostaining. The deposits are not PAS positive.

CLASSIC CJD

Several types of CJD can be distinguished on the basis of clinical and neuropathologic criteria. The main patterns of neuronal loss, astrocytosis, and spongiform change in CJD have been categorized as:

- cortical
- corticostriatal
- corticostriatocerebellar
- corticospinal
- corticonigral
- thalamic

It should, however, be emphasized that the distribution of lesions in individual cases may overlap these categories.

Recent studies have indicated that the pattern of disease is determined in part by the human PrP gene (*PRNP*) codon 129 haplotype (M/M, M/V, or V/V) and the PrPᴾ glycosylation pattern, as shown by the sizes of the PrPᴾ fragment on western blotting (type 1: small; or type 2: large) after proteinase K treatment. Four forms of sporadic CJD have been delineated:

- 129M/M homozygote with PrPᴾ type 1 (CJDM/M1) characterized by a rapid clinical course, with early dementia, myoclonus and periodic sharp waves on the EEG. Histologically, there is mild to moderate spongiosis and gliosis in the cerebral cortex, striatum, thalamus, and cerebellar cortex, with sparing of the brain stem, hippocampus, and hypothalamus. PrP deposition is mainly of the synaptic pattern, in areas of spongiosis.
- 129M/M homozygote with PrPᴾ type 2 (CJDM/M2) characterized by a long clinical course with dementia without myoclonus or periodic sharp waves. There is severe neuronal loss with status spongiosus, and PrP deposition is coarse rather than punctate.
- 129M/V heterozygote with PrPᴾ type 2 (CJDM/V2) characterized by cognitive and cerebellar signs. The deep cerebral nuclei, brain stem, and cerebellum are predominantly affected, with relative sparing of the neocortex. White matter is involved in disease of long duration.
- 129V/V homozygote with PrPᴾ type 2 (CJDV/V2) characterized by cerebellar signs early in the disease with late dementia. The deep cerebral nuclei, brain stem, and cerebellum are predominantly affected, with relative sparing of the neocortex. White matter is involved in disease of long duration.

GERSTMANN–SRAUSSLER–SCHEINKER DISEASE (GSS)

Several clinical conditions are encompassed by the designation GSS as defined by the presence of multicentric PrP amyloid plaques in the brain (**Fig. 32.21**):

- Ataxic GSS (*PRNP* PRO102LEU) in which ataxia is combined with varying degrees of dementia. Unicentric and multicentric amyloid plaques are present in the molecular layer of the cerebellar cortex and in smaller numbers in the cerebral cortex. Usually spongiform change is not prominent. The severity of neuronal loss from cerebral and cerebellar cortices is variable.

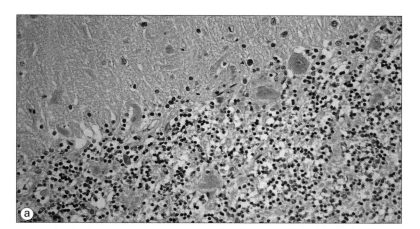
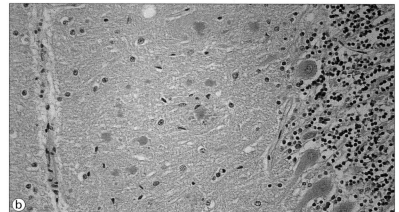
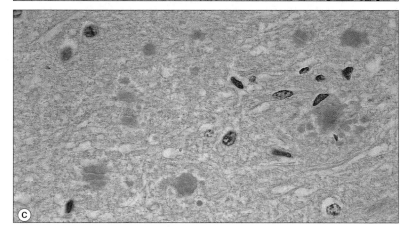

Fig. 32.21 Cerebellar plaques in GSS. Coarse granular clusters of eosinophilic plaque material are present in the cerebellar granule cell, Purkinje cell, and molecular layers. Some of the plaques have a typical multicentric appearance consisting of a large central accumulation with smaller adjacent deposits. The plaques have amyloid staining characteristics and react strongly with antibody to PrP. **(a)** Cerebellar plaques in cerebellar granule cell layer. **(b)** Plaques in the molecular layer. **(c)** Higher magnification view of plaques in the molecular layer.

- Telencephalic GSS (*PRNP* ALA117VAL) in which a dementia syndrome predominates, but ataxia has been the clinical presentation in one family. Multicentric and diffuse plaques are present in neocortical regions and occasionally in the cerebellum. Unicentric amyloid plaques are present in white matter. Spongiform change is absent. Severe neuronal loss and astrocytosis are evident in the basal ganglia and thalamus.

- NFT GSS (*PRNP* PHE198SER) or (*PRNP* GLN217ARG) in which there is a cognitive decline accompanying ataxia, and parkinsonism is a late feature. Multicentric and unicentric PrP amyloid plaques are seen in the neocortex and cerebellar cortex. There are Aβ plaques and tau-immunoreactive neurofibrillary tangles in a distribution compatible with early Alzheimer's disease. Plaques with combined Aβ and PrP immunoreactivities are a rare finding. Neuronal loss affects the neocortex and cerebellar cortex.

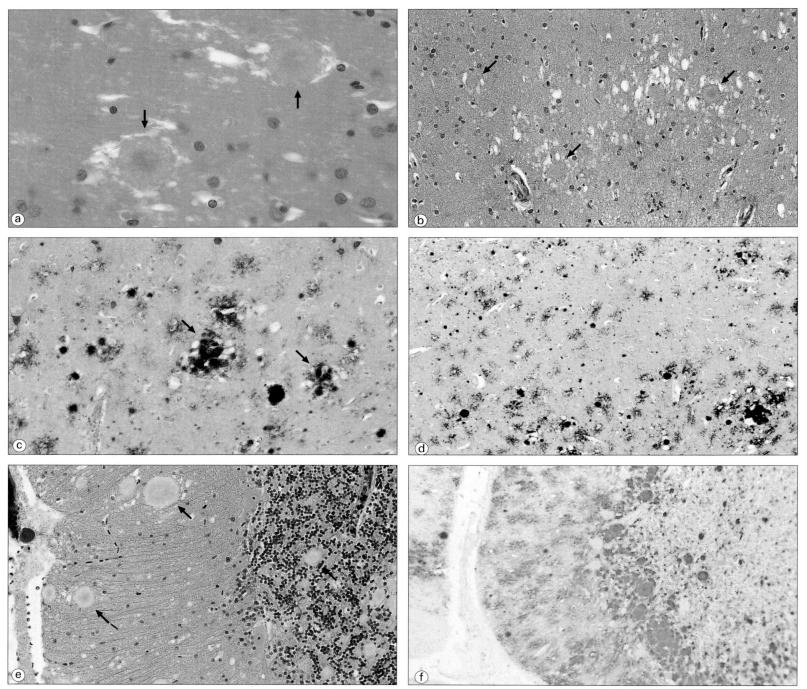

Fig. 32.22 vCJD. (a) The plaques of vCJD are typically of 'florid' type (arrows), consisting of an amyloid core with relatively coarse surrounding vacuoles in a pattern that has been likened to the petals of a daisy. **(b)** Plaques stained with phosphotungstic acid–hematoxylin (arrows). **(c)** The coarsely granular amyloid cores are strongly immunoreactive for PrP (arrows). **(d)** Finer granular deposits of PrP are also present. **(e)** Large numbers of plaques (arrows) are usually present in the cerebellum. (Phosphotungstic acid–hematoxylin) **(f)** The cerebellum shows abundant deposition of PrP on immunostaining.

- Progrssive spastic paraparesis GSS (*PRNP* PRO105LEU) in which a clumsy hand is an early feature. This is followed by gait disturbance, spastic paraparesis, and ataxia. Cognitive decline and dysarthria are late features. No spongiform change is seen. Plaques occur mainly in the cerebral cortex with less involvement of the cerebellum and basal ganglia.
- GSS (*PRNP* TYR145STOP) produces a slowly progressive dementia. The histology is characterized by amyloid plaques, tangles, and neuropil threads in the cerebral cortex.
- GSS (*PRNP* Octapeptide repeat 51–91) in which ataxia precedes dementia. Cerebellar plaques are found, with less involvement of the cerebral cortex. Spongiform change is present.

FATAL FAMILIAL INSOMNIA (FFI)

FFI is due to a PRNP 178ASN mutation in association with a methionine residue at codon 129. The pathologic features are:
- marked neuronal loss and gliosis in the thalamus
- inconsistent and mild neuronal loss and gliosis in the cerebral cortex
- inconsistent degeneration of the inferior olivary nuclei

The phenotype caused by the 178ASN mutation in the PrP is modified by the non-pathogenic polymorphism found at codon 129.
- if there is a methionine at 129, patients have the FFI phenotype
- if there is a valine at 129, patients develop the cortical pathology of familial CJD together with pathology in subcortical nuclei

It is believed that the 129 polymorphism has an effect on the rate of accumulation of the PrPP isoform.

NEW VARIANT CJD (vCJD)

vCJD has a distinct neuropathologic profile. There are typically numerous amyloid plaques in the cerebral cortex and cerebellum resembling those described in kuru. The plaques are often surrounded by vacuolation and have been termed florid plaques (**Fig. 32.22**). Spongiform change is most evident in the basal ganglia and thalamus.

Immunohistochemistry typically shows an abundant accumulation of PrP see Fig. 32.22f.

All vCJD samples show a distinctive pattern on Western blotting after proteinase K treatment. This has been termed a type 4 pattern and is characterized by a high proportion of diglycosylated PrP^P. The same pattern is produced by extracts from brains of BSE-infected cattle. These findings suggest that vCJD and BSE are caused by the same strain of agent.

IATROGENIC CJD

Iatrogenic CJD has been transmitted mainly by intramuscular administration of hormones (growth hormone or gonadotropin) derived from human cadaveric pituitary glands. The risk of contracting the disorder to those patients who have received human growth hormone is estimated at approximately 1:200. Disease has also been transmitted from human tissue grafts (cornea and dura) and by surgical instruments contaminated by infected brain tissue. In this variant, patients have a cerebellar syndrome and may later develop dementia.

There are typically widespread neuronal loss and spongiform change in the cerebellar cortex and to a lesser degree in the cerebral cortex. Plaques are common. PrP immunohistochemistry reveals heavy deposits in the cerebellum and a linear pattern of labeling in the cerebral cortex.

Many pituitary hormone recipients who have developed iatrogenic CJD have valine homozygosity at codon 129 and a type 2 pattern of PrP on western blotting after proteinase K digestion, but this is not the case for those CJD patients who received dural grafts.

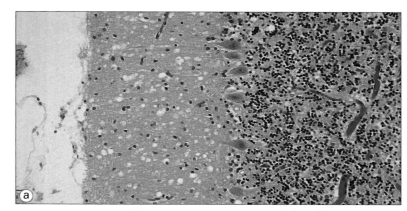
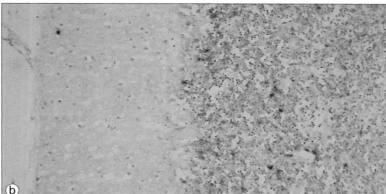
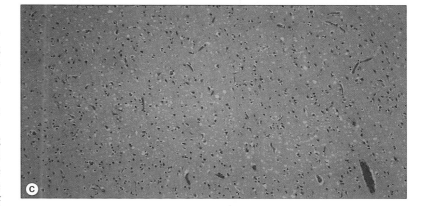

Fig. 32.23 Iatrogenic CJD. A recipient of human pituitary derived growth hormone, this patient developed ataxia followed by dementia. Spongiform change is present in the molecular layer of the cerebellum **(a)** and cerebral cortex **(c)**. Immunohistochemistry for PrP reveals scattered deposits in the cerebellum **(b)** and a linear pattern of immunoreactivity in the cerebral cortex **(d)**.

PANENCEPHALOPATHIC CJD

The panencephalopathic form of CJD is characterized by extensive involvement of white matter as well as cerebral cortex (**Fig. 32.24**). There are no published data concerning the *PRNP* codon 129 status in these patients, although it is noteworthy that white matter involvement is a recognized feature of some variants of classic CJD in which the codon 129 status has been determined (see p.32.9).

The brain generally shows severe atrophy. Marked neuronal loss and spongiform change in the cerebral cortex are associated with an intense astrocytosis. There is diffuse myelin pallor in the hemispheric white matter, which appears spongy and is accompanied by moderate astrocytosis and an accumulation of lipid in macrophages see Fig. 32.24. Coarse spongy cavities develop in the subcortical gyral crowns.

The basal ganglia and thalamus show severe neuronal loss and spongiform change with gliosis. The cerebellar granular cell layer is markedly depleted of neurons and the molecular layer correspondingly atrophic. Purkinje cells are relatively well preserved. The spinal cord shows distal degeneration of corticospinal tracts.

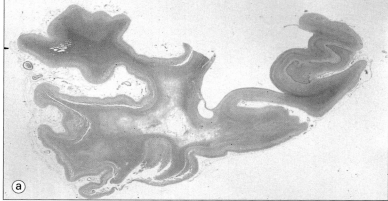
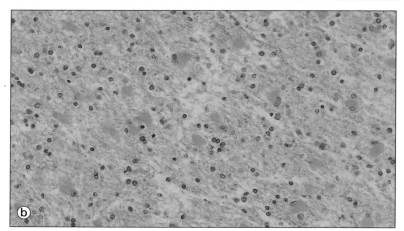
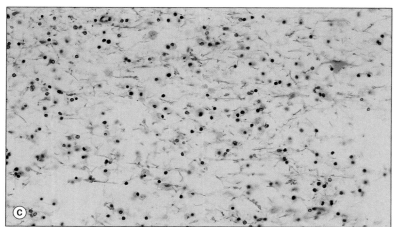

Fig. 32.24 Panencephalopathic CJD. (a) Severe white matter rarefaction and focal cavitation in panencephalopathic CJD. This patient had typical spongiform change in the basal ganglia and thalamus. **(b)** Marked reactive astrocytosis in the cerebral white matter. **(c)** Elsewhere the white matter is severely rarefied and contains scattered lipid-laden macrophages as well as reactive astrocytes. (Phosphotungstic acid–hematoxylin)

NECROPSY AND DECONTAMINATION PROCEDURES

- Cases of CJD are usually diagnosed antemortem and so the necropsy is undertaken with an appreciation of the potential risks.
- The main risk in the mortuary or laboratory is direct inoculation of infected tissue through a skin wound. Care should also be taken to avoid contamination of mucosal surfaces and the eyes. Tissues fixed in formalin and glutaraldehyde are potentially infective.
- The transmissable agent is classed as a category III* pathogen by the UK Advisory Committee on Dangerous Pathogens.

Necropsies should be conducted using precautions for containment of a prion disease for:

- Patients with a neurodegenerative disease if CJD has entered the differential diagnosis.
- Patients with a familial prion disease.
- Recipients of tissues from human cadavers (pituitary derived hormones or dura mater).

Necropsy to diagnosi of CJD can be carried out safely in a standard mortuary, but the following precautions should be taken:

- Care should be taken to avoid injury to mortuary personnel through innoculation.
- Personnel should wear eye and mouth protection, rubber gloves and cut proof gloves (e.g. chain mai gauntlets).
- Contamination of the work area should be minimized by covering surfaces with non-permeable plastic sheets and using absorbent pads to contain body-fluids.
- The brain should be removed by sawing through the skull with the head and saw encosed in a large transparent polythene bag.
- Tissues should be preserved in formalin (although this does not inactivate the agent).
- All disposable and contaminated articles should be destroyed by incineration according to accepted protocols for dealing with hazardous clinical waste.

Disinfection and contamination

- Conventional disinfection procedures are ineffective against the agent that causes prion disease, but tissues can be rendered non-infective by immersion of 5mm thick blocks in 95–100% formic acid for 1 hour. This allows inrestricted handling in the laboratory.
- In the mortuary of laboratory, instruments and surfaces can be decontaminated by immersion or application of 2N sodium hydroxide for 1 hour. Glassware can be cleaned in sodium hypochlorite (20,000ppm). Porous load steam autoclaving at 132°C for 4.5 hours can also be used.

REFERENCES

Budka H *et al.* (1995) Tissue handling in suspected Creutzfeldt–Jakob disease (CJD) and other human spongiform encephalopathies (prion diseases). *Brain Path* **5**: 319–322.

Budka H *et al.* (1995) Neuropathological diagnostic criteria for Creutzfeldt–Jakob disease and other human spongiform encephalopathies (prion diseases). *Brain Path* **5**: 459–466.

DeArmond, SJ and Prusiner, SB (1997) Prion Diseases. In Graham D, Lantos P (eds) *Greenfield's Neuropathology.* 6th Edition. Volume 2 pp 235–271. London: Arnold.

Kretzschmar HA *et al.* (1997) Cell death in prion disease. *Neural Trans* (Supp))191–210.

National CJD Survellance Unit and the Department of Epidemiology and Population Sciences (1995) *London School of Hygiene and Tropical Medicine Creutzfeldt–Jakob Disease Surveillance in the United Kingdom. Fourth Annual Report.*

Prusiner SB, DeArmond SJ (1994) Prion diseases and neurodegeneration. *Ann Rev Neurosci* **17**: 311–339.

Parchi P, *et al.* (1996) Molecular basis of phenotypic variability in sporadic Creutzfeldt–Jakob disease. *Ann Neurol* **39**: 767–778.

Roberts GW, Clinton J (1992) Prion disease: the spectrum of pathology and diagnositic considerations. In Prusiner SB, Collinge J , Anderton B , Powell J (eds) *Prion Disease.* pp. 214–240.

Will RG, *et al.* (1996) A new variant of Creutzfeldt–Jakob disease in the UK. *Lancet* **347**: 921–925.

33 Thalamic and pallidal degenerations, neuroaxonal dystrophy, and autonomic failure

THALAMIC DEGENERATIONS

Thalamic degeneration is a feature of several multisystem neurodegenerative disorders (**Fig. 33.1**), but can also rarely occur in a 'pure' form.

PURE THALAMIC ATROPHY
MACROSCOPIC AND MICROSCOPIC APPEARANCES
There is bilateral symmetric involvement of the thalamic nuclei with neuronal loss and astrocytic gliosis in the absence of inflammation or vascular disease. Atrophy of the inferior olives has been described in some cases.

PURE THALAMIC ATROPHY

- This occurs mainly in young adults, and can cause:
  - Behavioral disturbances: apathy, emotional lability, hypersomnia, stereotyped behavior.
  - Memory disturbance progressing to dementia.
  - Movement disorder: akinetic rigid syndrome, ataxia, choreoathetosis.

DIFFERENTIAL DIAGNOSIS OF PURE THALAMIC ATROPHY

- The conditions listed in Fig. 33.1 should be excluded. These include fatal familial insomnia, which has a primary thalamic pattern of involvement and is a genetic form of prion disease (see Chapter 32).
- Neuronal loss from the thalamus has been described in patients who have undergone leukotomy.

PALLIDAL DEGENERATIONS

The grouping together of pallidal degenerations is based on the morphologic finding of degeneration centered on the globus pallidus, either alone or in combination with degeneration of the subthalamic nucleus or substantia nigra. They have been subdivided according to the regions of the brain showing pathologic changes (**Fig. 33.2**). Clinically, these conditions are associated with a variety of movement disorders, with or without dementia. Some are familial while others occur as sporadic disorders.

It is difficult to evaluate the nosologic status of many of the cases described in the literature as their relationship to disorders that can now be better defined by molecular and immunohistochemical techniques is uncertain. In particular, cases of dentatorubropallidoluysial atrophy (DRPLA) (see chapter 29), spinocerebellar atrophies (see chapter 29), multiple system atrophy (see chapter 28), and diseases characterized by the ubiquitinated inclusions seen in ALS (see chapter 27) are probably included in most of the historic series. Once these entities are excluded, a group of pallidal degenerations remains that can be classified on a purely descriptive basis, although it is not clear to what extent they represent distinct diseases.

Diseases in which thalamic degeneration may be prominent

- multiple system atrophy (Glial cytoplasmic inclusions)
- spinocerebellar degenerations
- Wernicke's encephalopathy
- Huntington's disease
- Creutzfeldt–Jakob disease
- Menkes' syndrome
- membranous lipodystrophy
- neuroaxonal dystrophy
- fatal familial insomnia

Fig. 33.1 Diseases in which thalamic degeneration may be prominent.

DIFFERENTIAL DIAGNOSIS OF PALLIDAL DEGENERATIONS

- These include the neuroaxonal dystrophies (see below), multiple system atrophy, DRPLA, and ALS.
- A diagnosis of pallidal degeneration should not be made if there are dystrophic axonal swellings, inclusions of multiple system atrophy, or extramotor inclusions of ALS.

Pallidal degenerations

Juvenile pallidal degeneration	
Age of onset	• First and second decades
Clinical features	• Variable mental retardation, movement disorders (dystonia, rigidity, choreoatheosis), and sensory abnormalities
Neuropathology	• Loss of neurons from the globus pallidus, especially the external segment • Loss of myelinated fibers from the pallidoluysian tract • Mild gliosis of the subthalamic nucleus
Adult pallidal degeneration	
Age of onset	• After second decade
Clinical features	• Bradykinesia without rigidity • Dystonia of neck and hands
Neuropathology	• Selective neuronal loss from, and gliosis of, globus pallidus • Loss of myelinated fibers from the pallidoluysian tract • Mild gliosis of subthalamic nucleus
Pallidoluysian degeneration	
Clinical features	• Extrapyramidal movement disorder, dystonia, cognitive decline
Neuropathology	• Neuronal loss from, and gliosis of, the globus pallidus and subthalamic nucleus
Pallidonigroluysial degeneration	
Clinical features	• Extrapyramidal movement disorder, supranuclear gaze palsy
Neuropathology	• Degeneration of external and internal segments of the globus pallidus, subthalamic nucleus, ventrolateral thalamic nuclei, and substantia nigra
Pallidopontonigral degeneration	
Inheritance	• Autosomal dominant, linked to chromosome 17
Age of onset	• In the fifth decade
Clinical features	• Parkinsonism with dystonia, frontal lobe dementia, and pyramidal dysfunction
Neuropathology	• Severe neuronal loss from, and gliosis of, globus pallidus, pontine tegmentum, and substantia nigra • Mild involvement of the caudate nucleus and the putamen
Pallidonigrospinal degeneration	
Age of onset	• 17–54 years
Clinical features	• Extrapyramidal movement disorder with cognitive decline leading to dementia • Amyotrophy
Neuropathology	• Neuronal loss from globus pallidus, substatia nigia, and spinal anterior horns • Variable loss of neurons from subthalamic nucleus, pontine tegmentum • Variable degeneration of corticospinal tracts

Fig. 33.2 Pallidal degenerations.

NEUROAXONAL DYSTROPHY

Classification

Several conditions, grouped as neuroaxonal dystrophies, are characterized pathologically by the presence of axonal swellings, which are thought to develop as a result of neuronal dysfunction leading to distal axonal degeneration. In most cases, the nature of the neuronal dysfunction and the pathogenesis of the axonal swelling are poorly understood. Neuroaxonal dystrophy occurs in three contexts (**Fig. 33.3**).

MICROSCOPIC APPEARANCES

Dystrophic axonal swellings can be identified in sections stained with hematoxylin and eosin as rounded or elongated eosinophilic structures varying from 20–120 μm in diameter (**Fig. 33.4a,b**). Some dystrophic axons contain an intensely stained eosinophilic core surrounded by a paler zone (**Fig. 33.4c**). The swollen axons can be demonstrated by silver impregnation techniques (**Fig. 33.4d**). In toluidine-blue-stained resin sections, the swellings are seen to contain granular material (**Fig. 33.4e**). Electron microscopy shows this to consist of mitochondria, electron-dense lysosome-related bodies, tubulomembranous structures, and amorphous matrix material (**Fig. 33.4f**). Generally, relatively few neurofilaments are present and those that are may be displaced towards the periphery of the axon. Immunoreactivity for neurofilament protein and ubiquitin is largely confined to axonal swellings smaller than 30 μm in diameter (**Fig. 33.5**). Iron-containing and lipofuscin-like pigment may accumulate in axonal spheroids (**Fig. 33.6**), leading to the descriptive term pigment-spheroidal dystrophy.

PHYSIOLOGIC NEUROAXONAL DYSTROPHY

Dystrophic axons are a relatively common normal finding in certain parts of the CNS, particularly in the elderly. The main sites are:
- gracile and cuneate nuclei in the medulla (**Fig. 33.7a**).
- zona reticulata of the substantia nigra (**Fig. 33.7b**).
- inner segment of the globus pallidus.

In most instances there is little associated pigment. Dystrophic axons also accumulate with age in the peripheral sympathetic ganglia.

Classification of neuroaxonal dystrophic processes

Physiologic neuroaxonal dystrophy: normal brain aging
• Gracile and cuneate nuclei • Globus pallidus • Substantia nigra • Spinal anterior homs
Primary neuroaxonal dystrophy: diseases in which the main pathology is neuroaxonal dystrophy
• Infantile neuroaxonal dystrophy • Late infantile, juvenile, and adult neuroaxonal dystrophy • Neuroaxonal leukodystrophy • Hallervorden–Spatz disease • Nasu–Hakola disease • Giant axonal neuropathy
Secondary neuroaxonal dystrophy: accentuation of physiologic neuroaxonal dystrophy in other disease processes
• Neurodegenerative disease • Metabolic disease • Infective disease

Fig. 33.3 Classification of neuroaxonal dystrophic processes.

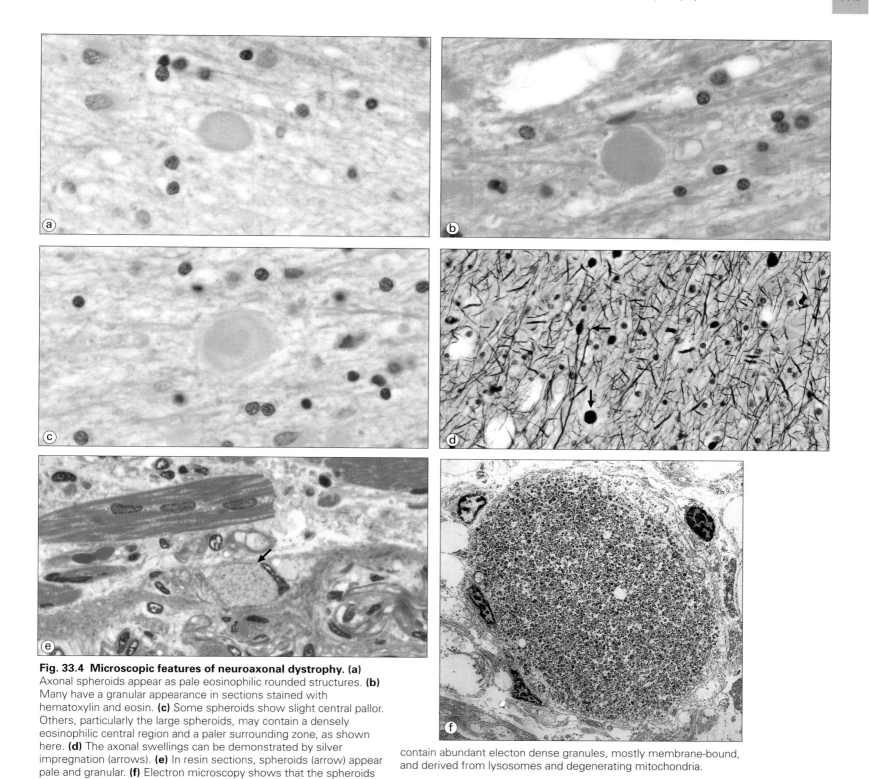

Fig. 33.4 Microscopic features of neuroaxonal dystrophy. (a) Axonal spheroids appear as pale eosinophilic rounded structures. **(b)** Many have a granular appearance in sections stained with hematoxylin and eosin. **(c)** Some spheroids show slight central pallor. Others, particularly the large spheroids, may contain a densely eosinophilic central region and a paler surrounding zone, as shown here. **(d)** The axonal swellings can be demonstrated by silver impregnation (arrows). **(e)** In resin sections, spheroids (arrow) appear pale and granular. **(f)** Electron microscopy shows that the spheroids contain abundant electon dense granules, mostly membrane-bound, and derived from lysosomes and degenerating mitochondria.

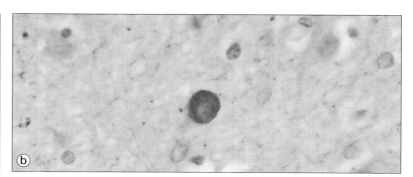

Fig. 33.5 Immunoreactivity of dystrophic axonal swellings. (a) Axonal swellings can be detected by immunohistochemistry for ubiquitin. **(b)** They can also be detected by immunohistochemistry for neurofilament protein. Strong immunoreactivity is generally seen only in small spheroids.

PRIMARY NEUROAXONAL DYSTROPHY

There are six diseases in which dystrophic axonal swellings are the principal pathologic abnormality:
- infantile neuroaxonal dystrophy (Seitelberger's disease)
- late infantile, juvenile, and adult neuroaxonal dystrophy
- neuroaxonal leukodystrophy
- Hallervorden–Spatz disease
- Nasu–Hakola disease
- giant axonal neuropathy

INFANTILE NEUROAXONAL DYSTROPHY
MACROSCOPIC AND MICROSCOPIC APPEARANCES
The cerebrum and cerebellum usually appear atrophic and the ventricles dilated. Axonal spheroids and reactive astrocytic gliosis are widely distributed in both the central and peripheral nervous system (**Fig. 33.8**). Degeneration of the corticospinal and spinobulbar tracts is usually prominent.

Diagnosis can be made by brain, peripheral nerve, conjunctival, skin, or rectal biopsy. Axonal swellings should be looked for by electron microscopy.

LATE INFANTILE, JUVENILE, AND ADULT NEUROAXONAL DYSTROPHY
This manifests with rigidity, ataxia, dysarthria, motor weakness, and psychiatric disorders, and, later, dementia.

MACROSCOPIC AND MICROSCOPIC APPEARANCES
Macroscopically and histologically, the appearances overlap those of Hallervorden–Spatz disease (see below). Neurofibrillary tangles or cortical and subcortical Lewy bodies may be present.

NEUROAXONAL LEUKODYSTROPHY
This is a very uncommon condition with only a few cases reported in the literature. Reported cases have been of adult onset, but the phenotype may be wider. Clinically, it manifests with neurobehavioral disturbance leading to dementia.

INFANTILE NEUROAXONAL DYSTROPHY

- Autosomal recessive inheritance.
- Early clinical features (1–2 years of age) are weakness, hypotonia, and areflexia.
- Later clinical features (2–6 years of age) are rigidity, spasticity, cerebellar ataxia, deafness, blindness, and cognitive decline.
- Most patients die before six years of age.
- An autosomal recessive neuroaxonal dystrophy due to lysosomal α-N-acetylgalactosaminidase deficiency has been described.

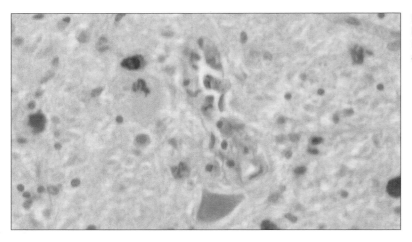

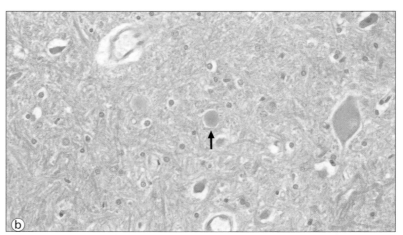

Fig. 33.6 Pigment accumulation in spheroids. Spheroids may contain brown-colored pigment, which is a mixture of lipofuscin-like material and iron. The iron is demonstrated in this section stained by Perls' method and appears blue in color.

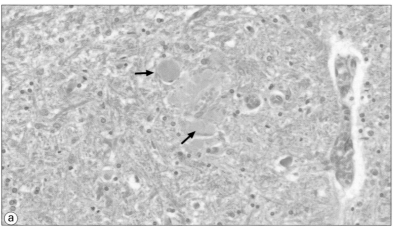

Fig. 33.7 Physiologic neuroaxonal dystrophy. (a) Pale eosinophilic axonal swellings (arrows) in the gracile nucleus of an elderly person. **(b)** In the substantia nigra, axonal swellings (arrow) are typically more eosinophilic.

MACROSCOPIC AND MICROSCOPIC APPEARANCES

There is cerebral atrophy with ventricular dilatation, and softening and gray discoloration of the white matter. Histology reveals severe loss of myelin from the hemispheric white matter, with astrocytic gliosis and numerous axonal swellings (**Fig. 33.9a–f**). Smaller numbers of dystrophic axonal swellings are present in gray matter areas, especially the cerebral cortex (**Fig. 33.9g**). There is distal tract degeneration in the spinal cord, that particularly involves the corticospinal tracts and posterior columns.

HALLERVORDEN–SPATZ DISEASE
MACROSCOPIC AND MICROSCOPIC APPEARANCES

The globus pallidus and pars reticularis of the substantia nigra appear shrunken, and rust-brown in color (**Fig. 33.10a**). Histology shows neuronal loss, astrocytic gliosis, and accumulation of iron-containing pigment in these regions, which also contain large numbers of axonal swellings (**Fig. 33.10b–d**). Spheroids may also be seen in the cerebral cortex and the brain stem nuclei (**Fig. 33.10e,f**). Some patients have associated Lewy body pathology, some have associated neurofibrillary tangles. Pigment can be found in the renal tubular epithelium.

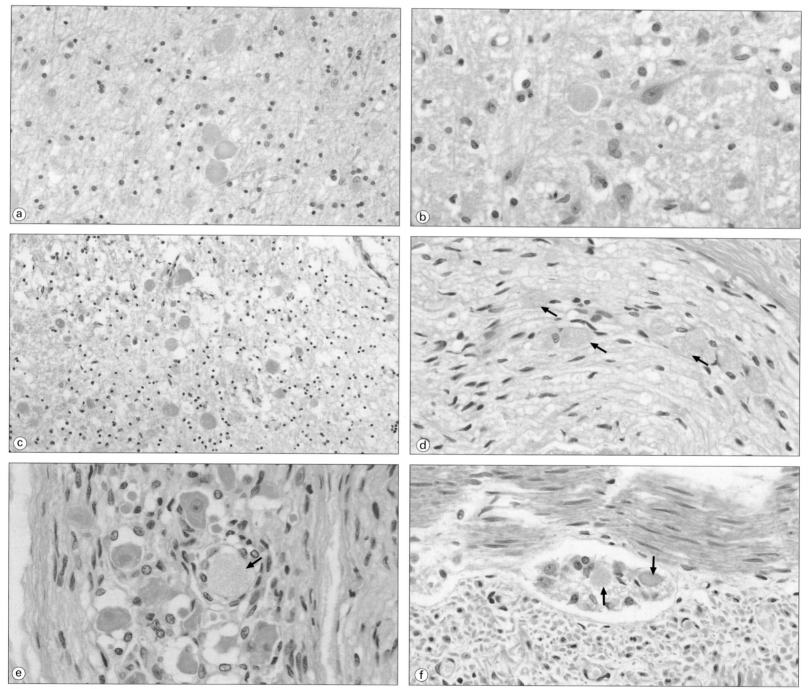

Fig. 33.8 Infantile neuroaxonal dystrophy. (a) Axonal spheroids are widely distributed in both white and gray matter in the CNS, as shown here in the hemispheric white matter. **(b)** Axonal spheroids in the basal ganglia. **(c)** Axonal spheroids are especially prominent in long tracts in the spinal cord. **(d)** Dystrophic axonal swellings (arrows) composed of granular eosinophilic material are also seen in peripheral nerves. **(e)** Dystrophic axonal swellings (arrowhead) and a demyelinating neuron (arrow) in sympathetic ganglia. **(f)** Dystrophic axonal swellings (arrows) in the myenteric plexus of the gut. In the CNS, the formation of spheroids is followed by loss of myelin, neuronal degeneration, and astrocytic gliosis.

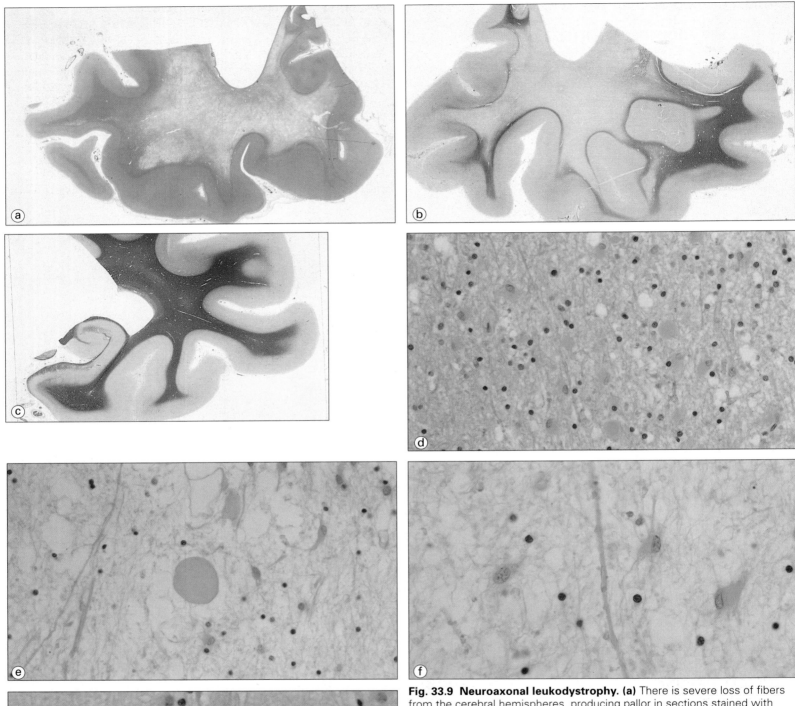

Fig. 33.9 Neuroaxonal leukodystrophy. (a) There is severe loss of fibers from the cerebral hemispheres, producing pallor in sections stained with hematoxylin and eosin. **(b)** The severe loss of fibers from the cerebral hemispheres also produces pallor in sections stained for myelin. The subcortical fibers are spared. **(c)** In a personally studied case, the temporal lobes were also relatively spared, as shown here. **(d)** Mildly affected regions show axonal spheroids with relative preservation of fiber density. **(e)** In severely affected regions, there are scattered spheroids amidst few preserved axons. **(f)** Astrocytic gliosis of white matter is prominent in severely affected white matter. **(g)** Small numbers of spheroids (arrow) are seen in the cerebral cortex.

HALLERVORDEN–SPATZ DISEASE

- Autosomal recessive inheritance is probable in many cases, but a gene has not yet been identified.
- Patients affected before 15 years of age:
  - develop a gait disorder with rigidity of the legs, and dystonia
  - progression of disease leads to motor slowing, dysarthria, cognitive decline, and, frequently, choreoathetosis
  - mean survival is 11 years.
- Patients affected in later life:
  - develop an extrapyramidal movement disorder

- show progressive cognitive decline, leading to dementia
- Computerized tomographic (CT) scans show high-signal lesions in the globus pallidus on both sides.
- Magnetic resonance imaging (MRI) (T_2-weighted) shows low signal in the globus pallidus with a central small area of hyperintensity (the 'eye of the tiger' sign).
- Some patients have associated hypoprebetalipoproteinemia, acanthocytosis, and retinitis pigmentosa (HARP syndrome).

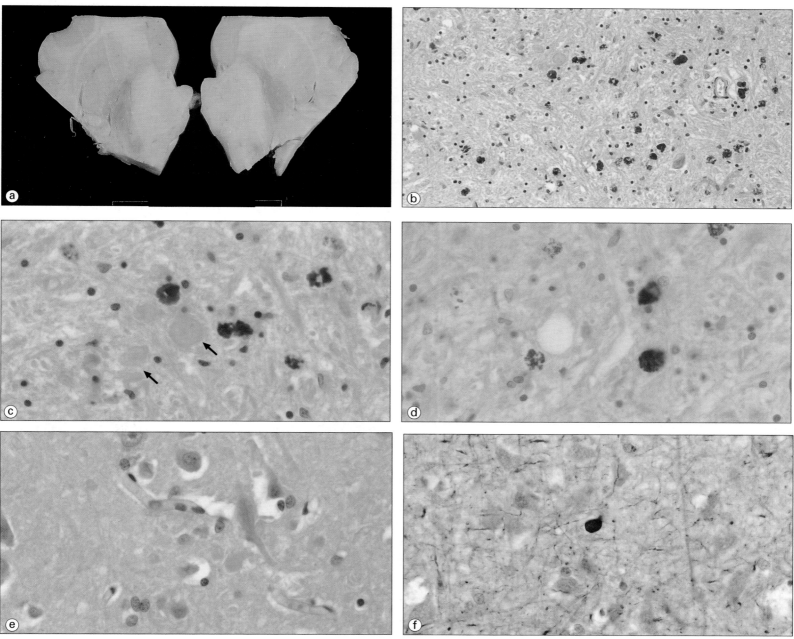

Fig. 33.10 Hallervorden–Spatz disease. (a) Macroscopically, the globus pallidus is rust-brown and atrophic. **(b)** The globus pallidus shows neuronal loss and gliosis and a conspicuous accumulation of pigment, seen as darkly stained material. **(c)** Closer examination reveals rounded eosinophilic axonal spheroids (arrows). **(d)** Pigment is present in surviving neurons, within spheroids, and in astrocytes. Some of the pigment, mostly around blood vessels, appears to be extracellular. The pigment contains lipofuscin, neuromelanin, and iron, which appears blue in this section by Perls' method. **(e)** Small numbers of spheroids can be seen in the cerebral cortex. **(f)** The spheroids in the cerebral cortex can be highlighted by silver impregnation, or immunohistochemistry for neurofilamant protein, as shown here.

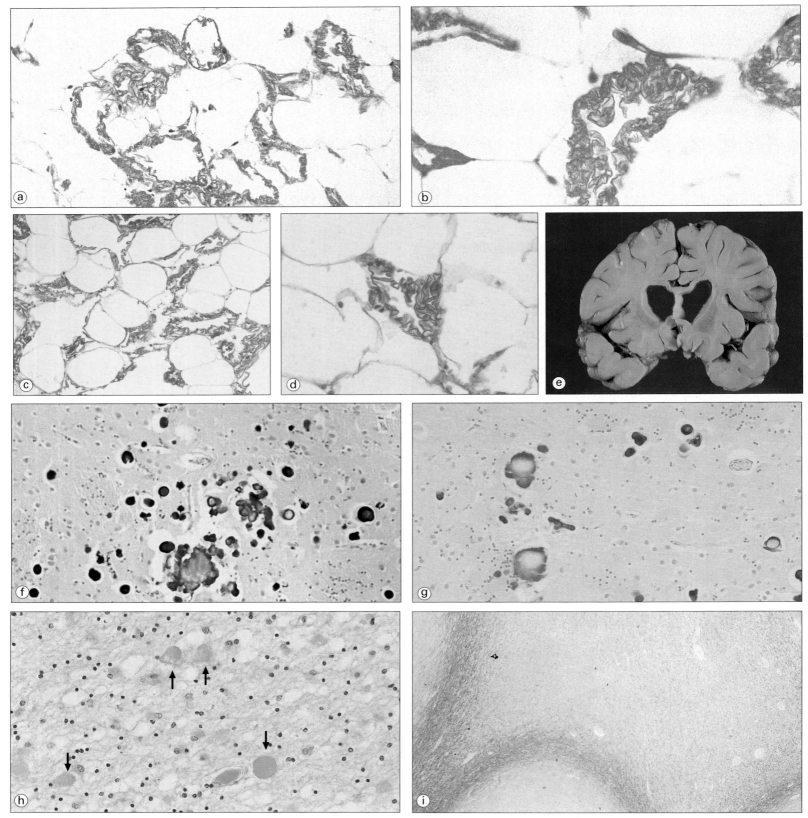

Fig. 33.11 Nasu–Hakola disease. (a) Histology reveals membranocystic lesions in adipose tissue, including that of bone marrow. The lesions are characterized by marked thickening and wrinkling of the plasma membrane of adipocytes. **(b)** At a higher magnification the complex infolding of the adipocyte membrane can be better appreciated. **(c)** This is well demonstrated on periodic acid–Schiff (PAS) staining. Individual lesions appear to coalesce to produce larger microcysts. In subcutaneous fat this degenerative change may be associated with dystrophic mineralization. **(d)** Higher magnification highlights the complex infolding of adipocyte membrane. **(e)** The brain shows atrophy with ventricular dilatation. There is softening and loss of hemispheric white matter. **(f)** The basal ganglia are typically severely shrunken and densely mineralized. Sections of the basal ganglia show atrophy, neuronal loss, astrocytic gliosis, microcysts, and severe mineralization. **(g)** The mineral deposits contain iron, which stains blue in sections stained by Perls' method. **(h)** The hemispheric white matter appears rarefied due to loss of myelinated fibers, and contains many axonal spheroids (arrows). Foci of mineralization may also be found. **(i)** There is relative sparing of subcortical fibers, stained blue in this preparation. (Luxol fast blue/cresyl violet)

NASU–HAKOLA DISEASE

This disorder is also called polycystic lipomembranous osteodysplasia with sclerosing leukoencephalopathy.

MACROSCOPIC AND MICROSCOPIC APPEARANCES

Adipocytes in subcutaneous tissue, bone marrow, and elsewhere show membranocystic (lipomembranous) lesions (**Fig. 33.11**). There is considerable loss of myelinated fibers from the hemispheric white matter, which contains many axonal spheroids. Severe neuronal loss with mineralization is seen in the basal ganglia, and in some cases, the thalamus (see Fig. 33.11f). Peripheral nerves may also be affected.

GIANT AXONAL NEUROPATHY
MACROSCOPIC AND MICROSCOPIC APPEARANCES

The peripheral nerves contain swollen axons with closely packed neurofilaments. There is gray discoloration and atrophy of the deep white matter in the cerebrum (**Fig. 33.12a**), the cerebellum, and the long tracts in the spinal cord. The brain and spinal cord contain many dystrophic axonal swellings, particularly in the corticospinal tracts, middle and inferior cerebellar peduncles, and posterior columns of the spinal cord (**Fig. 33.12b**). Smaller numbers of axonal swellings are present in the cerebral cortex (**Fig. 33.12c–e**) and basal ganglia. Numerous Rosenthal fibers are present in the white matter (**Fig. 33.12f**) and may

GIANT AXONAL NEUROPATHY

- Autosomal recessive disorder of unknown etiology.
- Most patients have tightly curled or kinky hair.
- Slowly progressive weakness and sensory loss commence within the first few years of life.
- By the start of the second decade most patients have developed spasticity, cerebellar ataxia, and dementia in addition to the peripheral neuropathy.
- A giant axonal neuropathy that is also autosomal recessive but may be genetically distinct has been described in a Tunisian kindred, in which the peripheral neuropathy is associated with prominent distal amyotrophy, brisk reflexes, and bulbar signs. Kinky hair has not been a feature.

NASU–HAKOLA DISEASE

- Autosomal recessive disorder of unknown etiology.
- Most reported patients have been from Japan and Scandinavia, with rare cases from elsewhere.
- Onset is non-neurologic in the second decade, with repeated bone fractures caused by multiple bone cysts, which are best seen in the small bones of the hands and feet.
- In the third decade patients develop neurobehavioral abnormalities and parkinsonism, progressing to dementia.
- Imaging shows cerebral atrophy with degeneration of the cerebral white matter and marked mineralization of the basal ganglia.
- There may be mineralization of soft tissues resembling calcinosis cutis.

cluster around blood vessels in a pattern resembling that of Alexander's disease (**Fig. 33.12g**) (see chapter 5). Occasional large multinucleated astrocytes may be seen (**Fig. 33.12h**). Abnormal accumulations of intermediate filaments have been noted in Schwann cells, fibroblasts, melanocytes, endothelial, and Langerhans' cells in some cases. Electron microscopy has shown longitudinal grooving of the kinky hairs.

SECONDARY NEUROAXONAL DYSTROPHY

The physiologic neuroaxonal dystrophy that affects certain regions of the CNS in the elderly (see p. 33.4) may be accentuated in:
- Parkinson's disease.
- Wilson's disease.
- chronic alcoholic liver disease.

More widespread neuroaxonal dystrophy may be a feature of several metabolic and other systemic disorders including:
- vitamin E deficiency (see chapter 21), particularly in association with cystic fibrosis, congenital biliary atresia, ataxia with isolated vitamin E deficiency caused by mutations in α-tocopherol transfer protein, and Bassen–Kornzweig syndrome (abetalipoproteinemia).
- Niemann–Pick disease type C.
- Zellweger's syndrome.
- human T cell leukemia/lymphoma virus-1 (HTLV-1) infection.

Dystrophic axonal swellings and focal white matter necrosis are also features of methotrexate leukoencephalopathy (see chapter 25) and the multifocal necrotizing leukoencephalopathy that occurs in several other clinical contexts (see chapter 22).

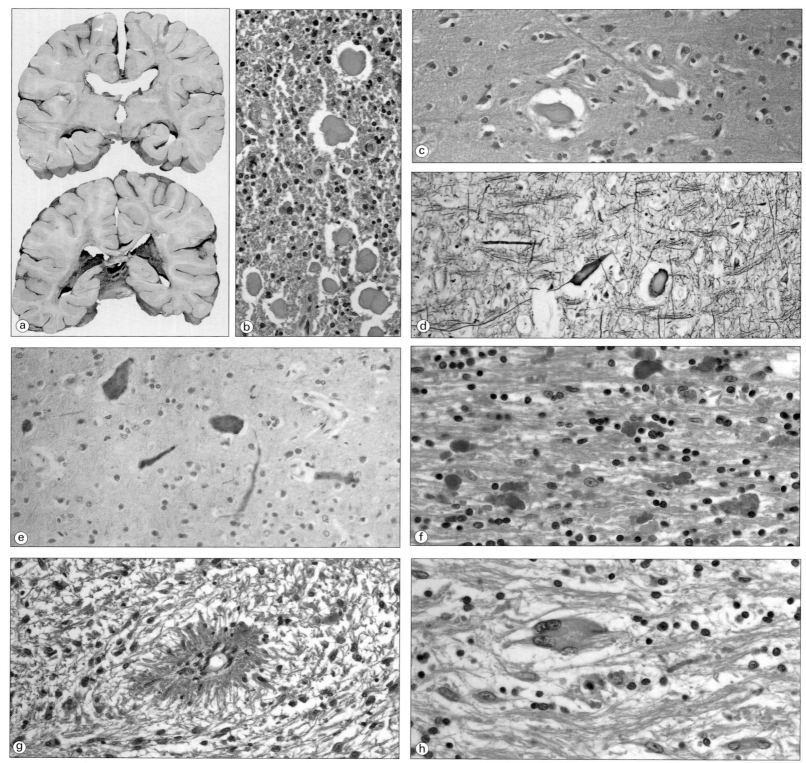

Fig. 33.12 Giant axonal neuropathy. (a) Shrinkage and gelatinous gray discoloration of the white matter in longstanding giant axonal neuropathy. The periventricular and parasagittal frontal white matter is most severely affected. **(b)** Numerous dystrophic axonal swellings in the posterior columns of the cervical spinal cord. **(c)** Scattered axonal swellings in the cerebral cortex in sections stained with hematoxylin and eosin. **(d)** Scattered axonal swellings in the cerebral cortex in sections stained by Bielschowsky's silver impregnation (toned). **(e)** Scattered axonal swellings in the cerebral cortex in sections stained with antibody to neurofilament protein. **(f)** The white matter contains large numbers of deeply eosinophilic Rosenthal fibers. **(g)** The clustering of Rosenthal fibers around blood vessels may simulate that of Alexander's disease. **(h)** Large multinucleated astrocyte in the centrum semiovale in giant axonal neuropathy.

CENTRAL AUTONOMIC FAILURE

Introduction and classification

Autonomic failure can be divided into primary and secondary types (**Fig. 33.13**). Diabetes mellitus is the commonest cause of autonomic failure. Of the remaining patients, about 50% have a primary autonomic failure and the other 50% autonomic failure secondary to an identifiable cause.

Primary central forms of autonomic failure are divided into those associated with parkinsonism (Shy–Drager syndrome) and the subgroup of pure progressive autonomic failure.

SHY–DRAGER SYNDROME

This is a syndrome of sympathetic insufficiency (the manifestations of which include chronic orthostatic hypotension, urinary incontinence, and absence of sweating) and parkinsonism. Although sometimes regarded as synonymous with a subtype of multiple system atrophy, Shy–Drager syndrome can also occur in patients who have Lewy body pathology:

- In both multiple system atrophy and Lewy body-associated disease, autonomic dysfunction is related to loss of cells from the intermediolateral column of the spinal cord (**Fig. 33.14a–c**).
- In multiple system atrophy, the typical glial cytoplasmic inclusions are widely distributed (**Fig. 33.14d,e**), supraspinal autonomic nuclei may be affected, and characteristic abnormalities are present in the substantia nigra and other regions of the brain (see chapter 28).

- In Lewy body-associated disease, there are also degenerative changes with Lewy bodies in the substantia nigra and elsewhere in the brain (see chapter 28), and in the peripheral sympathetic ganglia.

PURE PROGRESSIVE AUTONOMIC FAILURE

Pure progressive autonomic failure may be central or peripheral:
- Central disease is due to Lewy body pathology in the absence of clinical nigral involvement, or multiple system atrophy pathology in the absence of clinical involvement of other systems.
- Peripheral disease is associated with biochemical evidence of a low plasma norepinephrine (noradrenaline) concentration.

BRADBURY–EGGLESTON SYNDROME

This syndrome is a clinical diagnosis (of exclusion) used to describe patients who have pure autonomic failure with no other neurologic features. Some patients later develop features of parkinsonism and can then be classified as having Shy–Drager syndrome, while others have a low plasma norepinephrine concentration in keeping with a loss of postganglionic sympathetic efferent neurons.

Classification and causes of autonomic failure
Primary autonomic failure
• multiple system atrophy   • Lewy body disease   • progressive autonomic failure due to postganglionic pathology   • dopamine β-hydroxylase deficiency   • Bradbury–Eggleston syndrome (idiopathic)
Secondary autonomic failure

• structural lesions of central pathways in corticolimbic, hypothalamic, brain stem or spinal regions
 • Wernicke's encephalopathy
 • baroreceptor failure
 • botulism
 • acute autonomic neuropathy
 • peripheral neuropathy
   • diabetic
   • amyloid
   • inflammatory
   • alcoholic
   • toxic and drug-related
   • chronic renal failure
   • paraneoplastic
   • connective tissue disease
   • acute intermittent porphyria
   • familial neuropathy

Fig. 33.13 Classification and causes of autonomic failure.

NECROPSY IN AUTONOMIC FAILURE

Clinical information should be sought concerning:
- diabetes mellitus
- alcoholism
- renal failure
- connective tissue disease
- familial peripheral nerve disease

Blocks for histology should include samples from:
- brain and spinal cord
- peripheral nerve
- autonomic ganglia from sympathetic chain
- adrenal glands
- vagus nerve
- dorsal root ganglia

Examination of the CNS should concentrate on identifying:
- Lewy body pathology
- glial cytoplasmic inclusions of multiple system atrophy

Systemic and peripheral nerve examination should concentrate on excluding:
- peripheral neuropathy (particularly diabetic neuropathy, inflammatory neuropathy, and amyloid)

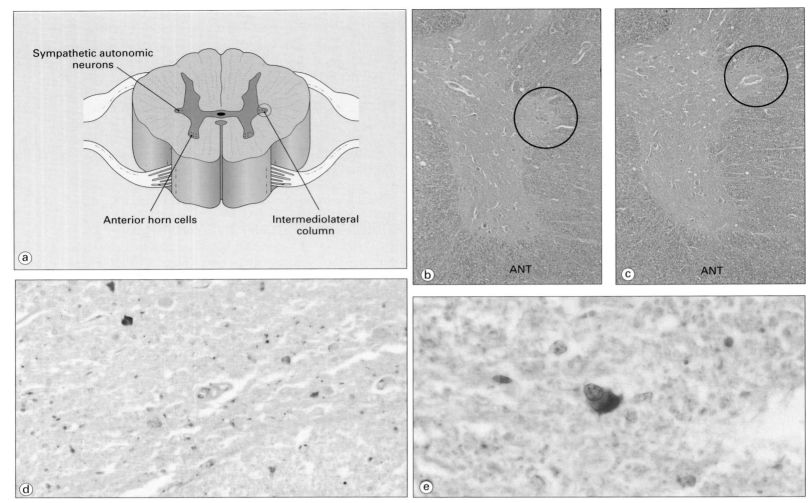

Fig. 33.14 Spinal autonomic neurons in autonomic failure. (a) The intermediolateral column contains preganglionic sympathetic neurons. **(b)** The intermediolateral group of neurons (in ring) is found in the lateral column in the thoracic spinal cord (ANT=anterior). They are preganglionic sympathetic neurons. The number of intermediolateral column neurons is greater in the upper thoracic cord segments than in the lower ones. **(c)** In central autonomic failure, these intermediolateral column neurons are reduced in number thoughout the thoracic cord and there is mild astrocytic gliosis. Because of the variability in the number of intermediolateral column neurons at any one level, counts should be obtained from several levels before a loss of preganglionic sympathetic neurons can be diagnosed. **(d)** In autonomic failure caused by multiple system atrophy, small numbers of glial cytoplasmic inclusions can be found in the intermediolateral column, as shown in these sections immunostained for ubiquitin. **(e)** MSA inclusion stained with anti-tau antibody.

REFERENCES

Antoine JC *et al.* (1985) Hallervorden–Spatz disease with Lewy bodies. *Rev Neurol Paris* **141**: 806–809.

Axelsson R *et al.* (1984) Hereditary diffuse leukoencephalopathy with spheroids. *Acta Psychiatr Scand* **314**: 225–228.

Eidelberg D *et al.* (1987) Adult onset Hallervorden–Spatz disease with neurofibrillary pathology. *Brain* **110**: 993–1013

Elleder M *et al.* (1985) Niemann–Pick disease type C. Study on the nature of the cerebral storage process. *Acta Neuropathol* **66**: 325–336.

Gray F *et al.* (1985) Luyso-pallido-nigral atrophy and amyotrophic lateral sclerosis. *Acta Neuropathol* **66**: 78–82.

Higgins JJ *et al.* (1992) Hypoprebetalipoproteinemia, acanthocytosis, retinitis pigmentosa, and pallidal degeneration (HARP syndrome). *Neurology* **42**: 194–198.

Jellinger K. (1986) Pallidal, pallidonigral and pallidoluysionigral degenerations including association with thalamic and dentate degenerations. *Handbook of Clinical Neurology: Extrapyramidal Disorders.* Vinken P and Bryan G (eds) pp. 445–464. Amsterdam: Elsevier.

Martin J. (1975) Thalamic degenerations. *Handbook of Clinical Neurology. Extrapyramidal disorders.* Vinken P and Bryan G (eds) pp. 587–604. Amsterdam: Elsevier.

McLeod JG, Tuck RR. (1987) Disorders of the autonomic nervous system: Part 1. Pathophysiology and clinical features. *Ann Neurol* **21**: 419–430.

Miyazu K *et al.* (1991) Membranous lipodystrophy (Nasu–Hakola disease) with thalamic degeneration: Report of an autopsied case. *Acta Neuropathol* **82**: 414–419.

Robertson D, Robertson RM. (1994) Causes of chronic orthostatic hypotension. *Arch Intern Med* **154**: 1620–1624.

Seitelberger F. (1986) Neuroaxonal dystrophy: its relation to aging and neurological diseases. In P Vinken, G Bruyn, H Klawans (eds) *Extrapyramidal Disorders.* pp. 391–415. Amsterdam: Elsevier Scientific.

Wang AM *et al.* (1990) Schindler disease: the molecular lesion in the alpha-N-acetylgalactosaminidase gene that causes an infantile neuroaxonal dystrophy. *J Clin Invest* **86**: 1752–1756.

Wijker M *et al.* (1996) Localization of the gene for rapidly progressive autosomal dominant parkinsonism and dementia with pallido-ponto-nigral degeneration to chromosome 17q21. *Hum Mol Genet* **5**: 151–154.

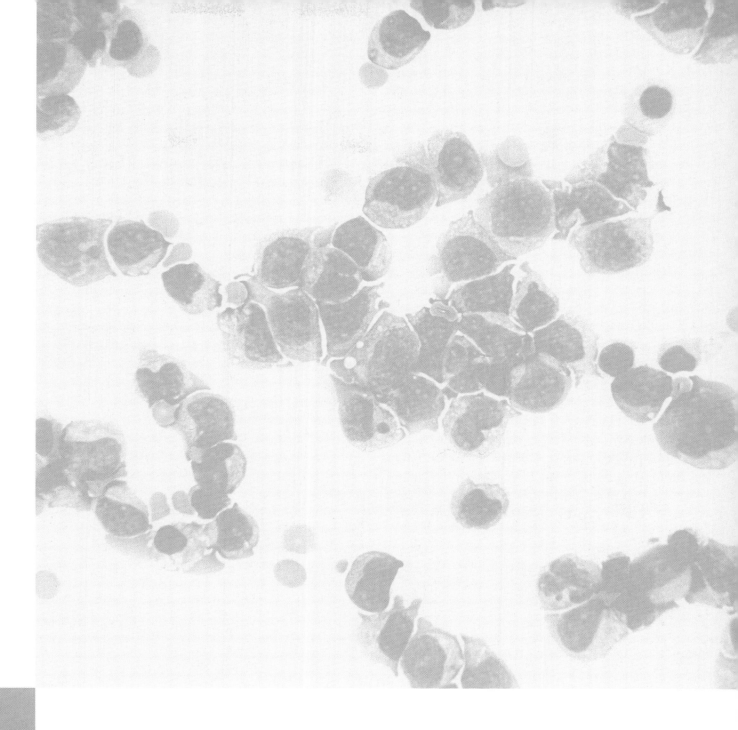

10 Neoplasms

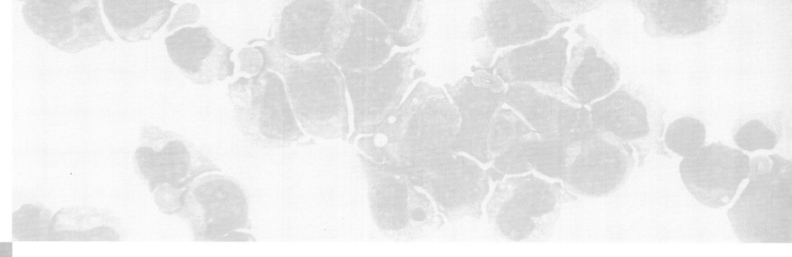

34 *Classification and general concepts of CNS neoplasms*

The opening chapter of this section considers general clinicopathologic aspects of CNS neoplasms and the role of the pathologist in their management. The clinical, biologic, genetic, and histologic characteristics of the principal categories of CNS neoplasms are dealt with in the subsequent chapters in this section. These chapters also include advice on discriminating between neoplasms with similar histologic appearances.

CNS NEOPLASMS

Primary CNS neoplasms account for:
- ~ 2% of all cancers.
- ~ 20% of cancers in children under 15 years of age.

Most primary CNS neoplasms are neuroepithelial (**Fig. 34.1**). The proportion of CNS neoplasms that is due to spread from a primary neoplasm outside the nervous system varies greatly (14–40%) between reports. Selection bias confounds many epidemiologic studies that rely solely on necropsy data or series from tertiary referral centers.

Most primary CNS neoplasms are sporadic and of unknown etiology. Fewer than 5% are associated with hereditary syndromes that predispose to neoplasia (**Fig. 34.2**). Other factors (**Fig. 34.3**) are implicated in only a small proportion of cases.

The clinical presentations of CNS neoplasms depend largely on their site (**Fig. 34.4**) and nature (see Fig. 34.1). Terminal events are usually related to raised intracranial pressure (**Figs 34.5, 34.6**).

CNS NEOPLASMS

CNS neoplasms present with:
- epilepsy (focal or generalized)
- focal neurologic deficits
- symptoms and signs of raised intracranial pressure
- symptoms and signs of hydrocephalus

Location will determine the symptoms and signs of focal epilepsy and neurologic deficit

Symptoms and signs of raised intracranial pressure include:
- headache (particularly postural and nocturnal or early morning)
- vomiting (particularly children)
- clouding of consciousness and coma
- papilledema

Neoplasms and cysts that often present with hydrocephalus include:
- any posterior fossa neoplasm (particularly primitive neuroectodermal tumor and ependymoma)
- pineal gland neoplasms
- subependymal giant cell astrocytoma
- hypothalamic pilocytic astrocytoma
- central neurocytoma
- colloid cyst of the third ventricle

Fig. 34.1 Neoplasms of the CNS. (The figures represent a synthesis of several sources of data and are approximate.)

Neoplasms of the CNS					
Intracranial neoplasms		Intracranial neoplasms – patients aged > 15 yrs		Intracranial neoplasms – patients aged ≤ 15 yrs	
Glioblastoma and anaplastic astrocytoma	35%	Glioblastoma and anaplastic astrocytoma	35%	Glioblastoma and anaplastic astrocytoma	4%
Astrocytoma	13%	Astrocytoma	12%	Astrocytoma	44%
Other neuroepithelial neoplasms	8%	Other neuroepithelial neoplasms	8%	Other neuroepithelial neoplasms	15%
Meningiomas	17%	Meningiomas & nerve sheath tumors	25%	Meningiomas & nerve sheath tumors	3%
PNETs	3%	PNETs	2%	PNETs	24%
Nerve sheath tumors	8%	Other neoplasms	18%	Other neoplasms	10%
Other neoplasms	16%				

Although understanding of the biology of CNS neoplasms has improved significantly in the last decade alongside knowledge of the mechanisms of neoplastic transformation, therapeutic advances have yet to reverse what is for most CNS neoplasms a poor prognosis. Only about 50% of patients with a CNS neoplasm are alive one year after diagnosis.

Inheritable syndromes carrying an increased risk for CNS neoplasms

Syndrome	Gene locus	Gene	Type(s) of CNS neoplasm
Neurofibromatosis type 1	17q11	NF1	neurofibroma; malignant nerve sheath tumor; optic nerve glioma; meningioma
Neurofibromatosis type 2	22q12	NF2	schwannoma; meningioma; ependymoma
Tuberous sclerosis	9q34/16p13	TSC1/TSC2	subependymal giant cell astrocytoma
Von Hippel–Lindau	3p25	VHL	hemangioblastoma
Li–Fraumeni syndrome	17q13	p53	glioma
Gorlin's syndrome	9q31	?	medulloblastoma
Turcot's syndrome	5q21	APC	astrocytoma; glioblastoma; medulloblastoma
Cowden's disease	10q23	PTEN	dysplastic gangliocytoma of cerebellum
Multiple endocrine neoplasia type 1	11q13	?	pituitary adenoma

Fig. 34.2 Inheritable syndromes carrying an increased risk for CNS neoplasms.

Factors in the etiology of CNS neoplasms

1a Sex:
   • gliomas are commoner (60:40) in men
   • meningiomas are commoner (67:33) in women

1b An association exists in women between the development of breast carcinoma and meningioma; both tumors may express sex hormone receptors

2 Exposure to ionizing radiation has been implicated in the genesis of:
   • meningiomas
   • gliomas
   • nerve sheath tumors

3a Primary CNS lymphoma is associated with immunodeficiency

3b Epstein–Barr virus has been found in a very high proportion of primary CNS lymphomas from immunocompromised patients

4 Nitroso compounds, particularly nitrosoureas, cause CNS neoplasms in experimental animals, yet evidence to implicate these compounds in the genesis of human CNS neoplasms has not been forthcoming.

5 No *convincing* evidence has linked CNS neoplasms with:
   • trauma
   • occupation
   • diet
   • electromagnetic fields

Fig. 34.3 Factors in the etiology of CNS neoplasms.

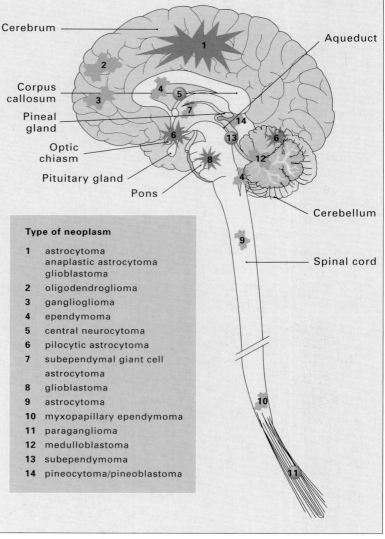

Type of neoplasm

1 astrocytoma
   anaplastic astrocytoma
   glioblastoma
2 oligodendroglioma
3 ganglioglioma
4 ependymoma
5 central neurocytoma
6 pilocytic astrocytoma
7 subependymal giant cell astrocytoma
8 glioblastoma
9 astrocytoma
10 myxopapillary ependymoma
11 paraganglioma
12 medulloblastoma
13 subependymoma
14 pineocytoma/pineoblastoma

Fig. 34.4 Common locations of various neuroepithelial neoplasms .

RAISED INTRACRANIAL PRESSURE

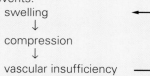

- As an intracranial neoplasm grows and edema accumulates in tissues around it, the contents of the skull, which behaves as a rigid box, are compressed.
- Within the skull the brain occupies approximately 1400 ml, cerebrospinal fluid (CSF) occupies 100–200 ml, and blood occupies 100–150 ml.
- Displacement of CSF (from the cranial compartment to the spinal compartment) and a reduction in blood volume in the cerebral veins compensate initially for the mass effect of a neoplasm. After this compensatory phase, intracranial pressure (ICP) rises quickly.
- In infants, the skull may enlarge because sutures and fontanelles have not fused.
- Mass effect from a neoplasm produces a vicious circle of events:

  swelling
  ↓
  compression
  ↓
  vascular insufficiency

This combination of events exacerbates the rise in ICP and leads to herniation of brain tissue from the affected intracranial compartment to another, in which the pressure is lower. Any obstruction of CSF pathways produces hydrocephalus which exacerbates the abnormalities.

Types of herniation

- Central (transtentorial): herniation of the diencephalon through the tentorium.
- Parahippocampal: herniation of the medial part of the temporal lobe across the tentorium (or uncal herniation, if only the anteromedial part of the temporal lobe is involved).
- Subfalcine: herniation of the cingulate gyrus beneath the falx.
- Tonsillar: herniation of the cerebellar tonsils through the foramen magnum (may follow central herniation).
- Superior cerebellar: herniation of the cerebellum upwards through the tentorium (posterior fossa neoplasms).

Blood vessels that may be compressed during herniation

- The microvasculature may be compressed at any site of increased pressure.
- The anterior cerebral artery may be compressed against the falx.
- The posterior cerebral artery may be compressed against the tentorium.

FALSE LOCALIZING SIGNS

Certain false localizing signs (so-called because they do not indicate the true location of the neoplasm) are associated with the compression of structures by the diencephalon displaced by the mass effect of a neoplasm.

- the oculomotor nerve being distorted or compressed by the herniated uncus, or by the posterior cerebral artery as it is displaced downwards by parahippocampal or central transtentorial herniation.
- the abducens nerve being compressed against the petrous ligament.
- ipsilateral hemiparesis may result from compression of the cerebral peduncle against the tentorium.
- posterior cerebral artery territory infarction may follow compression of the artery against the tentorium.

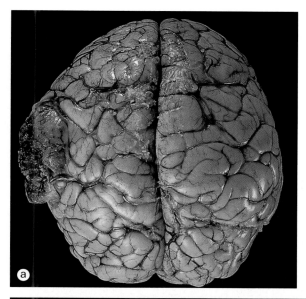

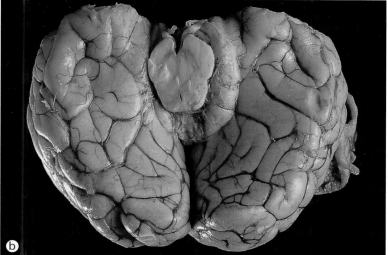

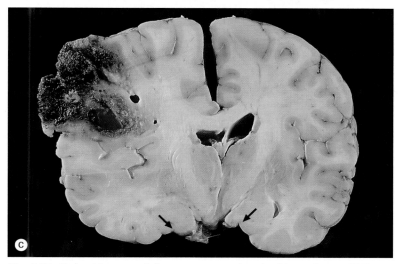

Fig. 34.5 Raised intracranial pressure associated with a primary CNS neoplasm. (a) Fatal brain swelling associated with a large left frontoparietal glioblastoma and resulting in flattened compacted cerebral gyri. Brain weight was 1680 g. **(b)** Examination of the undersurface of the brain revealing moderate herniation of the right parahippocampal gyrus and marked herniation of the left uncus and parahippocampal gyrus. **(c)** A coronal section showing the hemorrhagic glioblastoma and asymmetric swelling of the cerebrum. There is displacement of midline structures to the right, downwards displacement of the diencephalon, and distortion of part of the left cingulate gyrus secondary to subfalcine herniation. Grooves are present (arrows) on the inferomedial aspect of the temporal lobes where these have been indented by the edge of the tentorium.

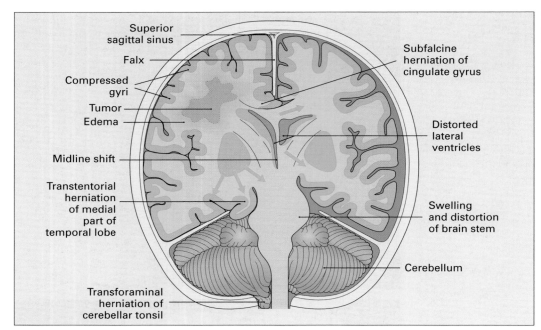

Fig. 34.6 The mass effects of a cerebral neoplasm. Tumor and associated edema distort the normal anatomy of the brain, eventually producing fatal raised intracranial pressure.

THE PATHOLOGIST AND CNS NEOPLASMS

Communication of relevant clinical and radiologic details to the pathologist is often helpful in preoperative planning and intraoperative management, and may be essential for accurate diagnosis.

The clinical details that may help the pathologist to narrow the differential diagnosis include:

- age
- sex
- family history (e.g. of syndromes predisposing to CNS neoplasms)
- relevant medical history (e.g. of neoplasia)
- duration of presenting symptoms
- site of neoplasm

At operation, neurosurgeons can provide information about the macroscopic appearance of a neoplasm and its relationship to adjacent normal structures. It may not be possible to preserve this relationship during the surgery and the pathologist is often presented with tissue fragments, which can be interpreted only in the light of an explanation from the surgeon as to their anatomic interrelationship. Useful histologic information, even a firm diagnosis, may be obtained intraoperatively by examination of touch preparations, smears, or cryostat sections (**Figs. 34.7, 34.10**).

More detailed examination of the tissue, including immunohistochemistry and electron microscopy, may be undertaken later after it has been fixed. Immunohistochemistry may aid the pathologist by demonstrating the production of proteins indicative of cellular ontogeny or proliferative activity (**Figs 34.8, 34.9**).

Although developments in immunohistochemistry have reduced the role of electron microscopy in the diagnosis of neoplasms, the detection of ultrastructural features that reveal the origins of particular types of neoplastic cells is still occasionally useful.

The pathologist not only makes the diagnosis, but also provides information about a neoplasm's likely biologic behavior and response to adjuvant therapy. The pathologist will often have responsibility for providing tissue for the molecular genetic assessment of CNS neoplasms. The impact of this on diagnosis and therapy in the future will almost certainly increase. Although some molecular genetic analysis is feasible on paraffin-embedded formalin-fixed tissue, frozen tissue should be retained if sufficient material is available, particularly if there are unusual clinical features or a family history of neoplasia.

Postmortem examination of CNS neoplasms (**Fig. 34.11**) provides

Perioperative pathologic assessment of CNS mass lesions

The aims of perioperative pathologic assessment of CNS mass lesions are to establish whether:

- sufficient material has been obtained for diagnostic purposes (including supplementary studies, such as electron microscopy).
- a neoplastic process is present.
- the course of the operation will be determined by a particular diagnosis.
- total removal of a neoplasm has been achieved, where this is desired.

Fresh tissue may be examined by three methods:
- touch preparation
- smear
- frozen section

Touch preparation:

A fragment of tissue is dabbed several times on a slide, the preparation is air-dried, and can be stained by various methods (haematoxylin and eosin / toluidine blue / Giemsa). This approach is valuable if only a limited quantity of tissue is available.

Smear:

A small quantity of soft tissue is squashed between two slides (**Fig. 34.10**), and the material is smeared across the touching surfaces of the two slides before brief fixation in alcohol. The tissue is then stained with toluidine blue, or hematoxylin and eosin.

Smear preparations are particularly good for assessment of glial tumors.

Frozen section:

Tissue is snap-frozen in liquid nitrogen, 5 μm sections are cut on a cryostat, and subsequently stained. Hematoxylin and eosin are appropriate for staining frozen sections, but a hematoxylin/van Gieson or a reticulin preparation takes little additional time and may be a useful adjunct.

Frozen sections are particularly good for firm specimens that are difficult or impossible to smear. These include many vasoformative neoplasms and craniopharyngiomas, and some schwannomas and meningiomas.

Freshly resected tissue should be regarded as potentially infectious and handled in a safety cabinet. If the clinical details suggest a significant risk of infection from the specimen, avoid using a cryostat. The preparation of tissue smears in a cabinet carries few hazards and is likely to provide the required information.

Fig. 34.7 Perioperative pathologic assessment of CNS mass lesions.

information on the histologic aspects of the entire neoplasm, the inter-action between neoplastic cells and surrounding normal tissues, and the effects of treatment.

The most practical way for a pathologist to provide information about a neoplasm's histopathology and anticipated behavior is to conform to a recognized scheme of classifying CNS neoplasms. The World Health Organization's classification of CNS neoplasms (**Fig. 34.13**) is the product of international consensus and combines elements of classifications based on ontogenesis (e.g. that of Bailey and Cushing) and measures of cytologic atypia (e.g. that of Ringertz).

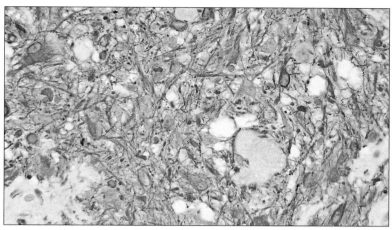

Fig. 34.8 Immunohistochemistry reveals protein production indicative of cellular onotogeny. Astrocytic cells in a ganglioglioma are highlighted with an antibody to GFAP.

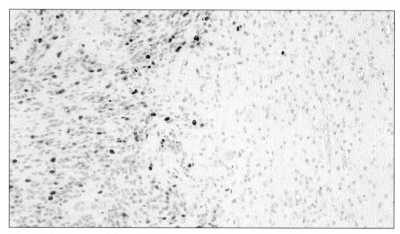

Fig. 34.9 Immunohistochemistry reveals protein production indicative of proliferative activity. The growth fraction in different regions of this ependymoma can be assessed with an antibody to Ki-67.

Necropsy examination of a patient with a CNS neoplasm

- A general rather than limited (CNS) examination is desirable, looking for:
  - evidence of systemic metastasis from a primary CNS neoplasm
  - the location of a primary systemic neoplasm when the CNS neoplasm is secondary
  - stigmata of any hereditary disorder that has induced a CNS neoplasm
  - endocrine effects associated with a pituitary adenoma / sellar tumor (hypopituitarism)
- The relationship between any CNS neoplasm and adjacent bony structures should be examined.
- A sellar neoplasm should be studied after removal of the pituitary fossa en bloc. The whole specimen can be examined histologically after decalcification.
- A neoplasm in the auditory meatus should be studied after removal of a wedge of petrous temporal bone containing the internal auditory meatus and inner ear (**Fig. 34.12**).
- The brain and spinal cord should each be removed intact, and fixed by suspension in an appropriate fixative (e.g. 10% neutral buffered formalin) after the fresh brain has been weighed.

Fig. 34.11 Necropsy examination of a patient with a CNS neoplasm.

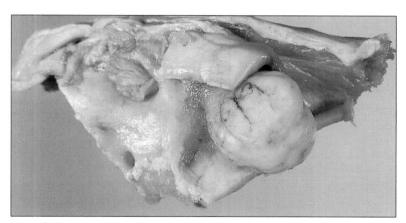

Fig. 34.12 Assessment of the relationship of a neoplasm to adjacent bony structure. A wedge of temporal bone containing the internal auditory meatus and showing a schwannoma of the eighth cranial nerve.

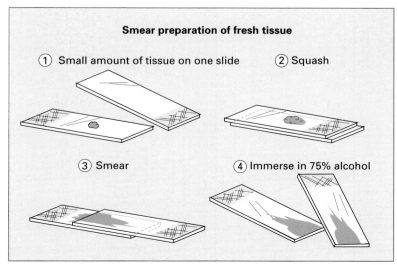

Smear preparation of fresh tissue

① Small amount of tissue on one slide   ② Squash

③ Smear   ④ Immerse in 75% alcohol

Fig. 34.10 Smear preparation of fresh tissue.

World Health Organization classification of CNS neoplasms (1993)

Tumors of neuroepithelial tissue

Astrocytic tumors
- Astrocytoma
  Variants:
    Fibrillary
    Protoplasmic
    Gemistocytic
- Anaplastic astrocytoma
- Glioblastoma
  Variants:
    Giant cell glioblastoma
    Gliosarcoma (spindle-cell glioblastoma)
- Pilocytic astrocytoma
- Pleomorphic xanthoastrocytoma
- Subependymal giant cell astrocytoma

Oligodendroglial tumors
- Oligodendroglioma
- Anaplastic oligodendroglioma

Ependymal tumors
- Ependymoma
  Variants:
    Cellular
    Papillary
    Clear cell
- Anaplastic ependymoma
- Myxopapillary ependymoma
- Subependymoma

Mixed gliomas
- Oligoastrocytoma
- Anaplastic oligoastrocytoma

Choroid plexus tumors
- Choroid plexus papilloma
- Choroid plexus carcinoma

Neuroepithelial tumors of uncertain origin
- Astroblastoma
- Polar spongioblastoma
- Gliomatosis cerebri

Neuronal and mixed neuronal-glial tumors
- Gangliocytoma
- Dysplastic gangliocytoma of cerebellum (Lhermitte-Duclos)
- Desmoplastic infantile ganglioglioma
- Dysembryoplastic neuroepithelial tumor
- Ganglioglioma
- Anaplastic ganglioglioma
- Central neurocytoma
- Paraganglioma of the filum terminale
- Olfactory neuroblastoma (esthesioneuroblastoma)

Pineal parenchymal tumors
- Pineocytoma
- Pineoblastoma
- Mixed / transitional pineal tumors

Embryonal tumors
- Medulloepithelioma
- Neuroblastoma
  Variant:
    Ganglioneuroblastoma

Tumors of neuroepithelial tissue (continued)

- Ependymoblastoma
- Primitive neuroectodermal tumors (PNETs)
    Medulloblastoma
    Variants:
      Desmoplastic medulloblastoma
      Medullomyoblastoma
      Melanotic medulloblastoma

Tumors of cranial and spinal nerves

- Schwannoma (Neurilemmoma, Neurinoma)
  Variants:
    Cellular
    Plexiform
    Melanotic
- Neurofibroma
  Variants:
    Circumscribed (solitary)
    Plexiform

- Malignant nerve sheath tumor (Neurofibrosarcoma)
  Variants:
    Epithelioid
    MNST with divergent mesenchymal and / or epithelial differentiation
    Melanotic

Tumors of the meninges

Tumors of meningothelial cells
- Meningioma
  Variants:
    Meningothelial
    Fibrous (fibroblastic)
    Transitional (mixed)
    Psammomatous
    Angiomatous
    Microcystic
    Secretory
    Clear cell
    Chordoid
    Lymphoplasmacyte-rich
    Metaplastic
- Atypical meningioma
- Papillary meningioma
- Anaplastic (malignant) meningioma

Mesenchymal, non-meningothelial tumors
Benign neoplasms
- Osteocartilaginous tumors
- Lipoma
- Fibrous histiocytoma
Malignant neoplasms
- Hemangiopericytoma
- Chondrosarcoma
  Variant:
    Mesenchymal chondrosarcoma
  Malignant fibrous histiocytoma
  Rhabdomyosarcoma
  Meningeal sarcomatosis

Tumors of the meninges

Primary melanotic lesions
- Diffuse melanosis
- Melanocytoma
- Malignant melanoma
  Variant:
    Meningeal melanomatosis

Tumours of uncertain histogenesis
- Hemangioblastoma

Lymphomas and hemopoietic neoplasms

- Malignant lymphomas
- Plasmacytoma
- Granulocytic sarcoma

Germ cell tumors

- Germinoma
- Embryonal carcinoma
- Yolk sac tumor (Endodermal sinus tumor)
- Choriocarcinoma
- Teratoma
  Variants:
    Immature
    Mature
    Teratoma with malignant transformation
- Mixed germ cell tumors

Cysts and tumor-like lesions

- Rathke cleft cyst
- Epidermoid cyst
- Dermoid cyst
- Colloid cyst of the third ventricle
- Enterogenous cyst
- Neuroglial cyst
- Granular cell tumor (Choristoma, Pituicytoma)
- Hypothalamic neuronal hamartoma
- Nasal glial heterotopia
- Plasma cell granuloma

Tumors of the sellar regin

- Pituitary adenoma
- Pituitary carcinoma
- Craniopharyngioma
  Variants:
    Adamantinomatous
    Papillary

Local extensions from regional tumors

- Paraganglioma (Chemodectoma)
- Chordoma
- Chondroma
- Chondrosarcoma
- Carcinoma

Metastatic tumors

Fig. 34.13 World Health Organization classification of CNS neoplasms.

REFERENCES

Batra SK, Rasheed BA, Bigner SH, Bigner DD. (1994) Oncogenes and anti-oncogenes in human central nervous system tumors. *Laboratory Investigation.* **71**: 621–637.

Burger PC. (1995) Revising the World Health Organization (WHO) Blue Book. Histological typing of tumors of the central nervous system. *Journal of Neuro-Oncology.* **24**: 3–7.

Burger PC Scheithauer BW. (1995) *Tumors of the Central Nervous System. Third edition.* Armed Forces Institute of Pathology. *Atlas of Tumor Pathology. Volume 10.*

Kallio M, Sankila R, Jaaskelainen, J Karjalainen T. A population based study on the incidence and survival rates of 3857 glioma patients diagnosed from 1953 to 1984. *Cancer* **68**: 1394–1400.

Langford LA. (1996) Central nervous system neoplasms: indications for electrom microscopy. *Ultrastructural Pathology.* **20**: 35–46.

Lantos PL, VandenBerg SR, Kleihues P. (1997) Tumors of the nervous system. In Graham DI and Lantos PL eds. *Greenfield's Neuropathology. Sixth edition.* pp.583–879 London: Arnold.

Preston-Martin S. (1996) Epidemiology of primary CNS neoplasms. *Neuroepidemiology* **14**: 273–290.

Russell DS, Rubinstein LJ. (1989) *Pathology of Tumours of the Nervous System. Fifth edition.* London: Edward Arnold, 1989.

Scheithauer BW. Central nervous system and pituitary. In EG Silva, BB Kraemer (eds) *Intraoperative Pathologic Diagnosis.* Baltimore: Williams and Williams.

Taratuto AL, Sevlever G, Piccardo P. (1991) Clues and pitfalls in stereotactic biopsy of the central nervous system. *Arch Pathol Lab Med* **115**: 596–602.

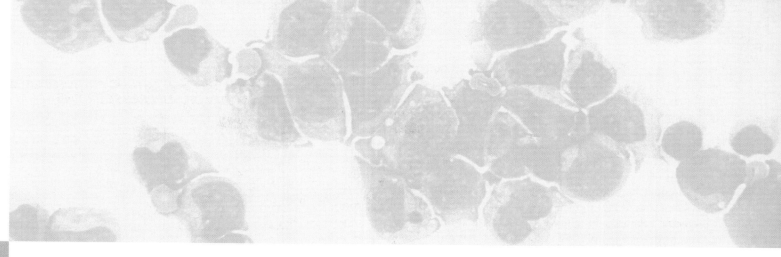

35 Astrocytic neoplasms

Glial cells give rise to most primary central nervous system (CNS) neoplasms (gliomas), and neoplasms are derived from each class of glial cell (i.e. astrocyte, oligodendrocyte, and ependymal cell). Astrocytic neoplasms are considered in this chapter and other gliomas in chapter 36. Astrocytic neoplasms listed in the World Health Organization (WHO) classification are:

- astrocytoma (fibrillary, protoplasmic, and gemistocytic)
- anaplastic astrocytoma
- glioblastoma
- pilocytic astrocytoma
- pleomorphic xanthoastrocytoma (PXA)
- subependymal giant cell astrocytoma (SEGA).

The first three (i.e. astrocytoma, anaplastic astrocytoma, and glioblastoma) form an interrelated subgroup:

- They share genetic abnormalities and a propensity to invade surrounding CNS tissue in a diffuse manner.
- Fibrillary, protoplasmic, and gemistocytic astrocytomas tend to progress to become anaplastic astrocytomas and glioblastomas.

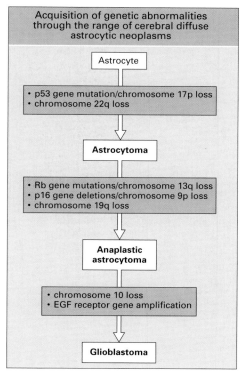

Fig. 35.1 Acquisition of genetic abnormalities through the range of diffuse astrocytic neoplasms.

Gliomatosis cerebri and meningeal gliomatosis are particularly widely infiltrative forms of astrocytic neoplasm and are also considered in this chapter. Desmoplastic infantile astrocytoma (DIA) is a rare neoplasm that shares clinical and pathologic features with the desmoplastic infantile ganglioglioma (DIGG) and is usually grouped with DIGG (see chapter 37). The astrocytic elements of both types of neoplasm share the same histologic features, but the DIA does not contain ganglion cells.

ASTROCYTOMA, ANAPLASTIC ASTROCYTOMA, AND GLIOBLASTOMA

These constitute a spectrum of diffusely invading astrocytic neoplasms that occur throughout the CNS. The term 'diffuse astrocytic neoplasms' is sometimes used for these, to distinguish them from the pilocytic astrocytoma and other rarer forms of localized astrocytic neoplasm (-pleomorphic xanthoastrocytoma and subependymal giant cell astrocytoma). The diffuse astrocytic neoplasms are commonest in the cerebrum in adults and brain stem in children. They are uncommon in the cerebellum and spinal cord. The glioblastoma has the highest incidence of any primary neuroepithelial neoplasm, accounting for approximately 50% of intracranial gliomas.

ANAPLASTIC TRANSFORMATION AND GRADING OF ASTROCYTIC NEOPLASMS

An important characteristic of the astrocytoma is its propensity for anaplastic transformation: 50–75% (in different series) of fibrillary astrocytomas progress to anaplastic astrocytomas or, ultimately, glioblastomas. This progression is associated with the acquisition of genetic abnormalities (**Fig. 35.1**). For example, p53 mutations are found in 25–35% of fibrillary astrocytomas, anaplastic astrocytomas, and glioblastomas, and are considered to be an early event in neoplastic progression. In contrast, loss of loci on chromosome 10 occurs almost exclusively in glioblastomas.

DIFFUSE ASTROCYTIC NEOPLASMS

- often present with epilepsy.
- commonly produce neurologic deficits and symptoms and signs of raised intracranial pressure at a later stage.
- generally produce cranial nerve palsies before long tract signs if in the brain stem.

Molecular genetic studies have revealed differences between glioblastomas that arise from astrocytomas (secondary) and those that arise *de novo* (primary) (**Fig. 35.2**).

Several grading systems have been applied to diffuse astrocytic neoplasms (**Fig. 35.3**). These use histologic parameters to separate the range of astrocytic neoplasms into three or four tiers, providing some indication of biologic behavior. Although there are some differences in the applied parameters, there is a broad correspondence between the systems and WHO nomenclature. Use of the WHO nomenclature is preferred because ambiguity may occur when the grading system is not specified, for example, the term 'grade 2' has different implications for treatment and prognosis in the St Anne/Mayo and Kernohan systems (**Fig. 35.4**). In addition, there is no evidence to suggest that grading systems offer any advantage over WHO nomenclature. Various clinical and pathologic variables, including histologic diagnosis, are prognostic indicators in astrocystic neoplasms (**Fig. 35.5**)

CEREBRAL DIFFUSE ASTROCYTIC NEOPLASMS AND THE p53 TUMOR SUPPRESSOR GENE

- 25–35% of these neoplasms have a p53 gene mutation.
- 45–75% show immunohistochemically demonstrable accumulation of p53 protein.
- A high p53 immunolabelling index correlates with the presence of a p53 mutation.
- Accumulation of wild-type p53 protein is not explained by alterations in the *mdm*-2 gene.
- Accumulation of p53 protein does not correlate with prognosis.

Characteristics of 2 subsets of glioblastoma

	Primary	Secondary
Mean age at biopsy§ (years)	55	39
p53 mutation present	10%	67%
Positive p53 IHC	37%	97%
p53 immunolabeling index†	low	high
Positive EGF receptor IHC	63%	10%

§		biopsy of glioblastoma
IHC		immunohistochemistry
†		this is not an absolute discriminator

(a)

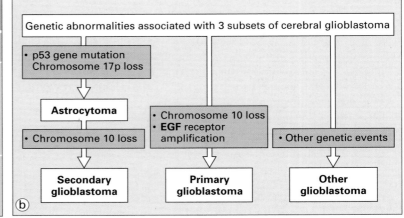

(b)

Fig. 35.2 Cerebral glioblastoma. (a) Characteristics of two subsets of glioblastoma. **(b)** Genetic abnormalities associated with three subsets of cerebral glioblastoma. Adapted from results von Deimling A. and Louis D.

Fig. 35.3 Comparison of grading systems.

Comparison of grading systems

WHO classification	WHO grade§	Kernohan¶	Ringertz	St Anne/Mayo#
Astrocytoma	II	1	astrocytoma	2
Anaplastic astrocytoma	III	2	intermediate*	3
Glioblastoma	IV	3 & 4	glioblastoma	4

§	grade 1 neoplasms are pilocytic astrocytomas
¶	grade 1 neoplasms include pilocytic astrocytomas
#	grade 1 neoplasms are very rare
*	astrocytoma with focal anaplasia

St Anne/Mayo grading system for diffuse astrocytic neoplasms

Each of the following scores 1 point:

- Nuclear atypia
- Mitoses
- Capillary endothelial proliferation
- Necrosis

Grade = score + 1, to a maximum grade of 4

Fig. 35.4 St Anne/Mayo grading system for diffuse astrocytic neoplasms.

Prognostic indicators in astrocytic neoplasms

- Age
- Karnofsky performance score
- Histologic diagnosis (WHO/grading system)
- Microcysts in astrocytoma
- Ki-67 labeling index (not independent of histologic grading in some studies)

Fig. 35.5 Prognostic indicators in astrocytic neoplasms.

ASTROCYTOMA
MACROSCOPIC APPEARANCES
In the postmortem brain, cerebral astrocytomas diffusely expand the white matter, sometimes distorting the overlying gray matter. The neoplasm is poorly demarcated (**Fig. 35.6**). An abnormal texture and slight discoloration of the white matter may be the only clues to its presence. Some neoplasms are gelatinous or tough and therefore more obvious. Astrocytomas of the brain stem and spinal cord expand normal tissues in a fusiform fashion. Brain stem astrocytomas are frequently centered on the pons and may encircle the basilar artery. Spinal cord astrocytomas may be associated with a syrinx.

MICROSCOPIC APPEARANCES
A diagnosis of astrocytoma is relatively easy if there is plenty of biopsied tissue: it can be distinguished from non-neoplastic lesions or normal brain by the presence of microcysts, the abnormally high nuclear:cytoplasmic ratio, and the presence of cells with pleomorphic and hyperchromatic nuclei (**Fig. 35.7**). Most are astrocytomas of the fibrillary type and are composed of cells with a small indistinct soma that form a dense meshwork of fine branching cytoplasmic processes.

If there is only limited material from a stereotactically obtained biopsy, the diagnosis may be difficult, especially if the biopsy is from the edge of the neoplasm. Infiltrated brain may be relatively undisturbed at the infiltrating edge of the neoplasm, so subtle cytologic differences must be sought to identify the neoplastic cells. Their cytoplasm may blend with the fibrillary background and the diagnosis is made on the basis of the nuclear characteristics and uneven distribution of the infiltrating cells. Immunohistochemistry with p53 antibodies may assist in the identification of astrocytoma. Cells in some astrocytomas show nuclear accumulation of p53, which is neither a feature of normal tissue nor non-neoplastic lesions with the notable exception of progressive multifocal leukoencephalopathy in which some infected oligodendrocytes label with p53 antibodies.

The rare protoplasmic astrocytoma (**Fig. 35.8**) is usually located superficially and composed of cells with small round nuclei and scanty perinuclear cytoplasm. The cytoplasmic processes are sparse and microcystic spaces are prominent. Larger cysts are also common .

Cells with abundant glassy deep-pink cytoplasm and eccentrically placed nuclei predominate in gemistocytic astrocytomas (**Fig. 35.9**). These neoplasms have a slightly poorer prognosis than other astrocytomas. Some gemistocytic astrocytomas contain mitoses and should be placed in the category of anaplastic astrocytoma (**Fig. 35.10**).

Most astrocytomas, and particularly gemistocytic astrocytomas, show immunoreactivity for glial fibrillary acidic protein (GFAP) and S-100 protein. However, GFAP immunoreactivity is scant or absent in protoplasmic astrocytomas.

GLIOMATOSIS CEREBRI
This is characterized by very widespread infiltration of the CNS by small cells. Typically a large proportion of the cerebrum is involved and this is sometimes accompanied by spread of neoplastic cells into the brain stem and even the spinal cord. Differentiating gliomatosis cerebri from

DIFFERENTIAL DIAGNOSIS OF ASTROCYTOMA

- Astrocytosis is generally characterized by an *even* distribution of reactive astrocytes with stellate processes. In addition, astrocyte hypertrophy is more evident than astrocyte hyperplasia, hypercellularity is exceptional, and microcysts are rarely seen.
- Demyelination is characterized by loss of myelin with preservation of axons, many lipid-containing CD68-positive macrophages, and macrophages in perivascular spaces.
- Infarction is characterized by lipid-containing CD68-positive macrophages and reactive astrocytosis.
- Oligodendroglioma is characterized by artefactual perinuclear halos, uniform round nuclei, minigemistocytic cells, and delicate branching vasculature.
- Pilocytic astrocytoma is characterized by a biphasic appearance with microcystic areas and fascicles, piloid cells, Rosenthal fibers, and characteristic neovascularization.

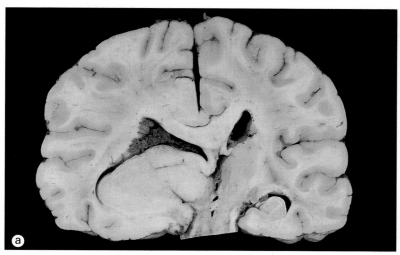

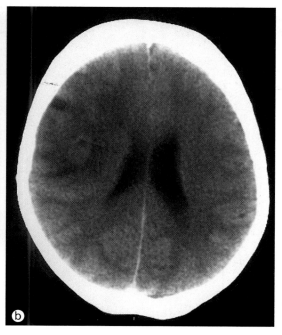

35.6 Astrocytoma. (a) An astrocytoma diffusely invades the cerebrum producing distortion and expansion of normal structures. The neoplasm produces midline shift and is poorly demarcated. **(b)** CT scan. A poorly defined mass in the right frontal lobe has lower density than the surrounding cerebrum and has produced midline shift. (Courtesy of Dr JS Millar, Wessex Neurological Center).

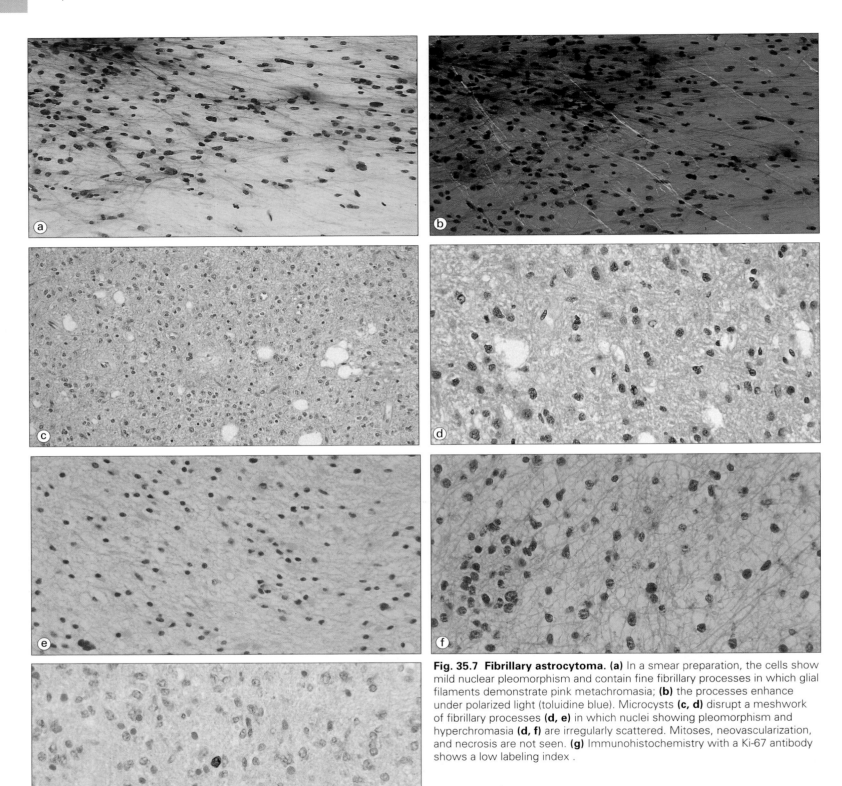

Fig. 35.7 Fibrillary astrocytoma. (a) In a smear preparation, the cells show mild nuclear pleomorphism and contain fine fibrillary processes in which glial filaments demonstrate pink metachromasia; **(b)** the processes enhance under polarized light (toluidine blue). Microcysts **(c, d)** disrupt a meshwork of fibrillary processes **(d, e)** in which nuclei showing pleomorphism and hyperchromasia **(d, f)** are irregularly scattered. Mitoses, neovascularization, and necrosis are not seen. **(g)** Immunohistochemistry with a Ki-67 antibody shows a low labeling index .

a large infiltrating astrocytic neoplasm can be difficult because no strict criteria distinguish these entities, the difference being one of degree. Neuroimaging studies may suggest the diagnosis, but confirmation is often obtained only at necropsy.

MACROSCOPIC AND MICROSCOPIC APPEARANCES

Gliomatosis cerebri produces diffuse expansion of at least one cerebral lobe (**Fig. 35.11a**). A moderate increase in cell density is seen in regions infiltrated by neoplastic cells, which have mildly pleomorphic, elongated nuclei and indistinct cytoplasm (**Fig. 35.11b**). Neoplastic cells tend to cluster around neurons and in subpial and perivascular spaces. Mitoses are sparse, and microvascular proliferation, necrosis, and destruction of existing structures are not generally seen.

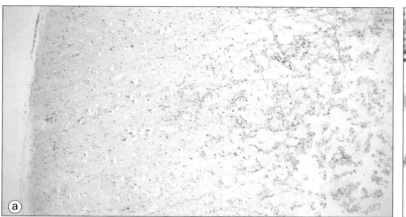

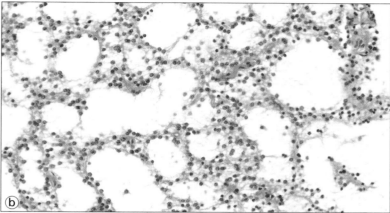

Fig. 35.8 Protoplasmic astrocytoma. (a) The neoplasm is quite superficially located, partly within the cerebral cortex. **(b)** At higher magnification the neoplasm is seen to consist of cells with small, round nuclei and relatively sparse cytoplasmic processes. Microcysts are a prominant feature.

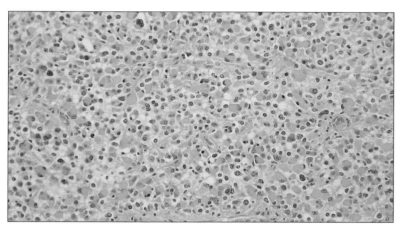

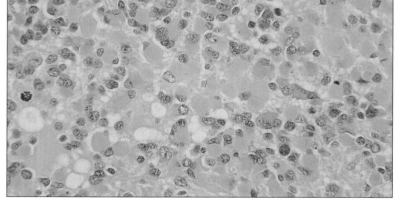

Fig. 35.9 Gemistocytic astrocytoma. This consists largely of plump cells with glassy pink cytoplasm.

Fig. 35.10 Anaplastic astrocytoma containing many gemistocytic cells. The presence of mitoses puts this astrocytoma into the anaplastic category.

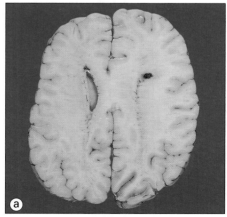

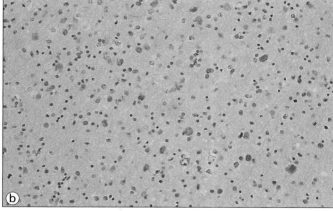

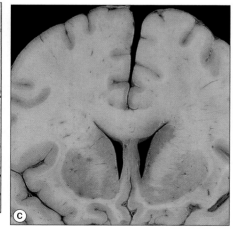

Fig. 35.11 Gliomatosis cerebri. (a) The brain is diffusely enlarged with some asymmetry of the cerebral hemispheres. Histology from this case **(b)** revealed a diffuse infiltrate of neoplastic glia and reactive changes in almost all cerebral lobes.**(c)** Another example demonstrates marked thickening of the corpus callosum. (Courtesy of Dr T Moss, Frenchay Hospital, Bristol)

MENINGEAL GLIOMATOSIS

Meningeal gliomatosis is characterized by the wide distribution of neoplastic cells with an astrocytic or oligodendroglial morphology (see chapter 36) within the leptomeninges, which produces meningeal thickening and entrapment of nerve roots and blood vessels. In most reported examples, there is focal involvement of the parenchyma, and this is thought to be the source of the disseminated neoplasm.

ANAPLASTIC ASTROCYTOMA

Anaplastic transformation of an astrocytoma is often heralded by:

- the development of rapidly worsening neurologic symptoms and signs.

- enhancement of the tumor in computerized tomographic scans of the brain.

The prognosis is significantly poorer than for astrocytoma (**Fig. 35.12**).

MACROSCOPIC AND MICROSCOPIC APPEARANCES

Anaplastic transformation may be associated with little discernible macroscopic change in an astrocytoma. Some histologic features of an astrocytoma are exaggerated in an anaplastic astrocytoma (**Figs. 35.13–35.15**): cytologic and nuclear pleomorphism may therefore be more pronounced, the nuclear:cytoplasmic ratio is increased, and mitoses are evident. Neovascularisation is enhanced, but glomeruloid microvascular proliferation with multiple layers of cells (see below) is a characteristic of glioblastomas.

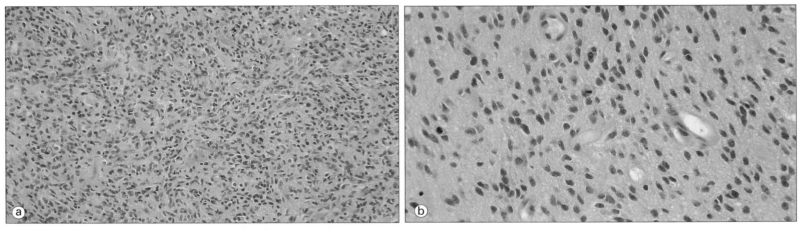

Diffuse cerebral astrocytic neoplasms			
	Astrocytoma	Anaplastic astrocytoma	Glioblastoma
Mean age at biopsy (years)	36	40	53
Median survival (months)	80	21	11

Fig. 35.12 Age at presentation and prognosis of diffuse astrocytic neoplasms.

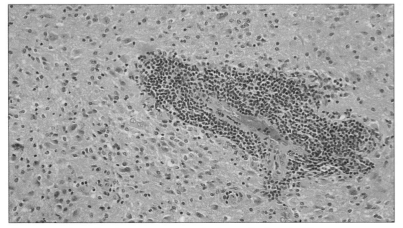

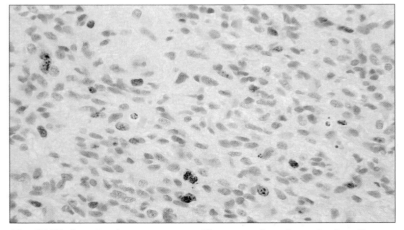

Fig. 35.13 Anaplastic astrocytoma. (a) An increased nuclear:cytoplasmic ratio and **(b)** mitotic figures are the principal characteristics that distinguish anaplastic astrocytoma from astrocytoma.

Fig. 35.14 Anaplastic astrocytoma. Perivascular lymphoid aggregates are not unusual in astrocytic neoplasms.

Fig. 35.15 Anaplastic astrocytoma. The proportion of neoplastic cells with Ki-67 immunoreactivity is on average greater in anaplastic astrocytomas than in astrocytomas. A moderately high labeling index is seen here.

GLIOBLASTOMA

Glioblastomas arise *de novo* or represent the endpoint of neoplastic progression from an astrocytoma. Separation of these two types of glioblastoma is justified on clinical and genetic grounds, but they are indistinguishable histologically (see Fig. 35.2).

MACROSCOPIC APPEARANCES

An infiltrating glioblastoma dramatically distorts the normal anatomy of the fixed postmortem brain (**Figs 35.16–35.18**). Foci of cyst formation, necrosis, and hemorrhage are admixed with mucoid gray neoplastic tissue. The neoplasm often extends to distant parts of the brain along white matter tracts and this can give it a multicentric appearance. Glioblastomas quite commonly appear as a spherical mass with a necrotic center, which is seen on CT imaging as a ring of contrast-enhancing tissue around a region of low attenuation. This appearance mimics an abscess, but the center of the glioblastoma is usually filled with straw-colored fluid and scanty necrotic debris rather than pus. Glioblastomas occasionally spread through cerebrospinal fluid pathways.

DIFFERENTIAL DIAGNOSIS OF GLIOBLASTOMA

If only a small amount of tissue is available for histologic examination, the infiltrative behavior and neuroepithelial nature of a glioblastoma may not be obvious. Glioblastoma must then be distinguished from metastatic carcinoma and lymphoma.

- Glioblastoma is generally immunoreactive for GFAP, but metastatic carcinoma and lymphoma are not.
- Lymphoma is immunoreactive for CD45, but glioblastoma and metastatic carcinoma are not. (N.B. Anaplastic large cell (Ki-1) lymphoma may not be immunoreactive for CD45, but may express epithelial membrane antigen (EMA): it is distinguished by its immunoreactivity for CD30.)
- Metastatic carcinoma often expresses EMA, but this is very rare in glioblastoma (exceptional metaplastic examples showing glandular differentiation) and lymphoma (see above).
- Metastatic carcinoma often expresses cytokeratins, while glioblastomas show scant focal immunoreactivity with some antibodies to cytokeratins, and lymphoma shows no reactivity.

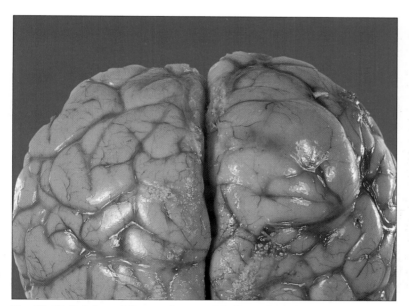

Fig. 35.16 Bulging of the cerebrum with distortion of gyri due to an underlying glioblastoma.

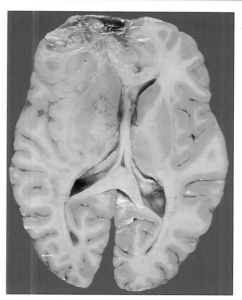

Fig. 35.17 Glioblastoma. A horizontal section through the cerebrum reveals distortion of the normal architecture and foci of necrosis and hemorrhage.

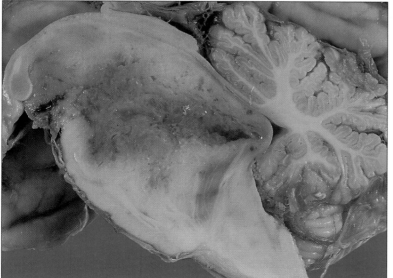

Fig. 35.18 Glioblastoma in the brain stem. A sagittal section shows the enlargement of the entire brain stem and foci of necrosis and hemorrhage centered on the pons.

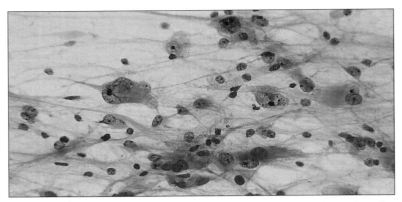

Fig. 35.19 Striking cytologic pleomorphism in a smear preparation of a glioblastoma. (Toluidine blue)

MICROSCOPIC APPEARANCES

Intraneoplasmal and interneoplasmal heterogeneity is characteristic of the glioblastoma (**Figs 35.19, 35.20**). Although some areas of a glioblastoma will have the histologic appearance of an astrocytoma or anaplastic astrocytoma, necrosis and microvascular proliferation are key features separating glioblastoma from the other two diffuse astrocytic neoplasms (**Fig. 35.21**). Microvascular proliferation is due to segmental or glomeruloid hyperplasia of capillary lining cells such that some no longer abut the lumen. The term 'endothelial hyperplasia' is also used, but some of the hyperplastic cells express smooth muscle actin and may be pericytes. Cellular pleomorphism in glioblastoma may be more extreme than that in anaplastic astrocytoma, with giant cells being seen in some examples (**Fig. 35.22**, see also Fig. 35.20b). Glioblastomas containing many giant cells ('giant cell glioblastomas') tend to be more circumscribed than classic glioblastomas, but there is no evidence to indicate that this variant has a distinct biologic behavior.

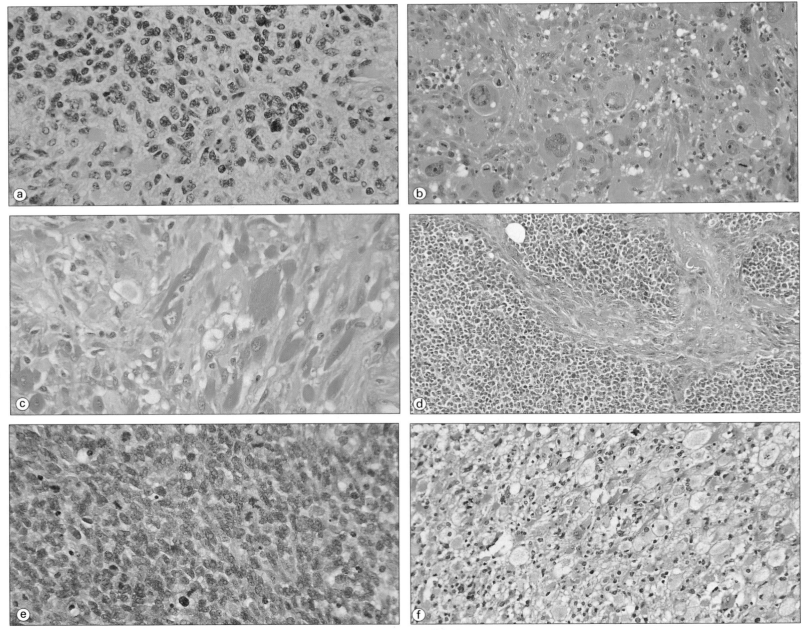

Fig. 35.20 Extraordinary diversity of histologic appearance characterizes the glioblastoma. **(a)** Variable nuclear:cytoplasmic ratio and a minority of cells with an astrocytic morphology are often seen. **(b)** Gross cytologic pleomorphism. **(c)** Cells may contain deeply eosinopilic masses. **(d)** and **(e)** A small cell component resembling PNET may be mixed with other histologic patterns and usually contains many mitoses. **(f)** Xanthomatous cells are common. The glioblastoma should, however, be distinguished from the pleomorphic xanthoastrocytoma (see box on page 35.18), which has a much better prognosis.

In some glioblastomas (sometimes referred to as gliosarcomas) neoplastic spindle-shaped cells with pericellular reticulin may dominate the histology or form a dual population with astrocytic cells (**Fig. 35.23**). Glioblastomas and gliosarcomas share the same biologic behavior and genetic abnormalities.

GFAP immunoreactivity in glioblastomas is variable, but those cells with an astrocytic morphophenotype are generally positive.

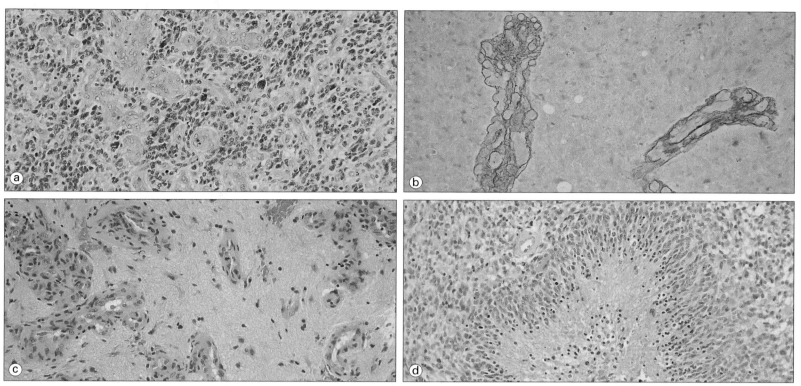

Fig. 35.21 Glioblastoma. In addition to diverse cytologic features, the glioblastoma is characterized by a distictive neovascularisation and micronecrosis. **(a)** Buds of capillary endothelial proliferation are seen among neoplastic cells, and **(b)** can be highlighted by a reticulin preparation. **(c)** Neovascularization may be induced in brain adjacent to a glioblastoma. **(d)** Pseudopalisading of cells around necrosis is sometimes seen.

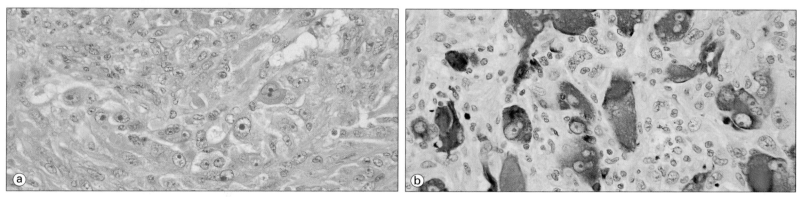

Fig. 35.22 Cellular pleomorphism in glioblastomas. (a) Cells with a large nucleus and a single prominent nucleolus may be present in glioblastomas as illustrated here. **(b)** The cells seen in (a) bear some resemblance to neurons, but are usually strongly immunoreactive for GFAP as demonstrated here.

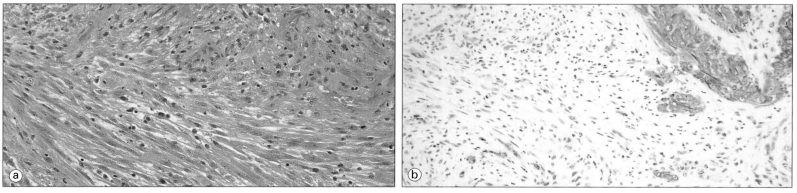

Fig. 35.23 Spindle cell glioblastoma. (a) Elongated cells are arranged in fascicles; mitotic figures are readily found in these sarcomatoid neoplasms which also contain foci of astrocytic cells. **(b)** The astrocytic cells are immunoreactive for GFAP whereas the spindle-shaped cells frequently are not.

Immunoreactivity for vimentin is more widespread and many glioblastomas are focally immunoreactive for S-100.

Glioblastomas previously treated with radiotherapy may be paucicellular and exhibit considerable cytologic atypia. Calcification and hyaline vascular thickening are seen (**Fig. 35.24**). Delayed coagulative necrosis may produce a marked mass effect. Positron emission tomography (PET) scanning is useful for distinguishing radionecrosis from recurrent neoplasm. Pseudopalisading of cells around the necrosis indicates recurrent glioblastoma.

PILOCYTIC ASTROCYTOMA

Pilocytic astrocytomas should be distinguished from the diffuse astrocytic neoplasms because they:
- do not share their genetic abnormalities.
- do not infiltrate surrounding tissue in the same manner.
- rarely progress to an anaplastic form.
- have a predilection for sites rarely involved by other astrocytic neoplasms.
- have a better prognosis.

MACROSCOPIC APPEARANCES

The pilocytic astrocytoma is relatively well circumscribed. It often has a heterogeneous consistency with firm or mucoid areas. Focal calcification may be present. A pilocytic astrocytoma sometimes forms a mural nodule in association with a cyst. Invasion of the subarachnoid space may be evident.

MICROSCOPIC APPEARANCES

Pilocytic astrocytomas typically have a biphasic appearance. Some parts of the neoplasm consist of elongated cells arranged in compact fascicles. Elsewhere the cells are stellate, with fine branching cytoplasmic processes that enclose a meshwork of microcysts (**Fig. 35.25a**). The two components are present to varying degrees, and the microcystic component may be lacking in some pilocytic astrocytomas from older patients (**Fig. 35.25b**). A lobulated pattern is sometimes seen. The nuclei of the neoplastic cells in some areas are round and perinuclear clearing in these cells can mimic the appearance seen in an oligodendroglioma (**Fig. 35.25g**). Invasion of surrounding tissues is limited to a narrow border zone around the neoplasm. Pilocytic astrocytomas may spread into perivascular and subarachnoid spaces, but do not disseminate through CSF pathways. Nuclear pleomorphism and hyperchromasia are usually present in a small proportion of cells, but carry no prognostic significance and represent a degenerative change, rather like that seen in schwannomas (**Fig. 35.25d**). Mitoses are rare, and areas of necrosis should prompt consideration of other diagnoses. Rosenthal fibers and intracellular eosinophilic globules (granular bodies) are classic features and may be abundant (**Fig. 35.25c**), but are sometimes difficult to find in neoplasms from adult patients. Groups of neoplastic cells may be separated by strands of fibrovascular tissue that can be quite broad. Delicate thin-walled blood vessels may form small tangles (**Fig. 35.25e, f**). True glomeruloid endothelial proliferation is occasionally found, but does not have an adverse prognostic significance in these neoplasms.

Most cells in all pilocytic astrocytomas label with antibodies to GFAP. Ultrastructural examination reveals abundant cytoplasmic intermediate filaments.

Pilocytic astrocytomas occasionally become anaplastic. Increased cytologic pleomorphism in association with mitoses and areas of micronecrosis in an otherwise typical pilocytic astrocytoma are signs of this progression, which is associated with rapid recurrence (**Fig. 35.25h**).

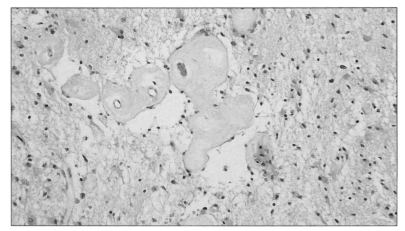

Fig. 35.24 Thickened blood vessel walls in a paucicellular glioblastoma previously treated with radiotherapy.

PILOCYTIC ASTROCYTOMA

- This tumor occurs mainly in children and young adults.
- The sites of predilection are: cerebellum, optic nerve, optic chiasm/hypothalamus/third ventricle, temporal lobe.
- Cerebral pilocytic astrocytomas tend to affect an older group of patients than do those of the cerebellum, optic chiasm or optic nerve.
- Pilocytic astrocytomas rarely arise in the brain stem (although this may be secondarily infiltrated) and are very rare in the spinal cord.
- Optic nerve pilocytic astrocytoma may be associated with neurofibromatosis type 1.

PILOCYTIC ASTROCYTOMA

- Pilocytic astrocytomas overexpress specific neurofibromatosis type 1 gene transcripts.
- Pilocytic astrocytomas do not contain 17p deletions.
- Approximately 20% of pilocytic astrocytomas show loss of chromosome 17q.

DIFFERENTIAL DIAGNOSIS OF PILOCYTIC ASTROCYTOMA

- Extensive gliosis with Rosenthal fibers may mimic a pilocytic astrocytoma and may surround other neoplasms, particularly craniopharyngiomas in the hypothalamus and hemangioblastomas in the cerebellum. A thorough examination of resected tissue is crucial for establishing the diagnosis.
- Distinguishing pilocytic astrocytoma from fibrillary astrocytoma has implications for treatment and prognosis. It may be helpful to bear in mind that they tend to occur at different sites (see text). Fibrillary astrocytomas do not have the biphasic appearance typical of pilocytic astrocytomas, Rosenthal fibers are unusual in fibrillary astrocytomas, and neovascularization typical of pilocytic astrocytomas is not seen in fibrillary astrocytomas.

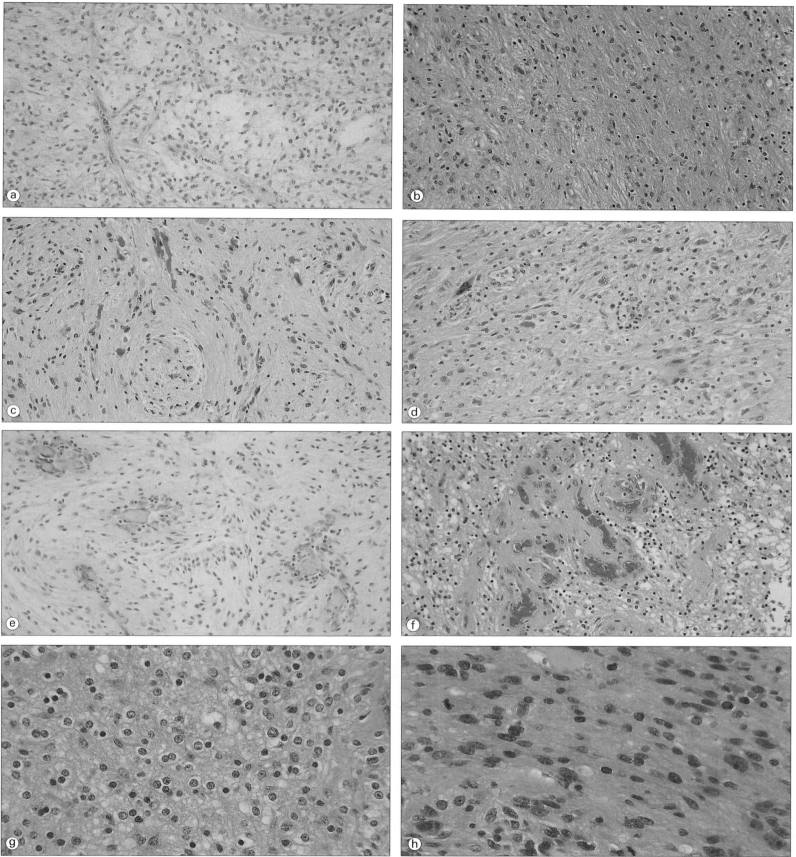

Fig. 35.25 Pilocytic astrocytoma. (a) Microcysts are seen among oval, spindle-shaped and stellate cells. **(b)** Compact arrangement of elongated cells is more typical of some examples. **(c)** Spindle-shaped cells may be arranged in fascicles and Rosenthal fibers may be numerous. **(d)** Foamy (xanthomatous) cells may be scattered among the astrocytic cells.

(e) and **(f)** Neovascularization is distinctive in pilocytic astrocytomas, and is not an indicator of anaplastic transformation. **(g)** Oligodendrocyte-like cells may be seen in some examples . **(h)** Anaplasia is uncommon in pilocytic astrocytomas and is evinced by mitotic activity in association with micronecrosis and an increased nuclear:cytoplasmic ratio.

PLEOMORPHIC XANTHOASTROCYTOMA (PXA)

This is a distinctive astrocytic neoplasm that is generally situated superficially in the cerebrum of children and young adults. Genetic studies indicate that it should be separated from the spectrum of diffuse cerebral astrocytic neoplasms. Although PXAs occasionally progress to become aggressive neoplasms, behaving like glioblastomas, they generally have a more favorable prognosis than diffuse astrocytomas.

MACROSCOPIC AND MICROSCOPIC APPEARANCES

PXA frequently forms a mural nodule within a cyst, and may be calcified. As its name implies, this neoplasm may show considerable cytologic pleomorphism (**Fig. 35.26a**). Many cells are large and have abundant eosinophilic cytoplasm; cytoplasmic lipid droplets are found with variable frequency. Nuclear pleomorphism and hyperchromasia are evident in some cells. Mitoses are rarely found. Necrosis is absent. Unlike most gliomas, it contains moderately dense pericellular reticulin (**Fig. 35.26b**).

PXA shows focal immunoreactivity for GFAP (**Fig. 35.26c**). Immunolabeling for S-100 is widespread. A subpopulation of cells without the typical features of ganglion cells shows immunoreactivity for neuronal proteins such as synaptophysin and neurofilaments.

The presence of necrosis indicates neoplastic progression and usually accompanies a significant mitotic count. In these circumstances, glioblastoma and malignant fibrous histiocytoma enter the differential diagnosis.

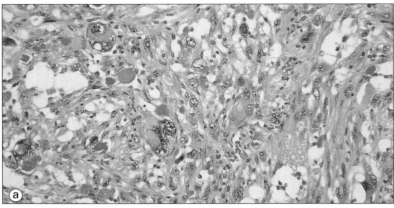

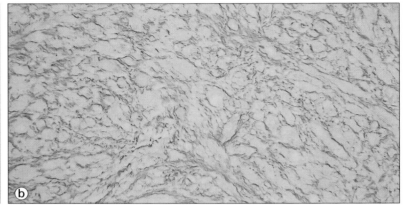

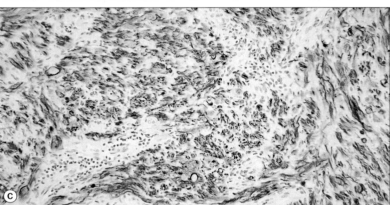

Fig. 35.26 Pleomorphic xanthoastrocytoma. (a) This neoplasm shows marked cytologic pleomorphism. **(b)** The reticulin pattern is characteristically dense. **(c)** There is variable immunoreactivity for GFAP.

PLEOMORPHIC XANTHOASTROCYTOMA

- presents mainly in children and young adults, initially with epilepsy.
- is predominantly a superficial supratentorial neoplasm.
- occurs most commonly in the temporal lobe.
- is typically associated with a cyst, which is evident on neuroimaging.
- has a much more favorable prognosis than anaplastic astrocytoma or glioblastoma.

PLEOMORPHIC XANTHOASTROCYTOMA

- PXAs very rarely contain mutations of the p53 gene, or show evidence of EGF receptor amplification.
- PXAs do not show loss of chromosomes 10 or 19q.

DISTINGUISHING PXA FROM GLIOBLASTOMA

PXA:

- has distinctive clinical and radiologic features (see clinical box).
- exhibits extensive pericellular reticulin.
- contains intracellular eosinophilic protein droplets.
- includes neoplastic cells with a neuronal immunophenotype.
- usually contains few mitotic figures.
- contains areas of necrosis only when undergoing progression to an anaplastic form.
- does not share the genetic abnormalities of a glioblastoma.

TUBEROUS SCLEROSIS COMPLEX (TSC) AND SUBEPENDYMAL GIANT CELL ASTROCYTOMA (SEGA)

TSC consists of multiple hamartomatous and occasionally neoplastic abnormalities, which tend to present at different ages (Fig. 35.27). It may be familial or sporadic. CNS manifestations include:

- Tubers (predominantly cerebral).
- Focal cerebellar abnormalities (including tubers).
- Subependymal nodules.
- SEGA.

MACROSCOPIC AND MICROSCOPIC APPEARANCES

Cortical tubers manifest as firm indistinct expansions of the gray matter and underlying white matter (Fig. 35.28). Cortical dysplasia, neuronal heterotopia, and gliosis are evident microscopically. Vascularity is often increased. Scattered within the tubers are large cells with cytologic and immunohistochemical characteristics of both glia and neurons. Tubers may contain foci of calcification. Tubers

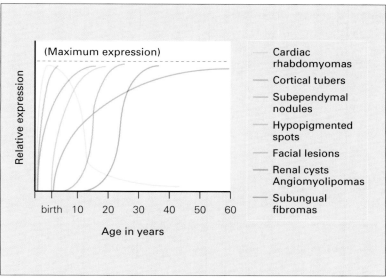

Fig. 35.27 Age of onset for common lesions of tuberculosis sclerosis coplex

TUBEROUS SCLEROSIS COMPLEX

- TSC has a prevalence of approximately 1/10,000.
- When familial, TSC shows autosomal dominant inheritance with high penetrance.
- TSC is commonly sporadic (approximately 60% of cases).
- Nearly all patients have CNS lesions, but 30–90% of patients in different series have CNS symptoms and signs.
- TSC is associated with SEGA in only 5% of patients.
- Epilepsy, mental retardation, hydrocephalus secondary to nodules or SEGA, and symptoms and signs related to SEGA, are manifestations of the varied CNS lesions.
- TSC can also manifest with cardiac rhabdomyomas, pulmonary lymphangioleiomyomatosis, retinal hamartomas, renal cysts, renal angiomyolipomas, fibrous dysplasia of bone, facial angiofibromas, subungual fibromas, hypopigmented macules.

GENETICS OF TUBEROUS SCLEROSIS COMPLEX

- TSC shows linkage to the *TSC*-1 gene on chromosome 9q34 in approximately 50% of families.
- In approximately 50% of families, TSC is due to mutations of *TSC*-2, a putative tumor suppressor gene on chromosome 16p13 that has recently been shown to encode a widely expressed 180 kD protein that causes activation of Rap1-GAP.

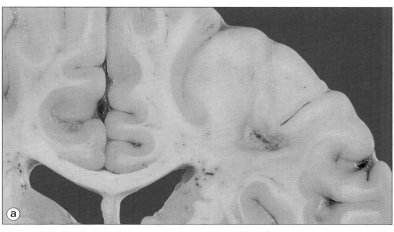
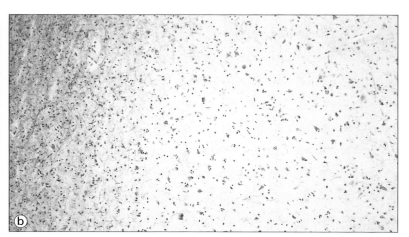

Fig. 35.28 Cortical tuber in a patient with TSC. (a) There is expansion of the gyrus and loss of definition in the gray/white matter interface. (b) Cortical dysplasia at the site of a tuber. (Luxol fast blue/cresyl violet)

occasionally occur in the cerebellum, where focal atrophy, dystrophic calcification, and focal loss of Purkinje and internal granular cells may also be evident (**Fig. 35.29**).

Subependymal nodules occur mainly around the lateral ventricles (**Fig. 35.30**), particularly in the region of the foramen of Monro. Enlargement of a subependymal nodule signals the development of a SEGA.

SEGA: A well-defined soft mass of gray tissue protrudes into the ventricle. Calcification may be present. At the microscopic level, most cells are oval or elongated and have abundant glassy eosinophilic cytoplasm and a large eccentric nucleus (**Fig. 35.31a,b**). Many have a glial immunophenotype (**Fig. 35.31c**), but some express neuronal antigens and others have an indeterminate nature. Mitoses are unusual. Capillary endothelial proliferation and necrosis are exceptional, and should prompt consideration of a glioblastoma.

The SEGA is predominantly exophytic and does not invade surrounding parenchyma in the manner of diffuse astrocytic neoplasms.

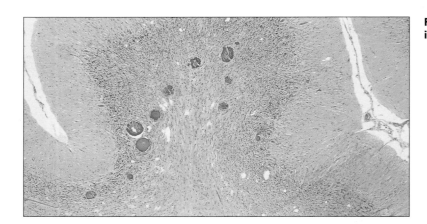

Fig. 35.29 Cerebellar atrophy with focal calcification and loss of internal granular cells in TSC.

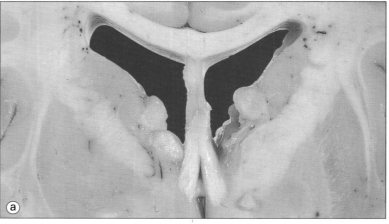

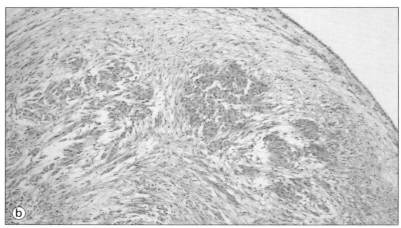

Fig. 35.30 Subependymal nodules in TSC. (a) Subependymal nodules around the lateral ventricles. **(b)** Swirled arrangement of spindle-shaped cells in a subependymal nodule.

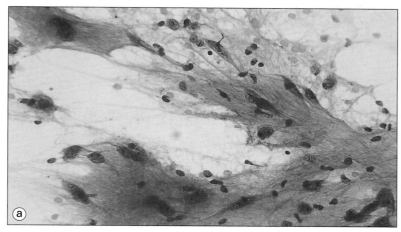

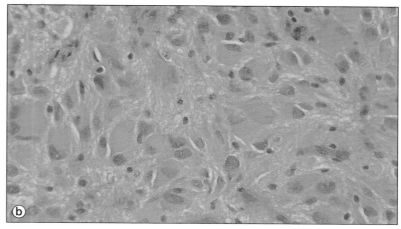

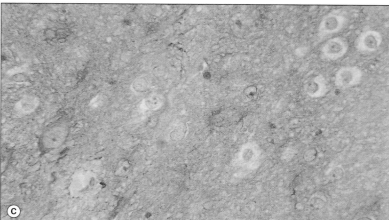

Fig. 35.31 SEGA associated with TSC. (a) Cytologic pleomorphism is evident in this smear preparation. **(b)** Large cells with eccentric nuclei are evident in this histologic section. **(c)** Only some of the large cells label with antibodies to GFAP.

REFERENCES

Burger PC, Vogel FS, Green SB, Strike TA. (1985) Glioblastoma multiforme and anaplastic astrocytoma. *Cancer* 56: 1106–1111.

Burger PC. (1996) Pathology of brain stem astrocytomas. *Pediatric Neruosurgery* 24:35–40.

Collins PV, James CD. (1993) Gene and chromosomal alterations associated with the development of human gliomas. *FASEB Journal* 7:926–930.

Daumas-Duport C, Scheithauer B, O'Fallon J, Kelly P. (1988) Grading of astrocytomas. A simple and reproducible method. *Cancer* 62: 2152–2165.

Ellison DW, Steart PV, Bateman AC, Pickering RM, Palmer JD, Weller RO. (1995) Prognostic indicators in a range of astrocytic tumours: an immunohistochemical study with Ki-67 and p53 antibodies. *Journal of Neurology, Neurosurgery, and Psychiatry* 59: 413–419.

Garcia DM, Latifi HR, Simpson JR, Picker S. (1989) Astrocytomas of the cerebellum in children. *Journal of Neurosurgery* 71: 661–664.

Kepes JJ. (1993) Pleomorphic xanthoastrocytoma; the birth of a diagnosis and a concept. *Brain Pathology* 3: 269–274.

Kim TS, Halliday AL, Hedley-Whyte ET, Convery K. (1991) Correlates of survival and the Daumas-Duport grading system for astrocytomas. *J Neurosurg* 74: 27–37.

Lantos PL, VandenBerg SR, Kleihues P. (1997) Tumors of the nervous system. In: Graham DI, Lantos PL, ed. *Greenfield's Neuropathology*. 6th ed. London; Arnold. p 583–879.

Lopes MB, Altermatt HJ, Scheithauer BW, VandenBerg Sr. (1996) Immunohistochemical characterization of subependymal giant cell astrocytomas. *Acta Neuropathologica* 91: 386–375.

Louis DN. (1994) The p53 gene and protein in human brain tumours. *Journal of Neuropathology and Experimental Neurology* 53: 11–21.

Louis DN. (1997) A molecular genetic model of astrocytoma histopathology. *Brain Pathology* 7: 755–764.

Plate KH, Breier G, Weich HA, Mennel HD, Risau W. (1994) Vascular endothelial growth factor and glioma angiogenesis: coordinate induction of VEGF receptors, distribution of VEGF protein and possible in vivo regulartory mechanisms. *International Journal of Cancer* 59: 520–529.

Powell SZ, Yachnis AT, Rorke Lb, Rojiani AM, Eskin TA. (1996) Divergent differentiation in pleomorphic xanthoastrocytoma. *American Journal of Surgical Pathology* 20:80–85.

VandenBerg SR. Current diagnostic concepts of astrocytic tumours. (1992) *Journal of Neuropathology and Experimental Neurology* 51: 644–657.

VandenBerg SR. (1993)Desmoplastic infantile ganglioglioma and desmoplastic cerebral astrocytoma of infancy. *Brain Pathology* 3: 275–281.

von Deimling A, Louis DN, Wiestler OD. (1995) Molecular pathways in the formation of gliomas. *Glia* 15: 328–338.

Wienecke R, Konig A, DeClue JE (1995) Identification of tuberin, the tuberous sclerosis-2 product. Tuberin possesses specific Rap1GAP activity. *J Biol Chem* 270: 16409–16414.

Yaziji H, Massarani-Wafai R, Gujrati M, Kuhns JG, Martin AW, Parker JC. (1996) Role of p53 immunohistochemistry in differentiation reactive gliosis from malignant astrocytlesions. *The American Journal of Surgical Pathology* 20: 1086–1090

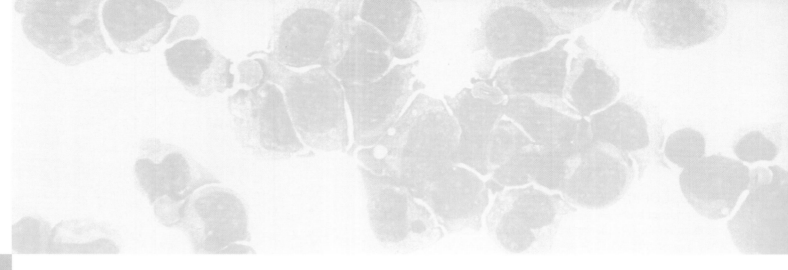

36 Non-astrocytic gliomas

Various non-astrocytic glial neoplasms are considered in this chapter, including oligodendrogliomas, ependymomas, and mixed gliomas. The astroblastoma and primitive (polar) spongioblastoma appear in the World Health Organization (WHO) classification under the heading of 'neuroepithelial tumors of uncertain etiology'. These neoplasms are extremely rare and because their histologic features are found focally in other gliomas, some authors have queried the justification of classifying astroblastomas and spongioblastomas as distinct entities. The astroblastoma exhibits pseudorosettes and perivascular hyalinization. The nuclei of astroblastoma cells are rounder and their perivascular cytoplasmic processes shorter and broader than those of ependymomas, with which this neoplasm can be confused. Polar spongioblastomas are characterized by uniform elongated cells arranged in ranks so that adjacent nuclei are aligned. This arrangement of nuclei, sometimes described as 'rhythmic nuclear palisading', may also be seen in oligodendrogliomas (see Fig. 36.7c), pilocytic astrocytomas, and neuroblastomas.

OLIGODENDROGLIOMAS

Oligodendrogliomas usually present in adulthood, but sometimes only after a long history of epilepsy. They show a broad range of behaviors. Some neoplasms with bland cytologic features grow extremely slowly, but anaplastic oligodendrogliomas behave aggressively. Attempts to categorize this heterogeneity in grading systems have been partially successful (**Fig. 36.1**), but most support the view that two broad categories are sufficient (**Fig. 36.2**). These correspond to 'oligodendroglioma' and 'anaplastic oligodendroglioma' in the WHO classification.

Studies of the genetic abnormalities of oligodendrogliomas indicate that they are distinct from those of diffuse astrocytic neoplasms.

MACROSCOPIC APPEARANCES

Oligodendrogliomas have a variety of macroscopic appearances. Small examples may be difficult to locate in resection specimens. Distortion of

---

St Anne/Mayo grading system for oligodendrogliomas
Each of the following scores 1 point:
• Nuclear atypia
• Mitoses
• Capillary endothelial proliferation
• Necrosis
Grade = score + 1, to a maximum grade of 4

Fig. 36.1 St Anne/Mayo grading system for oligodendrogliomas.

Prognostic indicators in oligodendrogliomas
• Age
• Pathologic distinction between St Anne/Mayo grades 1/2 and 3/4
• Pathologic distinction between oligodendroglioma and anaplastic oligodendroglioma
• Ki-67 labeling index

Fig. 36.2 Prognostic indicators in oligodendrogliomas.

SURVIVAL OF PATIENTS WITH OLIGODENDROGLIOMAS GRADED ACCORDING TO THE ST ANNE/MAYO SYSTEM

	Grades 1 & 2	Grades 3 & 4
Median survival (years)	10	4
Five-year survival (%)	75	41
Ten-year survival (%)	46	20

OLIGODENDROGLIOMAS

- constitute 7–10% of primary intracranial neoplasms.
- occur with equal incidence in males and females.
- occur most often in the frontal lobe.
- occur most frequently in patients aged 30–50 years.
- are more chemosensitive than most other gliomas.
- are more prone to hemorrhage than other gliomas.

the normal cortical gray and white matter interface and discoloration of tissue provide clues to their location (**Fig. 36.3**). Other neoplasms are more obvious, appearing as moderately well-circumscribed, gray masses. The propensity of superficial oligodendrogliomas to invade the subarachnoid space may produce a neoplasm that sits partially on the cortical surface of the cerebrum.

MICROSCOPIC APPEARANCES

Oligodendrogliomas are composed of uniform cells (**Fig. 36.4**). These readily infiltrate gray matter, but tend to produce a more abrupt edge in white matter (**Fig. 36.5**). A lobular architecture is sometimes seen and microcysts may be prominent. Small foci of dystrophic calcification are

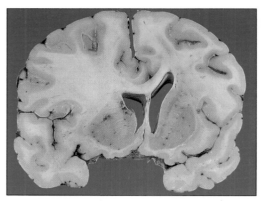

Fig. 36.3 Oligodendroglioma. The infiltrating neoplasm expands the gyri and deep white matter in the frontal lobe, distorting the striatum and lateral ventricles and causing subfalcine herniation of the cingulate gyrus.

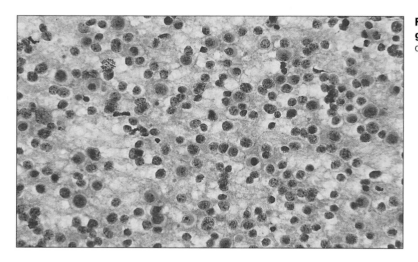

Fig. 36.4 Perioperative smear preparations of oligodendrogliomas generally reveal little cytologic pleomorphism. The round nuclei and ill-defined cytoplasm are typical. (Toluidine blue)

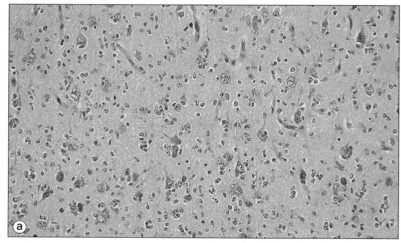

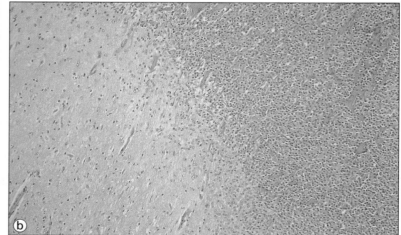

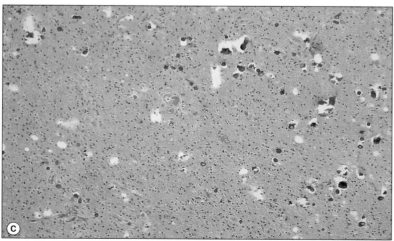

Fig. 36.5 Oligodendroglioma. (a) Cerebral cortex diffusely infiltrated by oligodendroglioma. **(b)** A relatively distinct border to the neoplasm may be observed in white matter. **(c)** Dystrophic calcification is a common feature.

usually found, often at the edge of the neoplasm or in infiltrated gray matter. A delicate vasculature consisting of branching capillaries runs through typical oligodendrogliomas (**Fig. 36.6**).

Cytoplasm is rather sparse and not easily identifiable in some cells. Artefactual clearing of the cytoplasm is common in fixed paraffin-embedded material, particularly when fixation is delayed, and gives a 'fried-egg' appearance to the cells (**Fig. 36.7a**). The nuclei are round and usually contain speckled chromatin. A single small nucleolus may be present. Cells occasionally adopt an elongated form (**Fig. 36.7d**),

but the nuclei retain their uniformity. Some cells, termed 'minigemisto-cytes', have eccentrically placed nuclei and eosinophilic cytoplasm that is immunoreactive for glial fibrillary acidic protein (GFAP) (**Fig. 36.8**). Invasion of the subarachnoid space is common (**Fig. 36.9**). Mitoses are rare, except in neoplasms with other anaplastic characteristics such as cytologic pleomorphism and areas of necrosis (**Fig. 36.10**).

Immunohistochemistry with antibodies to GFAP generally reveals labeling of only a small proportion of cells (**Fig. 36.11**). Immunoreactivity for myelin-specific proteins is rare.

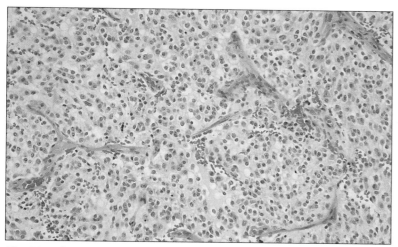

Fig. 36.6 Oligodendroglioma. A network of delicate bifurcating capillaries is typical.

GENETIC ASPECTS OF OLIGODENDROGLIOMAS, OLIGOASTROCYTOMAS AND EPENDYMOMAS

Common genetic features of oligodendrogliomas and oligoastrocytomas

- Loss of heterozygosity for markers on chromosome 1p
- Loss of heterozygosity for markers on chromosome 19q

Genetic features of oligodendrogliomas

- Very infrequent p53 mutations
- Frequent EGF-receptor overexpression that is not due to gene amplification

Genetic features of ependymomas

- Frequent loss of chromosome 22
- Very infrequent NF2 mutations
- Very infrequent p53 mutations

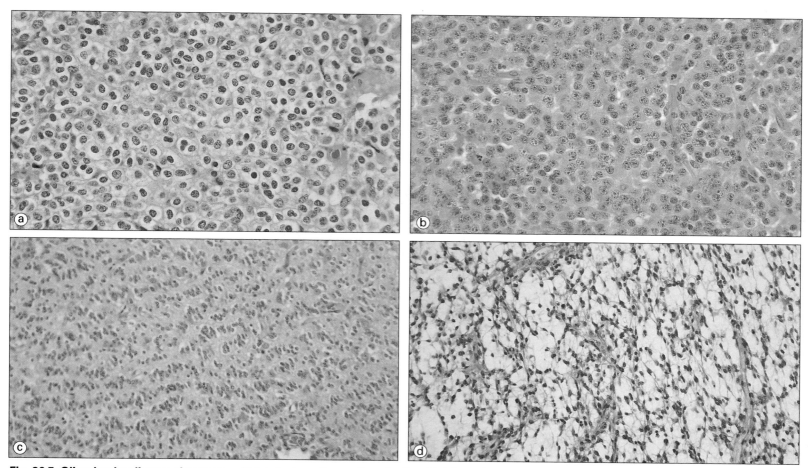

Fig. 36.7 Oligodendrogliomas show several histologic patterns. Round cells with **(a)** or without **(b)** artefactual clearing of the cytoplasm. **(c)** Rhythmic nuclear palisading reminiscent of a polar spongioblastoma. **(d)** Loosely arranged elongated cells with small round nuclei.

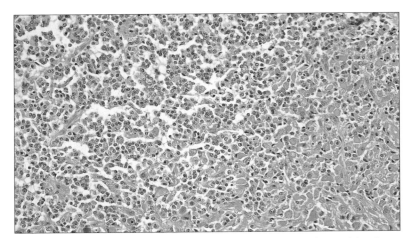

Fig. 36.8 Oligodendroglioma. Foci of small oval 'minigemistocytic' cells with eosinophilic cytoplasm and an eccentric, round nucleus. These are seen in some oligodendrogliomas. The nuclear form is similar to that in the round cells. These foci do not indicate a diagnosis of mixed glioma.

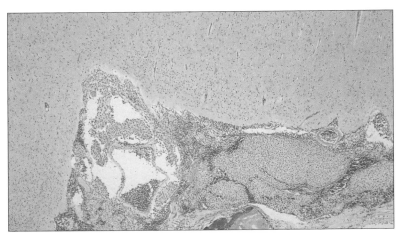

Fig. 36.9 Oligodendroglioma. Invasion of the subarachnoid space.

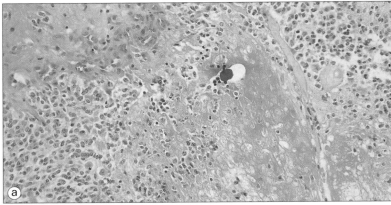

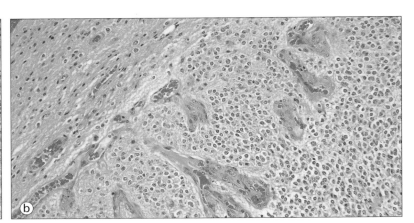

Fig. 36.10 Anaplastic oligodendroglioma. Increased cytologic pleomorphism **(a)**, capillary endothelial proliferation **(b)** and **(c),** and micronecrosis **(a)** and **(c)** are evident in these neoplasms which have an aggressive biologic behavior.

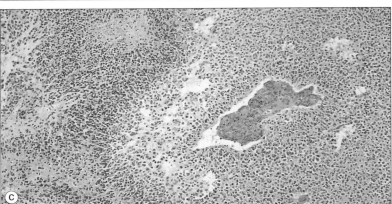

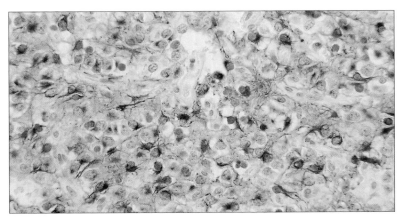

Fig. 36.11 Oligodendroglioma. Immunoreactivity for GFAP is variable in oligodendrogliomas.

DIFFERENTIAL DIAGNOSIS OF OLIGODENDROGLIOMA

Non-neoplastic conditions

- Macrophages in infarcts or demyelination can appear as scattered or grouped cells with small round nuclei and clear cytoplasm, but in contrast to neoplastic oligodendrocytes macrophages have a slightly granular cytoplasm, which contains lipid and periodic acid–Schiff positive material, and are immunoreactive for CD68.

Fibrillary astrocytoma

- Oligodendrogliomas and fibrillary astrocytomas may have somewhat similar appearances.
- Nuclei in astrocytomas are oval and show obvious pleomorphism.
- Astrocytomas do not contain cells with perinuclear halos or a network of fine branching capillary vessels.

Pilocytic astrocytoma, glioblastoma, medulloblastoma with a nodular pattern, central neurocytoma, and dysembryoplastic neuroepithelial tumor (DNT)

- Neoplastic oligodendrocyte-like cells (OLCs) can occur in these conditions.
- If adequate tissue is available for histology, the typical appearances of pilocytic astrocytoma and glioblastoma are generally present around areas with OLCs.
- Nodular medulloblastomas and central neurocytomas may show immunoreactivity for synaptophysin, which is not a feature of oligodendrogliomas.
- DNT has a nodular architecture. The nodules sometimes contain cells surrounding or within a mucoid matrix. Ganglion cells may be scattered among the OLCs.

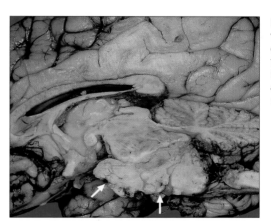

Fig. 36.12 A fourth ventricular ependymoma. This tumor has distorted the brain stem and formed an exophytic ventral mass (arrows).

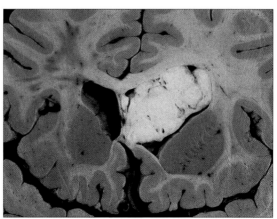

Fig. 36.13 Subependymoma.

EPENDYMOMAS

Gliomas derived from oncogenetic events in cells that manifest ependymal differentiation are divided by the WHO classification into:

- Ependymoma (variants: cellular, papillary, clear cell).
- Anaplastic ependymoma.
- Myxopapillary ependymoma.
- Subependymoma.

The first of these (classic ependymomas) generally present as intracranial neoplasms in childhood. Myxopapillary ependymomas, which have a more indolent behavior than classic ependymomas, nearly always present as spinal neoplasms in adulthood. Subependymomas are often incidental necropsy findings.

MACROSCOPIC APPEARANCES

Classic ependymomas grow as demarcated soft gray masses that are generally related to the ventricular system. In the posterior fossa, they may fill the fourth ventricle and pass through its exit foramina (**Fig. 36.12**).

Myxopapillary ependymomas appear as well-defined, lozenge-shaped neoplasms among the cauda equina, which they tend to envelop. Spontaneous hemorrhage into these neoplasms is quite common.

Subependymomas are firm lobulated intraventricular masses and are found predominantly in the fourth ventricle (**Fig. 36.13**).

EPENDYMOMAS

Intracranial ependymomas

- constitute 6–9% of primary CNS neoplasms.
- generally present in young children, with a mean age at presentation of 4 years.
- comprise 30% of primary CNS neoplasms in children less than 3 years of age.
- occur either infratentorially (60%) or supratentorially (40%).

Spinal ependymomas

- generally belong to the myxopapillary category.
- are frequently related to the conus or filum terminale.
- usually present in patients aged 20–40 years.
- are associated with syringomyelia.
- are associated with type 1 neurofibromatosis when occurring at multiple foci.

Subependymomas

- are generally found in the fourth and lateral ventricles.
- present with hydrocephalus or may be asymptomatic.

MICROSCOPIC APPEARANCES

Ependymomas are generally composed of uniform cells with indistinct cytoplasmic borders and round or oval nuclei (**Fig. 36.14**). The nuclear:cytoplasmic ratio varies; it is usually high, but infrequent nodules of densely packed cells may be scattered throughout paucicellular areas (**Fig. 36.15**). Cells in these nodules may show more nuclear pleomorphism than surrounding cells, and an increased mitotic count. Foci of micronecrosis may be present in classic ependymomas.

The pseudorosette is a perivascular anuclear zone of fibrillary processes that taper towards the vessel (**Fig. 36.16**). Pseudorosettes are a hallmark of ependymomas, but ependymal rosettes with a central lumen and a halo of neoplastic cells may also be found, although less consistently (**Fig. 36.17**). Rosettes and gland-like canals are manifestations of epithelial differentiation in ependymomas.

Some ependymomas contain elongated cells with an astrocytic morphology and have been referred to as tanycytic ependymomas (**36.18**), though this histologic pattern is not recognized by the WHO classification as a distinct variant.

Cellular ependymomas contain cells with a high nuclear:cytoplasmic ratio (**Fig. 36.19**). Few pseudorosettes are present, and cellular

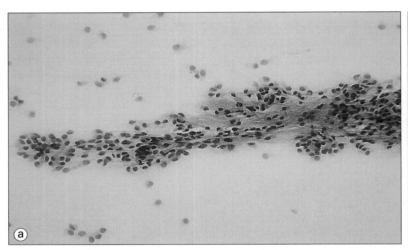

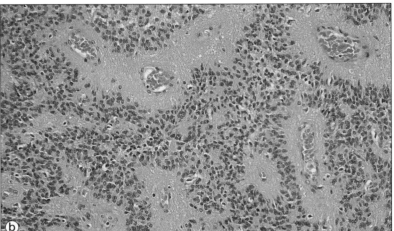

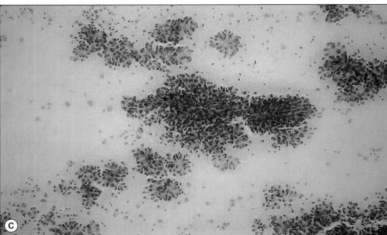

Fig. 36.14 Classic ependymoma. (a) Smear preparation showing cells with oval nuclei and fine cytoplasmic processes. (Toluidine blue) **(b)** Sheets of small uniform cells with a moderately high nuclear:cytoplasmic ratio are interrupted by pseudorosettes around blood vessels. **(c)** Smear preparations often contain perivascular pseudorosettes. True rosettes, as illustrated in this figure, are much less common.

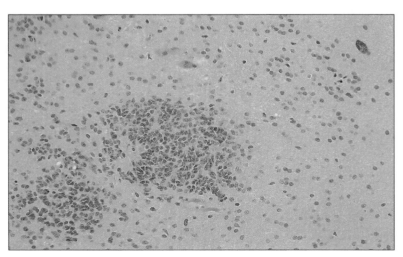

Fig. 36.15 Classic ependymoma. The nuclear:cytoplasmic ratio is low in some ependymomas but, as here, nodules of densely packed cells are then sometimes evident in paucicellular areas. Cells in these nodules tend to show more pleomorphism and mitoses than cells elsewhere.

ependymomas do not contain paucicellular areas. Differentiating this variant from anaplastic ependymomas is difficult, and depends on the identification of marked cytologic pleomorphism, capillary endothelial proliferation, and abundant necrosis in the latter.

Rarely, intraventricular ependymomas exhibit a papillary pattern and choroid plexus papilloma (CPP) then enters the differential diagnosis (**Fig. 36.20**). Papillary ependymomas do not have a subepithelial basement membrane over a fibrovascular core like the CPP, while the

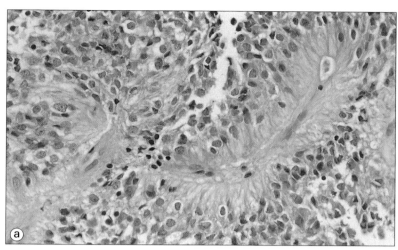

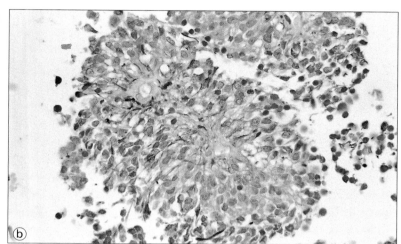

Fig. 36.16 Ependymal pseudorosettes. (a) These are characterized by fine cellular processes that taper towards the blood vessel. **(b)** The processes are immunoreactive for GFAP.

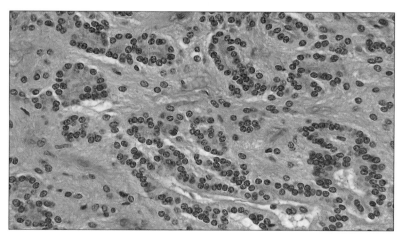

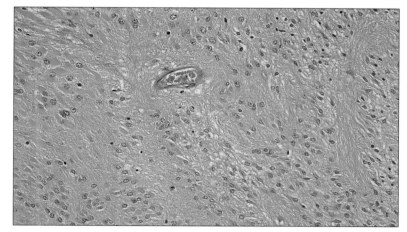

Fig. 36.17 Canals and true rosettes. These structures are found in only a minority of ependymomas.

Fig. 36.18 Ependymoma containing elongated cells with fibrillary cytoplasm. These neoplasms contain no true rosettes, but may be identified by the presense of pseudorosettes.

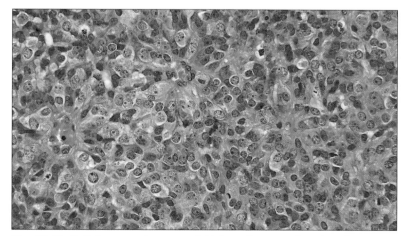

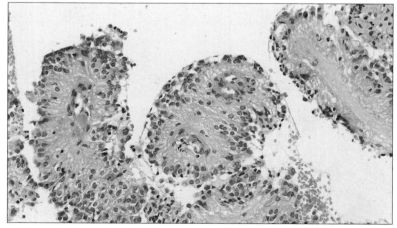

Fig. 36.19 Cellular ependymoma. A high nuclear:cytoplasmic ratio characterizes the cells of this neoplasm, and pseudorosettes are sparse.

Fig. 36.20 Papillary ependymoma. This neoplasm showed many papillary structures that, in cross section, consisted of pseudorosettes surrounded by uniform cells. Note the absence of a basement membrane beneath the circumferentially arranged cells. This pattern must not be confused with the artefactual pseudopapillae sometimes produced in section of classic ependymoma.

CPP does not contain pseudorosettes with tapering GFAP-positive processes.

Clear cell ependymoma may be confused with an oligodendroglioma, but the presence of pseudorosettes should declare its identity (**Fig. 36.21**).

Criteria for the diagnosis of anaplastic ependymoma are rather subjective. Necrosis and capillary endothelial proliferation may be widespread in anaplastic ependymoma (**Fig. 36.22**). The WHO classification emphasizes atypical cytologic features (i.e. nuclear pleomorphism and a very high nuclear:cytoplasmic ratio) in its diagnosis. It is important to note that no histologic feature of ependymomas correlates reliably with prognosis.

Myxopapillary ependymomas consist of uniform cells, which show either epithelial or glial differentiation (**Fig. 36.23**). They usually have monomorphic round nuclei and mitoses are rare. The regions of glial

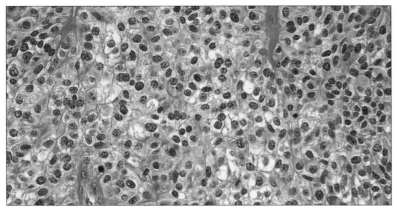

Fig. 36.21 Clear cell ependymoma. This may mimic an oligodendroglioma. Round cells with cytoplasmic clearing may be widespread in some ependymomas. Site and the presence of pseudorosettes help to distinguish this variant from oligodendroglioma.

DIFFERENTIAL DIAGNOSIS OF EPENDYMOMA

Astrocytoma, medulloblastoma, cerebral neuroblastoma, central neurocytoma, microcystic meningioma

- The presence of pseudorosettes with fine fibrillary GFAP-positive processes is the key to differentiating ependymomas from these neoplasms which can occur in the same region and may be confused with ependymoma if biopsied tissue is limited.
- In these neoplasms either pseudorosettes do not occur or fibrillary perivascular structures are immunoreactive for synaptophysin.

Paraganglioma of the filum terminale, schwannoma

- It may occasionally be difficult to distinguish a myxopapillary ependymoma from these neoplasms which occur in the same region.
- Paragangliomas can be distinguished by their immunoreactivity for chromogranin and synaptophysin and the arrangement of cells in nests or cords surrounded by reticulin.
- Schwannomas can be distinguished by pericellular reticulin.

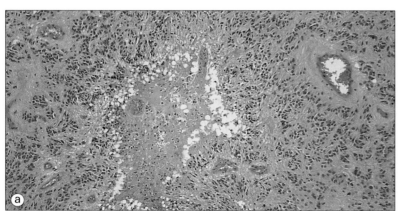

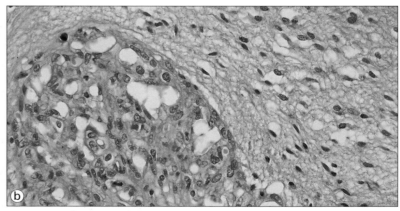

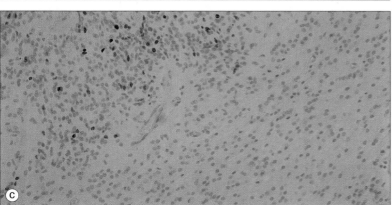

Fig. 36.22 Anaplastic ependymoma. (a) Micronecrosis and **(b)** capillary endothelial proliferation are not uncommon in classic ependymomas but are widespread in anaplastic ependymomas. The WHO criteria for anaplastic ependymoma are met when these features accompany marked cytologic abnormalities. **(c)** Immunohistochemistry with a Ki-67 antibody typically shows a high labelling index in areas with a high nuclear:cytoplasmic ratio.

differentiation contain cells with elongated fibrillary processes. The myxopapillary regions, which are responsible for the name of the neoplasm, consist of clusters of cuboidal or columnar cells separated by pools of mucin, often with a central small blood vessel. The epithelial cells may be arranged in papillary fronds around the vascular core and surrounding mucin.

Subependymomas are composed of cells with fairly uniform, round or oval nuclei and scanty perinuclear cytoplasm. The cells are clustered

in small, sparsely scattered groups and separated by broad bands of closely packed fibrillary processes. Microcysts are a common finding (**Fig. 36.24**). Mitoses are absent.

Ependymomas label with antibodies to GFAP (**Fig. 36.25**). Focal immunoreactivity for cytokeratins and epithelial membrane antigen is sometimes seen around canals. Ultrastructural examination reveals microvilli and cilia on the luminal surfaces, and zonulae adherentes (**Fig. 36.26**).

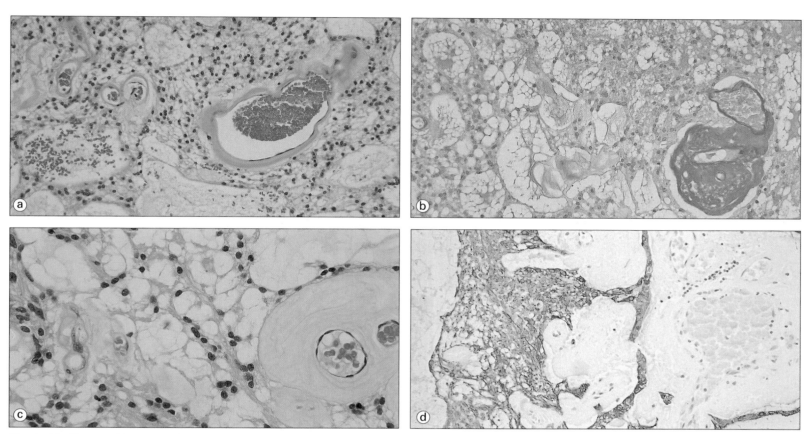

Fig. 36.23 Myxopapillary ependymoma. (a) and **(b)** Loosely arranged cells with delicate fibrillary cytoplasm surround pools of mucin in this myxopapillary ependymoma. (b, PAS/Alcian blue) **(c)** Blood vessels sometimes have markedly thickened walls. **(d)** The fibrillary cytoplasm is immunoreactive for GFAP.

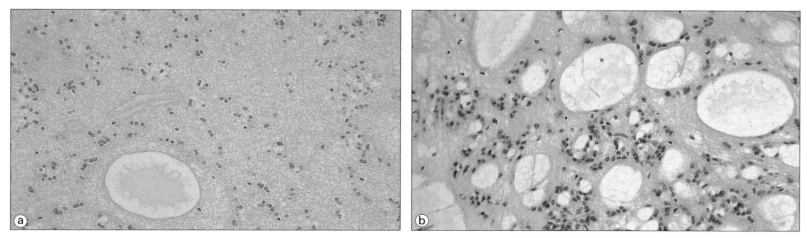

Fig. 36.24 Subependymoma. (a) Small groups of nuclei are surrounded by masses of fibrillary processes. **(b)** Clusters of microcysts in a subependymoma.

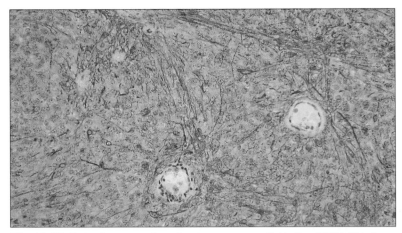

Fig. 36.25 Ependymoma showing immunoreactivity for GFAP. This is most pronounced in the fine cytoplasmic processes, particularly those that converge onto blood vessels.

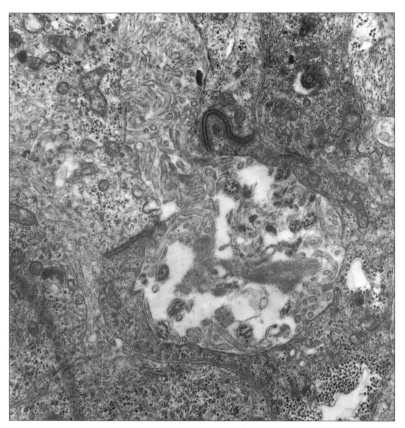

Fig. 36.26 Ependymoma. Microvilli and cilia are evident in this electron micrograph.

MIXED GLIOMAS

Mixed gliomas are composed of two types of neoplastic glia, but the diagnostic criteria are difficult to define. A diagnosis of mixed glioma should be reserved for neoplasms with separate regions of morphologically distinct cells. Many astrocytomas contain a few cells reminiscent of those in oligodendrogliomas, and vice versa, but such an admixture does not qualify for the term mixed glioma.

In practice, mixed gliomas are rare, and of the theoretic combinations oligoastrocytoma, ependymoastrocytoma, and oligoependymoma, the oligoastrocytoma clearly predominates (**Fig. 36.27**).

The oligodendroglial and astrocytic areas in oligoastrocytomas share genetic abnormalities that align these neoplasms with oligodendrogliomas.

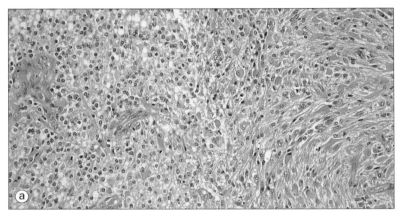

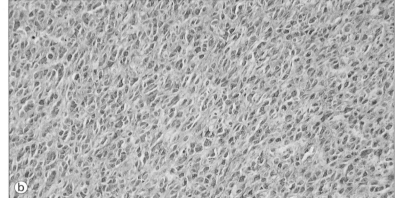

Fig. 36.27 Mixed glioma; oligoastrocytoma. (a) Oligodendroglial differentiation and distinct astrocytic differentiation are seen in one neoplasm. **(b)** Immunoreactivity for GFAP is usually evident, but the ubiquitous pattern here should be distinguished from the circumscribed dense cytoplasmic immunoreactivity of oligodendroglioma cells that show minigemistocytic differentiation.

REFERENCES

Duncan JA, Hoffman HJ, (1995) Intracranial ependymomas. In: Kaye AH, Laws ER, ed. *Brain tumours.* New York: Churchill Livingstone pp 493–504.

Kashima T, Vinters HV, Campagnoni AT. (1995) Unexpected expression of intermediate filament protein genes in human oligodendroglioma cell lines. *Journal of Neuropathology and Experimental Neurology* 54: 23–31.

Kraus JA, Koopmann J, Kaskel P, *et al.* (1995) Shared allelic losses on chromosomes 1p and 19q suggest a common origin of oligodendroglioma and oligoastrocytoma. *Journal of Neuropathology and Experimental Neurology* 54: 91–5.

Macdonald DR. (1994) Low-grade gliomas, mixed gliomas, and oligodendrogliomas. *Seminars in Oncology* 21: 236-48.

Mork SJ, Lindegaard K-F, Halvorsen TB, *et al.* (1985) Oligodendroglioma: incidence and biological behaviour in a define population. *Journal of Neurosurgery* 63: 881–889.

Mork SJ, Halvorsen TB, Lindegaard K-F, Eide GE. (1986) Oligodendroglioma. Histologic evaluation and prognosis. *Journal of Neuropathology and Experimental Neurology* 45: 65–78.

Nakagawa Y, Perentes E, Rubinstein LJ. (1986) Immunohistochemical characterization of oligodendrogliomas. An analysis of multiple markers. *Acta Neuropathologica* 72: 15–22.

Nazar GB, Hoffman JH, Becker LE, Jenkin D, Humphreys RP, Hendrick EB. (1990) Infratentorial ependymomas in childhood: prognostic factors and treatment. *Journal of Neurosurgery* 72: 408–417.

Ransom DT, Ritland SR, Kimmel DW, *et al.* (1992) Cytogenetic and loss of heterozygosity studies in ependymomas, pilocytic astrocytomas, and oligodendrogliomas. *Genes, Chromosomes & Cancer* 5:348–56.

Shaw EG, Scheithauer BW, O'Fallen JR, Tazelaar HD, Davis DH. (1992) Oligodendrogliomas: the Mayo Clinic experience. *Journal of Neurosurgery* 76: 428–434.

Shaw EG, Scheithauer BW, O'Fallon JR, Davis DH. (1994) Mixed oligoastrocytomas: a survival and prognostic factor analysis. *Neurosurgery* 34: 577–82.

von Deimling A, Louis DN, Wiestler OD. (1995) Molecular pathways in the formation of gliomas. *Glia* 15: 328–38.

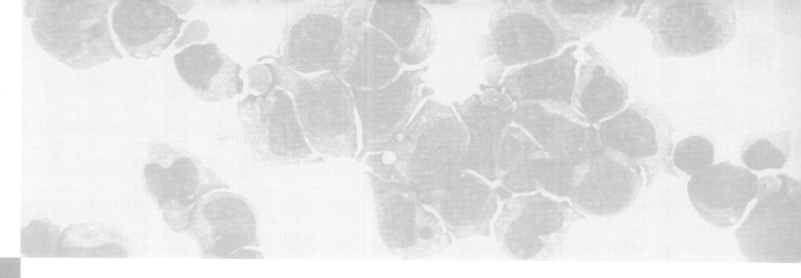

37 *Neuroepithelial neoplasms displaying neuronal features*

Neoplastic cells with morphologic and/or immunohistochemical characteristics of neurons may occur in neuroepithelial neoplasms as:
- Large ganglion cells.
- Small but well-differentiated neurocytes.
- Poorly differentiated, proliferating neuroblasts.

Neuroblasts may be present in embryonal neoplasms such as primitive neuroectodermal tumors (PNETs), and predominate in neuro-blastomas (see Chapter 38) and ganglioneuroblastomas. Ganglion cells or neurocytes form a significant component of:
- Ganglion cell neoplasms (i.e. gangliocytoma, ganglioglioma, anaplastic ganglioglioma).
- Desmoplastic infantile ganglioglioma (DIGG).
- Central neurocytoma.
- Paraganglioma of the filum terminale.
- Dysembryoplastic neuroepithelial tumor (DNT).
- Dysplastic gangliocytoma of the cerebellum (Lhermitte–Duclos disease).
- Hypothalamic neuronal hamartoma.

Most of these 'neuronal tumors' are characterized by a slow or negligible rate of growth.

The nature of the DNT and dysplastic gangliocytoma of the cerebellum is controversial. It has been suggested that they may be choristomas (i.e. the result of non-neoplastic proliferation of histologically normal but aberrantly situated tissue elements) rather than neoplasms.

GANGLION CELL NEOPLASMS

With the exception of rare anaplastic variants, ganglion cell neoplasms have a moderately good prognosis, because they are moderately well circumscribed and grow slowly.

MACROSCOPIC APPEARANCES
Ganglion cell neoplasms (**Fig. 37.1**) are firm and gray, and frequently contain flecks of calcification and cysts. They may appear as a mural nodule in a large cyst.

MICROSCOPIC APPEARANCES
Neoplastic 'ganglion' cells look like large neurons, possessing a round nucleus, prominent nucleolus, and Nissl substance. Ganglion cell neoplasms exhibit a range of histologic appearances; ganglion cells may either dominate the histologic picture or be part of a polymorphic population of cells.

Gangliocytomas consist of disorganized ganglion cells set against a lacy, fibrillary background containing a few reactive astrocytes (**Fig. 37.2**). Groups of ganglion cells may appear in nests enclosed by fibrovascular septa. In some cases, extensive desmoplasia may surround elongated cells that have a neuronal immunophenotype. Neoplastic ganglion cells possess abnormal processes and some have double nuclei. Small round cells with large nuclei and a prominent

GANGLION CELL NEOPLASMS

- usually present in the first three decades with epilepsy.
- have a predilection for the temporal lobe.
- frequently cause complex partial seizures.
- often form a cyst with a mural nodule.
- are associated with congenital abnormalities in 5% of cases.

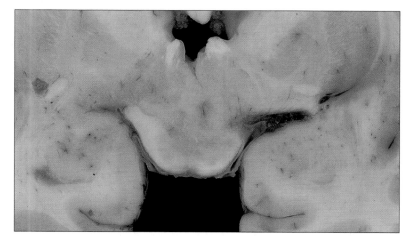

Fig. 37.1 Ganglioglioma. Invasion and expansion of midline and medial temporal structures are evident.

DIFFERENTIAL DIAGNOSIS OF GANGLION CELL NEOPLASMS

Diagnostic difficulty sometimes surrounds the separation of ganglion cell neoplasms from gliomas that diffusely invade gray matter or from other neuroepithelial neoplasms that contain large cells with prominent nucleoli.

In making a diagnosis, consider the following:

- **Are neoplastic ganglion cells present?** Neoplastic ganglion cells do not show the uniform orientation and orderly arrangement of neurons in the cerebral cortex, may be identified away from gray matter in the deep white matter or subarachnoid space (though sparsely scattered neurons are normally found in the white matter), and have abnormal cytologic characteristics, including double nuclei.
- **Not all large cells with large nuclei and prominent nucleoli are ganglion cells.** Similar cells are found in giant cell glioblastoma, pleomorphic xanthoastrocytoma, and subependymal giant cell astrocytoma of tuberous sclerosis. Check the immunophenotype of the cells. Ganglion cells are immunoreactive for synaptophysin and neurofilament proteins, but are not immunoreactive for glial fibrillary acidic protein (GFAP).
- **Mitoses are exceptional in gangliogliomas.** The presence of scattered mitoses in limited biopsy material indicates either infiltration of gray matter by an anaplastic astrocytoma or rare anaplastic transformation of a ganglioglioma. In either event, the prognosis is much worse than that of a ganglioglioma or an astrocytoma.

nucleolus represent a further neuronal phenotype encountered in these neoplasms (**Fig. 37.2**).

Gangliogliomas contain neoplastic glial cells, which may greatly outnumber the ganglion cells. Neoplastic glia in gangliogliomas may have an obvious astrocytic morphology, but some ganglion cell neoplasms contain cells with an indeterminate nature (**Figs 37.3, 37.4**). Some gangliogliomas manifest as pilocytic astrocytomas with a ganglion cell component. Eosinophilic globules and neovascularization may be evident. Degenerative cytologic changes take the form of nuclear pleomorphism and hyperchromasia.

Ganglion cell neoplasms may spread in the subarachnoid space and be associated with perivascular lymphocytes. Finding a mitotic figure in a ganglion cell neoplasm is exceptional. If there are mitoses accompanying cytologic pleomorphism in a ganglioglioma, the possibility of anaplastic transformation should be considered. This unusual event involves the glial component, and occurs in less than 10% of gangliogliomas.

The ganglion cells are immunoreactive for synaptophysin and neurofilament proteins (see Fig. 37.4), and electron microscopy reveals dense-core synaptic vesicles.

Small round cells with a high nuclear:cytoplasmic ratio and nuclear hyperchromasia are combined with ganglion cells in the ganglioneuroblastoma (**Fig. 37.5**). Mitoses and apoptosis are usually identifiable among the small cells. Recognition of the embryonal elements is important because their presence confers a much poorer prognosis.

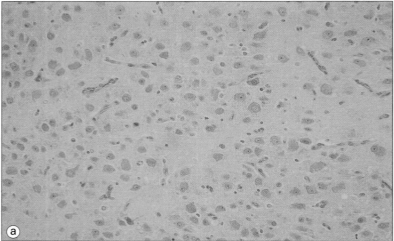

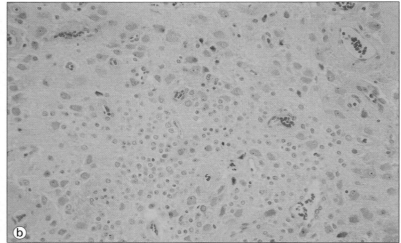

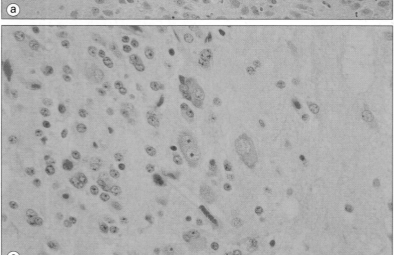

Fig. 37.2 Gangliocytoma. (a) and **(b)** This neoplasm is composed of admixed regions of large and small cells with round vesicular nuclei, prominent nucleoli, and, in the periphery of the cytoplasm, basophilic Nissl substance. **(c)** Some ganglion cells contain double nuclei.

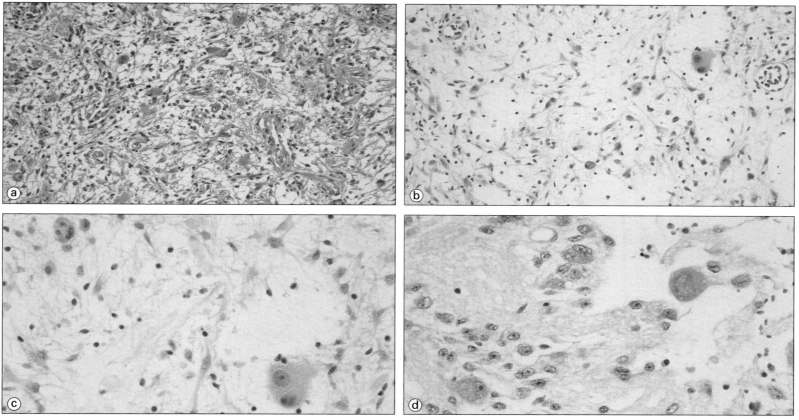

Fig. 37.3 Ganglioglioma. (a) Ganglion cells are seen among disorganized neoplastic cells with an astrocytic morphology. **(b)** Microcysts in another part of the same neoplasm. **(c)** Some neoplastic ganglion cells contain two nuclei. **(d)** The histogenesis of some cells is unclear. Here, some cells are not readily classified as neuronal or glial.

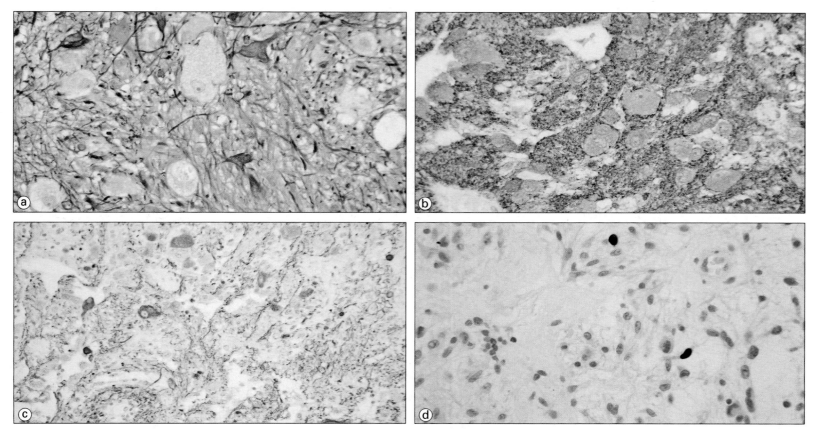

Fig. 37.4 Ganglioglioma. (a) Ganglion cells are surrounded by the processes of astrocytic cells that are immunoreactive for GFAP. **(b)** The cytoplasm of ganglion cells and a meshwork of neuritic processes are immunoreactive for synaptophysin. **(c)** The cell bodies of ganglion cells and some fine processes are also immunoreactive for neurofilament protein. **(d)** The low growth fraction of a ganglioglioma is illustrated by the paucity of Ki-67-labeled nuclei.

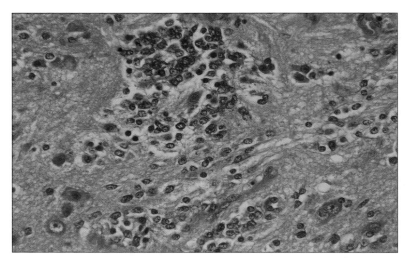

Fig. 37.5 Ganglioneuroblastoma. A closely packed group of small neuroblastoma cells with hyperchromatic nuclei is seen among ganglion cells.

DIFFERENTIAL DIAGNOSIS OF DIGG

- DIGG is closely related to the desmoplastic cerebral astrocytoma of infancy, which shares the clinical and histologic features of DIGG, but contains no cells with neuronal differentiation.
- DIGG shows some similarity to the pleomorphic xanthoastrocytoma, which is uncommon in infancy, has a predilection for the temporal lobe, and contains large pleomorphic cells lacking a neuronal immunophenotype.

DESMOPLASTIC INFANTILE GANGLIOGLIOMA (DIGG)

The DIGG is a supratentorial neuroepithelial neoplasm of infancy with a good prognosis.

MACROSCOPIC APPEARANCES

The desmoplastic nature of DIGGs gives them a firm texture. Part of the neoplasm may lie in the subarachnoid space. Cysts are usually evident, and a single cyst may occupy a large volume of brain.

MICROSCOPIC APPEARANCES

In areas of prominent desmoplasia, neoplastic cells are spindle-shaped with elongated hyperchromatic nuclei (**Fig. 37.6**). In some regions, spindle-shaped cells and desmoplasia may give way to plump astrocytic cells. Ganglion cells with large nucleoli are found within the neoplasm and can be numerous, mimicking a ganglioglioma. There may be a very small number of mitoses with a normal configuration.

Immunohistochemistry shows that many cells express GFAP. Synaptophysin and neurofilament antibodies label ganglion cells and some cells without obvious neuronal morphology. Ultrastructural examination reveals that many of the astrocytic cells have a prominent basal lamina.

DESMOPLASTIC INFANTILE GANGLIOGLIOMA

- usually presents in infants under 1 year of age.
- is usually a large superficial neoplasm of the cerebrum.
- is usually associated with a cyst.

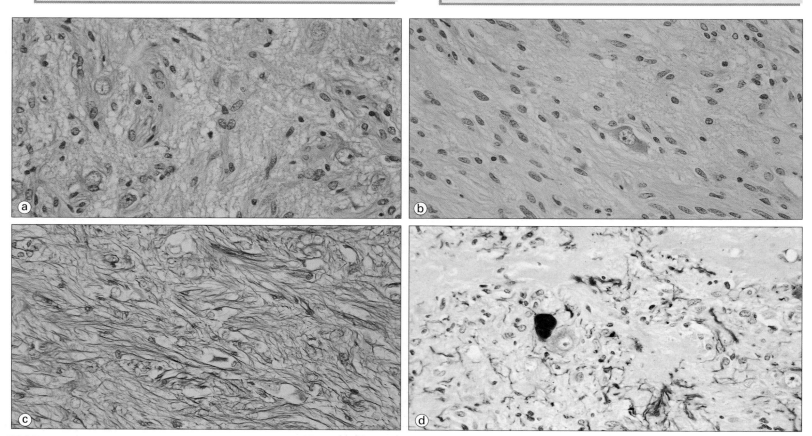

Fig. 37.6 Desmoplastic infantile ganglioglioma. Ganglion cells are scattered among cells with fibrillary cytoplasm and oval nuclei that have either **(a)** a random or **(b)** a fascicular arrangement. **(c)** Dense reticulin surrounds cells. **(d)** Ganglion cells and some fine processes show immunoreactivity for neurofilament protein.

CENTRAL NEUROCYTOMA

Before the neuronal immunohistochemical and ultrastructural characteristics of the central neurocytoma were recognized, this slowly growing neoplasm was usually termed an 'intraventricular oligodendroglioma' or an 'ependymoma of the foramen of Monro' (**Fig. 37.7**). A central neurocytoma is typically located immediately adjacent to the lateral or third ventricle, but there are a few reports of central neurocytomas elsewhere in the CNS.

MACROSCOPIC AND MICROSCOPIC APPEARANCES

The central neurocytoma is a soft, well-circumscribed neoplasm that often contains flecks of calcification. It consists of monotonous round to oval cells which contain fibrillary cytoplasm and round nuclei with finely granular chromatin (**Fig. 37.8**). A fixation artefact giving a 'fried egg' appearance to the cells is sometimes seen. The sheet of neoplastic cells is divided by anuclear fibrillary zones, which contain capillaries. Mitotic figures are seldom seen. Ganglion cells are rarely present, but evince the neuronal origin of the neoplasm.

Immunohistochemistry reveals synaptophysin in the cell bodies and fibrillary matrix. GFAP antibodies label reactive astrocytes and a few neoplastic cells in some neoplasms. Neurofilament protein is demonstrable in the occasional ganglion cell. Ultrastructurally, the cells contain microtubules and a few dense-core secretory vesicles.

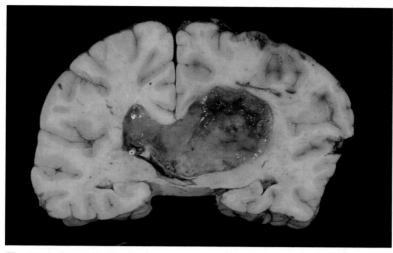

Fig. 37.7 Central neurocytoma. A coronal section through the cerebrum at the level of the hippocampus reveals a circumscribed, fleshy tumor in the ventricles.

CENTRAL NEUROCYTOMAS

- are midline neoplasms located predominantly in the vicinity of the septum pellucidum.
- cause hydrocephalus.
- usually present in young adults.

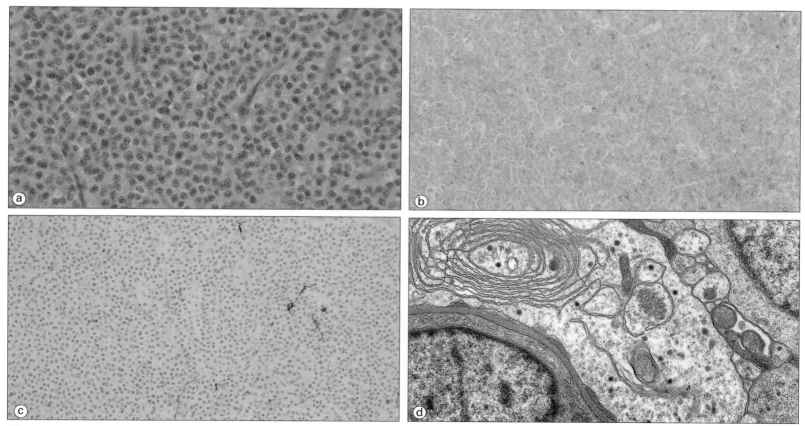

Fig. 37.8 Central neurocytoma. (a) A sheet of cells with uniform, round nuclei. This is typical of the central neurocytoma. **(b)** The cells show immunoreactivity for synaptophysin. **(c)** A few reactive astrocytes expressing GFAP. The neoplastic cells are rarely GFAP-positive. **(d)** Ultrastructural view of a central neurocytoma revealing dense-core synaptic vesicles.

PARAGANGLIOMA OF THE FILUM TERMINALE

This neoplasm shares the pathologic features of other extra-adrenal paragangliomas. It generally occurs in adults, and usually presents with sciatica. Significant pressor amine secretion has not been reported.

MACROSCOPIC AND MICROSCOPIC APPEARANCES

Paraganglioma of the filum terminale is an encapsulated neoplasm arising from the filum terminale or lumbosacral roots and forming a lozenge-shaped structure. It appears richly vascular and may be cystic. Microscopically, nests of polyhedral cells with granular cytoplasm are surrounded by a delicate fibrovascular network (**Fig. 37.9**). Some cytologic pleomorphism may be apparent, but is of no biologic significance. Nuclei contain stippled chromatin. Ganglion cells may make up a large proportion of the cells (gangliocytic paraganglioma).

Immunoreactivity for synaptophysin and chromogranin is present, and ultrastructural examination reveals dense-core granules. Sustentacular cells at the periphery of the cell nests are immunoreactive for S-100.

PARAGANGLIOMA AND EPENDYMOMA

Paraganglioma of the filum terminale and myxopapillary ependymoma may occur at the same site. Typical examples of each are readily distinguished, but sometimes their appearances can be similar. The diagnosis is then readily resolved by immunohistochemistry or electron microscopy.

- The ependymoma is immunopositive for GFAP, whereas the paraganglioma is immunopositive for synaptophysin.
- Ultrastructurally, the paraganglioma contains dense-core vesicles.

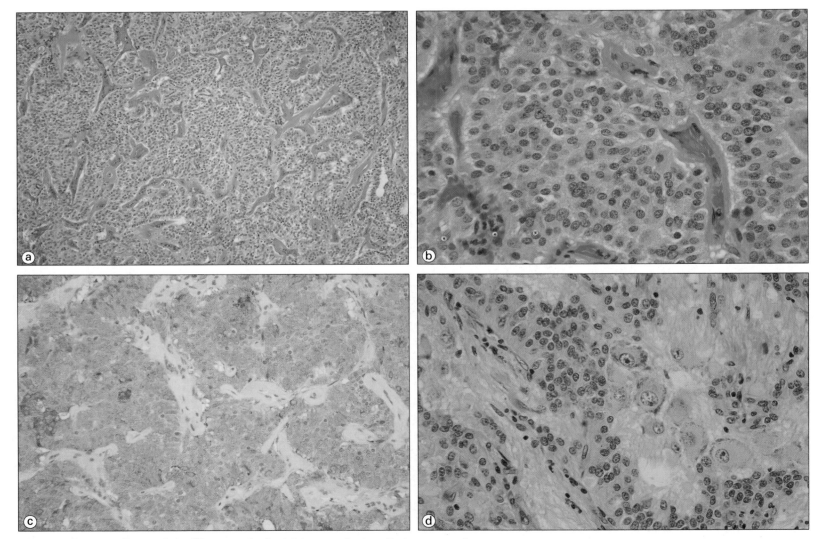

Fig. 37.9 Paraganglioma of the filum terminale. (a) A network of capillaries surrounds nests of uniform cells with stippled chromatin. **(b)** The same neoplasm at higher magnification. **(c)** Strong synaptophysin immunoreactivity of the tumor cells. **(d)** Paraganglioma containing numerous ganglion cells.

DYSEMBRYOPLASTIC NEUROEPITHELIAL TUMOR (DNT)

The DNT is a recently recognized supratentorial lesion. Recurrence after surgical resection is rare, and whether DNTs are truly neoplastic is still uncertain.

MACROSCOPIC AND MICROSCOPIC APPEARANCES

DNTs are composed of a mixed population of neuroepithelial cells and display a distinctive multinodular architecture. They may occupy a small or a large area of cerebral cortex, and involved gyri are often protuberant.

DYSEMBRYOPLASTIC NEUROEPITHELIAL TUMOR

- occurs mainly in the temporal lobe.
- usually presents in children or young adults.
- usually presents with simple or complex partial seizures which may becomne intractable.

The histologic hallmarks of the DNT are glial nodules and masses of oligodendrocyte-like cells (OLCs) which are usually dispersed around mucinous cysts (**Figs 37.10, 37.11**). The glial nodules contain astrocytic cells which are sometimes admixed with OLCs. The nodules are more cellular than the surrounding regions, and may resemble a pilocytic or fibrillary astrocytoma. Elsewhere, OLCs form small groups or columns showing little variation in shape or size. Cells with a typical neuronal morphology are scattered among the OLCs, and sometimes appear suspended within the mucinous cysts. The microcysts contain acid mucopolysaccharides, but this feature is not specific for DNTs. Some DNTs lack microcysts but have the typical nodular architecture.

The surrounding cortex, which may show discrete areas of dysplasia, is diffusely invaded by OLCs, but perineuronal satellitosis is not a prominent feature. Dystrophic calcification may be seen, but mitoses are very rarely encountered.

Immunohistochemistry and ultrastructural examination reveal that only few OLCs have neuronal or astrocytic features. However, the larger cells in the glioneuronal element are immunoreactive for neuronal markers, such as synaptophysin and neurofilament proteins.

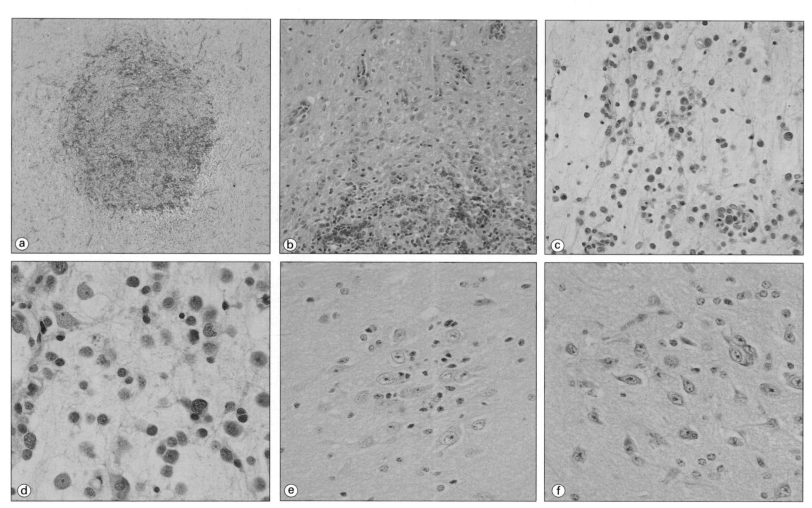

Fig. 37.10 Dysembryoplastic neuroepithelial tumor. (a) Nodular cluster of cells in a DNT. **(b)** OLCs are typical of DNTs, but cells with an astrocytic morphology are also present as demonstrated here. **(c)** OLCs appear in festoons against a mucinous background. **(d)** OLCs are admixed with larger cells that show neuronal features. **(e)** A cluster of neurons and small OLCs is seen away from the main tumor mass. **(f)** Cortical dysplasia in association with a DNT.

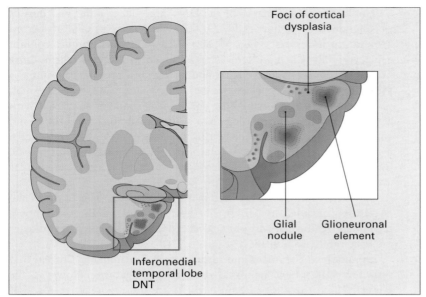

Foci of cortical
dysplasia

Glial
nodule

Glioneuronal
element

Inferomedial
temporal lobe
DNT

Fig. 37.11 DNT. This neoplasm sometimes contains glial nodules in addition to the specific glioneuronal elements and focal areas of cortical dysplasia. Nodules may contain cells with an astrocytic or oligodendroglial morphophenotype. Astrocytomatous nodules may resemble pilocytic or fibrillary astrocytomas. Glial nodules may occur in normal cortex away from the glioneuronal element.

DYSPLASTIC GANGLIOCYTOMA OF THE CEREBELLUM

The dysplastic gangliocytoma of the cerebellum (Lhermitte–Duclos disease) is a choristoma (see p. 37.1). Its growth is thought to be related to hypertrophy rather than replication of the constituent cells.

MACROSCOPIC AND MICROSCOPIC APPEARANCES

The folia within a dysplastic gangliocytoma of the cerebellum appear abnormally thickened (**Fig. 37.12a**). Enlarged abnormal neurons replace internal granule cells, distorting the normal cerebellar architecture (**Fig. 37.12b**). The cells are immunoreactive for synaptophysin and neurofilaments and their axons in the molecular layer are often myelinated. There are a loss of Purkinje cells and rarefaction or cavitation of white matter in the core of affected folia.

DYSPLASTIC GANGLIOCYTOMA OF THE CEREBELLUM

- usually presents with raised intracranial pressure in young adults.
- is associated with megalencephaly, polydactyly, Cowden's syndrome (multiple hamartoma–neoplasia syndrome), and multiple cutaneous schwannomas.

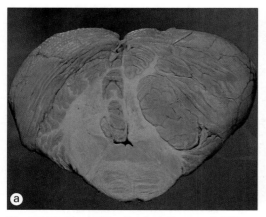
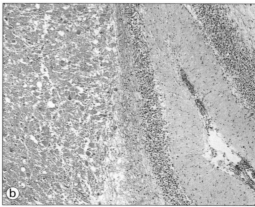
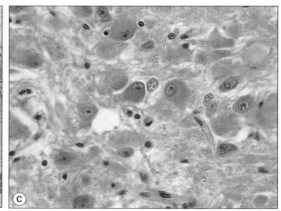

Fig. 37.12 Lhermitte–Duclos disease. (a) The cerebellum displays a markedly abnormal architecture. **(b, c)** Widened folia contain huge ganglion cells that replace internal granule cells; demarcation from relatively normal tissue may be abrupt.

HYPOTHALAMIC NEURONAL HAMARTOMA

This non-neoplastic lesion is composed of ganglion cells arranged singly and in clusters against a fibrillary neuroepithelial background and is usually evident as a small mass ventral to the hypothalamus. Generally it is asymptomatic, but rarely it may produce endocrine syndromes such as precocious puberty, which result from the capacity of the ganglion cells to secrete hypothalamic hormones in an aberrant fashion.

REFERENCES

Burger PC, Scheithauer BW (1994) Neuronal and glio-neuronal tumors. In *Tumors of the Central Nervous System*. pp. 163–191. Washington: Armed Forces Institute of Pathology. (J Rosai (ed.) *Atlas of Tumor Pathology. Volume 10.*)

Daumas-Duport C (1993) Dysembryoplastic neuroepithelial tumors. *Brain Pathology* **3**: 285–295.

Felix I, Bilbao JM, Asa SL, Tyndel F, Kovacs K, Becker LE (1994) Cerebral and cerebellar gangliocytomas: a morphological study of nine cases. *Acta Neuropathologica* **88**: 246–251.

Hirose T, Scheithauer BW, Lopes MB, VandenBerg SR (1994) Dysembryoplastic neuroepithelial tumour (DNT): an immunohistochemical and ultrastructural study. *J Neuropath Exp Neurol* **53**: 184–195.

Raymond AA, Halpin SF, Alsanjari N, Cook MJ *et al.* (1994) Dysembryoplastic neuroepithelial tumour: features in 16 patients. *Brain* **117**: 461–475.

VandenBerg SR, May EE, Rubinstein LJ, Herman MM *et al.* (1987) Desmoplastic supratentorial neuroepithelial tumours of infancy with divergent differentiation potential ('desmoplastic infantile gangliogliomas'). *J Neurosurg* **66**: 58–71.

Von Deimling A, Janzer R, Kleihues P, Wiestler OD (1990) Patterns of differentiation in central neurocytoma. An immunohistochemical study of eleven biopsies. *Acta Neuropathol Berl* **79**(5): 473–479.

EMBRYONAL NEUROEPITHELIAL NEOPLASMS

Embryonal (primitive) neuroepithelial neoplasms make up 4–5% of central nervous system (CNS) neoplasms. Their features include:
- A predominance in children.
- A tendency to disseminate through cerebrospinal fluid (CSF) pathways.
- A dominant population of small undifferentiated cells.
- High mitotic indices and widespread apoptosis.
- A potential for divergent neuroepithelial differentiation.

CLASSIFICATION

In the World Health Organization (WHO) classification of CNS neoplasms, the embryonal neuroepithelial neoplasms are:
- Primitive neuroectodermal tumor (PNET), including medulloblastoma and its variants: desmoplastic medulloblastoma, medullomyoblastoma, and melanotic medulloblastoma.
- Neuroblastoma and ganglioneuroblastoma.
- Ependymoblastoma.
- Medulloepithelioma.

Though placed among pineocytic neoplasms in the WHO classification, the pineoblastoma (chapter 39) is also considered to belong to the family of embryonal neoplasms.

Classification of embryonal neoplasms is controversial. On the basis of shared histologic characteristics and similar biologic behavior, embryonal neoplasms at different sites throughout the CNS have been grouped under the term PNET. This viewpoint postulates that PNETs share a common oncogenic process and arise from progenitor cells that have the potential for considerable histologic heterogeneity. However, there is an opposing viewpoint that neoplastic transformation of cells at particular sites in the CNS produces embryonal neoplasms with sufficiently distinctive histologic and clinical attributes to justify their separation in tumor classifications. Analyzing molecular genetic abnormalities in these neoplasms may help to clarify their relationships.

The WHO classification proposes the term PNET for a CNS neoplasm that resembles the medulloblastoma of the posterior fossa which is frequently undifferentiated but may show divergent differentiation. Other embryonal neuroepithelial neoplasms are separated from PNETs because they have:
- Restricted differentiation (i.e. neuroblastoma, ependymoblastoma, pineoblastoma).
- A unique architecture that resembles the primitive medullary epithelium of the neural tube (i.e. medulloepithelioma).

PNETs may occur at any site in the CNS, but the majority occurs in the cerebellum as medulloblastomas. Other embryonal neoplasms occur predominantly in the cerebrum.

EMBRYONAL NEUROEPITHELIAL NEOPLASMS

Medulloblastoma:
- represents about 5% of intracranial neoplasms.
- represents about 25% of childhood CNS neoplasms.
- represents about 90% of childhood CNS PNETs.
- can present at any age, but 50% occur in patients less than 10 years of age.
- generally arises from the vermis and fills the fourth ventricle.
- may be located laterally in the posterior fossa.
- may spread through CSF pathways.

Ependymoblastoma:
- is an extremely rare neoplasm.
- nearly always presents in children under 5 years of age.
- can be congenital.
- can affect any level of the CNS.
- has a very poor prognosis.

Neuroblastoma:
- is a very rare neoplasm.
- occurs mainly in patients under 20 years of age.
- is usually supratentorial.
- is associated with a median survival of 4 years.
- commonly disseminates through CSF pathways.

Medulloepithelioma:
- is an extremely rare neoplasm.
- nearly always presents in children under 5 years of age, and most patients are under 1 year.
- can be congenital.
- shows no bias towards either sex.
- generally presents as a deep-seated supratentorial mass.
- may occupy a large volume of one hemisphere.
- has a median survival of 8 months.

MACROSCOPIC APPEARANCES

The macroscopic appearances of different embryonal neoplasms are similar. Most are well-circumscribed, pink or gray neoplasms with areas of hemorrhage, necrosis, or calcification (**Fig. 38.1**). Neuroblastomas and medulloepitheliomas sometimes contain cysts.

The texture of embryonal neoplasms varies. Some are soft, but medulloblastomas in the lateral posterior fossa and most neuroblastomas tend to be firm because they contain areas of desmoplasia. Neoplastic cells commonly metastasize through the CSF pathways (**Fig. 38.2**).

MICROSCOPIC APPEARANCES
PNET (medulloblastoma)

PNETs are mainly composed of undifferentiated cells with hyperchromatic nuclei and sparse cytoplasm (**Fig. 38.3**). Although typically small and round, the nuclei may measure up to 20 μm or more in diameter and have contours that are focally flattened or even slightly indented. In some areas, the cells may contain a little more cytoplasm and the nuclei are set in a scanty fibrillary, eosinophilic background. Many PNETs do not show any morphologic or immuno-histochemical evidence of neuronal or glial differentiation, and ultra-structural examination supports the view that most cells in PNETs are undifferentiated. Mitoses and apoptotic bodies are plentiful in regions where the nuclear:cytoplasmic ratio is high. Microscopic foci or large areas of necrosis may be present. PNET cells have a tendency to spread along the pial surface of the brain, invading the underlying parenchyma in columns.

GENETIC ASPECTS OF MEDULLOBLASTOMAS

- Nearly all medulloblastomas are sporadic.
- Allelic losses on 17p (17p13.3–17pter) occur in about 50% of medulloblastomas.
- Less than 5% of medulloblastomas have p53 mutations.
- An isochromosome for 17q occurs in about 30% of medulloblastomas.
- Allelic losses on 9q occur in a few medulloblastomas.
- Allelic losses on 9q may be a particular feature of desmoplastic medulloblastomas.
- c-*myc* is amplified or overexpressed in only a few medulloblastomas.
- N-*myc* is not elevated in medulloblastomas.

SYNDROMES FEATURING MEDULLOBLASTOMAS

- **Gorlin's (basal cell nevus) syndrome**, which is characterized by basal cell carcinomas, ovarian fibromas, and developmental defects, shows autosomal dominant inheritance, and features medulloblastomas in 3–5% of patients. The syndrome occurs in 1–2% of patients with medulloblastomas. The gene is localized to chromosome 9q31.
- **Turcot's syndrome**, which includes medulloblastoma, astrocytic neoplasms, familial polyposis, and colonic carcinoma.

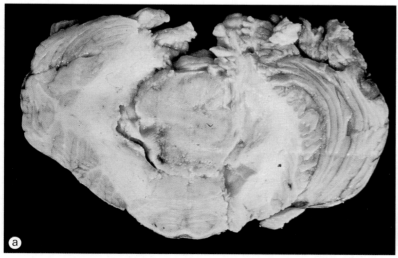
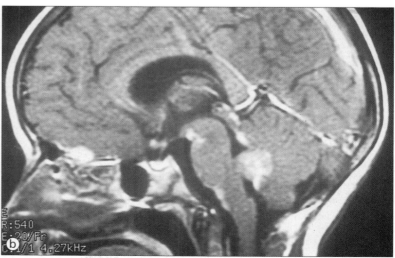

Fig. 38.1 PNET (medulloblastoma). (a) A soft homogeneous mass destroys the vermis and occupies the fourth ventricle.
(b) A sagittal midline MR image through the brain showing a PNET in the posterior fossa between the cerebellum and brainstem. (Courtesy of Dr JS Millar, Wessex Neurological Center)

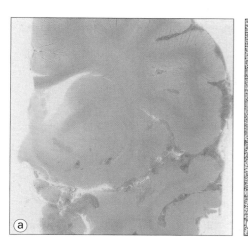

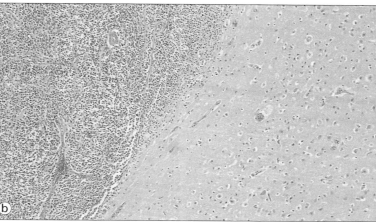

Fig. 38.2 PNET in the subarachnoid space.
(a) Extensive infiltration of the subarachnoid space by basophilic cells from a PNET. Several distinct parenchymal deposits are also present. **(b)** From the same case a mass of small cells fills the subarachnoid space and has begun to invade the pial surface of the cerebrum.

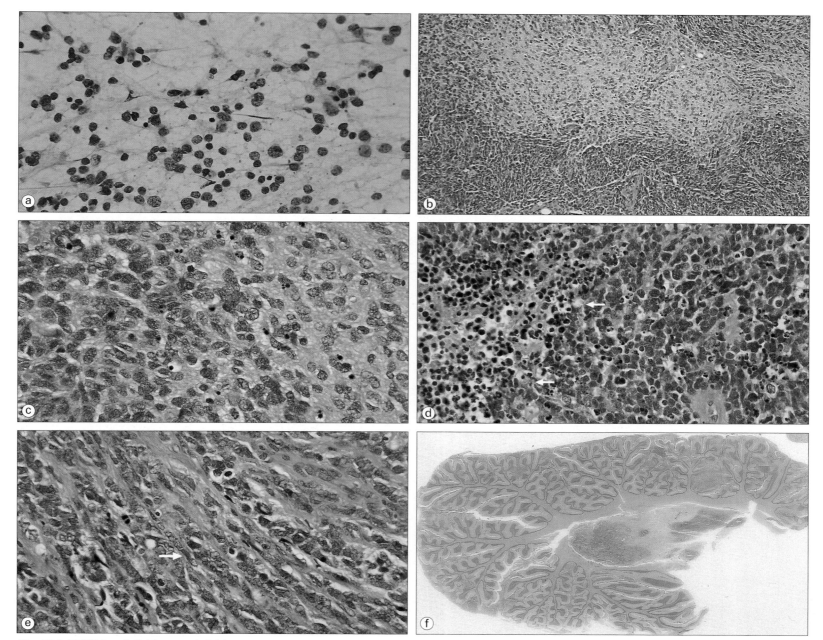

Fig. 38.3 PNET (medulloblastoma). (a) A smear preparation showing scattered bare hyperchromatic nuclei. (Toluidine blue) **(b)** A monotonous sheet of densely packed small cells is interrupted by an area where cells have a lower nuclear:cytoplasmic ratio. **(c)** Abundant mitoses and apoptotic bodies as seen here are typical features of PNET. Note the variation in nuclear size and shape. **(d)** Micronecrosis. **(e)** Focal desmoplasia constraining the cells into cords and files. Note the nuclear molding (arrow), which is a common finding in these neoplasms. **(f)** Multiple cerebellar deposits and meningeal spread of cells from a PNET. Note the invasion of cortex underlying the infiltrated leptomeninges.

Neuronal differentiation may take the form of rosettes that lack a central canal or capillary (Homer–Wright rosettes). Small neurons or ganglion cells are rare (**Fig. 38.4**). Groups of small cells without obvious neuronal morphology may show immunoreactivity for synaptophysin (**Fig. 38.4c**), but only ganglion cells label with neurofilament protein antibodies. Ultrastructural examination reveals secretory granules in a few larger cells.

Neoplastic cells with a typical astrocytic morphology are not found in PNETs, but the cytoplasm of some small neoplastic cells may occasionally be immunoreactive for GFAP (**Fig. 38.5**).

In searching for focal neuroepithelial differentiation, care should be taken to distinguish reactive astrocytes (**Fig. 38.6**) and entrapped native neurons from neoplastic cells. The prognostic significance of divergent neuroepithelial differentiation is not clear. Some studies have shown a poor outcome for patients with neoplasms that show glial differentiation as defined by immunoreactivity for GFAP.

DIFFERENTIAL DIAGNOSIS OF MEDULLOBLASTOMA

- Unlike a medulloblastoma, an ependymoma usually arises from the floor of the fourth ventricle and shows widespread pseudorosettes and GFAP immunoreactivity, but does not show focal immunoreactivity for synaptophysin.
- Unlike a medulloblastoma, a glioblastoma of the cerebellum contains many cells with an astrocytic morphophenotype, and a glomeruloid microvasculature, but does not show focal immunoreactivity for synaptophysin.

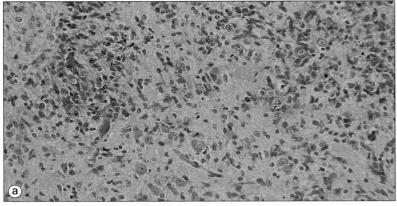

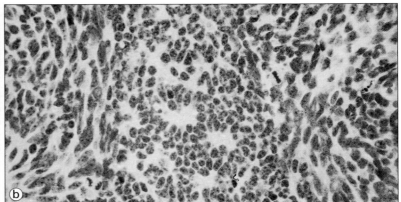

Fig. 38.4 Neuronal differentiation in a PNET. (a) Ganglion and neurocytic cells in a PNET are a rare manifestation of neuronal differentiation. **(b)** Rosette (Homer–Wright) formation. (Courtesy of Dr T Revesz, Institute of Neurology, London, U.K.) **(c)** There is prominent synaptophysin immunoreactivity in some cells of this medulloblastoma.

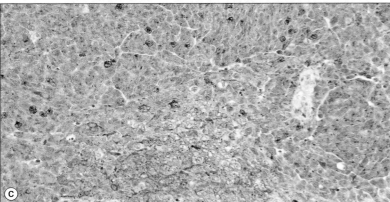

Fig. 38.5 Glial differentiation in a PNET. In a minority of PNETs, GFAP immunoreactivity is a feature of scattered neoplastic cells; in this case, GFAP-positive cells surround nodules in which GFAP-negative cells predominate.

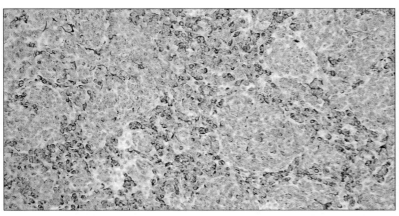

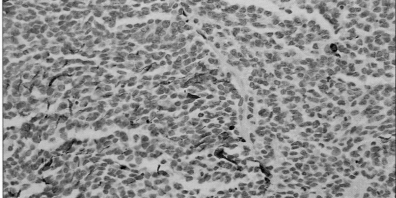

Fig. 38.6 PNET. The GFAP-positive processes of scattered reactive astrocytes are commonly found in PNETs and should not be mistaken for glial differentiation.

COLLINS' RULE FOR A CHILD WITH A PNET

Collins' rule:
- states that the period of risk for recurrence = the child's age at diagnosis + 9 months.
- applies to over 95% of children under 8 years of age with a medulloblastoma, provided the neoplasm appears to have been eradicated by surgery and radiotherapy.

Variants of medulloblastoma: Desmoplasia is common in embryonal neuroepithelial neoplasms, particularly when their cells invade the leptomeninges, but the desmoplastic variant of medulloblastoma is also characterized by distinctive reticulin-free 'islands' of monomorphic round cells among the reticulin-rich areas. Cells in the islands often have a lower nuclear:cytoplasmic ratio than surrounding cells, and their monotonous appearance matches that of the central neurocytoma. The histology of this variant merges with that of less desmoplastic, nodular medulloblastomas (**Fig. 38.7**). Neuronal differentiation is often prominent in nodular medulloblastomas. In some series, desmoplastic and nodular medulloblastomas have had a better outcome, but this has not been a consistent finding.

Focal melanin production (**Fig. 38.8**) and evidence of striated muscle differentiation (**Fig. 38.9**) can both occur in medulloblastomas, creating the variants melanotic medulloblastoma and medullomyoblastoma.

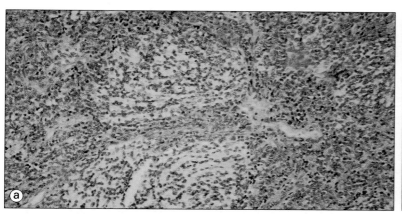
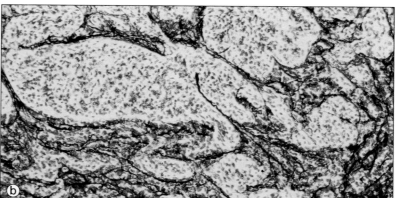

Fig. 38.7 Nodular (desmoplastic) medulloblastoma. (a) Groups of neoplastic cells are surrounded by fibrous septa which are highlighted **(b)** by reticulin. Cells within the nodules tend to have a lower nuclear:cytoplasmic ratio than cells elsewhere. (Courtesy of Dr T Revesz, Institute of Neurology, London, U.K.)

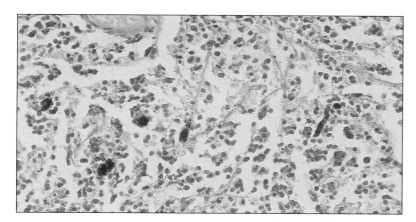

Fig. 38.8 Melanotic medulloblastoma. This shows focal melanin production in a medulloblastoma.

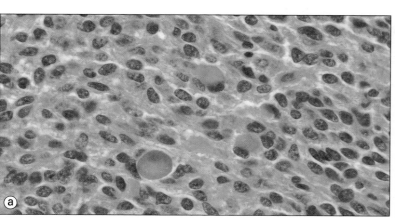
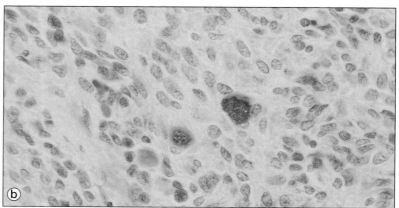

Fig. 38.9 Medullomyoblastoma. (a) Scattered large cells have abundant eosinophilic cytoplasm and eccentric nuclei. **(b)** These cells typically show immunoreactivity for myoglobin.

A pleomorphic large-cell variant of medulloblastoma is also recognized (**Fig. 38.10**) and has a poor prognosis.

Neuroblastoma and ganglioneuroblastoma
The rare neuroblastoma may occur anywhere in the CNS, but most reported cases have been supratentorial (**Fig. 38.11**). In common with PNETs, the neuroblastoma consists of small cells with sparse cytoplasm, hyperchromatic nuclei, and a high mitotic count. It exhibits focal neuronal differentiation in the form of Homer–Wright rosettes and scattered immunoreactivity for neurofilament protein, class III β-tubulin, and synaptophysin.

Neoplastic cells with the cytologic features of small or large neurons may be found in areas containing cells with a reduced nuclear:cytoplasmic ratio. If these cells are widespread, the neoplasm should be termed a ganglioneuroblastoma (**Fig. 38.12**). Desmoplasia may be found in neuroblastomas, particularly if there is invasion of the leptomeninges.

Ependymoblastoma
The ependymoblastic rosette is the key diagnostic feature of ependymoblastomas, which like other embryonal neuroepithelial neoplasms consist mainly of undifferentiated small cells (**Fig. 38.13**). Ependymoblastic rosettes are composed of multiple layers of small cells with hyperchromatic nuclei that surround a circular or elongated lumen. The lumen has a prominent internal limiting membrane, and mitotic figures are readily found in the rosettes. The rosettes label with antibodies to vimentin, and occasionally with antibodies to GFAP.

Anaplastic ependymoma differs from ependymoblastoma because it contains typical pseudorosettes rather than ependymoblastic rosettes and usually shows glomeruloid capillary endothelial proliferation. Both types of neoplasm have a high mitotic rate and foci of necrosis.

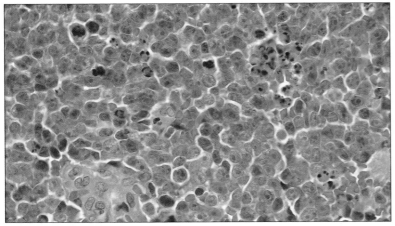

Fig. 38.10 Large-cell variant of medulloblastoma.

DIFFERENTIAL DIAGNOSIS OF NEUROBLASTOMA

- Unlike the glioblastoma, the cerebral neuroblastoma generally presents in childhood and shows focal synaptophysin immunoreactivity. The glioblastoma is characterized by some cells with an astrocytic morphophenotype and a glomeruloid microvasculature. These are not features of neuroblastoma.
- Unlike the cerebral neuroblastoma, the desmoplastic infantile ganglioglioma presents as a superficial cortical neoplasm with a cyst and shows widespread GFAP immunoreactivity. It also has a dense reticulin pattern, which is not always a feature of a cerebral neuroblastoma.
- Unlike the central neurocytoma, the cerebral neuroblastoma shows many mitoses, focal desmoplasia, and necrosis. A central neurocytoma is usually intraventricular; a cerebral neuroblastoma may occasionally involve periventricular tissue.

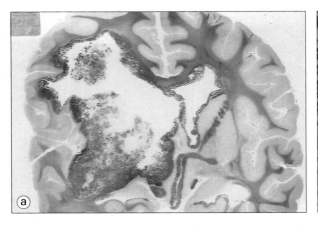

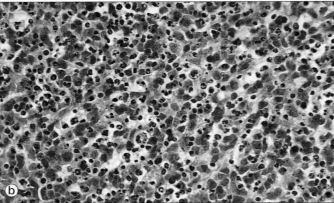

Fig. 38.11 Neuroblastoma. (a) This neuroblastoma has destroyed a large part of one cerebral hemisphere and has spread beneath the ependyma. (Luxol fast blue/cresyl violet) **(b)** A sheet of uniform cells contains abundant apoptotic bodies.

Fig. 38.12 Ganglioneuroblastoma. Widespread ganglionic differentiation was seen in this neuroblastoma. This neoplasm tends to behave like a PNET rather than a gangliocytic neoplasm.

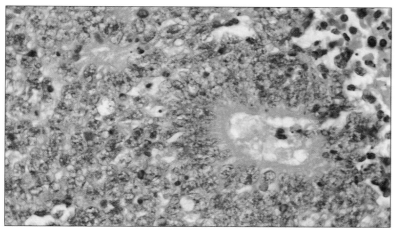

Fig. 38.13 Ependymoblastoma. Otherwise appearing as a PNET, this neoplasm contains rosettes composed of multiple layers of cells with a high nuclear:cytoplasmic ratio.

Medulloepithelioma

The defining histologic attribute of the medulloepithelioma is an arrangement of tightly packed multilayered cells into tubules that resemble embryonic neural tube. Convoluted ribbons and papillary structures may also be seen (**Fig. 38.14**). The tubules have a periodic acid–Schiff (PAS)-positive external basement membrane, and, in some cases, PAS-positive material that may resemble a basement membrane on their luminal aspect. The neoplastic cells have hyperchromatic nuclei and very scanty cytoplasm, and the mitotic count is high.

The primitive epithelium does not label with antibodies to GFAP or synaptophysin, but focal glial and neuronal differentiation is occaisonally detected in other regions of the neoplasm. Elongated cells with tapering processes and immunoreactivity for GFAP, ependymoblastic rosettes, neuroblastic rosettes, and ganglion cell formation have all been described in medulloepitheliomas. Mesenchymal differentiation has been reported in some examples, and very rarely manifests as bone, cartilage, or striated muscle.

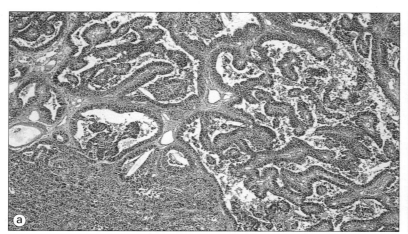

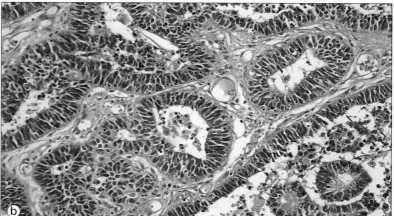

Fig. 38.14 Medulloepithelioma. (a) A papillary architecture is sometime seen in medulloepitheliomas, bringing choroid plexus neoplasms into the differential diagnosis. **(b)** Tubules of cells with hyperchromatic nuclei mimic primitive neural tube, and are characteristic of medulloepithelioma.

REFERENCES

Albrecht S, von Deimling A, Pietsch T *et al.* (1994) Microsatellite analysis of loss of heterozygosity on chromosomes 9q, 11p and 17p in medulloblastomas. *Neuropath App Neurobiol* **20**(1): 74–81.

Batra SK, McLendon RE, Koo JS *et al.* (1995) Prognostic implications of chromosome 17p deletions in medulloblastomas. *J Neuro Oncol* **24**(1): 39–45.

Brown WD, Tavare CJ, Sobel EL, Gilles FH (1989) Medulloblastoma and Collins' law: a critical review of the concept of a period of risk for tumor reccurence and patient survival. *Neurosurgery* **36**(4): 691–697.

Caccamo DV, Herman MM, Rubenstein LJ (1989) An immunohistochemical study of the primitive and maturing elements of human cerebral medulloepitheliomas. *Acta Neuropathologica* **79**: 248–254.

Fung K-M, Trojanowski JQ (1995) Animal models of medulloblastomas and related primitive neuroectodermal tumors. A review. *J Neuropathol Exp Neurol* **54**: 285–296.

Katsetos CD, Burger PC (1994) Medulloblastoma. *Seminars Diag Pathol* **11**: 85–97.

Lasorella A, Iavarone A, Israel MA (1995) Differentiation of neuroblastoma enhances bcl-2 expression and induces alteration of apoptosis and drug resistance. *Cancer Research* **55**: 4711–4716.

Packer RJ (1995) Brain tumors in children. *Current Opinion in Pediatrics* **7**(1): 64–72.

Rorke LB, Gilles FH, Davis RL, Becker LE. (1985) Revision of the world health Organization classification of brain tumors for childhood brain tumors. *Cancer* **56**: 1869–1886.

Rorke LB *et al.* (1997). Primitive neuroectodermal tumors of the central nervous system. *Brain Patholoy* **7**: 765–784.

Schofield D, West DC, Antony DC, Marshal R, Sklar J (1995) Correlation of loss of heterozygosity at chromosome 9q with histological subtype in medulloblastomas. *American J Pathol* **146**(2): 472–480.

Triche TJ (1990) Neuroblastoma and other childhood neural tumors: a review. *Pediat Pathol* **10**: 175–193.

VandenBerg SR, Herman MM, Rubinstein LJ (1987) Embryonal central neuropithelial tumors: current concepts and future challenges. *Cancer and Metastasis Reviews* **5**: 343–364.

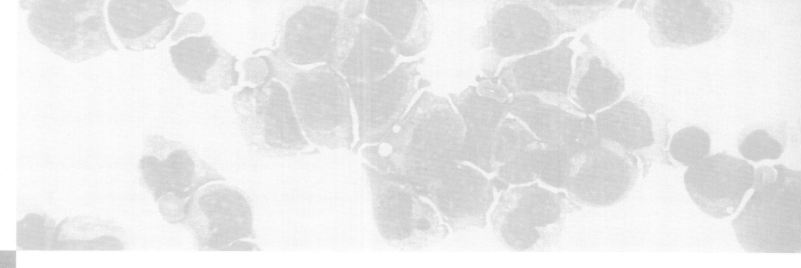

39 Neoplasms of the pineal gland

Neoplasms discussed in this chapter are pineocytic neoplasms and primary central nervous system (CNS) germ cell neoplasms. Nearly all primary CNS germ cell neoplasms arise in the pineal or suprasellar regions.

NEOPLASMS IN THE PINEAL GLAND

These may present with:
- raised intracranial pressure due either to mass effect or aqueduct compression and subsequent hydrocephalus
- brain stem compression, producing Parinaud's syndrome, other gaze palsies, nystagmus, ataxia, or long tract signs
- endocrine dysfunction related to hydrocephalus and rarely to neoplastic infiltration of the hypothalamus

PINEOCYTIC NEOPLASMS

- Approximately 40% of pineocytic neoplasms are pineocytomas, 40% are pineoblastomas, and 20% are mixed or intermediate pineocytic neoplasms.
- Patients presenting with pineocytic neoplasms are mostly in their third or fourth decade.
- There is an equal incidence of pineocytic neoplasms in males and females.
- Pineoblastomas occur at a younger mean age (approximately 20 years of age) than pineocytomas (approximately 40 years of age).
- Rarely, pineoblastomas are associated with bilateral retinoblastomas in children.
- Classic pineocytomas respond relatively well to surgery and focal radiotherapy.
- Other pineocytic neoplasms may metastasize through cerebrospinal fluid (CSF) pathways, and show a variable response to surgery and adjunctive therapies.

PINEOCYTIC NEOPLASMS

The developed pineal gland consists of nests of pinealocytes enclosed by fibrovascular septa. Pinealocytes are neuroepithelial cells, contain abundant secretory granules, and have elongated processes with club-like endings that extend towards blood vessels. Melatonin and serotonin are the major products of the pineal gland and, like cells in the retina, pinealocytes can produce S antigen. The different types of pineocytic neoplasm are:
- pineocytoma
- mixed pineocytic tumor
- intermediate pineocytic tumor
- pineoblastoma

The term pinealoma should no longer be used.

MACROSCOPIC APPEARANCES

Pineocytomas are firm gray neoplasms. Pineoblastomas are softer and sometimes gelatinous in texture and may contain areas of hemorrhage and necrosis. Although both types of neoplasm may be circumscribed, pineocytomas usually compress surrounding tissues (**Fig. 39.1**), while pineoblastomas tend to infiltrate the midbrain, third ventricle, or sometimes the thalamus and hypothalamus. Pineoblastomas frequently disseminate throughout the CNS along CSF pathways.

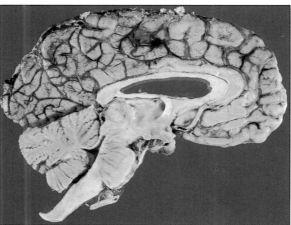

Fig. 39.1 Pineocytoma. Arising from the pineal gland, this neoplasm has invaded and distorted the rostral brain stem.

MICROSCOPIC APPEARANCES

Pineocytoma

The pineocytoma consists predominantly of small monomorphic cells set in a fibrillary background (**Fig. 39.2**). The cells are generally arranged in sheets, though a nodular pattern may be evident. A characteristic feature is the formation of pineocytomatous rosettes, which are relatively large zones of fine, fibrillary processes surrounded by an oval arrangement of neoplastic cell nuclei (see **Fig. 39.6**). The neoplastic cells generally resemble the cells of normal pineal gland, with their argyrophilic processes which may have club-like terminal expansions. Their processes express synaptophysin, and at the ultrastructural level contain microtubules and a few dense core vesicles. Some cells label with antibodies to S antigen.

Cytologic pleomorphism, manifesting occasionally as giant cells with misshapen, hyperchromatic nuclei, may be found in scattered groups of cells. Provided these cells are not accompanied by mitoses and other atypical cells with a high nuclear:cytoplasmic ratio, they are not thought to be an adverse prognostic sign. Ganglion cells may be found in some pineocytomas.

Cells in a pineocytoma may be immunoreactive for neurofilament proteins (**Fig. 39.3**). Immunolabeling for GFAP is confined to reactive astrocytes. Electron microscopy reveals cilia with a 9 + 0 configuration as well as dense core vesicles.

Mixed pineocytic and intermediate pineocytic tumors

Mixed and intermediate pineocytic tumors occupy a middle ground between pineocytoma and pineoblastoma:

- The mixed pineocytoma/pineoblastoma is characterized by groups of small, rapidly proliferating cells in a neoplasm which otherwise has the architecture and cytology of a pineocytoma. The small, 'blast' cells confer the behavioral properties of a pineoblastoma upon this neoplasm.
- The intermediate pineocytic tumor is characterized by a range of atypical cells with a variable nuclear:cytoplasmic ratio. The well-differentiated features of the pineocytoma, including pineocytomatous rosettes, are missing, as are large numbers of 'blast' cells. Ganglion cells and giant cells are occasionally found. Immunoreactivity for neuronal markers may be prominent (**Fig. 39.3**). This variant sometimes metastasizes throughout the CNS.

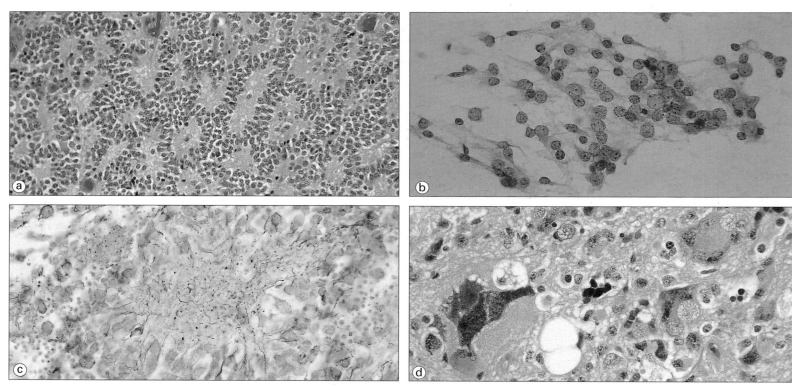

Fig. 39.2 Pineocytoma. (a) Pineocytomatous rosettes dominate this region of a typical pineocytoma. **(b)** In a smear preparation, the cells of this pineocytoma are characterized by uniformity, delicate cytoplasmic processes, and tiny nucleoli. **(c)** Silver impregnation of the neuritic processes in a pineocytomatous rosette. **(d)** Cytologic pleomorphism as marked as here may be seen in pineocytomas, and mixed or intermediate pineocytic neoplasms. In an otherwise typical pineocytoma with pineocytomatous rosettes, but without mitoses and focal increases in nuclear:cytoplasmic ratio, it is not thought to be an adverse prognostic sign.

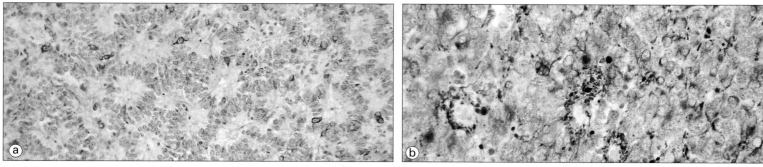

Fig. 39.3 Immunoreactivity for neurofilament protein in pineocytic neoplasms. (a) Widespread staining is seen in this pineocytoma. **(b)** This intermediate tumor is strongly immunopositive.

Pineoblastoma

The pineoblastoma resembles the medulloblastoma, and has been grouped with other embryonal neoplasms of neuroepithelial lineage in the broad category of primitive neuroectodermal tumors (chapter 38).

It contains round or polyhedral cells with a high nuclear:cytoplasmic ratio, arranged in sheets (**Fig. 39.4**). Mitoses and apoptotic bodies are generally plentiful. Neuroblastic (Homer–Wright) and Flexner–Wintersteiner rosettes may be found, but pineocytomatous rosettes are not a feature of the typical pineoblastoma (**Fig. 39.6**). Necrosis and hemorrhage are common, while melanin is a rare finding. Immunoreactivity for neuronal markers may be local or widespread (**Fig. 39.5**), and pineoblastomas may label with antibodies to retinal S-antigen.

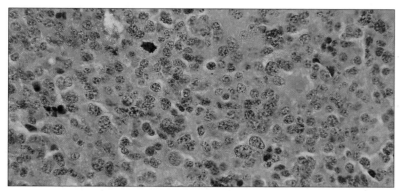

Fig. 39.4 Pineoblastoma. Monomorphic round cells with a high nuclear:cytoplasmic ratio and hyperchromatic nuclei are evident.

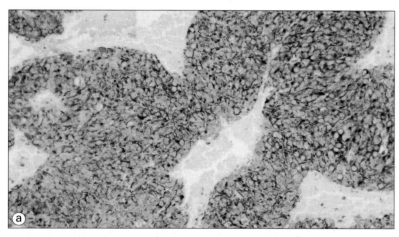

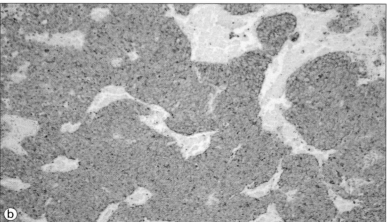

Fig. 39.5 Pineoblastoma. Lobules of neoplastic cells have labeled with antibodies (**a**) to neurofilament protein, and (**b**) to synaptophysin.

PINEAL CYST

A pineal cyst is a common finding at necropsy. Although it distorts the pineal gland, it rarely causes symptomatic compression of other structures.

MICROSCOPIC APPEARANCES

The pineal cyst has a thin wall composed of dense glial tissue containing Rosenthal fibers. Surrounding pineal gland may appear compressed.

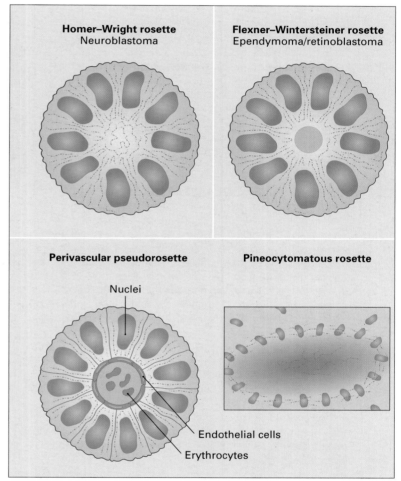

Fig. 39.6 Rosettes in CNS neoplasms. Diagrammatic representation of rosette-like structures in CNS neoplasms. The pineocytomatous rosette is larger than the rest.

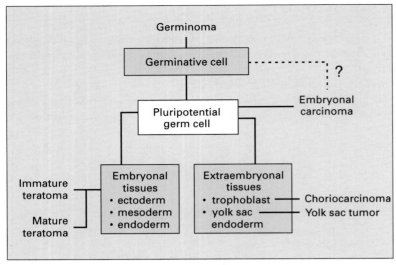

Fig. 39.7 Hypothetical scheme for the derivation of GCTs.

PRIMARY CNS GERM CELL NEOPLASMS

Primordial germ cells disseminate widely throughout the developing embryo. However, most germ cell tumors (GCTs) arise in:
- the gonads
- the diencephalon, mainly in the pineal and suprasellar regions
- the mediastinum

The pathology and biology of CNS GCTs are very similar to those of gonadal GCTs, and the World Health Organization (WHO) classification of GCTs at the different sites listed above is the same (given that the terms seminoma (testis), dysgerminoma (ovary), and germinoma are interchangeable). A germinoma must first be differentiated from a nongerminomatous GCT because germinomas are particularly sensitive to radiotherapy. Nongerminomatous GCTs range from slowly growing mature teratomas to undifferentiated neoplasms that grow and spread rapidly. GCTs recognized in the WHO classification of neoplasms of the CNS are germinomas, embryonal carcinomas, yolk sac tumors (endodermal sinus tumor), choriocarcinomas, teratomas (mature, immature, and with malignant transformation – usually carcinoma or sarcoma), and mixed GCTs (**Fig. 39.7**).

    Gliomas, meningiomas, and metastatic neoplasms may all occur in the region of the pineal gland, but are considered elsewhere.

BIOPSY OF PINEAL GLAND MASSES

- The ease with which a pineal mass is diagnosed depends partly upon the amount of tissue obtained. Often the pathologist is presented with a tiny piece of tissue and it is then important not to overstate any conclusions.
- In addition to hematoxylin and eosin, histochemical preparations should include periodic acid–Schiff, reticulin (to assess lobularity), and silver impregnation (to demonstrate neuritic processes).
- Histology may reveal an obvious pathologic process, but be prepared to cut many sections for immunohistochemistry.
- Useful antibodies for assessing pineocytic neoplasms are those to synaptophysin, neurofilament protein, glial fibrillary acidic protein, and Ki-67.
- Useful antibodies for assessing germ cell neoplasms are those to low molecular weight cytokeratin, placental alkaline phosphatase, α-fetoprotein (AFP), and β-human chorionic gonadotropin (β-HCG).
- If possible, keep a small piece of tissue for ultrastructural examination.

Diagnostic difficulties when only a small amount of tissue is available

- Monomorphic round cells in a fibrillary background containing no mitoses may be normal pineal gland, pineocytoma, or central neurocytoma (from third ventricle). Dystrophic calcification favors pineal gland. Lobularity of the pineal gland may be lost when it is compressed. Many pineocytomatous rosettes indicate a diagnosis of pineocytoma. Pineocytoma contains zonulae adherens junctions, unlike the neurocytoma.
- Elongated cells with fibrillary processes plus scattered Rosenthal fibers may be seen in a pineal cyst or a pilocytic astrocytoma. Dense gliosis is seen at the edge of a pineal cyst. Nuclear pleomorphism and hyperchromasia, microcystic areas, and neovascularization favor a diagnosis of pilocytic astrocytoma.

CNS GERM CELL TUMORS

- GCTs comprise germinomas (approximately 50%), teratomas (20%), mixed GCTs (25%), and pure nonteratomatous nongerminomatous GCTs (5%).
- At presentation 75% of patients are 10–20 years of age, and 95% are under 33 years of age.
- Germinomas occur most commonly around puberty.
- Choriocarcinomas and teratomas tend to present earlier (i.e. before puberty).
- GCTs show no familial tendency.
- The male:female ratio of pineal region GCTs is 2:1.
- Diabetes insipidus as a presenting symptom is most commonly associated with a suprasellar germinoma.
- GCTs may metastasize throughout the CSF pathways (negative CSF cytology does not exclude this) and outside the CNS (this is more common for nongerminomatous than germinomatous GCTs).
- GCTs are often treated without biopsy if serum or CSF markers (AFP, β-HCG) are raised.
- If a mixed GCT is treated with radiotherapy or chemotherapy on the basis of raised markers it may relapse as a symptomatic teratoma (growing teratoma syndrome).

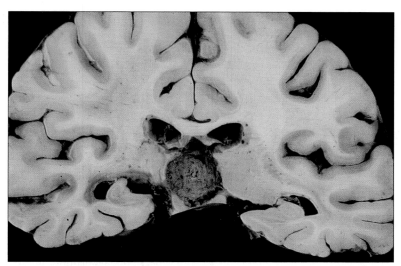

Fig. 39.8 Pineal germinoma.

GERMINOMAS
MACROSCOPIC APPEARANCES

Germinomas are generally soft, friable, and well-circumscribed masses (**Fig. 39.8**). Diffuse invasion of adjacent structures is unusual, but may occur, simulating a glioma. Cysts may be present.

MICROSCOPIC APPEARANCES

Pineal and suprasellar germinomas have the same histologic features as ovarian dysgerminomas and testicular seminomas. Groups of plump, round neoplastic cells with prominent nucleoli are surrounded by aggregates of reactive T lymphocytes (**Fig. 39.9**). The neoplastic cells often have clear, glycogen-rich cytoplasm. They label with antibodies to placental alkaline phosphatase. Granulomatous inflammation may be seen, and in small biopsies can cause confusion with sarcoidosis and tuberculosis.

The occurrence of isolated syncytiotrophoblastic giant cells reacting with antibodies to the β-subunit of human chorionic gonadotrophin has no prognostic significance in germinomas. However, if the β-HCG concentration is slightly raised in the CSF, an assiduous search should be undertaken for additional non-germinomatous elements. Similarly, an elevated α-fetoprotein (AFP) level indicates a probable diagnosis of mixed GCT.

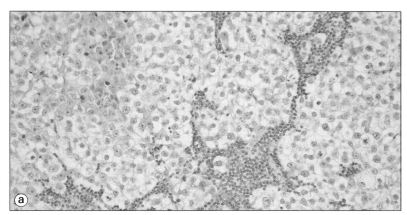

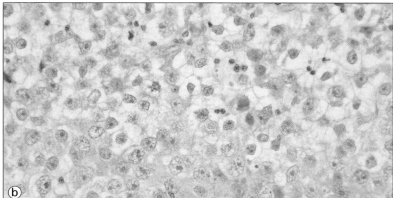

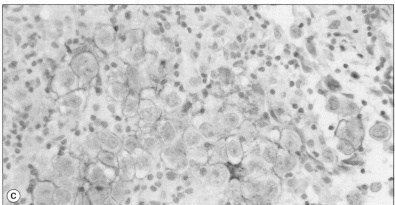

Fig. 39.9 Germinoma. (a) Sheets of large cells with clear cytoplasm are separated by thin fibrovascular septa containing infiltrates of lymphocytes. **(b)** Prominent nucleoli are seen in the nuclei of large cells. **(c)** Plasmalemmal placental alkaline phosphatase immunoreactivity of the large cells is characteristic.

EMBRYONAL CARCINOMA, YOLK SAC TUMOR, AND CHORIOCARCINOMA

Examples of nongerminomatous GCTs with a pure histologic picture of embryonal carcinoma, yolk sac tumor, or choriocarcinoma are rare. Mixed GCTs predominate. Elevation of the levels of β-HCG or AFP in CSF or blood strongly suggests the presence of one of these neoplasms.

MICROSCOPIC APPEARANCES
Embryonal carcinoma

This appears microscopically as sheets of large, moderately pleomorphic cells with a glandular, cribriform, papillary or solid arrangement. Clear cytoplasm may be a feature of some cells. Mitoses and necrosis are evident. Immunohistochemistry reveals scattered reactivity for low molecular weight cytokeratins (**Fig. 39.10**), and cells may occasionally label with antibodies to placental alkaline phosphatase, β-HCG, and AFP (see Fig. 39.13).

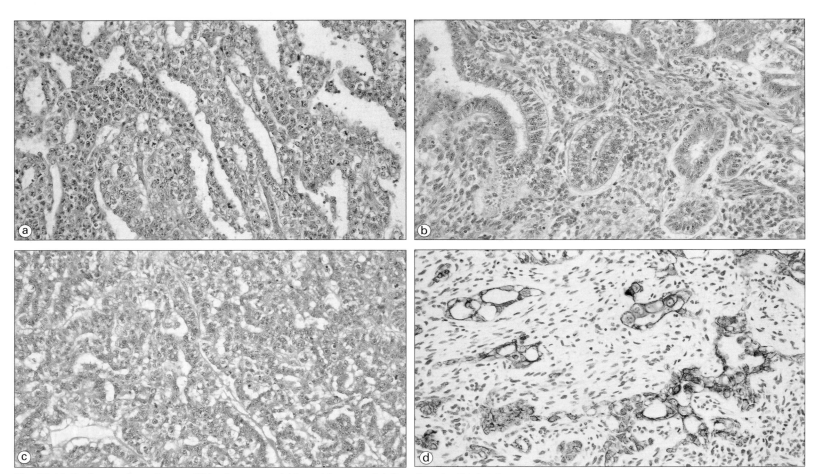

Fig. 39.10 Embryonal carcinoma. This shows a variable architecture. **(a)** Broad cords. **(b)** Acini. **(c)** A cribriform pattern. **(d)** Focal cytokeratin immunoreactivity is characteristically present.

Yolk sac tumor

Cells in a yolk sac tumor are arranged in a loose or lacy pattern and may have clear cytoplasm. The neoplasm is characterized by Schiller–Duval and eosinophilic bodies (**Fig. 39.11**). The eosinophilic bodies are PAS-positive and often contain AFP. Yolk sac tumor is generally less pleomorphic than embryonal carcinoma.

Choriocarcinomas

Choriocarcinomas contain syncytiotrophoblastic giant cells and cytotrophoblastic elements that show a bilaminar pattern (**Fig. 39.12**). Foci of hemorrhage and necrosis are usual. The syncytiotrophoblasts are immunoreactive for β-HCG.

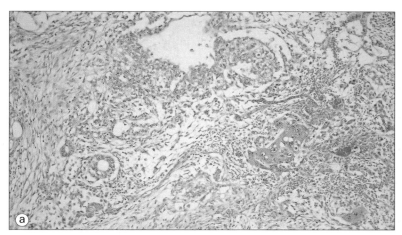

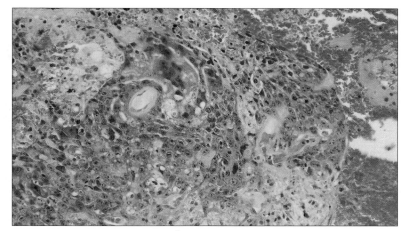

Fig. 39.12 Choriocarcinoma. This neoplasm contained islands of giant and small cells surrounded by areas of hemorrhage.

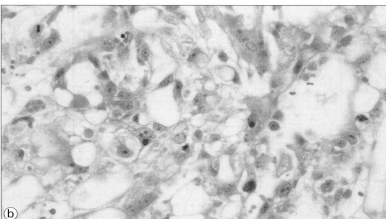

Immunohistochemistry of germ cell tumors

	PLAP	Low molecular weight CK	AFP	β-HCG
Germinoma#	+	±	–	–
Embryonal carcinoma*	±	+	±	±
Yolk sac neoplasma†	±	+	+	±
Choriocarcinoma	±	+	±	+

+	focally immunoreactive
±	may be focally immunoreactive
–	not immunoreactive
PLAP	placental alkaline phosphatase
CK	cytokeratins
AFP	α-feto protein
β-HCG	β-human chorionic gonadotropin
#	giant cells show immunoreactivity with antibodies to β-HCG
*	no immunoreactivity with antibodies to vimentin
†	immunoreactivity with antibodies to α-1-antitrypsin

Fig. 39.13 Immunohistochemistry of germ cell tumors.

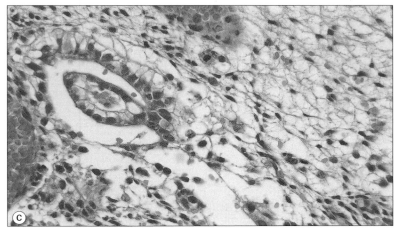

Fig. 39.11 Pineal yolk sac tumor. (a) This shows the typical lacy architecture. **(b)** Eosinophilic bodies which are PAS-positive and immunoreactive for AFP. **(c)** Schiller–Duval body.

TERATOMAS
MACROSCOPIC AND MICROSCOPIC APPEARANCES

Differentiated teratomas are well circumscribed and usually have a lobulated or partly cystic appearance. They may contain a mixture of tissues derived from three embryonic cell lines (i.e. ectoderm, mesoderm, and endoderm). Mature teratomas contain only adult tissues (**Fig. 39.14**), whil embryonic tissues predominate in immature teratomas. Disorganized embryonic neuroepithelial tissue is commonly seen, often as a cluster of rosettes. Malignant transformation of a mature teratoma to carcinoma (**Fig 39.15**) or sarcoma may rarely occur.

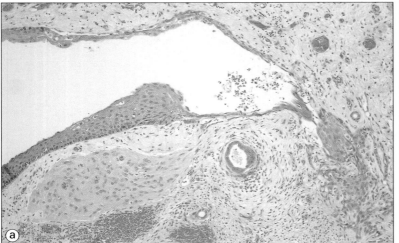

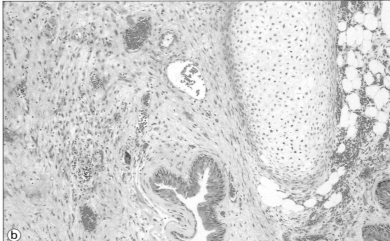

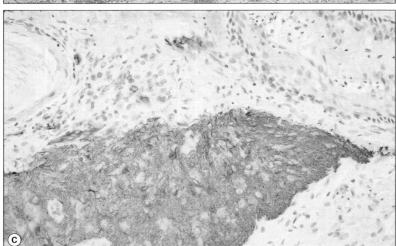

Fig. 39.14 Mature teratoma. (a, b) A variety of tissue types is present, including **(c)** neuroepithelial tissue that is immunoreactive for GFAP.

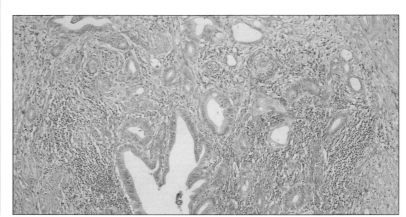

Fig. 39.15 An adenocarcinoma in a teratoma. Carcinomas and sarcomas occur very rarely in a teratoma.

REFERENCES

Baumgartner JE, Edwards MS. (1992) Pineal tumors. *Neurosurg Clin N Am* 3: 853–862.

Bjornsson J, Scheithauer BW, Okazaki H, Leech RW. (1985) Intracranial germ cell tumors: pathobiological and immunohistochemical aspects of 70 cases. *J Neuropath Exp Neurol* 44: 32–46.

Borit A, Blackwood W, Mair WG. (1980) The separation of pineocytoma from pineoblastoma. *Cancer* 45: 1408–1418.

Burger PC, Scheithauer BW, Vogel FS. (1991) Neoplasms of the pineal region. In *Surgical Pathology of the Nervous System and its Coverings*. pp. 503–568. Edinburgh: Churchill Livingstone.

Horowitz MB, Hall WA. (1991) Central nervous system germinomas. *Arch Neurol* 48: 652–657.

Schild SE *et al.* (1993) Pineal parenchymal tumors. Clinical, pathologic, and therapeutic aspects. *Cancer* 72: 870–880.

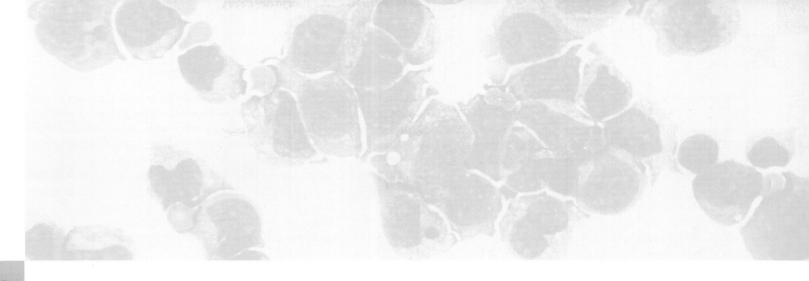

40 *Choroid plexus neoplasms*

CHOROID PLEXUS NEOPLASMS

The choroid plexus (CP) is a specialized epithelium that secretes cerebrospinal fluid (CSF) and is sited in the ventricles of the brain. Most neoplasms of CP are papillomas (CPPs), but some show the cytologic and behavioral characteristics of carcinomas (CPCs). CPCs are rare and mostly occur in children.

MACROSCOPIC APPEARANCES
CPPs are well-circumscribed neoplasms with a stippled surface that reflects their papillary structure (**Fig. 40.1**). In contrast, CPCs invade local structures. Both types of neoplasm can be highly vascular, and CPCs frequently contain foci of hemorrhage.

MICROSCOPIC APPEARANCES
CPPs resemble normal CP histologically and are characterized by a columnar epithelium resting on a delicate fibrovascular network and forming multiple papillary projections (**Figs 40.2, 40.3**). However, CPPs can be distinguished from CP because they have:
- a more columnar epithelium
- an increased nuclear:cytoplasmic ratio
- nuclear pleomorphism and hyperchromasia
- (sparse) mitotic figures.

Common histologic features found in both CPPs and CP include dystrophic calcification, xanthomatous change, and focal glial differentiation with areas of glial fibrillary protein (GFAP) immunoreactivity.

CHOROID PLEXUS NEOPLASMS

CP neoplasms:
- constitute approximately 0.5% of CNS neoplasms, approximately 3% of childhood CNS neoplasms, and may be congenital.
- occur over a wide age range, but over 50% are present before 2 years of age.
- are predominantly in the lateral ventricles in children.
- are nearly always in the fourth ventricle in adults.
- are frequently associated with hydrocephalus due to blocked CSF drainage pathways ± increased CSF production.

GENETIC FACTORS AND CP NEOPLASMS

CP neoplasms:
- have been reported in Li–Fraumeni syndrome and von Hippel–Lindau syndrome.
- are induced in transgenic mice by the large T antigen of simian virus 40.
- rarely contain mutations of the p53 tumor suppressor gene.

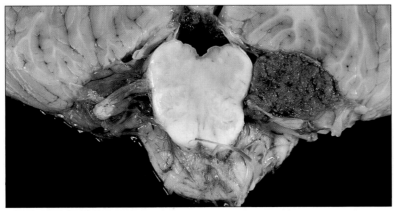

Fig. 40.1 CPP. The cerebellopontine angle is an unusual site for a CPP, nearly all are intraventricular.

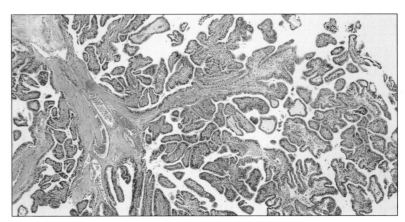

Fig. 40.2 CPP. A papillary architecture is evident on histology.

Uncommon histologic features in CPPs are glandular metaplasia, oncocytic change, pigmentation, chondroid metaplasia, and osseous metaplasia. Cytologic atypia may be more advanced in some CPPs (**Fig. 40.4**), and can progressively worsen in recurrent neoplasms. In addition to well-differentiated areas, atypical CPPs show foci of:

• cellular pleomorphism
• nuclear hyperchromasia
• moderate mitotic activity.

The presence of these features is not an infallible guide to prognosis. Atypical CPPs can be completely resected, and rarely CPPs with bland cytologic features disseminate through CSF pathways. However, it is prudent to carry out more frequent postoperative checks on patients with atypical CPPs.

CPCs are characterized by marked architectural and cytologic atypia. They invade adjacent structures, have a high mitotic index, and contain foci of necrosis (**Figs 40.5, 40.6**). Poorly differentiated CPCs may retain only small areas of papillary architecture.

Immunohistochemistry reveals that most cells in CPPs label with antibodies to cytokeratins (**Fig. 40.7**), S-100, and vimentin. CPPs also show focal GFAP immunoreactivity. Antibodies to transthyretin label CP neoplasms, but are not entirely specific to these neoplasms. Antibodies to carbonic anhydrase can also be useful in identifying CP neoplasms.

Ultrastructural examination may reveal features of CP in the neoplasms (i.e. cilia, apical junctions, apical microvilli, and a basement membrane around the cell's basal surface).

CHOROID PLEXUS NEOPLASMS

CPP:
• is distinguished from **normal CP** on architectural and cytologic grounds
• is distinguished from **papillary ependymomas** by a prominent PAS-positive basement membrane beneath the epithelium, widespread immunolabeling with cytokeratin antibodies, only scanty focal GFAP immunoreactivity, and the absence of pseudorosettes

CPC:
• may be difficult to distinguish from some primitive (embryonal) neuroepithelial neoplasms, anaplastic ependymoma, and undifferentiated germ cell neoplasms in children
• can be distinguished from **medulloepithelioma** because medulloepithelioma contains multilayered ribbons of primitive cells with very scanty cytoplasm and numerous apoptotic bodies, and is not immunoreactive for cytokeratin
• can be distinguished from **anaplastic ependymoma** because pseudorosettes and rosettes are not found in CPC and CPC shows widespread immunolabeling with cytokeratin antibodies
• can be distinguished from **embryonal carcinoma** because embryonal carcinoma has a predominantly sheet-like or trabecular architecture and may label with antibodies to placental alkaline phosphatase
• can be distinguished from **metastatic papillary carcinoma** in adults by the clinical features (i.e. patient's age, site of the neoplasm, a history of a non-CNS primary neoplasm), and because CPC may express transthyretin and/or S-100 in addition to cytokeratins, and, in many cases, shows focal immunoreactivity for GFAP

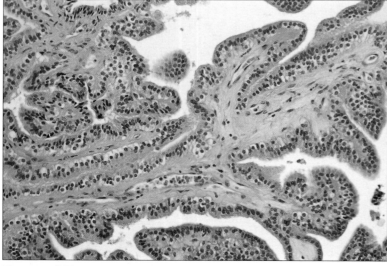

Fig. 40.3 CPP. A layer of cuboidal cells rests on a fibrovascular stroma.

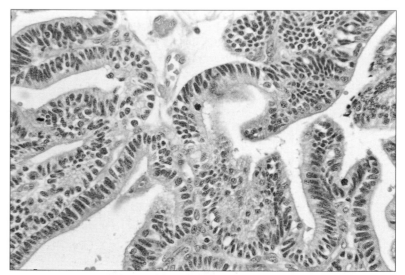

Fig. 40.4 CPP with mild atypia and scattered mitoses.

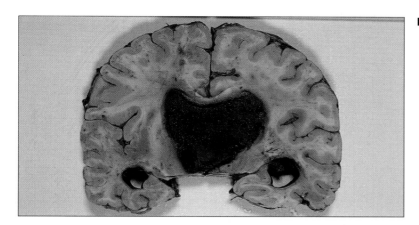

Fig. 40.5 CPC. A large, hemorrhagic mass fills the ventricles.

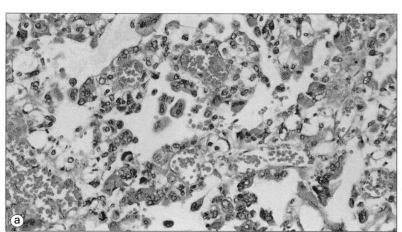

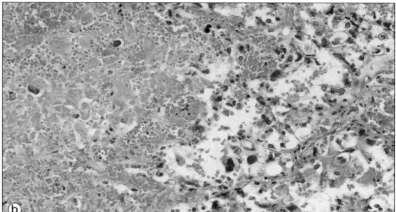

Fig. 40.6 CPC. (a) Marked cytological pleomorphism and **(b)** areas of necrosis.

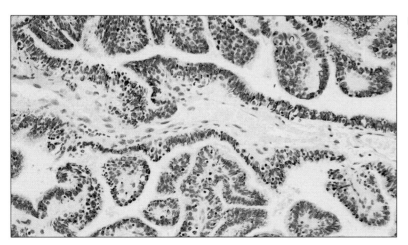

Fig. 40.7 CPP. The epithelium immunolabels with an antibody to low molecular weight cytokeratins.

REFERENCES

Furness PN, Lowe J, Tarrant GS (1990) Subepithelial basement membrane deposition and intermediate filament expression in choroid plexus neoplasms and ependymomas. *Histopathology* **16**: 251–255.

Ho DM, Wong TT, Liu HC (1991) Choroid plexus tumors in childhood. Histopathologic study and clinico-pathological correlation. *Child's nervous system* 7: 437–441.

Newbould MJ, Kelsey AM, Arango JC, Ironside JW, Birch J (1995) The choroid plexus carcinomas of childhood: histopathology, immunocytochemistry and clinicopathological correlations. *Histopathology* **26**: 137–143.

Packer RJ *et al.* (1992) Choroid plexus carcinoma of childhood. *Cancer* **69**: 580–585.

Paulus W, Jänisch W (1990) Clinicopathological correlations in epithelial choroid plexus neoplasms: a study of 52 cases. *Acta Neuropath* **80**: 635–641.

van Dyke TA (1993) Tumors of the choroid plexus. In Levine AJ, Schmidek HH (eds.) *Molecular genetics of nervous system tumors.* pp287–301. New York: Wiley-Liss.

41 Primary CNS lymphomas

CNS lymphomas may be primary or secondary:

- Primary CNS lymphomas (PCNSLs) are non-Hodgkin's lymphomas that are confined to the brain or spinal cord at presentation. Most involve the cerebrum, but approximately 10% present in the cerebellum, and a few originate in the brain stem or spinal cord. Over 80% of PCNSLs are diffuse large B cell lymphomas, but differ from systemic diffuse large B cell lymphomas in their behavior, optimum management, and prognosis.
- Secondary CNS lymphomas spread to the brain or spinal cord from a primary site outside the nervous system. They are commoner than PCNSLs as 5–10% of systemic lymphomas involve the CNS, often occupying the subarachnoid space. Leukemias share this predilection for the meninges.

Some lymphomas are epidural or vertebral in location and impinge on the CNS by neoplastic growth or vertebral collapse. Plasmacytomas and multiple myeloma in the thoracic and cervical vertebrae are common examples. Mediastinal lymphomas can also cause spinal cord compression. Many of the mediastinal lymphomas are high-grade B cell neoplasms.

CONDITIONS ASSOCIATED WITH PCNSL

Primary immunodeficiency syndromes

- Wiskott–Aldrich syndrome.
- X-linked lymphoproliferative syndrome.
- Severe combined immunodeficiency.
- Ataxia–telangiectasia.

Secondary immunodeficiency states

- HIV infection.
- Immunosuppressive therapy following organ transplantation.
- Hodgkin's disease.

Other disorders

- A few reports have linked PCNSL with autoimmune multisystem disorders such as Sjögren's syndrome, systemic lupus erythematosus, and rheumatoid arthritis.
- Epstein–Barr virus is implicated in the pathogenesis of PCNSL in all immunocompromised patients and 15–20% of immunocompetent patients.

CNS lymphomas respond rapidly to steroid therapy. Although this effect is transient, widespread apoptosis of lymphoma cells results in a marked reduction in tumor mass. Such shrinkage can compromise the yield of stereotactic biopsies and apoptosis their diagnostic use. Early biopsy is therefore recommended.

Cytologic examination of the cerebrospinal fluid (CSF) is often useful for both preliminary assessment and follow-up of the patient.

EPIDEMIOLOGIC AND CLINICAL ASPECTS OF PCNSL

- PCNSL accounts for 2–3% of intracranial neoplasms.
- PCNSL accounts for approximately 1% of non-Hodgkin's lymphomas.
- The incidence of PCNSL in both immunocompetent and immunocompromised patient groups has increased since 1985.
- Peak incidence is seen in the sixth and seventh decades in immunocompetent patients, and in the fourth decade in immunocompromised patients.
- PCNSL is slightly more common in males than females (i.e. 3:2 ratio).
- T cell PCNSL presents in a younger age group than B cell PCNSL.

- PCNSL presents as a space-occupying lesion causing raised intracranial pressure, focal neurologic deficit, or epilepsy.
- Angiotropic large-cell lymphoma presents with fluctuating confusion, transient ischemic attacks, or a rapid dementia.
- PCNSL is evident as irregular, sometimes multifocal, contrast-enhancing masses on CT scans or MRI.
- The radiologic appearances of PCNSL may mimic a high-grade glioma or toxoplasmosis in immunocompromised patients.
- A poor prognosis is characteristic despite a reported increase in median survival in some studies that have used combination radiotherapy and chemotherapy.
- There is a poorer prognosis in patients over 60 years of age and in those with a preoperative Karnovsky score of less than 70, a family history of cancer in first-degree relatives, or an immunocompromised status.
- Survival does not appear to be correlated with histologic features.

MACROSCOPIC APPEARANCES

PCNSL in the postmortem brain is often multifocal. The lesions appear quite well demarcated despite microscopic infiltration of surrounding tissue (**Figs 41.1, 41.2**). The affected brain tissue is softened, gray or brown in color, and may be focally hemorrhagic. Infiltrated meninges appear thick, and subependymal intraventricular spread may manifest as areas of irregularity and softening.

MICROSCOPIC APPEARANCES

Many PCNSLs are characterized by sheets of lymphoma cells separated by areas of necrosis. The cells tend to invade the walls of small cerebral blood vessels and accumulate in perivascular spaces (**Fig. 41.3**). This produces a characteristic lacy pattern of reduplicated perivascular reticulin (**Fig. 41.4**), which is evident even in necrotic tissue. Small-cell PCNSLs tend to be more infiltrative and less necrotic than large-cell PCNSLs. At its infiltrative edge, PCNSL diffusely invades CNS tissue,

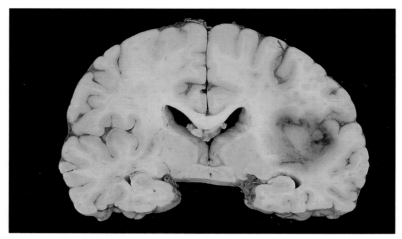

Fig. 41.1 PCNSL. A necrotic and hemorrhagic lesion in the cerebrum.

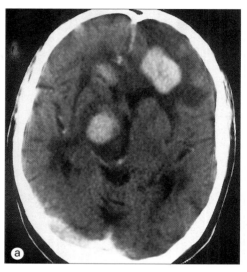

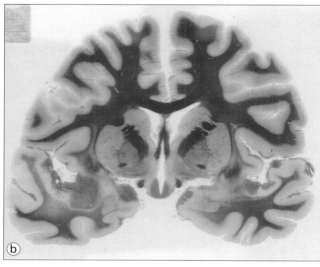

Fig. 41.2 Multifocal lesions in PCNSL.
(a) CT scan with contrast enhancement. (Courtesy of Dr JS Millar, Wessex Neurological Center) **(b)** Whole cerebral slice. (Luxol fast blue/cresyl violet)

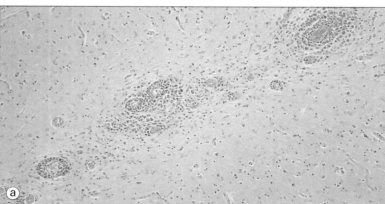

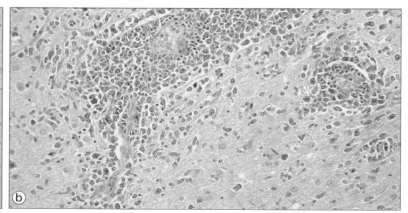

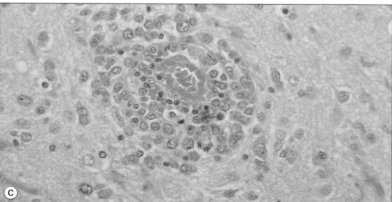

Fig. 41.3 PCNSL. (a) Perivascular neoplastic cells in the cerebal cortex at the edge of a large B cell lymphoma. **(b)** Large neoplastic cells spread from the perivascular spaces into the parenchyma. **(c)** Small reactive lymphocytes mixed with larger neoplastic cells around a cerebral blood vessel.

mimicking a glioma (**Fig. 41.5**). Like some neuroepithelial neoplasms, PCNSL also spreads through the subarachnoid space and invades the pial surface of the brain. Meningeal and intraventricular spread can be extensive (**Fig. 41.6**, see also Fig. 41.2b).

Polymorphous diffuse large B cell lymphomas account for more than 80% of PCNSLs. They contain cells resembling centroblasts and immunoblasts which are mixed with smaller cells, including reactive T cells (**Fig. 41.7**), and there are many mitotic figures and apoptotic bodies.

Less than 10% of PCNSLs are B cell lymphomas with lymphocytic or lymphoplasmacytoid cytology. Cells in these neoplasms are more monomorphic than those in their high-grade counterparts (**Fig. 41.8**).

T cell PCNSLs are very rare, and comprise monomorphic and pleomorphic neoplasms (**Fig. 41.9**).

The infiltrated brain parenchyma shows reactive changes such as astrocytosis and an increase in activated microglia. These changes may be florid and can lead to a misdiagnosis of an inflammatory rather than a neoplastic disorder.

The neoplastic cells of the rare CNS angiotropic lymphoma (previously termed malignant angioendotheliomatosis), which is usually a large B cell lymphoma, fill the lumina of small cerebral vessels and invade the surrounding parenchyma in only a few places (**Fig. 41.10**). These neoplasms tend to cause vascular occlusion and hemorrhagic infarcts. Most are systemic lymphomas that preferentially affect the CNS and the skin.

Immunohistochemistry with a panel of antibodies allows characterization of PCNSLs (**Fig. 41.11**). PCNSL may be distinguished from gliomas and metastatic small-cell carcinomas by immunolabeling of neoplastic cells with an antibody to CD45 (leukocyte common antigen).

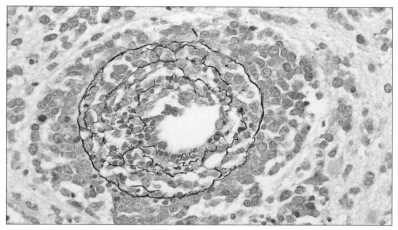

Fig. 41.4 PCNSL. Reticulin outlines the expanded perivascular space in PCNSL.

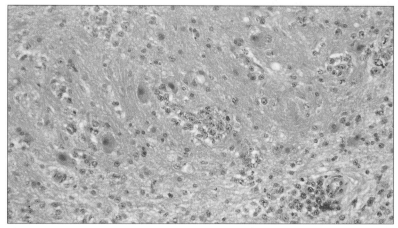

Fig. 41.5 Large B cell lymphoma of the cerebellum. Neoplastic cells have infiltrated the dentate nucleus.

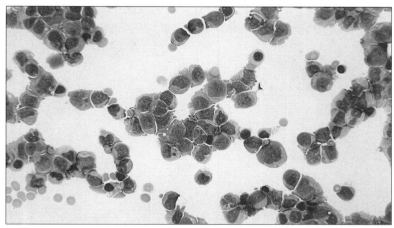

Fig. 41.6 CSF from a patient with PCNSL. Meningeal involvement with invasion of the subarachnoid space is common in PCNSL.

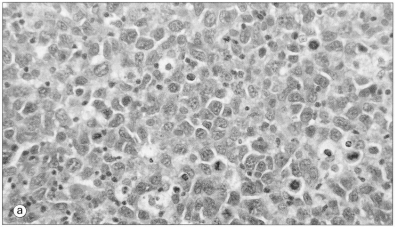

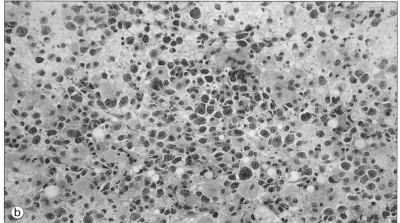

Fig. 41.7 Large B cell PCNSL. (a) Polymorphous cells are seen, some of which resemble centroblasts and centrocytes.
(b) Perioperative smear preparation of a biopsy of PCNSL from a patient with AIDS and multiple cerebral masses.

B cell lymphomas can be differentiated from T cell lymphomas by antibodies to the following antigens:

- CD79a (B cell marker).
- CD20 (B cell marker).
- CD3 (T cell marker).
- CD45Ro (T cell marker).

Immunohistochemistry with antibodies to κ and λ light chains may demonstrate light chain restriction in some lymphomas, though interpretation of these preparations can be difficult. Epstein–Barr virus may be demonstrated in some PCNSLs by immunohistochemistry or in-situ hybridization (**Fig. 14.12**).

Populations of neoplastic lymphoid cells may be revealed using the polymerase chain reaction to detect clonal immunoglobulin or T cell receptor gene rearrangements. All B cell PCNSLs examined so far have been clonal.

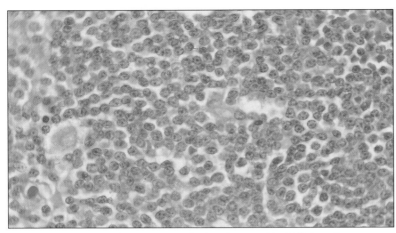

Fig. 41.8 Lymphoplasmacytoid PCNSL. Cells in this CNS lymphoma are smaller than those in other B cell PCNSLs, and some cells show plasmacytic differentiation

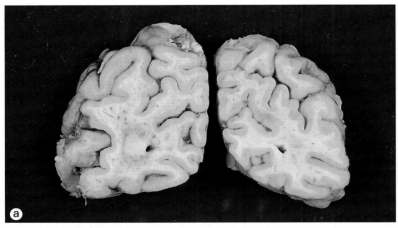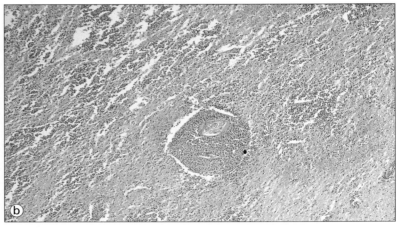

Fig. 41.9 T cell PCNSL in a patient with AIDS. (a) A circumscribed mass of cream-colored tumor lies next to the occipital horn of the left lateral ventricle. **(b)** Neoplastic cells infiltrate the cerebrum.

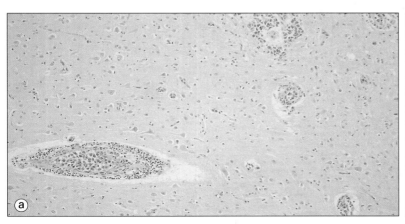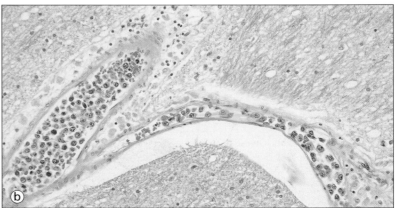

Fig. 41.10 Angiotropic large B cell lymphoma (a) and **(b)** Intravascular neoplastic lymphoid cells are evident, and perivascular lymphocytes are also present. Some neoplastic cells have invaded the brain around one blood vessel, but this is an uncommon finding.

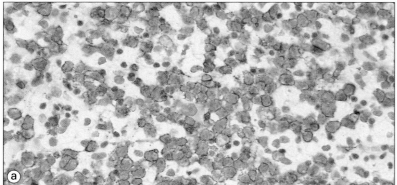

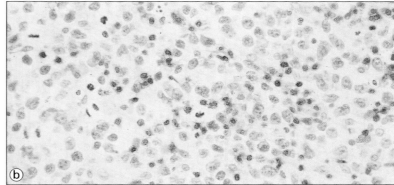

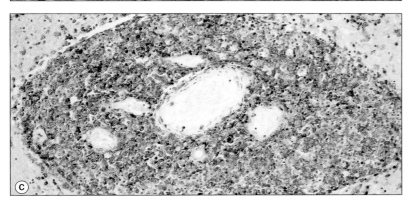

Fig. 41.11 PCNSL. (a) Antibody to CD20 labelling neoplastic cells in a B cell lymphoma. **(b)** Antibody to CD3 labelling reactive T cells in a B cell lymphoma. **(c)** Antibody to CD45Ro labelling neoplastic cells in a T cell lymphoma.

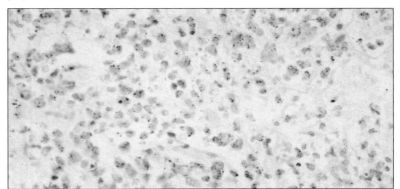

Fig. 41.12 Epstein–Barr virus in PCNSL. Revealed by *in situ* hybridisation. (Courtesy of Dr J Geddes, Royal London Hospital, U.K.)

DIFFERENTIAL DIAGNOSIS OF PCNSL

In the perioperative period

Without the benefit of immunohistochemistry, CNS lymphoma can be difficult to distinguish from oligodendroglioma and metastatic small-cell carcinoma. Features that may help to distinguish these neoplasms in cytologic preparations and frozen sections are:
- PCNSL: dispersed cells in a smear preparation, nuclei with prominent single or multiple nucleoli, many apoptotic bodies, a distinctive perivascular distribution.
- Oligodendroglioma: clumps of cells attached by fine fibrillary processes to small blood vessels, dystrophic calcification.
- Small-cell carcinoma: scattered clumps of cells in a smear preparation, dispersed nuclear chromatin, neoplastic cells that do not tend to invade surrounding brain.

In the postoperative period

With the aid of immunohistochemistry, PCNSL is readily distinguished from oligodendroglioma and metastatic small-cell carcinoma, and the histology of large B cell lymphomas is characteristic. Features that may help to distinguish small-cell lymphomas from encephalitis are listed below, but both conditions may coexist in immunosuppressed patients.
- Inflammatory infiltrates are generally more polymorphous and contain mature plasma cells.
- Perivascular lymphocytes are evident in both pathologic processes, but the vascular invasion shown by lymphomas is not a feature of encephalitis.
- A search for viral inclusions or *Toxoplasma* may be rewarding.
- Gene rearrangement studies and microbiologic investigations may support histologic assessment.

REFERENCES

Chappell ET, Guthrie BL, Orenstein J (1992) The role of stereotactic biopsy in the management of HIV-related focal brain lesions. *Neurosurgery* **30**: 825–829.

Grove A, Vyberg M (1993) Primary leptomeningeal T cell lymphoma: a case and a review of primary T cell lymphoma of the central nervous system. *Clinical Neuropathology* **12**: 7–12.

Harris NL, Jaffe ES, Stein H *et al.* (1994) A revised European-American classification of lymphoid neoplasms: a proposal from the international lymphoma study group. *Blood* **84**: 1361–1392.

Isaacson PG and Norton AJ. (1994) Lymphomas of the nervous system. In *Extranodal Lymphomas*. pp. 217–227. Edinburgh: Churchill Livingstone.

Morgello S (1995) Pathogenesis and classification of primary central nervous system lymphoma: an update. *Brain Path* **5**: 383–393.

Schwecheimer K *et al.* (1994) Polymorphous high-grade B-cell lymphoma is the predominant type of spontaneous primary cerebral malignant lymphoma. *Am J Surg Path* **18**: 931–937.

Tomlinson FH *et al.* (1995) Primary intracerebral malignant lymphoma: a clinicopathological study of 89 patients. *J Neurosurg* **82**: 558–566.

van der Valk P (1996) Central nervous system lymphomas. *Curr Diagn Pathol* **3**: 45–52.

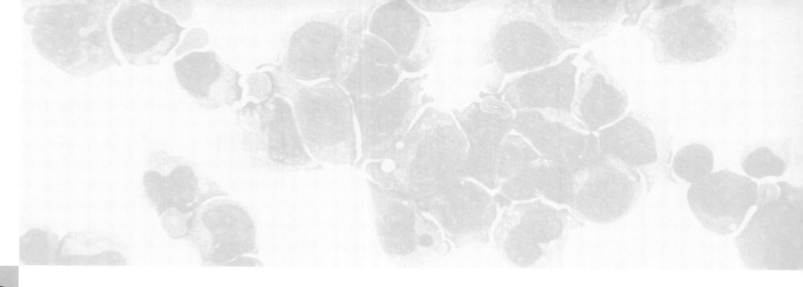

42 *Peripheral nerve sheath neoplasms*

Neoplasms derived from cells that surround peripheral nerves may present with central nervous system (CNS) symptoms and signs when they arise at a proximal site. The three main groups of these neoplasms are schwannomas (neurilemmomas), neurofibromas, and malignant nerve sheath tumors (MNSTs; neurofibrosarcomas). Nearly all cranial nerve sheath neoplasms and most peripheral nerve sheath tumors in the spinal canal are schwannomas. All three groups are associated with neurofibromatosis (NF).

SCHWANNOMAS

Schwannomas are slowly growing neoplasms composed of Schwann cells. Solitary schwannomas with effects on the CNS occur on cranial (Figs 42.1, 42.2) and spinal nerve roots; rarely they are found in the substance of the brain or spinal cord. Melanotic schwannomas have a predilection for spinal nerve roots. The plexiform schwannoma is rare and occurs in the skin. Unlike the plexiform neurofibroma, it is not associated with NF.

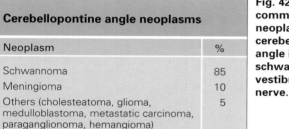

Cerebellopontine angle neoplasms	
Neoplasm	%
Schwannoma	85
Meningioma	10
Others (cholesteatoma, glioma, medulloblastoma, metastatic carcinoma, paraganglionoma, hemangioma)	5

Fig. 42.1 The commonest neoplasm of the cerebellopontine angle is a schwannoma of the vestibulocochlear nerve.

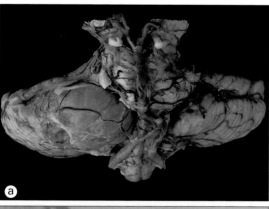
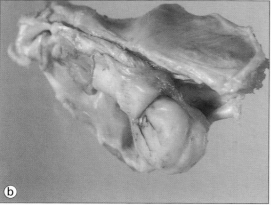

Fig.42.2 Vestibulocochlear nerve schwannomas.
(a) A partly cystic schwannoma in the cerebellopontine angle indents the brain stem. Flattened fascicles of vestibulocochlear nerve run over the surface of the neoplasm.
(b) A schwannoma sits at the mouth of the internal auditory meatus.

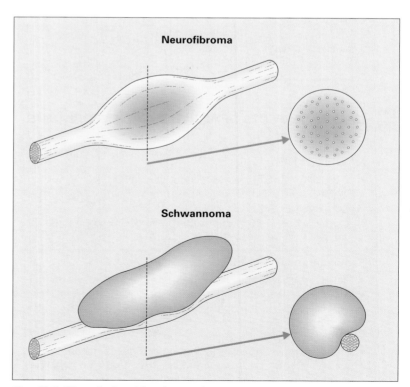

Fig. 42.3 The relationship of neurofibroma and schwannoma to associated nerve. The neurofibroma incorporates axons, but the schwannoma forms from the side of the nerve (see Fig. 42.4).

GENETICS OF NEUROFIBROMATOSIS TYPE 1 (NF1)

- The NF1 gene is on chromosome 17q11.
- NF1 shows autosomal dominant inheritance with almost complete penetrance.
- About 50% of cases represent new mutations. The prevalence of NF1 is approximately 1:3000.
- The NF1 gene product is neurofibromin, which is a guanosine triphosphatase-activating protein that influences cell proliferation and differentiation, and is abundant in Schwann cells and neurons.

NF1

Neoplasms associated with NF1

- Neurofibromas (all types)
- Malignant nerve sheath tumors
- Optic nerve gliomas
- Rhabdomyosarcomas
- Pheochromocytomas
- Carcinoid tumors

Clinical criteria for diagnosing NF1

Two or more of the following clinical features must be present to fulfil current diagnostic criteria for NF1:
- At least two solitary neurofibromas or one plexiform neurofibroma
- At least six café-au-lait spots larger than 5 mm diameter (pre-puberty) or larger than 15 mm diameter (post-puberty)
- At least two Lisch nodules
- Optic glioma (pilocytic astrocytoma)
- Osseous lesions (sphenoid dysplasia, pseudoarthrosis, or spinal deformity)
- Axillary freckling
- A family history of a first-degree relative with NF1 fulfilling the above criteria

GENETIC ASPECTS OF NERVE SHEATH NEOPLASMS

MNSTs and NF1

- 30–50% of MNSTs are associated with NF1.
- For NF1 patients, the lifetime risk of developing a MNST is approximately 2%.
- Approximately 5–10% of plexiform neurofibromas in patients with NF1 progress to MNST.

Schwannomas and NF2

- Patients with NF2 may have bilateral vestibular schwannomas.
- Sporadic schwannomas frequently show NF2 gene mutation plus allelic loss in the other chromosome (22q).

Carney's complex

- This autosomal dominant syndrome comprises melanotic schwannomas, spotty pigmentation, cardiac or skin myxomas, and endocrine overactivity (Cushing's syndrome or acromegaly).

GENETICS OF NEUROFIBROMATOSIS TYPE 2 (NF2)

- The NF2 gene is on chromosome 22q12.
- NF2 shows autosomal dominant inheritance with high penetrance.
- About 50% of cases represent new mutations.
- The prevalence of NF2 is approximately 1:40,000.
- The NF2 gene product is merlin, which is associated with membrane and cytoskeletal structures.

NF2

Neoplasms associated with NF2

- Schwannomas
- Neurofibromas
- Ependymomas
- Other gliomas
- Meningiomas (may be multiple)

(Plexiform neurofibromas are not found in NF2, and malignant progression of associated nerve sheath neoplasms is very rare.)

Clinical criteria for NF2

One of the following four clinical presentations is needed to fulfil current diagnostic criteria for NF2:
- Bilateral vestibular schwannomas
- First-degree relative with NF2 plus one vestibular nerve schwannoma
- First-degree relative with NF2 plus two of the following:
     meningioma
     schwannoma
     glioma
     neurofibroma
     posterior subcapsular lens opacity
- Two of the following:
     unilateral vestibular nerve schwannoma
     multiple meningiomas
     multiple schwannomas
     glioma
     neurofibroma
     posterior subcapsular lens opacity
     cerebral calcification

CNS SCHWANNOMAS

Cranial schwannomas

- constitute about 8% of intracranial neoplasms
- are most common in the fifth and sixth decades
- arise predominantly from the vestibular branch of the eighth cranial nerve
- sometimes encroach upon the vestibular ganglion
- sometimes occur on the fifth cranial nerve

Spinal schwannomas

- predominantly arise from sensory nerve roots
- are most common in the lumbosacral region
- are mainly intradural and extramedullary
- adopt a dumb-bell shape as they grow through the vertebral foramen
- may be multiple in NF2

MACROSCOPIC APPEARANCES

Schwannomas are composed of nodular rubbery tissue, which has a variegated cut surface. Yellow and gray areas may be interspersed with hemorrhagic foci or cysts. The neoplasm has a capsule and the nerve from which the schwannoma arises may be splayed over the surface of the neoplasm (**Figs 42.3, 42.4**).

MICROSCOPIC APPEARANCES

Two histologic patterns predominate (**Figs 42.5–42.7**):

- Antoni A areas, in which spindle-shaped cells with rod-shaped nuclei and dense pericellular reticulin are arranged in compact intertwining fascicles.
- Antoni B areas, in which stellate or spindle-shaped cells with smaller, more hyperchromatic nuclei, tenuous cytoplasmic processes, and scanty surrounding reticulin are loosely arranged in a myxoid stroma.

There may be conspicuous palisading of nuclei. Verocay bodies are a characteristic feature (**Fig. 42.8**). Thickened blood vessels with hyaline walls and clumps of hemosiderin-laden or foamy macrophages are

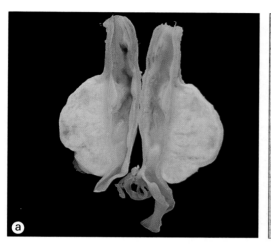

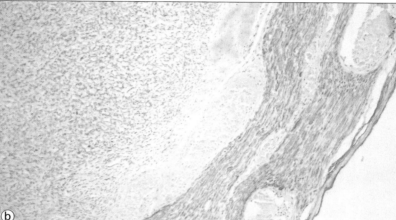

Fig. 42.4 The relationship between schwannoma and peripheral nerve.
(a) A schwannoma forms from the side of a nerve without disturbing its integrity. **(b)** An antibody to neurofilament protein labels axons in a nerve alongside a schwannoma.

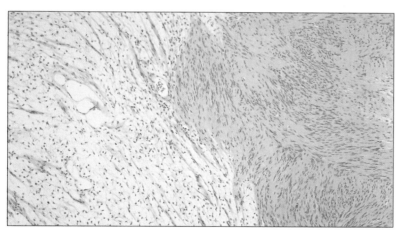

Fig. 42.5 Schwannoma. Adjacent Antoni A (right) and B (left) areas.

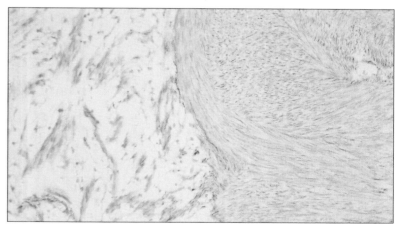

Fig. 42.6 Schwannoma. Abundant pericellular reticulin in an Antoni A area. Section adjacent to that in Fig. 42.5.

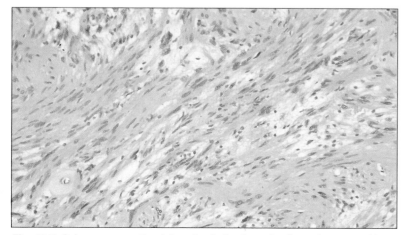

Fig. 42.7 Schwannoma. Fascicles of spindle-shaped cells are interrupted by small myxoid areas. Note the small blood vessels with markedly thickened walls.

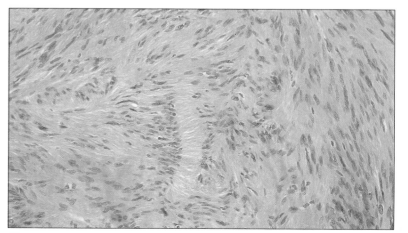

Fig. 42.8 Verocay body. This consists of sequential nuclear palisades separated by an anuclear area.

CEREBELLOPONTINE ANGLE (CPA) NEOPLASMS

Schwannomas make up the vast majority of CPA neoplasms (see Fig. 42.1), but two other CPA neoplasms (fibroblastic meningioma and astrocytoma of the brain stem or cerebellum) may be confused with schwannomas. Histologic features that distinguish these neoplasms include:

- **The reticulin pattern.** The reticulin in a fibroblastic meningioma can be extensive, but rarely surrounds each cell to produce the dense pattern seen in schwannomas.
- **Immunohistochemistry**. Most astrocytomas are GFAP-positive, but schwannomas are very rarely GFAP-positive. Schwannomas, but not meningiomas, label uniformly with S-100 antibodies.
- **Ultrastructural examination.** Schwannomas have a pericellular basal lamina (unlike most astrocytic, melanocytic and meningothelial neoplasms) and lack both the densely packed bundles of intermediate filaments that are seen in many astrocytic neoplasms and the desmosomes of meningiomas.

common findings (**Fig. 42.9**). Mitoses, if present, are sparse.

A small proportion of schwannomas contains melanin (**Fig. 42.10**), and melanotic schwannomas may contain epithelioid cells.

The presence of cells with misshapen hyperchromatic nuclei in many otherwise cytologically bland schwannomas is thought to be a manifestation of degenerative (or 'ancient') change (**Fig. 42.11**).

Cellular schwannomas rarely affect the CNS (**Fig. 42.12**). They show a marked preponderance of Antoni A areas that contain cells with a high nuclear:cytoplasmic ratio. Mitotic figures are evident. Xanthomatous foci may be seen. The cellular schwannoma can be distinguished from MNSTs by its circumscribed shape and fibrous capsule, hyalinized blood vessels, and small but distinct myxoid areas.

The term schwannosis refers to a reactive, usually ectopic, proliferation of Schwann cells. In the CNS it has a predilection for the dorsal root entry zone and perivascular spaces in the spinal cord or brain stem. Schwannosis is usually related to previous focal injury, but may occur in association with a schwannoma of the dorsal nerve root.

Immunohistochemically, schwannomas label with antibodies to S-100 and vimentin. Immunoreactivity for glial fibrillary acidic protein (GFAP) is rarely convincing. Melanotic variants label with S-100 and HMB-45 antibodies. Schwannomas have a pericellular basal lamina and this differentiates them from melanocytic neoplasms.

Malignant progression of a schwannoma is extremely rare, but has occurred in some melanotic schwannomas of the sympathetic chain.

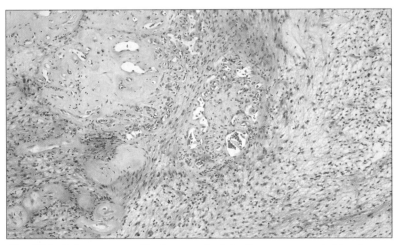

Fig. 42.9 Schwannoma. Hyaline paucicellular tissue surrounds blood vessels in a schwannoma.

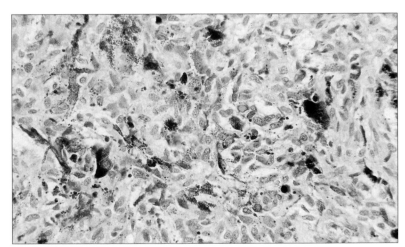

Fig. 42.10 Melanotic schwannoma.

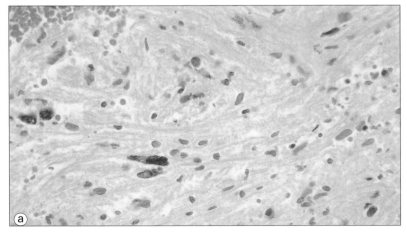

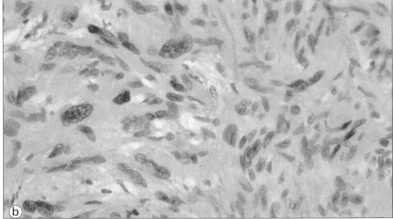

Fig. 42.11 Nuclear hyperchromasia and pleomorphism in a schwannoma. These are common findings in schwannomas and, if there are no mitoses, are thought to be degenerative. **(a)** Nuclear hyperchromasia. **(b)** Nuclear pleomorphism.

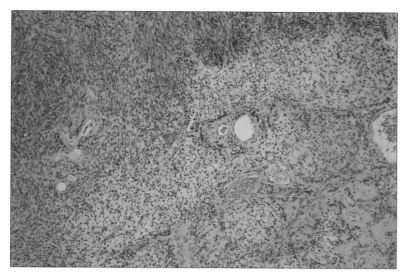

Fig. 42.12 Cellular schwannoma. A high nuclear:cytoplasmic ratio and scattered mitoses are present in some areas, but this neoplasm retains the architectural pattern of a schwannoma with Antoni A and B areas, and contains thick-walled blood vessels.

NEUROFIBROMAS

Neurofibromas may be:
- dermal, producing a nodular lesion in the skin
- intraneural, occurring as solitary or plexiform tumors

They rarely affect the CNS, and then usually in the context of NF (**Fig. 42.13**). Involvement of a plexus or large nerve trunks by plexiform neurofibromas is pathognomonic of NF1. In contrast, the rare plexiform schwannoma that occurs mainly in the skin is not associated with NF1. Neurofibromas grow slowly and arise within the endoneurium. They consist largely of Schwann cells, but fibroblasts and pericytes are also significant components.

MACROSCOPIC APPEARANCES

Solitary intraneural neurofibromas are usually oval gray or tan-colored neoplasms with a smooth shiny surface covered by a delicate pseudocapsule. Neurofibromas are not cystic and do not contain the xanthomatous areas seen in schwannomas. Solitary neurofibromas incorporate and expand the nerve from which they arise, whereas schwannomas grow away from the edge of the nerve (see Fig. 42.3).

Plexiform neurofibromas expand several nerves in a plexus or fascicles in a nerve trunk (**Fig. 42.14**). Irregular swellings give the nerve trunks the appearance of a ginger root.

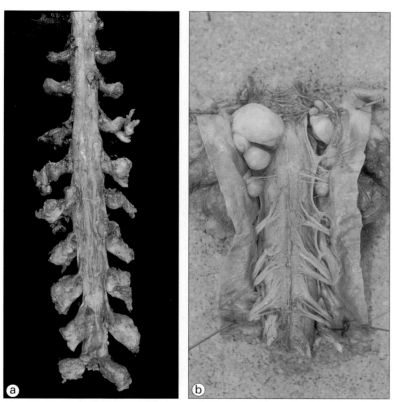

Fig. 42.13 Neurofibromatosis type 1. Multiple thoracolumbar **(a)** and cervical root **(b)** nerve sheath tumors in a patient with NF1.

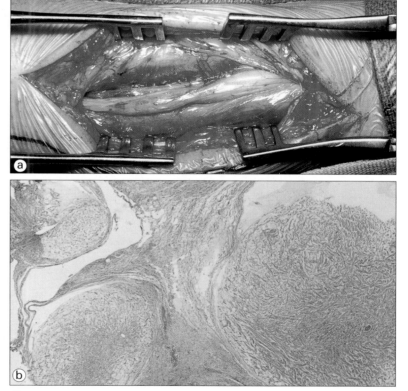

Fig. 42.14 Plexiform neurofibroma. (a) Intraoperative exposure of swollen nerve trunks that form part of a plexiform neurofibroma. **(b)** Histology of a plexiform neurofibroma reveals diffuse infiltration of multiple adjacent fascicles by neoplastic cells. (Hematoxylin/van Gieson)

MICROSCOPIC APPEARANCES

Neurofibromas are circumscribed, but not encapsulated. Their wavy spindle-shaped cells lie in a mucoid matrix or between bundles of collagen (**Fig. 42.15**). Many cells have nuclei with a serpentine form.

Immunohistochemical and ultrastructural studies suggest that neurofibromas are composed of several types of cell: fibroblasts and pericytes are mixed with Schwann cells, and mast cells may be scattered through the neoplasm. Neoplastic cells infiltrate nerve fascicles rather than displacing them (**Fig. 42.16**).

Cytologic pleomorphism and nuclear hyperchromasia may be degenerative, but such changes should be regarded with suspicion in neurofibromas. These cytologic features indicate anaplasia if there are mitoses (even only a few) or if they are seen in a neurofibroma from a patient with NF1. Anaplasia tends to become more extensive in successive biopsies from recurrent neoplasms, marking their progression to MNSTs.

Neurofibromas are immunoreactive for vimentin, but S-100 immunoreactivity is patchy, reflecting the scattered distribution of Schwann cells (**Fig. 42.17**).

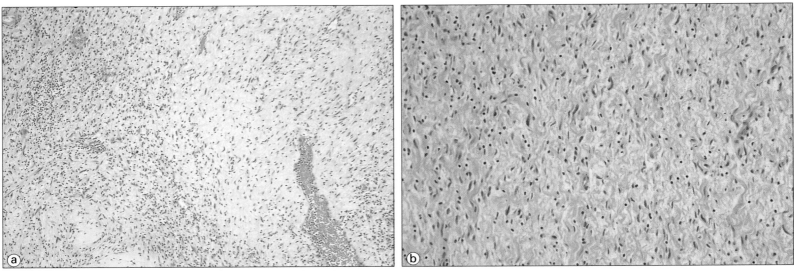

Fig. 42.15 Neurofibroma. (a) and **(b)** This nerve sheath tumor is composed of haphazardly arranged cells with wavy nuclei and variable amounts of cytoplasm. Scattered lymphocytes are also present in this case.

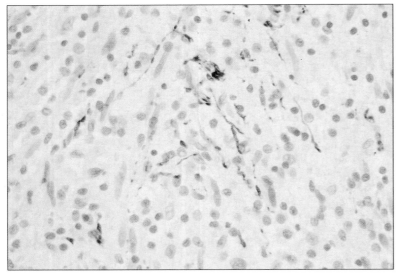

Fig. 42.16 Neurofibroma. Axons in the infiltrated nerve are immunolabeled with an antibody to neurofilaments. The axons are widely separated by the neoplastic cells.

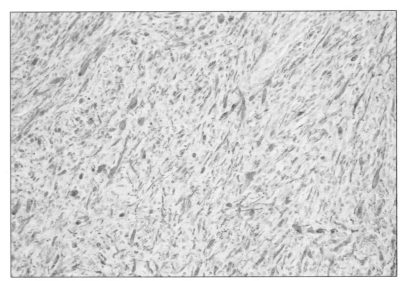

Fig. 42.17 Neurofibroma. The neoplastic Schwann cells are immunolabeled with an antibody to S-100 protein.

MALIGNANT NERVE SHEATH TUMORS

MNSTs that affect the CNS usually arise close to the spinal cord, from the cervical or brachial plexuses. Intracranial examples have been reported, and most commonly arise from the trigeminal nerve. Malignant transformation of plexiform neurofibromas in patients with NF1 is heralded by rapid enlargement, increasing neurologic deficit, and pain.

MACROSCOPIC APPEARANCES

MNSTs infiltrate and expand nerve trunks, producing fusiform swellings, and may invade surrounding soft tissues, resulting in a poorly defined border. They may contain areas of necrosis and hemorrhage.

MICROSCOPIC APPEARANCES

Fascicular and storiform patterns are typical. The nuclear:cytoplasmic ratio is high and mitotic figures are easily found (**Fig. 42.18**). Nuclear palisading is infrequent. Foci of necrosis are often evident. The waviness of the cell nuclei may be maintained, at least in some parts of the tumor.

About 10% of MNSTs show metaplasia. Mesenchymal tissues: skeletal muscle (triton tumor), bone, and cartilage may be present (**Fig. 42.19**).

Epithelial differentiation may result in the formation of clusters of glands. An epithelioid variant accounting for 5% of cases and consisting of round cells with prominent nucleoli can be mistaken for a carcinoma or malignant melanoma (**Fig. 42.20**). Very occasionally, MNSTs contain melanin, and rarely an MNST may arise from a melanotic schwannoma.

Immunohistochemical studies reveal that 30–50% of MNSTs do not label with S-100 antibodies, and in some MNSTs such immunolabeling is only patchy. Epithelioid MNSTs do not label with cytokeratin antibodies.

Approximately 50% of MNSTs have the ultrastructural features of Schwann cell differentiation.

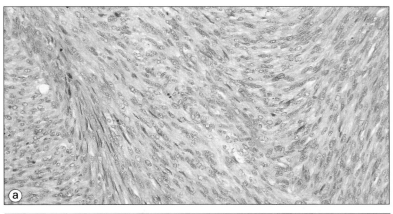

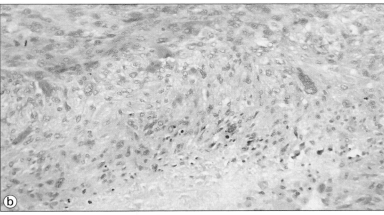

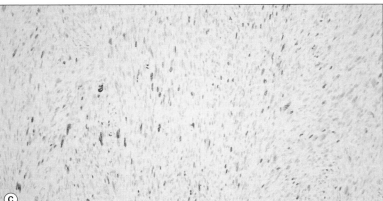

Fig. 42.18 MNST. (a) A higher nuclear:cytoplasmic ratio and mitotic count than in a schwannoma are found in this neoplasm. **(b)** Cytologic pleomorphism and micronecrosis are additional features. **(c)** The growth fraction, as indicated by Ki-67 immunoreactivity, is high.

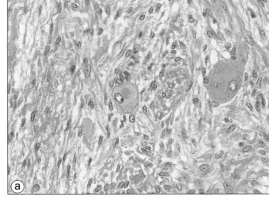

Fig. 42.19 Triton tumor. This variant of MNST is characterized by large cells with deeply eosinophilic cytoplasm **(a)**, in which cross-striations may occasionally be seen. These cells are immunoreactive for myoglobin **(b)**.

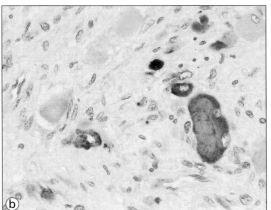

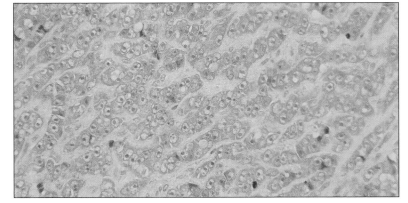

Fig. 42.20 Epithelioid MNST. Cords of round cells with prominent nuclei predominate in this variant.

REFERENCES

Enzinger FM, Weiss SW. In *Soft Tissue Tumors* (eds. Enzinger FM, Weiss SW). Third Edition. St. Louis: Mosby. Benign tumors of peripheral nerves: pp. 821–888. Malignant tumours of peripheral nerves: pp. 889–928.

Fletcher CD, Davies SE, McKee PH (1987) Cellular schwannoma: a distinct pseudosarcomatous entity. *Histopathology* 11: 21–35.

Louis DN, Ramesh V, Gusella JF (1995) Neuropathology and molecular genetics of neurofibromatosis type 2 and related tumors. *Brain Pathol* 5: 163–172.

von Deimling A, Krone W, Menon AG (1995) Neurofibromatosis type 1: pathology, clinical features and molecular genetics. *Brain Pathology* 5: 153–162.

Wanebo JE *et al.* (1993) Malignant peripheral nerve sheath tumors. A clinicopathological study of 28 cases. *Cancer* 71: 1247–1253.

Wick MR, Swanson PE, Scheithauer BW, Manivel JC (1987) Malignant peripheral nerve sheath tumor. An immunohistochemical study of 62 cases. *Am J Clin Path* 87: 425–433.

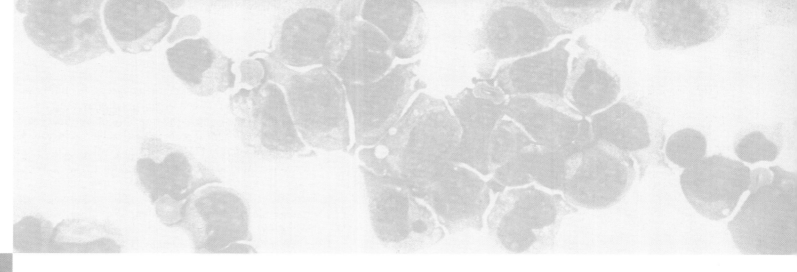

43 Meningiomas

MENINGIOMAS

Meningiomas arise from meningothelial (arachnoid) cells in the leptomeninges. These cells have both epithelial and mesenchymal characteristics, which are shown by meningiomas in a spectrum of diverse histologic appearances. The World Health Organization (WHO) classification recognizes several variants of meningioma (**Fig. 43.1**). Differentiation towards the epithelial end of the histologic spectrum is represented by the meningothelial and secretory variants. Differentiation towards the mesenchymal end of the spectrum is represented by the fibrous and metaplastic variants.

Meningiomas occur throughout the central nervous system (CNS), but have a predilection for certain sites (**Fig. 43.2**). Unusual sites include the ventricles and the epidural space. Depending on its location, a meningioma can grow for a prolonged period and to a considerable size before producing symptoms and signs. It may lead to increased intracranial pressure, loss of CNS function, or epilepsy. Some meningiomas are incidental postmortem findings (**Fig. 43.3**).

The site of a meningioma and any involvement of local structures are major prognostic factors because they affect surgical accessibility and therefore whether complete removal can be achieved.

Approximately 15% of meningiomas that appear to have been completely resected recur.

Histologic assessment of a meningioma provides some information about its biologic behavior. An increased tendency to recur and a shorter interval to recurrence are properties of meningiomas that show malignant architectural and cytologic features. Such features are

MENINGIOMAS

- The incidence of meningiomas rises with age.
- Asymptomatic meningiomas are often found at necropsy in elderly people.

Relative incidence:

- ~ 15% of intracranial neoplasms are meningiomas.
- ~ 25% of intraspinal neoplasms are meningiomas.
- ~ 10% of meningiomas are multiple.

Location:

- ~ 15% of intracranial meningiomas are infratentorial.
- ~ 15% of meningiomas are intraspinal.

Female:male gender bias:

- 3:2 for intracranial meningiomas.
- 10:1 for intraspinal meningiomas.
- Anaplastic meningiomas affect males and females equally.

Associations:

- Previous radiotherapy.
- Estrogen-dependent neoplasms. (breast carcinoma and endometrial carcinoma).
- Neurofibromatosis type 2.
- Castleman's syndrome. (for chordoid and lymphoplasmacyte-rich meningiomas).
- Polyclonal gammopathies. (for lymphoplasmacyte-rich meningiomas).
- Meningiomas are *not* associated with trauma.

WHO classification of meningiomas
Meningioma
Meningothelial
Fibrous
Transitional
Psammomatous
Angiomatous
Microcystic
Secretory
Clear cell
Chordoid
Lymphoplasmacyte-rich
Metaplastic
Atypical meningioma **Papillary meningioma** **Anaplastic (malignant) meningioma**

Fig. 43.1 WHO classification of meningiomas.

present in atypical and, to a greater extent, in anaplastic meningiomas, and develop progressively in meningiomas that recur several times. Infiltration of the brain is the most important histologic predictor of a high likelihood of local recurrence (see below). Other features are less reliable in predicting behavior. Even cytologically bland meningiomas can behave in a locally aggressive manner.

Not all meningeal neoplasms are meningiomas. Metastatic neoplasms (see chapter 46), hemangiopericytomas (see chapter 45), hemangioblastomas (see chapter 45), melanocytic neoplasms (see chapter 45), and various mesenchymal neoplasms (see chapter 45) may be located in the meninges. The term angioblastic meningioma, previously used for angiomatous meningiomas, hemangiopericytomas, and hemangioblastomas, is obsolete. Meningeal hemangiopericytomas share the histology of hemangiopericytomas outside the CNS and do not have the molecular genetic abnormalities of meningiomas.

MACROSCOPIC APPEARANCES

Meningiomas arising around the cerebral convexities are generally spherical because they can displace underlying brain (**Fig. 43.4**). The

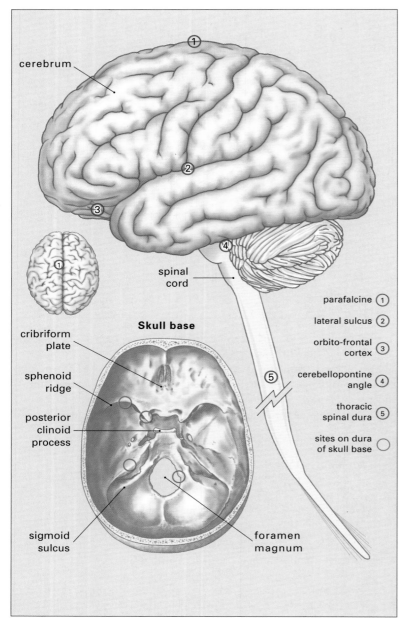

Fig. 43.2. **Sites of predilection for meningiomas.**

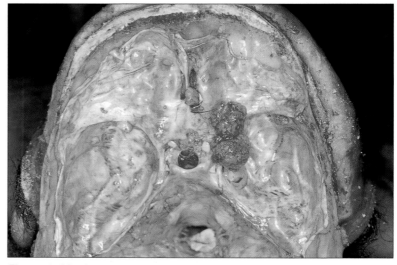

Fig. 43.3 **Meningiomas on the sphenoid ridge and olfactory groove.** These meningiomas were an incidental postmortem finding.

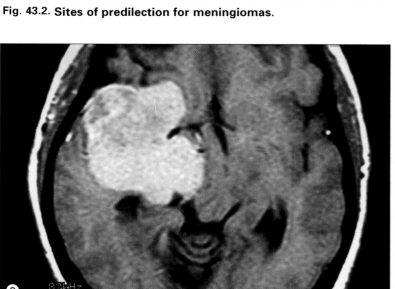

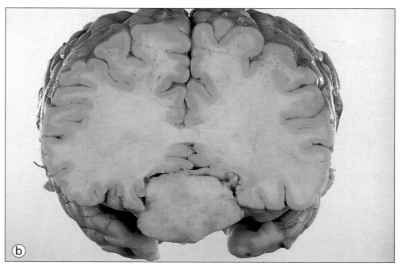

Fig. 43.4 **Meningioma. (a)** A contrast-enhanced MR scan showing a large sphenoid wing meningioma. (Courtesy of Dr JS Millar, Wessex Neurological Center) **(b)** A midline tumor has compressed the inferior part of the frontal lobes.

shape of other meningiomas is constrained by their location; for example, optic nerve meningiomas are fusiform. Meningiomas occasionally envelop rather than displace adjacent CNS structures (**Fig. 43.5**). Some meningiomas, particularly those on the sphenoid ridge, grow as plaques within the dura (en plaque meningioma).

Most meningiomas have a smooth or slightly lobulated surface and a rubbery consistency (**Fig. 43.6**). They are usually solid on sectioning, but may have a soft, granular texture, and there may be obvious interlacing bands of fibrous tissue. Rarer variants may have specific macroscopic features: for example, the microcystic meningioma has a gelatinous texture and the psammomatous meningioma feels gritty.

The attached dura should be inspected for separate nodules of neoplasm, and the relationship between dura and tumor should be examined histologically (**Fig. 43.7**). Invasion of adjacent bone may be evident at operation, and pieces of bone may be submitted for examination (**Fig. 43.8**). The infiltrated bone often shows hyperostosis, a feature that can, however, occur adjacent to meningiomas even in the absence of bony invasion.

MICROSCOPIC APPEARANCES

Meningiomas exhibit a wide range of histologic patterns. Furthermore, a single meningioma may show a combination of patterns. The meningothelial, transitional, and fibrous variants predominate, forming a histologic continuum that should be regarded as prototypical of this neoplasm because their features appear, to a greater or lesser extent, in other variants as well.

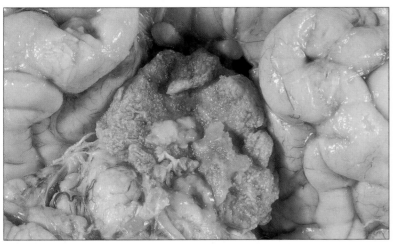

Fig. 43.5 Clival meningioma. This tumor has enveloped the brain stem.

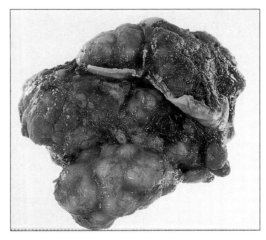

Fig. 43.6 Formalin-fixed meningioma. The tumor has a lobular appearance.

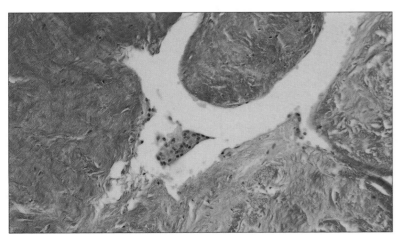

Fig. 43.7 Meningiomas may invade local structures. This relationship should be assessed histologically. In this case, a group of cells from a meningioma is present in a dural blood vessel. The vascular invasion does not signify a risk of distant metastasis. (Hematoxylin/van Gieson)

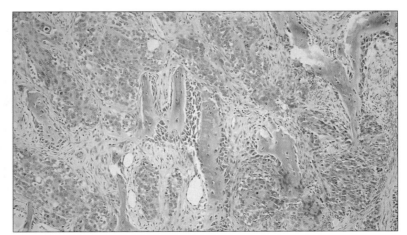

Fig. 43.8 Meningiomas may invade the skull. In this example, a meningioma invades the temporal bone. This behavior is not restricted to atypical and anaplastic meningiomas.

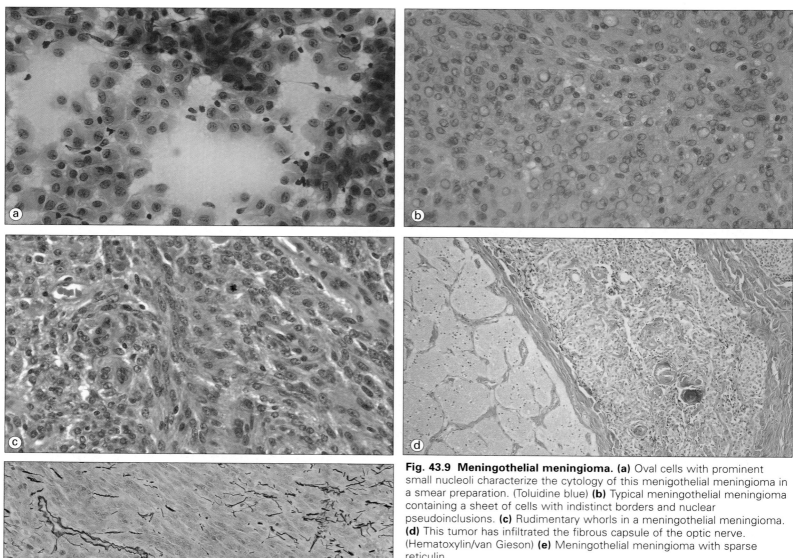

Fig. 43.9 Meningothelial meningioma. (a) Oval cells with prominent small nucleoli characterize the cytology of this menigothelial meningioma in a smear preparation. (Toluidine blue) **(b)** Typical meningothelial meningioma containing a sheet of cells with indistinct borders and nuclear pseudoinclusions. **(c)** Rudimentary whorls in a meningothelial meningioma. **(d)** This tumor has infiltrated the fibrous capsule of the optic nerve. (Hematoxylin/van Gieson) **(e)** Meningothelial meningioma with sparse reticulin.

Meningothelial meningiomas consist of sheets or lobules of oval cells that form rudimentary meningothelial whorls in a few places. The cytologic borders are indistinct. Single small nucleoli and nuclear pseudoinclusions formed by invaginations of the nuclear membrane are common (**Fig. 43.9**).

Fibrous meningiomas consist of spindle-shaped cells associated with variable amounts of pericellular collagen (**Fig. 43.10**).

Meningothelial and fibrous areas are combined in transitional meningiomas, which also contain widespread whorls and scattered psammoma bodies (**Fig. 43.11**).

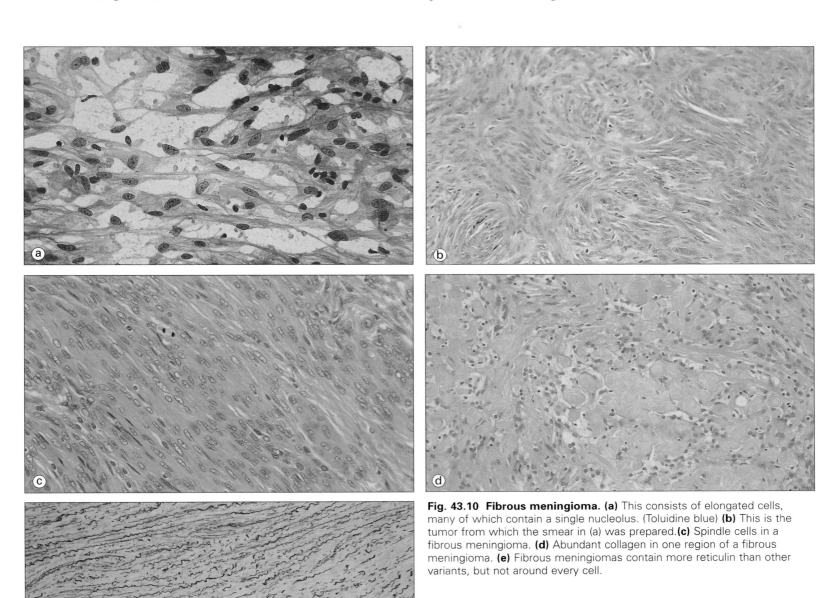

Fig. 43.10 Fibrous meningioma. (a) This consists of elongated cells, many of which contain a single nucleolus. (Toluidine blue) **(b)** This is the tumor from which the smear in (a) was prepared. **(c)** Spindle cells in a fibrous meningioma. **(d)** Abundant collagen in one region of a fibrous meningioma. **(e)** Fibrous meningiomas contain more reticulin than other variants, but not around every cell.

The criteria for diagnosing these variants of meningioma are subjective and a clear distinction is not always possible. This is also true for other variants of meningioma. For example, psammomatous meningioma is not defined by a specific density of psammoma bodies.

Focal cytologic pleomorphism in association with large hyperchromatic nuclei and in the absence of an increased mitotic count may be seen in classic meningiomas and does not indicate a worse prognosis.

Foci of foamy (xanthomatous) cells are frequently found in menin-giomas (**Fig. 43.12**), and should not be mistaken for micronecrosis.

Other variants of meningioma (**Fig. 43.13**) have distinctive architectural and cytologic features which are usually combined with the prototypical histology described above (**Figs 43.14–43.22**). No prognostic significance is attached to the diagnosis of particular variants, with the possible exception of the clear cell meningioma which has an increased tendency to recur, but it is useful to recognize them because they can resemble a range of other CNS neoplasms (see below).

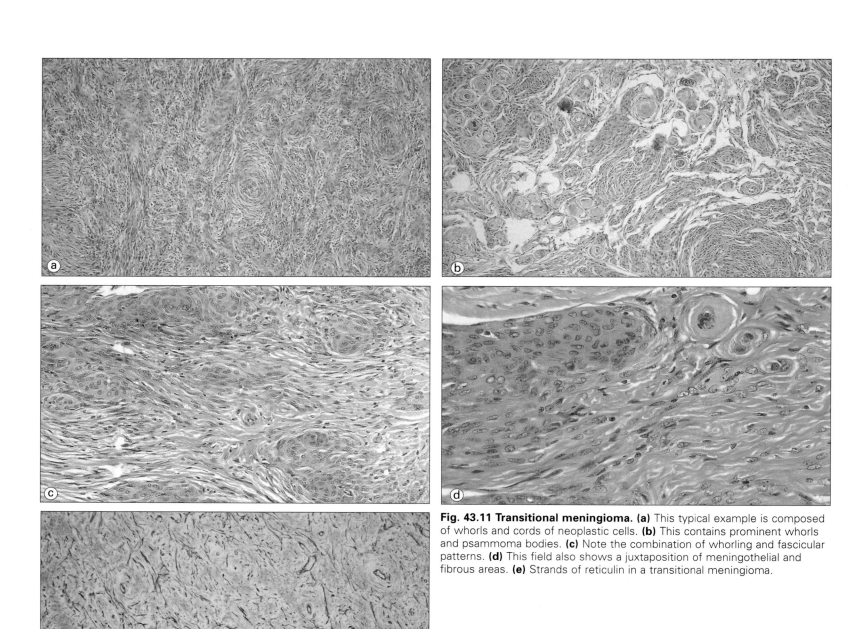

Fig. 43.11 Transitional meningioma. (a) This typical example is composed of whorls and cords of neoplastic cells. **(b)** This contains prominent whorls and psammoma bodies. **(c)** Note the combination of whorling and fascicular patterns. **(d)** This field also shows a juxtaposition of meningothelial and fibrous areas. **(e)** Strands of reticulin in a transitional meningioma.

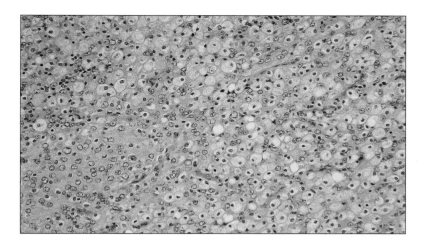

Fig. 43.12 Foci of foamy (xanthomatous) cells. These are found in many variants of meningioma.

Characteristics of variants of classic meningiomas

Psammomatous

- A transitional meningioma with many psammoma bodies.
- Intraspinal, orbital, and olfactory groove meningiomas are often psammomatous.

Angiomatous

- Multiple blood vessels of varying size among groups of meningothelial cells.
- Vessels tend to have thickened, hyaline walls.
- Intervening neoplastic cells show moderate nuclear pleomorphism.

Microcystic

- Characterized by cytoplasmic processes separated by extracellular fluid to produce a lacy meshwork of microcysts.
- Contains groups of thick-walled blood vessels and foamy cells.
- Moderate nuclear pleomorphism.
- Sparse whorls and psammoma bodies.

Secretory

- Charcterized by PAS-positive globular inclusions within intracytoplasmic lumina lined by microvilli. The microvilli are not usually discernible except by electron microscopy.
- Surrounding cells are immunoreactive for cytokeratins.

Clear cell

- Characterized by sheets and lobules of elongated cells with abundant intracytoplasmic glycogen.
- Sparse whorls and psammoma bodies.
- Hyalinization may be prominant.

Chordoid

- Lobulated and meningothelial patterns.
- Characterized by columns of cells in a mucoid stroma and scattered lymphoplasmacytoid infiltrates.

Lymphoplasmacyte-rich

- Abundant lymphocytes and plasma cells appear as an inflammatory infiltrate.
- May show germinal centres.
- May be associated with chordoid variant.

Metaplastic

- Shows mesenchymal differentiation (i.e lipomatous, cartilaginous, osseous).

Fig. 43.13 Characteristics of variants of classic meningiomas.

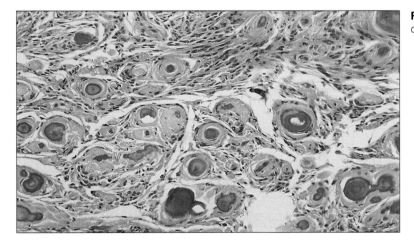

Fig. 43.14 Psammomatous meningioma. This consists of numerous compact whorls that contain psammoma bodies.

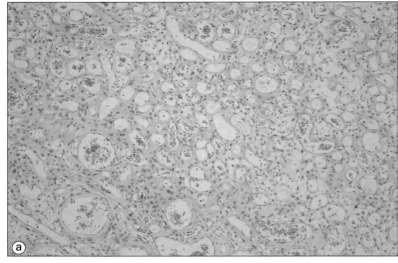

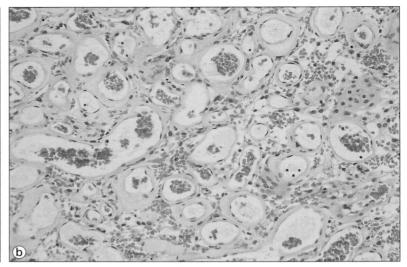

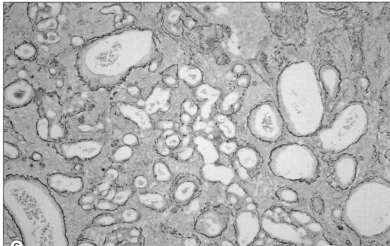

Fig. 43.15 Angiomatous meningioma. (a) Blood vessels are strikingly prominent. **(b)** Groups of neoplastic cells lie between thick-walled vessels. **(c)** A reticulin preparation highlights the numerous blood vessels.

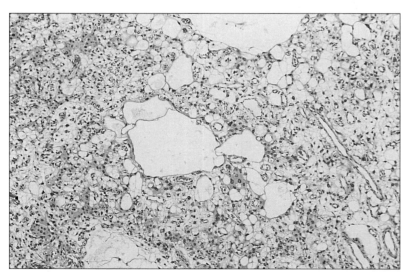

Fig. 43.16 Microcystic meningioma. Cystic spaces are widespread among the cells of this neoplasm.

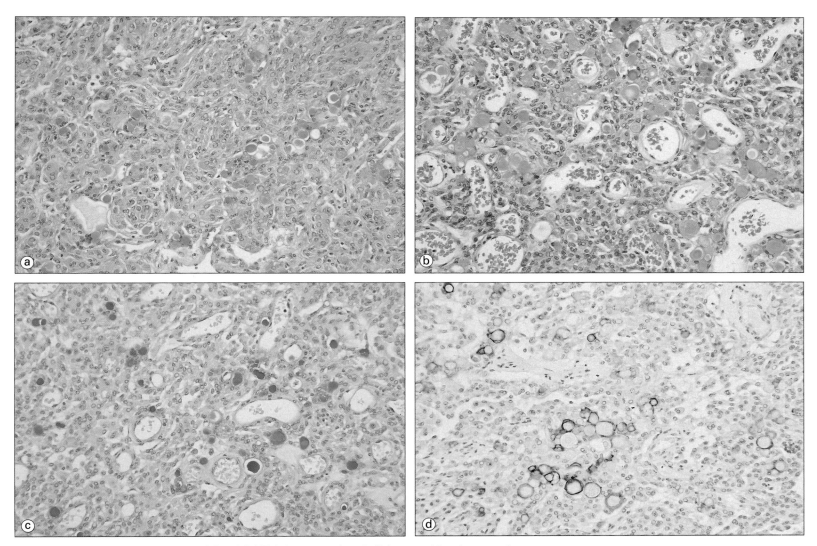

Fig. 43.17 Secretory meningioma. (a) and **(b)** This has a meningothelial or transitional pattern, but some of the cells contain eosinophilic globules. **(c)** The globules are PAS-positive. **(d)** The cells that secrete and enclose the globules show cytokeratin immunoreactivity.

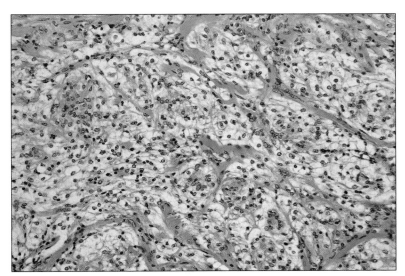

Fig. 43.18 Clear cell meningioma. Groups of clear cells are divided by fibrous septae which were particularly prominent in some areas of this neoplasm.

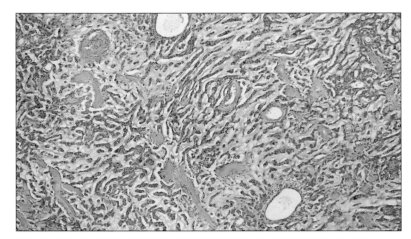

Fig. 43.19 Chordoid meningioma. An abundant myxoid matrix surrounds small strands of meningothelial cells. This appearance mimics the histology of a chordoma, but this neoplasm can be distinguished from a meningioma by widespread immunoreactivities for S-100 and cytokeratins and its tendency to permeate bone.

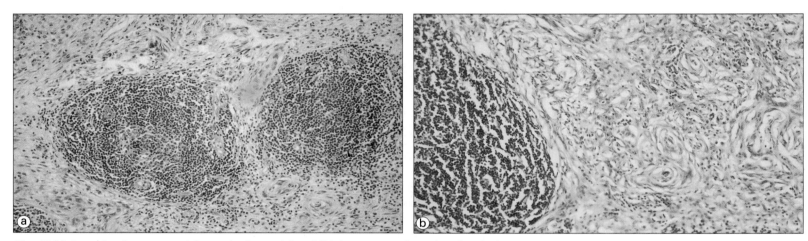

Fig. 43.20 Lymphoplasmacyte-rich meningioma. (a) and **(b)** Aggregates of mononuclear leukocytes are evident in this variant which otherwise shows the histology of a classic meningioma. (Courtesy of Dr. T Revesz, Institute of Neurology, London, U.K.)

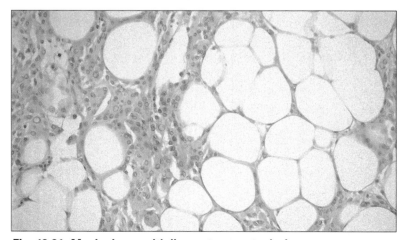

Fig. 43.21 Meningioma with lipomatous metaplasia.

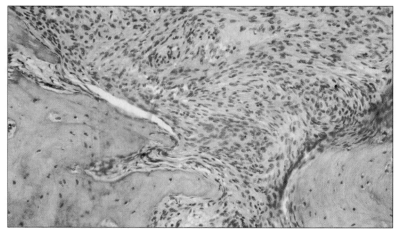

Fig. 43.22 Metaplastic bone in a meningioma. (Courtesy of Dr T Revesz, Institute of Neurology, London, U.K.)

Atypical, anaplastic, and papillary meningiomas exhibit histologic characteristics that reflect their aggressive biologic behaviors. These characteristics include a high mitotic count and groups of cells with a high nuclear:cytoplasmic ratio. Atypical and anaplastic meningiomas are situated on a histologic continuum from prototypical meningioma to sarcoma of meningothelial origin. The papillary meningioma (**Fig. 43.23**) is, however, set apart as a rare and distinctive neoplasm. It is characterized by monomorphic oval cells with a high nuclear:cytoplasmic ratio and a high mitotic count, prominent (pseudo)rosettes of tumor cells around blood vessels, a delicate reticulin pattern between cells, and sparse whorls and psammoma bodies.

A diagnosis of anaplastic meningioma indicates a strong likelihood of local recurrence and infiltration. However, distant metastasis of meningiomas is very rare except in the case of papillary meningiomas, which may metastasize through the cerebrospinal fluid pathways and occasionally outside the CNS.

The WHO classification lists histologic features to be assessed when considering a diagnosis of atypical or anaplastic meningioma (**Figs 43.24–43.26**), but the distinctions are rather subjective. Grading systems in which scores are allotted to the presence and extent of six histologic characteristics that can be correlated with the degree of malignancy have been assessed by Jääskeläinen and Mahmood (**Fig. 43.27**), and show a reasonable correlation with clinical behavior.

PAPILLARY MENINGIOMA

- is found particularly in young patients.
- exhibits aggressive biologic behavior with invasion of adjacent structures.
- has a high frequency of (late) metastasis.

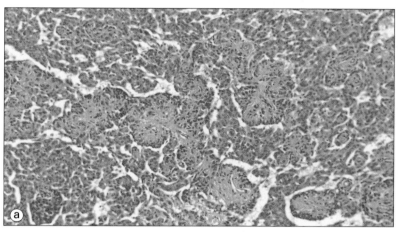

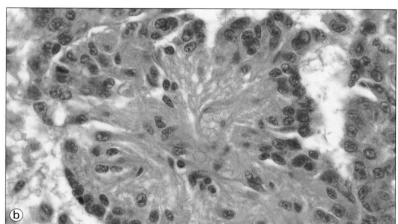

Fig. 43.23 Papillary meningioma. (a) This example consists of rather ill-defined papillary structures with perivascular clusters of meningioma cells. **(b)** Cells form a pseudorosette around a capillary.

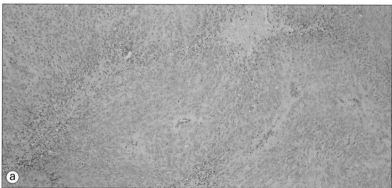

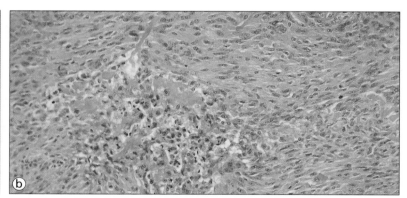

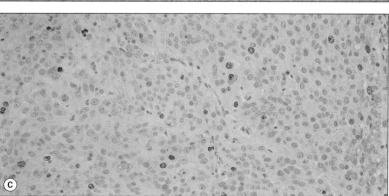

Fig. 43.24 Atypical meningioma. (a) This contains foci of micronecrosis and lacks whorls or well-defined lobules. **(b)** There are scattered mitoses, cellular pleomorphism, and micronecrosis. **(c)** Many of the nuclei label with a Ki-67 antibody.

Invasion of the brain is a particularly adverse prognostic feature and should be diagnosed with care. Indentation of the pial surface does not signify invasion, but invasion is present when fingers of tumor breach the pial surface to invade the parenchyma or perivascular space. Invasion of the brain is accompanied by reactive changes such as astrocytosis (**Fig. 43.28**).

Immunohistochemistry: Meningiomas are immunoreactive for vimentin (**Fig. 43.29**), and most meningiomas, particularly those with epithelial qualities, immunolabel with antibodies to epithelial membrane antigen (EMA) (**Fig. 43.30**). Fibrous meningiomas tend to show only focal labeling for EMA. Approximately 25% of meningiomas show focal immunoreactivity for cytokeratins. The neoplastic cells surrounding the characteristic globules in secretory meningiomas label strongly with antibodies to cytokeratin (see Fig. 43.18c). Some meningiomas contain scattered cells that are immunoreactive for S-100 protein. There is no immunoreactivity for GFAP.

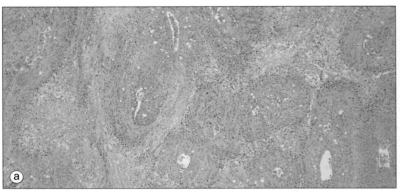

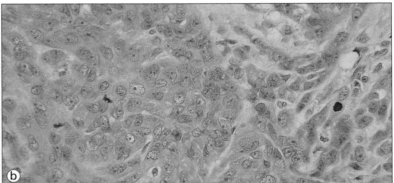

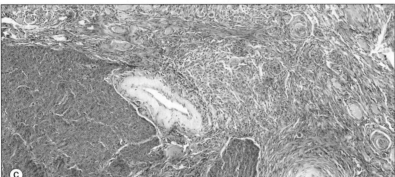

Fig. 43.25 Anaplastic meningioma. (a) This example has large areas of necrosis and marked cellular pleomorphism. **(b)** Note the nuclear pleomorphism, prominent nucleoli, and abundant mitoses. **(c)** This neoplasm contains a focus of anaplastic change characterized by a loss of whorls and a reduced nuclear:cytoplasmic ratio.

1993 WHO criteria for classifying meningiomas as atypical or anaplastic (malignant)	
Atypical meningioma	Anaplastic (malignant) meningioma
• Frequent mitoses • Increased cellularity • Small cells with high nuclear:cytoplasmic ratio • Small cells with prominent nucleoli • Patternless growth • Areas of necrosis	• Cytologic abnormalities exceeding those in atypical meningiomas • Abundant necrosis.

Fig. 43.26 1993 WHO criteria for classifying meningiomas as atypical or anaplastic (malignant).

Criteria for classifying meningiomas as atypical or anaplastic (malignant)

Features to score (0–3):	Jääskeläinen			Mahmood		
	Total score	Category	5 yr RR*	Total score	Category	5 yr RR*
• Loss of architecture • Increased cellularity • Nuclear pleomorphism • Mitoses • Necrosis • Brain invasion	0–2	Benign	3%	0–4	Benign	2%
	3–6	Atypical	38%	5–11	Atypical	50%
	7–11	Anaplastic	78%	>11	Malignant	33%
	>11	Sarcomatous				
	* 5 yr. RR = 5 year recurrence rate					

Fig. 43.27 Criteria for classifying meningiomas as atypical or anaplastic (malignant). From Jääskeläinen *et al.* (1986) *Surg Neurol* **25**: 233–242 and Mahmood *et al.* (1993) *Neurosurgery* **33**: 955–963.

DIFFERENTIAL DIAGNOSIS OF MENINGIOMA

Variant	Differential diagnosis	Distinguishing features
• Meningothelial meningioma	• Carcinoma	• is much more commonly and diffusely immunoreactive for cytokeratins. • usually shows more anaplasia and mitotic activity. • has more clearly defined cytoplasmic margins. • may have more prominent nucleoli.
	• Melanocytic neoplasm	• is frequently immunoreactive for S-100 and HMB-45. • is not immunoreactive for EMA. • may contain melanosomes on ultrastructural examination. • has more clearly defined cytoplasmic margins. • may have more prominent nucleoli.
	• Glioma	• shows a diffuse pattern of brain infiltration. • is usually immunoreactive for GFAP. • is not immunoreactive for EMA.
• Fibrous meningioma	• Astrocytoma • Schwannoma	• as above for differentiating glioma from meningothelial meningioma. • shows a pericellular reticulin pattern. • is diffusely immunoreactive for S-100. • is not immunoreactive for EMA.
• Angiomatous meningioma	• Arteriovenous malformation • Hemangiopericytoma	• shows an absence of meningothelial cells. • includes entrapped gliotic brain tissue. • is not immunoreactive for EMA. • has a pericellular basal lamina. • shows no desmosomes on electron microscopy.
• Microcystic meningioma	• Astrocytoma • Hemangioblastoma	• as above for differentiating glioma from meningothelial meningioma. • is not immunoreactive for EMA. • reveals a characteristic arrangement of stromal cells and capillaries. • contains no junctions on electron microscopy.
• Clear cell meningioma	• Renal cell carcinoma	• is usually immunoreactive for cytokeratins.
• Chordoid meningioma	• Chordoma	• shows widespread immunoreactivity for S-100 protein and cytokeratins. • permeates bone.
• Papillary meningioma	• Ependymoma • Carcinoma • Choroid plexus carcinoma	• as above for differentiating glioma from meningothelial meningioma. • as above for differentiating carcinoma from meningothelial meningioma. • is usually immunoreactive for cytokeratins, transthyretin, and carbonic anhydrase.

MENINGIOMAS AND PROGESTERONE RECEPTORS

- More than 75% of meningiomas express progesterone receptors.
- Antibodies to progesterone receptor label the nucleus and cytoplasm.
- Inverse relationships between progesterone receptor immunolabeling and cytologic atypia and between progesterone receptor immunolabeling and Ki-67 labeling indices have been shown in *some* studies.

GENETIC ABNORMALITIES IN MENINGIOMAS

- Monosomy of chromosome 22 is the most common cytogenetic abnormality in meningiomas.
- ~ 70% of meningiomas show loss of heterozygosity for chromosome 22q markers.
- 25–75% of meningiomas (in different series) contain inactivating mutations of the neurofibromatosis type 2 (NF2) gene.
- Allelic losses on chromosome 22q frequently accompany NF2 mutation.
- NF2 mutations occur in about 75% of fibrous and transitional meningiomas.
- NF2 mutations occur in about 25% of meningothelial meningiomas.
- Progression to atypical and anaplastic meningiomas correlates with additional allelic losses involving chromosomes 1p, 10, and 14q.

The proportion of neoplastic cells labeled by Ki-67 antibodies and other cell cycle specific markers is greater in atypical and anaplastic meningiomas than in prototypical meningiomas. In some series Ki-67 labeling indices have correlated with the rapidity of recurrence.

Ultrastructural features of meningiomas include interdigitating processes, intermediate filaments, desmosomes, and hemidesmosomes. Intercellular collagen deposition is found in fibrous variants.

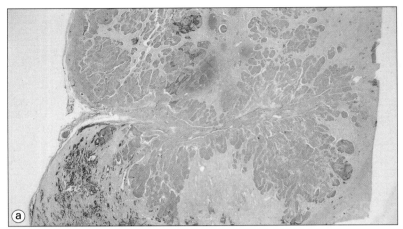
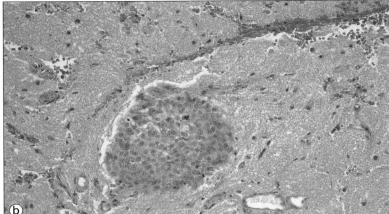

Fig. 43.28 Invasion of brain by meningioma. (a) This neoplasm extensively infiltrates the brain where **(b)** groups of cells have elicited a surrounding reactive astrocytosis.

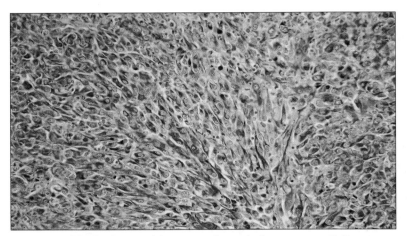
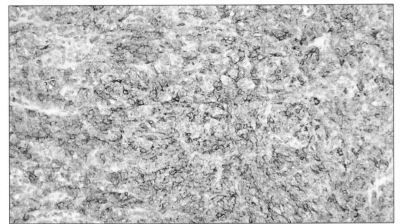

Fig. 43.29 Meningioma with strong vimentin immunoreactivity. This is typical of meningiomas.

Fig. 43.30 Meningioma immunostained for EMA.

REFERENCES

Kepes JJ. (1986) Presidential address: the histopathology of meningiomas. A reflection of origins and expected behaviour. *J Neuropathol Exp Neurol* **45**: 95–107.

Lantos PL, VandenBerg SR, Kleihues P. (1996) Tumors of the meninges. In Graham DI, Lantos PL (eds). Greenfield's *Neuropathology Vol. 2*. pp 727–752. London: Edward Arnold.

Maier H, Ofner D, Hittmair A, Kitz K, Budka H. (1992) Classic, atypical, and anaplastic meningioma: three histopathological subtypes of clinical relevance. *J Neurosurg* **77**: 616–623.

Ng HK. (1994) Atypical and malignant meningioma: any easy diagnostic criteria? *Adv Anat Pathol* **1**: 44–48.

Ruttledge MH, Sarrazin J, Rangaratnam S, Phelan CM *et al.* (1994) Evidence for the complete inactivation of the NF2 gene in the majority of sporadic meningiomas. *Nature Genet* **6**: 180–184.

Scheithauer BW. (1990) Tumors of the meninges: proposed modifications of the World Health Organization classification. *Acta Neuropathol* **80**: 343–354.

Schmidek HH. (1991) *Meningiomas and their surgical management*. Philadelphia: WB Saunders.

Simon M, von Deimling A, Larson JJ, Wellenreuther R *et al.* (1995) Allelic losses on chromosomes 14, 10, and 1 in atypical and malignant meningiomas: a genetic model of meningioma progression. *Cancer Res* **55**: 4696–4701.

Smith DA, Cahill DW. (1994) The biology of meningiomas. *Neurosurg Clin N Am* **5**: 201–215.

Wellenreuther R, Kraus JA, Lenartz D, Menon AG *et al.* (1995) Analysis of the neurofibromatosis 2 gene reveals molecular variants of meningioma. *Am J Pathol* **146**: 827–832.

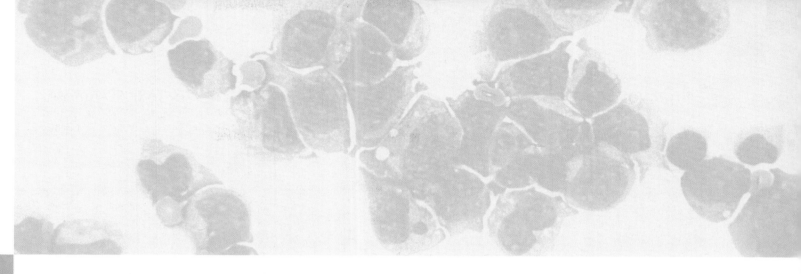

44 Neoplasms in the region of the pituitary fossa

Neoplasms in the region of the pituitary fossa may arise in the pituitary gland itself, the sphenoid bone that surrounds the fossa, or the suprasellar region (**Figs 44.1, 44.2**). Structures in the suprasellar region and adjacent to the pituitary fossa include the hypothalamus, optic chiasm, nasal sinuses, and cavernous sinuses and their contents.

Common neoplasms in this region are:

- pituitary adenomas
- meningiomas

Uncommon neoplasms in this region are:

- craniopharyngiomas
- germinomas
- metastatic carcinomas
- astrocytomas

Other neoplasms are rare.

The pituitary gland weighs about 600 mg and consists mainly of the adenohypophysis (anterior lobe) and the neurohypophysis (posterior lobe) (**Figs 44.3–44.5**); the pars intermedia is poorly developed in man.

Adenomas are the commonest neoplasms in the pituitary gland and are derived from cells in the adenohypophysis. Neoplasms of neurohypophyseal origin are very rare.

PITUITARY ADENOMAS

Pituitary adenomas are derived from secretory cells in the adenohypophysis. Some adenomas secrete peptides in an unregulated manner and may therefore produce abnormal endocrine effects in addition to causing mass effects in the region of the pituitary fossa (**Fig. 44.6**).

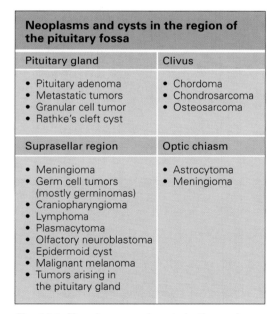

Neoplasms and cysts in the region of the pituitary fossa	
Pituitary gland	**Clivus**
• Pituitary adenoma • Metastatic tumors • Granular cell tumor • Rathke's cleft cyst	• Chordoma • Chondrosarcoma • Osteosarcoma
Suprasellar region	**Optic chiasm**
• Meningioma • Germ cell tumors (mostly germinomas) • Craniopharyngioma • Lymphoma • Plasmacytoma • Olfactory neuroblastoma • Epidermoid cyst • Malignant melanoma • Tumors arising in the pituitary gland	• Astrocytoma • Meningioma

Fig. 44.1 Neoplasms and cysts in the region of the pituitary fossa.

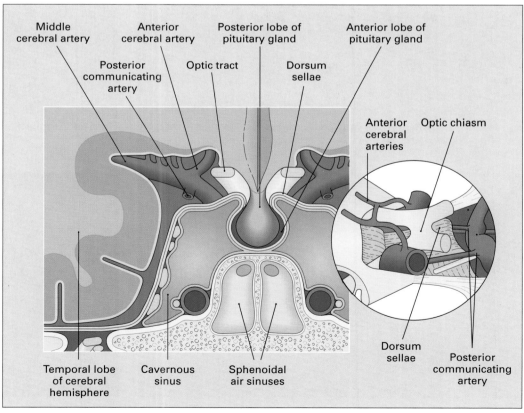

Fig. 44.2 Anatomic relationships of the pituitary gland.

PITUITARY PEPTIDES

Secretory cells in the adenohypophysis synthesize six major peptide hormones:
- Somatotrophs synthesize growth hormone (GH).
- Lactotrophs (mammotrophs) synthesize prolactin (PRL).
- Corticotrophs synthesize corticotropin (ACTH).
- Thyrotrophs synthesize thyrotropin (TSH).
- Gonadotrophs synthesize follicle stimulating hormone (FSH) and luteinizing hormone (LH).

TSH, FSH, and LH are glycoproteins composed of a common α subunit and different β subunits. The cross-reactivity sometimes seen with antibodies to these peptides is due to the considerable homology between the β subunits.

The neurohypophysis is continuous with the infundibular stalk and the median eminence. Its two major peptide hormones are synthesized in the supraoptic and para-ventricular nuclei of the hypothalamus and are:

- Oxytocin.
- Vasopressin.

GENETICS OF PITUITARY ADENOMAS

- Pituitary adenomas are associated with multiple endocrine neoplasia (MEN) type 1, which also comprises neoplasms of pancreatic islet cells and hyperplasia and neoplasms of the parathyroid glands, and is linked to a candidate tumor suppressor gene on chromosome 11q13. Less than 3% of patients with pituitary adenomas have MEN 1, but 25% of patients with MEN 1 have a pituitary adenoma.
- Nearly all pituitary adenomas are monoclonal.
- Some GH adenomas contain an activating mutation in the α-subunit of the Gs protein.
- Deletions in the region of a candidate tumor suppressor gene on chromosome 11q13 are found in approximately 20% of sporadic adenomas.
- Mutations of the p53 and retinoblastoma tumor suppressor genes have not been demonstrated.

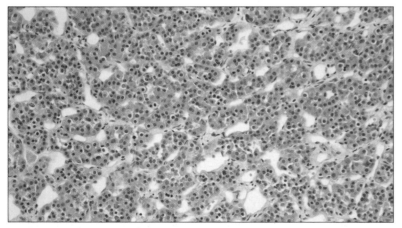

Fig. 44.3 Normal adenohypophysis. Nests of round or polyhedral cells, and an intervening network of vascular sinusoids are evident.

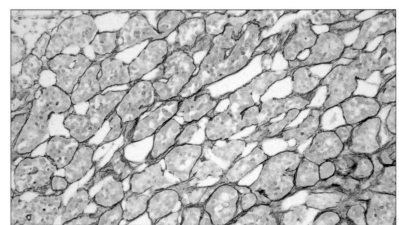

Fig. 44.4 Normal adenohypophysis. Cell nests are surrounded by reticulin.

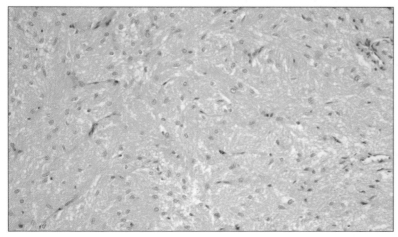

Fig. 44.5 Normal neurohypophysis. This consists of non-myelinated hypothalamohypophyseal nerve fibers and a meshwork of capillaries adjacent to which the fibers terminate. Also present are specialized astrocytes (pituicytes).

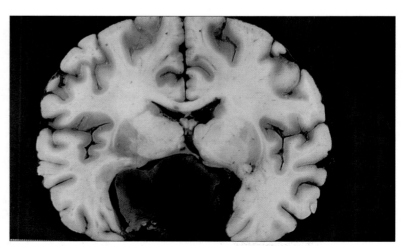

Fig. 44.6 Pituitary adenoma. Large, hemorrhagic pituitary adenoma producing distortion of surrounding structures.

MACROSCOPIC APPEARANCES

Pituitary adenomas are soft and have a beige or cream color. Discussion between the neurosurgeon and pathologist at the time of operation sometimes raises the possibility of an alternative diagnosis (e.g. a tough mass is more likely to be a meningioma).

By convention, macroadenomas and microadenomas have diameters above and below 10 mm respectively. Most microadenomas diagnosed in life are ACTH-cell adenomas and PRL-cell adenomas presenting early with endocrine effects. Histopathologic assessment of surgically treated microadenomas requires a thorough examination of all submitted tissue.

MICROSCOPIC APPEARANCES

The histology of pituitary adenomas is varied. Many adenomas consist of small, oval, or polyhedral cells. These may be arranged in monotonous sheets or show a variety of acinar, papillary, trabecular, or other patterns (**Figs 44.7–44.9**). The nuclei of neoplastic cells are generally round or oval and contain the stippled chromatin typical of neuroendocrine neoplasms. Tiny nucleoli may be evident. Cytologic pleomorphism and mitotic figures may be present, but do not necessarily signify aggressive biologic behavior (**Fig. 44.10**). Invasion of local structures (**Fig. 44.11**), particularly the dura, is common, even by adenomas with bland cytologic features.

Dystrophic calcification and eosinophilic (amyloid) bodies are strongly associated with prolactinomas (**Fig. 44.12**). Long-term treatment of prolactinomas with bromocriptine before surgical resection produces fibrosis.

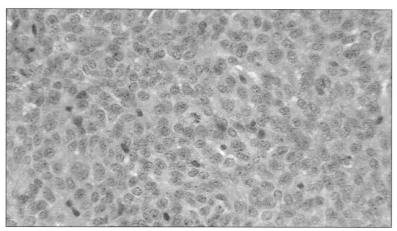

Fig. 44.7 Pituitary adenoma. A monotonous sheet of cells is typical.

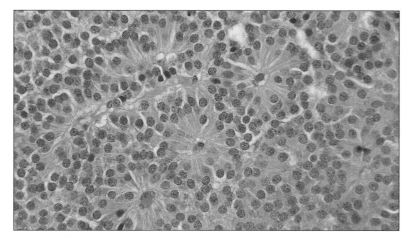

Fig. 44.8 Pituitary adenoma. A vascular network is seen between cells, some of which have formed pseudorosettes.

PITUITARY ADENOMAS

- are the commonest neoplasms in the region of the pituitary fossa, and represent 10–15% of intracranial neoplasms.
- have an incidence ranging from 1–15/100,000 in different populations.
- are most common in the third to sixth decades.
- show a female:male ratio of approximately 2:1 in younger patients.
- may be an incidental finding in approximately 10% of elderly people according to some necropsy series (40% of these neoplasms are prolactinomas).
- may present with the effects of increased peptide production (i.e. acromegaly or gigantism due to excess GH, Cushing's syndrome due to excess ACTH, amenorrhea, galactorrhea, or impotence due to excess PRL, hyperthyroidism due to excess TSH).
- may present with mass effects (i.e. headache, compression of the optic chiasm, (other) cranial nerve palsies, compression of the hypothalamus, hypopituitarism, pituitary infarction). Pituitary peptide deficiencies preceding complete hypopituitarism tend to occur in sequence (i.e. GH → FSH / LH → TSH → ACTH).
- may present acutely with mass effects when they undergo infarction or hemorrhage.

Non-neoplastic causes of infarction (pituitary apoplexy)
- Postpartum hemorrhage (Sheehan's syndrome).
- Raised intracranial pressure.
- Poorly controlled anticoagulation.

Prolactinomas
- commonly present in young women as microadenomas because amenorrhea is an early hormonal effect.
- tend to be larger and have a higher incidence of dural invasion in men and older women.
- result in increased serum PRL concentrations, which correlate with the size of the adenoma.
- can compress the pituitary stalk and thereby compromise transport of PRL inhibitory factor (dopamine) to the adenohypophysis, resulting in an elevated PRL level ('stalk effect'), but PRL concentrations seldom exceed 200 mg/l in these circumstances.
- usually present with acromegaly if the tumor is a PRL and GH mixed cell adenoma or mammosomatotroph adenoma.

ACTH-cell adenomas
- result in serum ACTH and cortisol concentrations that correlate poorly with their size.
- are occasionally clinically silent despite labeling with antibodies to ACTH.

Pituitary adenomas with an above-average tendency to aggressive behavior
- Acidophil stem cell adenoma.
- Sparsely granulated GH-cell adenoma.
- Sparsely granulated ACTH-cell adenoma.

Crooke's hyaline change describes the development of a zone of glassy agranular cytoplasm around the nuclei of non-adenomatous corticotrophs in patients with elevated corticosteroid concentrations due to an ACTH-cell adenoma, a systemic ACTH-producing neoplasm, an adrenal neoplasm or exogenous corticosteroid adminstration (**Fig. 44.13**). This appearance results from a massive accumulation of keratin microfilaments.

A small proportion of null-cell adenomas comprises oncocytomas (**Fig. 44.14**). The (arbitrary) ultrastructural criterion for a diagnosis of oncocytoma is that more than 10% of the cell volume must be occupied by mitochondria. ACTH-cell adenomas occasionally show oncocytic change.

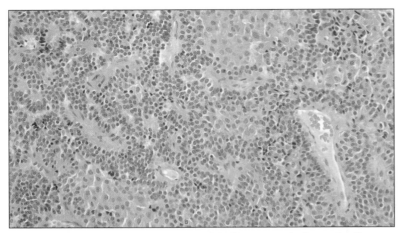

Fig. 44.9 Pituitary adenoma composed of two populations of cells. The larger cells were immunoreactive for GH.

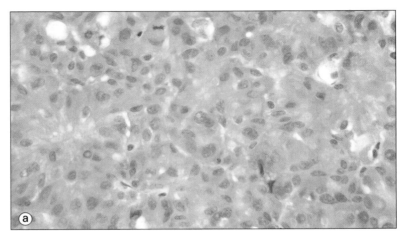

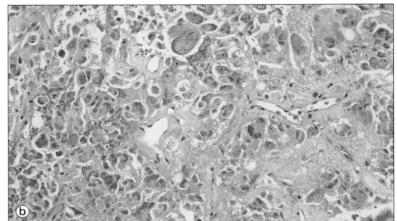

Fig. 44.10 Pituitary adenoma. (a) and **(b)** Cytologic pleomorphism and mitotic figures may be present and do not necessarily signify aggressive behavior.

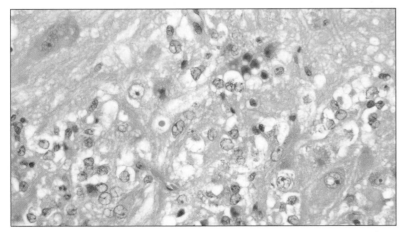

Fig. 44.11 Entrapped hypothalamic neurons at the invading edge of a suprasellar adenoma. Adenomas containing neoplastic ganglion cells are recorded but are extremely rare.

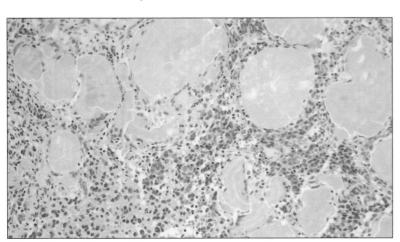

Fig. 44.12 Large masses of eosinophilic amyloid bodies in a prolactinoma. (Courtesy of Dr J Geddes, Royal London Hospital, U.K.)

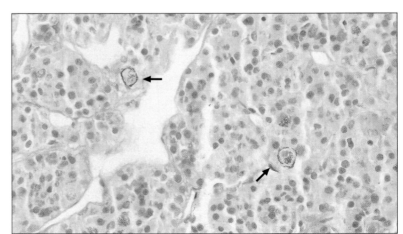

Fig. 44.13 Crooke's hyaline change. Basophilic cytoplasm in corticotrophs is displaced by amorphous material. Perinuclear material has displaced the magenta cytoplasmic granules in the corticotrophs (arrows). (Orange/fuschia/green)

Immunohistochemistry and electron microscopy: Immunohistochemistry to assess the production of peptide hormones (**Figs 44.15–44.19**) is used with electron microscopy (**Figs 44.20, 44.21**) to classify pituitary adenomas. The various pituitary trichrome stains are useful for demonstrating normal adenohypophysis, but of limited value for distinguishing different types of adenoma. Immunolabelling of a hormone in adenoma cells does not necessarily signify that it is secreted in a physiologically active form. Pituitary adenomas label with antibodies to synaptophysin, chromogranin-A, and low molecular weight cytokeratins (**Fig. 44.22**).

Invasive adenomas and adenomas that recur have a higher growth fraction as assessed by Ki-67 antibodies.

A diagnosis of pituitary carcinoma requires evidence of metastasis: either discontinuous spread of neoplasm within the CNS or spread outside the CNS. Pituitary carcinomas can produce any pituitary peptide.

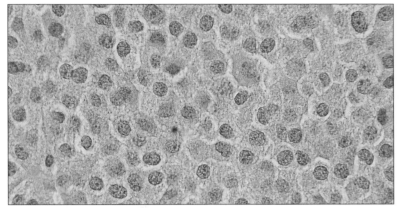

Fig. 44.14 Pituitary oncocytoma. The uniform cells in this adenoma exhibit cytoplasmic granularity and eosinophilia. (Courtesy of Dr S van Duinen, Academisch Ziekenhuis, Leiden)

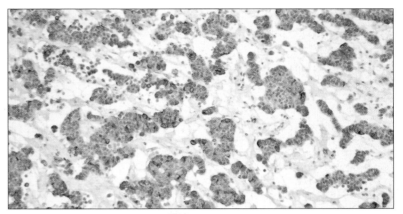

Fig. 44.15 Pituitary adenoma. Immunohistochemical demonstration of prolactin synthesis.

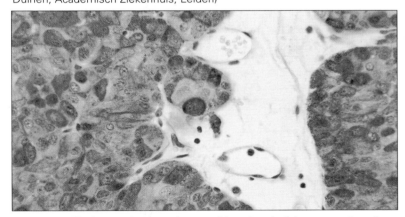

Fig. 44.16 Pituitary adenoma. Immunohistochemical demonstration of ACTH synthesis.

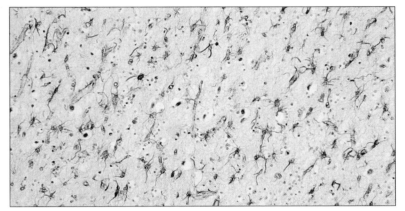

Fig. 44.17 Cells in a mammosomatotroph adenoma labeled with a GH antibody.

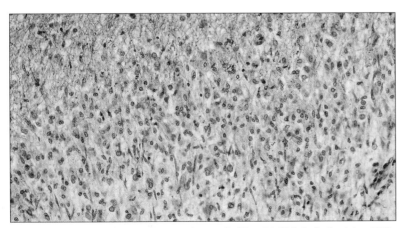

Fig. 44.18 Cells in the adenoma shown in Fig. 44.17 labeled with a PRL antibody.

Pituitary adenomas classified by peptide production		
Peptide		Percentage of total*
PRL		25
GH	densely granulated†	6
	sparsely granulated†	3
ACTH		12
FSH / LH		8
TSH		1
PRL + GH	mammosomatotroph adenoma	2
PRL + GH	acidophil stem cell adenoma	2
PRL + GH	mixed cell adenoma	5
GH + TSH ± α-subunit ± PRL and FSH + LH ± TSH ± α-subunit ± GH ± PRL		10
Null-cell adenoma		25
Others		1

* a synthesis of figures from several series
† on ultrastructural examination

Fig. 44.19 Pituitary adenomas classified by peptide production.

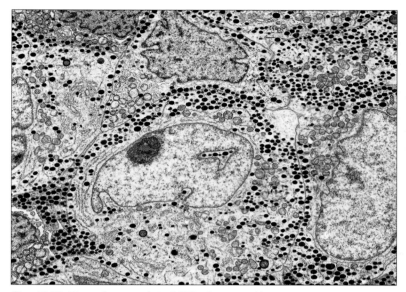

Fig. 44.20 Densely granulated GH adenoma. Numerous secretory granules of varying size are evident.

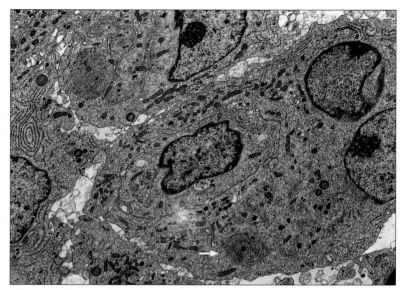

Fig. 44.21 Sparsely granulated GH adenoma. The fibrous body (arrow) is a consistent feature in this neoplasm which contains few secretory granules.

ULTRASTRUCTURAL EXAMINATION OF PITUITARY ADENOMAS

- Ultrastructural examination is most useful for further classification of GH-cell and combined PRL-cell plus GH-cell adenomas.
- Sparsely granulated GH-cell adenomas tend to be larger and more difficult to remove, grow more rapidly, and occur in younger patients than densely granulated GH-cell adenomas.
- Sparsely granulated GH-cell adenomas **(Fig. 44.21)** contain collections of intermediate filaments and smooth endoplasmic reticulum (fibrous bodies).
- Ultrastructural differences between prolactinomas do not signify differences in behavior.
- Ultrastructural examination is required for a definitive diagnosis of acidophil stem cell adenoma, which has poorly developed rough endoplasmic reticulum, giant mitochondria, fibrous bodies, inconspicuous Golgi apparatus, and few secretory granules.
- The mammosomatotroph adenoma, which like the acidophil stem cell adenoma comprises cells that immunolabel for both GH and PRL, contains abundant secretory granules.

Immunohistochemical profiles of neoplasms in the region of the pituitary fossa

	Pituitary adenoma	Metastatic carcinoma	Meningioma	Germinoma	Neuroblastoma	Malignant melanoma	Lymphoma	Chordoma	Glioma
Pituitary hormones	+/–	–	–	–	–	–	–	–	–
Cytokeratins	+	+	–/+ (a)	–/+	–	–	–	+/–	–
Epithelial membrane antigen	–	+/–	+/–	–	–	–	–/+ (b)	+	–
Vimentin	–	–/+	+	+/–	–	+	–/+	+	+
Carcinoembryonic antigen	–	–/+	– (a)	–	–	–	–	–/+	–
Leukocyte common antigen	–	–	–	–	–	–	+	–	–
S-100	–	– (c)	–/+	–	– (d)	+	–	+	+/–
HMB-45	–	– (c)	–	–	–	+	–	–	–
Neurofilament proteins	–	–	–	–	–/+	–	–	–	–
Synaptophysin	+	– (c)	–	–	+/–	–	–	–	–
GFAP	–	–	–	–	–	–	–	–	+/–
Placental alkaline phosphatase	– (c)	– (c)	–	+	–	–	–	–	–

+ Nearly always immunoreactive
– No immunoreactivity
+/– Majority of cases immunoreactive
–/+ Minority of cases immunoreactive
(a) Focal immunoreactivity in secretory meningiomas
(b) Immunoreactive in some anaplastic large cell lymphomas and lymphomas that show plasma cell differentiation
(c) Some immunoreactive examples recognized
(d) Immunoreactive sustentacular cells are present in some olfactory neuroblastomas

Fig. 44.22 Immunohistochemical profiles of neoplasms in the region of the pituitary fossa.

PITUITARY ADENOMAS

Pituitary adenomas must be distinguished from normal adenohypophysis, other neoplasms in the region of the pituitary fossa, and non-neoplastic masses in the region of the pituitary fossa.

Secretory cells in the adenohypophysis
- generally form a mixed population, though different cell types predominate in different regions (see Fig. 44.29).
- are arranged in nests surrounded by a network of reticulin (see Fig. 44.4).

Adenomas
- lose the normal pattern of nested cells.
- lack a honeycomb pattern of reticulin.
- usually contain cells with a higher than normal nuclear:cytoplasmic ratio.
- may contain mitotic figures.
- can sometimes be distinguished by a uniform pattern of immunolabeling with antibodies to pituitary peptides.

Other neoplasms in the region of the pituitary fossa
- These can generally be diagnosed by conventional histology.
- Immunohistochemistry may be helpful, especially for small biopsies (see Fig. 44.22).
- Metastases from primary neoplasms outside the CNS are found mainly in the neurohypophysis, but can present in the adenohypophysis where their identification may be difficult (**Figs 44.23–44.25**). It is important to distinguish carcinomas from native squamous cell nests (**Fig. 44.26**) that are present in approximately 30% of normal pituitaries in the pars tuberalis and hypophyseal stalk, do not disrupt the normal acinar reticulin pattern, are cytologically bland, without mitoses or pleomorphism, and often coexist with gonadotroph cells.

INFLAMMATORY DISEASES THAT MAY PRESENT AS A MASS LESION IN THE PITUITARY FOSSA

Lymphocytic hypophysitis (Fig. 44.27)
- occurs almost exclusively in women.
- usually occurs in pregnancy or the postpartum period.
- often presents with pituitary insufficiency.
- is characterized by a mixed infiltrate of inflammatory cells, mainly lymphocytes.

CNS sarcoidosis (see Chapter 16)
- is often associated with systemic sarcoidosis.
- preferentially affects structures in the suprasellar region.
- produces non-caseating, granulomatous inflammation with multinucleated giant cells.

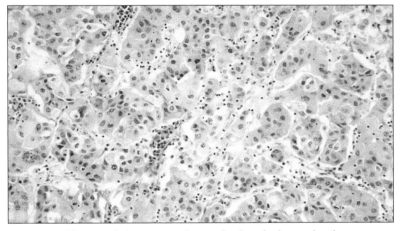

Fig. 44.23 Metastatic breast carcinoma in the pituitary gland.

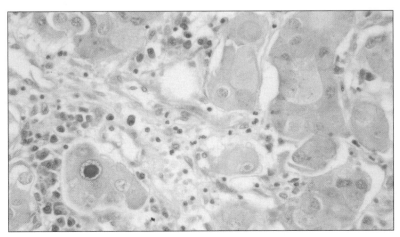

Fig. 44.24 Intracytoplasmic mucin in the metastatic breast carcinoma featured in Fig. 45.24. (Periodic acid–Schiff/Diastase+)

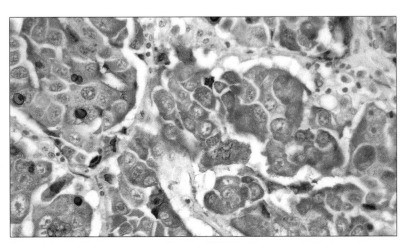

Fig. 44.25 Cells immunoreactive for EMA in the metastatic breast carcinoma featured in Fig. 45.24.

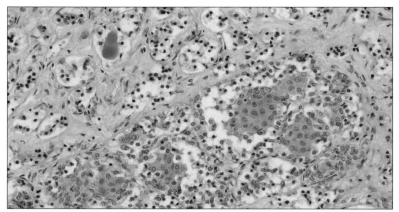

Fig. 44.26 Squamous cell nests in the pars tuberalis. This is a normal finding.

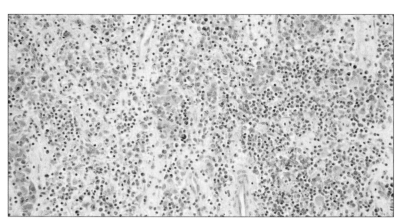

Fig. 44.27 Lymphocytic hypophysitis. Cells of the adenohypophysis are separated by an inflammatory infiltrate consisting mainly of lymphocytes.

PITUITARY HYPERPLASIA

Pituitary hyperplasia (**Figs 44.28**) may be nodular or diffuse. Nodular hyperplasia is characterized by enlarged cell nests and can be demonstrated in a reticulin preparation. Diffuse hyperplasia may not be obvious, requiring an appreciation of the uneven distribution of cells in the adenohypophysis (**Figs 44.29**) and cell counts to make the diagnosis.

Conditions associated with pituitary hyperplasia	
It is difficult to make a confident histologic diagnosis of pituitary hyperplasia which may occur in:	
Cells affected	**Associated conditions**
Lactotroph	Pregnancy, lactation, estrogen therapy
Corticotroph	Neoplasms producing CRH, Addison's disease
Thyrotroph	Chronic primary hypothyroidism
Somatotroph	Neoplasms producing GH-releasing hormone
Gonadotroph	Klinefelter's syndrome
In some cases the stimulus for hyperplasia remains obscure.	

Fig. 44.28 Conditions associated with pituitary hyperplasia.

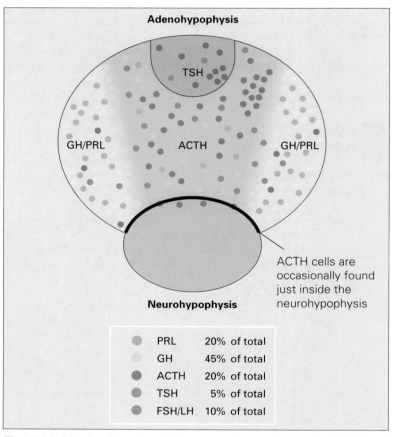

Fig. 44.29 Distribution of peptide-containing cells in the adenohypophysis.

CRANIOPHARYNGIOMAS

Craniopharyngiomas are slow-growing epithelial neoplasms in the suprasellar region and there are two variants:
- Adamantinomatous.
- Papillary.

These variants have both common and differentiating histopathologic features. Transitional forms exist, but attempts should be made to distinguish the two main variants, which have different outcomes: papillary neoplasms are more readily resected and recur less often.

The histogenesis of craniopharyngiomas is not established. Adamantinomatous neoplasms closely resemble the adamantinoma of the jaw and the calcifying odontogenic cyst. Papillary neoplasms may be related to Rathke's cleft cyst, which can show marked squamous metaplasia.

MACROSCOPIC APPEARANCES

An admixture of cystic and solid components is characteristic (**Figs 44.30–44.32**), and there is sometimes a smooth lobulated capsule. The solid tissue often contains foci of calcification and the cysts may contain a thick liquid that has been likened to machine oil. The papillary craniopharyngioma tends to be uncalcified and more circumscribed than the adamantinomatous type.

MICROSCOPIC APPEARANCES

Features of the adamantinomatous craniopharyngioma (**Figs 44.33–44.36**) include:
- Groups of squamous cells, often surrounded by a peripheral palisade of columnar cells.
- Intercellular accumulations of fluid that separate the cells in some parts of the neoplasm.
- Cohesive clusters or sheets of keratinized anuclear 'ghost' cells.
- Calcification, which may progress to metaplastic bone formation.
- Cholesterol clefts, which are often related to necrotic debris within the cysts.

Papillary craniopharyngiomas (**Fig 44.37**) consist of groups of squamous cells, which may form keratin pearls. Cysts are infrequent and an adamantinomatous pattern is absent. There are no nodules of keratinized 'ghost' cells and calcification is rare.

The surrounding brain parenchyma is usually densely gliotic (**Fig. 44.38**) and may contain many Rosenthal fibers. Leakage of cyst contents may provoke an inflammatory reaction, which includes multinucleated giant cells. (see **Fig. 44.36**)

CRANIOPHARYNGIOMAS

- account for approximately 2% of all intracranial neoplasms and 5–10% of childhood intracranial neoplasms.
- show a peak incidence in children aged 5–10 years, but also occur in adults.
- tend to be adamantinomatous when they occur in a child and adamantinomatous or papillary when they occur in an adult.
- present with symptoms and signs due to increased intracranial pressure, compression of the optic pathways (causing visual dysfunction), and compression of the hypothalamus or pituitary (leading to endocrine dysfunction).

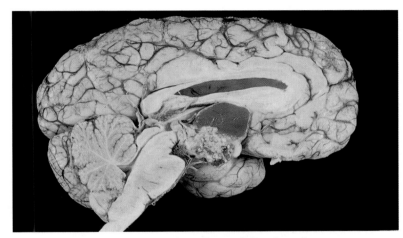

Fig. 44.30 This craniopharyngioma has solid and cystic components, and disrupts the diencephalon.

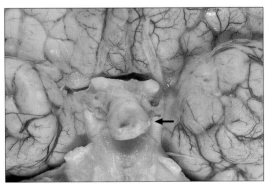

Fig. 44.31 A craniopharyngioma (arrow) bulging from the tuber cinereum.

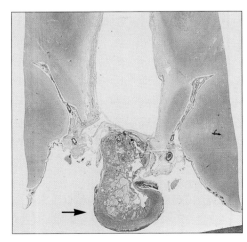

Fig. 44.32 Histology of the craniopharyngioma shown in Fig. 45.31 (arrow). (Hematoxylin and van Gieson)

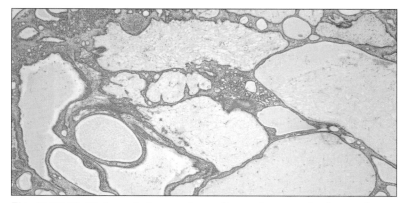

Fig. 44.33 Multiple cysts in an adamantinomatous craniopharyngioma.

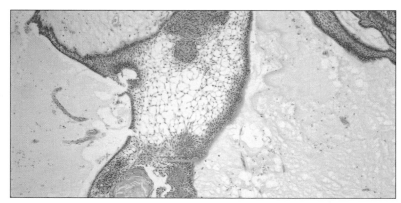

Fig. 44.34 Adamantinomatous craniopharyngioma. A loose matrix (stellate reticulum) is due to intercellular fluid accumulation.

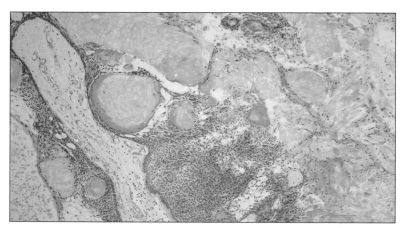

Fig. 44.35 Adamantinomatous craniopharyngioma. Sheets and nodules of keratinized 'ghost' cells are evident.

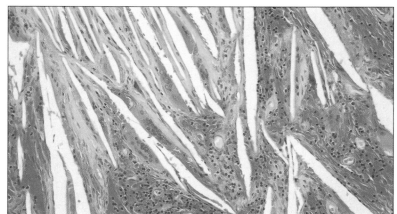

Fig. 44.36 Multinucleated giant cells surround cholesterol clefts in a craniopharyngioma.

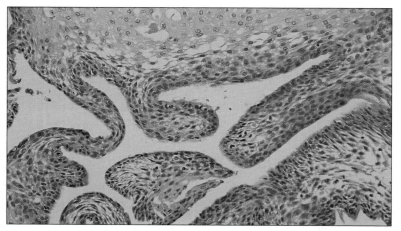

Fig. 44.37 Papillary craniopharyngioma.

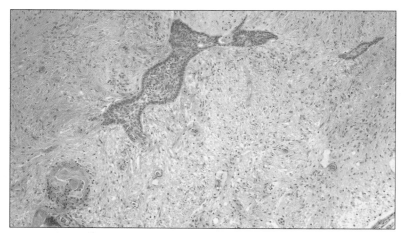

Fig. 44.38 Craniopharyngiomas elicit a gliotic reaction in surrounding tissues.

RATHKE CLEFT CYST

Small cysts lined by cuboidal epithelium in the pars intermedia of the pituitary gland are remnants of Rathke's pouch and can enlarge to produce a Rathke cleft cyst. This may be an incidental postmortem finding, but can produce endocrine or visual abnormalities if large enough.

MACROSCOPIC AND MICROSCOPIC APPEARANCES

Rathke cleft cysts usually have a thin wall and mucinous contents. The cyst is lined by cuboidal or columnar epithelium, which may be ciliated (**Fig. 44.39**). Peptide-containing cells may be found in the epithelium, and there may be squamous metaplasia and some goblet cells. Squamous metaplasia can produce a similar histologic picture to that of the papillary craniopharyngioma. Microscopic cysts with a similar appearance are occasionally found in pituitary adenomas.

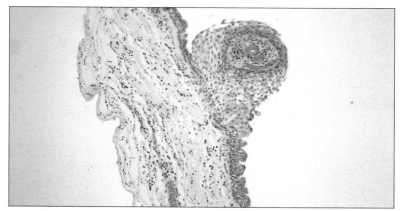

Fig. 44.39 Rathke's cleft cyst. The cyst is lined by a simple columnar epithelium which is cross-cut in places.

GRANULAR CELL NEOPLASM OF THE INFUNDIBULUM

Granular cells in the infundibulum or neurohypophysis are thought to be of glial origin. Symptomatic neoplasms of these cells are rare. Asymptomatic tiny groups of granular cells in this region, sometimes called choristomas, are more common.

MACROSCOPIC AND MICROSCOPIC APPEARANCES

A granular cell neoplasm of the infundibulum is a well-circumscribed, soft, homogeneous neoplasm that may straddle the diaphragma sellae. Choristomas and granular cell neoplasms share cytologic features (**Fig. 44.40**). Their oval cells contain finely granular, eosinophilic, strongly PAS-positive cytoplasm. In larger neoplasms the cells may be arranged in fascicles. There is little nuclear pleomorphism and mitotic figures are not found.

CRANIOPHARYNGIOMA

The craniopharyngioma must be distinguished from several cystic suprasellar lasions: epidermoid and dermoid cysts (chapter 45), pilocytic astrocytomas (chapter 35), and the Rathke's cleft cyst.

Epidermoid and dermoid cysts

- The epidermoid cyst is characterized by an epithelium containing prominent keratohyalin granules and an orderly maturation of squamous cells with formation of keratin flakes.
- The dermoid cyst is rare in the region of the pituitary fossa and contains dermal adnexal structures.

Pilocytic astrocytoma

- Florid reactive astrocytosis and Rosenthal fibers in a biopsy taken adjacent to rather than within a craniopharyngioma may simulate a pilocytic astrocytoma.
- Cholesterol clefts or giant cells suggest a craniopharyngioma.
- Microcystic areas, loosely arranged astrocytic cells, and degenerative, atypical nuclear features support the diagnosis of pilocytic astrocytoma.

Rathke's cleft cyst

- Prominent squamous metaplasia in the epithelium of these cysts may mimic the squamous nests in papillary craniopharyngiomas.
- The radiologic and operative findings may help because papillary craniopharyngiomas are rarely cystic.

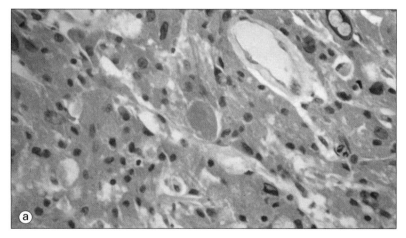

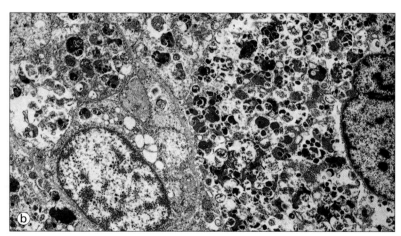

Fig. 44.40 Granular cell neoplasm. (a) Cytoplasmic granularity and small nuclei characterize the histology of this neoplasm. **(b)** Electron microscopy reveals abundant lysosomes.

REFERENCES

Burger PC, Scheithauer BW, Vogel FS (1991) Region of the sella turcica. In *Surgical Pathology of the Nervous System and its Coverings.* pp. 503–568. Edinburgh: Churchill Livingstone.

Horvath E (1994) Ultrastructural markers in the pathologic diagnosis of pituitary adenomas. *Ultrastructural Pathology* 18:171–179.

Horvath E, Scheithauer BW, Kovacs K. Lloyd RV. (1997) Regional neuropathology: hypothalamus and pituitary. In *Greenfield's Neuropathology* (Sixth edition) vol. 1. Eds Graham DI and Lantos PL. p. 1007–1094. Arnold: London.

Kovacs K, Horvath E (1986) *Tumors of the Pituitary Gland. Second edition.* Washington: Armed Forces Institute of Pathology. (Atlas of Tumor Pathology vol. 21).

Lloyd RV, Scheithauer BW, Kovacs K, Roche PC (1996). The immunophenotype of pituitary adenomas. *Endocrine Pathology* 7:145-150.

Spada A, Vallar L, Faglia G (1994) Cellular alterations in pituitary tumors. *Eur J Endocrinol* 130(1): 43–52.

Thapar K, Horvath E, Kovacs K, Muller PJ (1992) Pituitary adenomas: recent advances in classification, histopathology, and molecular biology. *Diagn Oncol* 2: 145–167.

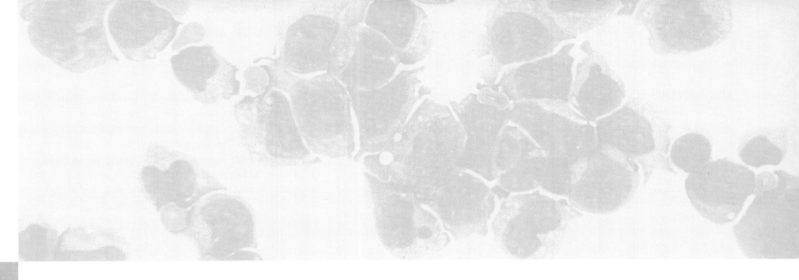

45 *Miscellaneous CNS neoplasms and cysts*

Neoplasms in this diverse group and covered in this chapter are:
- mesenchymal non-meningothelial neoplasms
- primary melanocytic neoplasms
- hemangioblastoma
- heterogeneous cysts and neoplasm-like entities

MESENCHYMAL NON-MENINGOTHELIAL NEOPLASMS

This group includes benign and malignant neoplasms, many of which are located in the meninges. Those discussed below are osteocartilaginous neoplasms of the meninges, lipoma, hemangiopericytoma, sarcoma, and the sarcoma variant, meningeal sarcomatosis.

OSTEOCARTILAGINOUS NEOPLASMS OF THE MENINGES

Benign osteocartilaginous neoplasms of the meninges are rarely encountered, unlike ossification of the parasagittal meninges, which is a common incidental postmortem finding. Discrete bony nodules composed of osteocytes are very rare and may contain cartilage (osteochondroma). Chondromas of the meninges usually present as a nodular mass over the cerebral convexities and are composed of well-differentiated chondrocytes.

LIPOMA

CNS lipomas are rare. They occur preferentially in the anterior part of the corpus callosum (usually in association with its partial agenesis – see chapter 3), over the quadrigeminal plate, in the cerebellopontine angle, at the base of the brain, and in the spinal cord. Lipomas of the lumbosacral cord are sometimes associated with neural tube defects.

MACROSCOPIC AND MICROSCOPIC APPEARANCES

Lipomas are soft yellow masses (**Figs 45.1, 45.2**) and usually encroach upon adjacent structures. They are composed of mature lipocytes, but rarely they contain other ectopic tissues such as striated muscle and cartilage. Spinal examples may be poorly circumscribed and occasionally have prominent blood vessels (angiolipoma).

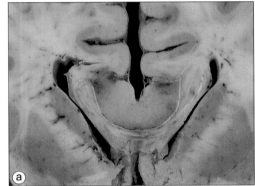
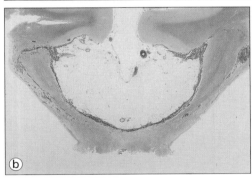

Fig. 45.1 Lipoma of the corpus callosum. (a) A mass of adipose tissue lies above the callosum. **(b)** Histology of the lipoma in (a), showing mature adipocytes. Note the thinning and typical distortion of the ventral part of the corpus callosum. (Phosphotungstic acid–hematoxylin)

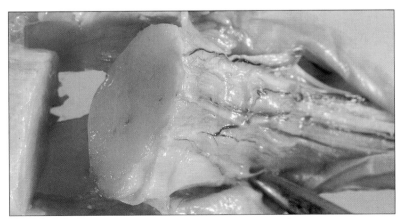

Fig. 45.2 Lipoma of the spinal cord. Diffuse enlargement and yellow discoloration of the spinal cord are evident.

HEMANGIOPERICYTOMA

CNS hemangiopericytomas occur mainly in the intracranial meninges and were once regarded as an angioblastic variant of meningioma. However, they share the histologic features of hemangiopericytomas outside the nervous system and do not have the genetic abnormalities characteristic of meningiomas such as NF2 gene mutations. Unlike meningiomas, hemangiopericytomas show no clear predilection for either sex. They occur in a younger age group than meningiomas, and have a tendency to recurrence and late metastasis.

MACROSCOPIC AND MICROSCOPIC APPEARANCES

Hemangiopericytomas are usually spherical and discrete, but may invade the skull. They have a firm and homogeneous texture. Microscopically, many hemangiopericytomas are characterized by a uniform histologic appearance (**Fig. 45.3**) with a sheet-like arrangement of cells having a high nuclear:cytoplasmic ratio. The cells are interspersed with many tiny capillaries, and a few larger, slightly gaping, vascular channels that may have a branching appearance. Other characteristics include focal lobularity, paucicellular areas, and dense pericellular reticulin. Diffuse fibrosis is sometimes seen. Mitoses are readily found, but foci of necrosis are uncommon. Cytologic pleomorphism and a high mitotic count are usually associated with rapid growth and aggressive behavior.

Immunohistochemistry reveals reactivity for vimentin, but no labeling with antibodies to epithelial membrane antigen which can help in distinguishing these neoplasms from meningiomas. Antibodies to markers of vascular endothelium such as factor VIII and *Ulex europaeus* lectin label only the endothelium of the vascular channels. CD34 antibodies label some of the neoplastic cells.

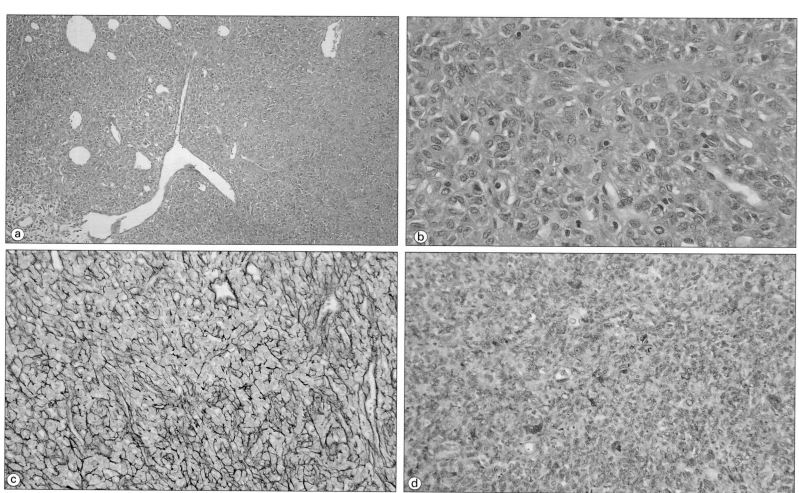

Fig. 45.3 Hemangiopericytoma. (a) This is characterized at low magnification by a sheet of neoplastic cells interspersed with dilated blood vessels. One of the blood vessels in this field has a typical 'stag horn' shape. **(b)** At higher magnification, smaller vascular channels can be discerned between the closely packed cells, which have oval or asymmetrically tapered nuclei and a high nuclear:cytoplasmic ratio. Mitoses are evident.

(c) Hemangiopericytomas have a dense reticulin pattern and this feature helps to distinguish them from meningiomas. **(d)** Cytologic pleomorphism and a high mitotic count are shown by some hemangiopericytomas and are usually associated with rapid growth and particularly aggressive behavior.

SARCOMAS

Primary sarcomas of the CNS are rare, though angiosarcoma, fibrosarcoma, malignant fibrous histiocytoma, and unclassifiable sarcomas have all been described. Chondrosarcomas and osteosarcomas arising in the skeleton around the CNS may cause neurologic problems (see p 46.1). Many sarcomas are associated with previous radiotherapy, usually 10–15 years earlier.

MACROSCOPIC AND MICROSCOPIC APPEARANCES

Sarcomas are generally composed of anaplastic spindle-shaped cells (**Fig. 45.4**). There are usually abundant mitoses and foci of necrosis. Individual histologic characteristics sometimes allow subclassification:
- A vasoformative pattern is seen in angiosarcomas.
- Fascicles arranged in a 'herring-bone' pattern are typical of fibrosarcomas.

Immunohistochemistry and electron microscopy may also identify patterns of differentiation.

Many sarcomas are based in the meninges. The term meningeal sarcomatosis is used when neoplastic cells infiltrate widely in the meninges. This process usually occurs in children and young adults.

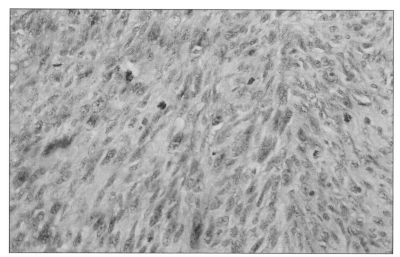

Fig. 45.4 Meningeal sarcoma. Pleomorphic spindle-shaped cells and many mitoses are seen.

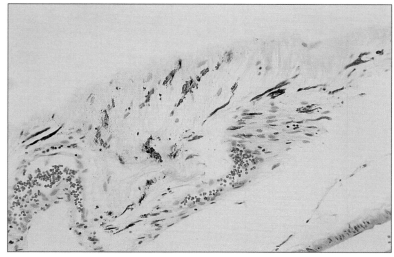

Fig. 45.5 Meningeal melanocytes.

MELANOCYTIC NEOPLASMS

Melanocytes are normally present in the leptomeninges (**Fig. 45.5**) and give rise to various lesions recognized by the World Health Organization (WHO) classification of CNS neoplasms. These are:
- diffuse melanosis
- melanocytoma
- malignant melanoma and its variant, malignant melanomatosis

Metastatic malignant melanomas greatly outnumber primary melanocytic neoplasms.

Diffuse proliferations of leptomeningeal melanocytes may be associated with large cutaneous nevi and a predisposition to malignant melanoma. This is known as neurocutaneous melanosis (Touraine syndrome), which is an autosomal dominant condition.

Melanin also occurs in a variety of CNS neoplasms, including schwannomas, ependymomas, embryonal neoplasms, and some pineal neoplasms.

MACROSCOPIC AND MICROSCOPIC APPEARANCES

Primary melanocytic neoplasms may be diffuse or nodular. Diffuse melanosis appears as discoloration of the leptomeninges. However, widespread involvement of the meninges in this way may be part of a malignant process that is also characterized by meningeal thickening, discontinuous spread, and invasion of underlying brain. Nodular neoplasms are most commonly sited in the posterior fossa, but may occur in any part of the neuraxis. Melanocytomas tend to be intraspinal.

Diffuse melanosis and melanocytoma are characterized by a nest-like pattern of oval cells or uniform spindle-shaped cells. Mitoses are not found. Melanin may be abundant.

Obvious malignant melanomas (**Fig. 45.6**) show cytologic atypia, an increased mitotic count, and necrosis, and invade adjacent structures. Neoplasms showing intermediate histology between those of melanocytoma and malignant melanoma may be difficult to classify.

Melanocytic neoplasms are immunoreactive for vimentin, and most label with S-100 and HMB-45 antibodies. Ultrastructural examination reveals melanosomes. A pericellular basal lamina is lacking, and melanocytic neoplasms can therefore be distinguished from melanotic schwannomas.

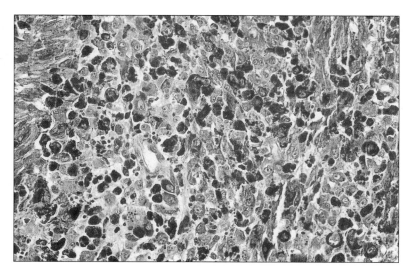

Fig. 45.6 Meningeal malignant melanoma. Many of the pleomorphic neoplastic cells contain melanin. This was a primary meningeal neoplasm; survival after diagnosis was 7 months.

HEMANGIOBLASTOMA

The hemangioblastoma is a neoplasm of uncertain histogenesis that is associated with von Hippel–Lindau syndrome (VHL). It has a predilection for the posterior fossa, but may also involve the brain stem and spinal cord. Rare supratentorial examples are usually attached to the dura, and these neoplasms have occasionally been grouped with hemangiopericytomas and termed 'angioblastic meningiomas'. However, although microcystic meningiomas may resemble hemangioblastomas, there is no evidence that hemangioblastomas and meningiomas are related histogenetically.

MACROSCOPIC APPEARANCES

Cerebellar hemangioblastomas frequently present as cysts with a mural nodule (**Fig. 45.7**), and their vascular nature imparts a red color to the nodule. The mural nodule is composed of clusters of neoplastic cells and may be minute. Surgical specimens of cyst wall should be examined carefully for neoplastic cells.

Other hemangioblastomas are globular. The discrete nature of most of these neoplasms facilitates complete resection, though some hemangioblastomas recur even when surgery appears to have been successful.

HEMANGIOBLASTOMAS

- account for approximately 2% of intracranial neoplasms
- account for approximately 7% of posterior fossa neoplasms
- usually present in patients aged 20–40 years
- are slightly more common in males
- are usually sited in a cerebellar hemisphere but can occur in the brain stem, spinal cord or rarely in the cerebrum
- may be multiple
- when in the posterior fossa, usually present with hydrocephalus
- when in the spinal cord, may cause syringomyelia
- cause polycythemia in 10% of cases as a result of inappropriate production of erythropoietin
- are associated with von Hippel–Lindau syndrome

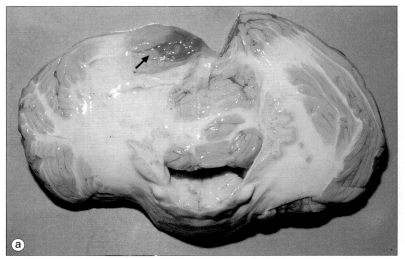

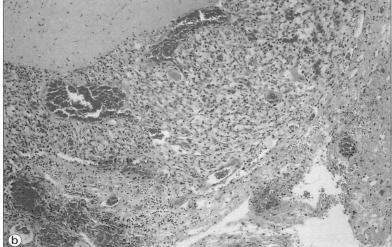

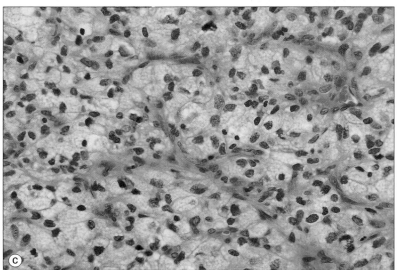

Fig. 45.7 Hemangioblastoma. (a) A red nodule is present on the superomedial aspect of the cerebellar hemisphere (arrow). (Courtesy of Dr. T Revesz, Institute of Neurology, London) **(b)** This histologic field shows a vascular neoplasm abutting brain tissue. **(c)** Lipid-containing interstitial cells dominate the histology of this hemangioblastoma.

MICROSCOPIC APPEARANCES

Hemangioblastomas comprise two cell populations which are combined in varying proportions (see Fig. 45.7):

- One population consists of endothelial cells and pericytes, which form a dense network of small vascular channels.
- The other population consists of interstitial cells, which contain lipid and variable amounts of glycogen and which often show nuclear pleomorphism and hyperchromasia.

Mitoses are uncommon. Mast cells may be present.

Hemangioblastomas are associated with marked reactive changes in the surrounding brain. Reactive astrocytosis and Rosenthal fiber formation are evident in the cyst wall and may divert the pathologist into considering a diagnosis of pilocytic astrocytoma.

Immunohistochemistry does not reveal the origin of the interstitial cells, which fail to label with antibodies to either vascular or epithelial markers. Ultrastructural examination has also failed to identify distinctive cytologic features that would establish a specific histogenesis.

VON HIPPEL–LINDAU SYNDROME (VHL)

- VHL is an autosomal dominant disorder with approximately 90% penetrance.
- The VHL gene is on chromosome 3p and is probably a tumor suppressor gene.
- One or more of: CNS hemangioblastoma, retinal angioma, renal cysts, renal cell carcinoma, pancreatic cysts, pheochromocytoma, or epididymal cystadenoma, may occur in affected members of a family with VHL.
- Minimal diagnostic criteria are: retinal angioma or CNS hemangioblastoma, plus one VHL abnormality in an immediate family member.
- Families may be grouped according to whether pheochromocytomas are present or absent.
- Nearly all families with pheochromocytomas have missense mutations of the VHL gene.
- ~20% of pheochromocytomas are associated with VHL.

RENAL CELL CARCINOMA AND HEMANGIOBLASTOMA

- It may be difficult to distinguish hemangioblastoma from metastatic renal cell carcinoma, which may also be a feature of VHL.
- Renal cell carcinoma may be confirmed by imaging the kidneys and is generally immunoreactive for cytokeratins and epithelial membrane antigen.

CYSTS

Benign cysts occur at several sites in and around the CNS (**Fig. 45.8**) and the cysts considered in this chapter are: epidermoid and dermoid cysts, colloid cyst of the third ventricle, enterogenous cyst, ependymal cyst, and arachnoid cyst.

EPIDERMOID AND DERMOID CYSTS

Epidermoid cysts are mainly intracranial. The cerebellopontine angle, parasellar region, and cranial diploë are common sites. Intraspinal examples are uncommon accounting for only 5% of cases.

Dermoid cysts are less common than epidermoid cysts (1:4). They are midline cysts, usually occurring in the region of the fontanelle, fourth ventricle, or cauda equina.

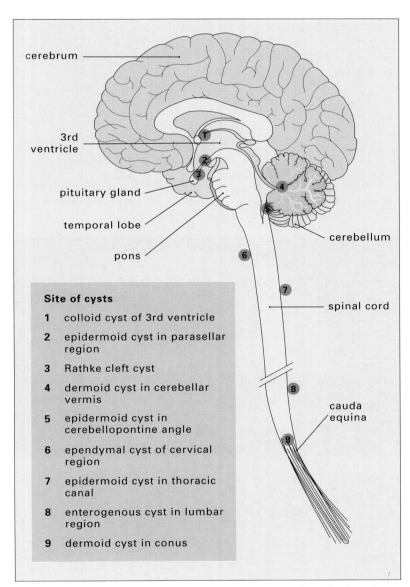

Site of cysts

1. colloid cyst of 3rd ventricle
2. epidermoid cyst in parasellar region
3. Rathke cleft cyst
4. dermoid cyst in cerebellar vermis
5. epidermoid cyst in cerebellopontine angle
6. ependymal cyst of cervical region
7. epidermoid cyst in thoracic canal
8. enterogenous cyst in lumbar region
9. dermoid cyst in conus

Fig. 45.8 Cysts around the midline of the brain and the spinal cord.

MACROSCOPIC APPEARANCES

Epidermoid cysts have a smooth gray surface and friable waxy material inside. They usually envelop adjacent structures. In contrast, dermoid cysts are usually well demarcated from surrounding structures. A smooth wall encases soft, greasy material, which may contain hairs.

MICROSCOPIC APPEARANCES

Both epidermoid (**Fig. 45.9**)and dermoid (**Fig. 45.10**) cysts are lined by stratified squamous epithelium. The central eosinophilic material is formed from degenerate keratinocytes plus secretions from sebaceous glands in the case of the dermoid cyst. The dermoid cyst is distinguished by the presence of adnexal appendages such as sebaceous glands and hair follicles.

COLLOID CYST OF THE THIRD VENTRICLE

The origin of this cyst is unknown; however, the colloid cyst shares an immunohistochemical profile with cysts that show endodermal differentiation (enterogenous cyst). It is considered to be congenital, but usually presents in people aged 20–50 years.

Colloid cyst of the third ventricle is a cause of recurrent headache because it intermittently obstructs the flow of CSF at the level of the foramen of Monro. It occasionally causes sudden death if the obstruction does not resolve spontaneously.

MACROSCOPIC AND MICROSCOPIC APPEARANCES

Nearly all colloid cysts are found in the anterior part of the third ventricle (**Fig. 45.11**), though some examples are located in the posterior part of

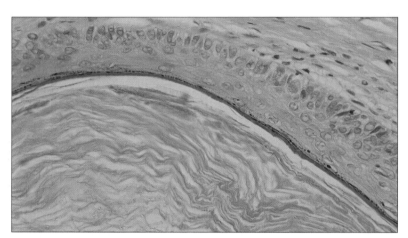

Fig. 45.9 Epidermoid cyst. Maturing and keratinizing squamous epithelium lines this epidermoid cyst. Note the granular cell layer.

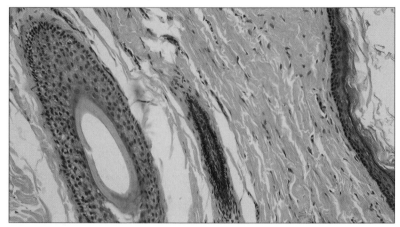

Fig. 45.10 Dermoid cyst. Beneath the squamous epithelium is a hair folicle. Unlike epidermoid cysts, dermoid cysts contain adnexal structures.

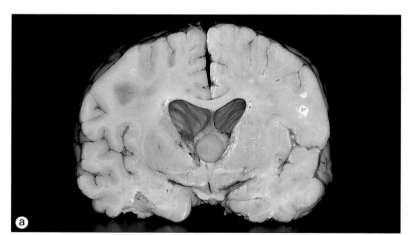

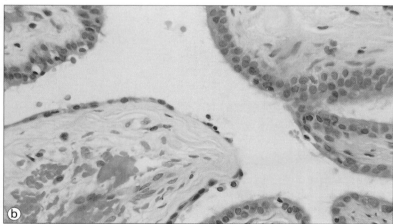

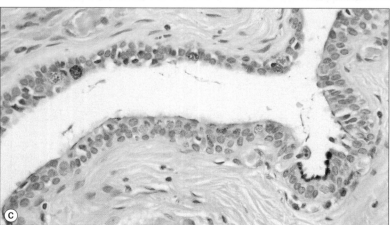

Fig. 45.11 Colloid cyst. (a) Colloid cyst of the third ventricle producing enlarged lateral ventricles (hydrocephalus). **(b)** The simple epithelium of a colloid cyst. **(c)** There are mucin-containing goblet cells in the epithelium of this colloid cyst. (Periodic acid–schiff–diastase)

the third ventricle and rare examples have been reported in the lateral and fourth ventricles. They are usually lined by a single layer of columnar cells, some of which are ciliated or contain mucin (see Fig. 45.10c).

ENTEROGENOUS CYST

This rare cyst has also been called a neurenteric, epithelial-lined, respiratory, or endodermal cyst. Most are intradural, extramedullary, intraspinal cysts, though very rare examples are intracranial. Some intraspinal examples are associated with developmental abnormalities, for example bony defects in the vertebrae and duplications in the gastrointestinal tract.

MACROSCOPIC AND MICROSCOPIC APPEARANCES

Endodermal cysts are simple fluid-filled sacs. Their thin walls are lined by a columnar or cuboidal epithelium (**Fig. 45.12**) which covers a connective tissue stroma. Goblet cells are readily found, but ciliation is a variable feature. Squamous metaplasia is sometimes seen.

EPENDYMAL CYST

This neuroglial cyst may be intraparenchymal, intraventricular, or leptomeningeal. The columnar epithelium which resembles ependyma may be ciliated, but does not contain goblet cells, and shows focal immunoreactivity for GFAP. A thin basement membrane can usually be demonstrated.

ARACHNOID CYST

Arachnoid cysts occur in the intracranial and intraspinal leptomeninges, particularly in the region of the temporal operculum. Other sites include the cerebellopontine angle, quadrigeminal region, and cisterna magna. Entrapment of CSF within the cyst occasionally causes symptoms of a mass lesion.

MACROSCOPIC AND MICROSCOPIC APPEARANCES

Arachnoid cysts are lined by a layer of meningothelial cells (**Fig. 45.13**). They may be multilocular. The meningothelial cells are neither ciliated nor immunoreactive for GFAP.

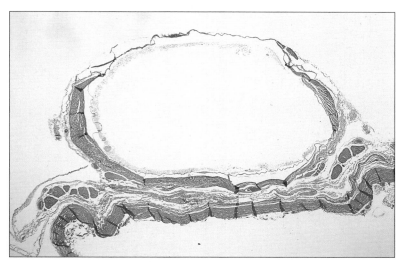

Fig. 45.12 Enterogenous cyst. This enterogenous cyst displaced and compressed the spinal cord at T11.

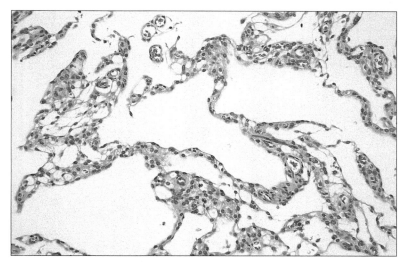

Fig. 45.13 Multilocular arachnoid cyst.

REFERENCES

Budka H. (1974) Intracranial lipomatous hamartomas (intracranial "lipomas"). *Acta Neuropathalogica* **28**:205–222.

Burger PC, Scheithauer BW. (1994) Benign cystic lesions. In *Tumors of the Central Nervous System. Third edition*. pp. 355–370. Bethesda: Armed Forces Institute of Pathology. (J Rosai (ed.) *Atlas of Tumour Pathology. Volume 10*).

Friede RL, Yasargil MG. (1977) Supratentorial intracerebral epithelial (ependymal) cysts: review, case reports, and fine structures. *J. Neurol. Neurosurg. Psychiat.* **40**: 127–137.

Inoue T, Matsushima T, Fukui M, Iwaki T, Takeshita I, Kuromatsu C. (1988) Immunohistochemical study of intracranial cysts. *Neurosurgery* **23**: 576–581.

Joseph JT *et al*. (1995) NF2 gene analysis distinguishes hemangiopeicytoma from meningioma. *American Journal of Pathology* **147**:1450–1455.

Lach B, Scheithauer BW, Gregor A, Wick MR. (1993) Colloid cysts of the third ventricle. A comparative immunohistochemical study of neuraxis cysts and choroid plexus epithelium. *J. Neurosurg.* **78**: 101–111.

Lantos PL, VandenBerg SR, Kleihues P. (1997) Cysts and tumor-like conditions. In *Greenfield's Neuropathology* (Sixth edition). Eds Graham DI and Lantos PL. p. 780–787. Arnold: London.

Netsky MG. (1988) Epidermoid tumors. Review of the literature. *Surg. Neurol.* **29**: 477–483.

Neumann HP, Lips CJ, Hsia YE, Zbar B. (1995) Von Hippel–Lindau syndrome. *Brain Pathology* **5**: 181–193.

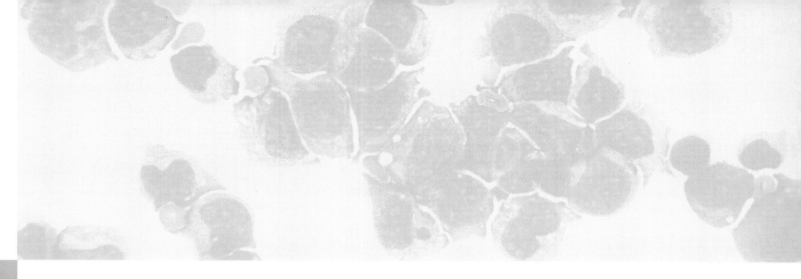

46 *Neoplasms that spread to the CNS*

Primary neoplasms of the skull and spine may impinge upon the CNS, and (primary) neoplasms in other organs may metastasize to the CNS, its coverings, or its bony surroundings (**Fig. 46.1**). In this chapter, neoplasms that spread to the CNS will be illustrated in three categories:

- Neoplasms within osteocartilaginous tissues surrounding the CNS.
- Secondary meningeal neoplasms.
- Secondary neoplasms in the brain and spinal cord.

Neoplasms that spread to the CNS, particularly intracerebral and intravertebral metastases, are common. Their reported incidence varies widely, and reflects whether authors have surveyed necropsy data or clinicopathologic data from centers that deal with different aspects of patient care (neurosurgery, radiotherapy, hospice care). The frequency of secondary CNS neoplasms also varies widely with the site of primary neoplasm (**Fig. 46.2**).

SECONDARY CNS NEOPLASMS

- account for approximately 15% of intracranial neoplasms (in neurosurgical centres).
- are present in approximately 30% of patients with disseminated cancer.
- present most frequently in the sixth and seventh decades.
- are solitary in approximately 50% of patients.
- are derived most commonly (40% of patients) from primary neoplasms in the lung.
- present before the primary neoplasm in approximately 15% of patients.

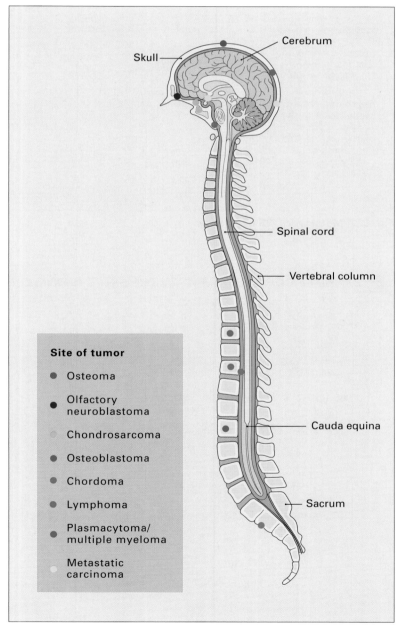

Site of tumor

- Osteoma
- Olfactory neuroblastoma
- Chondrosarcoma
- Osteoblastoma
- Chordoma
- Lymphoma
- Plasmacytoma/ multiple myeloma
- Metastatic carcinoma

Fig. 46.1 Neoplasms encountered by the pathologist in the skull and spine

NEOPLASMS IN TISSUES SURROUNDING THE CNS

Primary and secondary neoplasms of the skull and spine produce symptoms and signs by destroying bone and compressing nervous system structures, either elements of the CNS or proximal cranial and spinal nerves. Similar problems are caused on rare occasions when mediastinal and retroperitoneal neoplasms invade the extradural space around the spinal cord.

Secondary carcinoma is the commonest neoplasm to impinge upon the CNS from surrounding structures, but other types of neoplasm at these sites behave similarly. Diagnosis is facilitated by consideration of the patient's past medical history, assessment of hematologic indices, and a range of imaging studies, in conjunction with histologic examination of biopsies (**Figs 46.3–46.16**).

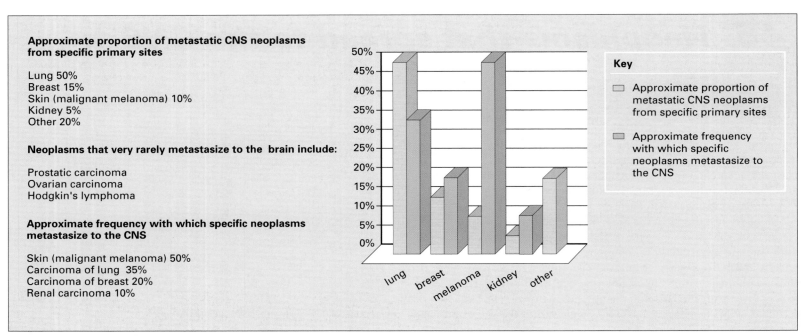

Approximate proportion of metastatic CNS neoplasms from specific primary sites

Lung 50%
Breast 15%
Skin (malignant melanoma) 10%
Kidney 5%
Other 20%

Neoplasms that very rarely metastasize to the brain include:

Prostatic carcinoma
Ovarian carcinoma
Hodgkin's lymphoma

Approximate frequency with which specific neoplasms metastasize to the CNS

Skin (malignant melanoma) 50%
Carcinoma of lung 35%
Carcinoma of breast 20%
Renal carcinoma 10%

Key

☐ Approximate proportion of metastatic CNS neoplasms from specific primary sites

☐ Approximate frequency with which specific neoplasms metastasize to the CNS

Fig. 46.2 Metastatic CNS neoplasms.

EXAMPLES OF NEOPLASMS IN THE SKULL, SPINE, OR EPIDURAL SPACE THAT MAY INVOLVE THE CNS

- Secondary (metastatic)
  Carcinoma
  Sarcoma
  Malignant melanoma

- Hodgkin's and non-Hodgkin's lymphoma

- Plasmacytoma (plasmacytic lymphoma)/multiple myeloma

- Chordoma

- Paraganglioma (glomus jugulare)

- Osteoblastoma

- Osteosarcoma (with or without Paget's disease)

- Chondrosarcoma

- Giant cell neoplasm of bone

- Langerhans' cell histiocytosis

- Olfactory neuroblastoma

- Ewing's tumor

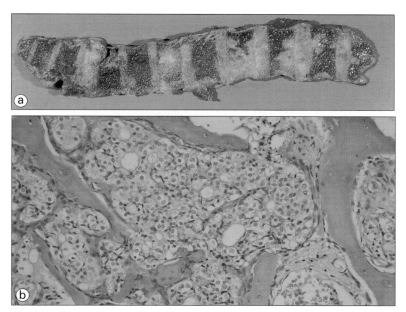

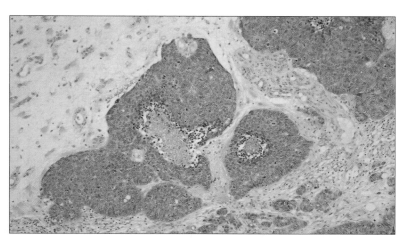

Fig. 46.4 Part of a carcinoma of the ethmoid sinus that had invaded the anterior fossa. These groups of undifferentiated cells contain areas of necrosis.

Fig. 46.3 Metastatic carcinoma in the spine. (a) Multiple deposits of metastic carcinoma are present in the vertebrae. **(b)** This shows a vertebral deposit of adenocarcinoma from a primary neoplasm in the prostate gland that presented with cord compression. An acinar structure is evident. Common secondary carcinomas in the spine are from primary sites in the breast, lung, and prostate gland. Prostatic carcinoma that has metastasized to bone is commonly osteoblastic, in contrast to metastases from other carcinomas, which tend to be osteolytic.

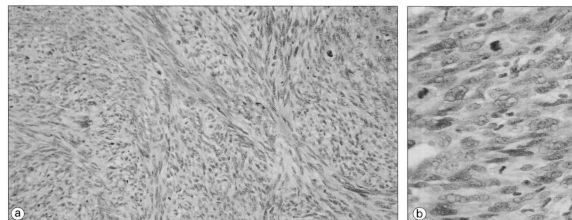

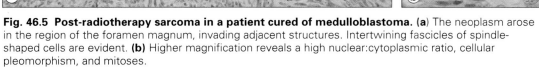

Fig. 46.5 Post-radiotherapy sarcoma in a patient cured of medulloblastoma. (a) The neoplasm arose in the region of the foramen magnum, invading adjacent structures. Intertwining fascicles of spindle-shaped cells are evident. **(b)** Higher magnification reveals a high nuclear:cytoplasmic ratio, cellular pleomorphism, and mitoses.

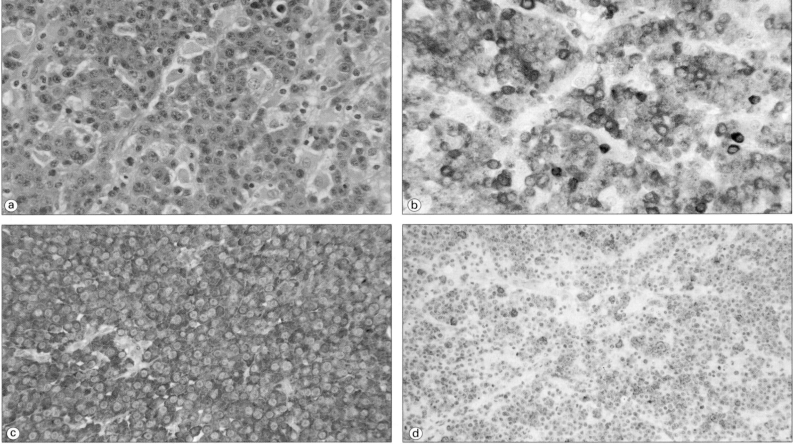

Fig. 46.6 Plasmacytic lymphoma (plasmacytoma). (a) This lymphoreticular neoplasm shows plasma cell differentiation and was a solitary lesion in the spine, causing local pain and compression of CNS structures. About 50% of solitary osseous plasmacytic lymphomas progress to multiple myeloma, which is the commonest primary neoplasm within bone to cause CNS symptoms. **(b)** This plasmacytic lymphoma labelled with an antibody to CD79a, a pan-B cell marker. **(c)** Light chain restriction can sometimes be demonstrated in plasmacytic lymphoma/multiple myeloma by immunohistochemistry. In this case, cells labelled with a λ antibody (as shown here), but not a κ antibody. **(d)** Plasmacytic lymphoma may rarely react with antibodies to epithelial membrane antigen (as shown here), leading potentially to an erroneous diagnosis of metastatic carcinoma. Normal plasma cells are immunoreactive for EMA. CD79a antibodies are helpful in this situation because they should not label carcinomas.

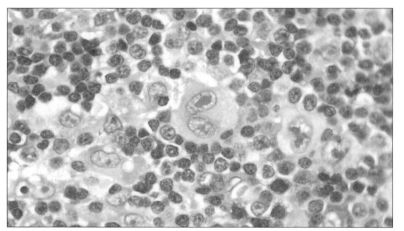

Fig. 46.7 Hodgkin's disease. Hodgkin's disease rarely spreads to the CNS, which is exceptional as a site of clinical presentation. Dural metastases are occasionally seen, but extradural infiltration around the thoracic spine is the commonest manifestation. The cell in the centre of this field is a classic Reed-Sternberg cell. (Courtesy of Dr A Ramsay, Southampton)

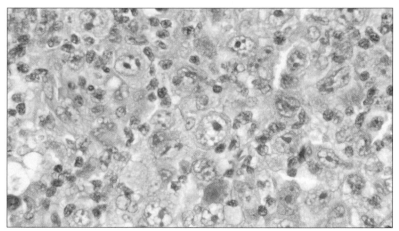

Fig. 46.8 Non-Hodgkin's lymphoma. NHL in the posterior mediastinum and spine may cause cord compression. Extradural deposits spreading from the posterior mediastinum are frequently large B cell lymphomas. This example is a monomorphic centroblastic lymphoma. (Courtesy of Dr A Ramsay, Southampton)

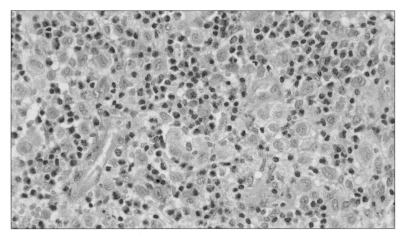

Fig. 46.9 Langerhans' cell histiocytosis (eosinophilic granuloma). This occured as a single focus in the skull. Langerhans' cells have oval grooved nuclei and pink cytoplasm. Eosinophils are frequently present. Langerhans' cells tend to cluster and are immunoreactive for S-100.

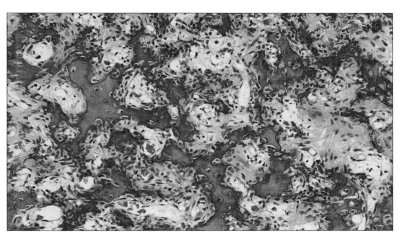

Fig. 46.10 Osteoblastoma. This neoplasm shows male predominance and has a predilection for the spine. Cells between scattered bony trabeculae tend to have an epithelioid appearance. Distinction from osteosarcoma can be difficult. Sheets of cells between sparse matrix and invasion of pre-existing bone favor a diagnosis of osteosarcoma.

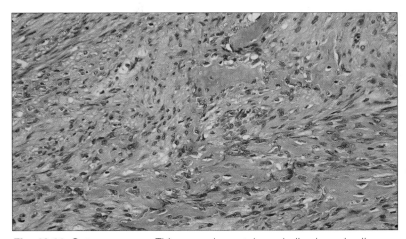

Fig. 46.11 Osteosarcoma. This example contains spindle-shaped cells, some of which have pleomorphic, hyperchromatic nuclei. An area of unmineralized osteoid surrounds cells in half of this illustration.

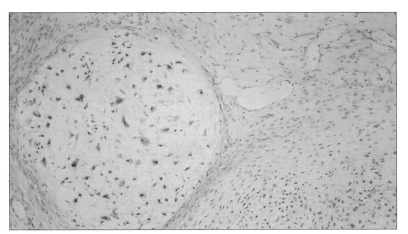

Fig. 46.12 Chondrosarcoma. This may involve the bones of the skull, impinging upon the brain and cranial nerves to cause neurologic symptoms and signs. These cartilaginous neoplasms are graded according to the degree of nuclear pleomorphism and hyperchromasia. Unlike chordomas, chondrosarcomas do not immunolabel with antibodies to epithelial markers such as cytokeratins and epithelial membrane antigen.

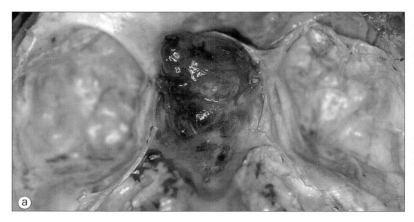

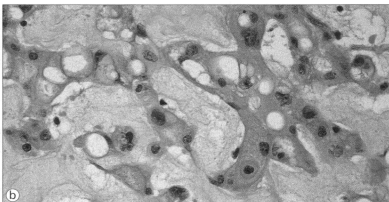

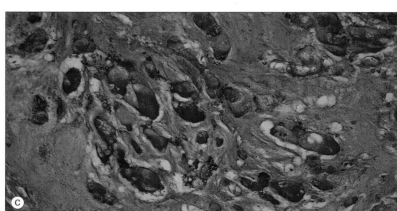

Fig. 46.13 Chordoma. (a) About 80% of chordomas arise in the sacrum or the clivus. This clival chordoma extends into the pituitary fossa and presented with visual field defects and pituitary disfunction. The foci of dark grey-brown discoloration are due to hemorrhage at the time of biopsy. **(b)** The neoplasm consists of strands of cells with vacuolated cytoplasm (physaliphorous cells) **(c)** The neoplastic cells contain abundant glycogen, stained here with PAS, and are surrounded by a matrix of mucinous, alcianophilic material. (PAS/alcian blue)

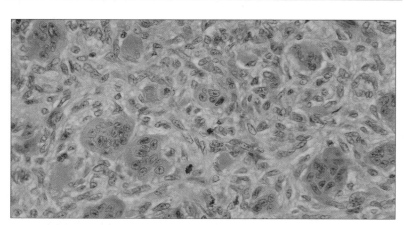

Fig. 46.14 Giant cell neoplasm of bone (osteoclastoma). This is moderately common in the sacrum, but is uncommon in the spine above this site, and is a rare finding in the skull. It can be a locally aggressive neoplasm and has two components: multinucleated giant cells and oval or elongated stromal cells (as shown here). It is important to remember that other lesions of bone such as osteosarcoma, osteoblastoma, aneurysmal bone cyst, and hyperparathyroidism may contain giant cells.

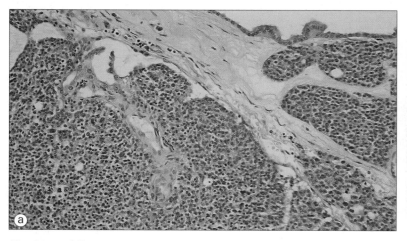

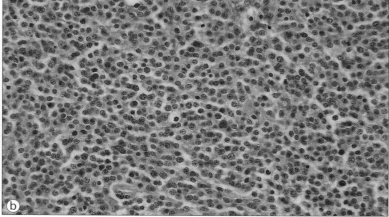

Fig. 46.15 Olfactory neuroblastoma. This is a rare neoplasm that arises at any age in the region of the cribriform plate and spreads into the cranial and nasal cavities. Its monomorphic, round cells are arranged in sheets or lobules. A neuronal phenotype is disclosed in a few examples by the presence of neuroblastic rosettes. Immunohistochemistry reveals variable reactivity for synaptophysin, neurofilament proteins and chromogranin A. Immunoreactivity for cytokeratins is exceptional, and these neoplasms lack immunoreactivity for epithelial membrane antigen. **(a)** Groups of basophilic cells invade soft tissues beneath the respiratory epithelium. **(b)** Small, round cells are typical of these neoplasms.

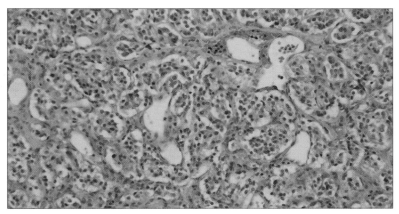

Fig. 46.16 Paraganglioma (of the glomus jugulare). Most paragangliomas in the region of the middle ear arise from the jugular bulb and invade the petrous temporal bone. They are more common in women than men. Approximately 20% spread to the cranial cavity, despite surgery. In this case nests of small, uniform cells are surrounded by a vascular stroma. The cells within the nests are immunoreactive for chromogranin-A, and S-100 antibodies immunolabel the sustentacular cells around the periphery of the nests.

SECONDARY MENINGEAL NEOPLASMS

Secondary neoplasms in the meninges may form discrete nodules or be disseminated within CSF pathways (**Figs 46.17–46.24**). Nodules of neoplasm compress underlying CNS tissue, producing focal symptoms and signs. Neoplasms that diffusely invade the subarachnoid space tend to spread throughout CSF pathways, producing hydrocephalus and raised intracranial pressure by blocking CSF drainage. Cranial nerve palsies are also a common manifestation of this process. In these cases, cytologic examination of CSF is often diagnostic. More than one sample is sometimes required to demonstrate neoplastic cells in the CSF.

NEOPLASMS THAT SHOW A PROPENSITY TO SPREAD WITHIN THE SUBARACHNOID SPACE

- Neuroepithelial neoplasms (PNET, ependymoma, choroid plexus carcinoma)
- Carcinoma (stomach, lung, breast)
- Leukemia (acute lymphoblastic leukemia, acute myeloblastic leukemia)
- Lymphoma (especially as a late feature of high-grade neoplasms)
- Malignant melanoma

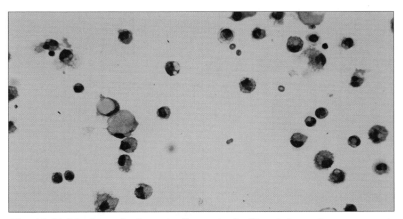

Fig. 46.17 Meningeal adenocarcinomatosis. Signet ring cells are present in the cerebrospinal fluid (CSF).

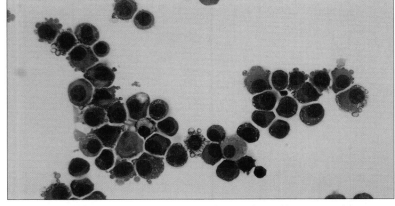

Fig. 46.18 Meningeal carcinomatosis. Disseminated breast carcinoma has invaded the CSF pathways. There are clumps of pleomorphic cells with hyperchromatic nuclei in the CSF. One cell contains intracytoplasmic mucin.

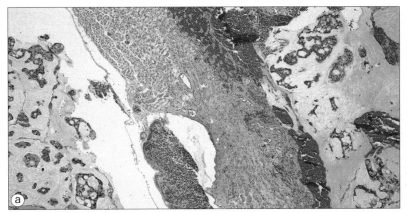

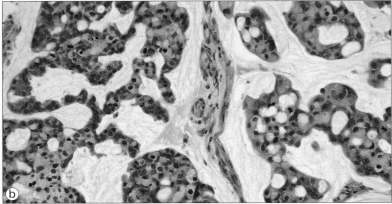

Fig. 46.19 Metastatic carcinoma of breast in the leptomeninges around the spinal cord. (a) The carcinoma has surrounded a spinal nerve root. **(b)** Higher magnification discloses abundant mucin around and within the cells.

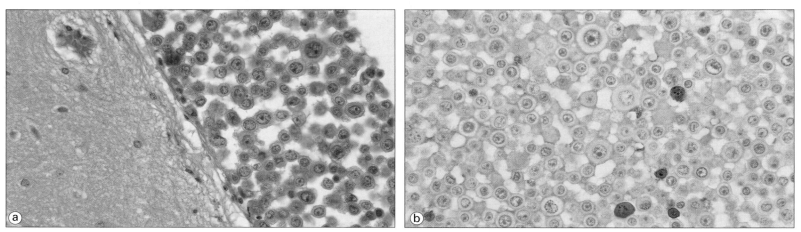

Fig. 46.20 Metastatic malignant melanoma in the cerebral leptomeninges. (a) Cells are present in the subarachnoid space over the pial surface of the cerebral cortex. **(b)** The neoplastic cells label with an antibody to S-100 protein.

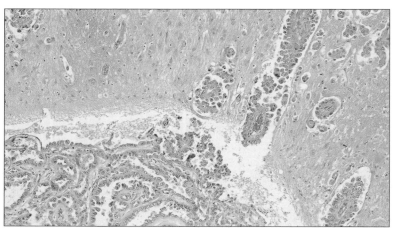

Fig. 46.21 Metastatic carcinoma in the cerebral leptomeninges. In this example, there is invasion of the superficial cerebral cortex along perivascular spaces.

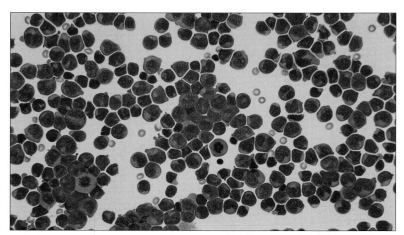

Fig. 46.22 Meningeal involvement by acute myeloid leukemia.

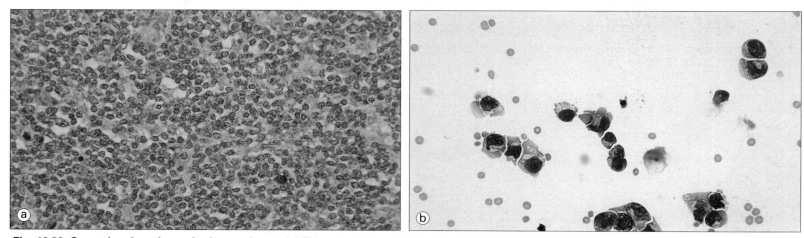

Fig. 46.23 Secondary lymphoma in the meninges. (a) This non-Hodgkin's lymphoma was centred on the dura. **(b)** Meningeal lymphomatosis.

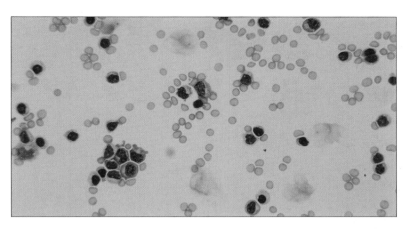

Fig. 46.24 Multiple myeloma involving CSF pathways. Disseminated plasma cell tumors frequently involve the vertebrae from where they can spread into the leptomeninges, in addition to causing spinal cord compression.

SECONDARY NEOPLASMS IN THE CNS

Solitary or multiple deposits of secondary neoplasm (**Figs. 46.25- 46.33**) may occur in the parenchyma of the CNS and present with symptoms and signs of raised intracranial pressure, focal neurologic deficit, and epilepsy. Secondary carcinomas from primary sites in the lung and breast are commonest (see Fig. 46.2). Neoplasms that show a particular tendency to spread to the CNS, such as malignant melanoma (see Fig. 46.2), usually present with multiple deposits (**Fig. 46.25**).

MACROSCOPIC APPEARANCES

Neoplastic deposits may occur anywhere, but are rare in the brain stem and spinal cord (**Fig. 46.26**). Watershed areas and the gray/white matter interface in the cerebrum are typical sites. Metastatic neoplasms form spherical masses in the brain and surrounding edema is evident. The deposits may be firm or have a soft, mucoid, or necrotic center. Hemorrhage into the neoplasm is most characteristic of malignant melanoma or choriocarcinoma, and is relatively common in metastatic renal carcinoma. Intraparenchymal foci of hemorrhage in association with intravascular and perivascular neoplastic cells are a rare feature of leukemia. Malignant melanoma may show obvious pigmentation.

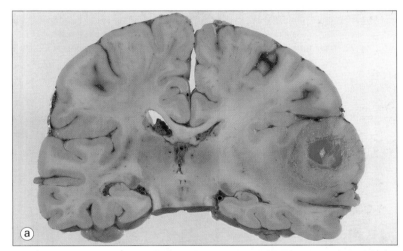

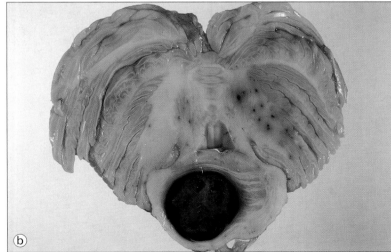

Fig. 46.26 Metastatic neoplasms in the CNS. (a) A solitary metastasis in the right temporal lobe is associated with edema and midline shift. The center of the neoplasm is necrotic. **(b)** A hemorrhagic metastatic neoplasm in the pons. This is an unusual site for a metastasis: approximately 2% of metastases are in the brain stem.

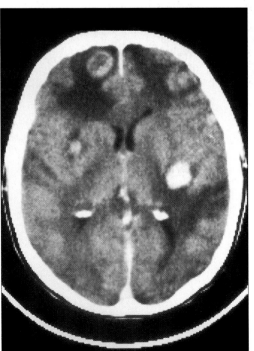

Fig. 46.25 Metastatic malignant melanoma in the cerebrum. Neuroimaging shows several contrast-enhancing masses surrounded by edema.(Courtesy of Dr JS Millar, Wessex Neurological Centre)

MICROSCOPIC APPEARANCES

The edge of the neoplasm is usually well demarcated from adjacent brain, which generally contains reactive astrocytes, variable edema, and in some cases, inflammation. Occasionally, secondary neoplasms invade the brain diffusely mimicking a primary neoplasm: malignant melanoma and squamous cell carcinoma are most often associated with this phenomenon (**Fig. 46.29**). Specific morphophenotypes and immunophenotypes allow the pathologist to establish a likely primary site for the neoplasm (**Figs. 46.30** and **46.31**), but a firm diagnosis may be impossible.

Metastatic carcinoma is occasionally encountered in the stalk of the pituitary gland, often from a primary neoplasm in the breast (**Fig. 46.32**). This should not be confused with squamous metaplasia, that often occurs in this part of the pituitary (see chapter 44).

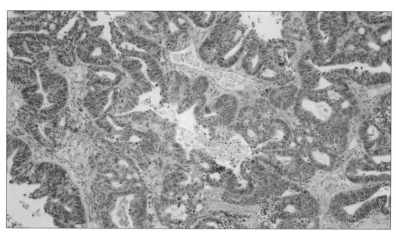

Fig. 46.27 Metastatic adenocarcinoma. Glandular structures are a feature of this neoplasm. Cytological atypia and mucin were present. The primary site was colon.

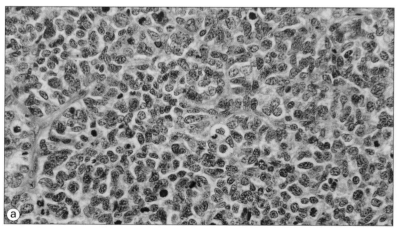

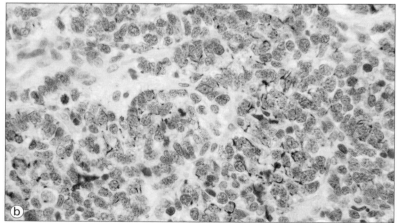

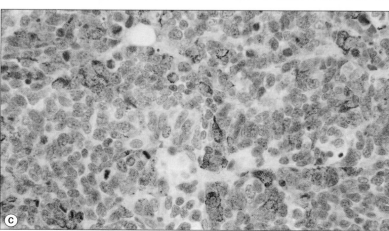

Fig. 46.28 Metastatic small cell lung carcinoma (SCLC). (a) This neoplasm is composed of small round and oval cells. The cytology and frequent mitoses and apoptotic bodies produce a resemblance to PNET, from which SCLC may be distinguished by its immunoreactivities for low molecular weight cytokeratins (**b**) and chromogranin (**c**).

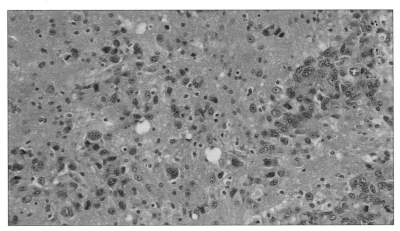

Fig. 46.29 Poorly differentiated metastatic carcinoma invading brain. Although most metastatic neoplasms are sharply demarcated from brain tissue, malignant melanomas and some poorly differentiated squamous carcinomas show diffuse infiltration.

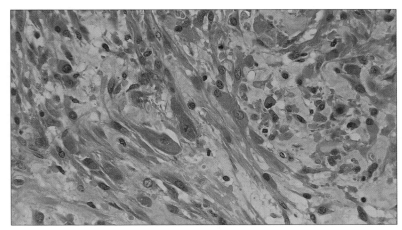

Fig. 46.30 Metastatic rhabdomyosarcoma. Sarcomas represent a very small proportion of CNS metastases.

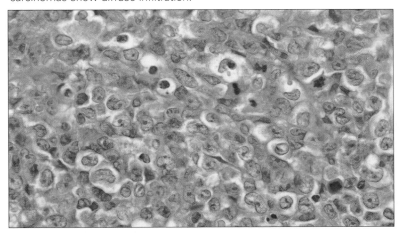

Fig. 46.31 Granulocytic sarcoma. This is a localized tumour of myeloid cells which may present before or after an acute myeloid leukemia. It is rare in the CNS.

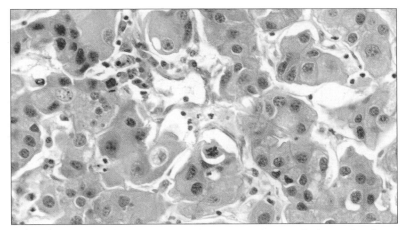

Fig. 46.32 Metastatic carcinoma of the breast in the pituitary gland. Rarely, metastatic neoplasms lodge in the stalk of the pituitary or in the neurohypophysis

REFERENCES

Barnes L, Kapadia SB (1994) The biology and pathology of selected skull base tumors. *J Neurooncology* 20: 213–240.

Burger PC, Scheithauer BW (1994) Metastatic and secondary neoplasms. In: Rosai J (ed.) *Atlas of tumor pathology*, volume 10. pp. 415–428. Washington: Armed Forces Institute of Pathology.

Henson RA, Urich H. (1982) *Cancer and the nervous system*. Oxford: Blackwell.

Mills SE, Frierson HF (1985) Olfactory neuroblastoma. *American Journal of Surgical Pathology* 9: 317–327.

Olson ME, Chernik NL, Posner JB (1974) Infiltration of the leptomeninges by systemic cancer. *Arch Neurol*. 30: 122–137.

Patchell RA. (1991) Brain metastases. *Neurol Clin* 9: 817–824.

Posner JB, Chernick NL (1978) Intracranial metastases for systemic cancer. *Advances in Neurology* 18: 579–592.

Russell DS, Rubinstein LF (1989) Secondary tumors of the nervous system. In: *Pathology of tumours of the nervous system* pp. 809–854. London: Edward Arnold.

Sawaya R, Bindal RK. (1995) Metastatic brain tumors. In: Kaye AH, Laws ER Jr. (eds) *Brain tumors*. pp. 923–946. Edinburgh: Churchill Livingstone.

47 *Paraneoplastic disorders*

Patients with a primary neoplasm remote from the CNS may develop neurologic symptoms and signs as a consequence of:

- Spread of the neoplasm to the nervous system (see Chapter 46).
- Systemic metabolic and hemodynamic disturbances (**Fig. 47.1**).
- Infections secondary to immunosuppression produced by lymphoreticular neoplasms (**Fig. 47.2**).
- Side effects of cancer therapy (**Fig. 47.3**).
- Production of antibodies that simultaneously target antigens on neurons and neoplastic cells (**Fig. 47.4**), which is the subject of this chapter.

Although the autoimmune diseases that constitute the paraneoplastic syndromes are generally initiated by systemic neoplasms, most can also occur in the absence of demonstrable neoplasm.

Paraneoplastic syndromes are rare, affecting less than 1% of patients with cancer. They may involve the CNS, peripheral nervous system, or produce a myopathy. The principal CNS paraneoplastic syndromes are:

- Paraneoplastic encephalomyelitis (PEM).
- Paraneoplastic cerebellar degeneration (PCD).
- Opsoclonus–myoclonus.

Cancer-related systemic disorders producing CNS symptomatology

Metabolic/endocrine disorders	Potential etiology
Hepatic failure	Liver metastases
Hypoglycemia	Consumption of glucose by disseminated sarcoma
Hyponatremia	Syndrome of inappropriate ADH secretion
Hypercalcemia	Bony metastases / inappropriate parathyroid hormone production
Cushing's syndrome	Inappropriate (ectopic) ACTH production
Wernicke–Korsakow syndrome	Thiamine deficiency secondary to emesis
Vascular disorders	**Potential etiology**
Encephalopathy / infarction – hyperviscosity	Waldenstrom's macroglobulinemia
Infarction–hypercoagulability state	Mucin-secreting adenocarcinomas
Infarction	Polycythemia rubra vera
Embolic infarction	Marantic endocarditis
Hemorrhage	Reduced coagulation factors in hepatic failure
Hemorrhage	Thrombocytopenia in bone marrow failure

Fig. 47.1 Cancer-related systemic disorders producing CNS symptomatology.

CNS infections particularly associated with lymphomas, leukaemias, and myeloma

Organism	Particular clinical association
Varicella–zoster virus encephalitis	Hodgkin's disease
Herpes simplex virus encephalitis	Hodgkin's disease
Cytomegalovirus encephalitis	Acute lymphoblastic leukemia
Progressive multifocal leukoencephalopathy (JC papovavirus)	Various
Listeria infection Streptococcal meningitis	Post-splenectomy
Toxoplasmosis	Lymphoma
Cryptococcal meningoencephalitis CNS aspergillosis	Various

Fig. 47.2 CNS infections particularly associated with lymphomas, leukemias, and myeloma.

CNS side-effects of cancer treatment

Radiotherapy

- encephalopathy
- delayed myelopathy
- hypothalamic/pituitary disturbances
- oncogenesis – mainly meningioma, sarcoma, rarely glioma

Chemotherapy

- encephalopathy and/or myelopathy (particularly after BCNU, L-asparaginase, intrathecal methotrexate)
- cerebellar disorder (cytosine arabinoside)

Fig. 47.3 CNS side-effects of cancer treatment.

Two or more nervous system paraneoplastic syndromes may coexist, being produced by the same antibody (e.g. encephalomyelitis and sensory neuronopathy produced by anti-Hu antibody).

Evidence for an autoimmune process is provided by the demonstration of:

- an inflammatory process around targeted neurons.
- antibodies directed against syndrome-specific neurons and neoplastic cells.
- neuronal antibodies present at higher titer in the cerebrospinal fluid than the serum.

Although the demonstration of antineuronal antibodies has provided clinicians with a useful diagnostic test, it is clear that not all patients with paraneoplastic syndromes have detectable antibodies, and paraneoplastic syndromes may be caused by antibodies other than those that have been characterized to date. For example, in PCD:

- Polyclonal immunoglobulin G (IgG) anti-Purkinje cell (anti-Yo) antibodies targeted against 62 kD and 34 kD proteins are associated almost exclusively with carcinomas of the breast and ovary.
- Antineuronal antibodies with characteristics distinct from anti-Yo or unidentified antibodies are associated with carcinoma of the lung and Hodgkin's disease.

Immunogenic paraneoplastic disorders affecting the nervous system

Central nervous system	Peripheral nervous system
Encephalomyelitis (PEM)	Sensory/autonomic ganglioneuronopathy
Cerebellar cortical degeneration (PCD)	Sensory/sensorimotor neuropathy
Retinopathy	Lambert–Eaton myesthenic syndrome
Opsoclonus–myoclonus	Acute inflammatory demyelinating polyneuropathy

CNS syndrome	Antibody [1]	Antigen	Target	Associated neoplasm(s)
PEM [2]	Anti-Hu	35 - 40 kD	Neuronal nuclei	Small-cell (anaplastic) carcinoma of lung (80%) Neuroblastoma Rhabdomyosarcoma
PCD	Anti-Yo	34 kD & 62 kD	Purkinje cells	Ovarian carcinoma Breast carcinoma
Retinopathy	CAR	20 kD & 65 kD	Retinal ganglion cells	Small-cell (anaplastic) carcinoma of lung
Opsoclonus –myoclonus	Anti-Ri	55 kD & 80 kD	Neuronal nuclei	Breast carcinoma Neuroblastoma Small-cell (anaplastic) carcinoma of lung

[1] Antibody predominantly associated with syndrome; an identical paraneoplastic syndrome may occur with other antibodies / no detectable antibody.
[2] Often associated with sensory / autonomic ganglioneuronopathy

Fig. 47.4 Immunogenic paraneoplastic disorders affecting the nervous system.

PARANEOPLASTIC ENCEPHALOMYELITIS

MACROSCOPIC AND MICROSCOPIC APPEARANCES

The histologic features of PEM are similar to those of viral encephalitis and myelitis. Neuronal loss, astrocytosis, and an increase in activated microglia are accompanied by an inflammatory infiltrate that consists mainly of lymphocytes and plasma cells and is concentrated in perivascular spaces (**Fig. 47.5**). The extent of the inflammation is variable and correlates poorly with neuronal loss. Inflammation affects gray matter, but secondary degeneration of white matter tracts can result. A leptomeningitis is nearly always present. No macroscopic abnormalities may be discerned.

Regions of the cerebrum, brain stem, cerebellum, spinal cord, and optic nerve may be affected alone or in combination.
- Cerebral PEM is mainly confined to the medial temporal and inferior frontal structures, insular cortex, and cingulate gyrus (limbic encephalitis).
- The medulla is particularly affected in brain stem encephalitis.
- Inflammation in the cerebellum is characteristically leptomeningeal or deep, affecting the dentate nucleus, but sparing the cortex. There is therefore only partial overlap with the histology of cerebellar cortical degeneration.

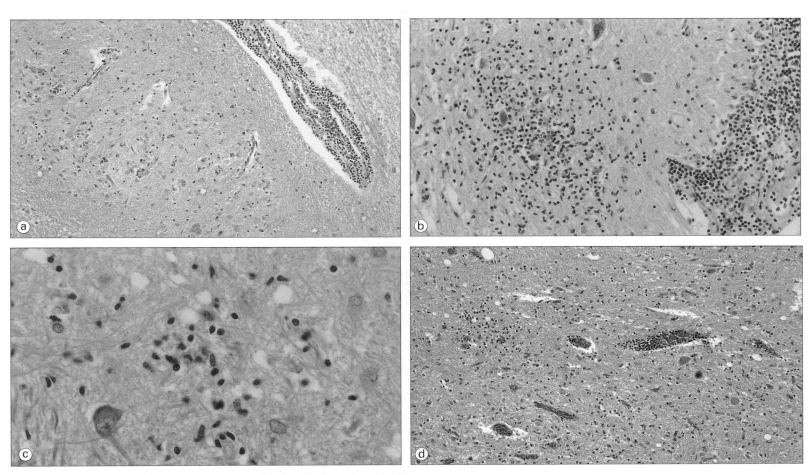

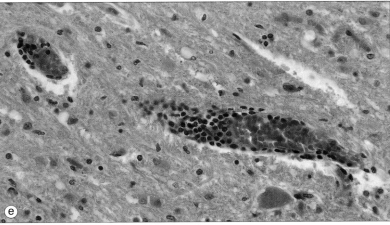

Fig. 47.5 Paraneoplastic encephalomyelitis. (a), (b) and **(c)** Perivascular lymphocytic cuffing, neuronophagia and gliosis are seen in the brainstem. **(d)** There is a diffuse lymphocytic infiltrate in the cervical cord. **(e)** Higher power view of perivascular lymphocytic cuffing, infiltration by microglia, and reactive astrocytosis.

- Myelitis may involve the entire cord or only a few segments, generally in the cervical or lumbar regions (see Fig. 47.5).

Some cases of PEM are combined with a sensory neuronopathy characterized by ganglionitis, loss of ganglion cells, and secondary degeneration of dorsal column fibers (**Figs 47.6**).

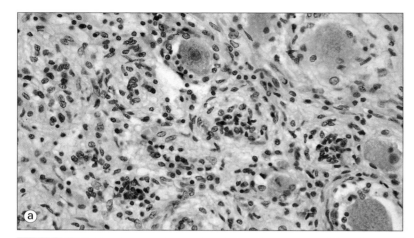

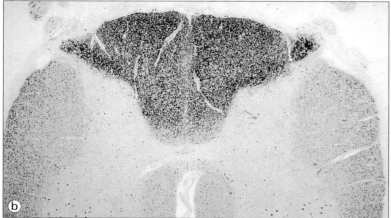

Fig. 47.6 Paraneoplastic ganglioneuronopathy. (a) The dorsal root ganglion is infiltrated by lymphocytes and contains scattered nodules of Nageotte marking sites of ganglion cell degeneration. **(b)** A Marchi preparation reveals degeneration of dorsal column fibers in association with the sensory ganglioneuronopathy illustrated in (a).

PARANEOPLASTIC CEREBELLAR DEGENERATION (PCD)

MACROSCOPIC AND MICROSCOPIC APPEARANCES

Mild cerebellar atrophy is occasionally observed, but there is generally no macroscopic abnormality in PCD. Histologically a severe loss of Purkinje cells is evident throughout most of the cerebellar cortex, and is accompanied by variable loss of granule cells, activated microglia, and Bergmann gliosis (**Fig. 47.7**). An infiltrate of mononuclear leukocytes may be seen in the cortex, and there may be perivascular aggregates of lymphocytes and a leptomeningitis. However, inflammation may be sparse or absent, despite a severe loss of Purkinje cells. In a minority of cases of PCD, there is patchy loss of neurons accompanied by inflammation in other regions of the brain, indicating some overlap with PEM.

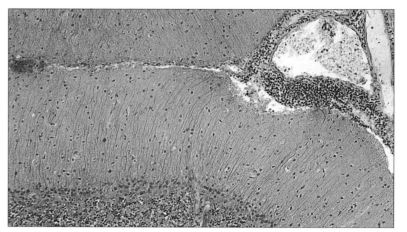

Fig. 47.7 PCD. Purkinje cells are absent, the number of Bergmann astrocytes is increased, and there is isomorphic gliosis of the molecular layer. (Phosphotungstic acid/hematoxylin)

PARANEOPLASTIC OPSOCLONUS–MYOCLONUS

There is no distinctive histologic feature of paraneoplastic opsoclonus–myoclonus. Approximately 50% of cases show a variable degree of Purkinje cell loss. Neuronal loss and inflammatory cells have been reported in the brain stem, but a single location does not appear to be involved in all cases.

REFERENCES

Dalmau J, Graus F, Rosenblum MK, Posner JB (1992) Anti-Hu associated paraneoplastic encephalomyelitis/sensory neuronopathy. *Medicine* 71:59–72.

Dalmau J, Posner JB (1994) Neurologic paraneoplastic antibodies (anti-Yo; anti-Hu, anti-Ri): the case for a nomenclature based on antibody and antigen specificity. *Neurology* 44: 2241–2246.

Dropcho EJ (1995) Autoimmune central nervous system paraneoplastic disorders: mechanisms, diagnosis, and therapeutic options. *Ann Neurol* 37(**S1**): S102–S113.

Henson RA, Urich H (1982) *Cancer and the Nervous System*. Oxford: Blackwell Scientific Publications.

Peterson K, Rosenblum MK, Kotanides H, Posner JB (1992) Paraneoplastic cerebellar degeneration. *Neurology* 42: 1931–1937.

Posner JB (1992) Pathogenesis of central nervous system paraneoplastic syndromes. *Rev Neurol* 148: 502–512.

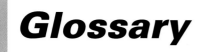

Glossary

ACA	anterior cerebral artery
ACTH	adrenocorticotropic hormone
AD	Alzheimer's disease
ADCA	autosomal dominant cerebellar ataxia
ADEM	acute disseminated encephalomyelitis
AFP	α-fetoprotein
AHL	acute hemorrhagic leukoencephalopathy
AIDS	acquired immunodeficiency syndrome
ALD	adrenoleukodystrophy
APLAs	antiphospholipid antibodies
APP	amyloid precursor protein
AR	autosomal recessive
AT	ataxia–telangiectasia
AVM	arteriovenous malformation
AZT	zidovudine
BCNU	1,3-bis(2-chloroethyl)-1-nitrosourea
BH	brain hemorrage
BSE	bovine spongiform encephalopathy
BSL	Binswanger's subcortical arteriosclerotic leukoencephalopathy
CAA	cerebral amyloid angiopathy
CADASIL	cerebral autosomal dominant arteriopathy with subcortical infarcts and leukoencephalopathy
CBD	corticobasal degeneration
CDG1	carbohydrate-deficient glycoprotein syndrome type 1
CERAD	Consortium to Establish a Registry for Alzheimer'sDisease
CGA	giant cell arteritis
CJD	Creutzfeldt–Jakob disease
CMV	cytomegalovirus
CP	choroid plexus
CPA	cerebellopontine angle
CPCs	choroid plexus carcinoma
CPEO	chronic progressive external ophthalmoplegia
CPH	choroid plexus hemorrhage
CPM	central pontine myelinolysis
CPP	choroid plexus papilloma
CSF	cerebrospinal fluid
CT	computerized tomography
CVT	cerebral venous thrombosis
DAI	diffuse axonal injury
DFT	dementia of frontal type
DIA	desmoplastic infantile astrocytoma
DIGG	desmoplastic infantil ganglioglioma
DLB	dementia with Lewy bodies
DNT	dysembryoplastic neuroepithelial tumor
DRPLA	dentatorubropallidoluysial atrophy
EBV	Epstein–Barr virus
EDH	extradural hemorrhage
ELISA	enzyme-linked immunosorbent assay
EMA	epithelial membrane antigen
FA	Friedreich's ataxia
FFI	fatal familial insomnia
FMD	fibromuscular dysplasia
FMR1	fragile X mental retardation type 1 gene

FSH	follicle stimulating hormone
GABA	gamma-aminobutyric acid
GAGs	glycosaminoglycans
GCT	germ cell tumor
GFAP	glial fibrillary acidic protein
GH	growth hormone
GSS	Gerstmann–Sraussler–Scheinker disease
HAM	human T cell leukemia/lymphotropic virus-1-associated myelopathy (tropical spastic paraparesis)
HD	Huntington's disease
HIV	human immunodeficiency virus
HLA	human leukocyte antigen
HSE	herpes simplex encephalitis
HSV	herpes simplex virus
HTLV-1	human T cell leukemia/lymphotropic type 1virus
IA	infectious (mycotic) aneurysm
IBSN	infantile bilateral striatal necrosis
IL	interleukin
INAD	infantile neuroaxonal dystrophy
INH	isonicotinic acid hydrazide
IVH	intraventricular hemorrhage
KSHV	Kaposi's sarcoma-associated herpesvirus
KSS	Kearns–Sayre syndrome
LH	luteinizing hormone
LHON	Leber's hereditary optic neuropathy
MAO	monoamine oxidase
MCA	middle cerebral artery
MCBs	membranous cytoplasmic bodies
MELAS	mitochondrial myopathy, encephalopathy, lactic acidosis, and stroke-like episodes
MERRF	myoclonic epilepsy with ragged red fibers
MGNE	microglial nodule encephalitis
MHC	major histocompatibility complex
MJD	Machado–Joseph disease
MLD	metachromatic leucodystrophy
MND	motor neuron disease
MNGIE	myoneurogastrointestinal encephalopathy syndrome
MNST	malignant nerve sheath tumor
MPDP	1-methyl-4-phenyl-2,3-dihydropyridinium
MPP+	1-methyl-4-phenylpyridinium
MPS	mucopolysaccharidosis
MPTP	1-methyl-4-phenyl-1,2,3,6-tetrahydropyridine
MRI	magnetic resonance imaging
MS	multiple sclerosis
MSA	multiple system atrophy
mtDNA	mitochondrial DNA
NADPH	nicotinamide–adenine dinucleotide phosphate
NARP	neuropathy, ataxia, and retinitis pigmentosa
NCL or CLN	neuronal ceroid lipofuscinosis
NFT	neurofibrillary tangle
NF	neurofibromatosis
NT	neuropil thread
OLC	oligodendrocyte-like cell
OPCA	olivopontocerebellar atrophy

OPLL	ossification of the posterior longitudinal ligament
PACNS	primary angiitis of the CNS
PAS	periodic acid–Schiff
PBP	progressive bulbar palsy
PCA	posterior cerebral artery
PCD	paraneoplastic cerebellar degeneration
PCNSL	primary CNS lymphomas
PCR	polymerase chain reaction
PD	Parkinson's disease
PEM	paraneoplastic encephalomyelitis
PET	positron emission tomography
PHF	paired helical filament
PLS	primary lateral sclerosis
PMA	progressive muscular atrophy
PMD	Pelizaeus–Merzbacher disease
PML	progressive multifocal leukoencephalopathy
PNDC	progressive neuronal degeneration of childhood
PNET	primative neuroectodermal tumor
PNU	N-3-pyridylmethyl-N′-p-nitrophenyl urea
POLIP	polyneuropathy, ophthalmoplegia, leukoencephalopathy and intestinal pseudo-obstruction
PPA	primary progressive aphasia
PRL	prolactin
PSP	progressive supranuclear palsy
PXA	pleomorphic xanthoastrocytoma
rRNA	ribosomal RNA
SACD	subacute combined degeneration
SAH	subarachnoid hemorrhage
SBMA	spinobulbar muscular atrophy
SCA	spinocerebellar ataxia
SCLC	small cell lung carcinoma
SDH	subdural hemorrhage
SEGA	subependymal giant cell astrocytoma
SEH	subependymal germinal plate/matrix hemorrhage
SLE	systemic lupus erythematosus
SMA	spinal muscular atrophy
SPECT	single photon emission computed tomography
SPH	subpial hemorrhage
SSPE	subacute sclerosing panencephalitis
TCE	trichlorethylene
TIA	transient ischemic attack
TNF	tumor necrosis factor
tRNA	transfer RNA
TSC	tuberous sclerosis complex
TSH	thyroid stimulating hormone
TTP	thrombotic thrombocytopenic purpura
vCJD	new variant CJD
VEE	Venezuelan equine encephalitis
VHL	von Hippel–Lindau syndrome
VZV	Varicella–Zoster virus
WHO	World Health Organization
WMN	white matter necrosis
ZWS	Zellweger syndrome

Index

Chapters in *Neuropathology* are numbered individually. Numbers following a chapter in the index refer to that chapter, i.e. 25.3,5,6 corresponds to 25.3, 25.5 and 25.6.